DSM-IV Sourcebook

Volume 3

Lake Oswego Public Library
706 Fourth Street
Lake Oswego, Oregon 97034

DSM-IV Sourcebook

Volume 3

Edited by

Thomas A. Widiger, Ph.D.
Allen J. Frances, M.D.
Harold Alan Pincus, M.D.
Ruth Ross, M.A.
Michael B. First, M.D.
Wendy Davis, Ed.M.

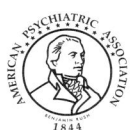

Published by the American Psychiatric Association
Washington, D.C.

Note: The authors have worked to ensure that all information in this book concerning drug dosages, schedules, and routes of administration is accurate as of the time of publication and consistent with standards set by the U.S. Food and Drug Administration and the general medical community. As medical research and practice advance, however, therapeutic standards may change. For this reason and because human and mechanical errors sometimes occur, we recommend that readers follow the advice of a physician who is directly involved in their care or the care of a member of their family.

The findings, opinions, and conclusions of this report do not necessarily represent the views of the officers, trustees, all members of the task force, or all members of the American Psychiatric Association. The views expressed are those of the authors of the individual chapters. Task force reports are considered a substantive contribution of the ongoing analysis and evaluation of problems, programs, issues, and practices in a given area of concern.

Copyright © 1997 American Psychiatric Association
ALL RIGHTS RESERVED
Manufactured in the United States of America on acid-free paper
First Edition 00 99 98 97   4 3 2 1
American Psychiatric Association
1400 K Street, N.W., Washington, DC 20005

Library of Congress Cataloging-in-Publication Data
(Revised for vol. 3)
DSM-IV sourcebook.
  Developed by the DSM-IV Task Force of American
Psychiatric Association.
  Includes bibliographical references and index.
  1. Diagnostic and statistical manual of mental
disorders. 2. Mental illness—Classification.
3. Mental illness—Diagnosis. I. Widiger, Thomas A.
II. American Psychiatric Association. Task Force on
DSM-IV. III. Title: DSM-4 sourcebook. [DNLM: 1. Mental
Disorders—classification. 2. Psychiatry—nomenclature.
WM 15 D277 1994]
RC455.2.C4D754 1994   616.89′075   93-48304
ISBN 0-89042-065-3 (v. 1)
ISBN 0-89042-069-6 (v. 2)
ISBN 0-89042-073-4 (v. 3)

British Library Cataloguing in Publication Data
A CIP record is available from the British Library.

Contents

Contributors xv

Preface xxvii

Acknowledgments xxxv

SECTION I
DISORDERS USUALLY FIRST DIAGNOSED IN
INFANCY, CHILDHOOD, OR ADOLESCENCE (PART I)

Introduction to Section I
Disorders Usually First Diagnosed in Infancy, Childhood, or
Adolescence (Part I) 3
    Magda Campbell, M.D.

Chapter 1
Autistic Disorder 15
    Peter Szatmari, M.D., F.R.C.P.C.

Chapter 2
Rett's Syndrome: A Subtype of Pervasive Developmental Disorder? 25
    Luke Y. Tsai, M.D.

Chapter 3
Childhood Disintegrative Disorder 35
    Fred R. Volkmar, M.D.

Chapter 4
Pervasive Developmental Disorder Not Otherwise Specified 43
    Peter Szatmari, M.D., F.R.C.P.C.

Chapter 5
Early-Onset Schizophrenia 55
    John S. Werry, M.D.

Chapter 6
Should Social Skills Deficits Be Included as a Primary Diagnostic
Criterion for Learning Disorders? 67
    Steven R. Forness, Ed.D.

Chapter 7
Language and Speech Disorders 79
    Rhea Paul, Ph.D., Lorian Baker, Ph.D., Donald J. Cohen, M.D.,
    Paula Tallal, Ph.D., and Dorothy Aram, Ph.D.

Section II
Disorders Usually First Diagnosed in Infancy, Childhood, or Adolescence (Part II)

Introduction to Section II
Disorders Usually First Diagnosed in Infancy, Childhood, or
Adolescence (Part II) 95
    David Shaffer, M.D., Thomas A. Widiger, Ph.D., and
    Harold A. Pincus, M.D.

Chapter 8
Attention-Deficit/Hyperactivity Disorder: A Review of Diagnostic Issues . . 111
    Keith McBurnett, Ph.D.

Chapter 9
Comorbidity of Attention-Deficit/Hyperactivity Disorder 145
    Joseph Biederman, M.D., Jeffrey H. Newcorn, M.D., and
    Susan Sprich, B.A.

Chapter 10
Attention-Deficit Disorder Without Hyperactivity 163
　Benjamin B. Lahey, Ph.D., Caryn L. Carlson, Ph.D., and
　Paul J. Frick, Ph.D.

Chapter 11
Oppositional Defiant Disorder and Conduct Disorder 189
　Benjamin B. Lahey, Ph.D., Rolf Loeber, Ph.D., Herbert C. Quay, Ph.D.,
　Paul J. Frick, Ph.D., and James Grimm, M.D.

Chapter 12
Feeding and Eating Disorders of Infancy or Early Childhood 211
　Fred R. Volkmar, M.D., and Linda C. Mayes, M.D.

Chapter 13
Anxiety Disorders of Childhood or Adolescence 221
　Rachel G. Klein, Ph.D., Nancy Kaplan Tancer, M.D., and
　John S. Werry, M.D.

Chapter 14
Elective Mutism 241
　Nancy Kaplan Tancer, M.D., and Rachel G. Klein, Ph.D.

Chapter 15
Reactive Attachment Disorder 255
　Fred R. Volkmar, M.D.

Chapter 16
The Nosological Status of Depression in Children and Adolescents 265
　Adrian Angold, M.B., B.S., M.R.C.Psych.

Chapter 17
Suicide in Childhood and Adolescence 279
　Robert A. King, M.D., G. Davis Gammon, M.D.,
　Cynthia R. Pfeffer, M.D., and Donald J. Cohen, M.D.

Chapter 18
Adjustment Disorder in Children and Adolescents 291
　Jeffrey H. Newcorn, M.D., and James Strain, M.D.

Chapter 19
Trichotillomania 303
    Ronald M. Winchel, M.D.

Chapter 20
Gender Identity Disorder 317
    Susan J. Bradley, M.D., Ray Blanchard, Ph.D., Susan Coates, Ph.D.,
    Richard Green, M.D., J.D., Stephen B. Levine, M.D.,
    Heino F. L. Meyer-Bahlburg, Dr. rer. nat., Ira B. Pauly, M.D., and
    Kenneth J. Zucker, Ph.D.

Chapter 21
Sibling Rivalry: Diagnostic Category or Focus of Treatment? 327
    Fred R. Volkmar, M.D., and Alice S. Carter, Ph.D.

SECTION III
EATING DISORDERS

Introduction to Section III
Eating Disorders 335
    B. Timothy Walsh, M.D.

Chapter 22
Subtyping Anorexia Nervosa 339
    Maria DaCosta, M.D., and Katherine A. Halmi, M.D.

Chapter 23
Diagnostic Criteria for Bulimia Nervosa 355
    G. Terence Wilson, Ph.D.

Chapter 24
Subtyping of Bulimia Nervosa 361
    James E. Mitchell, M.D.

Chapter 25
Importance of Attitudes Regarding Shape and Weight to the
Diagnosis of Bulimia Nervosa 375
    Paul E. Garfinkel, M.D.

Chapter 26
Forms of Overeating Not Meeting DSM-III-R Behavioral Criteria:
Pathological Overeating 379
    Michael J. Devlin, M.D., and B. Timothy Walsh, M.D.

SECTION IV
THE DSM-IV MULTIAXIAL SYSTEM

Introduction to Section IV
The DSM-IV Multiaxial System 393
    Janet B. W. Williams, D.S.W.

Chapter 27
Axis III: Relationship Between Psychiatric Syndromes and
Medical Disorders 401
    *Alan M. Gruenberg, M.D., Martin Rosenzweig, M.D., and
    Reed Goldstein, Ph.D.*

Chapter 28
Axis IV 409
    Andrew E. Skodol, M.D.

Chapter 29
A Proposed Axis for Social Supports 423
    *Cheryl S. Cohen, M.S., Janet B. W. Williams, D.S.W., and
    Judith G. Rabkin, Ph.D., M.P.H.*

Chapter 30
Revising Axis V for DSM-IV: A Review of Measures of Social
Functioning 439
    *Howard H. Goldman, M.D., Ph.D, Andrew E. Skodol, M.D., and
    Tamara R. Lave, B.A.*

Chapter 31
Patterns of Course of Illness 459
    Juan E. Mezzich, M.D., Ph.D., and Miguel R. Jorge, M.D., Ph.D.

Chapter 32
On Measuring Syndromic Severity 487
    Juan E. Mezzich, M.D., Ph.D., and Patrick F. Sullivan, M.D.

Chapter 33
Defense Mechanisms 503
    Andrew E. Skodol, M.D., and J. Christopher Perry, M.P.H., M.D.

Section V
Family/Relational Problems

Introduction to Section V
Family/Relational Problems 521
    Allen J. Frances, M.D., John F. Clarkin, Ph.D., and Ruth Ross, M.A.

Chapter 34
Relational Problem Related to a Mental Disorder or
General Medical Condition 531
    Michael J. Goldstein, Ph.D., Angus M. Strachan, Ph.D., and
    Lyman C. Wynne, M.D., Ph.D.

Chapter 35
Parent Inadequate Discipline 569
    P. Chamberlain, Ph.D, J. B. Reid, Ph.D., J. Ray, B.A.,
    D. Capaldi, Ph.D., and P. Fisher, Ph.D.

Chapter 36
Marital and Family Communication Difficulties 631
    John F. Clarkin, Ph.D., and David J. Miklowitz, Ph.D.

Chapter 37
Partner Relational Problems With Physical Abuse 673
    K. Daniel O'Leary, Ph.D., and Neil S. Jacobson, Ph.D.

Chapter 38
Sibling Relational Problems 693
    Michael D. Kahn, Ph.D., and Genevieve Monks, M.A.

Chapter 39
Physical Abuse and Neglect of Children 713
    John F. Knutson, Ph.D., and Helen A. Schartz, Ph.D.

Chapter 40
Incest 805
    Sandra Kaplan, M.D., and David Pelcovitz, Ph.D.

Section VI
Cultural Issues for DSM-IV

Introduction to Section VI
Cultural Issues for DSM-IV 861
    Juan E. Mezzich, M.D., Ph.D., Arthur Kleinman, M.D.,
    Horacio Fabrega Jr., M.D., Delores L. Parron, Ph.D., Byron J. Good, Ph.D.,
    Keh-Ming Lin, M.D., M.P.H., and Spero M. Manson, Ph.D.

Chapter 41
Culture in DSM-IV 867
    Arthur Kleinman, M.D., Delores L. Parron, Ph.D.,
    Horacio Fabrega Jr., M.D., Byron J. Good, Ph.D., and
    Juan E. Mezzich, M.D., Ph.D.

Chapter 42
Cultural Considerations in the Classification of
Mental Disorders in Children and Adolescents 873
    Glorisa Canino, Ph.D., Ian Canino, M.D., and William Arroyo, M.D.

Chapter 43
Cultural Considerations on Cognitive Impairment Disorders 885
    Keh-Ming Lin, M.D., M.P.H., and Horacio Fabrega Jr., M.D.

Chapter 44
Culture and Substance-Related Disorders 893
    Joseph Westermeyer, M.D., Ph.D., and Glorisa Canino, Ph.D.

Chapter 45
Cultural Considerations in the Diagnosis of Schizophrenia and
Related Disorders and Psychotic Disorders Not Otherwise Classified 901
    Marvin Karno, M.D., and Janis H. Jenkins, Ph.D.

Chapter 46
Cultural Considerations in the Diagnosis of Mood Disorders 909
    Spero M. Manson, Ph.D.

Chapter 47
Culture and the Anxiety Disorders 925
   Peter J. Guarnaccia, Ph.D., and Laurence J. Kirmayer, M.D.

Chapter 48
Cultural Considerations for Somatoform Disorders 933
   Laurence J. Kirmayer, M.D., and Mitchell Weiss, M.D., Ph.D.

Chapter 49
Impact of Culture on Dissociation: Enhancing the
Cultural Suitability of DSM-IV 943
   Carlos A. González, M.D., Roberto Lewis-Fernández, M.D.,
   Ezra E. H. Griffith, M.D., Roland Littlewood, M.B., D.Phil., M.R.C.Psych.,
   and Richard J. Castillo, Ph.D.

Chapter 50
Cultural Issues and Sexual Disorders 951
   Dona Davis, Ph.D., and Gilbert Herdt, Ph.D.

Chapter 51
Eating Disorders: A Cross-Cultural Review 959
   Cheryl Ritenbaugh, Ph.D., M.P.H., Catherine Shisslak, Ph.D.,
   Nicolette Teufel, Ph.D., Tina K. Leonard-Green, M.S., R.D., and
   Raymond Prince, Ph.D.

Chapter 52
Culture and the Diagnosis of Adjustment Disorders 969
   Janis H. Jenkins, Ph.D., and J. David Kinzie, M.D.

Chapter 53
Cultural Factors and Personality Disorders 975
   Renato D. Alarcon, M.D., M.P.H., and Edward F. Foulks, M.D., Ph.D.

Chapter 54
On Culturally Enhancing the DSM-IV Multiaxial Formulation 983
   Juan E. Mezzich, M.D., Ph.D., and Byron J. Good, Ph.D.

Chapter 55
The "Culture-Bound Syndromes" and DSM-IV 991
  Charles C. Hughes, Ph.D., Ronald C. Simons, M.D., and
  Ronald M. Wintrob, M.D.

Chapter 56
Religious or Spiritual Problems 1001
  Francis G. Lu, M.D., David Lukoff, Ph.D., and Robert Turner, M.D.

Index 1017

Contributors

Renato D. Alarcon, M.D., M.P.H. Department of Psychiatry and Behavioral Sciences, Emory University School of Medicine, Atlanta, Georgia

Adrian Angold, M.B., B.S., M.R.C.Psych. Assistant Professor of Psychiatry, Developmental Epidemiology Program, Department of Psychiatry, Duke University Medical Center, Durham, North Carolina

Dorothy Aram, Ph.D. Chair, Department of Communication Disorders, Emerson College, Boston, Massachusetts

William Arroyo, M.D. Division of Child and Adolescent Psychiatry, University of Southern California, Los Angeles, California

Lorian Baker, Ph.D. Professor (Ret.), Department of Child Psychiatry, University of California at Los Angeles, Los Angeles, California

Joseph Biederman, M.D. Chief, Joint Program in Pediatric Psychopharmacology, Massachusetts General Hospital, McLean Hospital, and Associate Professor of Psychiatry, Harvard Medical School, Boston, Massachusetts

Ray Blanchard, Ph.D. Gender Identity Clinic, Clarke Institute of Psychiatry, Toronto, Ontario, Canada

Susan J. Bradley, M.D. Chair, DSM-IV Subcommittee for Gender Identity Disorders, and Psychiatrist-in-Chief, Hospital for Sick Children, Toronto, Ontario, Canada

Magda Campbell, M.D. Professor of Psychiatry, New York University Medical Center, New York, New York

Glorisa Canino, Ph.D. Professor of Pediatrics and Director, Behavioral Sciences Research Institute, University of Puerto Rico School of Medicine, San Juan, Puerto Rico

Ian Canino, M.D. Associate Clinical Professor and Deputy Director Child Psychiatry Training, Columbia University College of Physicians and Surgeons, New York, New York

D. Capaldi, Ph.D. Oregon Social Learning Center, Eugene, Oregon

Caryn L. Carlson, Ph.D. Associate Professor of Psychology, University of Texas, Austin, Texas

Alice S. Carter, Ph.D. Child Study Center and Department of Psychology, Yale University, New Haven, Connecticut

Richard J. Castillo, Ph.D. Associate Professor of Psychology, University of Hawaii—West Oahu, Pearl City, Hawaii

P. Chamberlain, Ph.D. Oregon Social Learning Center, Eugene, Oregon

John F. Clarkin, Ph.D. Professor of Clinical Psychology, Department of Psychiatry, Cornell University Medical College, and Director of Psychology, The New York Hospital—Cornell Medical Center, Westchester Division, White Plains, New York

Susan Coates, Ph.D. Childhood Gender Identity Center, Department of Psychiatry, St. Luke's—Roosevelt Hospital Center, New York, New York

Contributors

Cheryl S. Cohen, M.S. New York State Psychiatric Institute, and Ferkauf Graduate School of Psychology, Yeshiva University, New York, New York

Donald J. Cohen, M.D. Irving B. Harris Professor of Child Psychiatry, Pediatrics, and Psychology, and Director, Yale Child Study Center, New Haven, Connecticut

Maria DaCosta, M.D. Associate Professor of Psychiatry, Hillside Hospital—OPD, Glenoaks, New York

Dona Davis, Ph.D. Department of Social Behavior, University of South Dakota, Vermillion, South Dakota

Michael J. Devlin, M.D. Assistant Professor of Clinical Psychiatry, Columbia University College of Physicians and Surgeons, and Research Psychiatrist, New York State Psychiatric Institute, New York, New York

Horacio Fabrega Jr., M.D. Professor of Psychiatry and Anthropology, and Director, Medical Student Education, University of Pittsburgh School of Medicine, Western Psychiatric Institute and Clinic, Pittsburgh, Pennsylvania

P. Fisher, Ph.D. Oregon Social Learning Center, Eugene, Oregon

Steven R. Forness, Ed.D. Department of Psychiatry and Biobehavioral Sciences, University of California at Los Angeles, Los Angeles, California

Edward F. Foulks, M.D., Ph.D. Department of Psychiatry and Neurology, Tulane University School of Medicine, New Orleans, Louisiana

Allen J. Frances, M.D. Chairman, Department of Psychiatry, Duke University Medical Center, Durham, North Carolina; and Chair, Task Force on DSM-IV, American Psychiatric Association, Washington, DC

Paul J. Frick, Ph.D. Associate Professor of Psychology, University of Alabama, Tuscaloosa, Alabama

G. Davis Gammon, M.D. Assistant Clinical Professor of Child Psychiatry, Yale Child Study Center, New Haven, Connecticut

Paul E. Garfinkel, M.D.   Professor and Chair of Psychiatry, University of Toronto, and President, Clarke Institute of Psychiatry, Toronto, Ontario, Canada

Howard H. Goldman, M.D., Ph.D.   Professor of Psychiatry, University of Maryland School of Medicine, Baltimore, Maryland

Michael J. Goldstein, Ph.D.   Professor of Psychology and Psychiatry, Department of Psychology, University of California at Los Angeles, Los Angeles, California

Reed Goldstein, Ph.D.   The Dave Garroway Laboratory for the Study of Depression, The Institute of Pennsylvania Hospital, and the Department of Psychiatry, University of Pennsylvania School of Medicine, Philadelphia, Pennsylvania

Carlos A. González, M.D.   Assistant Clinical Professor, Department of Psychiatry, Yale University School of Medicine; and Chief, Crisis Intervention Service, Griffin Hospital, Derby, Connecticut

Byron J. Good, Ph.D.   Professor of Social Medicine and Anthropology, Harvard University, Cambridge, Massachusetts

Richard Green, M.D., J.D.   Department of Psychiatry, University of California at Los Angeles, Los Angeles, California

Ezra E. H. Griffith, M.D.   Professor, Department of Psychiatry, Yale University School of Medicine, and Director, Connecticut Mental Health Center, New Haven, Connecticut

James Grimm, M.D.   Western Psychiatric Institute and Clinic, Pittsburgh, Pennsylvania

Alan M. Gruenberg, M.D.   The Dave Garroway Laboratory for the Study of Depression, The Institute of Pennsylvania Hospital, and the Department of Psychiatry, University of Pennsylvania School of Medicine, Philadelphia, Pennsylvania

Peter J. Guarnaccia, Ph.D.   Associate Professor, Department of Human Ecology, Cook College and Institute for Health, Health Care Policy and Aging Research, Rutgers University, New Brunswick, New Jersey

Contributors

Katherine A. Halmi, M.D. Professor of Psychiatry, Cornell University Medical College, New York Hospital—Westchester Division, White Plains, New York

Gilbert Herdt, Ph.D. Committee on Human Development, University of Chicago, Chicago, Illinois

Charles C. Hughes, Ph.D. Professor, Department of Family and Preventive Medicine and Department of Anthropology, University of Utah, Salt Lake City, Utah

Neil S. Jacobson, Ph.D. Department of Psychology, University of Washington, Seattle, Washington

Janis H. Jenkins, Ph.D. Departments of Anthropology and Psychiatry, Case Western Reserve University, Cleveland, Ohio

Miguel R. Jorge, M.D., Ph.D. Chair of the Department of Psychiatry, Escola Paulista de Medicina, Brazil; and Fulbright-CNPq Scholar, University of Pittsburgh, Pittsburgh, Pennsylvania

Michael D. Kahn, Ph.D. Professor and Associate Director, Doctoral Program in Clinical Psychology, University of Hartford, West Hartford, Connecticut

Sandra Kaplan, M.D. Associate Chairman, Department of Psychiatry for Child and Adolescent Psychiatry, North Shore University—Cornell University Medical College, and Associate Professor of Clinical Psychiatry, Cornell University Medical College, Manhassat, New York

Marvin Karno, M.D. Department of Psychiatry and Biobehavioral Sciences, University of California at Los Angeles, Los Angeles, California

Robert A. King, M.D. Associate Professor of Child Psychiatry, Yale Child Study Center, New Haven, Connecticut

J. David Kinzie, M.D. Department of Psychiatry, Oregon Health Sciences University School of Medicine, Portland, Oregon

Laurence J. Kirmayer, M.D. Professor and Director, Division of Social and Transcultural Psychiatry, McGill University, and Director, Culture and Mental Health Research Unit, Department of Psychiatry, Sir Mortimer B. Davis Jewish General Hospital, Montreal, Quebec, Canada

Rachel G. Klein, Ph.D. Professor of Clinical Psychology, Columbia University College of Physicians and Surgeons and New York State Psychiatric Institute, New York, New York

Arthur Kleinman, M.D. Professor and Chairman of Social Medicine, Professor of Psychiatry and Anthropology, Harvard University, Cambridge, Massachusetts

John F. Knutson, Ph.D. Professor, Department of Psychology, The University of Iowa, Iowa City, Iowa

Benjamin B. Lahey, Ph.D. Professor of Psychiatry, University of Chicago Pritzker School of Medicine, Chicago, Illinois

Tamara R. Lave, B.A. Haverford College, Haverford, Pennsylvania

Tina K. Leonard-Green, M.S., R.D. Department of Family and Community Medicine, University of Arizona, Tucson, Arizona

Stephen B. Levine, M.D. Department of Psychiatry, Case Western Reserve University, University Hospital, Cleveland, Ohio

Roberto Lewis-Fernández, M.D. Lecturer on Social Medicine, Department of Social Medicine, Harvard Medical School, Boston, Massachusetts; and Co-Investigator, Behavioral Sciences Research Institute, University of Puerto Rico, San Juan, Puerto Rico

Keh-Ming Lin, M.D., M.P.H. Professor of Psychiatry and Director, Research Center on the Psychobiology of Ethnicity, Harbor—UCLA Medical Center, Torrance, California

Roland Littlewood, M.B., D.Phil., M.R.C.Psych. Professor of Anthropology and Psychiatry, University College Centre for Medical Anthropology, Department of Anthropology, University College, London, England

Rolf Loeber, Ph.D. Professor of Psychiatry and Epidemiology, University of Pittsburgh School of Medicine, Pittsburgh, Pennsylvania

Francis G. Lu, M.D. Clinical Professor of Psychiatry, Department of Psychiatry, University of California, San Francisco, California

David Lukoff, Ph.D. Professor of Psychology, Saybrook Institute, San Francisco, California

Spero M. Manson, Ph.D. Professor, Department of Psychiatry, School of Medicine, University of Colorado Health Sciences Center, and Professor and Director, National Center for American Indian and Alaska Native Mental Health, University of Colorado, Denver, Colorado

Linda C. Mayes, M.D. Gessel Associate Professor of Pediatrics, Yale University, New Haven, Connecticut

Keith McBurnett, Ph.D. Assistant Professor, Pediatrics, Child Development Center, University of California, Irvine, Newport Beach, California

Heino F. L. Meyer-Bahlburg, Dr. rer. nat. Program of Developmental Psychoendocrinology, Division of Child Psychiatry, New York State Psychiatric Institute, New York, New York

Juan E. Mezzich, M.D., Ph.D. Professor of Psychiatry and Epidemiology, University of Pittsburgh, Pittsburgh, Pennsylvania

David J. Miklowitz, Ph.D. Assistant Professor of Psychology, Department of Psychology, University of Colorado, Boulder, Colorado

James E. Mitchell, M.D. Professor, Department of Psychiatry, University of Minnesota Medical School, Minneapolis, Minnesota

Genevieve Monks, M.A. Doctoral Program in Clinical Psychology, University of Hartford, West Hartford, Connecticut

Jeffrey H. Newcorn, M.D. Director, Division of Child and Adolescent Psychiatry, and Associate Professor of Psychiatry and Pediatrics, Mount Sinai School of Medicine, New York, New York

K. Daniel O'Leary, Ph.D. Department of Psychology, State University of New York at Stony Brook, Stony Brook, New York

Delores L. Parron, Ph.D. Associate Director for Special Populations, National Institute of Mental Health, Rockville, Maryland

Rhea Paul, Ph.D. Professor, Speech and Hearing Sciences Program, Portland State University, and Director, Portland Language Development Project, Portland, Oregon

Ira B. Pauly, M.D. Department of Psychiatry, University of Nevada School of Medicine, Reno, Nevada

David Pelcovitz, Ph.D. Chief Psychologist, Division of Child and Adolescent Psychiatry, North Shore University—Cornell University Medical College, and Clinical Associate Professor of Psychology in Psychiatry, Cornell University Medical College, Manhassat, New York

J. Christopher Perry, M.P.H., M.D. Associate Professor in Psychiatry, McGill University, and Director of Research, Department of Psychiatry, Sir Mortimer B. Davis—Jewish General Hospital, Montreal, Quebec, Canada

Cynthia R. Pfeffer, M.D. Professor of Psychiatry, Cornell University Medical Center, New York Hospital—Westchester Division, White Plains, New York

Harold A. Pincus, M.D. Deputy Medical Director and Director, Office of Research, American Psychiatric Association, Washington, DC

Raymond Prince, Ph.D. Department of Psychiatry, McGill University, Montreal, Quebec, Canada

Herbert C. Quay, Ph.D. Professor of Psychology (Emeritus), University of Miami, Miami, Florida

Judith G. Rabkin, Ph.D., M.P.H. Professor of Clinical Psychology (in Psychiatry), Columbia University College of Physicians and Surgeons, and Research Scientist, New York State Psychiatric Institute, New York, New York

J. Ray, B.A. Oregon Social Learning Center, Eugene, Oregon

J. B. Reid, Ph.D. Oregon Social Learning Center, Eugene, Oregon

Cheryl Ritenbaugh, Ph.D., M.P.H. Department of Family and Community Medicine, University of Arizona, Tucson, Arizona

Martin Rosenzweig, M.D. The Institute of Pennsylvania Hospital Department of Psychiatry, and the Department of Psychiatry, University of Pennsylvania School of Medicine, Philadelphia, Pennsylvania

Ruth Ross, M.A. Science Writer, DSM-IV, and Managing Editor, Journal of Practical Psychiatry and Behavioral Health, Independence, Virginia

Helen A. Schartz, Ph.D. Department of Psychology, Southwest Missouri State University, Springfield, Missouri

David Shaffer, M.D. Irving Philips Professor of Child Psychiatry, Director, Division of Child and Adolescent Psychiatry, Columbia University College of Physicians and Surgeons, New York, New York

Catherine Shisslak, Ph.D. Department of Family and Community Medicine, University of Arizona, Tucson, Arizona

Ronald C. Simons, M.D. Professor, Department of Psychiatry, Michigan State University, East Lansing, Michigan; and Clinical Professor, Department of Psychiatry and Behavioral Sciences, University of Washington, St. Louis, Missouri

Andrew E. Skodol, M.D. Professor of Clinical Psychiatry, Columbia University College of Physicians and Surgeons, and Research Psychiatrist, New York State Psychiatric Institute, New York, New York

Susan Sprich, B.A. Clinical Fellow in Psychology, Psychiatry Department, Massachusetts General Hospital, Boston, Massachusetts

Angus M. Strachan, Ph.D. Associate Clinical Professor of Psychology, Department of Psychology and Psychiatry, University of California at Los Angeles, Los Angeles, California

James Strain, M.D. Professor of Psychiatry and Director, Division of Behavioral Medicine and Consultation Psychiatry, Mount Sinai School of Medicine, New York, New York

Patrick F. Sullivan, M.D. Senior Psychiatric Resident, University of Pittsburgh, Pittsburgh, Pennsylvania

Peter Szatmari, M.D., F.R.C.P.C. Associate Professor, Department of Psychiatry, McMaster University, Chedoke—McMaster Hospitals, Center for the Study of Children at Risk, Hamilton, Ontario, Canada

Paula Tallal, Ph.D. Director, Center for Molecular and Behavioral Neuroscience, Rutgers University, Newark, New Jersey

Nancy Kaplan Tancer, M.D. Chief of Child and Adolescent Psychiatry, Bergen Pines County Hospital, Paramus, New Jersey

Nicolette Teufel, Ph.D. Department of Family and Community Medicine, University of Arizona, Tucson, Arizona

Luke Y. Tsai, M.D. Professor and Service Chief, Child and Adolescent Psychiatry Service, Department of Psychiatry, University of Michigan Medical Center, Ann Arbor, Michigan

Robert Turner, M.D. Assistant Clinical Professor of Psychiatry, Department of Psychiatry, University of California, San Francisco, California

Fred R. Volkmar, M.D. Harris Associate Professor of Child Psychiatry, Pediatrics, and Psychology, Yale University, Child Study Center, New Haven, Connecticut

B. Timothy Walsh, M.D. Professor of Clinical Psychiatry, Columbia University College of Physicians and Surgeons, and Director, Eating Disorders Research Unit, New York State Psychiatric Institute, New York, New York

Mitchell Weiss, M.D., Ph.D. Senior Scientist, Swiss Tropical Institute, Department of Public Health and Epidemiology, Basel, Switzerland

John S. Werry, M.D. Emeritus Professor of Psychiatry, University of Auckland, Auckland, New Zealand

Joseph Westermeyer, M.D., Ph.D. Department of Psychiatry, University of Minnesota, Minneapolis, Minnesota

Thomas A. Widiger, Ph.D. Professor, Department of Psychology, University of Kentucky, Lexington, Kentucky

Janet B. W. Williams, D.S.W. Professor of Clinical Psychiatric Social Work (in Psychiatry and Neurology), Columbia University College of Physicians and Surgeons, and Deputy Chief, Biometrics Research Department, New York State Psychiatric Institute, New York, New York

G. Terence Wilson, Ph.D. Graduate School of Applied and Professional Psychology, Rutgers University, Busch Campus, Piscataway, New Jersey

Ronald M. Winchel, M.D. New York State Psychiatric Institute and Columbia University College of Physicians and Surgeons, New York, New York

Ronald M. Wintrob, M.D. Professor, Department of Psychiatry, Brown University, and Department of Psychological Medicine, Christchurch School of Medicine, Providence, Rhode Island

Lyman C. Wynne, M.D., Ph.D. Professor of Psychiatry, School of Medicine and Dentistry, University of Rochester, Rochester, New York

Kenneth J. Zucker, Ph.D. Child and Adolescent Gender Identity Clinic, Child and Family Studies Centre, Clarke Institute of Psychiatry, Toronto, Ontario, Canada

Preface

DSM-IV Sourcebook: Volumes 1–3—Literature Reviews

For more than 5 years, the Task Force on DSM-IV and members of the DSM-IV Work Groups participated in a comprehensive effort of empirical review leading to the publication of the fourth edition of the American Psychiatric Association's *Diagnostic and Statistical Manual of Mental Disorders* (DSM-IV). The *DSM-IV Sourcebook* chronicles these efforts and their results, documenting the rationale and empirical support for the text and criteria sets presented in DSM-IV. The major emphasis in the DSM-IV process has been on empirical review and documentation (Frances et al. 1990; Pincus et al. 1992), and the *Sourcebook*, to be published in four volumes, is an important means of presenting that documentation. The first three volumes contain the DSM-IV literature reviews and summarize the DSM-IV Work Groups' efforts that led to the publication of the *DSM-IV Options Book* (American Psychiatric Association 1991). The fourth volume will contain summaries of the rationale for the final decisions of each Work Group, along with the results of the DSM-IV data reanalyses and DSM-IV field trials.

The *DSM-IV Sourcebook* is the culmination of a process that began in September 1987, when the American Psychiatric Association (APA) Committee on Psychiatric Diagnosis and Assessment met to explore possible timetables for the publication of DSM-IV. Because of the work already proceeding on the 10th edition of the International Classification of Diseases (ICD-10) by the World Health Organization (1992), the Committee concluded that work should also begin on DSM-IV to allow for mutual influence and convergence of the two systems (Frances et al. 1989). From the outset, the Committee recommended that review of the empirical evidence on diagnostic issues—often stimulated by the publication of DSM-III (American Psychiatric Association 1980) and DSM-III-R (American Psychiatric Association 1987)—be the centerpiece for the development of DSM-IV.

In May of 1988, the Board of Trustees of the APA appointed a Task Force to undertake the preparation of DSM-IV. Thirteen Work Groups were formed, each chaired by a member of the Task Force. These Work Groups covered the Anxiety Disorders; Child and Adolescent Disorders; Eating Disorders; Late Luteal Phase Dysphoric Disorder; Mood Disorders; the Multiaxial system; Delirium, Dementia, and Amnestic and Other Cognitive ("Organic") Disorders; Personality Disorders; Psychiatric System Interface Disorders (consisting of Somatoform, Factitious, Dissociative, Impulse Control, and Adjustment Disorders); Psychotic Disorders; Sexual Disorders; Sleep Disorders; and Substance-Related Disorders.

Two conferences were held to develop the process by which DSM-IV would be constructed. These conferences were attended by representatives of the DSM-IV Task Force; the various Work Groups; and expert consultants on the design, analysis, and review of empirical research. The first Methods Conference was held in August 1988 to discuss procedures for gathering and analyzing data from different studies to achieve a comprehensive and objective consideration of the empirical literature. The second Methods and Applications Conference was held in November 1988 to discuss in more detail procedures for reviewing research, for selecting validators for existing and proposed items, for conducting field trials, and for resolving the various issues that would be addressed by the respective Work Groups. It was decided that the development of DSM-IV should proceed through three interactive stages of empirical review and documentation: 1) literature reviews, 2) reanalyses of existing data sets, and 3) focused field trials (Widiger et al. 1991). The goal of this process was to maximize the impact of empirical research on the deliberations and decisions of the DSM-IV Work Groups and Task Force and to document the empirical support for the resulting recommendations and proposals (Frances et al. 1990; Pincus et al. 1992).

For any substantial revision of, addition to, or deletion from DSM-III-R to be considered for DSM-IV, it had to be accompanied by a review of the empirical and clinical literature (Widiger et al. 1990). Those conducting the reviews were to function as if they were consensus scholars (persons with no preconceptions who are fully aware of the clinical and research literature) (Cooper 1984). The reviews were to be not position papers arguing for particular proposals, but rather systematic, comprehensive, and objective overviews of the most relevant empirical research. These literature reviews are presented in the first three volumes of the *DSM-IV Sourcebook*.

The literature reviews also served to identify gaps and inadequacies within the literature on questions of crucial importance to the DSM-IV Work Groups. Fortunately, in many such instances, relevant existing data sets were available that had not yet been analyzed in a fashion that would provide useful answers. Therefore, the second stage of the DSM-IV development process was to obtain and reanalyze multiple data sets to address questions not answered in the published literature. This also allowed us to generate and pilot new proposals for criteria sets for DSM-IV (Widiger et al. 1991). These efforts were funded in part by the John D. and Catherine T. MacArthur Foundation, and the results will be presented in Volume 4 of the *DSM-IV Sourcebook*.

The culmination of the literature review and data reanalysis process was the publication of the *DSM-IV Options Book*. The purpose of the *Options Book* was both to present the major diagnostic issues, and options for dealing with them, that had been identified by the Task Force on DSM-IV and to encourage review, comments, and the contribution of additional available data. Summaries describing how the information from the literature reviews and data reanalyses aided the Task Force and Work Groups in developing these options are presented in the *Sourcebook*. It is hoped that the publication of this information will provide an explanation and documentation for the decisions made in DSM-IV.

The third stage of the DSM-IV development process was to perform focused field trials to assess the extent to which proposed revisions would actually improve the reliability and/or validity of criteria sets and to address the issues identified by the literature reviews. The field trials allowed the DSM-IV Work Groups to compare alternative options (usually DSM-III, DSM-III-R, ICD-10 research criteria, and the various proposals for DSM-IV that had been generated during the first two steps) and to study the possible impact of any suggested changes. Funding for the field trials was obtained from the National Institute of Mental Health in collaboration with the National Institute on Drug Abuse and the National Institute on Alcohol Abuse and Alcoholism. The results of the focused field trials and the rationale for the final decisions of the Work Groups and Task Force will also be presented in Volume 4 of the *DSM-IV Sourcebook*.

The culmination of this final stage in the DSM-IV development process was the publication of the *DSM-IV Draft Criteria* (American Psychiatric Association 1993). The purpose of this document was to invite review and comment on the proposed criteria before they appeared in DSM-IV. Readers were asked to help identify any mistakes, inconsistencies, oversights, unforeseen problems, potential for misuse, or boundary confusions.

In the rest of this Preface, we detail the organization and format of the literature reviews presented in the first three volumes of the *DSM-IV Sourcebook*. The introduction to Volume 4 will deal with issues specific to the data reanalyses and field trials.

The DSM-IV literature reviews are divided into three volumes, organized with respect to shared concerns and issues. Volume 1 presents the reviews for Substance-Related Disorders; Delirium, Dementia, and Amnestic and Other Cognitive Disorders (including a review on Mental Disorders Due to a General Medical Condition); Schizophrenia and Other Psychotic Disorders; Medication-Induced Movement Disorders; and Sleep Disorders. Volume 2 presents the reviews for the Mood Disorders, Late Luteal Phase Dysphoric Disorder, Anxiety Disorders, Personality Disorders, Psychiatric System Interface Disorders (consisting of Somatoform, Factitious, Dissociative, Impulse Control, and Adjustment Disorders), and Sexual Disorders.

The current volume, Volume 3, presents the reviews for Childhood Disorders, Eating Disorders, Multiaxial Issues, Family Relational Issues, and Cultural and Religious-Spiritual Issues. The literature reviews for the Childhood Disorders, Eating Disorders, and Multiaxial Issues were solicited by the respective DSM-IV Work Groups. The literature reviews for Family Relational Issues and Cultural and Religious-Spiritual Issues were solicited by the DSM-IV Task Force. In addition, the mandate for the authors of these reviews was modified. The authors of these reviews used the same format that was requested of all authors (presented below). However, they were also asked to critique DSM-III-R with respect to its consideration of family relational, cultural, and religious-spiritual issues. Therefore, the authors of these reviews were given more latitude to represent their own particular perspective rather than a consensus position. Their reviews may at times be inconsistent with the recommendations of the DSM-IV Task Force.

Each section of this volume of the *Sourcebook* begins with an introductory chapter that provides an executive summary of the material contained within that section as well as an overview of the activities and procedures of the respective Work Group, when applicable. This is followed by the individual literature reviews. In preparing the first three volumes of the *DSM-IV Sourcebook,* we have kept in mind that not all readers will be interested in all the fine points concerning every issue. For this reason, the introductory section for each set of reviews includes an executive summary of the important points in each review. For those interested in pursuing a subject in more detail, the individual reviews discuss the questions at hand in much greater depth and provide extensive reference sections.

The literature reviews from the Child and Adolescent Disorders Work Group are presented in two parts. This Work Group was responsible for reviewing proposals concerning the 46 diagnoses included within this section in DSM-III-R, proposals for new diagnoses to be included within this section, and proposals concerning diagnoses that are included within other sections of the manual that are relevant or apply to children and adolescents. As a result, their domain of responsibility was substantial. Therefore, the reviews for this Work Group are provided separately within the *Sourcebook* to facilitate their consideration. The first section provides the reviews for childhood autism (and the proposals for Rett's, childhood disintegrative, and pervasive developmental disorder not otherwise specified), early onset schizophrenia, social skills deficits, and language and speech disorders. The second section provides the reviews for the many other diagnoses that are relevant to children and adolescents.

Experts on the methodology of literature review provided guidelines for performing systematic, objective, and comprehensive evaluation of the available clinical research literature (Cooper 1984). The authors of the reviews were encouraged to follow an explicit format for conducting the review and presenting its findings. Successive drafts of each review were distributed widely to the advisers to each Work Group, who were specifically chosen to include individuals who represented a wide range of viewpoints on any given issue. Many of the reviews have also been published in revised form in professional and scientific journals and presented at conferences and meetings. We have encouraged the authors to publish and present their findings and interpretation to receive as much peer review and critical commentary as possible. This iterative process and the explicit format have been very helpful in identifying the various inadequacies, gaps, and biases that occurred in earlier drafts (e.g., failure to cover an important issue, a bias in the selection of studies, gaps in the coverage or presentation of the literature, disagreements concerning the interpretation of empirical findings, and failure to consider alternative options).

Each review contains the following sections: Statement of the Issues, Significance of the Issues, Method, Results, Discussion, and Recommendations (Widiger et al. 1990). The "Statement of the Issues" section outlines explicitly the issues being addressed in the review and keeps the review focused on the pertinent nosological questions. This section informs the reader of the focus and scope of the review.

The "Significance of the Issues" section frames the importance of the issue and discusses its clinical and/or empirical significance.

The "Method" section ensures replicability of the review and documents the extent to which the reviews were systematic and comprehensive in their coverage of the literature. This section indicates the types of studies that were considered and the ways they were identified with any explicit inclusion or exclusion criteria (e.g., requirements with respect to the populations sampled, the criteria sets used, how recently the study was conducted, and other methodological features). Authors were instructed to conduct computerized literature searches, to review specified journals systematically, and to solicit input from all the leading researchers in the field to minimize bias in the identification and consideration of studies that might result from the authors' own perspective on the literature.

The "Results" section provides an objective and thorough, yet succinct, summary of the findings most relevant to the issues. To facilitate a balanced presentation of the findings, the authors were discouraged from presenting their own conclusions or recommendations in this section.

The "Discussion" section addresses the implications of the clinical research findings for DSM-IV. Authors were encouraged to delineate and discuss all meaningful options for resolving the issues (including those they might not favor) and to outline the advantages and disadvantages of each option.

In the "Recommendations" section, the authors were encouraged to present their own recommendations for DSM-IV based on their review of the literature. In a few instances, these recommendations were not shared by the respective Work Group. In such cases, the recommendations were revised or the authors were requested to be explicit regarding their disagreements and to indicate the advantages and disadvantages of the various options. Authors were also encouraged to make suggestions for future research that would be helpful to the development of DSM-V.

It is unlikely that readers will agree with all the recommendations presented in these reviews. Many of the issues do not have clear or obvious solutions, and more or less plausible arguments can often be made for a variety of alternative viewpoints. Our efforts have been directed toward achieving solutions that reflect the available empirical data and provide an optimal balance among the various goals of the diagnostic process. The advance of fundamental understanding of mental disorders will undoubtedly provide much clearer (and probably often very different) answers to the questions raised here.

Thomas A. Widiger, Ph.D.
Allen J. Frances, M.D.
Harold Alan Pincus, M.D.
Ruth Ross, M.A.
Michael B. First, M.D.
Wendy Davis, Ed.M.

References

American Psychiatric Association: Diagnostic and Statistical Manual of Mental Disorders, 3rd Edition. Washington, DC, American Psychiatric Association, 1980

American Psychiatric Association: Diagnostic and Statistical Manual of Mental Disorders, 3rd Edition, Revised. Washington, DC, American Psychiatric Association, 1987

American Psychiatric Association: DSM-IV Options Book: Work in Progress 9/9/91. Washington, DC, American Psychiatric Association, 1991

American Psychiatric Association, Task Force on DSM-IV: DSM-IV Draft Criteria 3/1/93. Washington, DC, American Psychiatric Association, 1993
Cooper HM: The Integrative Research Review: A Systematic Approach, Vol 2. Beverly Hills, CA, Sage, 1984
Frances AJ, Widiger TA, Pincus HA: The development of DSM-IV. Arch Gen Psychiatry 46:373–375, 1989
Frances AJ, Pincus HA, Widiger TA, et al: DSM-IV: work in progress. Am J Psychiatry 147:1439–1448, 1990
Pincus HA, Frances AJ, Davis W, et al: DSM-IV and new diagnostic categories: holding the line on proliferation. Am J Psychiatry 149:112-117, 1992
Widiger TA, Frances AJ, Pincus HA, et al: DSM-IV literature reviews: rationale, process, and limitations. Journal of Psychopathology and Behavioral Assessment 12:189–202, 1990
Widiger TA, Frances AJ, Pincus HA, et al: Toward an empirical classification for the DSM-IV. J Abnorm Psychol 100:280–288, 1991
World Health Organization: The ICD-10 Classification of Mental and Behavioral Disorders: Clinical Descriptions and Diagnostic Guidelines. Geneva, Switzerland, World Health Organization, 1992

Acknowledgments

DSM-IV has been a team effort, with more than 1,000 people (and numerous professional organizations) helping us in its preparation. The Task Force on DSM-IV and Work Group members have worked hard and cheerfully throughout the demanding process of developing DSM-IV. Without their energy and expertise, this project would not have been possible.

Bob Spitzer has our thanks for his untiring efforts and unique perspective. Norman Sartorius, Michael Rutter, Darrel Regier, Lewis Judd, Fred Goodwin, and Chuck Kaelber were instrumental in facilitating a mutually productive interchange between the American Psychiatric Association (APA) and the World Health Organization. Dennis Prager, Peter Nathan, and David Kupfer helped us in developing a novel data reanalysis strategy that has been supported with funding from the John D. and Catherine T. MacArthur Foundation.

There are several individuals within APA who deserve special recognition. Mel Sabshin's special wisdom and grace made even the most tedious tasks seem worth doing. The APA Committee on Diagnosis and Assessment (chaired by Layton McCurdy) provided valuable direction and counsel. We also thank the APA Presidents (Drs. Fink, Pardes, Benedek, Hartmann, English, and McIntyre) and Assembly Speakers (Drs. Cohen, Flamm, Hanin, Pfaehler, and Shellow), who helped with the planning of our work. Carolyn Robinowitz and her staff in the APA Medical Director's office provided valuable assistance in the organization of the project.

The energy, intelligence, and scholarship of the authors of the DSM-IV literature reviews have surpassed our highest demands and expectations. Each review was read and commented on by many authorities in the field. Reviews often went through as many as half a dozen revisions. We would like to thank all those who contributed to this tremendous effort (in particular, the Work Group chairs, literature review authors, and commentators) for their unflagging efforts and good nature throughout this effort.

Excellent administrative and editorial support was provided by Myriam Kline, Gloria Miele, Sarah Tilly, Willa Hall, Kelly MacKinney, Helen Stayna, Nina Rosenthal, Susan Mann, Joanne Mas, Nancy Vettorello, Nancy Sydnor-Greenberg, Cindy Jones, Rebekah Brown, and Stacey Tipp, without whose help these volumes would have been impossible. Finally, we thank Ron McMillen, Claire Reinburg, Pam Harley, and Karen Sardinas-Wyssling for their expert production and editorial assistance.

We thank our patient readers. We hope that our efforts are useful to you.

Allen J. Frances, M.D.
Chair, Task Force on DSM-IV

Harold Alan Pincus, M.D.
APA Deputy Medical Director

Michael B. First, M.D.
Editor, DSM-IV Text and Criteria

Thomas A. Widiger, Ph.D.
Research Coordinator

Wendy Wakefield Davis, Ed.M.
Editorial Coordinator

Ruth Ross, M.A.
Science Writer

Section I

Disorders Usually First Diagnosed in Infancy, Childhood, or Adolescence (Part I)

Introduction to Section I

Disorders Usually First Diagnosed in Infancy, Childhood, or Adolescence (Part I)

Magda Campbell, M.D.

This section of the *DSM-IV Sourcebook* deals with the proposals made for DSM-IV with regard to pervasive developmental disorders, early onset schizophrenia, learning disorders, and language and speech disorders.

Pervasive Developmental Disorders

Pervasive developmental disorders, a new class of disorders, was introduced in DSM-III (American Psychiatric Association 1980) and included infantile autism (full syndrome, residual state), childhood onset pervasive developmental disorder, and atypical pervasive developmental disorder.

The term *pervasive developmental disorder* was retained in DSM-III-R (American Psychiatric Association 1987), although considerable changes were made: autistic disorder and pervasive developmental disorder not otherwise specified (PDDNOS) replaced the previous subtypes; the category was placed on Axis II; age at onset was removed as a criterion; 16 criteria (under the following three headings: qualitative impairment in reciprocal social interaction, qualitative impairment in verbal and nonverbal communication and in imaginative activity, and markedly restricted repertoire of activities and interests) were given for autistic disorder, of which at least 8 had to be present to diagnose autistic disorder; and atypical pervasive developmental disorder was replaced by PDDNOS.

The DSM-IV Work Group members responsible for studying the pervasive developmental disorders identified the following as the most pertinent issues for DSM-IV:

1. Moving pervasive developmental disorder from Axis II to Axis I
2. Age at onset for autistic disorder
3. The apparent overinclusiveness of the DSM-III-R criteria compared with other diagnostic criteria and clinical diagnosis and the excessive number of criteria
4. Inclusion of certain syndromes under PDDNOS that are given a discrete diagnostic status within the pervasive developmental disorder category in ICD-10 (World Health Organization 1990)

Literature reviews were solicited to address these issues.

Autistic Disorder

The literature review on the DSM-III-R criteria for autistic disorder by Szatmari (Chapter 1) provided a critical analysis of five studies with the goal of determining whether the psychometric properties of the criteria are appropriate and adequate for clinical practice, teaching, and research. Two studies were based on the DSM-III-R field trial data from which the diagnostic algorithm was developed (Siegel et al. 1989; Spitzer and Siegel 1990). In the Spitzer and Siegel report, the sensitivity and the specificity of the actual field trial data were very high (.86 and .80, respectively), although Siegel et al. reported lower sensitivity (.82) in their subsample. In the DSM-III-R field trial, of the various diagnostic algorithms, 2 from A, 1 from B, 1 from C, and 8 from the total of 16 criteria had shown the highest sensitivity (.86) and specificity (.80) and were most clinically meaningful. The data from the remaining three studies (Hertzig et al. 1989; Szatmari 1989; Volkmar et al. 1988) agreed among themselves but disagreed with the field trial data. Although sensitivity ranged from .90 to .97, specificity (.64–.82) and positive predictive value were low. Using DSM-III-R criteria, nearly 30% of patients in the replication samples were false positives, whereas in a general child development clinic more than 50% would be misdiagnosed as autistic (Szatmari, Chapter 1). Thus these studies have shown that the DSM-III-R criteria for autistic disorder were overinclusive as compared with clinical diagnosis or with DSM-III and that more stringent criteria are required to raise the threshold for the diagnosis. Children with mental retardation and those with developmental delays could easily be misdiagnosed as autistic by DSM-III-R criteria. Furthermore, there were too many criteria, and some were redundant (Siegel et al. 1989).

The deliberations of the Work Group resulted in the proposed criteria for autistic disorder presented in the *DSM-IV Options Book* (American Psychiatric Association 1991). Although the literature review did not specifically address the age-at-onset criterion, it was proposed that it be changed to "abnormal development prior to age three manifested by delays or abnormal functioning in social development, language used in social communication, or play." It was also proposed that autistic disorder be placed on Axis I because substantial evidence supports the validity of autistic disorder as an Axis I disorder of infancy and early childhood.

The following additional proposals were made:

1. That the number of criteria be reduced from 16 to perhaps 15.
2. That item A be changed to "gross and sustained impairment in social interaction" with 5 criteria that are in essence the DSM-III-R criteria, but with wording simplified and/or parenthetical examples deleted.
3. That item B be changed to "gross and sustained impairment in communication" and that the number of criteria be reduced from 6 to 5. Criterion B1 would encompass DSM-III-R criteria B1, B2, and B6 as follows "a delay in or the total absence of spoken language with markedly abnormal nonverbal communication." However, whereas DSM-III-R B1 and B2 were symptoms usually seen in low-functioning autistic persons and/or in very young autistic children, DSM-III-R criterion B6 clearly reflected language and communication deviances or problems in higher-functioning individuals ("marked impairment in the ability to initiate or sustain a conversation with others, despite adequate speech" [American Psychiatric Association 1987, p. 39]). It was also proposed that a new criterion (B4) be added: "failure to use social or emotional cues to regulate communication."

Although it was proposed that "gross and sustained" precede "impairment" in items A and B, it was suggested that "markedly" be deleted in item C and the C wording be changed from "markedly restricted repertoire of activities and interests" (American Psychiatric Association 1987, p. 39) to "restricted patterns of behavior, interest, and activities." It was proposed that the number of C criteria be reduced from 5 to 4, by combining DSM-III-R C3 and C4 into the proposed DSM-IV C1: "insistence on sameness (e.g., resistance to change, distress over small changes, interest in nonfunctional routines or rituals)."

Although Szatmari recommended in his literature review that poor language comprehension, a clinical feature that is often characteristically associated with autism, be incorporated in the language criterion, this proposal was not included in the *DSM-IV Options Book*. The majority of the Work Group agreed that poor language comprehension should not be included as a criterion in DSM-IV but should instead be discussed in the descriptive text accompanying the criteria.

Rett's Disorder

Because Rett's disorder is included in ICD-10, a literature review was undertaken to gather information on the internal and external validity of Rett's disorder to determine whether it should also be included in DSM-IV. Tsai (Chapter 2) identified 330 published articles in English on Rett's syndrome, 37 of which he considers in his chapter. Rett's syndrome was delineated and reported in a sample of 22 patients by Rett in 1966. The prevalence is estimated to be 1:10,000 to 1:15,000. Although all reported cases are in females, female sex is not proposed as an inclusion criterion because it is thought that there might be male patients with this syndrome who have not been diagnosed. Characteristically, the pre- and perinatal period is apparently normal; head circumference is normal at birth and so is psychomotor development in the first 6 months of extrauterine life. Deceleration of head growth starts between 5 months and 4 years. Purposeful hand skills are lost between 6 and 30 months and are replaced by hand stereotypies and mouthing. Severe impairment of language, apraxia/ataxia, and social withdrawal appear. Supportive criteria include respiratory difficulties and seizures. Scoliosis and motor deterioration are described in the final stages.

The hand stereotypies typically involve washing movements, bringing hands together (wringing/clapping), and wetting hands with saliva. These typical hand stereotypies and the early development and course differentiate Rett's disorder both from autistic disorder and from childhood disintegrative disorder. Furthermore, social withdrawal is less severe in Rett's syndrome than in autism and is perhaps transient.

Thus there is evidence supporting both the internal and external validity of Rett's syndrome. There are at least three sets of existing diagnostic criteria for the disorder (see Chapter 2). The proposed DSM-IV criteria are similar to those in ICD-10. Although Rett's disorder contains autistic features and can be considered as one of the pervasive developmental disorders, there is evidence in the published studies that certain physical and behavioral characteristics differentiate it from autism and from childhood disintegrative disorder. The inclusion of Rett's disorder in DSM-IV would allow for greater specificity in the differential diagnosis of nonautistic pervasive developmental disorders. Because the proposed DSM-IV criteria are close to those of ICD-10, the inclusion of this condition would increase the compatibility of DSM-IV with ICD-10.

Childhood Disintegrative Disorder

Childhood disintegrative disorder was also not included in DSM-III-R but was included in ICD-9 (World Health Organization 1978) (as disintegrative psychosis) and in ICD-10 (as other childhood disintegrative disorder, to be differentiated from Rett's syndrome). The literature review by Volkmar (Chapter 3) has shown evidence supporting both the external and internal validity of childhood disintegrative disorder. It was first described in 1908 by Heller, who called the condition dementia infantilis. Heller reported on six children who, following a normal or relatively normal development, showed regression and progressive deterioration with loss of speech and social skills associated with behavioral symptoms including stereotypies and hyperactivity. Although in some cases the loss of skills and cognitive deterioration was associated with central nervous system disease, in other cases such association was not clear or was altogether absent, or psychosocial influences seemed to be at work.

PDDNOS

The issue addressed in the literature review on PDDNOS by Szatmari (Chapter 4) was whether all pervasive developmental disorder subtypes not meeting the criteria for autistic disorder (Rett's disorder, childhood disintegrative disorder, Asperger's disorder, and atypical autism) should be included in the PDDNOS category, as in DSM-III-R, or listed as separate diagnostic categories, as in ICD-10. There was strong evidence based on the literature reviews by Tsai (Chapter 2) and Volkmar (Chapter 3) and clinical and research needs for including Rett's disorder and childhood disintegrative disorder as separate diagnostic categories in DSM-IV. The case was somewhat weaker for including Asperger's disorder and atypical autism as separate diagnoses, particularly given the presence of the PDDNOS category in the DSM system.

Asperger's Disorder

The literature review by Szatmari (Chapter 4) shows that the internal and external validity of Asperger's disorder has not been well established. This syndrome is considered to be a milder form of autism or a high-functioning autism; there is certainly overlap with autism (impairment in social interaction and restricted, repetitive behavior and interests). The problems are due mainly to the fact that there are no specified diagnostic criteria for Asperger's syndrome, with the result that investigators use different diagnostic criteria and different definitions. Schizoid disorder of childhood (Wolff and Barlow 1979) is similar, but quite a bit broader than Asperger's disorder. However, investigators do agree to some extent on the clinical phenomenology of Asperger's disorder and that differences do exist between high-functioning autistic subjects and those diagnosed as having Asperger's disorder (Gillberg 1989; Szatmari et al. 1989). Asperger's disorder differs from autism in the following ways:

- Lack of significant delay in language
- Lack of significant delay in cognitive development
- Greater verbal IQ scores than performance IQ scores
- Motor delays more variable than in autism
- Isolated special skills (often related to abnormal preoccupation) more common than in autism

- Later age at onset
- Higher intellectual functioning
- Less severe symptoms
- Presence of anxiety
- Speech characteristically tangential, repetitive, and pedantic (Wing 1981)

Asperger's disorder has the following similarities to autism:

- Some impairment in social interaction
- Restricted range of interest

Thus there is some evidence to support the distinctiveness of Asperger's syndrome from autism, and the literature review indicates that there is some agreement among researchers concerning phenomenology (see Chapter 4). Members of the Child Work Group recommended the inclusion of Asperger's disorder in DSM-IV. It has been suggested that the study of Asperger's syndrome and its differentiation from autism, schizophrenia, schizotypal personality disorder, and schizoid personality disorder is important in investigating the possible link between autistic disorder and schizophrenia and that including Asperger's in DSM-IV would contribute further to our understanding of schizophrenia and promote family studies of schizophrenia with onset in childhood (J. L. Rapoport, personal communication, October 22, 1992); a review is available elsewhere (Rutter and Garmezy 1983). Although the empirical evidence of validity is only partial, and it is unclear whether Asperger's disorder and high-functioning autism are the same, it seems justified to include Asperger's disorder as a separate condition to provide better and more individualized services (and treatment different from that for autism) for these children and to promote research in this area. Asperger's disorder is a lifelong disorder, and the characteristic features persist into adulthood. The members of the DSM-IV Work Group on autism/pervasive developmental disorder agreed that Asperger's disorder might have inadequate visibility if placed in PDDNOS (Rutter and Schopler 1992). The criteria for Asperger's disorder proposed in the *DSM-IV Options Book* are close to those in ICD-10.

Atypical Autism

In ICD-10, atypical autism is "a pervasive developmental disorder that differs from autism in terms of *either age of onset or of failure to fulfill all three sets of diagnostic criteria*" (World Health Organization 1990, p. 255). The inclusion of this category in DSM-IV would be justified as a means of identifying cases with atypical onset and of giving a diagnosis to those children who are subthreshold in terms of behavioral symptoms. Another option would be to include this category in PDDNOS as *PDDNOS (including atypical autism)*.

Schizophrenia With Onset in Childhood

The members of the Child Work Group responsible for schizophrenia identified the following issues for DSM-IV:

- Is schizophrenia with onset in childhood the same disorder as schizophrenia with onset in adulthood?
- If not, should a separate subcategory be included under schizophrenia for childhood onset presentations?
- Are amendments to criteria required for this age group?
- Do developmental factors influence the diagnosis in this age group?

Werry (Chapter 5) provided the Work Group with a critical review and analysis of the pertinent literature.

The diagnosis itself presented the greatest difficulty in this endeavor. With one or two exceptions, the distinction between childhood schizophrenia and autism was not made until the late 1970s. Because of this, fewer than 10 studies were considered for the literature review; all but one represented retrospective chart reviews.

In three reports, the diagnosis of schizophrenia was made by DSM-III criteria; in one, the diagnosis was made by DSM-III-R criteria. In a recent study (Spencer and Campbell 1994; Spencer et al. 1992), children ages 5–12 years were hospitalized and carefully studied; the structured interviews used included the Diagnostic Interview for Children and Adolescents—Revised (Reich and Welner 1990) and the Kiddie Schedule for Affective Disorders and Schizophrenia (Overall and Pfefferbaum 1982); the diagnosis of schizophrenia was made by DSM-III-R criteria. All the studies (both retrospective chart reviews and prospective studies) indicate that schizophrenia can be diagnosed in children between ages 6 and 12 years employing the same criteria as are used for older adolescents and adults. There is strong evidence that schizophrenia with onset in childhood is the same disorder as schizophrenia with onset in adulthood. The differences, usually seen in younger children or those with lower (borderline) IQs are quantitative rather than qualitative. The phenomenology seems to be influenced not only by IQ, but also by the level of language development. Delusions are less common in children than in adults, whereas visual hallucinations are more common in children than in adults. Unlike in adults, hallucinations are also reported in children in association with conditions other than schizophrenia or another psychotic disorder. In children under age 12, schizophrenia is more common in males than in females. It is unlikely that the diagnosis can be made reliably in children under the age of 5 years or in young retarded children.

In summary, it seems that the criteria for schizophrenia proposed for DSM-IV are appropriate for children, with one exception. Criterion B, describing impairment in functioning, should perhaps contain the statement that children may be unable to attend school or to function in school.

Learning Disorders

The deliberations of the Child Work Group studying learning disorders resulted in a number of proposals for DSM-IV. It was proposed that the name of the section be changed from "Academic Skills Disorder" to "Learning Disorders"; that developmental reading disorder be changed to reading disorder, developmental arithmetic disorder to mathematics disorder; and developmental expressive writing disorder to disorder of written expression. It was proposed that the wording of a number of criteria be changed to achieve greater clarity. The Work Group also undertook a literature review on social skills deficits.

Social Skills Deficits

The issue to be addressed by the members of the Work Group was whether social skills deficits should be included as a primary diagnostic criterion for learning disorders. There were only a few reports on this topic prior to 1980. The Interagency Committee on Learning Disabilities, formed in 1985, defined learning disabilities as a heterogeneous group of disorders characterized by marked problems in acquiring and using various cognitive abilities, including social skills (Interagency Committee on Learning Disabilities 1987). The pertinent literature supported the notion that many individuals with learning disabilities have difficulties in social relationships. However, the inclusion of "social skills" in the definition of learning disorder has been considered problematic by some, mainly because it allowed an individual to be diagnosed as having a learning disorder in the absence of any academic difficulties (e.g., reading disorder) solely on the basis of having deficient social skills. Furthermore, the inclusion of social difficulties as a primary diagnostic criterion in this definition of learning disorders contributed to the poor delineation between learning disorders and serious emotional disturbance under the Disabilities Education Act. Finally, the inclusion of social skills deficits as a primary diagnostic criterion was problematic because of its influence on the type of treatment provided to children and adolescents with learning disabilities.

In his literature review, Forness (Chapter 6) considered the following issues: the nature and origins of social skills deficits in this population, the extent (frequency) of the problem, comorbidity, comparisons with persons without learning disorders, and educational as well as therapeutic interventions. The literature review clearly shows that children and adolescents with learning disabilities often do have social skills problems. However, at present, there is no compelling evidence that social skills deficits should be viewed as an invariable or required feature of learning disorders that should be included in DSM-IV. As suggested by Forness, an additional reason social skills deficits should not be included as a diagnostic criterion in DSM-IV is that such inclusion would imply that psychiatric intervention will follow or is available.

Speech and Language Disorders

DSM-III-R included developmental articulation disorder, developmental expressive language disorder, and developmental receptive language disorder as "Language and Speech Disorders." The Work Group studying speech and language disorders addressed the following issues in their literature review (Paul et al., Chapter 7):

- Should both childhood onset speech disorders and those with onset in adulthood (e.g., voice disorder) be included in the Speech and Language Disorders section in DSM-IV?
- Is cluttering a language deficit or a disorder?
- Should the terminology for speech sound disorders be changed from deficits in motor output to that used in speech-language pathology, which reflects current theories regarding these motor manifestations as deficits of phonological representations and rule learning?
- Should voice disorder, a disorder recognized by the American Speech-Language and Hearing Association, be included in DSM-IV?
- What is the earliest age at which a speech or language disorder can be identified (this information is not provided in DSM-III-R)?
- Is there any receptive aphasia in childhood analogous to Wernicke's aphasia of adults?
- What inclusionary criteria can be used to define or delineate speech and language disorders in place of the exclusionary criteria of DSM-III-R?
- Do aphasias acquired in childhood require a separate status or should they be combined with developmental aphasias?
- Should elective mutism be included in the Speech and Language Disorders section?
- Can the continuity or comorbidity between expressive and receptive language

disorders and learning disorders be represented in DSM-IV, unlike in DSM-III-R, where they are placed as separate entities?

Based on their findings, the following proposals for DSM-IV were presented in the *DSM-IV Options Book*:

1. That the name of the section be changed to "Speech and Language Disorders," with the word developmental deleted from the names of all disorders in recognition of the fact that in some children these disorders are acquired.
2. That developmental receptive language disorder (DSM-III-R) be replaced by mixed receptive/expressive language disorder, because receptive language disorders are accompanied by expressive language problems.
3. That articulation disorder be changed to phonological disorder and the criteria reorganized and revised to conform to the terminology currently employed in speech-language pathology.
4. That voice disorder be considered for inclusion in DSM-IV. This newly proposed diagnostic category, usually with onset in adulthood, will be considered for inclusion to have a more complete representation of speech and language disorders and because psychological and emotional influences may play a role in the development of this disorder and behavioral as well as psychotherapeutic interventions are often employed in its treatment.
5. That cluttering be removed as a separate diagnosis and listed only as an associated feature of expressive and receptive language disorders because there is no evidence in the literature to support its validity as a separate diagnostic entity. There is some supportive evidence that cluttering can be viewed as a language deficit rather than only a speech problem.
6. That stuttering, which was listed in DSM-III-R, together with cluttering, as a speech disorder not elsewhere classified, be included as a separate diagnostic category with a specified set of criteria in the Speech and Language Disorders section of DSM-IV.
7. That elective mutism, which was listed in DSM-III-R under "Other Disorders of Infancy, Childhood, or Adolescence," be included under the Speech and Language Disorders section with expanded criteria.
8. That changes be made in the wording of certain criteria across disorders.
9. That, as shown, all disorders related to speech and communication be included in the Speech and Language Disorders section of DSM-IV, including those recognized by the American Speech-Language and Hearing Association.

Clearly, the revisions proposed in the *DSM-IV Options Book* reflect a strong influence of the American Speech-Language and Hearing Association.

References

American Psychiatric Association: Diagnostic and Statistical Manual of Mental Disorders, 3rd Edition. Washington, DC, American Psychiatric Association, 1980

American Psychiatric Association: Diagnostic and Statistical Manual of Mental Disorders, 3rd Edition, Revised. Washington, DC, American Psychiatric Association, 1987

American Psychiatric Association: DSM-IV Options Book: Work in Progress. Washington, DC, American Psychiatric Association, 1991

Gillberg C: Asperger's syndrome in 23 Swedish children. Dev Med Child Neurol 81:520–531, 1989

Heller T: Dementia Infantilis. Zeitschrift für die Erforschung & Behandlung des Jugendlichen Schwachsinns 2:141–165, 1908

Hertzig M, Snow ME, New E, et al: DSM-III and DSM-III-R: diagnosis of autism and PDD in a nursery school population. J Am Acad Child Adolesc Psychiatry 29:123–126, 1989

Interagency Committee on Learning Disabilities: Learning Disabilities: a Report to the U.S. Congress. Washington, DC, U.S. Department of Health & Human Services, 1987

Overall JE, Pfefferbaum B: The Brief Psychiatric Rating Scale for Children. Psychopharmacol Bull 18:10–16, 1982

Reich W, Welner Z: Diagnostic Interview for Children and Adolescents—Revised. St. Louis, MO, Washington University Press, 1990

Rett A: Ueber ein Cerebral-Atrophisches Syndrom bei Hyperammonamie. Vienna, Austria, Brüder Hollinek, 1966

Rutter M, Garmezy N: Developmental psychopathology, in Handbook of Child Psychology, Vol 4. Edited by Hetherington EM. New York, John Wiley, 1983, pp 775–911

Rutter M, Schopler E: Classification of pervasive developmental disorders: some concepts and practical considerations. J Autism Dev Disord 22:459–482, 1992

Siegel B, Vukicevic J, Elliott GR, et al: The use of signal detection theory to assess DSM-III-R criteria for autistic disorder. J Am Acad Child Adolesc Psychiatry 28:542–548, 1989

Spencer EK, Campbell M: Children with schizophrenia: diagnosis, phenomenology, and pharmacotherapy. Schizophr Bull 20:713–725, 1994

Spencer EK, Kafantaris V, Padron-Gayol MV, et al: Haloperidol in schizophrenic children: early findings from a study in progress. Psychopharmacol Bull 28:183–186, 1992

Spitzer RL, Siegel B: The DSM-III-R field trial of pervasive developmental disorder. J Am Acad Child Adolesc Psychiatry 29:855–862, 1990

Szatmari P: Differential diagnosis of Asperger's syndrome and autistic disorder using DSM-III-R. Paper presented at annual meeting of the American Academy of Child and Adolescent Psychiatry, New York, October 1989

Szatmari P, Bartolucci G, Bremner R, et al: A follow-up of high-functioning autistic children. J Autism Dev Disord 19:213–225, 1989

Volkmar FR, Bregman J, Cohen DJ, et al: DSM-III and DSM-III-R diagnoses of autism. Am J Psychiatry 145:1404–1408, 1988

Wing L: Asperger's syndrome: a clinical account. Psychol Med 11:115–130, 1981

Wolff S, Barlow A: Schizoid personality in childhood: a comparative study of schizoid, autistic, and normal children. J Child Psychol Psychiatry 20:29–46, 1979

World Health Organization: Mental Disorders: Glossary and Guide to Their Classification in Accordance With the Ninth Revision of the International Classification of Diseases. Geneva, Switzerland, World Health Organization, 1978

World Health Organization: ICD-10 Chapter V, Mental and Behavioral Disorders, Diagnostic Criteria for Research. Geneva, Switzerland, World Health Organization, 1990

Chapter 1

Autistic Disorder

Peter Szatmari, M.D., F.R.C.P.C.

Statement and Significance of the Issues

The objective of this chapter is to review critically the DSM-III-R (American Psychiatric Association 1987) criteria for autistic disorder. These criteria represent a significant departure from those outlined in DSM-III (American Psychiatric Association 1980). The rationale behind these changes has been well summarized elsewhere (Waterhouse et al. 1992) and is not reviewed here. In DSM-III-R, there are 16 criteria under three general headings: 1) qualitative impairments in two-way social interaction, 2) abnormalities in verbal and nonverbal communication and imaginative activities, and 3) a markedly restricted repertoire of activities and interests. Age at onset was dropped as an inclusion item. Within each criterion, examples are ordered by developmental level from youngest to oldest, and each criterion needs to be evaluated against the child's developmental level. The concern for this review is whether the psychometric properties of these criteria are sufficient for both clinical practice and research.

Method

At the time of writing, there were five data sets available to evaluate the psychometric properties of the DSM-III-R criteria for autistic disorder. These five studies, identified through a Medline search using the key words *autism* and *DSM-III-R*, as well as through consulting experts in the field, are: 1) the original field trial results (Spitzer and Siegel 1990), 2) the reevaluation of the Stanford sample in the field trial by Siegel et al. (1989), and the studies reported by 3) Volkmar et al. (1988), 4) Hertzig et al. (1989), and 5) Szatmari (1989). The studies were evaluated according to the following criteria adapted from Sackett et al. (1985):

1. Was there an assessment of reliability?

2. Were the criteria blindly compared with a "gold standard" using information collected independently?
3. Was a consecutive series of cases used, and did the control subjects have disorders frequently encountered in differential diagnosis?
4. Was the sample size large enough?
5. Was the cost of misclassification evaluated?

Results

The five studies are summarized in Table 1–1. In reviewing the studies, we considered sensitivity, specificity, positive predictive values, kappas, and likelihood ratios (the probability that a child actually has the diagnosis given that he or she is test positive). Where possible, 95% confidence intervals are calculated to see the extent to which the estimates obtained disagree.

Spitzer and Siegel (1990) studied 426 patients in the original field trial. Approximately half of the sample consisted of patients with autistic disorder. The rest had other types of pervasive developmental disorder and other mental disorders, including a substantial number of children with conduct disorder, anxiety disorders, and so on. Approximately 70% of the patients were male, and the median age ranged from 6 to 11 years for each group. The method of accrual of patients was not specified. The methodology for the field trial was as follows. Clinicians were asked to select a sample of individuals whom they considered (according to their best clinical judgment) to have autistic disorder as well as control subjects with other mental disorders. The same clinicians then evaluated these cases and filled out the 16 DSM-III-R criteria for autism. Various diagnostic algorithms were tried to arrive at the one that resulted in the highest sensitivity and specificity and was the most clinically meaningful. This algorithm turned out to include two criteria from the A criteria, one from the B criteria, and one from the C criteria, with a total of 8 of 16 criteria positive. This resulted in a sensitivity of .86, a specificity of .80, positive predictive value of .80, and a likelihood ratio of 4.3. There was no variation in measures of agreement by chronological age. It did appear, however, that specificity decreased when language was absent. There was no assessment of reliability, and the gold standard comparison was not done blindly. The comparison was probably independent in that the information used in filling out the DSM-III-R criteria was not used in the diagnosis of cases. The sample was not entirely appropriate in that a substantial proportion of control subjects did not have developmental disabilities. The sample was clearly large enough to obtain precise estimates, but there was no discussion of the costs of misclassification.

Siegel et al. (1989) reported on a subsample of 60 patients from their own

Table 1–1. Studies on autistic disorder

Study	N	Autism (%)[a]	Sensitivity	Specificity	Positive predictive value	Likelihood ratio	Kappa
Spitzer and Siegel 1990	574	47	.85 (.05)	.80 (.05)	.80 (.05)	4.3	.66
Siegel et al. 1989	60	38	.82 (.10)	.97 (.4)	.95 (.06)	27.3	.82
Volkmar et al. 1988	114	46	.90 (.05)	.64 (.09)	.68 (.09)	2.5	.53
Hertzig et al. 1989	112	28	.97 (.06)	.65 (.10)	.52 (.13)	2.8	.49
Szatmari 1989	81	29	.96 (.04)	.82 (.09)	.69 (.10)	5.3	.69

Note. Numbers in parentheses refer to ± 95% confidence intervals.
[a] According to gold standard assessment.

center who participated in the field trial. These 60 represented a consecutive series of cases, 75% of whom were mentally retarded. Most subjects were younger than 16 years old, but the breakdown by sex was not reported. Control subjects consisted of 11 individuals with childhood onset or atypical pervasive developmental disorder and 26 with other mental disorders, but with various developmental disabilities. The same methodology used in the field trial was carried out here—that is, clinicians identified autistic and nonautistic individuals according to their best clinical judgment. The 16 DSM-III-R criteria were evaluated in these subjects. The importance of this reevaluation of the field trial was that it used "receiver operating characteristic" curves to determine the most efficient diagnostic algorithm for making a diagnosis. These curves determined that items 1 and 13 alone resulted in a sensitivity of .82, specificity of .97, positive predictive value of .95, and a likelihood ratio of 27.3. A number of subanalyses were also carried out. The authors concluded that 1) several DSM-III-R criteria do not distinguish between case subjects and control subjects, 2) some criteria are more related to the degree of mental retardation, 3) some criteria are redundant and do not add new information, and 4) the sensitivity and specificity of the individual criteria are not uniform but vary dramatically. The finding that some criteria were more related to the degree of mental retardation than to diagnosis is interesting because it emphasizes the importance of matching for confounding variables. For example, if case and control subjects have different degrees of mental retardation, and *if* the diagnostic criteria are related to mental retardation, the sensitivity and specificity might be artificially high because case and control subjects are being distinguished on developmental level rather than on diagnostic criteria. For this evaluation, there was no assessment of reliability. The comparison was not done blind but was independent. The measures of agreement were very high, the sample was appropriate, and the confidence intervals around the measures were reasonable. There was no discussion of the cost of misclassification.

The study reported by **Volkmar et al. (1988)** represents the first independent attempt to replicate the sensitivity and specificity estimates obtained in the field trial. It is important to emphasize that the field trial and the Siegel et al. (1989) reevaluation were primarily attempts to *derive* diagnostic algorithms that maximized agreement between the diagnostic criteria and the gold standard. It is quite another thing to test independently that diagnostic algorithm in a new sample. It is for this reason that the Volkmar et al. study is of particular interest. The sample for this study included 114 individuals, 62 with autism and 52 with various developmental disabilities. The sample was a consecutive series of case subjects from a clinic and individuals from a school for autistic persons. Each case subject had been seen within 2 years of the evaluation. The gold standard in this instance was the best clinical judgment by the experienced clinician who did the original evaluation. Charts were reviewed by an independent team of clinicians, and the DSM-III-R criteria for pervasive developmental disorder were filled out. In this instance, sensitivity was .90, specificity was .64, and positive predictive value was .68. The likelihood ratio was 2.7. Case and control subjects differed on both age and IQ, so these may again be confounding variables in the analysis. Methodologically, this study is an improvement over previous investigations. First, excellent reliability was observed between raters. Second, the clinicians were blind to the gold standard diagnosis on the subjects but the assessment was not done independently—that is, the same information used in the gold standard to arrive at a diagnosis was also used by the clinicians rating the charts. The composition of case and control subjects was appropriate, and the sample was large enough for very precise estimates of agreement. The cost of misclassification was not discussed but the false positives were characterized. The major difference between this and other studies was the blinding of the raters. This appears to have a dramatic effect on specificity but little impact on sensitivity.

This study also looked at the psychometric properties of DSM-III criteria. Of 52 patients receiving a best-estimate diagnosis of autism, 42 met DSM-III criteria (sensitivity .81). For the 62 nonautistic control subjects, specificity was .94 (positive predictive value was .91, kappa = .75, and likelihood ratio was 12.6). It is apparent that the DSM-III criteria agree *better* with the best-estimate diagnosis than do the DSM-III-R criteria. Unfortunately, the steps used in the best-estimate approach are not specified. It is unclear, then, whether this agreement is due to the possibility that the best-estimate approach is, in fact, based on the DSM-III criteria.

In the fourth study, **Hertzig et al. (1989)** also reported results of a comparison of DSM-III and DSM-III-R criteria. In this study, 112 children, ranging from 23 to 66 months old, in a therapeutic preschool placement were evaluated. A DSM-III diagnosis was made at a case conference while the child was attending the nursery school. Data from the clinical records were abstracted and used to evaluate the DSM-III-R criteria. Thus, the same data were used in the evaluation of both criteria. The authors did not mention whether the DSM-III-R evaluation was blind to the DSM-III diagnosis; however, the reliability of ratings was reported. Compared with DSM-III, the DSM-III-R criteria have a sensitivity of .97, a specificity of .65, a positive predictive value of .52, a likelihood ratio of only 2.8, and a kappa value of .49.

The final study was reported by **Szatmari (1989)**. The sample consisted of a consecutive series of 78 children in whom there was a high index of suspicion of a pervasive developmental disorder. A semistructured interview was carried out with the parents. On the basis of this information, the 16 DSM-III-R criteria were filled out, but not used in further evaluation. At a case conference, all available information was pooled, including the psychiatric and pediatric assessments, speech and language evaluation, and psychometric evaluations. At the case conference, a clinical diagnosis was made based on the best clinical judgment of those individuals involved. The final diagnostic categories included 19 children with Asperger's syndrome, 23 high-functioning (nonretarded) autistic children, 17 children with mental retardation, and 19 children with developmental language disorders. IQs were not different among those with Asperger's syndrome, developmental language disorder, and autism. The children with mental retardation were somewhat older, and the children with language disorders were somewhat younger. All were outpatients. Comparing the DSM-III-R criteria with the gold standard clinical consensus resulted in a sensitivity of .96, specificity of .82, positive predictive value of .69, and likelihood ratio of 5.3. Once again there was no assessment of reliability, and the comparison with the gold standard was not blind. However, it was independent because the specific DSM-III-R criteria were not used in the consensus diagnosis. The case and control subjects were appropriate, the sample was large enough, and the cost of misclassifications was discussed.

Discussion

Of the five studies available for evaluating the DSM-III-R criteria for autistic disorder, two represent data from the original field trial from which the diagnostic algorithm was established. Three other studies represent attempts to replicate the sensitivity and specificity on a new sample. Only two of the five studies established reliability estimates, so the extent to which the psychometric properties in the other studies are compromised by low test-retest or interrater reliability is not known. Unfortunately, it is not possible to say that any of the five studies represent "grade A evidence" for the conclusions they present. None of the studies had *both* blind and independent comparisons between the DSM-III-R criteria and a gold standard. It is apparent from the confidence intervals that the original and replication samples also produced very different estimates for specificity. The original field trial results showed surprisingly high sensitivity, specificity, and likelihood ratios. The replication results support the high sensitivities but report lower specificities and lower positive predictive values. It should be mentioned that the lack of a blind, independent assessment would tend to *inflate* agreement between DSM-III-R criteria and the gold standard. As a result, these estimates of sensitivity and specificity should be seen as upper limits. It is impossible to say whether removing age at onset as a criterion has also had any effect on lowering specificity. The effect of age at onset on the psychometric properties of the criteria needs to be explored.

The replication samples report higher sensitivities than specificities. Under these circumstances, the positive predictive values are rather low (.52–.69). A positive predictive value of .7 suggests that of 10 individuals diagnosed as having autistic disorder according to the DSM-III-R criteria, only 7 have it according to a gold standard clinical assessment. More than 30% of case subjects diagnosed according to DSM-III-R criteria are false positives in these specialized clinics.

The effects of this low positive predictive value will be even more dramatic in nonspecialized clinics (Galen and Gambino 1975). For example, say 200 children a year are evaluated in a general child development clinic and assume that 10% (or 20 children) are truly autistic. Given that sensitivity and specificity will be constant across settings, we can estimate the positive predictive value of the DSM-III-R criteria in this clinic using the sensitivities and specificities obtained by one of our studies (take the Szatmari 1989 values as a compromise: sensitivity = .96, specificity = .82). The 2 × 2 table would look like Table 1–2. Thus, of 51 children (19 + 32) identified by DSM-III-R criteria as being autistic, only 37% (19 of 51) do, in fact, have the disorder. Well over half the children will be misdiagnosed as autistic in the general child development clinic. The cost of such misclassification is potentially quite high and suggests that modifying the diagnostic algorithm to maximize specificity (even at the expense of sensitivity) might be considered an option.

This combination of high sensitivity, low specificity, and potentially low positive predictive value could have a number of other important implications for research and clinical practice. First, autistic subjects diagnosed by DSM-III-R will be more heterogeneous in their clinical presentation. This is not necessarily wrong, but it does carry the assumption that the attempt to identify more homogeneous subtypes of autism on the basis of clinical features and etiology is not a worthwhile pursuit. It is true that valid subtypes have not yet emerged, but this may have more to do with the state of knowledge than with the true state of affairs. Second, this increased heterogeneity may make it more difficult to replicate research findings across studies, because it is likely that samples might differ considerably. Third,

Table 1–2. Diagnostic validity of DSM-III-R criteria for autistic disorder

Diagnosed by DSM-III-R	True diagnosis		Total
	Autistic disorder	Not autistic disorder	
Autistic disorder	19	32	51
Not autistic disorder	1	148	149
Total	20	180	

Note. Sensitivity = .96, specificity = .82, positive predictive value = .37, percentage agreement = 84, kappa = .45.

there is a real danger that many mentally retarded, purely developmentally delayed individuals will now be diagnosed as autistic simply because the DSM-III-R stipulation that the criteria be out of context of the child's developmental age is so hard to operationalize. For example, when are stereotypies, a restricted range of interests, or an inability to initiate and sustain a conversation developmentally inappropriate? Unfortunately, good data on these developmental milestones are lacking.

The study by Siegel et al. (1989) indicated that various DSM-III-R diagnostic items are redundant and that others are of varying sensitivity and specificity. This suggests that the 16 criteria could be simplified in some way to arrive at a more clinically manageable set without any loss of information. Furthermore, two studies indicate that the sensitivity and specificity of the items vary by both mental and chronological age. In future studies of the psychometric properties of the DSM-III-R criteria, it will be important to control for these confounding variables to make sure that the psychometric properties of the criteria are not influenced by differences in mental or chronological age.

Recommendations

In terms of face validity, the DSM-III-R criteria have two important advantages: a broader range of clinical manifestations is included, and developmental variations in the criteria are described. However, the diagnostic algorithm probably results in too low a specificity for research, education, or clinical practice. In essence, the algorithm acts more like screening criteria (which minimize the false negative rate) rather than diagnostic criteria (which should minimize the false positive rate).

There are several options:

1. Do nothing; sensitivities and specificities reported here are probably as good as any in child psychiatry.
2. Keep the criteria the same but change the text to improve clarity and add further examples.
3. Be more precise about developmental level and whether the number of criteria to be met should vary with the developmental level of the child, or the absence of speech.
4. Reintroduce age at onset as a diagnostic criterion to increase specificity.
5. Improve the specificity by increasing the threshold to 9 or 10 positive criteria, collapsing redundant criteria or eliminating those that do not add to the diagnosis, and making some items mandatory (e.g., 1 and 13 [Siegel et al. 1989]).
6. Some clinical features usually associated with autism are absent in the DSM-III-R criteria (e.g., poor language comprehension). Some consideration might be

given to including this item under the heading of "qualitative impairment in verbal and nonverbal communication."
7. "Lack of imaginative play" might more logically be placed under the third major heading, "markedly restricted repertoire of activities and interests," rather than with the communication items.
8. Finally, there has been some discussion whether autism and the other pervasive developmental disorders should be placed on Axis I or II. Although there is no question that pervasive developmental disorder is a developmental disorder, many Axis I disorders are *excluded* by the presence of pervasive developmental disorder (e.g., attention deficit). Insofar as pervasive developmental disorder takes precedence over these (unlike the other developmental disorders), perhaps it should be listed on Axis I.

References

American Psychiatric Association: Diagnostic and Statistical Manual of Mental Disorders, 3rd Edition. Washington, DC, American Psychiatric Association, 1980

American Psychiatric Association: Diagnostic and Statistical Manual of Mental Disorders, 3rd Edition, Revised. Washington, DC, American Psychiatric Association, 1987

Galen RS, Gambino SR: Beyond Normality: The Predictive Value and Efficiency of Medical Diagnoses. New York, John Wiley, 1975

Hertzig M, Snow ME, New E, et al: DSM-III and DSM-III-R: diagnosis of autism and PDD in a nursery school population. J Am Acad Child Adolesc Psychiatry 29:123–126, 1989

Sackett DL, Haynes RB, Tugwell P: The interpretation of diagnostic data, in Clinical Epidemiology: A Basic Science For Medicine. Toronto, Little, Brown, 1985, pp 59–138

Siegel B, Vukicevic J, Elliott GR, et al: The use of signal detection theory to assess DSM-III-R criteria for autistic disorder. J Am Acad Child Adolesc Psychiatry 28:542–548, 1989

Spitzer RL, Siegel B: The DSM-III-R field trial of pervasive developmental disorder. J Am Acad Child Adolesc Psychiatry 29:855–862, 1990

Szatmari P: Differential diagnosis of Asperger's syndrome and autistic disorder using DSM-III-R. Paper presented at annual meeting of the American Academy of Child and Adolescent Psychiatry, New York, October 1989

Volkmar FR, Bregman J, Cohen DJ, et al: DSM-III and DSM-III-R diagnoses of autism. Am J Psychiatry 145:1404–1408, 1988

Waterhouse L, Wing L, Spitzer R, et al: Pervasive developmental disorders: DSM-III to DSM-III-R. J Autism Dev Disord 22:535–549, 1992

Chapter 2

Rett's Syndrome: A Subtype of Pervasive Developmental Disorder?

Luke Y. Tsai, M.D.

Statement and Significance of the Issues

This literature review was undertaken because of the decision to include Rett's syndrome in ICD-10 (World Health Organization 1990) as a subcategory of pervasive developmental disorders. This decision sparked a number of significant controversies. Some discussions have centered on the diagnostic validity of Rett's syndrome; others have focused on the suitability of classifying Rett's syndrome as a mental disorder and as a subtype of pervasive developmental disorders. The objective of this literature review is to assess whether Rett's syndrome should also be included in DSM-IV as a subcategory of pervasive developmental disorders, with DSM-IV adopting a concept of pervasive developmental disorders that is similar to that described in the ICD-10 draft.

Method

A comprehensive computer search was done on PaperChase using the key word *Rett syndrome* to identify all relevant articles in English that were published from 1980 to 1992. More than 330 articles were identified. Papers reporting fewer than 10 cases were excluded from the final literature review, as were papers that dealt specifically with genetic, neurochemical, neuropathological, neurophysiological, neuroimaging, and other biological aspects of Rett's syndrome. The final literature review includes articles concerned with *Rett's syndrome delineation and definition* (Burd and Gascon 1988; Burd et al. 1991; Haas 1988; Hagberg 1989, 1992; Hagberg and Witt-Engerstrom 1986, 1987; Hagberg et al. 1985; Kerr and Stephenson 1985;

Kulz et al. 1990; Leiber 1985; Nomura and Segawa 1990a, 1990b; Oguro et al. 1990; Opitz and Lewin 1987; Perry 1991; Rapin 1992; Trevathan and Moser 1988; Trevathan and Naidu 1988; Tuchman et al. 1991; Van Acker 1991; Witt-Engerstrom 1990, 1992; Witt-Engerstrom and Hagberg 1990; Zappella 1992); *autistic traits in Rett's syndrome* (Gillberg 1987; Hagberg et al. 1983; Olsson 1987; Olsson and Rett 1985, 1990; Percy et al. 1988, 1990; Witt-Engerstrom and Gillberg 1987); and *Rett's syndrome atypical variants* (Coleman 1990; Goutieres and Aicardi 1986, 1987; Philippart 1990). The final review of the internal and external validity of Rett's syndrome, as well as the relationship between Rett's syndrome and infantile autism (a subtype of pervasive developmental disorders), was based on these 37 papers.

Results

Internal Validity of Rett's Syndrome

Rett's syndrome was originally described by Rett (1966), who reported (in German) his findings in 22 patients. However, Rett's syndrome did not gain wide recognition until 1983, when a series of 35 cases from a pool of French, Portuguese, and Swedish patients was reported in English (Haas 1988; Hagberg et al. 1983). Since then, the International Rett Syndrome Association (IRSA) was founded, international conferences on the syndrome have been held regularly, and at least four special medical journal issues (two in Japan and two in the United States) have been devoted to the delineation and classification of Rett's syndrome (Hagberg 1989).

Diagnostic criteria for Rett's syndrome were developed by a group representing the Centers for Disease Control (CDC), the American Association of University Affiliated Programs, and the IRSA (Trevathan and Moser 1988). This set of diagnostic criteria was developed based on the "Vienna criteria" for the diagnosis of Rett's syndrome (Hagberg et al. 1985) and was adopted by a panel of international experts at the 1984 Rett Syndrome Conference. The diagnostic criteria contain three categories: necessary criteria, supportive criteria, and exclusion criteria.

Necessary criteria.

1. Apparent normal prenatal and perinatal period
2. Apparent normal psychomotor development through the first 6 months (in some cases development may appear to be normal for up to 18 months)
3. Normal head circumference at birth
4. Deceleration of head growth between ages 5 months and 4 years
5. Loss of acquired purposeful hand skills between ages 6 and 30 months

6. Development of stereotypic hand movements such as hand wringing/squeezing, clapping/tapping, mouthing, and "washing"/rubbing automatisms appearing after purposeful hand skills are lost
7. Development of severely impaired expressive and receptive language
8. Presence of apparent severe psychomotor retardation
9. Appearance of gait apraxia and truncal apraxia/ataxia between ages 1 and 4 years
10. Temporal social withdrawal
11. Diagnosis tentative until age 2–5 years

Although "female sex" was considered by Hagberg et al. (1985) as one of the inclusion criteria of Rett's syndrome, the IRSA-CDC criteria do not include female sex as a necessary criterion. This decision was made with consideration of possible undiagnosed male cases (Trevathan and Moser 1988).

Supportive criteria.

1. Breathing dysfunction, such as periodic apnea during wakefulness, intermittent hyperventilation, breath-holding spells, and forced expulsion of air or saliva
2. Electroencephalogram abnormalities, including a slow-waking background and intermittent rhythmical slowing, epileptiform discharge, with or without clinical seizures
3. Seizures
4. Spasticity, often with associated development of muscle wasting
5. Dystonia
6. Peripheral vasomotor disturbances
7. Scoliosis
8. Growth retardation
9. Hypotrophic small feet

Although most Rett's syndrome patients display many of the supportive criteria, diagnosis is possible in the absence of all the supportive criteria, especially in young patients (Trevathan and Moser 1988).

Exclusion criteria.

1. Evidence of intrauterine growth retardation
2. Organomegaly or other signs of storage disease
3. Retinopathy at birth

4. Evidence of perinatally acquired brain damage
5. Existence of identifiable metabolic or other progressive neurological disorder
6. Acquired neurological disorders resulting from severe infections or head trauma

The presence of one or more of the exclusion criteria excludes the diagnosis of Rett's syndrome, regardless of whether all of the necessary criteria have been met in an individual patient (Trevathan and Moser 1988).

The IRSA-CDC diagnostic criteria for Rett's syndrome were restricted to include only typical patients, thereby ensuring a homogeneous patient population for future clinical and epidemiological research.

Using both the Vienna criteria and the IRSA-CDC criteria, the estimated prevalence is at least 1:10,000–15,000, based on Swedish (Hagberg and Witt-Engerstrom 1987), Scottish (Kerr and Stephenson 1985), and Portuguese (Hagberg and Witt-Engerstrom 1987) studies. Today, Rett's syndrome is known to exist in all races and probably all countries (Hagberg 1989). There are more than 1,500 recognized cases of Rett's syndrome worldwide. The many pathognomonic examples of its clinical expression have convinced clinicians of the existence of this unique syndrome.

External Validity of Rett's Syndrome

In the past, children with Rett's syndrome were frequently regarded as autistic (Olsson 1987; Olsson and Rett 1985, 1990; Percy et al. 1988). Witt-Engerstrom and Gillberg (1987) reported that 78% of children with Rett's syndrome have previously been diagnosed as having infantile autism. These reports raised a question in terms of the external validity of Rett's syndrome.

Several independent studies of behavioral observations had demonstrated qualitative and quantitative differences between Rett's syndrome patients and persons with autism. Gillberg (1987) used a comprehensive questionnaire containing a number of semistructured questions and 130 items concerned with early characteristics of perceptual, motor, and emotional development in children. Eight mothers of eight young Rett's syndrome girls (ages 3–9 years) were interviewed using the questionnaire. Although there was considerable overlap between early symptoms in Rett's syndrome and infantile autism, there were indications that certain features might be used to differentiate the two disorders. For example, there were three items typical of autism but rare in Rett's syndrome: 1) "played only with hard objects," 2) "did not like to be disturbed 'in her world,'" and 3) "very pleased when left completely to herself."

Olsson and Rett (1985) compared the behavior of girls with Rett's syndrome with that of patients with infantile autism. Visual, acoustic, tactile, and gustatory stimuli and social contact were used for the comparison. The following are behaviors that were observed only in the Rett's syndrome patients (not in the autistic patients): 1) slow movements plus hypoactivity; 2) uniform stereotypic movements of hands with a broad-base stance; 3) stereotypic "washing movements" of hands; 4) stereotypic wetting of hands with saliva; 5) stereotypic bringing together of hands; 6) consistent, isolated stretching and flexing of the middle finger joints; 7) episodic hyperventilation via mouth; and 8) no chewing. Among behaviors that are characteristic of autism, the following five traits were not seen in the Rett's syndrome patients: 1) predominant rejection of caressing and tenderness, 2) conspicuous physical hyperactivity in terms of continuous grabbing and concomitant locomobility, 3) excessive attachment to certain objects, 4) rotation of small objects, and 5) stereotypic playing habits. Olsson and Rett thus demonstrated that Rett's syndrome and autism could be differentiated based on behavioral observations.

Percy et al. (1988) analyzed motor and behavioral characteristics of 15 patients with Rett's syndrome. They found that children with Rett's syndrome differed from children with autism in having ataxia, breath-holding, hyperventilation, bruxism, simplicity of stereotypies, and hand apposition. On the other hand, the children with autism differed from those with Rett's syndrome in having overactivity, complex repetitive movements, and inappropriate vocalization. It is quite apparent that the course of Rett's syndrome is very different from that of autism, progressing to various forms of neurological impairment that are not seen in autism.

Other variables such as etiology, outcome, and response to treatment have not yet been studied systematically. Nonetheless, with increasing awareness of Rett's syndrome and its characteristic developmental profile, children with Rett's syndrome should have demonstrated the typical clinical features by 3–4 years of age and should be easily distinguishable from those with autism (Trevathan and Naidu 1988).

Chatterjee et al. (1990) did two blind studies on the plasma glycosphingolipids in patients with Rett's syndrome, patients with other developmental disorders, and control subjects from Baltimore, Maryland; Vienna, Austria; and Rostock, East Germany. The presence of an unusual glycosphingolipid was found in 70% of the patients with Rett's syndrome and in approximately 10% of those with other disorders. However, this glycosphingolipid was absent from the plasma of control subjects.

These data appear to suggest that Rett's syndrome has enough distinguishing features to warrant being considered a distinct diagnostic entity.

Relationship Between Rett's Syndrome and Pervasive Developmental Disorders

It is essential to recognize that Rett's syndrome is a progressive neurological disorder and that there is variability of clinical presentation depending on patient age and the stage of the disease. Cross-sectional findings at a single examination can easily lead to erroneous diagnostic association when the developmental profile is not analyzed (Hagberg 1989). Hagberg and Witt-Engerstrom (1986) proposed a four-stage model for classic Rett's syndrome.

1. Early-onset stagnation stage is present between age 6 months and 1½ years.
2. Rapid developmental regression stage usually appears at age 1–2 years.
3. Pseudostationary stage usually occurs at age 3–4 years, but can be delayed and persists for many years or even decades.
4. Late motor deterioration stage often occurs during school age or early adolescence.

Many investigators reported that "autistic features" developed during the rapid developmental regression stage (stage 2). These features include 1) no sustained interest in persons or objects; 2) stereotypic responses to environmental stimuli; 3) absent or very limited interpersonal contact; 4) manifestation of great anxiety and apparent fear when confronted with an unfamiliar situation or event without evident stimulation; 5) loss of already acquired elements of language; 6) stereotypic hand movements, especially "hand-washing" movements in front of the mouth or chest and rubbing motions of the hands; and 7) repetitive blows on the teeth, grabbing of the tongue, and other movements (Hagberg et al. 1983). It appears that at the early stage of Rett's syndrome, there are impairments in reciprocal social interaction and in patterns of communication. Stereotypic behaviors are also manifested. These are all the essential behavioral characteristics of pervasive developmental disorders.

Discussion

The key issue of this literature review is whether Rett's syndrome should be considered as a subtype of the pervasive developmental disorders in DSM-IV. Before a final decision on this issue can be reached, a number of conceptual issues regarding the definition of "autistic features in Rett's syndrome" require further discussion.

The definition of pervasive developmental disorders in DSM-III-R is given as a group of mental disorders

> characterized by qualitative impairment in the development of reciprocal social interaction, in the development of verbal and nonverbal communication skills, and in imaginative activity. Often there is a markedly restricted repertoire of

activities and interests, which frequently are stereotyped and repetitive. (American Psychiatry Association 1987, p. 33)

These qualitative abnormalities are a pervasive feature of the individual's functioning in all situations, although they vary in degree. With few exceptions, the conditions appear by age 5, and in most cases development is abnormal from infancy. There is usually, although not always, some degree of general cognitive impairment, but the disorders are defined in terms of *behavior* that is deviant for the individual's mental age.

At the early stage of Rett's syndrome, there are impairments in reciprocal social interaction and in patterns of communication. There is also manifestation of stereotypic behaviors. These are all the essential behavioral characteristics of pervasive developmental disorders. However, it is not clear whether these "behaviors" of Rett's syndrome are "deviant in relation to the individual's *mental age*." Although it is quite clear that all the Rett's syndrome patients continue to function in the range of severe to profound retardation, none of the studies on Rett's syndrome has provided information regarding the relationship between the mental age and the level of social and language/speech developments or impairments. Without such information, it is difficult to differentiate the "impairment of social interaction" in the Rett's syndrome patients from the "lack of appropriate play and social skills" usually noticeable in young preschool and primary school children with moderate or severe retardation. It is also difficult to refute the argument that the stereotyped hand movements in the Rett's syndrome patients are the "stereotyped self-stimulating behaviors" commonly seen in persons with severe or profound mental retardation.

Another issue that should be discussed is the course of Rett's syndrome and its relationship to pervasive developmental disorders. Although M. Rutter (personal communication, 1990) noted that older Rett's syndrome patients continued to exhibit "autistic features," some studies have reported that the autistic features of Rett's syndrome that appeared in late infancy tended to diminish or resolve in stage 3 (i.e., pseudostationary stage). Autistic traits, in fact, became less prominent than evidenced during the initial phase of the disorder in most of the patients who were followed at least until age 15 (Hagberg 1989; Hagberg et al. 1983). The ICD-10 draft (World Health Organization 1990), in describing Rett's syndrome, says that "*social interest tends to be maintained*" (p. 255) and that "*often social interactions develop later*" (p. 256). Gillberg (1987) reported that eye contact improved and sometimes became very intense. The girls with Rett's syndrome did not mind human interaction and did not usually protest if their world was "disturbed." The automatisms also tended to become slower and more simplified in adulthood. In fact, the IRSA-CDC criteria define the communication dysfunction and social withdrawal as "*temporal*" features. It is not clear whether "temporal" means that all Rett's syndrome patients eventually regain communicative and social skills that match their mental age. In other words, it is unclear whether Rett's syndrome patients at the late motor deterioration stage present a clinical picture that is commonly seen in immobile persons with severe/profound mental retardation instead of a picture seen in patients who are evaluated as having improved/residual pervasive developmental disorders. Because Rett's syndrome is a newly recognized disorder, many questions remain concerning the course of Rett's syndrome. Further follow-up studies are needed to resolve these questions.

Lastly, there have been reports of patients who did not satisfy all the official criteria, but presented several features suggestive of Rett's syndrome, especially *hand stereotypies, autism,* and *mental retardation.* These cases did not meet the criteria because either they lacked a history of normal development for several months followed by a period of definite deterioration, they had congenital or acquired encephalopathy of known cause, or they were males (Coleman 1990; Goutieres and Aicardi 1986, 1987; Philippart 1990). These cases do seem, however, to present cross-sectional features that are seen in pervasive developmental disorders. A controversial term, *forme fruste Rett's syndrome,* has been used by many clinicians to describe the atypical/abortive variants of Rett's syndrome. It is to be expected that more cases with variant forms of Rett's syndrome will be forthcoming.

Recommendations

On the basis of available empirical data, it would be extremely unsatisfactory to bury Rett's syndrome in the insufficiently defined manner of DSM-III-R—that is, to view Rett's syndrome as one of many medical conditions associated with autism or atypical autism. I support the Work Group's recommendation to include Rett's syndrome in DSM-IV as a distinct diagnostic entity to provide greater specificity in the differential diagnosis of pervasive developmental disorders. However, the reliability of the diagnosis has not been systematically studied. Some patients may present with abnormalities during the first 6 months, and it may be arbitrary to include Rett's syndrome and exclude other neuropsychiatric medical conditions associated with autistic features. For these reasons, the Work Group is also considering classifying Rett's syndrome as a pervasive developmental disorder not otherwise specified (American Psychiatric Association 1991).

Finally, if the Work Group decides to adopt Rett's syndrome as a subtype of pervasive developmental disorders, it should also consider including "atypical Rett's syndrome" as another subtype of pervasive developmental disorders.

References

American Psychiatric Association: Diagnostic and Statistical Manual of Mental Disorders, 3rd Edition, Revised. Washington, DC, American Psychiatric Association, 1987

American Psychiatric Association: DSM-IV Options Book: Work in Progress. Washington, DC, American Psychiatric Association, 1991

Burd L, Gascon GG: Rett syndrome: review and discussion of current diagnostic criteria. J Child Neurol 3:263–268, 1988

Burd L, Vesley B, Martsolf JT, et al: Prevalence study of Rett syndrome in North Dakota children. Am J Med Genet 38:565–568, 1991

Chatterjee S, Ghosh N, Goh KM, et al: Glycosphingolipids in patients with the Rett syndrome. Brain Dev 12:85–87, 1990

Coleman M: Is classical Rett syndrome ever present in males? Brain Dev 12:31–32, 1990

Gillberg C: Autistic syndrome in Rett syndrome: the first two years according to mother reports. Brain Dev 9:499–501, 1987

Goutieres F, Aicardi J: Atypical forms of Rett syndrome. Am J Med Genet 24:184–194, 1986

Goutieres F, Aicardi J: New experience with Rett syndrome in France: the problem of atypical cases. Brain Dev 9:502–505, 1987

Haas RH: The history and challenge of Rett syndrome. J Child Neurol 3 (suppl):S3–5, 1988

Hagberg BA: Rett syndrome: clinical peculiarities, diagnostic approach, and possible cause. Pediatr Neurol 5:75–83, 1989

Hagberg B: The Rett syndrome: an introductory overview 1990. Brain Dev 14 (suppl):S5–8, 1992

Hagberg BA, Witt-Engerstrom I: Rett syndrome: a suggested staging system for describing impairment profile with increasing age toward adolescence. Am J Med Genet 24:47–59, 1986

Hagberg BA, Witt-Engerstrom I: Rett syndrome: epidemiology and nosology—progress in knowledge 1986—a conference communication. Brain Dev 9:451–457, 1987

Hagberg BA, Aicardi J, Dias K, et al: A progressive syndrome of autism, dementia, ataxia, and loss of purposeful hand use in girls: Rett's syndrome: report of 35 cases. Ann Neurol 14:471–479, 1983

Hagberg B, Goutieres F, Hanefeld F, et al: Rett syndrome: criteria for inclusion and exclusion. Brain Dev 7:372–373, 1985

Kerr AM, Stephenson JBP: Rett's syndrome in the west of Scotland. BMJ 291:579–582, 1985

Kulz J, Rohmann E, Hobusch D: A study on the Rett syndrome in the GDR. Brain Dev 12:37–39, 1990

Leiber B: Rett syndrome: a nosological entity. Brain Dev 7:275–276, 1985

Nomura Y, Segawa M: Characteristics of motor disturbances of the Rett syndrome. Brain Dev 12:27–30, 1990a

Nomura Y, Segawa M: Clinical features of the early stage of the Rett syndrome. Brain Dev 12:16–19, 1990b

Oguro N, Momoi M, Nakamigawa T, et al: Multi-institutional survey of the Rett syndrome in Japan. Brain Dev 12:753–759, 1990

Olsson B: Autistic traits in the Rett syndrome. Brain Dev 9:491–498, 1987

Olsson B, Rett A: Behavioral observations concerning differential diagnosis between the Rett syndrome and autism. Brain Dev 7:281–289, 1985

Olsson B, Rett A: A review of the Rett syndrome with a theory of autism. Brain Dev 12:11–15, 1990

Opitz JM, Lewin SO: Rett syndrome: a review and discussion of syndrome delineation and syndrome definition. Brain Dev 9:445–450, 1987

Percy AK, Zoghbi HY, Lewis KR, et al: Rett syndrome: qualitative and quantitative differentiation from autism. J Child Neurol 3 (suppl):S65–S67, 1988

Percy A, Gillberg C, Hagberg B, et al: Rett syndrome and autistic disorders. Neurol Clin 8:659–676, 1990

Perry A: Rett syndrome: a comprehensive review of the literature. Am J Ment Retard 96:275–290, 1991

Philippart M: The Rett syndrome in males. Brain Dev 12:33–36, 1990

Rapin I: Discussion for the Rett syndrome symposium: the importance of rigorously defining one's level of investigation. Brain Dev 14 (suppl):S145, 1992

Rett A: Ueber ein Cerebral-Atrophisches Syndrome bei Hyperammonamie. Vienna, Austria, Brüder Hollinek, 1966

Trevathan E, Moser HW: Diagnostic criteria for Rett syndrome. Ann Neurol 23:425–428, 1988

Trevathan E, Naidu S: The clinical recognition and differential diagnosis of Rett syndrome. J Child Neurol 3 (suppl):S6–S16, 1988

Tuchman RF, Rapin I, Shinnar S: Autistic and dysphasic children, I: clinical characteristics. Pediatrics 88:1211–1218, 1991

Van Acker R: Rett syndrome: a review of current knowledge. J Autism Dev Disord 21:381–406, 1991

Witt-Engerstrom I: Rett syndrome in Sweden: neurodevelopment, disability, pathophysiology. Acta Paediatr Scand Suppl 369:1–60, 1990

Witt-Engerstrom I: Age-related occurrence of signs and symptoms in the Rett syndrome. Brain Dev 14 (suppl):S11–20, 1992

Witt-Engerstrom I, Gillberg C: Rett syndrome in Sweden. J Autism Dev Disord 17:149–150, 1987

Witt-Engerstrom I, Hagberg B: The Rett syndrome: gross motor disability and neural impairment in adults. Brain Dev 12:23–26, 1990

World Health Organization: ICD-10 Chapter V. Mental and Behavioral Disorders. Diagnostic Criteria for Research. Geneva, Switzerland, World Health Organization, 1990

Zappella M: The Rett girls with preserved speech. Brain Dev 14:98–101, 1992

Chapter 3

Childhood Disintegrative Disorder

Fred R. Volkmar, M.D.

Statement and Significance of the Issues

This review is concerned with classification of children who develop a pervasive developmental disorder after a relatively prolonged period of normal development. A specific diagnostic concept (disintegrative disorder/disintegrative psychosis) has been proposed for this condition and is included in ICD-9 (World Health Organization 1978) and ICD-10 (World Health Organization 1990) but not in DSM-III (American Psychiatric Association 1980) or in DSM-III-R (American Psychiatric Association 1987). Various terms have been used to refer to the condition; for purposes of simplicity, the term *childhood disintegrative disorder* is used in this review. Issues of primary concern for this review include

1. The use of the term in clinical practice.
2. Characteristics of cases reported.
3. The validity of the condition (particularly in relation to autism).
4. If the disorder is included in DSM-IV, should it be grouped within the pervasive developmental disorder class or as a dementia?
5. If the disorder is included in DSM-IV, how should it be named and defined?

The condition was first described by Heller (1908, 1930/1969), who described six children who exhibited severe developmental regression after a period of some years of normal development. Other cases were subsequently reported and diagnostic guidelines formulated. Over the years, the disorder has been variously named (e.g., dementia infantilis, Heller's syndrome, disintegrative psychosis, disintegrative disorder). The term *childhood disintegrative disorder* seems particularly apt (Corbett 1987) because the earlier term "disintegrative psychosis" reflected assumptions of continuity with adult psychotic conditions that were not justified.

The condition was included in ICD-9 and will be included in ICD-10. ICD-10 gives the following criteria for the disorder:

1. Apparently normal development for at least 2 years.
2. A definite loss of previously acquired skills in two of five areas: language, play, social skills and/or adaptive behavior, bowel and/or bladder function, and motor skills.
3. Qualitatively abnormal social and communicative functioning of a type similar to that observed in autism with repetitive patterns of interest/behavior.
4. By definition, the disorder is not attributable to other pervasive developmental disorders nor to elective mutism, schizophrenia, or acquired aphasia with epilepsy.

In DSM-III and DSM-III-R, the presumption was that the condition was more appropriately considered an organic brain syndrome. The position on "age at onset" of autism in DSM-III-R would also have complicated the use of the concept of childhood disintegrative disorder, because it was not specific about either the age or type of onset of the symptoms. A somewhat overlapping diagnostic concept (childhood onset pervasive developmental disorder) was included in DSM-III but not in DSM-III-R. Because the available research indicated that most children with childhood disintegrative disorder exhibited an "autistic-like" clinical picture (apart from the different history of a period of normal development), it appears likely that such children would meet criteria for autistic disorder in DSM-III-R. This would not have been the case with the DSM-III definition of infantile autism.

Method

For this review, relevant computer databases were searched from 1980 to 1990. Approximately 25 case reports or reviews were identified; citations from earlier studies were largely derived from these sources (e.g., Corbett 1987; Kurita 1988a; Rapin 1965). The bulk of the available literature consists of reviews or case reports that typically contain minimal follow-up information. The available information was variable, and the use of control or contrast groups (e.g., of autistic children) was uncommon. The task of reviewing the literature was also complicated by the various changes in the nomenclature used to describe the "childhood psychoses" over the past two decades. On the other hand, the disorder is quite rare so that, for purposes of the present review, a relatively large number of the available case reports could be abstracted and summarized.

Information was abstracted from the following case series/reports: Burd et al.

Table 3–1. Characteristics of disintegrative disorder cases

Variable	Cases 1908–1976 ($n = 48$)		Cases 1977–1990 ($n = 29$)		Entire sample ($N = 77$)	
Sex ratio (male:female)	35:12		26:3		61:15	
Age at onset (mean ± SD years)	3.42 ± 1.12		3.25 ± 1.61		3.36 ± 1.32	
Age at follow-up (mean ± SD years)	8.67 ± 4.14		14.25 ± 5.35		10.91 ± 5.39	
Symptoms (% of n cases)						
Speech deterioration/loss	100%	47	100%	29	100%	76
Social disturbance	100%	43	96%	28	99%	71
Stereotypy/resistance to change	100%	38	100%	25	100%	63
Overactivity	100%	42	89%	19	97%	61
Affective symptoms/anxiety	100%	17	94%	17	97%	34
Deterioration in self-help skills	94%	33	90%	20	92%	53

(1989); Corbett et al. (1977); Evans-Jones and Rosenbloom (1978 [follow-up for nine cases reported by Hill and Rosenbloom 1986]); Kurita (1985, 1988a, 1988b); and Volkmar and Cohen (1989). The variable case information made it difficult to ascertain how many of the 77 cases would meet ICD criteria for the disorder. Accordingly, cases were also subgrouped depending on whether the case was reported before 1977 ($n = 48$) or subsequently ($n = 29$). The latter cases generally used a concept very close to the ICD description of the disorder. In one series (Volkmar and Cohen 1989), ICD-10 criteria were used. Characteristics of the various cases identified for this review are presented in Table 3–1.

Results

Clinical Features

As shown in Table 3–1, the vast majority of cases exhibited a pattern of behavioral disturbance generally consistent with an "autistic-like" condition (Kurita 1988a). It appears that the majority of cases would likely meet DSM-III-R criteria for autistic disorder, particularly given the somewhat broader diagnostic concept employed in DSM-III-R (Volkmar and Cohen 1989). The cases differed from "classical" autism in that the period of normal development was quite prolonged and in terms of sex ratio (Lord et al. 1982). Language and communication skills, by definition, significantly declined, and both language expression and comprehension were severely affected. Intellectual functioning similarly deteriorated.

Prognosis

Information on prognosis is particularly relevant to the issue of whether the condition might best be considered a subtype of autism. Follow-up information was available in some cases and suggested that, generally, recovery was quite limited. In a few cases, a progressive neurological process was associated with a downhill course (Corbett et al. 1977). The course was static in about three-fourths of the cases, with some minimal improvement noted in a minority of cases. Approximately 40% of the subjects who had previously had the capacity to speak in sentences remained mute at follow-up, and most cases were moderately to severely mentally retarded.

Neurological Findings

The issue of associated neurological findings is particularly relevant to the issue of whether this condition might more properly be classified as a dementia. Heller (1908) suggested that disintegrative disorder was observed in the absence of apparent organic disease. As was true for infantile autism, this initial impression of no apparent "organicity" has been modified, because various organic conditions have been identified, and seizures develop in a minority of cases. The notion (e.g., as in DSM-III and DSM-III-R) that a progressive neurological process was likely to be observed in the majority of cases of the condition was not supported by examination of the available cases. Various neurological abnormalities (e.g., in encephalogram) and/or seizure disorder were noted and were similar to those observed in autistic children (Volkmar and Nelson 1990). With few exceptions, other laboratory studies failed to confirm the presence of a specific medical condition that could account for the condition (Volkmar and Cohen 1989), although it must be noted that the diagnosis of neurodegenerative disorders remains difficult (Corbett 1987; Rivinus et al. 1975; Wilson 1974) and the failure to find an underlying medical condition more likely reflects our ignorance of fundamental neurobiological mechanisms than the absence of "organic" factors. A similar problem exists for the diagnosis of autism.

Epidemiology

Epidemiological data are relevant to the validity of childhood disintegrative disorder as a condition distinct from autism. In one consecutive case series (although epidemiological data were sparse), the disorder was one-tenth as common as autism (Volkmar and Cohen 1989); in another, more truly epidemiological study, the prevalence of the disorder was .11/10,000 for males (Burd et al. 1989). Childhood disintegrative disorder appears to be much less frequent than autism as the latter condition is usually defined.

Discussion

Childhood disintegrative disorder appears to be a very rare condition with behavioral features, once the condition is established, similar to those observed in autism. It differs from autism in terms of clinical features, onset, course, and prognosis. Most autistic children do not exhibit an unequivocal period of normal development, although case recognition may be delayed by various factors such as higher IQ in the child or parental denial or lack of sophistication. In childhood disintegrative disorder, early development is much more clearly normal, or near normal. The pattern of developmental regression differs from that observed in autism or other ICD-10 pervasive developmental disorder categories such as Rett's syndrome and Asperger's syndrome (see Harper and Williams 1975). "Later onset" autism appears to have a significantly better long-term prognosis than childhood disintegrative disorder. Although various neurological findings are often observed, specific neurological disease processes are not typically identified, and, in most cases, the clinical picture is one of developmental stagnation rather than progressive intellectual decline. As in autism, the clinical features and course of the disorder suggest that some organic process is likely, although as Rutter (1985) noted, this remains a hypothesis, and precise neurobiological mechanisms have yet to be identified.

Recommendations

Various alternatives are available for DSM-IV. Continuation of the current DSM-III-R approach would entail minimal change in DSM-IV. Most cases of childhood disintegrative disorder would continue to receive a diagnosis of autistic disorder, with later age at onset specified as well as the appropriate diagnosis of mental retardation. Any neurological or other conditions possibly accounting for the disorder would be noted on Axis III. This approach has the disadvantages of being incompatible with ICD-10, failing to make the clinically meaningful distinction regarding characteristics of onset and ignoring a body of literature that suggests that the concept has validity apart from autism. This approach would also impede research on this disorder that might provide important evidence regarding underlying neurobiological processes.

An alternative would be to define the disorder as a pervasive developmental disorder not otherwise specified or as "atypical autism" (a concept included in ICD-10). This method would entail some change from DSM-III-R (because most cases would likely meet criteria for autistic disorder) and has several other disadvantages. It would include childhood disintegrative disorder in a broad and heterogeneous group, and it would have the usual disadvantages associated with negative definition (Corbett 1987). It would, however, offer an apparent compatibility with ICD-10, which does include an atypical autism category and allows for use of this category on the basis of atypical age at onset. Such an approach in DSM-IV would entail use of age at onset as a criterion, a change from DSM-III-R. Not all cases of disintegrative disorder would, however, exhibit age at onset past the level specified in ICD-10 for the atypical autism category.

A third option is formal inclusion of the disorder within the pervasive developmental disorder class. As summarized, this approach has the advantage of consistency with ICD-10 and can be supported on the basis of available data. If the disorder is included, compatibility with the ICD-10 definition is desirable. Although beyond the scope of the present review, the inclusion of other (nonautistic) pervasive developmental disorders will have relevance to the definition of childhood disintegrative disorder as well as to autism (i.e., if explicitly defined disorders in addition to autistic disorder are included in the pervasive developmental disorder class). This approach would mark a change from DSM-III-R. Although the data reviewed are obviously limited, there does appear to be sufficient evidence to warrant inclusion of the disorder in DSM-IV. Inclusion of the disorder would also enhance compatibility with ICD-10 and should facilitate both research and clinical service. Given the behavioral similarity to autism, inclusion within the pervasive developmental disorder class is appropriate. If the disorder is included, it will be necessary for clinicians to make reference both to present examination and to past history (a difference from DSM-III-R). Description of the pattern of onset and the differentiation of the disorder from autism will be important, but available data suggest that such a distinction can be reasonably made and that relatively few (and then typically the higher-functioning) children with autism would potentially present a later onset.

References

American Psychiatric Association: Diagnostic and Statistical Manual of Mental Disorders, 3rd Edition. Washington, DC, American Psychiatric Association, 1980

American Psychiatric Association: Diagnostic and Statistical Manual of Mental Disorders, 3rd Edition, Revised. Washington, DC, American Psychiatric Association, 1987

Burd L, Fisher W, Kerbeshian J: Pervasive disintegrative disorder: are Rett syndrome and Heller dementia infantilis subtypes? Dev Med Child Neurol 31:609–616, 1989

Corbett J: Development, disintegration, and dementia. Journal of Mental Deficiency Research 31:349–356, 1987

Corbett J, Harris R, Taylor E, et al: Progressive disintegrative psychosis of childhood. J Child Psychol Psychiatry 18:211–219, 1977

Evans-Jones LG, Rosenbloom L: Disintegrative psychosis in childhood. Dev Med Child Neurol 20:462–470, 1978

Harper J, Williams S: Age and type of onset as critical variables in early infantile autism. Journal of Autism and Childhood Schizophrenia 5:25–35, 1975

Heller T: Dementia infantilis. Zeitschrift für die Erforschung und Behandlung des Jugendlichen Schwachsinns 2:141–165, 1908

Heller T: Ueber dementia infantilis. Zeitschrift für Kinderforschung 37: 661–667, 1930 (reprinted in Modern Perspective in International Child Psychiatry. Edited by Howells JG. Edinburgh, Scotland, Oliver & Boyd, 1969, pp 610–616)

Hill AE, Rosenbloom L: Disintegrative psychosis of childhood: teenage follow-up. Dev Med Child Neurol 28:34–40, 1986

Kurita H: Infantile autism with speech loss before the age of thirty months. Journal of the American Academy of Child Psychiatry 24:191–196, 1985

Kurita H: The concept and nosology of Heller's syndrome: review of articles and report of two cases. Japanese Journal of Psychiatry and Neurology 42:785–793, 1988a

Kurita H: A case of Heller's syndrome with school refusal. J Autism Dev Disord 18:315–319, 1988b

Lord C, Schopler E, Revicki D: Sex differences in autism. J Autism Dev Disord 12:317–330, 1982

Rapin I: Dementia infantilis (Heller's disease), in Medical Aspects of Mental Retardation. Edited by Carter CH. Springfield, IL, Charles C Thomas, 1965, pp 760–767

Rivinus TM, Jamison DL, Graham PJ: Childhood organic neurological disease presenting as a psychiatric disorder. Arch Dis Child 50:115–119, 1975

Rutter M: Infantile autism and other pervasive developmental disorders, in Child and Adolescent Psychiatry: Modern Approaches. Edited by Rutter M, Hersov L. London, England, Blackwell, 1985, pp 545–566

Volkmar FR, Cohen DJ: Disintegrative disorder or "late onset" autism? J Child Psychol Psychiatry 30:717–724, 1989

Volkmar FR, Nelson D: Seizures disorders in autism. J Am Acad Child Adolesc Psychiatry 29:127–129, 1990

Wilson J: Investigation of degenerative disease of the central nervous system. Arch Dis Child 47:163–170, 1974

World Health Organization: Mental Disorders: Glossary and Guide to Their Classification in Accordance With the Ninth Revision of the International Classification of Diseases. Geneva, Switzerland, World Health Organization, 1978

World Health Organization: ICD-10 Chapter V: Mental and Behavioral Disorders: Diagnostic Criteria for Research. Geneva, Switzerland, World Health Organization, 1990

Chapter 4

Pervasive Developmental Disorder Not Otherwise Specified

Peter Szatmari, M.D., F.R.C.P.C.

Statement and Significance of the Issues

The purpose of this literature review is to assess the taxonomic validity of the diagnostic category *pervasive developmental disorder not otherwise specified* (PDDNOS), a term that describes children who have some of the characteristics of a pervasive developmental disorder but not enough to qualify for a diagnosis of autistic disorder. The issue that has prompted this literature review was the decision by the DSM-III-R (American Psychiatric Association 1987) Work Group on pervasive developmental disorder to use PDDNOS as a single residual category for all subtypes of pervasive developmental disorder other than autism (Waterhouse et al. 1992). The rationale for this was that subgroups on the pervasive developmental disorder spectrum, such as atypical autism and Asperger's syndrome, could not be reliably distinguished from autistic disorder and did not differ from that disorder in either etiologic variables or clinical course (Waterhouse et al. 1992). According to the DSM-III-R Work Group, therefore, there was insufficient evidence for the validity of other disorders on the pervasive developmental disorder spectrum to justify the establishment of separate diagnostic categories. The purpose of this literature review is to see whether these conclusions still hold in light of more recent empirical data.

The author was supported in the preparation of this chapter by grants from The Ontario Mental Health Foundation and National Health and Welfare Canada.

Method

A comprehensive search was carried out to identify all relevant articles in English, using a Medline computer search and consulting key references, fairly recent reviews (Gillberg and Gillberg 1989; Tantum 1988a, 1988b), and experts in the field. No papers were identified that dealt specifically with the term *PDDNOS*. Therefore, inclusion criteria for the search were expanded to include any article concerned with the following nonautistic subtypes of pervasive developmental disorder: *atypical autism, atypical pervasive developmental disorder, Asperger's syndrome, schizotypal personality disorder in children, schizoid disorders in children,* and *autistic psychopathy*. Papers that attempted to define subgroups of autistic children were also included if the use of *autism* was sufficiently broad and comprehensive.

The next step was to eliminate papers that did not allow for comparisons between autism and the proposed PDDNOS subtype. Thus, individual case studies were eliminated first. Case-series (i.e., without a control group of autistic subjects) descriptions were included if 1) they were of sufficient sample size (i.e., $N > 5$) and 2) were carried out in a rigorous fashion, allowing the reader to draw comparisons with autism. It must be emphasized, however, that case-series provide weak evidence for validity, because, once again, there is no comparison with autistic disorder. This type of design is useful chiefly in the absence of carefully done case-control studies.

Results

Twenty-one studies were identified that met the inclusion criteria: five case-series, eight case-control studies, four cross-sectional surveys, three follow-up studies, and one family history study. This literature review discusses clinical features, prevalence, etiology, and outcome of the various PDDNOS subtypes. Most of the literature discusses Asperger's syndrome or atypical children with pervasive developmental disorder who function at either a high or low level in terms of IQ. In this review, these categories are considered to be more specific subtypes of PDDNOS. From the data provided in these studies, unfortunately, it is not always clear which subtype is being investigated.

Clinical Features

Five case-series have described the clinical features of Asperger's syndrome (Gillberg and Gillberg 1989; Szatmari et al. 1989b; Tantum 1988a, 1988b; Wing 1981; Wolff and Chick 1980). These case-series show consistent similarities in their clinical descriptions. Most of the subjects were male, and, although their IQs were below normal, they did not fall in the severely or moderately retarded range. All authors agree that elements of the autistic triad are essential to the diagnosis: 1) various impairments in reciprocal social interaction, 2) deficits in verbal and nonverbal communication, and 3) a restricted range of imaginative activities. Generally speaking, the individuals with Asperger's syndrome are described as being eccentric and socially isolated, possessing bizarre interests or preoccupations yet demonstrating a high degree of verbal ability. The examples differ only slightly (e.g., whether motor clumsiness should be a diagnostic criterion). Wolff and Chick (1980), who described "schizoid" children (a disorder conceptually similar to Asperger's syndrome), emphasized personality traits such as hypersensitivity to criticism and rigidity of mental set. Although these are associated features in the other descriptions, such traits are not seen as essential. Thus, there seems to be reasonable agreement on the clinical features of Asperger's syndrome.

An alternative way to identify homogeneous and specific PDDNOS subtypes is to use multivariate techniques such as factor or cluster analysis. Instead of differentiating groups on the basis of categorical diagnostic criteria, these studies use dimensional indices (i.e., scores on socialization and communication scales) to cluster together children with similar symptom profiles. Evidence of internal validity is provided if more than one group of children with pervasive developmental disorder (i.e., an autistic and nonautistic group) can be empirically identified. The subgroups can then be evaluated for internal consistency (i.e., how homogeneous are they?) and for specificity (i.e., how different are the subgroups on their input parameters?).

Five studies have used cluster-analytic techniques to subclassify children with pervasive developmental disorder. In the earliest study, Prior et al. (1975) derived two clusters: a "Kanners" and "non-Kanners" (i.e., atypical pervasive developmental disorder) group. In general, the non-Kanners group had less severe symptoms across dimensions of socialization, communication, and repetitive activities and a later age at onset. Two other cluster-analytic studies used overlapping clinical samples and might be considered together (Dahl et al. 1986; Rescorla 1986, 1988). In the Rescorla (1988) study, the sample included, among other disorders, 79 autistic and "autistic-like" (the atypical pervasive developmental disorder group) children. Two clusters of children with pervasive developmental disorder emerged only when four, five, or six clusters were requested. In general, the autistic-like group was more developmentally mature and had more symptoms of anxiety than the autistic group.

Siegel et al. (1986) used a sophisticated procedure to cluster analyze 35 male and 11 female autistic and autistic-like subjects on the basis of behavior during a semistructured play situation. Four clusters emerged, three of which roughly correspond to 1) a classic "autistic" group, 2) an atypical pervasive developmental disorder group with mental retardation, and 3) a "schizoid" group. The classically autistic group was characterized by high scores on perseverative play and preoccupations with parts of objects. In addition, their language was mostly noncommunicative. The atypical pervasive developmental disorder group showed a high number of stereotypies and were usually without language altogether. The schizoid group, on the other hand, was characterized by less perseverative play and fewer stereotypies, but displayed odd speech, unusual ideas, and "disjointed" play. This third group appears to resemble closely the descriptions of Asperger's syndrome.

Szatmari et al. (1989a) performed a cluster analysis on 28 children with Asperger's syndrome and 25 individuals with high-functioning (i.e., nonretarded) autism matched on IQ. Dimensional scores on impairments in socialization, communication, and imaginative activities were used to separate the groups. A two-cluster solution showed good agreement with the clinical diagnosis (kappa = .52), indicating that multivariate classification techniques confirmed distinctions based on clinical diagnosis. A three-cluster solution was also derived that characterized a third "hybrid" group. This study suggests that among nonretarded PDDNOS children, two groups emerge: one with good language (Asperger's syndrome) and a second group similar to the receptive dysphasic children with autistic features described by others (Bartak et al. 1975; Paul et al. 1983).

Thus, all five multivariate studies agree that children with pervasive developmental disorder behaviors can be classified into at least two, and possibly three, more homogeneous subgroups. The problem with these multivariate techniques is that these are hypothesis "generating" rather than confirmatory. Homogeneous clusters can emerge even with randomly generated data, so that the results need to be replicated using other designs.

In fact, several studies have compared autistic and PDDNOS children on features of clinical presentation independent of the original diagnostic criteria (Fisher et al. 1987; Gillberg 1989; Szatmari et al. 1989a; Volkmar et al. 1988, 1989; Wing and Gould 1979). In these investigations, autistic and various PDDNOS subgroups are defined a priori and then compared on other clinical features. All studies, except the Wing and Gould survey, were able to find differences between the PDDNOS group (however defined) and the autistic disorder group. In general, these studies found that the atypical or PDDNOS group had better social responsiveness, fewer impairments in language development, and, more variably, a less restricted range of imaginative interests. In most instances, the atypical group shows fewer autistic traits than the autistic group, so that differences may be in severity rather than type. The only example of possibly qualitative differences is that the PDDNOS group can show more symptoms of anxiety (Rescorla 1988; Szatmari et al. 1989a) and schizotypal symptoms (Siegel et al. 1986; Szatmari et al. 1989a; Volkmar et al. 1988). Perhaps the most outstanding clinical difference is that, among the Asperger's syndrome or high-functioning type of PDDNOS, there is little or no evidence of deviant language development such as delayed echolalia, pronoun reversal, jargon speech, neologisms, or idiosyncratic word usage (Gillberg 1989; Szatmari et al. 1989a; Volkmar et al. 1988). Instead, the speech of individuals with Asperger's syndrome is most often characterized as tangential, pedantic, repetitive, or one-sided (Wing 1981).

Although the evidence for clinical differences is quite consistent across the study designs, many of the studies have methodological limitations. First, only two studies (Gillberg 1989; Szatmari et al. 1989a) matched Asperger's syndrome and autistic patients on IQ. In the other studies, the differences found between the groups could still be accounted for by confounding differences in developmental level or in severity, independent of IQ. Second, the measurement of dependent variables may not have been blind to diagnostic status. This would add a substantial source of bias that could exaggerate differences between the groups. Third, many of the dependent variables were associated with the diagnostic criteria, rendering the comparisons potentially circular. Nevertheless, these reports, and the multivariate cluster-analysis studies, are reasonably consistent in demonstrating clinical differences between autism and several PDDNOS subtypes.

Prevalence

Gillberg and Gillberg (1989) summarized four prevalence studies of Asperger's syndrome (Gillberg et al. 1982, 1986; Holstrom 1985 [cited in Gillberg and Gillberg 1989]; Wing and Gould 1979). Their estimate of prevalence rates of Asperger's syndrome without mental retardation is between 10 and 26 per 10,000. For Asperger's syndrome children with mild mental retardation, much lower rates were observed (i.e., between 0.4 and 1.7 per 10,000). There were no cases of Asperger's syndrome among moderately retarded children.

There are three studies of the prevalence of atypical pervasive developmental disorder with lower functioning. Burd et al. (1987) reported a prevalence rate of 1.16 per 10,000 for autism and 1.99 per 10,000 for "atypical pervasive developmental disorder" based on an administrative survey. In a total population of children in one urban and one rural area, Steffenburg and Gillberg (1986) reported rates of 4.5 per 10,000 for infantile autism and 2.2 per 10,000 for "autistic-like conditions." Much higher rates were observed by Wing and Gould (1979) in their epidemiological study of handicapped children with impairments in social interaction. They were able to identify 74 children (21 per 10,000) who fit the "autistic triad" (i.e., they had qualitative impairments in social interaction, deficits in communication, and a restricted range of imaginative activities). Of these children, 17 met the classic description of infantile autism. Another 57 were considered to have "atypical autism" (i.e., 16 per 10,000). Wing and Gould concluded that atypical autism is, in fact, three times more common than "classical autism." These prevalence studies indicate that children with PDDNOS do exist and are at least as common as those with autism, if not more common (assuming these rates can be replicated using proper survey methodology).

Etiological Markers

Thirteen studies have compared etiological markers in autism and PDDNOS subtypes: for the most part sex ratio, IQ, the presence of neurological disorders, and age at onset. Both cluster-analytic and case-control studies have explored this issue. Among the cluster-analytic studies, Siegel et al. (1986) reported that, compared with the autistic group, the atypical group with mental retardation (MR-PDDNOS) contained a higher proportion of females and showed greater developmental delays and lower IQ; no differences were observed in the number of pregnancy and birth complications. The "schizoid" group also contained more females, but showed higher IQ and fewer pregnancy and birth complications than the autistic group. Rescorla (1988) and Dahl et al. (1986) reported that the PDDNOS group also had higher IQ, but found a higher proportion of males. No other differences on a variety of psychosocial and developmental correlates were noted.

Ten case-control and cross-sectional survey studies compared autistic and PDDNOS groups on etiological markers. These can be divided into studies that sample PDDNOS from a retarded or a nonretarded population. Lower-functioning subjects (i.e., MR-PDDNOS) appear to have higher rates of organicity, lower IQ, and a higher proportion of females than the autistic group (Fisher et al. 1987; Gillberg and Steffenburg 1987; Steffenburg and Gillberg 1986; Wing and Gould 1979). The findings are different if one samples the PDDNOS group from a primarily nonretarded population. For example, Volkmar et al. (1988, 1989) reported that the PDDNOS group in their study included a higher proportion of males, a somewhat later age at onset, higher IQ, and less evidence of organicity. Wolff and Barlow (1979) found differences between an autistic and a schizoid group on measures of cognitive function. In contrast, Szatmari et al. (1989b, 1990) found no differences between IQ-matched Asperger's syndrome and autistic subjects on sex ratio, family history, organicity, or neuropsychological testing.

Perhaps the most comprehensive study of etiology was recently reported by Gillberg (1989). He compared 23 Asperger's syndrome children with IQ-matched autistic control subjects. The Asperger's syndrome group had a higher proportion of males, later onset, fewer pregnancy and birth complications, and fewer neurological disorders. These differences were not significant, however, and were of uncertain clinical importance. Gillberg concluded that Asperger's syndrome and autism differed little on etiological parameters. Perhaps the etiological differences previously reported by others between PDDNOS and autism (Siegel et al. 1986; Volkmar et al. 1988, 1989) may have been due to the fact that the autistic group was more severely retarded.

In addition, there appear to be no differences in family history. Delong and Dwyer (1988) found higher rates of Asperger's syndrome in the first- and second-degree relatives of nonretarded, compared with retarded, autistic individuals. This suggests that there may be a common genetic relationship between Asperger's syndrome and nonretarded autism.

Thus, the pattern of differences in etiological markers between autism and PDDNOS appears to depend on whether the latter group is retarded. The MR-PDDNOS group appears to include a larger number of subjects with identifiable neurological disorders and a higher number of females. Although the higher-functioning atypical and Asperger's syndrome subtypes of PDDNOS have higher IQ, more males, and later onset, it does appear that, if one matches Asperger's syndrome and autism on IQ, there are no major differences in etiology.

Outcome

Four studies have reported on outcome. Among a cohort of primarily retarded, atypical children with pervasive developmental disorder, Gillberg and Steffenburg (1987) reported worse outcome compared with children with autism. The other three studies reported on higher-functioning children with pervasive developmental disorder. Szatmari et al. (1989a) found that children with Asperger's syndrome spent significantly less time in special education classes than an IQ-matched autistic group. Two other follow-up studies of schizoid (Wolff and Chick 1980) and atypical (Sparrow et al. 1986) children, both uncontrolled, suggest that the diagnosis is stable over time (i.e., at follow-up the PDDNOS children are not diagnosed as autistic) and that the impairments in socialization and communication persist. Although there was no direct comparison with autism, these PDDNOS children appear to have better outcomes than those usually reported for high-functioning autistic individuals (Cantwell et al. 1989; Rumsey et al. 1985; Szatmari et al. 1989c). However, the definitive follow-up study comparing PDDNOS and autistic children matched on IQ remains to be done.

Discussion

Most studies report some differences between the autistic and PDDNOS groups, although in the studies of Steffenburg and Gillberg (1986), Wing and Gould (1979), and Gillberg (1989), these differences were minimal and hardly of clinical significance. These findings are stronger if one compares groups on clinical features rather than on putative etiological factors. The direction of etiological differences depends almost entirely on whether the PDDNOS sample is retarded. If retarded, the PDDNOS group (compared with an autistic group) tends to show more evidence of organicity, lower IQ, a higher number of females, and a worse outcome. If the PDDNOS group is primarily nonretarded (e.g., Asperger's syndrome, schizoid, or atypical pervasive developmental disorder), the group tends to demonstrate a higher male-to-female ratio, higher IQ, less severe symptomatology, more anxiety symptoms and, perhaps, a better outcome. Data on other etiological variables are unclear, but the Delong and Dwyer (1988) and Gillberg (1989) studies would have to be taken as reasonable evidence that both Asperger's syndrome and high-functioning autism share a common etiology, whereas MR-PDDNOS includes some cases with identifiable neurological disorder.

Three varieties of PDDNOS have been discussed in the literature: a lower-functioning atypical group, a higher-functioning atypical group, and Asperger's syndrome. The evidence that the clinical differences found between autism and these various PDDNOS subtypes carry any inferences with respect to etiology and clinical course is only suggestive and is based on only a few studies. Replication is obviously needed, with greater attention to matching IQ and to blind assessment of dependent variables. The outstanding issue is whether the differences demonstrated between autism and the atypical forms of pervasive developmental disorder are simply a function of severity or developmental level. Do the clinical differences still hold if the autistic and PDDNOS groups are matched on a measure of developmental level such as IQ? The Szatmari et al. (1989a, 1989b, 1990) and Gillberg (1989) studies suggest that they do for Asperger's syndrome, but further replication is needed. It is also not clear whether clinical differences exist between Asperger's syndrome and the higher-functioning atypical children with pervasive developmental disorder described by Volkmar et al. (1988), Siegel et al. (1986), and others. Clearly, studies are needed that investigate whether homogeneous subtypes of nonretarded children with pervasive developmental disorder exist.

One obstacle to a quick resolution of this issue is that the data on diagnostic validity conflict. There is some evidence that Asperger's syndrome and autism do not differ in etiology, but do have a different clinical presentation and clinical course. Is this sufficient to conclude that one disorder is different from the other, or are they the same? What criteria actually constitute the criteria for "same" and "different" when one is comparing related diagnostic categories? Should the criteria for taxonomic validity be different if one is considering subgroups of a more general category (e.g., pervasive developmental disorder) than when one compares conceptually different disorders (e.g., anxiety and conduct disorder)?

At this stage, the issue may be whether it is useful, even if not necessarily valid, to distinguish and characterize subtypes of PDDNOS for purposes of clinical practice, education, and research. Perhaps diagnostic validity should be a relative, not an absolute, concept. There may be instances when it is "valid" to combine Asperger's syndrome and autism, such as for genetic studies. There may be other instances when it is equally "valid" to consider them as separate, such as for follow-up studies. The key issue may be, "valid for what?"

An important principle to determine is whether DSM-IV should include disorders with suggestive, but limited, evidence of validity. The only way to answer this question is to assess the risks and benefits of inclusion. What would be the potential risks and benefits of setting out diagnostic criteria for atypical forms of pervasive developmental disorder?

Several potential risks include 1) introducing another DSM disorder with little empirical evidence of validity; 2) encouraging overdiagnosis (e.g., some hyperactive children or those with language delay may be diagnosed as Asperger's syndrome or atypical pervasive developmental disorder); and 3) "carving up" the autistic triad at false "joints" (i.e., Wing [1988] argued that the autistic triad be considered dimensions along which children with pervasive developmental disorder differ; by carving up these dimensions at false joints, we may lose this important concept).

On the other hand, potential benefits of inclusion include 1) stimulating research concerning PDDNOS children, 2) replacing terms such as *autistic-like* and providing a diagnostic label for families confused by their child's clinical picture, 3) providing educational and clinical resources to a previously unrecognized group, 4) giving more foundation to the notion of a group of disorders on the pervasive developmental disorder spectrum, 5) avoiding the potential overdiagnosis of PDDNOS among the mental retardation population by specifying criteria, and 6) promoting compatibility with ICD-10 (World Health Organization 1990).

Recommendations

The options for DSM-IV include

1. Do nothing other than changing the DSM-III-R text related to PDDNOS to be more informative based on this review.
2. Adopt the ICD-10 approach and identify Asperger's syndrome, atypical autism, Rett's syndrome, and so on, and specify diagnostic criteria. In the text of ICD-10, explicit recognition is made of the fact that subtypes such as Asperger's syndrome and atypical autism are of uncertain diagnostic validity. It would be important to acknowledge this in DSM-IV.
3. Selectively adopt the ICD-10 approach, adding fewer pervasive developmental disorder subtypes than ICD-10. For example, a lower-functioning and a

higher-functioning form of atypical pervasive developmental disorder would cover most of the children described in this literature review.
4. Instead of adding further subtypes to the classification of pervasive developmental disorder, the disorders discussed in this literature review could be identified as specific examples of PDDNOS with a brief description of clinical presentation.

Clearly further research is needed before a final resolution is possible. Priorities for research include 1) establishing the reliability of diagnostic criteria for Asperger's syndrome, atypical autism, and so on; 2) conducting prevalence studies of pervasive developmental disorder subtypes in both clinic and community samples; 3) initiating outcome studies to determine whether pervasive developmental disorder subtypes have a different natural history while controlling for potentially confounding factors such as IQ; 4) designing further etiological studies using brain imaging, neurotransmitter assays, and genetic designs; and 5) conducting treatment studies, controlling for IQ or severity, to see whether pervasive developmental disorder subtypes have a differential response to various treatment strategies.

References

American Psychiatric Association: Diagnostic and Statistical Manual of Mental Disorders, 3rd Edition, Revised. Washington, DC, American Psychiatric Association, 1987

Bartak L, Rutter M, Cox A: A comparative study of infantile autism and specific developmental receptive language disorder, I: the children. Br J Psychiatry 126:127–145, 1975

Burd L, Fisher W, Kerbeshian J: A prevalence study of pervasive developmental disorders in North Dakota. J Am Acad Child Adolesc Psychiatry 26:700–703, 1987

Cantwell DP, Baker L, Rutter M, et al: Infantile autism and developmental receptive dysphasia: a comparative follow-up into middle childhood. J Autism Dev Disord 19:19–32, 1989

Dahl EK, Cohen DJ, Provence S: Clinical and multivariate approaches to the nosology of pervasive developmental disorders. Journal of the American Academy of Child Psychiatry 25:170–181, 1986

Delong GR, Dwyer JJ: Correlation of family history with specific autistic subgroups: Asperger's syndrome and bipolar affective disorder. J Autism Dev Disord 18:593–600, 1988

Fisher W, Burd L, Kerbeshian J: Comparisons of DSM-III defined pervasive developmental disorders in North Dakota children. J Am Acad Child Adolesc Psychiatry 26:704–710, 1987

Gillberg C: Asperger's syndrome in 23 Swedish children. Dev Med Child Neurol 81:520–531, 1989

Gillberg C, Gillberg C: Asperger syndrome: some epidemiological considerations: a research note. J Child Psychol Psychiatry 30:631–638, 1989

Gillberg C, Steffenburg S: Outcome and prognostic factors in infantile autism and similar conditions: a population-based study of 46 cases followed through puberty. J Autism Dev Disord 17:273–288, 1987

Gillberg C, Rasmussen RP, Carlstrom G, et al: Perceptual, motor, and attentional deficits in six-year-old children: epidemiological aspects. J Child Psychol Psychiatry 23:131–144, 1982

Gillberg C, Persson E, Gurfman M, et al: Psychiatric disorders in mildly and severely mentally retarded urban children and adolescents. Br J Psychiatry 149:68–74, 1986

Paul R, Cohen DJ, Caparulo DK: A longitudinal study of patients with severe developmental disorders of language learning. Journal of the American Academy of Child Psychiatry 22:525–534, 1983

Prior M, Perry D, Gajzago C: Kanner's syndrome or early onset psychosis: a taxonomic analysis of 142 cases. Journal of Autism and Childhood Schizophrenia 5:71–80, 1975

Rescorla LA: Preschool psychiatric disorders: diagnostic classification and symptom patterns. Journal of the American Academy of Child Psychiatry 25:162–170, 1986

Rescorla L: Cluster analytic identification of autistic preschoolers. J Autism Dev Disord 18:475–492, 1988

Rumsey JM, Rapoport JL, Sceery WR: Autistic children as adults: psychiatric, social, and behavioural outcomes. Journal of the American Academy of Child Psychiatry 24:465–473, 1985

Siegel B, Anders TF, Ciaranello RD, et al: Empirically derived subclassification of the autistic syndrome. J Autism Dev Disord 16:275–294, 1986

Sparrow SS, Rescorla LA, Provence S, et al: Follow-up of "atypical" children. Journal of the American Academy of Child Psychiatry 25:180–185, 1986

Steffenburg S, Gillberg C: Autism and autistic-like conditions in Swedish rural and urban areas: a population study. Br J Psychiatry 149:81–87, 1986

Szatmari P, Bartolucci G, Bremner R, et al: A follow-up of high-functioning autistic children. J Autism Dev Disord 19:213–225, 1989a

Szatmari P, Bartolucci G, Bremner R: Asperger's syndrome and autism: comparisons on early history and outcome. Dev Med Child Neurol 31:709–720, 1989b

Szatmari P, Bremner R, Nagy J: Asperger's syndrome: a review of clinical features. Can J Psychiatry 34:554–560, 1989c

Szatmari P, Tuff L, Finlayson MAJ: Asperger's syndrome and autism: neurocognitive aspects. J Am Acad Child Adolesc Psychiatry 29:130–136, 1990

Tantum D: Asperger's syndrome. J Child Psychol Psychiatry 29:245–255, 1988a

Tantum D: Lifelong eccentricity and social isolation, II: Asperger's syndrome or schizoid personality disorder? Br J Psychiatry 153:783–791, 1988b

Volkmar FR, Cohen DJ, Hoshino Y, et al: Phenomenology and classification of the childhood psychoses. Psychol Med 18:191–201, 1988

Volkmar FR, Cohen DJ, Bergman JD, et al: An examination of social typologies in autism. J Am Acad Child Adolesc Psychiatry 28:82–86, 1989

Waterhouse L, Wing L, Spitzer R, et al: Pervasive developmental disorders (PDD): from DSM-III to DSM-III-R. J Autism Dev Disord 22:525–549, 1992

Wing L: Asperger's syndrome: a clinical account. Psychol Med 11:115–130, 1981

Wing L: The continuum of autistic characteristics, in Diagnosis and Assessment in Autism. Edited by Schopler E, Mesibov G. New York, Plenum, 1988, pp 91–110

Wing L, Gould J: Severe impairments of social interaction and associated abnormalities in children: epidemiology and classification. J Autism Dev Disord 9:11–29, 1979

Wolff S, Barlow A: Schizoid personality in childhood: a comparative study of schizoid, autistic, and normal children. J Child Psychol Psychiatry 20:29–46, 1979

Wolff S, Chick J: Schizoid personality in childhood: a controlled follow-up study. Psychol Med 10:85–100, 1980

World Health Organization: ICD-10 Chapter V: Mental and Behavioral Disorders: Diagnostic Criteria for Research. Geneva, Switzerland, World Health Organization, 1990

Chapter 5

Early-Onset Schizophrenia

John S. Werry, M.D.

Statement and Significance of the Issues

This review is concerned with schizophrenia during childhood or adolescence, termed *early-onset schizophrenia*. The subgroup of early-onset schizophrenia beginning before age 13 is termed very early-onset schizophrenia in preference to prepubertal, because puberty may begin before that age. The questions addressed are

1. Is early-onset schizophrenia the same disorder as in adults?
2. If similar, should early-onset schizophrenia (or the very early-onset schizophrenia subgroup) be a separate subcategory?
3. Are adjustments to the criteria required for children or adolescents?
4. Are there any other developmental issues affecting diagnosis?

Method

Previous reviews (Beitchman 1985; Eisenberg 1957; Kolvin and Berney 1990; Prior and Werry 1986) were canvassed and a Medline search undertaken to locate the small number of studies on early-onset schizophrenia. Only those in English, and, because of differences in classification, only those subsequent to 1970 (with one exception: Makita 1966) were included. Studies have been subject to usual methodological scrutiny, but, because of the very small number of studies, standards had to be relaxed somewhat. This should be borne in mind in evaluating the results.

The most critical methodological issue was diagnosis. Studies should use DSM-III (American Psychiatric Association 1980) criteria for schizophrenia or an equivalent psychotic state characterized by hallucinations, delusions, or other first-ranked symptoms. Unfortunately, most studies of "childhood schizophrenia"

An extended version of this review appeared in the *Journal of Autism and Developmental Disorders* 22:601–624, 1993.

between 1960 and 1975 were actually of autism or contained mixed groups of autistic and schizophrenic children (Prior and Werry 1986), and only two studies (Kolvin 1971; Makita 1966) distinguished between the two.

Because the studies by J. R. Asarnow and Ben-Meir (1988), J. R. Asarnow et al. (1988), R. F. Asarnow et al. (1989), Caplan et al. (1989, 1990), Russell et al. (1989), and Watkins et al. (1988) use the same subject pool, they are treated as a single set called the *UCLA group* and arbitrarily cited as Russell et al. (1989) except where specific findings of particular studies apply. Studies of any kind were very few, and there were only seven that were acceptable and addressed most of the critical issues above, although there were a few more that addressed one or two important points. The seven studies and their main features are summarized in Table 5–1.

It can be seen that most of the studies rely on informal methods, chart reviews, and consensus diagnosis by two psychiatrists. Although some kept data extractors blind or made simple reliability checks (e.g., Volkmar et al. 1988; Werry et al. 1991), only the UCLA group (Russell et al. 1989) observed high-quality data capture and reliability techniques. Two of the studies (Eggers 1978, 1989; Werry et al. 1991) were able to validate the diagnosis by long-term outcome and found a substantial error rate in initial diagnoses of schizophrenia, notably misclassification of bipolar and/or schizoaffective disorders. However, because both studies relied on diagnoses made well in the past, this error may not apply to the more recent studies that employ more exact diagnostic criteria. The concurrence of mood disorder and early-onset schizophrenia in the UCLA studies (J. R. Asarnow and Ben-Meir 1988; Russell et al. 1989) suggest, however, that strict adherence to DSM-III criteria may not have solved this problem, which is neither new nor confined to early-onset presentations (Carlson 1990; Joyce 1984).

Table 5–1 does not include a large ($N = 1,084$) study by Bettes and Walker (1987) of first-admission psychotic patients to age 19. Bettes and Walker offer valuable information, but only on developmental and gender aspects of symptoms in early-onset schizophrenia. They are cited, even though selection criteria were positive and negative schizophrenic symptoms rather than diagnosis. Four widely cited studies are not included because there was doubt about too many cases and details were often insufficient (Cantor et al. 1982; Garralda 1985; Jordan and Prugh 1971) or because follow-up (Werry et al. 1991) had shown high initial misclassification (Kydd and Werry 1981).

Results

The results are summarized in Table 5–2.

Nosological Similarity of Adult and Early-Onset Schizophrenia

Because the diagnosis of schizophrenia in DSM-III-R (American Psychiatric Association 1987) is based solely on three clinical criteria—symptomatology, severity of disturbance, and duration—proof of similarity rests on finding such criteria in children and adolescents. All studies show that DSM-III-R adult-type symptomatology of delusions, hallucinations, incoherence, catatonic behavior, and flat/inappropriate affect (usually accompanied by marked deterioration in function and a prodrome/active/residual phase lasting 6 months or more) can be found in children and adolescents.

Early-Onset Schizophrenia as a Subcategory

Subcategorization, except in residual schizophrenia, rests on which type of clinical symptomatology—paranoid, catatonic, disorganized, or none (i.e., undifferentiated)—predominates. Thus, an age-dependent variation in predominant clinical symptomatology could argue for a separate subcategory of early-onset schizophrenia. There seems to be some agreement across studies (Bettes and Walker 1987; Eggers 1978; Russell et al. 1989; Watkins et al. 1988; Werry et al. 1991) that well-formulated delusions are less frequent in early-onset schizophrenia, especially in very early-onset schizophrenia, although this is not unanimous (Green et al. 1984; Volkmar et al. 1988). All agree that hallucinations, thought disorder, and flattened/inappropriate affect are characteristic of early-onset schizophrenia. Catatonic symptoms seem infrequent in most studies (see also Spencer et al. 1991). However, only two studies (Eggers 1978; Werry et al. 1991) assigned subcategories, and they are in conflict, although the preponderance of undifferentiated subtypes in the latter is more consistent with the symptomatological picture in other studies.

Modification of Criteria

Although the diagnostic criteria seem to apply satisfactorily to children and adolescents, minor areas of misfit due to developmental differences would be expected. Many of the symptoms of schizophrenia are in language, thought, and cognition, all of which are affected by developmental stage. Not surprisingly, then, in early-onset schizophrenia, well-formed positive symptoms have been shown to become more evident with age (Bettes and Walker 1987; Caplan et al. 1990; Eggers 1978). Developmental language disorders, which are much more common than very early-onset schizophrenia, are characterized by "disorganized speech" (Cantwell and Baker 1987), a key symptom in adult schizophrenia. Hallucinations are found in nonschizophrenic children, in those with psychotic relatives, and in nonpsychotic disorders where they are not conspicuously different from those in schizo-

Table 5–1. Characteristics of early onset schizophrenia studies

Characteristics	Makita 1966	Kolvin 1971	Eggers 1978 (1989)	Green et al. 1984 (Green & Padron-Gayol 1986)	Volkmar et al. 1988	UCLA group[a]	Werry et al. 1991
Diagnosis							
Criteria	Adult type	First-rank symptoms Other schizophrenia symptoms	Bleulerian first-rank	DSM-III	DSM-III	DSM-III	DSM-III-R
Method	?Psychiatric exam	?Chart review, ?psychiatric exam, consensus	Chart review, follow-up, informants, discards at follow-up	Chart review, consensus	Chart review, blind consensus	Chart review, K-SADS/DICA etc. (kappa = .88)	Chart review, follow-up SCID, consensus checks, discards at follow-up
Comparison	Autism, COPDD	Autism	Schizoaffective	Autism, conduct	Autism, COPDD	STPD, depression Bipolar & comorbidity	
Sample[b]							
N	32	33	57 (41)	40 (24)	14	18–35	18
Male:female	?	2.66:1	1:1.28	2.33:1	?	2.6–2.2:1	1.5:1
Age at onset							
Range	10–15	?7–13+[c]	7–13	5–12	7–14	3–11	9–15

Age							
5–10	2	4[c]	11	36	7	24[c] (2<5)	1
11–12	1	6[c]	46	4	3	9[c]	5
13–15	29	23[c]	0	0	4	0	12
16+	0	—	0	0	0	0	0
Social class	?	All	?	No I,II	—	I,II 64%	All
Country	Japan	United Kingdom	Germany	United States	United States	United States	New Zealand

Note. Parentheses refer to second study by same author(s). K-SADS = Schedule for Affective Disorders and Schizophrenia—Children's Version. DICA = Diagnostic Interview for Children and Adolescents. SCID = Structured Clinical Interview for DSM-III. COPDD = childhood-onset pervasive developmental disorders. STPD = schizotypal personality disorder.

[a] J. R. Asarnow and Ben-Meir 1988; J. R. Asarnow et al. 1988; R. F. Asarnow et al. 1989; Caplan et al. 1989, 1990; Russell et al. 1989; Watkins et al. 1988.
[b] Source of the sample was a children's psychiatric clinic.
[c] Age seen; onset not stated.

Table 5–2. DSM-III-R diagnostic features of studies (%)

Diagnostic features	Makita 1966	Kolvin 1971	Eggers 1978 (1989)	Green et al. 1984 (Green & Padron-Gayol 1986)	Volkmar et al. 1988	UCLA group[a]	Werry et al. 1991
Delusions	?	57	?68 (rare < 10)	50	All	63	41
Hallucinations	?	81	Frequent		All	83	35
Auditory	?	81	Commonest	85	?	80	29
Visual	?	30	?50	48	?	37	6
Other	?	36	Sometimes	8	?	23	12
Thought disorder	Yes	60	?	80	?	40	24
Catatonic	Yes	?60–80	?Unusual	30	?	?	25
Flat/inappropriate affect	Yes	> 60	?	80	?	74	82
Changed function	Yes	?	Yes	Yes	Yes	Yes	Yes
Psychotic mood	?	?	Yes	?Yes	?Yes	Yes	Yes
Disorders excluded			At follow-up				At follow-up

Early-Onset Schizophrenia

	?	?No	?No	?Yes	?Yes	Yes	
Signs 6/12	?	?No	?No	?Yes	?Yes	Yes	90
Prodrome	?	?Unusual	?	?	?	50 (> 8)	Some
Residual phase	?	?	Most	?	?	?	
Subtypes							
Catatonic	A few	?	?4	?	?	?	25
Disorganized	Most	?	?14	?	?	?	6
Paranoid	?	?	?68	?	?	?	13
Undifferentiated	?	?	?14	?	?	?	47

Note. Parentheses refer to second study by same author(s). Question marks indicate uncertainty.
[a] J. R. Asarnow and Ben-Meir 1988; J. R. Asarnow et al. 1988; R. F. Asarnow et al. 1989; Caplan et al. 1989, 1990; Russell et al. 1989; Watkins et al. 1988.

phrenia (Burke et al. 1985; Garralda 1985; Rothstein 1981). Young children's fantasies or imaginings may be mistaken for delusions. However, children and adolescents with early-onset schizophrenia have multiple symptoms of schizophrenia and significant disability (Garralda 1985; Werry et al. 1991). Children do not have well-developed discursive speech, and symptoms that are based on well-developed speech are liable to be overlooked unless special techniques are used to elicit them (Caplan et al. 1989, 1990). Poverty of thinking does not differentiate nonschizophrenic and schizophrenic children, whereas loose associations and illogical thinking do. Thought insertion and thought echo appear to be rare in children (Garralda 1985; Spencer et al. 1991).

Most of the studies cited show that severe premorbid personality abnormality is very common (54%–86%) in very early-onset schizophrenia, and onset often occurs over a long period (Spencer et al. 1991). This makes defining prodromal and active phases and/or a marked change in function especially difficult in early-onset schizophrenia (Cantor et al. 1982; Kolvin 1971; Volkmar et al. 1988; Watkins et al. 1988), although not all authors agree (Green et al. 1984; Werry et al. 1991).

Other Diagnostic Issues

Concern has been expressed (Cantor et al. 1982; Kolvin 1971; Reid 1983; Volkmar et al. 1988; Watkins et al. 1988) that, because positive symptoms of schizophrenia are dependent on language, it is impossible to make the diagnosis in those too young or too handicapped to be proficient with language. However, the earliest age at which almost all studies have reported schizophrenia is 6 years, an age that is too old to support the contention that language or cognitive development artificially restricts the age at onset.

This does not address the problem of those children older than 5 years who lack sufficient language skills to describe schizophrenic symptoms. For example, in a review of psychiatric illness in developmentally disabled patients, Reid (1983) concluded that the diagnosis of schizophrenia in the nonverbal was impossible. So far, there has been no systematic study to see whether reliable behavioral indicators of schizophrenia might be developed for this group.

There are some issues in differential diagnosis. When language is present, the differential with autism may present difficulties because the children are discernibly odd, with abnormalities of speech and language. However, hallucinations and delusions are not seen in autism, and the developmental abnormality of autism begins before age 3 years and is much more pervasive than any seen in those who later develop schizophrenia (Kolvin 1971; Makita 1966). In rare cases, autism and schizophrenia can occur together (Petty et al. 1984; Watkins et al. 1988), although the onset of schizophrenia is later and the characteristic schizophrenic symptoms such as delusions, hallucinations, and formal thought disorder constitute a qualitative change in the clinical picture. Differentiating mood and schizoaffective disorder seems to present a special problem in children and adolescents because the more florid, ill-formed psychotic symptoms may be mistaken for schizophrenia (Apter et al. 1987; Carlson 1990; Eggers 1989; Garralda 1985; Werry et al. 1991). In fact, differentiation may be possible only at longer-term follow-up. Because of the lifelong history of abnormality common in early-onset schizophrenia, differentiating it from schizotypal disorder may be very difficult, particularly because the difference seems to be one of degree rather than type (Caplan et al. 1989, 1990; Russell et al. 1989; Watkins et al. 1988).

Discussion

There is general agreement that a clinical syndrome that resembles adult schizophrenia can be found in children and adolescents and that childhood schizophrenia should be considered as the same disorder as adult schizophrenia. There is insufficient evidence to show that any differences in symptomatology in early-onset schizophrenia are substantial, common, or specific enough that they cannot be encompassed within existing subcategories, although there has been little systematic study of this.

There are some developmental differences in symptomatology that have significance for diagnosis. Disorganized speech is as characteristic of developmental language disorders as of early-onset schizophrenia (Burke et al. 1985; Cantwell and Baker 1987; Garralda 1985; Rothstein 1981). Likewise, hallucinations are not specific to early-onset schizophrenia, although they are its commonest symptom. Thus, emphasis on these two symptoms in diagnosis would need to take account of their lack of diagnostic specificity in children. Poverty of thinking, thought insertion, other passivity phenomena, well-formed delusions, and those delusions with adult content such as religion or sexuality appear to be rare in children (Caplan et al. 1989, 1990; Russell 1992; Spencer et al. 1991), and, if they are included in the criteria, their infrequency in children would require some kind of disclaimer for early-onset schizophrenia and compensatory recognition of other more common key symptoms such as loosening of associations and hallucinations.

Because insidious onset and lifelong, highly abnormal personality are common in early-onset schizophrenia and especially so in very early-onset schizophrenia, both a dramatic change in function and well-defined prodromes may be difficult to observe and may create problems if these are critical inclusive criteria (Reid 1983; Russell 1992; Volkmar et al. 1988). However, because this problem of insidious onset is not peculiar to early-onset schizophrenia (e.g., it is also seen in simple schizophrenia and schizotypal disorder in adults), it is unlikely that special criteria for children in excess of those for adults would be required.

When language is absent or extremely restricted, as in very young children or severely developmentally disabled persons, a diagnosis of schizophrenia may be impossible (Cantor et al. 1982; Reid 1983), creating a problem of false negatives unless good behavioral indicators are developed. At the moment, there are insufficient data on what these might be to warrant inclusion as specific criteria to cover this contingency.

Autism may present a special difficulty in differential diagnosis, because children with early-onset schizophrenia have also usually been discernibly odd since birth. However, schizophrenic symptoms are not characteristic of autism, and the abnormality of development and impaired interpersonal relatedness are much more pervasive. Differentiating mood disorder with psychosis from early-onset schizophrenia is a particular problem (Carlson 1990; Werry et al. 1991), but this is also true in adults (Carlson 1990; Joyce 1984), and no special criteria for children and adolescents seem to be required for this.

Recommendations

1. Schizophrenia in children and adolescents should be regarded as the same disorder as in adults, requiring the same basic diagnostic criteria.
2. Current subcategories seem adequate for children and adolescents and require no adjustment.
3. Some minor adjustments in symptoms may be needed to take care of the developmental differences found especially in children as follows:
    3.1. The need for more than one prominent and persisting schizophrenic symptom (such as hallucinations, disorganized thinking, or delusions) should be emphasized to avoid misinterpretation of normal phenomena or nonspecific symptoms.
    3.2. Where "disorganized speech" is referred to, the phrase "in children, loose associations and illogical thinking" should be added to make this more specifically schizophrenic and avoid confusion with developmental language disorders. If disorganized speech is not a criterion, the phrase above should be added to assist in diagnosis in children.
4. The criterion requiring children with a previous history of autism to have prominent delusions or hallucinations should be continued.
5. The problems of insidious onset, lack of clear prodrome, and differential diagnosis from mood disorder with psychosis and from schizotypal disorder are not qualitatively different in children and adolescents but are especially frequent and conspicuous. Criteria addressing these issues should be formulated to be as clear as possible in the interests of children and adolescents.

References

American Psychiatric Association: Diagnostic and Statistical Manual of Mental Disorders, 3rd Edition. Washington, DC, American Psychiatric Association, 1980

American Psychiatric Association: Diagnostic and Statistical Manual of Mental Disorders, 3rd Edition, Revised. Washington, DC, American Psychiatric Association, 1987

Apter A, Bleich A, Tyano S: Affective and psychotic psychopathology in hospitalized adolescents. J Am Acad Child Adolesc Psychiatry 27:116–120, 1987

Asarnow JR, Ben-Meir S: Children with schizophrenia spectrum and depressive disorders: a comparative study of premorbid adjustment, onset pattern, and severity of impairment. J Child Psychol Psychiatry 29:477–488, 1988

Asarnow JR, Goldstein MJ, Ben-Meir S: Parental communication deviance in childhood onset schizophrenia spectrum and depressive disorders. J Child Psychol Psychiatry 29:825–838, 1988

Asarnow RF, Asarnow JR, Strandburg R: Schizophrenia: a developmental perspective, in Rochester Symposium on Developmental Psychology. Edited by Cicchetti D. New York, Cambridge University Press, 1989, pp 189–220

Beitchman JH: Childhood schizophrenia: a review and comparison with adult-onset schizophrenia. Psychiatr Clin North Am 8:793–814, 1985

Bettes BA, Walker E: Positive and negative symptoms in psychotic and other psychiatrically disturbed children. J Child Psychol Psychiatry 28:555–567, 1987

Burke P, Del Becarro M, McCauley E, et al: Hallucinations in children. J Am Acad Child Adolesc Psychiatry 24:71–75, 1985

Cantor S, Evans J, Pearce J, et al: Childhood schizophrenia: present but not accounted for. Am J Psychiatry 139:758–762, 1982

Cantwell DP, Baker L: Developmental Speech and Language Disorders in Children. New York, Guilford, 1987

Caplan R, Guthrie D, Fish B, et al: The Kiddie Formal Thought Disorder Rating Scales: clinical assessment, reliability and validity. J Am Acad Child Adolesc Psychiatry 28:408–416, 1989

Caplan R, Perdue S, Tanguay PE, et al: Formal thought disorder in childhood onset schizophrenia and schizotypal personality disorder. J Child Psychol Psychiatry 31:1103–1114, 1990

Carlson GA: Child and adolescent mania: diagnostic considerations. J Child Psychol Psychiatry 31:331–342, 1990

Eisenberg L: The course of childhood schizophrenia. Archives of Neurology and Psychiatry 78:69–83, 1957

Eggers C: Course and prognosis in childhood schizophrenia. Journal of Autism and Childhood Schizophrenia 8:21–36, 1978

Eggers C: Schizoaffective disorders in childhood: a follow-up study. J Autism Dev Disord 19:327–342, 1989

Garralda ME: Characteristics of the psychoses of late onset in children and adolescents. J Adolesc 8:195–207, 1985

Green WH, Campbell M, Hardesty AS, et al: A comparison of schizophrenic and autistic children. Journal of the American Academy of Child Psychiatry 23:399–409, 1984

Green WH, Padron-Gayol M: Schizophrenic disorder in childhood, in Biological Psychiatry 1985. Edited by Shagass C. Amsterdam, Netherlands, Elsevier, 1986, pp 1484–1486

Jordan K, Prugh DC: Schizophreniform psychoses of childhood. Am J Psychiatry 128:323–331, 1971

Joyce PR: Age of onset in bipolar affective disorder and misdiagnosis of schizophrenia. Psychol Med 14:145–149, 1984

Kolvin I: Studies in the childhood psychoses. Br J Psychiatry 118:381–419, 1971

Kolvin I, Berney TP: Childhood schizophrenia, in Handbook of Studies in Child Psychiatry. Edited by Tonge B, Burrows GD, Werry JS. Amsterdam, Netherlands, Elsevier, 1990, pp 123–136

Kydd RR, Werry JS: Schizophrenia in children under 16 years. J Autism Dev Disord 12:343–357, 1981

Makita K: The age of onset of childhood schizophrenia. Folia Psychiatrica et Neurologica Japonica 20:111–121, 1966

Petty LK, Ornitz EM, Michelman JD, et al: Autistic children who become schizophrenic. Arch Gen Psychiatry 41:129–135, 1984

Prior M, Werry JS: Autism, schizophrenia and allied disorders, in Psychopathological Disorders of Childhood, 3rd Edition. Edited by Quay HC, Werry JS. New York, John Wiley, 1986, pp 156–210

Reid AH: Psychiatry of mental handicap. J R Soc Med 76:587–592, 1983

Rothstein A: Hallucinatory phenomena in children. Journal of the American Academy of Child Psychiatry 20:623–635, 1981

Russell AT: Schizophrenia, in Assessment and Diagnosis of Child and Adolescent Psychiatric Disorders: Current Issues and Procedures. Edited by Hooper SR, Hynd GW, Mattison RE. Hillsdale, NJ, Lawrence Erlbaum Associates, 1992, pp 22–63

Russell AT, Bott L, Sammons C: The phenomenology of schizophrenia occurring in childhood. J Am Acad Child Adolesc Psychiatry 28:399–407, 1989

Spencer EK, Meeker W, Kafantaris V, et al: Symptom duration in schizophrenic children: DSM-III-R compared with ICD-10 criteria. Presented at the annual meeting of the American Academy of Child and Adolescent Psychiatry, San Francisco, CA, 1991

Volkmar FR, Cohen DJ, Hoshino Y, et al: Phenomenology and classification of the childhood psychoses. Psychol Med 18:191–201, 1988

Watkins JM, Asarnow RF, Tanguay P: Symptom development in childhood onset schizophrenia. J Child Psychol Psychiatry 29:865–878, 1988

Werry JS, McClellan JM, Chard L: Early onset schizophrenia, bipolar and schizoaffective disorders: a clinical and outcome study. J Am Acad Child Adolesc Psychiatry 30:457–465, 1991

Chapter 6

Should Social Skills Deficits Be Included as a Primary Diagnostic Criterion for Learning Disorders?

Steven R. Forness, Ed.D.

Statement of the Issues

The question for the Work Group on learning disorders (academic skills disorders) is whether social skills deficits should be listed as a primary diagnostic criterion for these disorders in DSM-IV. In this chapter, I address this issue by considering three questions: 1) What is the nature of social skills deficits in children or adolescents with learning disabilities? 2) What is the extent of such deficits in the population? and 3) What implications might there be in regard to intervention? These questions address the core issue that underlies assumptions behind such a proposed diagnostic criterion: just how integral are social skills deficits to the phenomenology of learning disabilities?

Significance of the Issues

The Interagency Committee on Learning Disabilities was formed in 1985 as a study group commissioned by Congress to review and assess the status of learning disabilities in this country. The committee was initially composed of representatives from several governmental agencies involved with persons with learning disabilities, but its subsequent report (Interagency Committee on Learning Disabilities 1987) was ultimately reviewed by organizations in the National Joint Committee on Learning Disabilities, all but one of which had difficulties with the definition of learning disabilities developed by the Interagency Committee on Learning Disabilities (Silver 1988). The definition refers to learning disabilities as a "generic term that refers to a heterogeneous group of disorders manifested by significant difficulties in the acquisition and use of listening, speaking, reading, writing, reasoning or mathematical abilities, or of social skills" (Interagency Committee on Learning Disabilities 1987, p. 3).

The addition of the phrase "or of social skills" is the most problematic aspect of the definition. It was apparently prompted by a relatively comprehensive review of available literature that was commissioned by the Interagency Committee on Learning Disabilities and suggested that many children or adolescents with learning disabilities have difficulty in establishing and maintaining satisfactory social relationships (Hazel and Schumaker 1987).

There are a number of potential problems with the use of social skills deficits as a diagnostic criterion for learning disorders (academic skills disorders) in DSM-IV, the first and foremost of which is that the wording of the definition might allow for an individual with difficulties in social skills, but without academic deficits, to be diagnosed as having a learning disorder. Thus a child or adolescent without any difficulties in reading, math, or other areas traditionally known as learning disorders could still be diagnosed as having a learning disorder. This child or adolescent could also presumably be placed in a learning disabilities program solely for treatment of his or her social disorder.

A second and somewhat related problem is that this definition might exacerbate a long-standing confusion between the category of learning disabilities and the category of serious emotional disturbance under Public Law 94-142: the Education of the Handicapped Act (now known as the Individuals With Disabilities Education Act). This act defines serious emotional disturbance, for example, by five diagnostic criteria, only one of which must be met to qualify a child or adolescent under this category for special education services. In fact, the first of these five criteria refers to an inability to learn that cannot be explained by intellectual, sensory, or health factors—a condition that is so similar as to be almost indistinguishable from learning disabilities. The problems with the serious emotional disturbance definition have been extensively documented elsewhere (Forness and Kavale 1989; National Mental Health and Special Education Coalition 1989), but the confusion between diagnostic criteria for serious emotional disturbance and learning disabilities is only exacerbated by the fact that a definition of major learning disabilities now includes social difficulties as a primary diagnostic criterion.

The third problem with inclusion of social skills deficits as a primary diagnostic criterion for learning disabilities would seem to rest with the issues surrounding the actual nature and extent of social skills deficits in children or adolescents with learning disabilities, along with related diagnostic or treatment implications.

Method

Computer searches were conducted on Medline and ERIC document retrieval, using a variety of key terms, but the yield of relevant citations was quite small compared with citations I already had on hand. The search was subsequently confined to learning disability journals (*Journal of Learning Disabilities, Learning Disability Quarterly, Learning Disability Research, Learning Disability Focus, Academic Therapy*); general special education or educational psychology journals (*Exceptional Children, Remedial and Special Education, Journal of Special Education, Teaching Exceptional Children, Behavioral Disorders, Journal of Psychoeducational Assessment, Journal of Educational Psychology, Psychology in the Schools, Journal of School Psychology*); selected psychology journals (*Child Development, Journal of Consulting and Clinical Psychology, Journal of Applied Behavioral Analysis, American Psychologist, Journal of Clinical Child Psychology, Journal of Applied Developmental Psychology, Journal of Child Psychology and Psychiatry*); and relevant psychiatry or medical journals (*American Journal of Orthopsychiatry, Journal of the American Academy of Child and Adolescent Psychiatry, Child Psychiatry and Human Development, Annals of Psychiatry, American Journal of Psychiatry, American Journal of Diseases of Children, Journal of Pediatrics*). The search covered the time period 1970–1990, although it should be noted that very little relevant literature appeared in this area prior to 1980, and some of the above journals were not even in existence prior to 1980. Recent comprehensive texts on learning disabilities were also reviewed. In each relevant article or textbook, secondary references were cross-checked, especially for those texts or articles published from approximately 1985 through 1990. The Interagency Committee on Learning Disabilities literature review (Hazel and Schumaker 1987) also served as a source for secondary citations.

Studies that dealt with the issue of comorbidity were also examined, especially if these dealt with either formally diagnosed learning disabilities or academic skills disorders as preexisting diagnoses or as secondary diagnoses (i.e., not directly caused by the primary diagnosis) to a primary psychiatric diagnosis (using DSM-III [American Psychiatric Association 1980] or other standard diagnostic criteria). As indicated later in this chapter, there is considerable confusion in the literature between the narrow term *social skills deficits* and the more inclusive concept of *social adjustment* in children with learning or related problems.

Results

Nature of Social Skills Deficits in Learning Disabilities

Speculation on phenomenology of social skills deficits within learning disabilities seems to focus on at least five hypotheses, although there is considerable disagreement as to which of these should be primary (Bender 1987a, 1987b; Gresham and Elliott 1989a, 1989b; Hazel and Schumaker 1987; La Greca 1981; G. G. Osman 1982; Wilchesky and Reynolds 1986).

The first hypothesis is that social skills deficits result from the same neurological dysfunction that is presumed to cause the child's or adolescent's academic difficulties. There are some problems with this hypothesis, as Gresham and Reschly (Gresham and Reschly 1988; Reschly and Gresham 1988) have argued, in that the connection between neurological dysfunction and specific social skills deficits would seem as difficult to establish as the connection between such dysfunctions and specific academic skills deficits. The nature of these social skills deficits, furthermore, seems to be quite similar across children and adolescents in various diagnostic categories (e.g., learning disabilities, behavior disorders, and mild mental retardation). Support for this hypothesis would seem to come, on the other hand, from review of certain language or related processing deficits associated with learning disabilities that seem to be at the core of difficulties in social communication, knowledge of social rules, and social strategies in children and adolescents with learning disabilities (Boucher 1986; Bryan 1982; Oliva and La Greca 1988; Renshaw and Asher 1983; Wiener 1980).

The second hypothesis is that social skills deficits in persons with learning disabilities are secondary (i.e., academic or learning problems lead to poor self-concept, rejection or isolation from peers, or other negative consequences that prevent the development of social skills). This has been considered the more traditional view of the origin of social skills deficits in learning disabilities (B. B. Osman 1987).

The third hypothesis involves social learning theory and states that children or adolescents with learning disabilities fail to "acquire" social skills due to lack of environmental opportunity to learn such skills or fail to "perform" the requisite social skills due to lack of opportunity or lack of reinforcement (Gresham 1988).

The fourth hypothesis relates to the possibility of a dysfunctional family system, not in the sense that parents are the cause of the child's social difficulties, but that, as with any other handicap, the stress of dealing with or adapting to a special child may lead to reduced effectiveness of the family as a social support system for the child (Amerikaner and Omizo 1984; Kronick 1978; Wilchesky and Reynolds 1986).

The fifth hypothesis, not widely mentioned by most authors in this area, concerns the issue of comorbidity. There is not only a clear overlap between learning disabilities and hyperactivity (Felton and Wood 1989; Goldstein 1987; Holoborow and Perry 1986; Lambert 1988; Margalit 1989; Shworm and Birnbaum 1989), but also a growing literature linking depression and learning disabilities (Forness 1988; Gerring and McCarthy 1988; Livingston 1985; Mokros et al. 1989; Rourke et al. 1989; Stevenson and Romney 1984). This suggests that the occurrence of social skill deficits found in persons with learning disabilities might coincide with the occurrence of other associated diagnoses found in this group.

None of these hypotheses has unequivocal empirical support nor are they an exhaustive list of the possibilities underlying social skill deficits in children or adolescents with learning disabilities. It should also be noted that most of the research in social skills has been published only recently (Gresham 1988; Gresham and Elliott 1989b).

Extent of Social Skills Deficits in Learning Disabilities

Although there may be disagreement on the nature of social skills deficits in this population, there is considerably less disagreement that social skills deficits do, in fact, occur in children or adolescents with learning disabilities. Research in this area is in the general context of studies on behavioral and social problems of youngsters with learning disabilities using direct observation (Bender 1985; Bryan 1974, 1978; Forness and Esveldt 1975; McKinney 1989; McKinney et al. 1975), sociometric measures (Bak et al. 1987; Bryan 1976; Bryan and Bryan 1978; Bursuck 1983; Horowitz 1981; Hoyle and Serafica 1988; Prillman 1981; Sabornie and Kauffman 1986; Sabornie et al. 1987–88), videotaped interactions (Bryan and Perlmutter 1979; Bryan et al. 1982; Pearl and Cosden 1982), teacher or parent questionnaires (Baum et al. 1988; Bruck and Hebert 1982; Epstein and Cullinan 1984; McConaughy and Ritter 1986; McKinney et al. 1982), and self-concept measures (Bender 1987b; Hiebert et al. 1982; Silverman and Zigmond 1983). It should be noted, however, that thoughtful reviews of this research suggest conflicting results, with a number of studies suggesting either no differences between samples of persons with learning disabilities and persons without learning disabilities or no characteristic differences between children or adolescents with learning disabilities and those with other related handicaps such as behavior disorders, mild mental retardation, or low achievement (Bryan 1986; Dudley-Marling and Edmiaston 1985; Wiener 1987).

It is also important to distinguish between studies of general social or behavioral difficulties of children with learning disabilities and those studies that specifically address *social skills deficits* in learning disabilities. There seems to be a rather confusing tendency in the available literature on learning disabilities to treat social or behavioral problems and social skills deficits as one and the same. The latter is generally a much smaller literature, both when considered within the learning disabilities field and also when compared with the amount of social skills research in related areas (e.g., in mental retardation or behavior disorders). It appears, furthermore, that social skill development may not be viewed as nearly as important as academic remediation (Cartledge et al. 1985).

Available evidence suggests that children or adolescents with learning disabilities may have social skills deficits, but not invariably so and perhaps not to a degree that is different from children with other handicaps. Gresham and Reschly (1986), for example, had teachers, parents, and peers rate social skills of children with learning disabilities and children without learning disabilities on measures of social skills and found that children with learning disabilities had significantly more difficulty in nearly all areas, including accepting authority, helping others, expressing feelings, and having a positive self-attitude. Cartledge et al. (1986), on the other hand, used some of the same measures and generally did not find significant differences on teacher ratings between matched pairs of subjects with and without learning disabilities; they also found no relationship within their sample between social empathy measures and social skills. There were also no differences between groups on empathy. Gresham et al. (1987) found that children with learning disabilities were significantly below children without learning disabilities in teacher-rated social skills but were not significantly below children with mild mental retardation or behavior disorders, as has been found by others (La Greca and Mesibov 1981; Schumaker et al. 1982).

Even those who claim that social skill deficits do exist in children with learning disabilities hasten to add that available social skills assessment instruments are often less than adequate or that assessment technology is only now beginning to be reliable (Gresham and Elliott 1990; Hazel and Schumaker 1987). Reviews of studies on social skills deficits in other handicapped children, where such research has traditionally been more focused, are also somewhat critical of existing methodology (Hollinger 1987; Mathur and Rutherford 1989; Nelson 1988; Schloss et al. 1986), although longitudinal data are beginning to verify the importance of social skill development in overall outcome (Walker et al. 1987).

Available evidence on these deficits has not yet answered the question of *prevalence* of social skill deficits in the learning disabilities population. Teacher estimates suggest that significant numbers of children with mild handicaps do indeed seem to have adequate social performance (Pullis 1985; Ray 1985). Social skill deficits, however, have been at least tentatively established to some degree in samples of children or adolescents with learning disabilities in nearly every study to date. Although there is little doubt that social or behavioral difficulties exist in this population, it is not yet completely established that these are mediated by deficits in social skills per se or that these social skill deficits are distinctly characteristic of children or adolescents with learning disabilities, at least when compared with children or adolescents with other handicaps of a similar nature.

Treatment or Intervention Implications

Treatment of social skill deficits in children or adolescents with learning disabilities has focused almost exclusively on educational rather than therapeutic interventions (i.e., direct instruction rather than psychotherapy) (Nelson 1988). Strain and Odom (1986) reviewed programs in this area and emphasized the need for pinpointing specific peer interactions that should be taught; arranging the physical environment to promote interaction; training and rewarding both peers and the target child for successive approximations of desired interaction; and evaluating the effectiveness of the program, including generalization of skills to other situations. Blackbourn (1989) demonstrated a program in which such generalization was systematically programed in boys with learning disabilities; Larson and Gerber (1987) developed a form of social metacognition to be used to enhance social skills training in delinquent children with learning disabilities. There is indeed a small but growing literature on effective intervention in social skills training with children and adolescents with learning disabilities (Bierman 1986; Hazel et al. 1982; La Greca and Mesibov 1979, 1981; Matson and Ollendick 1988; Vaughn et al. 1984, 1988) as well as a variety of proven social skills programs that can be adapted for use with children with learning disabilities (H. Hops, J. J. Guild, D. H. Fleischman, et al: PEERS [Procedures for Establishing Effective Relationship Skills]: Manual for Consultants, Eugene, OR, University of Oregon, Center for Behavioral Education of the Handicapped, unpublished manuscript, 1987; H. M. Walker, A. Street, B. Garrett, et al: RECESS [Reprogramming Environmental Contingencies for Effective Social Skills]: Manual for Consultants, Eugene, OR, University of Oregon, Center for Behavioral Education of the Handicapped, unpublished manuscript, 1978; Walker et al. 1983).

The difficulty with referencing social skills deficits as a diagnostic criterion in DSM-IV, however, is the implication that psychiatric treatment or other mental health interventions will necessarily follow. As implied, most treatments for social skill deficits not only are educative but are also routinely done in classrooms or other care settings rather than as an intervention that would be carried out directly by child or adolescent psychiatrists or other mental health professionals.

Discussion

It is clear, even from this cursory review, that social skills deficits are an important consideration in planning programs for children or adolescents with learning disabilities. Such deficits, however, seem not to be exclusively or inevitably characteristic of children or adolescents with learning disabilities; nor is it clear that social skills deficits per se are at the core of the social or emotional difficulties widely reported in this population. A variety of social skills problems are also ascribed to children or adolescents with hyperactivity, childhood depression, or related disorders (Cantwell and Carlson 1983; Henker and Whalen 1989; Kovacs 1989; Prior and Griffin 1985). Because these problems co-occur in large measure with learning disabilities, it is possible that such disorders alone account for significant numbers of social skills difficulties in those with learning disabilities, a hypothesis that remains as yet largely untested (Kistner and Gatlin 1989). If true, however, the treatment for such disorders is much more complex than social skills training (Forness and Kavale 1988); it would be a possible disservice to imply that such problems are an inherent difficulty in learning disabilities, at least to the extent implied by the Interagency Committee on Learning Disabilities definition.

Recommendations

That some children or adolescents with learning disabilities may have social skills difficulties is not at all in question, but the Interagency Committee on Learning Disabilities definition would seem to imply that a learning disability could be diagnosed if only social skills deficits (without accompanying academic deficits) were present. This does not seem to be an acceptable view to most professionals (Newcomer 1989; Silver 1988), nor does it seem warranted by evidence reviewed here. It would, therefore, seem unwise to include social skills deficits as a primary diagnostic criterion for learning disorders (academic skills disorders) as suggested by the Interagency Committee on Learning Disabilities definition. Such deficits should, however, be noted as associated (but not invariable) features of such disorders.

References

American Psychiatric Association: Diagnostic and Statistical Manual of Mental Disorders, 3rd Edition. Washington, DC, American Psychiatric Association, 1980

Amerikaner MJ, Omizo MM: Family interaction and learning disabilities. Journal of Learning Disabilities 17:540–543, 1984

Bak JJ, Cooper EM, Dobroth KM, et al: Special class placements as labels: effects on children's attitudes toward learning handicapped peers. Exceptional Children 54:151–155, 1987

Baum DD, Duffelmeyer F, Geelan M: Resource teacher perceptions of the prevalence of social dysfunction among students with learning disabilities. Journal of Learning Disabilities 21:380–381, 1988

Bender WN: Differential diagnosis based on the task-related behavior of learning disabled and low-achieving adolescents. Learning Disability Quarterly 8:261–266, 1985

Bender WN: Correlates of classroom behavior problems among learning disabled and nondisabled children in mainstream classes. Learning Disability Quarterly 10:312–324, 1987a

Bender WN: Secondary personality and behavioral problems in adolescents with learning disabilities. Journal of Learning Disabilities 20:280–285, 1987b

Bierman KL: Process of change during social skills training with pre-adolescents and its relation to treatment outcome. Child Dev 52:230–240, 1986

Blackbourn JM: Acquisition and generalization of social skills in elementary-aged children with learning disabilities. Journal of Learning Disabilities 22:28–34, 1989

Boucher CR: Pragmatics: the meaning of verbal language in learning disabled and nondisabled boys. Learning Disability Quarterly 9:285–294, 1986

Bruck M, Hebert M: Correlates of learning disabled students' peer inter-action patterns. Learning Disability Quarterly 5:353–362, 1982

Bryan TH: An observational study of classroom behaviors of children with learning disabilities. Journal of Learning Disabilities 7:16–34, 1974

Bryan TH: Peer popularity of learning disabled children: a replication. Journal of Learning Disabilities 11:307–311, 1976

Bryan TH: Social relationships and verbal interactions of learning disabled children. Journal of Learning Disabilities 11:107–115, 1978

Bryan TH: Social skills of learning disabled children and youth: an overview. Learning Disability Quarterly 5:332–333, 1982

Bryan TH: Self-concept and attributions of the learning disabled. Learning Disabilities Focus 1:82–89, 1986

Bryan TH, Bryan JH: Social interactions of learning disabled children. Learning Disability Quarterly 1:33–38, 1978

Bryan TH, Perlmutter B: Immediate impressions of LD children by female adults. Learning Disability Quarterly 1:33–38, 1979

Bryan JH, Bryan TH, Sonnefeld LJ: Being known by the company we keep: the contagion of first impressions. Learning Disability Quarterly 5:288–294, 1982

Bursuck WD: Sociometric status, behavior ratings and social knowledge of learning disabled and low-achieving students. Learning Disability Quarterly 6:329–338, 1983

Cantwell DP, Carlson GA: Affective Disorders in Childhood and Adolescence: an Update. New York, Spectrum, 1983

Cartledge G, Frew T, Zaharias J: Social skill needs of mainstreamed students: peer and teacher perceptions. Learning Disability Quarterly 8:132–140, 1985

Cartledge G, Stupay D, Kaczala C: Social skills and social perception of LD and nonhandicapped elementary-school students. Learning Disability Quarterly 9:226–234, 1986

Dudley-Marling CC, Edmiaston R: Social status of learning disabled children and adolescents: a review. Learning Disability Quarterly 8:189–204, 1985

Epstein MH, Cullinan D: Behavior problems of mildly handicapped and normal adolescents. Journal of Clinical Child Psychology 13:33–37, 1984

Felton RH, Wood FB: Cognitive deficits in reading disability and attention deficit disorder. Journal of Learning Disabilities 22:3–13, 1989

Forness S: School characteristics of children and adolescents with depression. Monographs in Behavioral Disorders 10:177–203, 1988

Forness S, Esveldt K: Classroom observation of learning and behavior problem children. Journal of Learning Disabilities 8:382–385, 1975

Forness SR, Kavale KA: Psychopharmacologic treatment: a note on classroom effects. Journal of Learning Disabilities 21:144–147, 1988

Forness S, Kavale K: Identification and diagnostic issues in special education: a status report for child psychiatrists. Child Psychiatry Hum Dev 19:279–301, 1989

Gerring JP, McCarthy LP: The Psychiatry of Handicapped Children and Adolescents: Managing Emotional and Behavioral Problems. Waltham, MA, College-Hill Press, 1988

Goldstein HS: Cognitive development in inattentive, hyperactive, and aggressive children: two- to five-year follow-up. J Am Acad Child Adolesc Psychiatry 26:214–221, 1987

Gresham FM: Social competence and motivational characteristics of learning disabled students, in The Handbook of Special Education: Research and Practice. Edited by Wang M, Reynolds M, Walberg H. Oxford, England, Pergamon, 1988, pp 283–302

Gresham FM, Elliott SN: Social skills assessment technology for LD students. Learning Disability Quarterly 12:141–152, 1989a

Gresham FM, Elliott SN: Social skills deficits as a primary learning disability. Journal of Learning Disabilities 22:120–124, 1989b

Gresham FM, Elliott SN: Social Skills Rating Scales. Circle Pines, MN, American Guidance Service, 1990

Gresham FM, Reschly DJ: Social skill deficits and low peer acceptance of mainstreamed learning disabled children. Learning Disability Quarterly 9:23–32, 1986

Gresham FM, Reschly DJ: Issues in the conceptualization, classification and assessment of social skills in the mildly handicapped, in Advances in School Psychology. Edited by Kratochwill T. Hillsdale, NJ, Lawrence Erlbaum Associates, 1988, pp 203–247

Gresham FM, Elliott SN, Black FL: Teacher-rated social skills of mainstreamed mildly handicapped and nonhandicapped children. School Psychology Review 16:78–88, 1987

Hazel JS, Schumaker JB: Social skills and learning disability. Paper presented at the National Conference on Learning Disabilities, Bethesda, MD, 1987

Hazel JS, Schumaker JB, Sherman JA, et al: Application of a group training program in social skills and problem solving skills to learning disabled and non-learning disabled youth. Learning Disability Quarterly 5:398–408, 1982

Henker B, Whalen CK: Hyperactivity and attention deficits. Am Psychol 44:216–223, 1989

Hiebert B, Wong B, Hunter M: Affective influences on learning disabled adolescents. Learning Disability Quarterly 5:334–343, 1982

Hollinger JD: Social skills for behaviorally disordered children as preparation for mainstreaming: theory, practice and new directions. Remedial and Special Education 8:17–27, 1987

Holoborow PL, Perry PS: Hyperactivity and learning difficulties. Journal of Learning Disabilities 29:426–430, 1986

Horowitz EC: Popularity, decentering ability, and role-taking skills in learning disabled and normal children. Learning Disability Quarterly 4:23–30, 1981

Hoyle GS, Serafica FC: Peer status of children with and without learning disabilities: a multimethod study. Learning Disability Quarterly 4:322–331, 1988

Interagency Committee on Learning Disabilities: Learning Disabilities: a Report to the US Congress. Washington, DC, US Department of Health and Human Services, 1987

Kistner JA, Gatlin D: Correlates of peer rejection among children with learning disabilities. Learning Disability Quarterly 12:133–140, 1989

Kovacs M: Affective disorders in children and adolescents. Am Psychol 2:209–215, 1989

Kronick D: An examination of the psychosocial aspects of learning disabled adolescents. Learning Disability Quarterly 1:86–93, 1978

La Greca A: Social behavior and social perception in learning disabled children: a review with implications for social skills training. J Pediatr Psychol 6:395–416, 1981

La Greca AM, Mesibov GB: Social skills intervention with learning disabled children: selecting skills and implementing training. Journal of Clinical Child Psychology 8:234–241, 1979

La Greca AM, Mesibov GB: Facilitating interpersonal functioning with peers in learning disabled children. Journal of Learning Disabilities 14:197–199, 1981

Lambert NM: Adolescent outcomes for hyperactive children: perspectives on general and specific patterns of childhood risk for adolescent educational, social, and mental health problems. Am Psychol 43:786–799, 1988

Larson KA, Gerber MM: Effects of social metacognitive training for enhancing overt behavior in learning disabled and low achieving delinquents. Except Child 54:201–211, 1987

Livingston R: Depressive illness and learning difficulties: research needs and practical implications. Journal of Learning Disabilities 18:518–522, 1985

Margalit M: Academic competence and social adjustment of boys with learning disabilities and boys with behavior disorders. Journal of Learning Disabilities 22:41–45, 1989

Mathur S, Rutherford R: Analysis of literature on social competence of behavioral disordered children and youth. Monographs in Behavioral Disorders 9:72–86, 1989

Matson JL, Ollendick TH: Enhancing Children's Social Skills. New York, Pergamon, 1988

McConaughy SH, Ritter DR: Social competence and behavioral problems of learning disabled boys aged 6–11. Journal of Learning Disabilities 19:39–45, 1986

McKinney JD: Longitudinal research on the behavioral characteristics of children with learning disabilities. Journal of Learning Disabilities 22:141–150, 1989

McKinney JD, Mason J, Perkerson K, et al.: Relationship between classroom behavior and achievement. Journal of Educational Psychology 67:198–203, 1975

McKinney JD, McClure S, Feagans L: Classroom behavior of learning disabled children. Learning Disability Quarterly 5:45–52, 1982

Mokros HB, Poznanski EO, Merrick WA: Depression and learning disabilities in children: a test of an hypothesis. Journal of Learning Disabilities 22:230–233, 1989

National Mental Health and Special Education Coalition: Statement to Senate Subcommittee on the Handicapped Regarding Reauthorization of Education of the Handicapped Act (Available from National Mental Health Association, 1021 Price Street, Alexandria, VA 22314–2917), 1989

Nelson CM: Social skills training for handicapped students. Teaching Exceptional Children 20:19–23, 1988

Newcomer PL: Comments on the Interagency Committee on Learning Disabilities definition of learning disabilities. Learning Disability Quarterly 12:140, 1989

Oliva AH, La Greca AM: Children with learning disabilities: social goals and strategies. Journal of Learning Disabilities 21:301–306, 1988

Osman BB: Promoting social acceptance of children with learning disabilities: an educational responsibility. Reading, Writing & Learning Disabilities 3:111–118, 1987

Osman GG: No One to Play With: The Social Side of Learning Disabilities. New York, Random House, 1982

Pearl RN, Cosden M: Sizing up a situation: LD children's understanding of social interaction. Learning Disability Quarterly 5:371–373, 1982

Prillman D: Acceptance of learning disabled students in the mainstream environment: a failure to replicate. Journal of Learning Disabilities 14:344–346, 1981

Prior M, Griffin M: Hyperactivity: Diagnosis and Management. London, England, Heinemann Medical Publishers, 1985

Pullis M: Temperament characteristics of LD students and their impact on decisions made by resource and mainstream teachers. Learning Disability Quarterly 8:104–123, 1985

Ray BM: Measuring the social position of the mainstreamed handicapped child. Except Child 52:57–62, 1985

Renshaw P, Asher S: Children's goals and strategies for social interaction. Merrill-Palmer Quarterly 29:353–374, 1983

Reschly DJ, Gresham FM: Adaptive behavior and the mildly handicapped, in Advances in School Psychology. Edited by Kratochwill T. Hillsdale, NJ, Lawrence Erlbaum Associates, 1988, pp 249–282

Rourke BJ, Young GC, Leenaars AA: A childhood learning disability that predisposes those afflicted to adolescent and adult depression and suicide risk. Journal of Learning Disabilities 22:169–175, 1989

Sabornie EJ, Kauffman JM: Social acceptance of learning disabled adolescents. Learning Disabilities Quarterly 9:55–60, 1986

Sabornie EJ, Kauffman JM, Ellis ES, et al: Bi-directional and cross-categorical social status of learning disabled, behaviorally disordered, and nonhandicapped adolescents. Journal of Special Education 21:39–56, 1987–88

Schloss PJ, Schloss CN, Wood CE, et al: A critical review of social skills research with behaviorally disordered students. Behavioral Disorders 12:11–15, 1986

Schumaker JG, Hazel JS, Sherman JA, et al: Social skill performances of learning disabled, non learning-disabled, and delinquent adolescents. Learning Disability Quarterly 5:409–414, 1982

Schworm RW, Birnbaum R: Symptom expression in hyperactive children: an analysis of observations. Journal of Learning Disabilities 22:35–40, 1989

Silver LB: A review of the federal government's interagency committee on learning disabilities report to the US Congress. Learning Disabilities Focus 3:73–80, 1988

Silverman RN, Zigmond N: Self-concept in learning disabled adolescents. Journal of Learning Disabilities 16:478–482, 1983

Stevenson DT, Romney DM: Depression in learning disabled children. Journal of Learning Disabilities 17:579–582, 1984

Strain PS, Odom SL: Peer social initiations: effective intervention for social skills development of exceptional children. Except Child 52:542–551, 1986

Vaughn SR, Ridley CA, Bullock DD: Interpersonal problem solving skills training with aggressive young children. Journal of Applied Developmental Psychology 5:213–223, 1984

Vaughn SR, Lancelotta GX, Minnis S: Social strategy training and peer involvement: Increasing peer acceptance of a female LD student. Learning Disabilities Focus 4:32–37, 1988

Walker HM, McConnell SR, Walker J, et al: ACCEPTS: A Curriculum for Effective Peer and Teacher Skills. Austin, TX, Pro-Ed, 1983

Walker HM, Shinn RE, O'Neill, et al: A longitudinal assessment of the development of antisocial behavior in boys: rationale, methodology, and first-year results. Remedial & Special Education 8:7–16, 1987

Wiener J: A theoretical model of the acquisition of peer relationships of learning disabled children. Journal of Learning Disabilities 13:42–47, 1980

Wiener J: Peer status of learning disabled children and adolescents: a review of the literature. Learning Disabilities Research 2:62–79, 1987

Wilchesky M, Reynolds T: The socially deficient LD child in context: a systems approach to assessment and treatment. Journal of Learning Disabilities 19:411–415, 1986

Chapter 7

Language and Speech Disorders

Rhea Paul, Ph.D., Lorian Baker, Ph.D., Donald J. Cohen, M.D., Paula Tallal, Ph.D., and Dorothy Aram, Ph.D.

Overview

In DSM-III-R (American Psychiatric Association 1987), one variety of speech disorder, developmental articulation disorder, was included under "Language and Speech Disorders," while another, stuttering, was included under "Speech Disorders Not Elsewhere Classified." For DSM-IV, it has been proposed that all disorders that pertain to speech be placed in one subsection. In addition, it has been proposed that all disorders of communication recognized by the American Speech-Language and Hearing Association as "Speech Disorders" (i.e., phonological disorder, voice disorder, and stuttering) be included in this subsection.

It has also been proposed that the name of the language disorders be changed from *specific developmental language disorders* to *specific language disorders of childhood* in DSM-IV. This change is proposed because some of the disorders discussed in the current draft are not developmental in nature but are acquired during childhood. This change in terminology would allow a broader range of disorders affecting language acquisition to be discussed and would provide a basis for differential diagnoses, when appropriate, among disorders of unknown origin and those with acute traumatic onset.

Statement and Significance of the Issues

Ten major issues concerning speech and language disorders have been identified for DSM-IV.

First, *should both child and adult speech disorders be included?* Although the disorders covered here usually occur in childhood, many have effects that extend into the adult years. Voice disorder may have its onset in adulthood.

Second, *should cluttering, considered a "Speech Disorder Not Elsewhere Classified" in DSM-III-R, be placed under speech disorders, or is it more properly considered a language deficit?* Current literature suggests that this disorder might have been misclassified in DSM-III-R.

Third, *should terminology for speech sound disorders be changed in DSM-IV to conform to the terminology currently in use in the field of speech-language pathology even if this terminology is less familiar to psychiatrists?* Terminology in use in the field of speech-language pathology reflects current theories about the bases of these disorders. Use in DSM-IV should perhaps conform to the most advanced thinking in relevant fields.

Fourth, *should voice disorder, which is not represented in DSM-III-R but has been identified by the American Speech-Language and Hearing Association as a speech disorder, be included in DSM-IV?* Voice disorders are common problems, and many have psychogenic components. It is therefore proposed that voice disorder be included in DSM-IV so that psychiatrists and other mental health professionals may have access to this diagnosis.

Fifth, *what is the earliest age at which language disorders can be identified?* Although DSM-III-R does not give guidelines for making these diagnoses before the preschool period, current research has provided data for identifying language disorders at an earlier age.

Sixth, *are there receptive language disorders in childhood that are analogous to Wernicke's aphasias in adults?* The terminology used in DSM-III-R reflects the notion that these disorders are analogous, but current neurological data dispute this claim.

Seventh, *are there any inclusionary criteria that can define language disorders, rather than the exclusionary criteria that were used in DSM-III-R?* Current research suggests that inclusionary criteria may assume more importance as new information accumulates. It is proposed that DSM-IV recognize this possibility.

Eighth, *should aphasias acquired in childhood be given separate diagnostic descriptions, or should they be incorporated within the broad category of language deficits seen in children?* This issue has been a matter of debate in the literature for years and should be addressed in DSM-IV.

Ninth, *should elective mutism be included as a childhood language disorder?* Elective mutism was included under "Other Disorders of Infancy, Childhood, or Adolescence" in DSM-III-R. Because this disorder affects communication, placing it with other communication disorders should be considered.

Tenth, *how can the known comorbidity between expressive and mixed receptive/expressive language disorders and learning disabilities be represented in DSM-IV when the two disorders are treated as independent conditions in the DSM?* DSM-III-R reflects earlier conceptualizations of these two disorders, but the current literature suggests that the closer connections between these disorders ought to be addressed in DSM-IV.

Method

The literature review for these disorders involved an examination of the most recent standard textbooks and research papers concerning diagnosis, classification, etiology, and epidemiology, as well as consultation with recognized experts in each of four areas: articulation, stuttering, voice, and language (Aronson 1985; Bloodstein 1987; Boone 1980; Darley and Spriestersbach 1991; Emerick and Hatten 1979; Fey 1986; Hixon et al. 1980; Lahey 1988; Lass et al. 1982; Leske 1981; Meitus and Weinberg 1983; Nation and Aram 1984; Prater and Swift 1984; Travis 1971; Wilson 1987). Because classification schemes for stuttering and voice are not a matter of great debate and are fairly well established within the field of speech-language pathology, the most current, well-agreed-on definitions were sought from the leading researchers and practitioners in the field; it is proposed that these be adopted without major changes. Issues in speech sound development are somewhat more in flux and are treated in more detail in this review. In addition, we reviewed the issue of the placement of cluttering by examining studies that referred to this condition and noting whether it was included under the rubric of "speech" or "language" and also explored how this disorder is handled in standard diagnostic texts in speech-language pathology.

The literature review on language disorders in childhood focused on research published since 1983, because literature available prior to that time was adequately represented in DSM-III-R. The review focused on studies in which subjects with language disorders were well defined in terms of the presence of frank neurological signs, IQ, and linguistic and nonlinguistic behavior. Studies using newer methodologies such as genetic approaches, analyses of perceptual skills, and newer language assessment instruments (e.g., the Vineland Adaptive Behavior Scales [Sparrow et al. 1984] and the Language Development Survey [Rescorla 1989]) were highlighted.

Results

Should both child and adult speech disorders be included? A review of standard texts in speech-language pathology (Andrews et al. 1983; Boone 1980; Conture 1990; Freeman 1982; Murray 1982; Perkins 1980) indicated that, in the case of stuttering and voice disorders, separate diagnostic schemes for children and adults are not the norm. Although the prevalence of these disorders differs at different ages, as noted under "Prevalence" in the proposed descriptive text to accompany the diagnostic criteria, the symptom picture needed to confer the diagnosis in children and adults is essentially the same. Because, according to current literature, most stuttering and voice disorders do emerge during these developmental periods, the decision not to exclude adults from the possibility of receiving these diagnoses should not affect their placement in DSM-IV.

Should cluttering, considered a "Speech Disorder Not Elsewhere Classified" in DSM-III-R, be placed under speech disorders, or is it more properly considered a language deficit? The symptom constellation frequently described as "cluttering" is placed variously in "speech disorders" and "language disorders" categories by different authors. C. Weiss et al. (1987) considered it a variant of a developmental phonological disorder. Perkins (1980) and Daly (1986) discussed it as a variant of stuttering. Freeman (1982) and D. Weiss (1964) discussed cluttering as a "central language imbalance" and pointed out its nonspeech characteristics, including syntactic difficulties; poor integration of thought processes; and reading, writing, and language formulation disorders. The American Speech-Language and Hearing Association does not list cluttering as a major diagnostic category.

Should terminology for speech sound disorders be changed in DSM-IV to conform to the terminology currently in use in the field of speech-language pathology even if this terminology is less familiar to psychiatrists? Since the mid-1970s, terminology used to describe disorders in the acquisition of speech sound production has shifted away from "articulation disorders" toward "phonological disorders." The reasons for this shift stem primarily from a reorientation of the theoretical bases for these disorders. Prior to 1968, when Chomsky and Halle published their landmark work, *Sound Pattern of English,* speech sound disorders were seen as problems in output patterns at the motokinesthetic level. With Chomsky and Halle's discussion of phonological rules as a set of underlying mental representations that govern the conceptual organization of sounds and their combinations as well as the production of motor patterns for speech, the conception of speech sound development and disorders changed. These phenomena began to be viewed as reflections of more abstract levels of rule learning and phonological representations. Thus, speech sound development was seen not only as the maturation of the articulators and the stabilization of motor patterns, but rather as the development of auditory images of words and the acquisition of abstract rules governing the possible sequence and distribution of sounds for the particular language being learned. Similarly, speech sound disorders came to be viewed not merely as evidence of faulty motor patterns or immature musculature, but as manifestations of deficits in the underlying representation of sounds in syllables and words and the failure to generate rules for sound production and combination that conformed to those of the ambient language (see Edwards and Shriberg 1983; Ingram 1976; Shriberg and Kwiatkowski 1980.) To accommodate this shift in perspective, a shift in terminology was also required.

Should voice disorder, which is not represented in DSM-III-R but has been identified by the American Speech-Language and Hearing Association as a speech disorder, be included in DSM-IV? Voice disorder is one of the three categories of speech disorder identified by the American Speech-Language and Hearing Association. Although some forms of voice disorder have bases in laryngeal pathology, a substantial portion of voice problems are considered "functional" or psychogenic, having no observable relationship to abnormal vocal fold morphology (Aronson 1985; Boone and McFarlane 1988). In fact, some studies show that close to one-third of patients with voice disorders have normal larynges on examination (Blakeley 1991), suggesting nonorganic etiologies. Further, many types of voice disorders show improvement with behavioral intervention (Boone and McFarlane 1988; Prater and Swift 1984), which is often used as an adjunct to medical or surgical treatment even in organically based disorders, both to help restore normal vocal function more quickly and to prevent behaviors that may have contributed to the original pathology. In addition, in cases of functional voice disorders, standard texts advocate the use not only of behavioral therapy but also of psychological counseling and psychotherapeutic discussion with the client to uncover and ameliorate the root psychological causes of these disorders (Aronson 1985; Boone and McFarlane 1988). Clinical studies (Hartman et al. 1989) suggest that both organic and psychogenic components may be present in some patients. In these cases, again, a combination of surgical, behavioral, and psychotherapeutic management is needed. In fact, some researchers (Allen et al. 1991) argue that even voice disorders with known laryngeal pathology (e.g., vocal nodules) should be treated without surgery with a combination of behavioral and psychotherapeutic management and argue that this approach is more effective in preventing recurrence.

What is the earliest age at which language disorders can be identified? A variety of studies of children with slow language development (Paul 1991; Rescorla 1989; Thal 1989) indicate that children who show significant discrepancies from normal language acquisition can be reliably identified by 24 months and that children so identified have a very high risk of persistent language delay, at least through the preschool period. These children have been further shown to differ from peers who speak normally on a variety of linguistic and nonlinguistic dimensions (Paul 1991; Thal 1991).

Are there receptive language disorders in childhood that are analogous to Wernicke's aphasias in adults? DSM-III-R described two types of specific developmental language disorder: expressive and receptive. Although there are language disorders in which receptive skills are involved, or in which receptive deficits appear to be primary, a child cannot develop an isolated receptive language disorder without there also being an effect on productive skills. Studies of children with primary receptive deficits (Aram and Nation 1982; Eisenson 1966; Paul et al. 1983; Tallal 1988) consistently report that productive deficits, distinct from those that might be seen in an adult with a Wernicke's aphasia, are associated with the comprehension disorder. Further, brain imaging data on subjects with receptive language deficits in childhood show that the neurological substrate for these disorders does not correspond to that found in adults with Wernicke's aphasia (Paul 1993).

Are there any inclusionary criteria that can define language disorders, rather than the exclusionary criteria that were used in DSM-III-R? The issue of inclusionary criteria has been raised by research conducted by Tallal (1988) and her colleagues. DSM-III-R diagnostic criteria for language disorders are based on traditional exclusionary principles—that is, identifying specific language disorders by ruling out other deficits that might cause communication handicaps, such as hearing impairment and mental retardation. The work of Tallal and her colleagues has raised the possibility that there are specific patterns of deficit that are associated with language disorders in children; however, these deficits are primarily in perceptual and motor domains and not in the linguistic behaviors themselves.

Should aphasias acquired in childhood be given separate diagnostic descriptions, or should they be incorporated within the broad category of language deficits seen in children? This issue is a matter of some controversy. Traditionally (Benton 1964), descriptions of developmental language disorders have been written to exclude disorders with any basis in identifiable neurological abnormality or central nervous system trauma (acquired aphasia in childhood). However, early descriptions of language disorders in childhood (Freud 1897; Guttman 1942) did not preclude frank neurological symptoms, but rather emphasized them in their characterization of the syndrome. Myklebust (1971) defined language disorders in the following way:

> Childhood aphasia refers to one or more significant deficits in essential processes as they relate to facility in the use of auditory language. Children having this disability demonstrate a discrepancy between expected and actual achievement in one or more of the following functions: auditory perception, auditory memory, integration, comprehension, expression. The deficits referred to are not the result of sensory, motor, intellectual or emotional impairment, nor to the lack of opportunity to learn. *They are assumed to derive from dysfunctions in the brain, though the evidence for such dysfunctioning may be mainly behavioral, rather than neurological, in nature.* (emphasis added) (p. 1186)

Thus, in this definition, frank neurological disorders do not preclude the diagnosis.

The ICD-10 (World Health Organization 1990) system does exclude one specific type of acquired aphasia, the Landau-Kleffner syndrome (Landau and Kleffner 1957), which involves a disorder with onset generally between ages 3 and 7 years, following a period of normal development and accompanied by paroxysmal abnormalities on the electroencephalogram. Other types of acquired aphasia in childhood, such as those accompanying head trauma or encephalitis, are not mentioned in ICD-10, leaving their diagnostic classification in doubt.

Few studies have addressed differences in behavioral profiles or outcome between children with language disorders with and without frank neurological involvement. Because studies that have examined performance in children with known neurological involvement have specifically excluded children with disorders of unknown origin (Alajouanine and L'Hermitte 1965; Bishop 1982; Van Dongen and Loonen 1977), direct comparisons are difficult to obtain. Thus the current literature provides little guidance on this point.

Should elective mutism be included as a childhood language disorder? Elective mutism is listed under "Other Disorders of Infancy, Childhood, or Adolescence" in DSM-III-R. There is some debate in the literature (Kratochwill 1981) as to whether to consider elective mutism as an anxiety disorder, and some advisers to the Work Group also expressed a preference for doing so. Research (Brown and Lloyd 1975; Fundudis et al. 1979; Kolvin and Fundudis 1981; Wilkins 1985), however, emphasizes that elective mutism is frequently associated with mild forms of specific expressive or mixed language disorders.

How can the known comorbidity between expressive and mixed receptive/expressive language disorders and learning disabilities be represented in DSM-IV when the two disorders are treated as independent conditions in the DSM? Numerous studies (Aram and Nation 1975, 1980; Hall and Tomlin 1978; Silva 1980; Stark et al. 1984; Strominger and Bashir 1977; Tallal 1988) have consistently shown a co-occurrence of specific language disorders of childhood and learning disorders. Tallal argued that it is the child's age rather than his or her neurological profile that differentiates specific language disorders and learning disorders.

Discussion

Should both child and adult speech disorders be included? A decision to exclude fluency and voice disorders in adults would allow these conditions to be referred to as "developmental." But because the disorders can, in fact, emerge or resurface in adulthood, even though they typically have their onset in childhood, the term *developmental* is simply inaccurate. Excluding fluency and voice disorders would also involve the loss of access to information about them in the developmental period in which they most commonly occur.

Should cluttering, considered a "Speech Disorder Not Elsewhere Classified" in DSM-III-R, be placed under speech disorders, or is it more properly considered a language deficit? There is a dearth of research on this condition, limiting the definitiveness of diagnostic, epidemiological, and prognostic information that could be included in DSM-IV. The few studies that have examined cluttering as a clinical entity (Hanson et al. 1986; Tiger et al. 1980) tend to see it in the context of problems in language formulation and expression, rather than as purely a speech problem.

Should terminology for speech sound disorders be changed in DSM-IV to conform to the terminology currently in use in the field of speech-language pathology even if this terminology is less familiar to psychiatrists? While "articulation disorders" implies an emphasis on motor output patterns, "phonological disorders" reflects the assumptions that underlying levels of representation may be involved. Shriberg and Kwiatkowski (1988) presented clinical evidence that phonological disorder is a more valid way of conceptualizing speech sound deficits.

Should voice disorder, which is not represented in DSM-III-R but has been identified by the American Speech-Language and Hearing Association as a speech disorder, be included in DSM-IV? Voice disorder could be excluded from this section of DSM-IV because it does not always emerge in childhood and because it is not typically thought of as a "mental" disorder. However, voice disorder is common in children and thought by many clinicians to have important psychogenic components. Further, it is frequently treated with a combination of behavioral and medical interventions.

What is the earliest age at which language disorders can be identified? Because federal legislation mandates services for children under the age of 3 years who are identified as having significant developmental disorders, it makes sense to encourage clinicians to identify such children so that they may take advantage of whatever intervention programs are available. Similarly, because it is known that toddlers with slow language development differ on a variety of linguistic and nonlinguistic dimensions from their peers who speak normally (Paul 1991), for research purposes it makes sense to be able to identify children in the earliest stages of language delay to provide longer-term follow-up studies and to investigate issues of prognosis at various ages.

Are there receptive language disorders in childhood that are analogous to Wernicke's aphasias in adults? To call these deficits "receptive" could misleadingly imply that they would be present in conjunction with intact language production. It is important to highlight the inevitable involvement of productive language skills in children with primary receptive disorders.

Are there any inclusionary criteria that can define language disorders, rather than the exclusionary criteria that were used in DSM-III-R? Although the findings of Tallal's (1988) group are important both for understanding the syndromes of specific language disorders and for identifying children for research studies, the difficulty of replicating the assessment of perceptual and motor behaviors in clinical

Language and Speech Disorders

settings, as well as the lack of psychometric data available for deciding when performance falls outside the normal range, precludes adopting a completely inclusionary scheme in DSM-IV. However, these findings may eventually have a great impact on the diagnosis and treatment of these disorders.

Should aphasias acquired in childhood be given separate diagnostic descriptions, or should they be incorporated within the broad category of language deficits seen in children? DSM-IV could, as other sources do, simply exclude language disorders of known neurological origin or those accompanied by "hard" neurological signs. However, the symptom manifestations of these disorders in children are not definitively different from those in children with language disorders of unknown origin. Further, the interventions required for both developmental and acquired disorders are very similar. Although it is crucially important to distinguish these two types for research purposes, their clinical pictures are more convergent.

Should elective mutism be included as a childhood language disorder? The major manifestation of this disorder is a restriction in the use of expressive language to communicate. As such, it needs to be differentiated from expressive language disorder. Placing these two diagnostic discussions in close proximity may facilitate that differentiation.

How can the known comorbidity between expressive and mixed receptive/expressive language disorders and learning disabilities be represented in DSM-IV when the two disorders are treated as independent conditions in the DSM? Although the connection between these disorders is strongly established in the literature and ought to be more strongly emphasized in DSM-IV, as yet it seems premature to subsume them into one category, because there may be certain forms of each that are independent of the other. Nevertheless, reference should be made to their connection in DSM-IV.

Recommendations

Should both child and adult speech disorders be included? Speech disorders should be included under developmental disorders in DSM-IV, with the notation that they can also be seen in adults. Voice disorder should not be called "developmental" because it may also emerge in adulthood. Developmental phonological disorders always do emerge in childhood. Although the diagnosis of developmental phonological disorder may be given to, for example, an adult with mental retardation, it is generally restricted to children.

Should cluttering, considered a "Speech Disorder Not Elsewhere Classified" in DSM-III-R, be placed under speech disorders, or is it more properly considered a language deficit? It is proposed that cluttering be described in the "Associated

Features" section of the text for childhood language disorders and not listed as a separate diagnostic category. It can be explained that the constellation of symptoms described is sometimes labeled as "cluttering," without saying that it is necessary to distinguish this constellation of symptoms as a distinct diagnostic entity.

Should terminology for speech sound disorders be changed in DSM-IV to conform to the terminology currently in use in the field of speech-language pathology even if this terminology is less familiar to psychiatrists? Current terminology referring to speech sound disorders as "phonological" should be adopted.

Should voice disorder, which is not represented in DSM-III-R but has been identified by the American Speech-Language and Hearing Association as a speech disorder, be included in DSM-IV? The inclusion of voice disorder in DSM-IV seems warranted because of its position as one of the three speech disorders recognized by the American Speech-Language and Hearing Association and because of the strong evidence for its association with psychogenic factors. Voice disorder should be included in the childhood section, even though it can emerge in adulthood, because it is common in children and manifests similarly across the life span.

What is the earliest age at which language disorders can be identified? Although DSM-III-R criteria set the lower limit for identification of expressive and receptive language as generally around age 3 years, it is suggested that in DSM-IV it be stated that identification is possible at 24 months.

Are there receptive language disorders in childhood that are analogous to Wernicke's aphasias in adults? Mixed receptive/expressive language disorder is proposed as the new label in DSM-IV for disorders that primarily affect receptive language development. This recommendation was made to highlight the fact that both modalities are virtually always involved.

Are there any inclusionary criteria that can define language disorders, rather than the exclusionary criteria that were used in DSM-III-R? It is recommended that the findings of Tallal's (1988) group be included under the "Associated Features" section of the text for expressive and mixed receptive/expressive language disorder. This placement will encourage clinicians to begin to take note of these features so that further data can be accumulated that will inform future research and diagnostic schemes for these populations.

Should aphasias acquired in childhood be given separate diagnostic descriptions, or should they be incorporated within the broad category of language deficits seen in children? It is recommended that two subtypes of these disorders be noted in the text of both expressive and mixed receptive/expressive language disorders of childhood: *developmental,,* referring to disorders of unknown origin, and *acquired,* referring to those with acute onset associated with a known neurological condition. Differences between these two subtypes can be discussed in terms of onset, prevalence, familial pattern, and so on. It is proposed that language disorders associated with frank neurological signs not be precluded from being diagnosed as specific language disorders of childhood to include the broadest range of disorders under this rubric. In the "Associated Features" section of the text, frank neurological signs or history that may be associated with the disorder in a particular patient can be noted, so that these children could be singled out for research purposes. This would encourage both researchers and clinicians to use the terms *developmental* and *acquired* as descriptive adjuncts to the DSM-IV diagnoses. Thus a child could be labeled as having a mixed receptive/expressive language disorder–acquired Landau-Kleffner type, or mixed receptive/expressive language disorder–acquired with history of encephalitis. In this way, important distinctions can be retained for the purpose of further investigations of these disorders, while allowing any child whose disorder primarily affects linguistic functioning to be given a diagnosis of specific language disorder of childhood, regardless of the cause.

Should elective mutism be included as a childhood language disorder? Because it is important to distinguish elective mutism from expressive language disorder and because elective mutism is a problem primarily affecting the ability to use language, the inclusion of this form of communication handicap within the childhood language and speech disorders framework appears justified.

How can the known comorbidity between expressive and mixed receptive/expressive language disorders and learning disabilities be represented in DSM-IV when the two disorders are treated as independent conditions in the DSM? It is recommended that the comorbidity between language and learning disorders be emphasized in the "Associated Features" section of the text for both expressive and mixed receptive/expressive language disorders.

References

Alajouanine T, L'Hermitte F: Acquired aphasia in children. Brain 88:653–662, 1965

Allen M, Pettit J, Sherblom J: Management of vocal nodules: a regional survey of otolaryngologists and speech-language pathologists. J Speech Hear Res 34:229–235, 1991

American Psychiatric Association: Diagnostic and Statistical Manual of Mental Disorders, 3rd Edition, Revised. Washington, DC, American Psychiatric Association, 1987

Andrews G, Craig A, Feyer A, et al: Stuttering: a review of research findings and theories circa 1982. J Speech Hear Disord 48:226–246, 1983

Aram DM, Nation JE: Patterns of language behavior in children with developmental language disorders. J Speech Hear Res 18:229–241, 1975

Aram DM, Nation JE: Preschool language disorders and subsequent language and academic difficulties. J Commun Disord 13:159–170, 1980

Aram DM, Nation JE: Child Language Disorders. St. Louis, MO, CV Mosby, 1982

Aronson A: Clinical Voice Disorders. New York, Thieme, 1985

Benton AL: Developmental aphasia and brain damage. Cortex 1:40–52, 1964

Bishop DVM: Comprehension of spoken, written and signed sentences in childhood language disorders. J Child Psychol Psychiatry 23:1–20, 1982
Blakeley R: Voice assessment without instrumentation. Seminars in Speech & Language 12:142–153, 1991
Bloodstein O: A Handbook of Stuttering. Chicago, IL, National Easter Seal Society, 1987
Boone D: Voice disorders, in Introduction to Communication Disorders. Edited by Hixon T, Shriberg L, Saxman J. Englewood Cliffs, NJ, Prentice-Hall, 1980
Boone D, McFarlane S: The Voice and Voice Therapy, 4th Edition. Englewood Cliffs, NJ, Prentice-Hall, 1988
Brown BJ, Lloyd H: A controlled study of children not speaking at school. Journal of the Association of Workers With Maladjusted Children 3:49–63, 1975
Chomsky N, Halle M:. Sound Pattern of English. Cambridge, MA, MIT Press, 1968
Conture E: Stuttering. Englewood Cliffs, NJ, Prentice-Hall, 1990
Daly D: The clutterer, in The Atypical Stutter: Principles and Practices of Rehabilitation. Edited by St. Louis KO. Orlando, FL, Academic Press, 1986
Darley F, Spriestersbach D: Diagnostic Methods in Speech-Language Pathology, 2nd Edition. Prospect Heights, IL, Waveland Press, 1991
Edwards ML, Shriberg L: Phonology: Applications in Communication Disorders. San Diego, CA, College Hill, 1983
Eisenson J: Perceptual disturbances in children with central nervous system dysfunction and implications for language development. British Journal of Disorders of Communication 1:21–32, 1966
Emerick L, Hatten J: Diagnosis and Evaluation in Speech Pathology, 2nd Edition. Englewood Cliffs, NJ, Prentice-Hall, 1979
Fey M: Language Intervention with Young Children. San Diego, CA, College Hill, 1986
Freeman F: Stuttering, in Speech, Language and Hearing. Edited by Lass N, McReynolds L, Northern J, et al. Philadelphia, PA, WB Saunders, 1982
Freud S: On Aphasia. New York, International Universities Press, 1897
Fundudis T, Kolvin I, Garside R: Speech Retarded and Deaf Children: Their Psychological Development. New York, Academic Press, 1979
Guttman E: Aphasia in children. Brain 65:205–219, 1942
Hall PK, Tomlin JB: A follow-up study of children with articulation and language disorders. J Speech Hear Disord 43:227–241, 1978
Hanson D, Jackson A, Hagerman R: Speech disturbances (cluttering) in mildly impaired males with Martin Bell/Fragile X syndrome. Am J Med Genet 23:195–206, 1986
Hartman D, Daily W, Morin K: A case of superior laryngeal nerve paresis and psychogenic dysphonia. J Speech Hear Disord 54:526–529, 1989
Hixon T, Shriberg L, Saxman J: Introduction to Communication Disorders. Englewood Cliffs, NJ, Prentice-Hall, 1980
Ingram D: Phonological Disability in Children. London, England, Edward Arnold, 1976
Kolvin I, Fundudis T: Elective mute children: psychological development and background factors. J Child Psychol Psychiatry 22:219–232, 1981
Kratochwill TR: Selective Mutism. New York, Lawrence Erlbaum Associates, 1981
Lahey M: Language Disorders and Language Development. New York, Macmillan, 1988
Landau W, Kleffner F: Syndrome of acquired aphasia with convulsive disorder in children. Neurology 7:523–530, 1957
Lass N, McReynolds L, Northern J, et al: Speech, Language and Hearing. Philadelphia, PA, WB Saunders, 1982

Leske M: Prevalence estimates of communication disorders in the US: speech disorders. ASHA 23:217–225, 1981

Meitus I, Weinberg B: Diagnosis in Speech-Language Pathology. Baltimore, MD, University Park Press, 1983

Murray T: Phonation: assessment, in Speech, Language and Hearing. Edited by Lass N, McReynolds L, Northern J, et al. Philadelphia, PA, WB Saunders, 1982

Myklebust H: Childhood aphasia: an evolving concept, in Handbook of Speech Pathology and Audiology. Edited by Travis LE. Englewood Cliffs, NJ, Prentice-Hall, 1971

Nation J, Aram D: Diagnosis of Speech and Language Disorders. San Diego, CA, College Hill, 1984

Paul R: Profiles of toddlers with slow expressive language development. Topics in Language Disorders 11:1–13, 1991

Paul R: Specific developmental language disorders, in Psychiatry, 2nd Edition, Vol 2. Edited by Michels R, Cavenar JO. Philadelphia, PA, JB Lippincott, 1993

Paul R, Cohen DJ, Caparulo B: A longitudinal study of patients with severe developmental disorders of language learning. Journal of the American Academy of Child Psychiatry 22:525–534, 1983

Perkins W: Disorder of speech flow, in Introduction to Communication Disorders. Edited by Hixon T, Shriberg L, Saxman J. Englewood Cliffs, NJ, Prentice-Hall, 1980

Prater R, Swift R: Manual of Voice Therapy. Boston, MA, Little, Brown, 1984

Rescorla L: The Language Development Survey: a screening tool for delayed language in toddlers. J Speech Hear Res 54:587–599, 1989

Shriberg L, Kwiatkowski J: Natural Process Analysis of Continuous Speech Samples. New York, John Wiley, 1980

Shriberg L, Kwiatkowski J: A follow-up study of children with phonologic disorders of unknown origin. J Speech Hear Disord 53:144–155, 1988

Silva P: The prevalence, stability and significance of developmental language delay in preschool children. Dev Med Child Neurol 22:768–777, 1980

Sparrow S, Balla D, Ciccetti D: Vineland Adaptive Behavior Scales. Circle Pines, MN, American Guidance Systems, 1984

Stark R, Bernstein L, Condino R, et al: Four year follow-up study of language impaired children. Annals of Dyslexia 34:49–68, 1984

Strominger A, Bashir A: A nine-year follow-up of 50 language delayed children. Paper presented at the annual meeting of the American Speech and Hearing Association, Chicago, IL, 1977

Thal D: Language and gesture in late talkers. Paper presented at the Society for Research in Child Development Biennial Meeting, Kansas City, MO, 1989

Thal D: Language and cognition in normal and late-talking toddlers. Topics in Language Disorders 11:33–42, 1991

Tallal P: Developmental language disorders, in Learning Disabilities: Proceedings of the National Conference. Edited by Kavanaugh J, Truss T. Parkton, MD, York Press, 1988

Tiger R, Irvine T, Reis R: Cluttering as a complex of learning disabilities. Language, Speech & Hearing Services in Schools 11:3–14, 1980

Travis L: Handbook of Speech Pathology and Audiology. Englewood Cliffs, NJ, Prentice-Hall, 1971

Van Dongen HR, Loonen MCB: Factors related to prognosis of acquired aphasia in children. Cortex 13:131–136, 1977

Weiss C, Gordon M, Lillywhite H: Articulatory and Phonologic Disorders. Baltimore, MD, Williams & Wilkins, 1987

Weiss D: Cluttering. Englewood Cliffs, NJ, Prentice-Hall, 1964

Wilkins R: A comparison of elective mutism and emotional disorders in children. Br J Psychiatry 146:198–203, 1985

Wilson D: Voice Problems of Children. Baltimore, MD, Williams & Wilkins, 1987

World Health Organization: ICD-10 Chapter V: Mental and Behavioral Disorders: Diagnostic Criteria for Research. Geneva, Switzerland, World Health Organization, 1990

Section II

Disorders Usually First Diagnosed in Infancy, Childhood, or Adolescence (Part II)

Introduction to Section II

Disorders Usually First Diagnosed in Infancy, Childhood, or Adolescence (Part II)

David Shaffer, M.D., Thomas A. Widiger, Ph.D., and
Harold A. Pincus, M.D.

This section of the *DSM-IV Sourcebook* covers the issues and diagnoses relevant to children and adolescents that were not covered in the previous section. We begin with an overview of proposed changes to the organization of the childhood and adolescent section of DSM, followed by a discussion of individual diagnoses and proposals.

Organization of Childhood and Adolescent Section

DSM-III (American Psychiatric Association 1980) and DSM-III-R (American Psychiatric Association 1987) include a section devoted to disorders that are usually first evident in infancy, childhood, or adolescence. DSM-II (American Psychiatric Association 1968) had included such a section, but it contained only seven diagnoses. One of the innovations of DSM-III was to give much more prominence to the disorders of childhood. The section was moved to the front of the manual in DSM-III and was expanded to include 44 disorders (46 disorders in DSM-III-R).

It is likely that this section will be retitled "Disorders Usually First Diagnosed in Infancy, Childhood, or Adolescence" in DSM-IV to more accurately reflect the organizing principle for this section (American Psychiatric Association 1991). It is important to note that this organization is not absolute. The disorders in this section are usually first evident in childhood or adolescence, but some individuals with these disorders may not in fact receive treatment until adulthood. In addition, the age at onset for many of the disorders included elsewhere in the manual can be during childhood or adolescence. The disorders included in the rest of the manual are therefore not exclusively "adult disorders." For example, mood, anxiety, sexual, and sleep disorders do occur during childhood or adolescence.

There are advantages and disadvantages to this organization of the child and adolescent disorders. The main advantage is that it facilitates the use of the manual by persons who specialize in the diagnosis and treatment of children and adolescents. A disadvantage is that it may discourage these clinicians from considering diagnoses that are included elsewhere in the manual and also discourage those who specialize in the diagnosis and treatment of adults from considering the diagnoses in the child and adolescent section of the manual. For example, the placement of major depressive disorder in the Mood Disorders section might contribute to its being overlooked in children (as if it were an "adult disorder,") and the placement of attention-deficit/hyperactivity disorder (ADHD) in the child/adolescent section of the manual might contribute to its being overlooked in adults (as if it were a "childhood disorder"). The diagnosis of mood disorders in children and adolescents is the focus of the review by Angold (Chapter 16), and the diagnosis of ADHD in adults is discussed in the review by Lahey et al. (Chapter 10).

Defining this section of the manual in terms of age at diagnosis could contribute to artificial distinctions, particularly in the case of the anxiety disorders. DSM-III-R provided no childhood mood disorders, but several childhood/adolescent anxiety disorders. The Task Force was concerned that anxiety disorders diagnosed in childhood should not be regarded as different from comparable disorders in adults (i.e., the diagnosis should not change arbitrarily when the person reaches the age of 18).

Several proposals have been offered to address this issue (American Psychiatric Association 1991). One option would be for the childhood anxiety disorders to be preempted by the "adult" anxiety disorders so that a childhood anxiety disorder diagnosis could be given only if the criteria were not met for any of the adult anxiety disorders. A second option would be to retain the section for Anxiety Disorders of Childhood or Adolescence, but to emphasize that the adult anxiety disorders should also be considered for children and adolescents. A third option would be to eliminate the Anxiety Disorders of Childhood or Adolescence section entirely, incorporating all the diagnoses into the adult Anxiety Disorder section. A related option is to incorporate a subset of the diagnoses into the adult anxiety disorders, with the most likely possibilities being avoidant disorder (which may represent a childhood/adolescent variant of social phobia) and overanxious disorder (which may represent a childhood/adolescent variant of generalized anxiety disorder). These options are discussed in the review by Klein et al. (Chapter 13).

Similarly, a proposal is also being considered for moving gender identity disorder out of the childhood section. The advantages of retaining it within the childhood/adolescent section are historical continuity and to emphasize its onset in children and adolescents. However, as indicated in the review by Bradley et al. (Chapter 20), it is perhaps misleading to suggest that there are distinct, different disorders of gender identity that occur in children and adults. It may be more accurate to indicate that it is a single disorder that varies in its expression through childhood, adolescence, and adulthood. It may be first diagnosed in a child or an adolescent, but is not confined or unique to childhood or adolescence, and in the Task Force's experience is most likely to be brought to clinical attention in early adulthood. Moving gender identity disorder to another section of the manual would also be more consistent with ICD-10 (World Health Organization 1990).

Likewise, some of the eating disorders included within the DSM-III-R section for Disorders Usually First Evident in Infancy, Childhood, or Adolescence are not usually first evident in infancy, childhood, or early adolescence, but rather in later adolescence and early adulthood (see the next section of this *Sourcebook*). Bulimia nervosa and anorexia nervosa have historically been the responsibility of the Eating Disorders Work Group, in part because these disorders are usually diagnosed, treated, and researched by persons who are not specialists in disorders of childhood and adolescence, but rather specialists in eating disorders.

Attention-Deficit Disorders

DSM-II introduced the diagnostic category "hyperkinetic reaction of childhood or adolescence." Reflecting research at the time that suggested that attention problems were central to the disorder, it was renamed attention-deficit disorder with hyperactivity in DSM-III (see McBurnett, Chapter 8). DSM-III attention-deficit disorder with hyperactivity required the presence of symptoms from three domains: inattention, impulsivity, and hyperactivity. In DSM-III-R, the name was changed to attention-deficit hyperactivity disorder, and criteria from these three domains were ordered into a single list of 14 symptoms, from which any 8 were required.

The validity and utility of the single list of symptoms is reviewed by McBurnett (Chapter 8). There does appear to be substantial empirical support for the presence of two separate factors or clusters of symptoms (e.g., inattention-disorganization and impulsivity-hyperactivity). The single DSM-III-R criteria set resulted in substantial heterogeneity and a concern among clinicians that the diagnosis could be made without the presence of one of the core components of the disorder. The DSM-III-R diagnosis of undifferentiated attention-deficit disorder does recognize the presence of ADHD without hyperactivity, but it is quite possible for some persons diagnosed with undifferentiated attention-deficit disorder to have more symptoms of hyperactivity than persons diagnosed with ADHD.

The review by Lahey et al. (Chapter 10) considers the validity of the distinction between DSM-III-R ADHD and DSM-III-R undifferentiated attention-deficit disorder. DSM-III included a diagnosis of attention-deficit disorder without hyperactivity in recognition of the finding that some persons with attentional difficulties lacked concomitant hyperactivity. DSM-III-R, however, required that this diagnosis be coded within undifferentiated attention-deficit disorder, a much broader, residual, and inherently heterogeneous diagnosis that lacked specific diagnostic criteria. Lahey et al. recommend that the distinction between attention-deficit disorder with hyperactivity and attention-deficit disorder without hyperactivity be recognized and propose a variety of ways in which this could be done. Two major options are to provide 1) two distinct diagnoses (i.e., attention-deficit disorder with hyperactivity and attention-deficit disorder without hyperactivity) that overlap in their diagnostic criteria, or 2) one diagnosis that is subtyped according to the predominance of the symptomatology. Although it is clear that there are children with predominant symptoms of inattention (American Psychiatric Association 1991; Lahey et al., Chapter 10), it is not clear whether this reflects the presence of a qualitatively distinct disorder from attention-deficit disorder with hyperactivity or a form of attention-deficit disorder with hyperactivity in which the symptoms of hyperactivity are not prominent. Different options for resolving this question will be considered in analyses of existing data sets and in a forthcoming field trial.

An additional issue for ADHD is its application to adults (McBurnett, Chapter 8). The DSM-III-R criteria for ADHD were better operationalized than DSM-III attention-deficit disorder with hyperactivity and made several references to specifically childhood activities (e.g., play). This improved the reliability of the diagnosis but complicated the application of the diagnosis across different ages. Furthermore, DSM-III-R provided for a single threshold requirement regardless of age. Clinicians working with adults with ADHD felt that adults had fewer symptoms than they had had during childhood, but were nevertheless impaired. It has been proposed that DSM-IV revise DSM-III-R items to be more applicable across different ages and/or alter the diagnostic threshold for different ages. The effect of age could also be appropriately addressed in the text discussion of the disorder in the proposed new organization of the text that will provide age-related features for each disorder.

One of the more controversial issues regarding DSM-III-R ADHD was its potential for overdiagnosis and labeling unimpaired children. This concern could be addressed by raising the threshold, but that could lead to a failure to diagnose children with ADHD who might benefit from clinical treatment. A proposal for DSM-IV is to require that each symptom occur "often" and that together they result in a significant impairment in social or academic (occupational) functioning or cause marked distress (American Psychiatric Association 1991).

Another approach to avoiding overdiagnosis is to require that the symptoms be evident in multiple settings (McBurnett, Chapter 8). To the extent that ADHD is in fact a disorder in the child, it should be evident across a variety of settings. However, as noted by McBurnett, individual diagnostic symptoms of ADHD may not be consistent across different settings, and it would not be reasonable to require each symptom to be present in more than one setting. An alternative would be to require that at least some criteria be met in different settings. ICD-10 allows cross-situationality to occur between a school setting and also a less structured home or even office setting.

A final issue for ADHD is its relationship to other disorders, particularly those within the Disruptive Behavior Disorders section of DSM-III-R: conduct disorder and oppositional defiant disorder (see Biederman et al., Chapter 9; McBurnett, Chapter 8). DSM-III had separate sections for attention-deficit disorder and conduct disorder and placed oppositional defiant disorder within the category for Other Disorders of Infancy, Childhood, or Adolescence. DSM-III-R grouped all three within the Disruptive Behavior Disorders section. This grouping was useful for differential diagnosis, because these three diagnoses may often be comorbid. However, the grouping was also problematic because it implied that disruption is a fundamental feature, symptom, or pathology of ADHD. One likely change for DSM-IV is to rename this section Disruptive Behavior and Attention-Deficit Disorders.

It has been proposed that DSM-IV acknowledge the frequent co-occurrence of ADHD and conduct disorder by providing a compound diagnosis with the symptoms of hyperactivity, inattention, and antisocial conduct. This proposal is reviewed by Biederman et al. (Chapter 9). A difficulty with this proposal is that ADHD can also co-occur with other disorders of childhood, and it may not be meaningful or accurate to develop hybrid diagnoses whenever such co-occurrences are observed. In addition, there appear to be different risk factors, course, and treatment implications for ADHD and conduct disorder. Although the presence of the symptoms of both disorders should certainly be recognized when this occurs, this may be better achieved by encouraging the diagnosis of both disorders.

Oppositional Defiant and Conduct Disorders

The DSM-III diagnosis of oppositional disorder was characterized by disobedient, negativistic, and provocative opposition to authority figures and was considered to be a childhood variant of the adult passive-aggressive personality disorder. The diagnosis was specifically excluded if there were violations of major age-appropriate societal norms. DSM-III-R modified the name to oppositional defiant disorder, changed the individual diagnostic criteria, raised the threshold for diagnosis, and characterized the disorder as involving an enduring pattern of oppositional, irritable, and defiant behavior. These revisions resulted in similarities between oppositional defiant disorder and conduct disorder, and the differentiation of the two disorders is an issue for DSM-IV.

One proposal for DSM-IV is to include lying, bullying, and physical fighting, which empirical work has shown are often seen in persons with oppositional defiant disorder (see Lahey et al., Chapter 11), as new criteria for the diagnosis. However, these items are currently within the diagnostic criteria for conduct disorder. Including them within the diagnostic criteria for oppositional defiant disorder may only further blur the boundary between oppositional defiant disorder and conduct disorder.

It has also been proposed that the distinction between oppositional defiant disorder and conduct disorder be abandoned altogether and that the two disorders be replaced with one diagnosis of "disruptive behavior disorder" that would be distinguished along three levels of severity and development (American Psychiatric Association 1991; Lahey et al., Chapter 11). There are data that suggest that many children with oppositional defiant disorder eventually meet the criteria for conduct disorder, and risk factors for the two disorders overlap. Oppositional defiant disorder may represent a less severe variant of the same disorder as conduct disorder. The three levels of disruptive behavior disorder might be mild (or oppositional defiant), moderate conduct, and severe conduct disorder (an additional option would be to have only two levels). There is little research indicating that oppositional defiant disorder is a childhood variant of passive-aggressive personality disorder.

However, there are a number of difficulties with this proposal. The revision would represent a substantial and perhaps fundamental change in the conceptualization of these disorders. Many children with oppositional defiant disorder do not eventually meet the criteria for conduct disorder, and subsuming oppositional defiant disorder under conduct disorder may be unnecessarily stigmatizing and misleading (e.g., suggesting that children with oppositional defiant disorder are at risk for developing adult antisocial personality disorder). In addition, drawing boundaries between the three levels in the absence of good epidemiological and natural history data would be arbitrary. The DSM-III-R criteria were already regarded as unnecessarily lengthy, complex, and cumbersome for clinical practice (American Psychiatric Association 1991), and the three levels proposed for DSM-IV could increase the complexity of the diagnosis even further.

If oppositional defiant disorder is retained as a separate diagnosis, then attention will also be given to differentiating it from normal oppositional behavior, which can be difficult during the preschool years and in adolescence. It has therefore been suggested that the criteria for oppositional defiant disorder include a requirement that the behavior results in significant impairment in social or academic (occupational) functioning.

DSM-III included two subtypes of conduct disorder: socialized versus unsocialized and aggressive versus nonaggressive. The differentiation between socialized and unsocialized behavior was clinically difficult and had questionable empirical support. However, there are now data to suggest that the earlier the age at onset, the more likely the disorder will be enduring (Lahey et al., Chapter 11), and it has been proposed that conduct disorder be subtyped according to age at onset. ICD-10 will include subtypes for socialized, unsocialized, and confined to family context.

An additional issue is whether the DSM-III-R conduct disorder criteria are appropriate for girls. There has been relatively little research on girls with conduct disorder, and existing diagnostic criteria draw largely from descriptions of males. For example, it may be the case that boys but not girls with conduct disorder force persons to engage in a sexual activity. Features of conduct disorder that have been noted in girls and that may be included are precocious alcohol and drug use (prior to age 13) and engaging in sexual activities to obtain money, goods, or drugs. Additional analyses of existing data sets and a field trial will evaluate these and other items that might be particularly helpful in identifying the presence of conduct disorder in girls (Lahey et al., Chapter 11).

Feeding and Eating Disorders

As indicated, it has been proposed to move bulimia nervosa and anorexia nervosa out of the Childhood and Adolescent Disorders section for DSM-IV. If this occurs, this subsection might be retitled "Feeding Disorders of Infancy or Early Childhood," and would include pica and rumination disorder of infancy, both of which were included in DSM-III-R, and possibly feeding disorder of infancy or early childhood, a new diagnosis proposed for DSM-IV.

The ICD-10 criteria for pica will be more restrictive than the DSM-III-R criteria. ICD-10 requires the eating of nonnutritive substances at least twice a week for at least 1 month, specifies that no other disorder except for "mental handicap" be present, and requires that the child be at least 2 years old with a mental age of at least 18 months (see Volkmar and Mayes, Chapter 12). DSM-III-R excluded autistic disorder and schizophrenia but, as Volkmar and Mayes suggest, this exclusion criterion was problematic because pica is sometimes observed in association with autism as a distinct clinical condition that warrants specific intervention. A proposal for DSM-IV is to require that the eating of nonnutritive substances be developmentally inappropriate.

Proposals for rumination disorder of infancy are 1) to change the name to rumination disorder because the symptom is also observed in older persons, particularly those with mental retardation; and 2) to delete the exclusion for nausea, which is difficult to establish in infancy (Volkmar and Mayes, Chapter 12). Volkmar and Mayes also note that the disorder may be more common in infants who lack the usual physiological barrier to reflux, and an additional proposal for DSM-IV is to exclude cases that are due to a medical condition, such as Sandifer's syndrome or esophageal reflux.

The proposed new diagnosis of feeding disorder of infancy or early childhood is often recognized in the clinical literature, where it is also described as "nonorganic failure to thrive" (Volkmar and Mayes, Chapter 12). This disorder has been described as a persistent failure to eat adequately with a failure to gain weight or a loss of weight. "Nonorganic failure to thrive" is also recognized by ICD-10, which makes no distinction between DSM-III-R rumination disorder and failure to thrive. If failure to thrive is included in DSM-IV as a diagnosis separate from rumination disorder, then it is likely that the requirement of a weight loss or failure to make expected weight gain for rumination disorder will be deleted.

Anxiety Disorders

As noted, the features of avoidant disorder are very similar to those of social phobia. It is not yet clear whether children and adolescents with avoidant disorder eventually develop avoidant personality disorder, and a closer examination of the two categories seems necessary. If these are similar conditions, it is misleading to provide two distinct diagnostic categories; if they are distinct, the diagnostic criteria for avoidant disorder should be revised to sharpen the distinction (American Psychiatric Association 1991). Children with excessive performance anxiety but no generalized social anxiety might receive the diagnosis of social phobia, whereas those with a more generalized social anxiety would be diagnosed with avoidant disorder (see Klein et al., Chapter 13). Another option would be to replace the diagnosis of avoidant disorder with social phobia and specify any age-specific features of social phobia in the diagnostic criteria or the text. This format would be consistent with the Mood Disorders and Schizophrenia sections of DSM and with ICD-10.

Similar issues apply to overanxious disorder, which shares many similarities with generalized anxiety disorder and may simply represent a childhood variant of this anxiety disorder. Because of the poorly operationalized criteria, its reliability has been inconsistent. Its co-occurrence with other disorders of childhood is substantial (Klein et al., Chapter 13). Proposals for DSM-IV are to revise the criteria for overanxious disorder to develop a more specific diagnosis that is distinct from generalized anxiety disorder or to indicate in DSM-IV that it is a childhood variant of generalized anxiety disorder. Klein et al. recommend that the diagnosis be retained but this has not yet been decided by the Work Group.

Klein et al. (Chapter 13) recommend only minor revisions to the diagnostic criteria for separation anxiety disorder. Adjustments for different developmental periods and gender were considered, but do not currently appear appropriate or necessary. However, it is recommended that some clarification of the symptomatology, such as including persistent concerns about the death of attachment figures, be provided. Klein et al. also recommend that the DSM-IV Task Force consider adopting the 4-week duration required in ICD-10 rather than the 2-week duration required in DSM-III-R.

Elective Mutism

In DSM-III-R, elective mutism was placed in a miscellaneous category in the Disorders Usually First Evident in Infancy, Childhood, or Adolescence section. A number of options are being considered for DSM-IV, as noted in the review by Tancer and Klein (Chapter 14). One option is to include elective mutism in the Speech and Language Disorders subsection because it clearly does involve an impairment in communication and is discussed in the differential diagnosis of disorders within this section. An additional option is to move it to the subsection for Anxiety Disorders of Childhood or Adolescence because substantial anxiety is often present in children with elective mutism. However, as noted by Tancer and Klein, this may be premature or presumptive. A third option is keep the diagnosis within the miscellaneous section.

Tancer and Klein also suggest excluding those cases in which the mutism is due to a lack of fluency in the language (e.g., recent immigrant children who are mute until they become familiar with the English language) and among children with a different speech and language disorder who are embarrassed to speak in public. An additional suggestion is to increase the minimum duration (Tancer and Klein, Chapter 14), because there are data suggesting that, in some instances, symptoms are quite transient. DSM-III-R provided no minimum duration, ICD-10 requires 6 months, Tancer and Klein suggest 3 months, and the Work Group proposed 1 month.

A final recommendation is to change the name of the disorder from elective to selective mutism because there is no evidence to support the suggestion that children with this disorder are expressing a deliberate preference not to speak. A diagnosis of "selective" mutism may be less presumptive and stigmatizing.

Reactive Attachment Disorder

The major issue for reactive attachment disorder is whether to continue to require the presence of pathological care. Pathological care was required in both DSM-III and DSM-III-R, but it is not included in the corresponding diagnosis within ICD-10, which allows the diagnosis to be made on the basis of the behavioral symptomatology. As indicated in the review by Volkmar (Chapter 15), the deletion of this requirement could be helpful when it is difficult or impossible to document the presence of early damaging experiences. Requiring early pathological care presumes an etiology for the disorder that is inconsistent with the behaviorally descriptive approach followed almost universally in DSM. On the other hand, the symptoms of the disorder overlap considerably with those of other diagnoses, and there is the risk that such a significant revision could lead to unwarranted etiological inferences for other quite common childhood behaviors.

Two subtypes, inhibited and disinhibited, are included in ICD-10. These are being considered for DSM-IV; they could provide useful distinctions for treatment and understanding and would not substantially alter the diagnostic criteria. Changes in wording are also proposed to improve the clarity and specificity of the diagnostic criteria.

Mood Disorders

DSM-III provided modified diagnostic criteria for a depressive episode in persons younger than age 6 years, including inferring the presence of depressive mood on the basis of persistently sad facial expressions, reducing the number of necessary criteria, allowing a failure to gain expected weight instead of requiring a loss in weight, allowing hypoactivity in place of psychomotor retardation, and allowing signs of apathy instead of loss of interest or pleasure in usual activities. However, as noted in the review by Angold (Chapter 16), there was no substantial empirical support for these changes.

DSM-III-R eliminated the age of 6 cutoff point (and the modifications associated with it), but also noted that irritability could be a primary mood in a depressive episode in children. This revision was supported by the experience of some clinicians, but again lacked systematic empirical support (Angold, Chapter 16). On the basis of his review of the literature, Angold suggests that it is not clear if the adult criteria for depression are optimal for diagnosing mood disorders in children, but that no other set of criteria appear to have sufficient empirical support at this time to warrant their formal recognition in DSM-IV.

Suicidality in Children and Adolescents

A new diagnosis of suicidality of childhood and adolescence is being considered for inclusion in DSM-IV (King et al., Chapter 17). The presence of suicidal ideation or behavior is a common reason for clinical assessment and intervention, and the inclusion of a discrete diagnosis of suicidality would highlight its importance and facilitate research.

The major concern regarding the proposal is that suicidality commonly occurs with other mental disorders, and the inclusion of a single-symptom diagnosis could lead to underreporting of those disorders.

One option being considered for DSM-IV is to provide additional nonmental disorder codes to recognize specifically the presence of suicidal ideation and behavior (American Psychiatric Association 1991). However, these codes could be used only if the suicidal behavior were not better accounted for by a mental disorder, which is the case with the clinical examples provided by King et al. (Chapter 17). An option that would not result in underreporting associated Axis I diagnoses would be to include a specific subtype of adjustment disorder with suicidal behavior (American Psychiatric Association 1991). This would highlight the central presence and importance of suicidal ideation and behavior in cases that do not meet criteria for another Axis I diagnosis.

Adjustment Disorder

As noted in the review by Newcorn and Strain (Chapter 18), adjustment disorder is one of the most frequently used diagnoses in children and adolescents. It is likely that the diagnosis is sometimes used to avoid the stigma of another Axis I diagnosis and sometimes to reflect the widespread clinical view that most childhood disorders are reactive to environmental stress. Newcorn and Strain consider the possibilities of providing more specific diagnostic criteria for children, but conclude that there are currently insufficient data to justify a distinct childhood variant. Their proposals for revising this diagnosis include extending the duration criterion to longer than 6 months if the duration of the stressor also persists; providing more specific examples of the nature of the stressors; and, within the "not otherwise specified" category, clarifying the distinctions between atypical or subthreshold conditions and adjustment disorder.

Trichotillomania

Trichotillomania is currently included in the DSM-III-R section for Impulse Control Disorders. The disorder is commonly used for children and is often first evident in childhood or adolescence. On the other hand, as indicated in the review by Winchel (Chapter 19), the disorder is often first diagnosed in adulthood, and it does appear to represent a disorder of impulse control.

One option that has been proposed is to include trichotillomania within the Anxiety Disorders section, as it often co-occurs with obsessive-compulsive disorder. However, this seems premature, because, as noted by Winchel (Chapter 19), it also occurs independently of this anxiety disorder, it occurs in the presence of other mental disorders, and it shares many features with disorders outside the Anxiety Disorders section. To differentiate it from other mental disorders, it has been proposed that a criterion be added to exclude hair-pulling, which is better accounted for by another mental disorder (American Psychiatric Association 1991). Winchel also recommends considering the addition of subtyping based on age at onset, but notes that the data may as yet be insufficient to warrant this distinction.

Gender Identity Disorder

DSM-III-R distinguishes between gender identity disorder of childhood; gender identity disorder of adolescence or adulthood, nontranssexual type (GIDAANT); and transsexualism. The review by Bradley et al. (Chapter 20) suggests that the distinctions may have been arbitrary, artificial, and cumbersome. The disorder does appear to have a different presentation in childhood than adulthood, but it appears to be the same disorder. When the disorder is first diagnosed in adults, it has usually been present since childhood. It may be more meaningful and useful to recognize the presence of one disorder, but provide different criteria for children and adults. The DSM-III-R transsexualism and GIDAANT categories are also quite similar, with the only distinction perhaps being the presence of a desire for surgical sex reassignment. Proposed criteria for this single gender identity disorder diagnosis are presented in Chapter 20 and the *DSM-IV Options Book* (American Psychiatric Association 1991). Further refinement is likely to occur with the pilot testing of these proposed criteria.

Bradley et al. also recommend a subtyping scheme based on sexual preference (i.e., sexually attracted to males, females, both, or neither). The sexual preference of the person with gender identity disorder clearly has important clinical and treatment implications.

The DSM-III-R criteria for gender identity disorder of childhood provided different criteria for boys and girls that Bradley et al. point out may have lacked adequate empirical support. Substantial revisions to the criteria have been proposed to address concerns regarding differentiating girls with gender identity disorder from healthy "tomboys" and to remedy inconsistencies across the criteria for boys and girls. A further proposal is to add a requirement for clinically significant impairment or distress to emphasize the presence of a mental disorder rather than simply a deviant or aberrant sexual behavior pattern. However, this criterion may be difficult to assess in young children.

Sibling Rivalry

ICD-10 will include a diagnosis of sibling rivalry disorder that is not currently recognized in DSM-III-R. A sibling rivalry disorder would involve a persistent and marked change in the behavior of a child that occurs in response to the birth of a sibling. There would be abnormally negative feelings of jealousy, tantrums, dysphoria, sleep disturbance, oppositionalism, or attention seeking that persist at least 4 weeks.

The major concern regarding this proposed diagnosis, as noted in the review by Volkmar and Carter (Chapter 21), is whether this reaction represents a mental disorder. The symptomatology is nonspecific, and its inclusion could contribute to an overdiagnosis of mental disorders in children who are having a difficult reaction to the birth of a sibling. Volkmar and Carter also suggest that many of the behaviors may be strongly related to the relationships within the family and should perhaps be understood in the context of the family rather than as a distinct mental disorder in the child. They recommend that DSM-IV include a nonmental disorder code (within the section for Other Conditions That May Be a Focus of Diagnosis and Treatment) to acknowledge the presence of sibling relational problems, because such problems may often be the focus of child or family therapy.

Identity Disorder

Identity disorder was introduced in DSM-III (and retained in DSM-III-R) to provide coverage for individuals in late adolescence who are becoming detached from family value systems and attempting to establish independent identities. It was considered a childhood or premorbid variant of borderline personality disorder. This diagnosis was included in DSM-III in the absence of any systematic research, and the diagnosis has not yet been the subject of systematic empirical research. There are a priori concerns that in some cases the symptomatology may represent normal developmental features and in others a manifestation of another, better established, mental disorder. A review of case materials provided for the Task Force's review by the American Society for Adolescent Psychiatry suggested that this was the case. The relationship to borderline personality disorder has not been established, and most adolescents who struggle with questions regarding their future, identity, and values do not develop this severe and highly dysfunctional personality disorder. It is therefore proposed that, in DSM-IV, the diagnosis of identity disorder be shifted to the section of the manual for Other Conditions That May Be a Focus of Diagnosis and Treatment until there is systematic research to support its validity as a mental disorder (American Psychiatric Association 1991).

Elimination Disorders

Only minor revisions were proposed for the elimination disorders: functional encopresis and functional enuresis (American Psychiatric Association 1991). Reviews were not obtained on these disorders because no substantive changes were proposed. One proposal is to modify the names of the primary and secondary subtypes because these terms are used elsewhere with a different meaning and purpose. A more appropriate subtyping for encopresis—because it affects treatment—is whether the condition is associated with constipation. Consideration is also being given to raising the age limit for functional enuresis to reflect the common clinical practice in which treatment is not usually started until age 7 years. However, nocturnal urinary incontinence that persists after age 5 is less likely to remit spontaneously and is more likely to be associated with additional behavioral and emotional symptoms (American Psychiatric Association 1991).

Tic Disorders

No significant changes are proposed for the tic disorders, other than to provide the definition of a tic within the diagnostic criteria (i.e., an involuntary, sudden, rapid, recurrent, nonrhythmic, stereotyped motor movement or vocalization), to delete the age at onset requirement, and to require a level of distress and/or impairment consistent with the general definition of mental disorder provided in the introduction to the manual. There is no reason to require that a tic disorder be evident prior to the age of 21. These disorders will usually first be diagnosed in childhood or adolescence, but they can also develop for the first time later in life.

References

American Psychiatric Association: Diagnostic and Statistical Manual of Mental Disorders, 2nd Edition. Washington, DC, American Psychiatric Association, 1968

American Psychiatric Association: Diagnostic and Statistical Manual of Mental Disorders, 3rd Edition. Washington, DC, American Psychiatric Association, 1980

American Psychiatric Association: Diagnostic and Statistical Manual of Mental Disorders, 3rd Edition, Revised. Washington, DC, American Psychiatric Association, 1987

American Psychiatric Association: DSM-IV Options Book: Work in Progress. Washington, DC, American Psychiatric Association, 1991

World Health Organization: ICD-10 Chapter V, Mental and Behavioral Disorders, Diagnostic Criteria for Research. Geneva, Switzerland, World Health Organization, 1990

Chapter 8

Attention-Deficit/Hyperactivity Disorder: A Review of Diagnostic Issues

Keith McBurnett, Ph.D.

Statement of the Issues

In preparing DSM-IV, we are to base proposed diagnostic changes to DSM-III-R (American Psychiatric Association 1987) on empirical reviews and reports (when these are available and pertinent), rather than solely on "expert opinion" or committee consensus. This approach is acknowledged (Barkley 1990b) to be one of the strengths of DSM and one of the advantages it may enjoy over the approach used for ICD. In support of proposed changes for diagnosing the attention-deficit disorders, two other reviews of diagnostic issues have been prepared that limit the scope of this chapter. Biederman et al. (Chapter 9, this volume) cover issues related to the comorbidity of attention-deficit/hyperactivity disorder (ADHD) with other disorders, particularly with conduct disorder. Lahey et al. (Chapter 10, this volume) cover issues related to the distinction between attention-deficit disorder with and without hyperactivity. In this chapter, I concentrate on the following six issues:

1. The subgrouping of ADHD symptoms
2. The applicability of the symptoms throughout the life span
3. The utility of additional symptoms that are not part of the current DSM-III-R ADHD criteria set
4. The threshold for the diagnosis
5. The specification of the environments in which the disorder should be assessed
6. Exclusion criteria

Another consideration in revising the DSM-III-R ADHD criteria for DSM-IV is that the new criteria should maximize as much as possible the correspondence with other diagnostic systems, particularly ICD-10 (World Health Organization 1990) (Shaffer et al. 1989). Correspondence between the two classification systems would facilitate record keeping for international health studies and research and would support greater generalizability of findings from studies using either diagnostic system.

Significance of the Issues

Issue 1: Symptom Grouping

DSM-II (American Psychiatric Association 1968) introduced the category of hyperkinetic reaction of childhood (or adolescence). In response to observations that attention problems nearly always accompany this disorder (e.g., Douglas and Peters 1979), the disorder was renamed attention-deficit disorder with hyperactivity in DSM-III (American Psychiatric Association 1980). To make the diagnosis under DSM-III, symptoms were required from three groups: inattention (three required), impulsivity (three required), and hyperactivity (two required). Under DSM-III-R, these three groups were collapsed (with some modifications) into a single list of 14 symptoms, from which any 8 were required to make the diagnosis of ADHD. There have been four major criticisms of the single symptom list:

1. A single list deprives the system of the mnemonic and heuristic value of multiple subgroups of symptoms and decreases the emphasis on impairment in multiple areas of psychopathology.
2. A single list does not correspond to empirical findings that at least two (and perhaps three) separate factors or clusters of ADHD symptoms exist.
3. A single list provides no basis for using hyperactivity symptoms in making the distinction between attention-deficit disorder with and without hyperactivity. If undifferentiated attention-deficit disorder (the vestigial category for DSM-III attention-deficit disorder without hyperactivity) is diagnosed by identifying fewer than 8 symptoms from a single symptom list, it is possible for a child with undifferentiated attention-deficit disorder to have more symptoms of hyperactivity than a child with ADHD.
4. Allowing any 8 symptoms from a list of 14 may result in considerable heterogeneity among cases. For example, two children, each exhibiting 8 ADHD symptoms, could share only 2 symptoms in common, yet receive the same diagnosis. It is possible that such cases may differ in other important ways (etiology, correlates, prognosis, treatment response) that would exacerbate the heterogeneity problem.

If symptoms are to be subgrouped, the leading options are for two groupings (inattention-disorganization and impulsivity-hyperactivity) or three groupings (inattention, impulsivity, and hyperactivity). The former approach of two factors may have better empirical support from factor-analytic and cluster-analytic studies. The latter approach of three factors has the advantages of greater historical continuity with DSM-III and possibly greater mnemonic utility for clinicians. Also, by grouping impulsivity symptoms separately, research on these symptoms may be stimulated.

Issue 2: Applicability of Symptoms and Symptom Descriptions Throughout the Life Span

The DSM-III-R symptoms for ADHD are in general more specific and narrowly defined than those for DSM-III ADHD. Although this language may increase the reliability of individual symptoms, it has led to some awkwardness in applying the symptoms to preschool children and to older adolescents and young adults. If a symptom description is age related and difficult to apply outside a portion of the age range, individuals outside that range may be underdiagnosed. One proposed solution to this problem has been to maintain symptom descriptions as general constructs, but to expand the specific behavioral examples to include items appropriate for different levels of development (Barkley 1990b; Shaffer et al. 1989).

A related issue concerns the appropriateness of using a fixed symptom count (or cutoff) across age levels. The significance of this issue includes the possible underidentification of older ADHD children, and the potential overidentification (classifying children without ADHD as having ADHD) of younger children. The problem of a fixed cutoff across the age range is not independent from the problem of applicability of individual symptoms across the age range, nor from the related problem (see issue 4) that some "symptoms" may be normatively more prevalent at younger ages and more rare or deviant at later ages.

In a more general sense, problems of symptom applicability, fixed cutoff, and prevalence extend beyond differences in developmental level. Difficulties similar to those just described arise also if symptoms vary in prevalence across genders or cultural groups or if symptoms differ in how characteristic they are of social roles associated with different genders or cultural groups.

Issue 3: Tests of New Symptoms

One recommendation for DSM-IV that emerged from the discussion of the DSM-III-R field trials of disruptive behavior disorders was that the symptom lists and cutoff scores be continually refined, with new symptoms being evaluated for incremental clarity, detail, and discriminative power. Several new symptoms have been proposed.

1. Three symptoms (acts without thinking, driven by a motor, runs about or climbs excessively) from the DSM-III list were withdrawn from the DSM-III-R ADHD list. Part of the rationale for not including these symptoms, particularly the first two, was that they were vague, inferential, and not tied to specific behaviors. The counterargument is that the choice to include symptoms is best made on empirical, not rational, grounds, and if the language describing a symptom is too vague for reliably identifying the symptom, the description should be operationalized. These symptoms were not included in the DSM-III-R field trials, and thus have not been tested for their utility along with the current list. Another symptom from the DSM-III list (has difficulty organizing work) has also been proposed for evaluation in the DSM-IV field trials, but with some modification to increase its applicability to more general situations (often has difficulty organizing goal-directed activities).
2. One symptom from the Yale Children's Inventory (Shaywitz et al. 1979, 1988)—confuses details—may have utility as a DSM-IV symptom, based on its strong loading (.77) with the attention scale of the inventory.
3. Attention-deficit disorder without hyperactivity has been associated with characteristics such as extreme forgetfulness, daydreaming, lethargy or hypoactivity, and sluggish cognitive tempo (Barkley 1990a; Barkley et al. 1990b; Lahey et al. 1985). It has been suggested that these items be included in the field trials to test whether they may help differentiate attention-deficit disorder without hyperactivity.

Issue 4: Clinical Threshold and Functional Impairment

Many of the symptoms of ADHD may be considered normal behaviors of childhood when they occur occasionally, in isolated settings, or for a limited developmental period. It is desirable for the diagnostic criteria to identify a statistically rare disorder that is functionally impairing and therefore warrants treatment, rather than to identify a highly prevalent condition that may include essentially normal personality variants.

In DSM-III-R, the features of ADHD are described in the text as *developmentally inappropriate degrees* of inattention, impulsiveness, and hyperactivity, in an effort to distinguish symptoms of clinical significance from behaviors that may be typical of many children of a given age. This notion is also stated in a note preceding the diagnostic criteria. Some of the symptoms include the qualifier "often" to avoid identifying occasional behaviors as symptoms, but this qualifier is not used consistently across symptoms. Proposed revisions include stating explicitly within each symptom group that the symptoms must be "inconsistent with developmental level" and adding the qualifier "often" to several symptoms to provide a consistent emphasis on high frequency.

In DSM-III-R, children can meet criteria for mild ADHD even if there is "only minimal or no impairment in school or social functioning." To help identify a disorder of low prevalence that warrants professional attention, and to ensure that no child that exhibits these patterns as part of normal development without clear impairment would be diagnosed with ADHD, it has been suggested that a requirement of functional impairment or marked distress be added.

Issue 5: Situational Presentation of Symptoms

This issue concerns whether the criteria should require symptoms to occur in multiple settings or in structured settings, rather than only in a single setting or only in the relatively unstructured home environment. One of the reasons for raising this issue is to help ensure, as for the previous issue, that the disorder is applied only to children with clinically significant functional impairment. Another reason is the contention that "true" ADHD cases are most likely to be symptomatic and most easily distinguishable in highly structured settings (Barkley 1985; Jacob et al. 1978; Luk 1985; Routh and Schroeder 1976). A third reason is that the ICD-10 category of hyperkinetic disorder requires symptom presentation in multiple settings, and inclusion of multiple-setting criteria would increase the correspondence between the two systems. Thus, a proposed revision in DSM-IV is to require symptoms to be present in a structured (school or occupational) environment, rather than only the home environment.

Issue 6: Primary Versus Secondary Status of ADHD Symptoms

Many of the symptoms of ADHD are nonspecific and can be manifested in other disorders. The diagnosis of ADHD is not intended to be given when the symptoms are part of, or secondary to, another disorder. In DSM-III-R, a criterion specifies that ADHD should not be diagnosed if the person meets criteria for a pervasive developmental disorder. In the text preceding the ADHD criteria, the importance of distinguishing ADHD hyperactivity and inattention from the psychomotor agitation and difficulty concentrating that occur in some mood disorders is discussed. In ICD-10, a criterion specifies that hyperkinetic disorder should not be diagnosed if the person meets criteria for pervasive developmental disorder, mania, depressive disorder, or anxiety disorder. It is suggested that ADHD not be diagnosed if the symptoms occur exclusively during the course of a pervasive developmental disorder, if the symptoms are due to substance intoxication or withdrawal, or if the symptoms are better accounted for by another disorder that may impair attention and involve psychomotor agitation or restlessness (e.g., major depressive disorder, schizophrenia, or generalized anxiety disorder).

Method

Although the rationale for each of the six issues warrants discussion in this chapter, only two of the issues were selected for the literature review using database searches. Several of the issues (issues 4, 6, and some aspects of 2) relate primarily to philosophical, logical, or pragmatic considerations, and the empirical literature provides little direction for deciding these issues. The utility of proposed new symptoms (issue 3) can be evaluated fairly only in an empirical test along with the existing symptom list. The problem of age-specific symptom cutoff points for the disorder is related but is somewhat tangential to the applicability of symptoms across the age range (issue 2). This problem was not addressed by a systematic database search, but some findings related to cutoffs and age were retrieved and are described in the results section.

Database searches were conducted to retrieve papers germane to the issue of symptom grouping (issue 1) and to the issue of situational versus pervasive symptom presentation (issue 5). A reference librarian searched the Medline and Psychinfo databases using all terms related to the disorder, such as *attention-deficit disorder, hyperkinesis,* and *minimal-brain-disorder*. The retrieved abstracts were reviewed, and those not judged pertinent were discarded. The results of each database search were supplemented by examining the reference lists of retrieved papers and by discussions with research colleagues.

Issue 1: Symptom Grouping

The Boolean logic used for these searches was designed to retrieve sources with any key word from the ADHD-related terms and a keyword from a group of terms related to factor analysis. Papers were reviewed only if they reported a factor analysis of items designed to represent DSM-III or DSM-III-R symptom lists. The extensive literature on the factor structure of several rating scales that do not closely approximate the symptom lists was therefore not included.

Issue 5: Situational Presentation of Symptoms

The Boolean logic used for these searches was designed to retrieve sources with any keyword from the ADHD-related terms and with either *pervasive* or *situational* as a keyword. Papers pertinent to the issue were tabulated if they reported a comparison of correlates or outcome between groups identified as situationally and pervasively hyperactive.

Results

Issue 1: Symptom Grouping

The chief empirical question related to this issue is the factor structure of ADHD symptomatology. Table 8–1 presents the seven studies that were found to have factor-analyzed items representing DSM-III ADHD or DSM-III-R ADHD symptoms. Within the seven studies, 10 samples of children were studied. Two of the samples participated in two separate factor analyses: in Lahey et al.'s (1988) clinic sample, teacher and clinicians' ratings were factor analyzed separately, and in Healey et al.'s (1993) sample, separate analyses were conducted for DSM-III and DSM-III-R items. Thus, a total of 12 factor analyses of symptoms were located, 10 of which used independent samples. Of these 12, the one analysis using a preschool sample found ADHD symptoms to be unidimensional for that age range (Bauermeister 1992). One analysis found ADHD symptoms to fit a three-factor solution (inattentive, hyperactive, impulsive) similar to the symptom categories from DSM-III (Lindgren et al. 1990). One analysis that included oppositional defiant disorder items resulted in a three-factor solution (oppositional-defiant, inattention, impulsivity-overactivity) for the ADHD items, with three ADHD symptoms (difficulty awaiting turn, interrupts or intrudes, engages in dangerous activities) showing primary loadings on the oppositional-defiant factor (Pelham et al. 1992).

Another analysis with school-age children that included oppositional defiant disorder items also resulted in an oppositional defiant disorder factor being extracted, but this analysis resulted in the ADHD symptoms fitting a two-factor solution (inattention-distractibility and hyperactivity-impulsivity) except for a single symptom that loaded with oppositional defiant disorder (Bauermeister 1992). Two of the analyses included "attention-deficit disorder without" items (e.g., sluggishness, drowsiness) in addition to the ADHD items. One of these (Bauermeister et al. 1992) resulted in a two-factor solution (inattention and hyperactivity-impulsivity). The other (Lahey et al. 1988), using clinician ratings rather than teacher ratings, yielded three factors, the third factor reflecting sluggish tempo factor. All but one of the ADHD items in that study loaded on the first two factors of motor hyperactivity-impulsivity and inattention-disorganization. Thus, of the 11 analyses with school-age children, 9 found that the ADHD symptoms (with the exception of one symptom in each of two studies) loaded on two factors—impulsivity-hyperactivity and inattention—even when the analyses contained other items that resulted in additional factors. Only one study (Lindgren et al. 1990) supported a DSM-III type three-factor structure for ADHD symptoms.

A further finding from Pelham et al. (1992) suggests that a two-factor division may provide greater utility by increasing the joint predictive power of symptoms across the two categories (using the ADHD diagnosis as the criterion). Within

Table 8–1. Studies reporting factor analyses of DSM ADHD or ADDH symptoms

Study	Subjects and source	Symptom determination	Factor-analytic procedure	Method (selection of number of factors)	Rotation	Results
Bauermeister 1992	Preschool sample: 665 Puerto Rican children ages 4–5 years from Head Start centers, preschool programs, and day care centers; school-age sample: 680 Puerto Rican children ages 6–16; both samples recruited by soliciting teacher referrals for learning, behavior, or emotional problems	Teacher-completed experimental scale composed of ADHD and oppositional defiant disorder symptoms worded similarly to DSM-III-R	Principal components analysis, followed by maximum likelihood analysis (yielded similar results)	Horn's (1965) test followed by plotting obtained eigenvalues against eigenvalues from random matrices of same data	Varimax and oblimin (oblique) rotations yielded similar results	Preschool sample: two-factor solution (oppositional defiant disorder, ADHD symptoms [ADHD symptoms were unidimensional]); school-age sample: three-factor solution (oppositional defiant disorder, inattention-distractability, hyperactivity-impulsivity); ADHD symptoms loaded almost entirely on latter two factors

Study	Sample	Items	Method	Extraction	Rotation	Solution
Bauermeister et al. 1992	614 Puerto Rican children ages 6–16 from epidemiological sample	Pool of teacher-rated items indicative of symptoms of DSM-III-R ADHD and attention-deficit disorder without hyperactivity/undifferentiated attention-deficit disorder, plus six items descriptive of sluggishness, drawn from Teacher Rating Form and School Behavior Inventory—Revised	Principal components	Factors with eigenvalues exceeding 1.0	Varimax	Two-factor solution (inattention, hyperactivity-impulsivity)
Hart et al., unpublished manuscript, 1992[a]	117 clinic-referred boys (clinic sample); 106 referred and non-referred children (mixed sample)	Clinic sample: parent and teacher DISC interviews; mixed sample: teacher-completed SNAP checklist	24 exploratory factor analyses were conducted for each sample (12 two-factor and 12 three-factor solutions); maximum likelihood provided best two-factor representation	Factors with eigenvalues exceeding 1.0	Varimax	Clinic-referred sample: two-factor solution (inattention-distractability, hyperactivity-impulsivity); mixed sample: two-factor solution (inattention-distractability, hyperactivity-impulsivity)

(continued)

Table 8–1. Studies reporting factor analyses of DSM ADHD or ADDH symptoms *(continued)*

Study	Subjects and source	Symptom determination	Factor-analytic procedure	Method (selection of number of factors)	Rotation	Results
Healey et al. 1993	85 nonreferred children recruited from New York City parochial school (grades 1–6), ages 6–12, primarily black and Hispanic	Teacher-completed experimental questionnaire composed of DSM-III ADDH and DSM-III-R ADHD items, rated on a 4-point scale	Principal components analyses conducted separately for DSM-III and DSM-III-R items	Factors with eigenvalues exceeding 1.0	Varimax	DSM-III symptoms: two-factor solution (hyperactivity-impulsivity, inattention); DSM-III-R symptoms: two-factor solution (hyperactivity-impulsivity, inattention)
Lahey et al. 1988	Community sample: 667 nonreferred children recruited from two elementary schools in Florida (grades K–5); clinic sample: 86 children ages 6–14, consecutive referrals to university psychology clinic in Georgia	Teacher-completed SNAP ratings of DSM-III symptoms for both samples; clinic sample was also rated by clinicians on an experimental scale consisting of attention-deficit disorder with hyperactivity items from DSM-III and DSM-III-R plus attention-deficit disorder without hyperactivity items (e.g., sluggish, daydreams, drowsy)	Principal components	Factors with eigenvalues exceeding 1.0	Varimax	Community sample: two-factor solution (inattention-disorganization, motor hyperactivity-impulsivity); clinic sample, teacher ratings: two-factor solution (inattention-disorganization, motor hyperactivity-impulsivity); clinic sample, clinician ratings: three-factor solution (motor hyperactivity-impulsivity, inattention-disorganization, sluggish tempo)

Lindgren et al. 1990	4,022 nonreferred elementary school children ages 6–12, screened to 1,285 rated with at least one symptom	Teacher-completed DSM-III-R Disruptive Behavior Disorders Checklist (worded closely to DSM-III-R)	Principal components	Factors with eigenvalues exceeding 1.0	Varimax	ADHD symptoms fit three-factor solution (inattentive, hyperactive, impulsive); total item pool fit six-factor solution (including oppositional, aggressive, delinquent)
Pelham et al. 1992	931 nonreferred children ages 5–14, recruited from regular classrooms	Teacher-completed Disruptive Behavior Disorders rating scale (worded closely to DSM-III-R); items endorsed by less than 5% of sample or rated "don't know" by 40% of sample were excluded (mostly conduct disorder items)	Principal components	Factors with eigenvalues exceeding 1.0	Varimax	Three-factor solution (oppositional-defiant, inattention, impulsivity-overactivity)

Note. ADHD = attention-deficit/hyperactivity disorder. ADDH = attention-deficit disorder with hyperactivity. DISC = Diagnostic Interview Scale for Children. SNAP = Swanson, Nolen, and Pelham scales.

[a] B. Hart, B. Applegate, B. Lahey, S. M. Green, P. J. Frick: Factor structure of ADHD: testing the final assumptions of the DSM-IV model, unpublished manuscript, 1992.

categories, however, combinations of impulsivity-hyperactivity symptoms netted greater increases in joint predictive power than combinations of inattention symptoms.

Symptom Cutoffs by Age

Concerns were raised in the report of the DSM-III-R field trial (Spitzer et al. 1990) that the cutoff of eight symptoms may be overly sensitive for very young children and undersensitive for adolescents. In that report, age ranges were set at 2–7, 8–11, and above 11 years. As a function of increasing age group, the sensitivity and specificity of the diagnostic criteria decreased. Barkley et al. (1990a) reported that by requiring only 6 of the 14 DSM-III-R ADHD symptoms among their adolescent group (mean age, 14.9 years), clinical severity was maintained at two standard deviations above the mean. Pelham et al. (1992) examined developmental differences in symptom expression using teacher endorsement of ADHD symptoms in a large, nonselected sample of boys grades K through 8. Although oppositional defiant disorder symptoms and conduct disorder symptoms varied in prevalence as a function of age, ADHD symptoms did not.

Issue 5: Symptoms Required in Structured Setting

This issue bears on two questions. First, should symptoms be reported in the school setting, and not just in the home, to restrict the diagnosis to "true cases" who are definitely impaired? If school symptoms are required, will this reduce the prevalence of ADHD? Based on the low concordance of parent and teacher reports (e.g., Achenbach et al. 1987), this requirement would be expected to restrict prevalence. Only one study has addressed this question by calculating the conditional probability of obtaining an ADHD diagnosis by teacher report of symptoms, given an ADHD diagnosis by parent report (Biederman et al. 1990). The positive predictive power of a parent-based diagnosis for a teacher-based diagnosis was found to be more than 90% in that study's clinic-referred sample. This suggests that in the typical setting in which diagnostic decisions are made, a diagnosis of ADHD based on parent report alone is unlikely to identify a child who would not receive the same diagnosis based on the teacher's report, were it available. However, this inference is made from a single study in which the base rates of parent-based and teacher-based ADHD diagnoses were very high.

The second question is whether children who are identified as symptomatic in the home setting but not the school setting differ in important respects from those who are symptomatic in school only or symptomatic in the home and school (Rapoport and Benoit 1975). The relatively large literature that examines this issue of pervasive versus situational hyperactivity is summarized in Table 8–2. Note that in the fourth column, the constitution of situationally hyperactive groups is

Table 8–2. Studies evaluating situational presentation of hyperactivity

Study	Subjects	Situational measure	Constitution of situational group	Situational versus pervasive	Situational versus control subjects
Beck et al. 1990	30 boys; 6–9 years; community-recruited hyperactive groups; 10 Per, 10 Sit, 10 control subjects	*Per:* > 15 Conners (1989) Hyperactivity Index, problem behavior in 50% of situations on Home Situations Questionnaire (Barkley 1990a) *Sit:* > 15 Conners Hyperactivity Index, problem behavior in 50% of situations on School Situations Questionnaire (Barkley 1990a)	7 of 10 home, 3 of 10 school; data pooled	*Sit = Per:* IQ, SES, marital status, Home Situations Questionnaire, parent aspects of maternal stress, self-rated maternal parenting competence, CBCL internalizing, Werry-Weiss-Peters (Routh et al. 1974), most measures of social skill and social anxiety from lab role-plays *Sit < Per:* Parent and teacher Conners Hyperactivity Index, School Situations Questionnaire, child aspects of maternal stress, CBCL externalizing	*Sit = Control:* IQ, SES, marital status, self-rated maternal parenting competence, CBCL internalizing, most measures of social skill and social anxiety from lab role-plays *Sit > Control:* Parent and teacher Conners Hyperactivity Index, Home and School Situations Questionnaires, parent and child aspects of maternal stress, CBCL externalizing, Werry-Weiss-Peters

(*continued*)

Table 8–2. Studies evaluating situational presentation of hyperactivity *(continued)*

Study	Subjects	Situational measure	Constitution of situational group	Situational versus pervasive	Situational versus control subjects
Boudreault et al. 1988	42 boys, 11 girls; 7.6–9 years; school-recruited hyperactive groups: 16 Per (2 girls), 9 Sit (1 girl), 28 control subjects (8 girls)	*Per:* > 90 percentile on teacher-rated Conners externalizing, teacher report of 3 inattention and 3 impulsivity symptoms consistent across 2 months *Sit:* > 90 percentile on teacher-rated Conners externalizing, parent endorsement of 3 inattention and 3 impulsivity symptoms consistent across 2 months	Proportion of home-only Sit to school-only Sit not reported; data pooled	*Sit = Per:* Global IQ and 3 IQ factors; reading achievement, visuomotor coordination	*Sit = Control:* Verbal IQ and 3rd IQ factor, reading achievement, visuomotor coordination *Sit < Control:* Global and nonverbal IQ

Study	Subjects	Setting	Findings
Campbell et al. 1977a	31 subjects followed up from Schleifer et al. 1975; 7 Per, 8 Sit (3 girls), 16 control subjects (2 girls); control subjects were originally matched on age, IQ, and SES; 31 additional children were recruited as classroom control subjects and matched on sex	See Schleifer et al. 1975	All Sit children were originally home only	$Sit = Per$: Teacher-rated activity, conduct problem, and attention-anxiety (Conners); all self-esteem variables (Coopersmith 1967); most child and teacher observational categories

$Sit < Per$: Teacher-rated inattention-passivity (Conners); coded observations of out-of-seat off-task

$Sit = Control$: Teacher-rated conduct problem, attention-anxiety, and inattention-passivity (Conners); all self-esteem variables (Coopersmith); most child and teacher observational categories

$Sit > Control$: Teacher-rated hyperactivity (Conners); coded negative teacher feedback following attention-seeking behavior |

(continued)

Table 8–2. Studies evaluating situational presentation of hyperactivity *(continued)*

Study	Subjects	Situational measure	Constitution of situational group	Situational versus pervasive	Situational versus control subjects
Campbell et al. 1977b	41 subjects followed up from Schleifer et al. 1975; 9 Per, 11 Sit (5 girls), 21 control subjects (2 girls); control subjects were originally matched on age, IQ, and SES; at follow-up, control subjects > hyperactive subjects on IQ	See Schleifer et al. 1975	All Sit children were originally home only	*Sit = Per:* Familiar figures, embedded figures, mother behaviors and most child behaviors in parent-child lab interactions; Peterson-Quay[a] socialized delinquency; most parent Conners factors; trend for Per children to show lower moral judgment *Sit < Per:* "Requests feedback" and "comments on performance" in parent-child interactions; parent Conners perfectionism *Sit > Per:* Peterson-Quay conduct problem, personality problem, and inadequacy-immaturity	*Sit = Control:* Familiar figures, embedded figures; mother and child behaviors in parent-child interactions; Peterson-Quay socialized delinquency; most parent Conners factors *Sit > Control:* Peterson-Quay conduct problem, personality problem, and inadequacy-immaturity; parent Conners conduct and learning problems

Attention-Deficit/Hyperactivity Disorder: A Review of Diagnostic Issues 127

Study	Sample	Per (P)	Sit (S)	Measures & Findings
Cohen and Minde 1983	42 boys, 7 girls; mean ages 5.5 years; clinic-referred and school-screened (community), control subjects matched on age, SES and IQ; 14 Per (13Per by parent/teacher report but not hyperactive in clinic, designated as C), 14 Sit 10 "normal" control subjects (N)	Per (P): Parent, teacher, and child interviews yield chronic cross-Sit symptoms, mean 1.5 teacher Conners, psychiatrist and psychometrist observations of symptoms in clinic. Clinically diagnosed hyperactive (C): Same as P, but not observed with symptoms in clinic. Sit (S): Only one source (parent or teacher) reported symptoms. Control subjects (N): Obtained from same classrooms as community subjects	Proportion of home-only Sit to school-only Sit not reported; data pooled	Note: Groups (S, P, C, N) are followed by subscripts (a, b, c); groups notated with the same subscripts do not differ significantly on the measures that follow

$S_a P_a C_a N_a$: Birth/developmental history, SES, Wechsler Preschool and Primary Scale of Intelligence IQ, familiar figures, Etch-a-Sketch test of motor impulsivity (but trend toward more impulsive errors by P), self-concept, social problem-solving skill, parent Conners conduct problem and anxiety factors, teacher Conners tension-anxiety factor; coded behavioral observations during mother-child interactions: Maternal approval (strong trend for greater approval in P), maternal specific suggestions and impulse control suggestions, maternal structuring (trend toward less structuring in P and C), child comments on performance and child requests for help

$S_a P_a C_a N_b$: Signs of slow development, incidence of broken homes, incidence of parental psychopathology and marital discord, parent-rated social-emotional problems (Richman and Graham 1971), teacher Conners hyperactivity factor [N is lower on these measures]

$S_{ab} P_a C_a N_b$: Parent Conners total scores, teacher Conners conduct problem factor [P,C > N] |

(continued)

Table 8–2. Studies evaluating situational presentation of hyperactivity (continued)

Study	Subjects	Situational measure	Constitution of situational group	Situational versus pervasive	Situational versus control subjects
				$S_aP_bC_{ab}N_{ab}$: Maternal negative feedback during interaction [P > S]	
				$S_aP_{ab}C_bN_b$: Maternal disapproval during interaction [S > C,N]	
				$S_{ab}P_cC_{ac}N_b$: Parent Conners impulsivity-hyperactivity factor [P > S,N low]	
				$S_{ab}P_{ab}C_aN_b$: Parent Conners learning problem factor [C > N]	
				$S_aP_bC_{ab}N_c$: Teacher Conners total scores [P > S > N]	
				$S_aP_aC_bN_c$: Teacher Conners inattention-passive factor [C > S,P > N]	
				Classroom observations were coded for a subset of the P and C groups, along with control subjects; for these measures:	

Study	Sample	Criteria	Groups	Measures/Notes
Goodman and Stevenson 1989	285 twin pairs; 13 years; community-recruited (epidemiological sample)	*Sit/home*: 3 or greater on mother-completed Rutter (1967) questionnaire *Sit/school*: 3 or greater on teacher-completed Rutter (1967) questionnaire *Per*: 3 or greater on both questionnaires	Not hyperactive (N): 376 (75.5%); home only (H): 63 (12.7%); school only (S): 36 (7.2%); Per (P): 23 (4.6%); Sit data not pooled (72 pairs dropped due to missing data)	P = C = N: Duration of bouts of play (on-task), duration of unoccupied and onlooker behavior (off-task), duration of talking to peers, duration of being talked to by peers, frequency of ignoring others, frequency of being ignored P > C = N: Duration of solitary play, rate of activity shifts, frequency of disruptive behavior, frequency of aggressive behavior P < C = N: Duration of parallel play *Note*: Groups (N, H, S, P) are followed by subscripts (a, b, c); groups notated with the same subscripts do not differ significantly on the measures that follow. $N_a H_a S_a P_a$: Gender, SES, Wechsler Intelligence Scale for Children, Revised 3rd factor, letter cancellation $N_a H_{ab} S_b P_b$: IQ $N_a H_{ab} S_{ab} P_b$: Percentage exhibiting reading and spelling retardation $N_a H_b S_a P_b$: Mother-rated Rutter total deviance score, excluding hyperactivity and adjusted for IQ (b indicates higher)

(continued)

Table 8–2. Studies evaluating situational presentation of hyperactivity *(continued)*

Study	Subjects	Situational measure	Constitution of situational group	Situational versus pervasive	Situational versus control subjects
				$N_aH_aS_bP_b$: Teacher-rated Rutter total deviance score, excluding hyperactivity and adjusted for IQ (b indicates higher)	
				$N_aH_aS_{ab}P_b$: Percentage of cases exceeding mother or teacher total deviance cutoff score	
				$N_aH_{ab}S_{bc}P_c$: Percentage of cases identified as antisocial, or mixed on mother or teacher questionnaire	
Klorman et al. 1983	24 boys, 4 girls; mean age 8.9 years; clinic-referred, 14 Per, 14 Sit, matched on gender, age, and IQ	*Per*: Physician recommendation for methylphenidate; rating from parent interview greater than 1.05 on Werry-Sprague Home Activity Scale (Werry and Sprague 1970); Conners Abbreviated Teacher Scale greater than 2 SDs above mean for grade level	7 of 14 home only, 2 of 14 school only, 5 of 14 did not meet criteria for either setting, but were physician-recommended for methylphenidate; data pooled	Because 36% of Sit group (as termed in this table; originally termed *borderline group*) did not exceed rating cutoff in either home or school setting, detailed results are not presented here; in general, drug effects were comparable for both groups	

Luk et al. 1991	61 boys, 6–12 years; clinic referred; 43 CPer (see right), 18 Per	*Sit*: Physician recommendation for methylphenidate, but failed to meet grading cutoff for home setting, school setting, or both

Per: School and parent report of restless, inattentive behavior, plus mother endorsement of hyperkinetic or attention-deficit/hyperactivity disorder diagnosis

CPer: Same criteria as Per plus hyperactivity observed in clinic interview | No true Sit-only group

Per = CPer: All demographic categories, marital and family relationship measures, most Conners teacher rating scores, Rutter parents questionnaire, Parental Account of Childhood Symptoms (Taylor et al. 1986), verbal IQ, figure cancellation (easy condition), familiar figures

Per < CPer: Conners teacher anxiety/tension, hyperactivity during interview, actometer readings, figure cancellation errors (difficult condition), Porteus Mazes questionnaire score, Continuous Performance Test wrong responses and reaction times, minor neurological deficits

Per > CPer: Performance and full IQ, Porteus Mazes quantitative score, Continuous Performance Test correct responses, clumsiness test performance |

(continued)

Table 8–2. Studies evaluating situational presentation of hyperactivity *(continued)*

Study	Subjects	Situational measure	Constitution of situational group	Situational versus pervasive	Situational versus control subjects
Rapoport et al. 1986	16 boys, mean age 8.5; clinic-referred, 8 Sit, 8 Per, matched on age	*Sit:* Teacher-rated Conners hyperactivity factor > 2 SDs above mean; parent-rated Conners hyperactivity factor < 1 SD above mean *Per:* Parent- and teacher-rated Conners hyperactivity factor > 2 SDs above mean	Sit group were all hyperactive in school setting only	*Sit = Per:* Most demographic variables; prevalence of attention deficit disorder subtype diagnoses; IQ, achievement and Continuous Performance Test scores, Conners hyperactivity ratings on ward; actometer counts, neurological status *Sit < Per:* Frequency of conduct disorder, trend toward lower verbal IQ and math achievement *Sit > Per:* More likely to be adopted, in foster care, or living with relative other than parent; greater frequency of specific developmental disorders	No control subjects

| Sandberg et al. 1978 | 14 boys, mean age 6.9 years; clinic-referred, 7 Sit, 7 Per, matched on age, IQ, and psychiatric diagnosis | *Sit*: Fell in lower range of larger clinic sample on one or more scores of parent-rated, teacher-rated, or directly observed hyperactivity

Per: Scores on Conners Teacher Questionnaire (> 11), Conners Parent Questionnaire (> 13), and coded observations of activity and attention fell in upper halves of scores from larger clinic sample | Proportions of home, school, and clinic hyperactivity not reported; data pooled | *Sit = Per*: Demographics, marital discord and parent psychopathology, physical anomalies, reading backwardness

Sit < Per: Matching familiar figures errors, neurological abnormalities

Sit > Per: Age at onset (earlier in Per) | No control subjects |

(continued)

Table 8–2. Studies evaluating situational presentation of hyperactivity *(continued)*

Study	Subjects	Situational measure	Constitution of situational group	Situational versus pervasive	Situational versus control subjects
Sandberg et al. 1980	226 boys, 5–9 years, mean age 6.6 years; community sample recruited from schools in inner London; high rates of psychosocioeconomic disadvantage	*Sit:* Hyperactivity scores from 3 measures were used to designate 3 non-exclusive Sit groups: Top 10% (*n* = 20) of sample on Conners Teacher Questionnaire; top 13% (*n* = 28) on Rutter Teacher Scale, top 8% (*n* = 16) on Conners Parent Questionnaire *Per:* Not used in comparisons because only 3 boys were rated high on hyperactivity by both parent and teacher	Comparisons were reported separately for 2 school-Sit groups and 1 home-Sit group	Sit groups were compared with remainder of sample not to each other or to a Per group	Sit groups did not differ from the rest of the sample on pre/perinatal complications, neurodevelopmental abnormalities, or minor physical anomalies; only the school-Sit groups were higher on social disadvantage index; among background factors of social disadvantage index, only the Rutter-defined school-Sit group exceeded its sample remainder on low social class, broken home, and single parent, and only the home-Sit group exceeded remainder of sample on mother's mental distress (particularly mother's malaise scores [Rutter et al. 1970])

Study	Sample	Definition	Comments	Results
Schachar et al. 1981	1,536 children, 10–11 years at entry and 14–15 years at follow-up; epidemiological sample (Isle of Wight): 1,285 control subjects (47.5% boys); 220 Sit (65% boys); 31 Per (74.2% boys)	*Sit:* Score of 3 or greater on hyperactivity factor of Rutter teacher or parent questionnaire *Per:* Score of 3 or greater on hyperactivity factor of Rutter teacher and parent questionnaire	Proportion of home versus school not reported for most analyses; data pooled for most comparisons	General trend of Per > Sit > Control on associated psychiatric disturbance, conduct versus emotional correlates, lower IQ and achievement, lower occupational status of father, ratio of boys *Sit = Per:* Parent-rated emotional and conduct disturbance *Sit < Per:* General psychiatric disturbance and persistence of disturbance (Rutter total scores), teacher-rated conduct disturbance, prevalence of cognitive impairment *Sit > Per:* Nonverbal intelligence, other cognitive measures, teacher-rated emotional disturbance *Sit = Control:* Prevalence of cognitive impairment, parent-rated emotional and conduct disturbance *Sit > Control:* Greater percentage of boys, general psychiatric disturbance and persistence of disturbance (Rutter total scores)

(continued)

Table 8–2. Studies evaluating situational presentation of hyperactivity *(continued)*

Study	Subjects	Situational measure	Constitution of situational group	Situational versus pervasive	Situational versus control subjects
Schleifer et al. 1975, study 1	48 boys, 6 girls, 3.3–4.8 years; clinic-referred hyperactive groups; control subjects matched on age, IQ, and SES; 10 Per, 18 Sit (3 girls), 26 control subjects (3 girls)	*Sit:* Parent visit to clinic with chief complaint of overactivity *Per:* Parent clinic visit without overactivity plus preschool teacher rating of extremely hyperactive	All 18 Sit children were home only, not a "problem in the nursery" (preschool)	*Sit = Per:* Familiar figures; mother-endorsed hyperactivity and aggression in psychiatric interview, mother-endorsed family psychopathology; coded observations and psychologist impressions during free play *Sit < Per:* Motor impulsivity; observations of away from seat during structured play *Sit > Per:* Embedded figures	*Sit = Control:* Embedded figures, motor impulsivity, coded observations and psychologist impressions during free play *Sit > Control:* Mother-endorsed hyperactivity and aggression in psychiatric interview

Study	Subjects	SES	Setting	Results	Limitations
Schleifer et al. 1975, study 2	26 hyperactive children from study 1; 10 Per, 16 Sit	Same as study 1	All 16 Sit children were home only	Sit = Per: All medication-induced changes; multivariate group × condition was nonsignificant; dependent measures included familiar figures, embedded figures, motor impulsivity, behavioral observations, and teacher rating	No control subjects

Note. Per = pervasive. Sit = situational. SES = socioeconomic status. CBCL = Child Behavior Checklist (Achenbach and Edelbrock 1983).
[a] D. Peterson, H. Quay: Manual for the Behavior Problems Checklist, unpublished manuscript, 1967.

described, including whether a particular group was hyperactive only at home or only at school. This column also reports whether data from home-only and school-only hyperactive children were pooled into a single group, which would defeat the present purpose of examining the distinctiveness of a home-only hyperactive group. Furthermore, as pointed out by Costello et al. (1991), when the data from home-only and school-only symptomatic cases is pooled into a single "situationally hyperactive" group and a dependent measure based on parent or teacher report is selected, the effect is to average symptomatic and nonsymptomatic children in each setting. The parent report will then show artifactual differences between pervasively and situationally hyperactive children in the home setting, as will the teacher report in the school setting, with the situational groups appearing less severe. The fifth and sixth columns report how situationally hyperactive children differ from pervasively hyperactive children and from control subjects, respectively. The relevant comparisons for this review are those between home-only hyperactive children and either school-only hyperactive children, pervasively hyperactive children, or nonhyperactive children. Differences between pervasively hyperactive children and control subjects are irrelevant to the proposed option and are well established. The Costello et al. report itself was not included in the table because the samples were regrouped and analyzed multiple times to demonstrate that no meaningful differences existed between school-only, home-only, and pervasively hyperactive children, except as an artifact of the informant.

Most of the studies in Table 8–2 pooled data from home-only and school-only cases, thus obscuring any distinct differences in the home-only group, even for those measures that are not derived from parent report. However, the situational group studied by Campbell et al. (1977a, 1977b) and Schleifer et al. (1975) was all symptomatic in the home only. At the time of initial evaluation (ages 3.3–4.8 years), these home-hyperactive children differed from control subjects on parent report of hyperactivity and aggression. They were indistinguishable from pervasively hyperactive children on most dependent measures, but the pervasive group was worse on a task of motor impulsivity, on a task of field independence, and on some behavioral observations. These groups did not differ in response to medication. This sample was followed into elementary school. At follow-up intervals, children who were originally identified as home-symptomatic only continued to be distinguished from control subjects by their worse scores on rating scales. They also continued to be distinguished from the pervasive children on some measures, but not always in the expected direction of being less deviant. In the sample reported by Goodman and Stevenson (1989), the home-only group differed from the school-only and pervasive groups on teacher ratings, whereas the school-only group differed from the home-only and pervasive group on parent ratings: the situation-by-informant confound discussed by Costello et al. (1991).

Discussion and Recommendations

As indicated previously, the existing literature was not searched with regard to several proposed changes that have predominantly logical or pragmatic rationales. These changes include revising symptom descriptions to increase flexibility of application across the age range, requiring symptoms to occur "often," requiring functional impairment or marked distress (criterion E), and specifying that the disorder is not secondary to other disorders. Determining symptom utility from a large pool of symptoms is a major empirical goal of the field trials.

The existing literature on the factor structure of DSM ADHD symptoms strongly supports the adoption of two categories of symptoms. In some studies, the inclusion of "sluggish tempo" items or oppositional defiant disorder/conduct disorder items has resulted in one or more ADHD items loading primarily on sluggish tempo or oppositional defiant disorder. Simultaneous factor analysis of all the disruptive behavior disorder symptoms in the field trials would provide a further guide to categorizing ADHD symptom groups. If the results are similar to those of Pelham et al. (1992) and some impulsivity items load on oppositional defiant disorder but not on ADHD, elimination or recategorization of these items may reduce some spurious comorbidity of ADHD and oppositional defiant disorder.

The small literature consulted on the issue of whether symptom cutoffs for ADHD should remain constant across ages is inconsistent (Barkley et al. 1990a; Pelham et al. 1992; Spitzer et al. 1990). As noted by Pelham et al. (1992), some studies using teacher ratings of ADHD items have often shown decreasing symptomatology over age, but others have not. Data from the field trials may be used to test whether a constant cutoff 1) identifies the disorder with similar rates of sensitivity and specificity, using the criterion of clinical diagnosis based on all information, in children at different ages; and 2) identifies similar proportions of children with similar degrees of impairment at different ages.

Finally, the literature does not provide clear justification for adopting a requirement that symptoms must be present in a structured setting (criterion D). On close inspection, the literature on pervasive versus situational hyperactivity is methodologically limited and provides only modest support for the distinction between home-only and pervasive hyperactivity. Most studies have relied on rating scales to define groups, and the effects of requiring clinical identification of symptoms in a structured setting are not clear. The Costello et al. (1991) analyses suggest that, on many important correlates, the various types of setting-defined hyperactivity do not differ from each other, but all differ significantly from nonhyperactive control subjects. Response to stimulants does not appear to differ between pervasively and situationally hyperactive children (Klorman et al. 1983; Schleifer et al.

1975). Preschoolers judged to be home-only hyperactive using preschool teacher information appear not to differ from their pervasively hyperactive peers on most school-based measures at 3-year follow-up (Campbell et al. 1977a). Pragmatically, it is sometimes difficult or impossible to obtain teacher reports (e.g., during school vacations, for preschoolers, for middle- or high-schoolers who do not have a teacher who knows them well, and in other situations), yet there is no justification in the literature that the unavailability of this information argues against making the ADHD diagnosis. In some cases, inattention and hyperactivity-impulsivity symptoms in the home setting are highly disruptive to family functioning and social development (e.g., Mash and Johnston 1983), yet symptoms in the school setting may be controlled by appropriate structure or tolerated by a charismatic and involved teacher. To rule out the ADHD diagnosis entirely in such a case—despite the behavioral deviance, functional impairment, and topographic similarity of home symptom presentation to ADHD—would result in another classification problem.

Although the literature does not provide strong support for *requiring* symptoms in a structured setting, some reports suggest that there may be some meaningful differences among groups with home, school, or pervasive symptom presentation. Thus, there appears to be a basis for further investigation of the validity of distinguishing among groups that present symptoms in different settings. A subtyping scheme such as home only, structured setting only, pervasive, and unspecified would standardize the subtyping procedure, stimulate research on these subtypes, and facilitate comparisons between DSM-IV and ICD-10 diagnoses of this disorder.

References

Achenbach TM, Edelbrock CS: Manual for the Child Behavior Checklist and Revised Child Behavior Profile. Burlington, VT, TM Achenbach, 1983

Achenbach TM, McConaughy SH, Howell CT: Child/adolescent behavioral and emotional problems: implications of cross-informant correlations for situational specificity. Psychol Bull 101:213–232, 1987

American Psychiatric Association: Diagnostic and Statistical Manual of Mental Disorders, 2nd Edition. Washington, DC, American Psychiatric Association, 1968

American Psychiatric Association: Diagnostic and Statistical Manual of Mental Disorders, 3rd Edition. Washington, DC, American Psychiatric Association, 1980

American Psychiatric Association: Diagnostic and Statistical Manual of Mental Disorders, 3rd Edition, Revised. Washington, DC, American Psychiatric Association, 1987

Barkley RA: The social interactions of hyperactive children: developmental changes, drug effects, and situational variation, in Childhood Disorders: Behavioral-Developmental Approaches. Edited by McMahon R, Peters R. New York, Brunner/Mazel, 1985, pp 218–243

Barkley RA: Attention Deficit Hyperactivity Disorder: A Manual for Diagnosis and Treatment. New York, Guilford, 1990a

Barkley RA: A critique of current diagnostic criteria for attention deficit hyperactivity disorder: clinical and research implications. J Dev Behav Pediatr 11:343–352, 1990b

Barkley RA, Fisher M, Edelbrock CS, et al: The adolescent outcome of hyperactive children diagnosed by research criteria, I: an 8-year follow-up study. J Am Acad Child Adolesc Psychiatry 29:546–557, 1990a

Barkley RA, Dupaul GJ, McMurray MB: Comprehensive evaluation of attention deficit disorder with and without hyperactivity as defined by research criteria. J Consult Clin Psychol 58:775–789, 1990b

Bauermeister J: Factor analyses of teacher ratings of attention-deficit hyperactivity and oppositional defiant symptoms in children aged four through thirteen years. Journal of Clinical Child Psychology 21:27–34, 1992

Bauermeister J, Alegria M, Bird H, et al: Are attentional-hyperactivity deficits unidimensional or multidimensional syndromes? empirical findings from a community survey. J Am Acad Child Adolesc Psychiatry 31:423–431, 1992

Beck S, Young G, Tarnowski K: Maternal characteristics and perceptions of pervasive and situational hyperactives and normal controls. J Am Acad Child Adolesc Psychiatry 29:558–565, 1990

Biederman J, Keenan K, Faraone S: Parent based diagnosis of attention deficit disorder predicts a diagnosis based on teacher report. J Am Acad Child Adolesc Psychiatry 29:698–701, 1990

Boudreault M, Thivierge J, Cote R, et al: Cognitive development and reading achievement in pervasive ADD, situational ADD, and control children. J Child Psychol Psychiatry 29:611–619, 1988

Campbell S, Endman M, Bernfield G: A three-year follow-up of hyperactive preschoolers into elementary school. J Child Psychol Psychiatry 18:239–249, 1977a

Campbell S, Schleifer M, Weiss G, et al: A two-year follow-up of hyperactive preschoolers. Am J Orthopsychiatry 47:149–162, 1977b

Cohen NJ, Minde K: The "hyperkinetic syndrome" in kindergarten children: comparison of children with pervasive and situational symptoms. J Child Psychol Psychiatry 24:443–455, 1983

Conners CK: Conners' Parent and Teacher Rating Scales. Toronto, Ontario, Multi-Health Systems, 1989

Coopersmith S: The Antecedents of Self-Esteem. San Francisco, CA, WH Freeman, 1967

Costello E, Loeber R, Stouthamer-Loeber M: Pervasive and situational hyperactivity—confounding effect of informant: a research note. J Child Psychol Psychiatry 32:367–376, 1991

Douglas VI, Peters KG: Toward a clearer definition of the attentional deficit of hyperactive children, in Attention and the Development of Cognitive Styles. Edited by Hale G, Lewis M. New York, Plenum, 1979, pp 173–248

Goodman R, Stevenson J: A twin study of hyperactivity, I: an examination of hyperactivity scores and categories derived from Rutter Teacher and Parent Questionnaires. J Child Psychol Psychiatry 30:671–689, 1989

Healey J, Newcorn J, Halperin J, et al: The factor structure of ADHD items in DSM-III-R: internal consistency and external validation. Journal of Abnormal Child Psychology 21:441–453, 1993

Horn JL: A rationale and test for the number of factors in factor analysis. Psychometrika 30:179–186, 1965

Jacob RG, O'Leary KD, Rosenblad C: Formal and informal classroom settings: effects on hyperactivity. J Abnorm Child Psychol 6:47–59, 1978

Klorman R, Salzman LF, Bauer LD, et al: Effects of two doses of methylphenidate on cross-situational and borderline hyperactive children's evoked potentials. Electroencephalogr Clin Neurophysiol 56:169–185, 1983

Lahey BB, Frame EL, Strauss CC: Teacher ratings of attention problems in children experimentally classified as exhibiting attention deficit disorders with and without hyperactivity. J Am Acad Child Adolesc Psychiatry 24:613–616, 1985

Lahey BB, Pelham W, Schaughency E, et al: Dimensions and types of attention deficit disorder. J Am Acad Child Adolesc Psychiatry 27:330–335, 1988

Lindgren S, Wolraich M, Stromquist A, et al: Re-examining attention deficit hyperactivity disorder. Paper presented at the 8th annual meeting of the Society for Behavioral Pediatrics, Denver, CO, September, 1990

Luk SL: Direct observation studies of hyperactive behaviors. J Am Acad Child Adolesc Psychiatry 24:338–344, 1985

Luk SL, Leung PWL, Yuen J: Clinic observations in the assessment of pervasiveness of childhood hyperactivity. J Child Psychol Psychiatry 32:833–850, 1991

Mash EJ, Johnston C: Sibling interactions of hyperactive and normal children and their relationship to reports of maternal stress and self-esteem. J Clin Child Psychol 12:91–99, 1983

Pelham WE, Gnagy EM, Greenslade KE, et al: Teacher ratings of DSM-III-R symptoms for the disruptive behavior disorders. J Am Acad Child Adolesc Psychiatry 31:210–218, 1992

Rapoport J, Benoit M: The relation of direct home observations to the clinic evaluation of hyperactive school age boys. J Child Psychol Psychiatry 16:141–147, 1975

Rapoport J, Donnelly D, Zametkin A, et al: Situational hyperactivity in a U.S. clinical setting. J Am Acad Child Adolesc Psychiatry 27:639–646, 1986

Richman N, Graham PJ: A behavioural screening questionnaire for use with three-year-old children: preliminary findings. J Child Psychol Psychiatry 12:5–33, 1971

Routh DK, Schroeder CS: Standardized playroom measures as indices of hyperactivity. J Abnorm Child Psychol 4:199–197, 1976

Routh DK, Schroeder CS, O'Tuama LS: Development of activity level in children. Developmental Psychology 10:163–168, 1974

Rutter M: A children's behaviour questionnaire for completion by teachers: preliminary findings. J Child Psychol Psychiatry 8:1–11, 1967

Rutter M, Tizard J, Whitmore K (eds): Education, Health and Behavior. London, England, Longmans, 1970

Sandberg S, Rutter M, Taylor E: Hyperkinetic disorder in psychiatric clinic attenders. Dev Med Child Neurol 20:279–299, 1978

Sandberg S, Wieselberg M, Shaffer D: Hyperkinetic and conduct problem children in a primary school population: some epidemiological considerations. J Child Psychol Psychiatry 21:293–311, 1980

Schachar R, Rutter M, Smith A: The characteristics of situationally and pervasively hyperactive children: implications for syndrome definition. J Child Psychol Psychiatry 22:375–392, 1981

Schleifer M, Weiss G, Cohen N, et al: Hyperactivity in preschoolers and the effect of methylphenidate. Am J Orthopsychiatry 45:38–50, 1975

Shaffer D, Campbell M, Cantwell D, et al: Child and adolescent psychiatric disorders in DSM-IV: issues facing the work group. J Am Acad Child Adolesc Psychiatry 28:830–835, 1989

Shaywitz S, Schnell C, Shaywitz B: Yale Children's Inventory (YCI): a newly developed instrument to assess children with attentional deficits and learning problems, I: scale development and psychometric properties. J Abnorm Child Psychol 47:223–233, 1979

Shaywitz SE, Shaywitz BA, Schnell SE, et al: Concurrent and predictive validity of the Yale Children's Inventory: an instrument to assess children with attentional deficits and learning disabilities. Pediatrics 81:562–571, 1988

Spitzer RL, Davies M, Barkley RA: The DSM-III-R field trial of disruptive behavior disorders. J Am Acad Child Adolesc Psychiatry 29:690–697, 1990

Taylor EA, Schachar R, Thorley G, et al: Conduct disorder and hyperactivity, I: separation of antisocial conduct in British child psychiatric patients. Br J Psychiatry 149:760–767, 1986

Werry JS, Sprague RL: Hyperactivity, in Symptoms of Psychopathology. Edited by Costello CG. New York, John Wiley, 1970, pp 397–417

World Health Organization: ICD-10 Chapter V: Mental and Behavioral Disorders: Diagnostic Criteria for Research. Geneva, Switzerland, World Health Organization, 1990

Chapter 9

Comorbidity of Attention-Deficit/ Hyperactivity Disorder

Joseph Biederman, M.D., Jeffrey H. Newcorn, M.D., and Susan Sprich, B.A.

Statement of the Issues

In recent years, evidence has been accumulating regarding the high level of comorbidity of attention-deficit/hyperactivity disorder (ADHD) with a number of disorders in culturally and regionally diverse epidemiological samples (Anderson et al. 1987; Bird et al. 1988; McGee et al. 1985), as well as in clinical samples (Biederman et al. 1992). In ICD-10 (World Health Organization 1990), there are separate diagnostic categories for hyperkinesis, conduct disorder, and the mixed category "hyperkinetic conduct disorder." However, DSM-III-R (American Psychiatric Association 1987) does not have a separate category for this comorbid condition and encourages the diagnosis of both disorders when they co-occur. This review addresses the question of how the comorbidity of ADHD should be handled in DSM-IV; specifically, whether a separate comorbid diagnosis for ADHD and conduct disorder is required, and how comorbidity of ADHD and other conditions should be considered in the hierarchical organization of the ADHD diagnosis.

Significance of the Issues

Comorbidity raises fundamental questions as to whether psychiatric disorders are discrete and independent disease entities (Hinshaw 1987). Comorbidity pervasively affects research and clinical practice as a result of its influence on diagnosis, prognosis, treatment, and health care delivery (Maser and Cloninger 1990). From the research perspective, the subgroup of patients with ADHD and a comorbid disorder may represent a more homogeneous subgroup within ADHD. From the clinical perspective, subgroups of patients with ADHD and a comorbid disorder may respond differentially to specific therapeutic approaches. From the public health perspective, the subgroup of patients with ADHD and a comorbid disorder may be at high risk for the development of severe psychopathology. Subgrouping of ADHD children may permit the development of early intervention strategies. This is particularly important in light of published long-term follow-up studies of ADHD children that indicate that a subgroup of ADHD subjects with comorbid disorders had a poorer outcome as evidenced by significantly greater social, emotional, and psychological difficulties (Gittelman and Mannuzza 1988; Weiss et al. 1985). Although the comorbidity of psychiatric disorders has been studied in adult psychiatry as a topic of major practical and theoretical significance (Maser and Cloninger 1990), research data on ADHD have only recently been analyzed taking comorbidity into account. Therefore, it remains to be determined whether research findings previously reported in samples of ADHD children are related to the ADHD itself, to the existence of comorbid disorders, or to the combination of both (Rutter 1989).

Several competing hypotheses have been proposed to account for patterns of comorbidity (Rutter 1989):

1. The comorbid disorders do not represent distinct entities but rather are the expression of the phenotypic variability of the same disorder.
2. Each of the comorbid disorders represents distinct and separate clinical entities.
3. The comorbid disorders share common vulnerabilities (Pauls et al. 1986)—genetic (genotype), psychosocial (adversity), or both.
4. The comorbid disorders may represent a distinct subtype (genetic variant) within a heterogeneous disorder (Pauls et al. 1986).
5. One syndrome may be an early manifestation of the comorbid disorder.
6. The development of one syndrome may increase the risk for the comorbid disorder.

Investigation of these issues should help to clarify the etiology, course, and outcome of ADHD.

The development of a conceptual model for understanding the high rate of comorbidity in ADHD is complicated by controversy regarding the validity of ADHD itself as a distinct clinical entity. Disagreements remain as to which of the multiple symptom domains represented in the ADHD criteria should be viewed as constituting the core deficit (i.e., inattention versus hyperactivity), the categorical or typological nature of the medically dominated diagnostic system versus a dimensional approach to classification, and whether pervasive or situational symptomatology should be required for diagnosis. For example, a number of European investigators have argued that evidence for the validity of ADHD is limited to a rather severe or pervasive type of the disorder (Rutter 1982; Taylor 1986; Taylor et al. 1986a, 1986b). Despite this controversy, an extensive body of literature derived from longitudinal follow-up studies (Gittelman et al. 1985; Loeber at al. 1988; Weiss et al. 1985), treatment studies (Barkley 1977), psychosocial and developmental correlates (Szatmari et al. 1989), and family-genetic studies of male probands (Biederman et al. 1986, 1992) and female probands (Faraone et al. 1991a) supports the concurrent and predictive validity of the broad conceptualization of ADHD as proposed in DSM-III (American Psychiatric Association 1980) and DSM-III-R.

Method

Despite the thousands of scientific articles, multiple review articles, books, and book chapters on ADHD published in the medical, psychological, and educational literature, little is known about its comorbidity. To this end, a systematic search was conducted of the psychiatric and psychological literature for empirical studies dealing with ADHD and comorbidity. The search terms included *hyperactivity, hyperkinesis, attention-deficit disorder,* and *ADHD,* cross referenced with *antisocial disorder (aggression, conduct disorder, antisocial disorder), depression (depression, mania, depressive disorder, bipolar), anxiety (anxiety disorder, anxiety), learning problems (learning, learning disability, academic achievement), substance abuse (alcoholism, drug abuse), mental retardation,* and *Tourette's disorder.* Because citation of every published article on this topic is beyond the scope of this review, we selected representative papers that described studies conducted with the most sophisticated methodology. Although the DSM-III-R definitions of ADHD and related disorders anchor this review, many of the studies described here use other means of classification, including DSM-II (American Psychiatric Association 1968), DSM-III, and dimensional descriptions of clinical syndromes. For simplicity of exposition, the names of DSM-III-R categories are used generically unless otherwise specified.

Results

Comorbidity of ADHD and Conduct Disorder

ADHD and conduct disorder have been found to co-occur in 30%–50% of cases in both epidemiological and clinical samples (Table 9–1). Whether ADHD and conduct disorder constitute separate symptom domains or diagnostic categories has been the topic of considerable debate (Hinshaw 1987; Lahey et al. 1980; Loney and

Milich 1982; Offord et al. 1979; Quay 1986a; Rutter 1983; Shapiro and Garfinkel 1986; Thorley 1984). Two central positions can be identified: 1) ADHD and conduct disorder are *indistinguishable* (complete overlap), or 2) they are either partially or completely *independent.*

The position that ADHD and conduct disorder are indistinguishable suggests

Table 9–1. Summary of representative studies of comorbid attention-deficit/hyperactivity disorder (ADHD) and antisocial disorders, mood disorders, and anxiety disorders

- **ADHD plus antisocial disorders** (conduct, oppositional, or antisocial personality disorders)

    27 studies (18 referred, 9 nonreferred) 1979–1991; age range, 4–25 years; 8,036 subjects.

    In ADHD, overlap with antisocial disorders ranged from 23% to 64% in referred and from 47% to 57% in nonreferred children.

    In antisocial disorders, overlap with ADHD was reported as 85% in one study of referred children and ranged from 35% to 47% in nonreferred children.

    All but one study reported at least some differences between ADHD and antisocial disorders.

    ADHD plus conduct disorder was a more severe subtype of ADHD.

- **ADHD plus mood disorders**

    18 studies (16 referred, 2 nonreferred) 1973–1989; age range, 4–33 years; 3,344 subjects.

    In ADHD, overlap with mood disorders ranged from 25% to 75% in referred and from 15% to 19% in nonreferred children.

    In mood disorders, overlap with ADHD was reported as 55% in one study of referred children and ranged from 30% to 57% in nonreferred children.

    78% of studies reported higher than expected rates of mood disorders in ADHD children.

- **ADHD plus anxiety disorders**

    11 studies (9 referred, 2 nonreferred) 1985–1991; age range, 4–23 year; 2,259 subjects.

    In ADHD, overlap with anxiety disorders ranged from 27% to 30% in referred children and from 8% to 26% in nonreferred samples.

    In anxiety disorders, overlap with ADHD was reported as 18% in one study of referred children and ranged from 18% to 24% in nonreferred children.

    All but two studies reported at least some overlap between ADHD and anxiety disorders.

Source. Adapted from Biederman J, Newcorn J, Sprich S: "Comorbidity of Attention Deficit Hyperactivity Disorder With Conduct, Depressive, Anxiety, and Other Disorders." *American Journal of Psychiatry* 148:564–577, 1991a.

that, given the measurement/diagnosis of either ADHD or conduct disorder, the identification of the other yields no additional information. Proponents of this position point to the similarities between children with ADHD and children with conduct disorder frequently reported in studies of correlates, outcome, and treatment responses (Barkley et al. 1989; Quay et al. 1987). Similarly, they point to intercorrelations between symptoms of ADHD and of conduct disorder (aggressive, disruptive, and noncompliant behaviors) often reported in factor-analytic studies of children with behavior disorders (Campbell and Werry 1986; Quay 1986a, 1986b). In addition, they cite a lack of significant differences in psychosocial, neurodevelopmental, and perinatal factors between ADHD children and children with conduct disorder (Sandberg et al. 1980).

Proponents of the independent position view ADHD and conduct disorder as either completely or partially independent. Support for this position can be derived from studies that compared patterns of familial aggregation, cognitive performance, and outcome between ADHD children and those with ADHD plus conduct disorder. Loney et al. (1981) found that symptoms of hyperactivity and aggression were not highly correlated and showed different patterns of concurrent and predictive validity, suggesting that they were separate dimensions. In those studies, the presence of conduct disorder in childhood, whether associated with ADHD or not, was significantly correlated with aggressive behavior and delinquency in adolescence. In contrast, childhood ADHD without conduct disorder was found to correlate with cognitive and academic deficits (Milich and Loney 1979; Stewart et al. 1980; Szatmari et al. 1989). Similar findings emerged from a recent follow-up study in a nonclinical sample (McGee et al. 1984a, 1984b). Other studies have demonstrated that the subgroup of ADHD children with an associated childhood onset conduct disorder has a more serious clinical course and poorer outcome than the subgroup of ADHD children without conduct disorder (August and Holmes 1984; August et al. 1983; Farrington et al. 1989; Milich et al. 1987; Reeves et al. 1987; Robins 1966).

Family studies have shown that childhood conduct disorder, and not ADHD, is associated with parental antisocial behaviors and alcoholism (August et al. 1983; Biederman et al. 1992; Faraone et al. 1991b; Stewart et al. 1980, 1981). Investigators have found that the familial risk for ADHD and antisocial disorders is highest among relatives of ADHD children with concomitant conduct disorder (Biederman et al. 1987; Sandberg et al. 1978; Singer at al. 1981). Several reports have also shown that a current or past history of ADHD is frequently reported among patients with alcohol dependence (Alterman et al. 1982; DeObaldia and Parsons 1984; Wood et al. 1983) and drug addiction (Cocores et al. 1987; Eyre et al. 1982). Because follow-up studies of children and adolescents diagnosed with conduct disorder are in agreement regarding the strong predictive power of conduct disorder for future psychiatric disorders, social adjustment problems, antisocial personality, alcoholism, and criminality (Robins 1966), it has been suggested that the delinquent behaviors and substance abuse often reported in follow-up studies of boys with ADHD (Gittelman et al. 1985; Weiss et al. 1985) may be linked to childhood antisocial disorders rather than to the syndrome of ADHD per se (August and Stewart 1983; Farrington et al. 1989; Mannuzza et al. 1989).

Two studies (Barkley et al. 1989; Klorman et al. 1988) examined the response to stimulants in ADHD children with and without associated conduct disorder and found that both groups of children showed a similar pattern of improvement with regard to ADHD symptoms. Although these two studies cannot help resolve the debate regarding the independence of ADHD and conduct disorder, they support the clinical relevance of diagnosing both ADHD and conduct disorder when the disorders co-occur.

Although debate continues as to whether ADHD is distinct from conduct disorder, the bulk of the evidence appears to indicate that ADHD and conduct disorder are at least partially independent dimensions or categories. ADHD and conduct disorder differ not only in their defining clinical features but also in external variables such as outcome (cognitive dysfunction for ADHD versus aggression, antisocial behaviors, substance abuse, and delinquency for conduct disorder), etiologic factors (familial aggregation), and psychosocial and developmental correlates. Data from treatment studies have thus far not resolved the debate. There is increasing evidence that children with ADHD + conduct disorder may have a particularly severe form of the disorder. Thus, subgrouping based on comorbidity with conduct disorder may be of potential value in determining which ADHD children have a more serious prognosis and different family-genetic risk factors and require specialized comprehensive therapeutic interventions.

Comorbidity With Oppositional Defiant Disorder

The nosologic status of oppositional defiant disorder, and consequently that of ADHD plus oppositional defiant disorder, remains unclear (Popper 1988; Werry et al. 1987). To date, only a few studies have generated data on oppositional defiant disorder. Some of these have grouped oppositional defiant disorder and conduct disorder together into a single antisocial behavioral category, making it difficult to draw conclusions about oppositional defiant disorder itself. The few studies available report an overlap of at least 35% between ADHD and oppositional defiant disorder, either alone or combined with conduct disorder, in both epidemiological (Anderson et al. 1987; Bird et al. 1988) and clinical (Biederman et al. 1992; Faraone et al. 1991b) studies of children and adolescents. Faraone et al. (1991b) demonstrated that DSM-III oppositional disorder itself is also familial, with the risk for oppositional disorder among relatives of DSM-III attention-deficit disorder + oppositional disorder probands being 3 times greater than the risk to relatives of attention-deficit disorder probands without oppositional disorder and nearly 10 times greater than the risk to relatives of control subjects. These data provide some evidence for the validity of DSM-III oppositional disorder.

In terms of severity of the clinical picture, the available data suggest that children with ADHD + oppositional defiant disorder may form an intermediate subgroup between those who have ADHD alone and those with ADHD + conduct disorder. For example, Faraone et al. (1991b) showed that although probands with DSM-III attention-deficit disorder + oppositional disorder had a higher rate of school dysfunction than those with attention-deficit disorder alone, this rate was lower than that of the attention-deficit disorder + conduct disorder subgroup. A similar pattern was observed for the risk for attention-deficit disorder and antisocial disorders among relatives of probands. Family members of probands with attention-deficit disorder + probands with oppositional disorder were at higher risk for antisocial disorders and attention-deficit disorder than relatives of probands with attention-deficit disorder alone, but at lower risk than relatives of attention-deficit disorder + conduct disorder probands. These findings are consistent with the hypothesis that oppositional defiant disorder may be a subsyndromal manifestation of conduct disorder.

Comorbidity With Mood Disorders

ADHD and mood disorders have been found to co-occur in 15%–75% of cases in both epidemiological (Anderson et al. 1987; Bird et al. 1988) and clinical (Biederman et al. 1991b; Jensen et al. 1988; Munir et al. 1987; Staton and Brumback 1981; Woolston et al. 1989) samples of children and adolescents. Some investigators, however, have not found higher-than-expected rates of mood disorders in ADHD children (Gittelman et al. 1985; Lahey et al. 1988; Stewart and Morrison 1973; Weiss et al. 1985). In clinical samples, the association between ADHD and mood disorders has been reported in studies of children with nonbipolar major depression and dysthymia (Alessi and Magen 1988), adolescents with bipolar disorder (Strober et al. 1988), and children with ADHD (Biederman et al. 1991b; Bohline 1985; Brown et al. 1988; Munir et al. 1987). Studies of high-risk children of parents with mood disorders have found high rates of ADHD (Keller et al. 1988; Orvaschel et al. 1988), and family studies of ADHD children have found a significantly higher rate of mood disorders in probands with ADHD and in their first-degree relatives compared with control children and their first-degree relatives (Biederman et al. 1987). Studies of adopted children diagnosed with ADHD showed high rates of major depressive disorder in their biological relatives compared with their adoptive relatives and the biological relatives of control subjects (Deutsch et al. 1982). Case reports have described individuals with a childhood history of ADHD who developed major affective disorders in later years (Dvoredsky and Stewart 1981). It is doubtful that the comorbidity between ADHD and mood disorders can be explained by ascertainment bias because high levels of comorbidity between ADHD and mood disorders have also been found in culturally and regionally diverse population-based epidemiological samples (Anderson et al. 1987; Bird et al. 1988; McGee et al. 1985).

Findings reported by Biederman et al. (1989, 1990) support the hypothesis that DSM-III attention-deficit disorder and major depressive disorder may share common familial vulnerabilities. Familial risk analyses revealed the following: 1) the risk for major depressive disorder among the relatives of patients with attention-deficit disorder was significantly higher than the risk to relatives of a comparison group of children without attention-deficit disorder, 2) the risk for major depressive disorder was the same among the relatives of attention-deficit disorder probands with and without major depressive disorder and significantly higher in both groups than the risk to relatives of control children, and 3) the two disorders did not co-segregate within families. These findings are consistent with the hypothesis that attention-deficit disorder and major depressive disorder may represent a different expression of the same etiologic factors responsible for the manifestation of attention-deficit disorder. The reasons why the shared genotype may have differing phenotypic expressions such as attention-deficit disorder, major depressive disorder, or attention-deficit disorder + major depressive disorder remain unknown.

Follow-up data of ADHD children as well as of children with major depressive disorder (Kovacs et al. 1984, 1988) strongly suggest that, although these disorders are individually associated with significant long-term psychiatric morbidity, their co-occurrence may be associated with a particularly poor outcome. In a study that evaluated predictors of suicide in adolescents, Brent et al. (1988) reported that adolescents who committed suicide had increased rates of bipolarity and ADHD in comparison with those who attempted suicide. Thus, the co-occurrence of ADHD and a mood disorder is suggestive of a subpopulation of ADHD children at higher risk for greater psychiatric morbidity, disability (Weinberg et al. 1989), and perhaps suicide than other ADHD children and adolescents without such comorbidity.

Comorbidity With Anxiety Disorders

A comorbid association of approximately 25% between ADHD and anxiety disorders has been found in epidemiological (Anderson et al. 1987; Bird et al. 1988) and clinical (Last et al. 1987) samples of children with anxiety disorders and children with ADHD (Biederman et al. 1992; Lahey et al. 1988; Munir et al. 1987; Pliszka 1989; Woolston et al. 1989). Investigators have also noted higher rates of ADHD in children of parents with anxiety disorders than in children of comparison groups (Sylvester et al. 1987). Lahey et al. (1987, 1988) noted that children with the DSM-III diagnosis of attention-deficit disorder without hyperactivity had higher rates of anxiety disorders than those with ADHD. An investigation of the familial interrelationship between ADHD and anxiety disorders (Biederman et al. 1991c) provides evidence for an association between the two disorders as follows: 1) the risk for anxiety disorders among the relatives of patients with ADHD was significantly higher than the risk to relatives of comparison children without ADHD, 2) the risk for anxiety disorders was significantly higher in relatives of probands with ADHD and anxiety disorders compared with relatives of ADHD children without anxiety disorders, and 3) co-segregation between ADHD and anxiety disorders within families could not be established. These findings suggest that ADHD and anxiety disorders transmit independently in families.

Comorbidity With Learning Disabilities

An overlap between ADHD and learning disabilities has been consistently reported in the literature. The reported degree of overlap ranges from as low as 10% (August and Holmes 1984; Halperin et al. 1984) to as high as 92% (Silver 1981). This variability is most likely due to differences in selection criteria, sampling, and measurement instruments, as well as inconsistencies in the criteria used to define both ADHD and learning disabilities in different studies (August and Garfinkel 1989; Halperin and Gittelman 1982). In addition to these inconsistencies in the definitions of learning disabilities and of ADHD, the academic dysfunction commonly associated with both conditions and the heterogeneity of the learning disabilities has led to widespread confusion about these disorders. Studies have consistently shown that ADHD children perform more poorly in school than control subjects, as evidenced by more grade repetitions, poorer grades in academic subjects, more placement in special classes, and more tutoring (Edelbrock et al. 1984; Lahey et al. 1984; Silver 1981; Weiss et al. 1979). Findings also indicate that ADHD children perform more poorly than control subjects on standard measures of intelligence and achievement (Campbell and Werry 1986). Follow-up studies have found that the academic and learning problems of ADHD children persist into adolescence and are associated with chronic underachievement and school failure (Gittelman et al. 1985; Weiss et al. 1985). It is still unknown whether school failure in ADHD children is related to the psychiatric picture of inattention and impulsivity (ADHD), cognitive deficits (learning disabilities), a combination of both factors (ADHD + learning disabilities), or perhaps other factors such as social disadvantage or demoralization and consequent decline in motivation (Campbell and Werry 1986).

The finding in some studies that learning disabilities is almost universally found among ADHD children (Silver 1981) led some authors to suggest that ADHD and learning disabilities may be indistinguishable (Prior and Sanson 1986). However, important differences exist in the defining characteristics of both disorders. Whereas ADHD is a behavioral syndrome with characteristic symptoms of inattentiveness, impulsivity, and hyperactivity, learning disabilities refer to a group of cognitive disorders thought to reflect perceptual handicaps in one or more basic cognitive processes and are manifested as disorders of language, reading, writing and spelling, or arithmetic. Moreover, many ADHD children are achieving adequately, and not all children with learning disabilities have ADHD, suggesting that the two disorders may be independent but can overlap in some individuals (Interagency Committee on Learning Disabilities 1987).

In an attempt to clarify the nature of the association between ADHD and learning disabilities, researchers have begun to compare subgroups of children with learning disabilities, ADHD, and ADHD + learning disabilities (Ackerman et al. 1979; Halperin et al. 1984). Although this approach holds promise, most studies have found few differences among subgroups. For example, Halperin et al. compared children with ADHD + learning disabilities (reading disability) with ADHD children to examine whether ADHD + learning disabilities constitutes a distinct subgroup of ADHD. Because the two groups did not differ behaviorally or in sociodemographic characteristics, the authors interpreted their findings as giving minimal support to the usefulness of subgrouping ADHD based on the presence of learning disabilities. In a study using a similar design and analytic approach, Ackerman et al. also failed to find differences between ADHD + learning disabilities versus ADHD children on measures of impulsivity and response to stimulants. It is important to stress, however, that although the children in these studies all shared the clinical features of ADHD, they may have differed in fundamental ways determined by the presence of learning disabilities and its correlates. The identification of these differences may have major clinical and educational significance, because the two disorders require different intervention approaches. Although more research is needed to evaluate further the nature of the association between ADHD and learning disabilities, the subgroup with ADHD + learning disabilities deserves special clinical and educational attention.

Comorbidity With Other Disorders

ADHD is generally considered to be three to four times more prevalent in children with mental retardation than in those with normal IQ scores (Epstein et al. 1986; Hunt and Cohen 1988; Koller et al. 1983; Russell 1988). In a study that analyzed the type of behavioral disturbance as a function of IQ (Koller et al. 1983), conduct disorder was found to be far more common than ADHD in boys with IQ > 50, but

ADHD and conduct disorder were equally prevalent in children with IQ < 50. In another study (Epstein et al. 1986), ADHD was found to be much more common in educable mentally retarded persons (IQ > 50) than in the general population. Russell noted that individuals with IQ < 50 may exhibit different types of psychiatric disorders than those with milder mental retardation. In addition, studies in which stimulant treatment has been shown to be effective in children with ADHD + mental retardation have been conducted only in populations with mild mental retardation (Chandler et al. 1988; Varley and Trupin 1982). These data are consistent with a definition of ADHD that allows comorbidity with mild mental retardation but imposes an IQ cutoff below which ADHD should not be diagnosed. Because ADHD appears to occur with increasing frequency in individuals with mental retardation, more work needs to be done to evaluate whether attention and activity problems in mentally retarded persons should be viewed as constituting ADHD or whether they are a consequence of having a low IQ.

Comorbidity of Tourette's syndrome and ADHD has been well documented. Approximately 60% of children and adolescents with Tourette's syndrome have been shown to have comorbid ADHD (Comings and Comings 1984, 1985, 1987; Pauls et al. 1986). Because the prevalence of ADHD is much higher than that of Tourette's syndrome, only a small percentage of ADHD children have comorbid Tourette's syndrome. Although the comorbidity figures from these studies are in close agreement, discrepant viewpoints have been proposed regarding their interpretation. Comings and Comings (1984, 1987) contended that there is a genetic relationship between Tourette's syndrome and ADHD, with a Tourette's syndrome gene (as yet unidentified) accounting for approximately 10%–30% of ADHD. Conversely, Pauls et al. disputed the conclusion that ADHD and Tourette's syndrome are genetically related. Identification of children at risk for the development of Tourette's syndrome within the larger ADHD population has important practical implications, because psychostimulant treatment has been associated with the development of Tourette's syndrome in some studies (Lowe et al. 1982) and may be contraindicated in children at high risk for Tourette's syndrome.

Comorbidity of ADHD and borderline personality disorder has been described by Andrulonis et al. (1982), who found that 25% of a group of 106 borderline patients with IQ > 80 had a current or past history of ADHD and/or learning disabilities. Similarly, Bellak (1979, 1985; Bellak et al. 1987) described a population of children whom he refers to as having "ADHD psychosis" who present with impulsive behavior, learning problems, mood lability, impaired judgment, disorganization, and intermittently poor reality testing. Successful treatment of comorbid ADHD plus borderline personality with methylphenidate (Hooberman and Stern 1984) and imipramine (Satel et al. 1988) has been described in case reports.

Discussion and Recommendations

There is increasing recognition that ADHD is a heterogeneous disorder with considerable and varied comorbidity. The weight of the available literature indicates the frequent co-occurrence of ADHD with conduct/oppositional, mood, anxiety, learning, and a number of other disorders in childhood, adolescence, and adulthood. The observed comorbidity does not appear to be either random or artifactual. Rather, specific patterns of symptoms and syndromes tend to occur together in individuals and families. Recent family-genetic data suggest that ADHD plus conduct disorder may be a distinct condition, characterized by different risk factors and clinical course. Thus far, however, the few available studies of pharmacological response have failed to demonstrate the predictive value of a separate ADHD + conduct disorder subtype. There is less reason to question whether a subtype of ADHD + anxiety disorder is required, because ADHD and anxiety disorders appear to be transmitted independently in family pedigrees. The fact that ADHD and depression appear to share common familial vulnerabilities raises as many questions about discriminant validity and natural history as comorbidity.

It is therefore our recommendation, on the basis of the literature reviewed, that DSM-IV continue to recommend that ADHD and the various conditions with which it presents comorbidly be diagnosed independently, using all appropriate diagnoses when indicated. Comorbidity with conduct disorder, oppositional defiant disorder, mood disorder, anxiety disorders, and specific developmental disorders (learning disabilities) should all be permitted. Although the resultant high level of comorbidity within ADHD may lead to problems in differential diagnosis, these difficulties are not likely to invalidate the diagnosis of ADHD. Rather, the continued ability to diagnose both conditions will lead to a further examination of the patterns and structure of observed comorbidity and could help to revise and improve existing methods of classification.

References

Ackerman PT, Elardo PT, Dykman RA: A psychosocial study of hyperactive and learning-disabled boys. J Abnorm Child Psychol 7:91–99, 1979

Alessi NE, Magen J: Comorbidity of other psychiatric disturbances in depressed, psychiatrically hospitalized children. Am J Psychiatry 145:1582–1584, 1988

Alterman AI, Petrarulo E, Tarter R, et al: Hyperactivity and alcoholism: familial and behavioral correlates. Addict Behav 7:413–442, 1982

American Psychiatric Association: Diagnostic and Statistical Manual of Mental Disorders, 2nd Edition. Washington, DC, American Psychiatric Association, 1968

American Psychiatric Association: Diagnostic and Statistical Manual of Mental Disorders, 3rd Edition. Washington, DC, American Psychiatric Association, 1980

American Psychiatric Association: Diagnostic and Statistical Manual of Mental Disorders, 3rd Edition, Revised. Washington, DC, American Psychiatric Association, 1987

Anderson JC, Williams S, McGee R, et al: DSM-III disorders in preadolescent children: prevalence in a large sample from the general population. Arch Gen Psychiatry 44:69–76, 1987

Andrulonis PA, Glueck BC, Stroebel CF, et al: Borderline personality subcategories. J Nerv Ment Dis 170:670–679, 1982

August GJ, Garfinkel BD: Behavioral and cognitive subtypes of ADHD. J Am Acad Child Adolesc Psychiatry 28:739–748, 1989

August GJ, Holmes CS: Behavior and academic achievement in hyperactive subgroups and learning-disabled boys. Am J Dis Child 138:1025–1029, 1984

August GJ, Stewart MA: Familial subtypes of childhood hyperactivity. J Nerv Ment Dis 171:362–368, 1983

August GJ, Stewart MA, Holmes CS: A four-year follow-up of hyperactive boys with and without conduct disorder. Br J Psychiatry 143:192–198, 1983

Barkley RA: A review of stimulant drug research with hyperactive children. J Child Psychol Psychiatry 18:137–165, 1977

Barkley RA, McMurray MB, Edelbrock CS, et al: The response of aggressive and nonaggressive ADHD children to two doses of methylphenidate. J Am Acad Child Adolesc Psychiatry 28:873–881, 1989

Bellak L: Schizophrenic syndrome related to minimal brain dysfunction. Schizophr Bull 11:523–527, 1979

Bellak L: ADD psychosis as a separate entity. Schizophr Bull 11:523–527, 1985

Bellak L, Kay SR, Opler LA: Attention deficit disorder psychosis as a diagnostic category. Psychiatr Dev 3:239–263, 1987

Biederman J, Munir K, Knee D, et al: A controlled family study of patients with attention deficit disorder and normal controls. J Psychiatr Res 20:263–274, 1986

Biederman J, Munir K, Knee D: Conduct and oppositional disorder in clinically referred children with attention deficit disorder: a controlled family study. J Am Acad Child Adolesc Psychiatry 26:724–727, 1987

Biederman J, Faraone S, Keenan K, et al: Family-genetic and psychosocial risk factors in DSM-III attention deficit disorder (abstract). Biol Psychiatry 25 (suppl):145A, 1989

Biederman J, Faraone SV, Keenan K, et al: Family-genetic and psychosocial risk factors in attention deficit disorder. J Am Acad Child Adolesc Psychiatry 29:526–534, 1990

Biederman J, Newcorn J, Sprich S: Comorbidity of attention deficit hyperactivity disorder with conduct, depressive, anxiety, and other disorders. Am J Psychiatry 148:564–577, 1991a

Biederman J, Faraone SV, Keenan K, et al: Evidence of familial association between attention deficit disorder and major affective disorders. Arch Gen Psychiatry 48:633–642, 1991b

Biederman J, Faraone SV, Keenan K, et al: Familial association between attention deficit disorder (ADD) and anxiety disorders. Am J Psychiatry 148:251–256, 1991c

Biederman J, Faraone SV, Keenan K, et al: Further evidence for family-genetic risk factors in attention deficit hyperactivity disorder (ADHD): patterns of comorbidity in probands and relatives in psychiatrically and pediatrically referred samples. Arch Gen Psychiatry 49:728–738, 1992

Bird HR, Canino G, Rubio-Stipec M, et al: Estimates of the prevalence of childhood maladjustment in a community survey in Puerto Rico. Arch Gen Psychiatry 45:1120–1126, 1988

Bohline DS: Intellectual and affective characteristics of attention deficit disordered children. J Learn Dis 18:604–608, 1985

Brent DA, Perper JA, Goldstein CE, et al: Risk factors for adolescent suicide: a comparison of adolescent suicide victims with suicidal inpatients. Arch Gen Psychiatry 45:581–588, 1988

Brown RT, Borden KA, Clingerman SR, et al: Depression in attention deficit-disordered and normal children and their parents. Child Psychiatry Hum Dev 18:119–132, 1988

Campbell SB, Werry JS: Attention deficit disorder (hyperactivity), in Psychopathologic Disorders of Childhood. Edited by Quay HC, Werry JS. New York, John Wiley, 1986, pp 111–155

Chandler M, Gualtieri CT, Fahs JJ: Other psychotropic drugs: stimulants, antidepressants, the anxiolytics, and lithium carbonate, in Psychopharmacology of the Developmental Disabilities. Edited by Aman MG, Singh DN. New York, Springer-Verlag, 1988

Cocores JA, Davies RK, Mueller PS, et al: Cocaine abuse and adult attention deficit disorder. J Clin Psychiatry 48:376–377, 1987

Comings DE, Comings BG: Tourette's syndrome and attention deficit disorder with hyperactivity: are they genetically related? J Am Acad Child Psychiatry 23: 138–146, 1984

Comings DE, Comings BG: Tourette syndrome: clinical and psychological aspects of 250 cases. Am J Hum Genet 37:435–450, 1985

Comings DE, Comings BG: A controlled study of Tourette syndrome, I: attention deficit disorder, learning disorders, and school problems. Am J Hum Genet 41:701–741, 1987

DeObaldia R, Parsons OA: Relationship of neuropsychological performance to primary alcoholism and self-reported symptoms of childhood minimal brain dysfunction. J Stud Alcohol 45:386–391, 1984

Deutsch CK, Swanson JM, Bruell JM, et al: Overrepresentation of adoptees in children with the attention deficit disorder. Behav Genet 12:231–238, 1982

Dvoredsky A, Stewart M: Hyperactivity followed by manic depressive disorder: two case reports. J Clin Psychiatry 42:212–214, 1981

Edelbrock C, Costello AJ, Kessler MD: Empirical corroboration of attention deficit disorder. Journal of the American Academy of Child Psychiatry 23:285–290, 1984

Epstein MH, Cullinan D, Polloway ED: Patterns of maladjustment among mentally retarded children and youth. American Journal of Mental Deficiency 91:127–134, 1986

Eyre SL, Rounsaville BJ, Kleber HD: History of childhood hyperactivity in a clinical population of opiate addicts. J Nerv Ment Dis 170:522–529, 1982

Faraone SV, Biederman J, Keenan K, et al: A family-genetic study of girls with DSM-III attention deficit disorder. Am J Psychiatry 148:112–117, 1991a

Faraone SV, Biederman J, Keenan K, et al: Separation of DSM-III attention deficit disorder and conduct disorder: evidence from a family-genetic study of American child psychiatric patients. Psychol Med 21:109–121, 1991b

Farrington DP, Loeber R, Van Kammen WB: Long-term criminal outcomes of hyperactivity-impulsivity-attention deficit and conduct problems in childhood, in Straight and Devious Pathways to Adulthood. Edited by Robins LN, Rutter MR. New York, Cambridge University Press, 1989, pp 62–81

Gittelman R, Mannuzza S: Hyperactive boys almost grown up, III: methylphenidate effects on ultimate height. Arch Gen Psychiatry 45:1131–1134, 1988

Gittelman R, Mannuzza S, Shenker R, et al: Hyperactive boys almost grown up. Arch Gen Psychiatry 42:937–947, 1985

Halperin JM, Gittelman R: Do hyperactive children and their siblings differ in IQ and academic achievement? Psychiatry Res 6:253–258, 1982

Halperin JM, Gittelman R, Klein DF, et al: Reading-disabled hyperactive children: a distinct subgroup of attention deficit disorder with hyperactivity. J Abnorm Child Psychol 12:1–14, 1984

Hinshaw SP: On the distinction between attentional deficits/hyperactivity and conduct problems/aggression in child psychopathology. Psychol Bull 101:443–463, 1987

Hooberman D, Stern TA: Treatment of attention deficit and borderline personality disorders with psychostimulants: case report. J Clin Psychiatry 45:441–442, 1984

Hunt RD, Cohen DJ: Attentional and neurochemical components of mental retardation: new methods for an old problem, in Mental Retardation and Mental Health: Classification, Diagnosis, Treatment Services. Edited by Stark JA, Menolasino FJ, Albarelli MH, et al. New York, Springer-Verlag, 1988

Interagency Committee on Learning Disabilities (eds): Learning Disabilities: A Report to the U.S. Congress. Washington, DC, Interagency Committee on Learning Disabilities, 1987

Jensen JB, Burke N, Garfinkel BD: Depression and symptoms of attention deficit disorder with hyperactivity. J Am Acad Child Adolesc Psychiatry 27:742–747, 1988

Keller MB, Beardslee W, Lavori PW, et al: Course of major depression in non-referred adolescents: a retrospective study. J Affect Disord 15:235–243, 1988

Klorman R, Brumaghim JT, Salzman LF, et al: Effects of methylphenidate on attention-deficit hyperactivity disorder with and without aggressive/noncompliant features. J Abnorm Psychol 97:413–422, 1988

Koller H, Richardson SA, Katz M: Behavior disturbance since childhood among a 5-year birth cohort of all mentally retarded young adults in a city. American Journal of Mental Deficiency 87:386–395, 1983

Kovacs M, Feinberg TL, Crouse N, et al: Depressive disorders in childhood, I: a longitudinal prospective study of characteristics and recovery. Arch Gen Psychiatry 41:229–237, 1984

Kovacs M, Paulauskas S, Gatsonis C, et al: Depressive disorders in childhood, III: a longitudinal study of comorbidity with and risk for conduct disorders. J Affect Disord 15:205–217, 1988

Lahey BB, Green KD, Forehand R: On the independence of rating hyperactivity, conduct problems, and attention deficits in children: a multiple regression analysis. J Consult Clin Psychol 48:566–574, 1980

Lahey BB, Schaughency EA, Strauss CC, et al: Are attention deficit disorders with and without hyperactivity similar or dissimilar disorders? Journal of the American Academy of Child Psychiatry 23:302–309, 1984

Lahey BB, Schaughency EA, Hynd GW, et al: Attention deficit disorder with and without hyperactivity: comparison of behavioral characteristics of clinic-referred children. J Am Acad Child Adolesc Psychiatry 26:718–723, 1987

Lahey BB, Pelham WE, Schaughency EA, et al: Dimensions and types of attention deficit disorder. J Am Acad Child Adolesc Psychiatry 27:330–335, 1988

Last CG, Strauss CC, Francis G: Comorbidity among childhood anxiety disorders. J Nerv Ment Dis 175:726–730, 1987

Loeber R, Brinthaupt VP, Green SM: Attention deficits, impulsivity, and hyperactivity with or without conduct problems: relationships to delinquency and unique contextual factors, in Behavior Disorders in Adolescence: Research, Intervention and Policy in Clinical and School Settings. Edited by MacMahon RJ, Peters RD. New York, Plenum, 1988

Loney J, Milich R: Hyperactivity, inattention, and aggression in clinical practice, in Advances in Developmental and Behavioral Pediatrics. Edited by Wolraich M, Routh D. Greenwich, CT, JAI Press, 1982, pp 113–147

Loney J, Kramer J, Milich RS: The hyperactive child grows up: predictors of symptoms, delinquency and achievement at follow-up, in Psychosocial Aspects of Drug Treatment for Hyperactivity. Edited by Gadow KD, Loney J. Boulder, CO, Westview Press, 1981, pp 381–416

Lowe TL, Cohen DJ, Detlor J: Stimulant medications precipitate Tourette's syndrome. JAMA 247:1168–1169, 1982

Mannuzza S, Gittelman-Klein R, Horowitz-Konig P, et al: Hyperactive boys almost grown up, IV: criminality and its relationship to psychiatric status. Arch Gen Psychiatry 46:1073–1079, 1989

Maser JD, Cloninger CR: Comorbidity of anxiety and mood disorders: introduction and overview, in Comorbidity of Mood and Anxiety Disorders. Edited by Maser JD, Cloninger CR. Washington, DC, American Psychiatric Press, 1990, pp 3–12

McGee R, Williams S, Silva PA: Background characteristics of aggressive, hyperactive and aggressive-hyperactive boys. Journal of the American Academy of Child Psychiatry 23:280–284, 1984a

McGee R, Williams S, Silva PA: Behavioral and developmental characteristics of aggressive, hyperactive and aggressive-hyperactive boys. Journal of the American Academy of Child Psychiatry 23:270–279, 1984b

McGee R, Williams S, Silva PA: Factor structure and correlate of ratings of inattention, hyperactivity, and antisocial behavior in a large sample of 9-year-old children from the general population. J Consult Clin Psychol 53:480–490, 1985

Milich R, Loney J: The role of hyperactive and aggressive symptomatology in predicting adolescent outcome among hyperactive children. J Pediatr Psychol 4:93–112, 1979

Milich R, Widiger TA, Landau S: Differential diagnosis of attention deficit and conduct disorders using conditional probabilities. J Consult Clin Psychol 55:762–767, 1987

Munir K, Biederman J, Knee D: Psychiatric comorbidity in patients with attention deficit disorder: a controlled study. J Am Acad Child Adolesc Psychiatry 26:844–848, 1987

Offord DR, Sullivan K, Allen N, et al: Delinquency and hyperactivity. J Nerv Ment Dis 167:734–741, 1979

Orvaschel H, Walsh-Allis G, Ye W: Psychopathology in children of parents with recurrent depression. J Abnorm Child Psychol 16:17–28, 1988

Pauls DL, Hurst CR, Kruger SD, et al: Gilles de la Tourette's syndrome and attention deficit disorder with hyperactivity: evidence against a genetic relationship. Arch Gen Psychiatry 43:1177–1179, 1986

Pliszka SR: Effect of anxiety on cognition, behavior, and stimulant response in ADHD. J Am Acad Child Adolesc Psychiatry 28:882–887, 1989

Popper CW: Disorders usually first evident in infancy, childhood or adolescence, in Textbook of Psychiatry. Edited by Talbott JA, Hales RE, Yudofsky SC. Washington, DC, American Psychiatric Press, 1988

Prior M, Sanson A: Attention deficit disorder with hyperactivity: a critique. J Child Psychol Psychiatry 27:307–319, 1986
Quay HC: Conduct disorder, in Psychopathologic Disorders of Childhood. Edited by Quay HC, Werry JS. New York, John Wiley, 1986a, pp 1–34
Quay HC: A critical analysis of DSM-III as a taxonomy of psychopathology in childhood and adolescence, in Contemporary Issues in Psychopathology. Edited by Millon T, Klerman G. New York, Guilford, 1986b, pp 151–165
Quay HC, Routh DK, Shapiro SK: Psychopathology of childhood: from description to validation. Annu Rev Psychol 38:491–532, 1987
Reeves JC, Werry JS, Elkind GS, et al: Attention deficit, conduct, oppositional, and anxiety disorders in children, II: clinical characteristics. J Am Acad Child Adolesc Psychiatry 26:144–155, 1987
Robins L (ed): Deviant Children Grown Up. Baltimore, MD, Williams & Wilkins, 1966
Russell AT: The association between mental retardation and psychiatric disorder: epidemiological issues, in Mental Retardation and Mental Health: Classification, Diagnosis, Treatment Services. Edited by Stark JA, Menolasino FJ, Albarelli MH, et al. New York, Springer-Verlag, 1988
Rutter M: Syndromes attributed to "minimal brain dysfunction" in childhood. Am J Psychiatry 139:21–33, 1982
Rutter M: Questions and findings on the concept of a distinct syndrome, in Developmental Neuropsychiatry. Edited by Rutter M. New York, Guilford, 1983
Rutter M: Isle of Wight revisited: twenty-five years of child psychiatric epidemiology. J Am Acad Child Adolesc Psychiatry 28:633–653, 1989
Sandberg ST, Rutter M, Taylor E: Hyperkinetic disorder in psychiatric clinic attenders. Dev Med Child Neurol 20:279–299, 1978
Sandberg ST, Wieselberg M, Shaffer D: Hyperkinetic and conduct problem children in a primary school population: some epidemiologic considerations. J Child Psychol Psychiatry 21:293–311, 1980
Satel S, Southwick S, Denton C: Use of imipramine for attention deficit disorder in a borderline patient. J Nerv Ment Dis 176:305–307, 1988
Shapiro SK, Garfinkel HD: The occurrence of behavior disorders in children: the interdependence of attention deficit disorder and conduct disorder. Journal of the American Academy of Child Psychiatry 25:809–819, 1986
Silver LB: The relationship between learning disabilities, hyperactivity, distractibility, and behavioral problems. Journal of the American Academy of Child Psychiatry 20:385–397, 1981
Singer SM, Stewart MA, Pulaski L: Minimal brain dysfunction: differences in cognitive organization in two groups of index cases and their relatives. J Learn Dis 14:470–473, 1981
Staton RD, Brumback RA: Non-specificity of motor hyperactivity as a diagnostic criterion. Percept Mot Skills 52:323–332, 1981
Stewart MA, Morrison JR: Affective disorders among the relatives of hyperactive children. J Child Psychol Psychiatry 14:209–212, 1973
Stewart MA, DeBlois CS, Cummings C: Psychiatric disorder in the parents of hyperactive boys and those with conduct disorder. J Child Psychol Psychiatry 21:283–292, 1980
Stewart MA, Cummings C, Singer S, et al: The overlap between hyperactive and unsocialized aggressive children. J Child Psychol Psychiatry 22:35–45, 1981

Strober M, Morrell W, Burroughs J, et al: A family study of bipolar I disorder in adolescence: early onset of symptoms linked to increased familial loading and lithium resistance. J Affect Disord 15:255–268, 1988

Sylvester CE, Hyde TS, Reichler RJ: The diagnostic interview for children and personality inventory for children in studies of children at risk for anxiety disorders or depression. J Am Acad Child Adolesc Psychiatry 26:668–675, 1987

Szatmari P, Boyle M, Offord DR: ADDH and conduct disorder: degree of diagnostic overlap and differences among correlates. J Am Acad Child Adolesc Psychiatry 28:865–872, 1989

Taylor EA: Childhood hyperactivity. Br J Psychiatry 149:562–573, 1986

Taylor E, Schachar R, Thorley G, et al: Conduct disorder and hyperactivity, I: separation of hyperactivity and antisocial conduct in British child psychiatric patients. Br J Psychiatry 149:760–767, 1986a

Taylor E, Everitt B, Thorley G, et al: Conduct disorder and hyperactivity, II: a cluster analytic approach to the identification of a behavioural syndrome. Br J Psychiatry 149:768–777, 1986b

Thorley G: Hyperkinetic syndrome of childhood: clinical characteristics. Br J Psychiatry 144:16–24, 1984

Varley CK, Trupin EW: Double-blind administration of methylphenidate to mentally retarded children with attention deficit disorder: a preliminary study. Am J Ment Defic 86:560–566, 1982

Weinberg WA, McLean A, Snider RL, et al: Depression, learning disability and school behavior problems. Psychol Rep 64:275–283, 1989

Weiss G, Hechtman L, Perlman T, et al: Hyperactives as young adults: a controlled prospective ten-year follow-up of 75 children. Arch Gen Psychiatry 36:675–681, 1979

Weiss G, Hechtman L, Milroy T, et al: Psychiatric status of hyperactives as adults: a controlled prospective 15-year follow-up of 63 hyperactive children. Journal of the American Academy of Child Psychiatry 24:211–220, 1985

Werry JS, Reeves JC, Elkind GS: Attention deficit, conduct, oppositional, and anxiety disorders in children, I: a review of research on differentiating characteristics. J Am Acad Child Adolesc Psychiatry 26:133–143, 1987

Wood D, Wender PH, Reimherr FW: The prevalence of attention deficit disorder, residual type, or minimal brain dysfunction, in a population of male alcoholic patients. Am J Psychiatry 140:95–98, 1983

Woolston JL, Rosenthal SL, Riddle MA, et al: Childhood comorbidity of anxiety/affective disorders and behavior disorders. J Am Acad Child Adolesc Psychiatry 28:707–713, 1989

World Health Organization: ICD-10 Chapter V: Mental and Behavioral Disorders: Diagnostic Criteria for Research. Geneva, Switzerland, World Health Organization, 1990

Chapter 10

Attention-Deficit Disorder Without Hyperactivity

Benjamin B. Lahey, Ph.D.,
Caryn L. Carlson, Ph.D., and
Paul J. Frick, Ph.D.

Statement and Significance of the Issues

The *DSM-IV Options Book* (American Psychiatric Association 1991) describes possible diagnostic criteria for attention-deficit disorder without hyperactivity (ADD/WO). The purposes of this chapter are to review evidence on the validity of such a diagnosis, to examine similarities to and differences from attention-deficit/hyperactivity disorder (ADHD), and to describe evidence relevant to the writing of specific diagnostic criteria for ADD/WO.

The publication of DSM-III (American Psychiatric Association 1980) provided a reconceptualization of the DSM-II (American Psychiatric Association 1968) diagnostic category of hyperkinetic reaction of childhood. Compared with DSM-II, the DSM-III criteria were far more specific and placed greater emphasis on inattention and impulsivity than on motor hyperactivity. This reconceptualization de-emphasized motor hyperactivity to the point that a subtype of the diagnosis was added for difficulties in inattention and impulsivity that were not accompanied by excessive motor activity. This diagnostic subtype, ADD/WO, had no counterpart in previous diagnostic nomenclatures, except perhaps for those children considered to exhibit minimal brain dysfunction who were normoactive or hypoactive (Clements and Peters 1962). Accordingly, no empirical literature existed at the time on ADD/WO, and the validity of the new type of attention-deficit disorder (ADD) was very much in question.

Since the publication of DSM-III in 1980, however, numerous studies have been conducted of children who meet DSM-III criteria for ADD/WO (Berry et al. 1985; C. L. Carlson, C. T. Alvarez, L. Needleman: Effects of task difficulty and reward on the cognitive styles of children with attention-deficit disorders with and without hyperactivity, unpublished manuscript, 1989; Conte et al. 1986; Edelbrock et al. 1984; Famularo and Fenton 1987; Frank and Ben-Nun 1988; Frick et al. 1991; Hynd et al. 1989, 1991; Lahey et al. 1987b; Maurer and Stewart 1980; Neeper et al. 1990; Saul and Ashby 1986; Ullman and Sleator 1985). Similarly, in a number of studies, nonreferred children considered to have ADD/WO according to experimental criteria based on DSM-III have been identified in school-based samples (Barkley et al. 1990, 1991; Carlson et al. 1986; King and Young 1982; Lahey et al. 1984; Pelham et al. 1981a; Sargeant and Scholton 1985a, 1985b). In addition, factor- and cluster-analytic studies of the symptoms of ADD have been conducted using large samples (E. A. Hart, B. B. Lahey, K. Hern, B. Applegate, and P. J. Frick: Dimensions and types of ADD: two replications, unpublished manuscript, 1991; Healy et al. 1987; Lahey et al. 1988; Pelham et al. 1992).

Most of the evidence on ADD/WO was not available when DSM-III-R (American Psychiatric Association 1987) was written, however. As a result, nagging questions about the validity of ADD/WO led to the downgrading of its status as a diagnostic entity in DSM-III-R. The original decision of the DSM-III-R committee was to eliminate the distinction between attention-deficit disorder with hyperactivity (ADD/H) and ADD/WO altogether and replace them with a single, uni- dimensional category termed *attention-deficit/hyperactivity disorder* (ADHD), which requires a child to display any 8 of 14 symptoms of inattention, impulsivity, and motor hyperactivity. In the final draft of DSM-III-R, however, a category of undifferentiated ADD was also included, to classify "disturbances in which the predominant feature is the persistence of developmentally inappropriate and marked inattention" (American Psychiatric Association 1987, p. 95).

These changes in DSM-III-R may have created diagnostic confusion in three ways. First, the use of the diagnostic category of undifferentiated ADD was tacitly discouraged by providing no diagnostic criteria for it. Second, the definition of ADHD is predicated on the assumption that symptoms of inattention are part of a single dimension that also includes impulsivity and motor hyperactivity, whereas the definition of undifferentiated ADD is based on the assumption that children can be deviant on symptoms of inattention alone. Third, it is likely that some children who would have been classified as ADD/WO would be classified as ADHD on the basis of their symptoms of inattention and impulsivity despite an absence of symptoms of motor hyperactivity (Lahey et al. 1990).

In this chapter, we review the existing research literature on ADD/WO with respect to the possible need to define a category of ADD/WO that is distinct from ADHD. Earlier reviews by Carlson (1986) and Lahey and Carlson (1991) addressed many of these same issues in more detail.

Method

Table 10–1 contains a summary of the studies reviewed, including a description of the source of subjects (clinic-referred or nonreferred school-based samples), number of subjects, subject selection criteria, and primary outcome measures. This literature contains both multivariate studies of the dimensions and types of ADD and studies comparing the maladjustment associated with ADD/WO and ADHD.

A cautionary note should be added before reviewing this literature. Although many of the studies cited used unadjusted DSM-III criteria for ADD/H and ADD/WO, many others used experimental criteria based on DSM-III. Whether a study should be included in the literature review was, therefore, a matter of judgment, because no data exist for judging the appropriateness of the various experimental criteria. It is likely, therefore, that the variability in findings in some areas of research on the ADD subtypes, such as cognitive characteristics, is due to variability in the experimental diagnostic criteria used.

Factor Analyses of ADD Symptoms

Perhaps the key question that must be resolved concerning the diagnosis of ADD concerns the number of dimensions of maladaptive behavior that underlie the disorder(s). The DSM-III definition of ADD was based on three hypothesized dimensions of ADD symptoms (inattention, impulsivity, and motor hyperactivity). As noted, the DSM-III-R definition of ADHD is based on the assumption of a single, unitary dimension of ADD symptoms; the definition of undifferentiated ADD assumes that inattention is distinct from impulsivity and motor hyperactivity. The most fundamental issue to be addressed concerning ADD diagnoses, therefore, is the number of dimensions of behavioral covariation among ADD symptoms.

Factor analyses of six samples in which the specific symptoms of ADD in DSM-III and DSM-III-R were used have been published. Lahey et al. (1988) conducted a factor analysis of teacher ratings of ADD symptoms. Two samples of children (667 nonreferred elementary school children and 86 children referred to a psychological evaluation center) were rated by their teachers on the SNAP (Swanson, Nolan, and Pelham) checklist (J. M. Swanson, W. J. Nolan, W. E. Pelham: A parent-teacher rating scale for operationalizing DSM-III symptoms of attention-deficit disorder, unpublished manuscript, 1981), and the clinic sample was also rated by clinicians on a set of 25 ADD symptoms that was derived from DSM-III, DSM-III-R, and a set of teacher rating scale items believed to be associated with ADD/WO. Separate factor analyses of teacher-completed SNAP checklists yielded two factors that were nearly identical for both the school-based and the clinic-referred samples. One factor consisted of all of the DSM-III motor hyperactivity items and the impulsivity items that referred most directly to the construct

Table 10–1. Summary of studies of attention-deficit disorder without hyperactivity

Study	Subjects	Source	Method of diagnosis	Assessment measures
Social, emotional, and behavioral characteristics				
Barkley et al. 1990	23 ADD/H, 17 ADD/WO	Clinic	Rating scales and clinical diagnosis	Rating scales, direct observations, and lab measures
Berry et al. 1985	94 ADD/H, 40 ADD/WO	Clinic	Rating scale	Rating scales and self-ratings
Carlson et al. 1987	36 ADD/H, 20 ADD/WO	Clinic	Structured diagnostic interviews	Peer sociometric
Edelbrock et al. 1984	18 ADD/H, 7 ADD/WO	Clinic	DSM-III diagnoses based on case histories	Rating scale
King and Young 1982	22 ADD/H, 9 ADD/WO	School	Rating scale and peer sociometrics	Rating scale
Lahey 1988	64 ADD/H, 39 ADD/WO	Clinic	Structured diagnostic interview	Parent, child, and teacher interview
Lahey et al. 1984	10 ADD/H, 20 ADD/WO	School	Rating scales	Rating scales and self-rating
Lahey et al. 1987b	41 ADD/H, 22 ADD/WO	Clinic	Structured diagnostic interview	Rating scales and self-rating
Maurer and Stewart 1980	52 ADD/WO	Clinic	Retrospective diagnosis	Parent interview items, files

Pelham et al. 1981a, 1981b	78 ADD/H, 36 ADD/WO	School	Rating scale	Rating scales and peer rating
Pliszka 1989	79 ADHD	Clinic	Rating scale, direct observation	
Pliszka 1992	107 ADHD	Clinic	Rating scale, direct observation, structured diagnostic interview	
Cognitive characteristics and academic underachievement				
Barkley et al. 1990	23 ADD/H, 17 ADD/WO	Clinic	Rating scales and clinical diagnosis	Rating scales, direct observations, and lab measures
Carlson et al. 1986	20 ADD/H, 15 ADD/WO	School	Rating scale	Cognitive test battery
Conte et al. 1986	8 ADD/H, 8 ADD/WO	Clinic	Rating scale and clinical diagnosis	Matching Familiar Figures Test and paired associate
Frank and Ben-Nun 1988	21 ADD/H, 11 ADD/WO	Clinic	Rating scale and school reports	Neuropsychological battery
Frick et al. 1991	97 ADD/H, 15 ADD/WO	Clinic	Structured diagnostic interview	Intelligence and academic achievement
Hynd et al. 1989	43 ADD/H, 22 ADD/WO	Clinic	Structured diagnostic interview	Reaction time, speeded classification task
Hynd et al. 1991	10 ADD/H, 10 ADD/WO	Clinic	Structured diagnostic interview	Intelligence and academic achievement

(continued)

Table 10–1. Summary of studies of attention deficit-disorder without hyperactivity *(continued)*

Study	Subjects	Source	Method of diagnosis	Assessment measures
Lahey et al. 1985	10 ADD/H, 20 ADD/WO	School	Rating scale	Teacher ratings of inattention
Neeper et al. 1990	148 ADD/H, 29 ADD/WO	Clinic	Structured diagnostic interview	Rating scale
Sargeant and Scholten 1985a, 1985b	8 ADD/H, 8 ADD/WO	School	Class observation, rating scale	Visual search task
Schaughency et al. 1988	43 ADD/H, 22 ADD/WO	Clinic	Structured diagnostic interview	Luria-Nebraska Neuropsychological Battery—Children's Revision
Medication outcome				
Barkley et al. 1991 (methylphenidate)	23 ADD/H, 17 ADD/WO		Clinic rating scales and clinical diagnosis	Rating scales, direct observations, lab measures
Famularo and Fenton 1987 (methylphenidate)	10 ADD/WO	Clinic	Structured diagnostic interview, school reports, rating scales	School grades
Saul and Ashby 1986 (pemoline)	21 ADD/H, 49 ADD/WO	Clinic	Rating scales	Rating scale
Ullman and Sleator 1985 (methylphenidate)	61 ADD/H, 13 ADD/WO	Clinic	Rating scale and clinical diagnosis	Rating scale

Factor analytic			
Hart et al., unpublished study, 1991	177 referred, 101 nonreferred	Clinic, school	Structured diagnostic interview and rating scale
Healy et al. 1987	85 nonreferred	School	Rating scale
Lahey et al. 1988	677 nonreferred, 63 referred	School, clinic	Rating scales, structured diagnostic interview
Pelham et al. 1992	931 nonreferred	School	Rating scale

Note. ADD/H = attention-deficit disorder with hyperactivity. ADD/WO = attention-deficit disorder without hyperactivity. ADHD = attention-deficit/hyperactivity disorder.

of impulsivity (e.g., "acts before thinking"). The second factor consisted of all of the inattention items and those impulsivity items in DSM-III that described disorganization and difficulty in finishing tasks.

Factor analyses of the clinicians' ratings also yielded inattention-disorganization and motor hyperactivity-impulsivity factors that were very similar to the factors derived from the SNAP ratings. In addition, a third factor was extracted that was composed of items that were not part of the DSM-III or DSM-III-R symptom lists, but were thought to characterize ADD/WO (e.g., "sluggish" or "forgetful"). All of the items loading most strongly on this third factor were not DSM-III symptoms and, therefore, were not included in the SNAP checklist items.

Healy et al. (1987) performed a similar factor analysis of teacher-completed SNAP checklists on a nonreferred sample of 85 children ages 6–13 years, but their version of the SNAP included both DSM-III and DSM-III-R symptoms of ADD (which were analyzed separately). The results of their factor analysis of DSM-III symptoms of ADD were nearly identical to those of Lahey et al. (1988). In addition, factor analysis of DSM-III-R symptoms yielded two similar factors, although they were less distinct than when DSM-III symptoms were analyzed.

Hart et al. (unpublished manuscript, 1991) performed a factor analysis of symptoms of ADD in two new samples (reported in Lahey and Carlson 1991). The first sample was a mixed group composed of 106 children ages 6–13 years, including 46 who were referred to a psychological evaluation center and 60 nonreferred school children. A principal components analysis of teacher-completed SNAP checklist items resulted in a two-factor solution that provided a clear replication of the earlier findings by Lahey et al. (1988). The ADD symptoms on the SNAP factored into two dimensions, one composed of inattention and disorganization symptoms and another composed of motor hyperactivity and impulsivity symptoms.

Hart et al. (unpublished manuscript, 1991) conducted additional factor analyses of parent and teacher responses to all questions concerning DSM-III and DSM-III-R symptoms of ADD on an updated version of the National Institute of Mental Health Diagnostic Interview Schedule for Children (Costello et al. 1984) for a second sample of 177 clinic-referred children, ages 7–12 years. The results of the factor analysis of teacher reports closely match the findings of previous studies. The analysis of parent reports of symptoms also yielded inattention-disorganization and motor hyperactivity-impulsivity factors, but the two factors were less distinct than in the factor analyses of teacher reports.

Pelham et al. (1992) reported the results of a factor analysis of teacher ratings of DSM-III-R symptoms of ADD and oppositional defiant disorder in 931 boys in regular education classrooms, grades kindergarten through eight. In addition to a factor on which oppositional symptoms had their primary loadings, a factor composed of inattention symptoms and a factor composed of motor hyperactivity and impulsivity symptoms were extracted.

The results of the six factor analyses reviewed in this section are summarized in Table 10–2. The segregation of symptoms into two factors was quite consistent for most symptoms. Only three symptoms failed to show a consistent pattern of unique factor loadings across at least five of the six studies ("difficulty sticking with a play activity," "excessive shifting from one activity to another," and "frequently engages in physically dangerous activities"). Indeed, engaging

Table 10–2. Summary of factor segregation of DSM-III and DSM-III-R attention-deficit disorder symptoms

- Symptoms with consistent unique loadings on the inattention-disorganization factor
    Difficulty organizing things
    Difficulty finishing tasks
    Difficulty following through on instructions
    Often loses things
    Easily distracted[a]
    Does not seem to listen[a]
    Difficulty concentrating/sustaining attention[a]
    Needs a lot of supervision[b]

- Symptoms with consistent unique loadings on the motor hyperactivity-impulsivity factor
    Excessive running or climbing
    Difficulty playing quietly
    Talks excessively
    Interrupts or intrudes
    Always on the go/driven by a motor
    Acts before thinking
    Calls out in class
    Difficulty staying seated
    Fidgets and squirms
    Difficulty waiting for turn
    Blurts out answers

- Symptoms with weak or inconsistent loadings
    Difficulty sticking with a play activity
    Excessive shifting of activities
    Engages in physically dangerous acts

[a]Symptoms with superscripts segregated consistently only when teachers were the respondents. All other symptoms segregated consistently; no symptoms segregated consistently based on parent reports only.
[b]Segregates consistently only when teachers were the respondents and only when samples were clinic-referred.

in dangerous activities never loaded uniquely on one factor.

The results of these factor analyses of the specific symptoms used in DSM-III and/or DSM-III-R not only are consistent with one another but also are consistent with the much larger literature on the factor analysis of standardized teacher and parent rating scales. As reviewed comprehensively by Quay (1986), factors similar to the inattention-disorganization and motor hyperactivity-impulsivity factors have been extracted in a large number of studies using a variety of scales with diverse samples.

Cluster Analytic Studies

The finding that ADD symptoms consistently factor into two dimensions suggests that it may be possible to identify two syndromes of ADD. On the other hand, the identification of two dimensions does not necessarily imply that there are two syndromes of ADD; all children who are judged to be in need of treatment could be deviant on both dimensions. Fortunately, this issue has been addressed using the technique of cluster analysis.

Lahey et al. (1988) subjected the two dimensions of ADD derived from the factor analysis of best-estimate clinicians' ratings (inattention-disorganization and motor hyperactivity-impulsivity) to cluster analysis. In that factor analysis, items reflecting sluggishness and drowsiness were also included to investigate additional hypotheses about ADD/WO. These items formed a sluggish tempo factor that was entered in the cluster analysis. The cluster analysis yielded two profiles of ADD based on different patterns of deviance on these three factors. One profile was high on inattention-disorganization and motor hyperactivity-impulsivity, but low on the sluggish tempo factor (resembling ADHD), and the second profile was low on motor hyperactivity-impulsivity, but high on both the inattention-disorganization and sluggish tempo dimensions (resembling ADD/WO). Not only did these two profiles resemble the two forms of ADD, but 75% of the children who had been independently given the DSM-III diagnosis of ADD/H fell in the first cluster, and 95% of the children given the diagnosis of ADD/WO fell in the second cluster.

Similarly, Hart et al. (unpublished manuscript, 1991) subjected the two dimensions of inattention-disorganization and motor hyperactivity-impulsivity based on factor analysis of teacher Diagnostic Interview Schedule for Children interviews to cluster analysis. As in Lahey et al. (1988), the analysis yielded two clear profiles of ADD: one in which the children were deviant on both inattention-disorganization and motor hyperactivity-impulsivity, and a second profile in which the children were deviant on only the inattention-disorganization dimension. Also like the earlier study (Lahey et al. 1988), there was a significant correspondence between the profiles yielded by the cluster analysis and best-estimate clinical diagnoses (based on both parent and teacher reports of symptoms). Indeed, all 15 children in the sample receiving a diagnosis of ADD/WO fell in the cluster that was deviant on only the inattention-disorganization factor.

Thus, there is now considerable taxometric evidence that the symptoms of ADD are multidimensional. Factor-analytic studies consistently indicate that covariation among the symptoms of ADD reflects two dimensions. One dimension consists of symptoms descriptive of motor hyperactivity and impulsive behavior, whereas the second dimension consists of symptoms describing inattention, disorganization, and difficulty completing tasks. Although this two-factor structure is more distinct when teachers are the informants, it is found for parent reports as well. It is important to note that, when scores on these two factors are subjected to cluster analysis, the two resulting profiles of deviance correspond well to DSM-III diagnoses of the two types of ADD. Additional evidence is needed before deciding whether ADD/WO is consistently characterized by sluggish tempo.

Comparisons of ADD/WO and ADHD

The phenomenological description of children with ADD/WO provided by recent studies rather consistently suggests that ADD/WO differs from ADHD in clinically important ways. This evidence is reviewed to determine if sufficient support exists to make a clinical distinction between separate categories of ADD/WO and ADHD in DSM-IV.

Emotional and behavioral correlates of ADD/WO and ADHD. A number of studies of both clinic-referred and school-identified samples suggest that children with ADD/WO differ from children with ADHD in terms of disruptive behavior and emotional problems. Pelham et al. (1981b) used a battery of teacher and peer ratings to compare experimentally defined groups with ADD identified from a school-based sample of children in kindergarten through the fifth grade. The SNAP checklist was used experimentally to classify 78 children as exhibiting ADHD (two standard deviations above the mean on hyperactivity, inattention, and impulsivity ratings) and 36 children as exhibiting ADD/WO (two standard deviations above the mean on inattention and impulsivity ratings and less than two standard deviations above the mean on hyperactivity ratings). Teachers rated children with ADHD significantly higher on the conduct problem factor of the Behavior Problem Checklist (Quay and Peterson 1975) and the SNAP impulsivity factor than children with ADD/WO. In addition, girls with ADD/WO were rated as more socially withdrawn by peers than girls with ADHD.

Using a school-based sample, Lahey et al. (1984) compared children experimentally classified as exhibiting the two ADDs (10 ADHD, 20 ADD/WO, and 20 nondisabled control children) on a battery of teacher, peer, and self-ratings. Groups with ADD were classified based on the Revised Behavior Problem Checklist

(Quay and Peterson 1983). Children with ADHD were required to score one standard deviation above the mean on both the attention problem-immaturity and motor excess factors, and children with ADD/WO were required to score one standard deviation above the mean on the attention problem-immaturity factor but less than one standard deviation above the mean on the motor excess factor. Teachers rated children with ADD/WO significantly higher on anxiety-withdrawal and nominated them as being more shy and socially withdrawn than nondisabled control children. Compared with control subjects, children with ADHD received significantly higher ratings on conduct disorder, socialized aggression, and psychotic behavior and were nominated by teachers as being more aggressive and guiltless.

The findings of these studies of experimentally classified school-based samples are useful because school-based samples are not subject to the referral biases that characterize clinic-referred samples. However, teacher rating scales and structured diagnostic interviews classify somewhat different groups of subjects (Lahey et al. 1987a, 1987b), and one cannot be confident that nonreferred samples exhibit maladaptive levels of the syndromes, even when using norm-referenced rating scales. Therefore, it is essential that studies also be conducted using children who are judged to be in need of clinical services. Fortunately, a number of such studies have been carried out, and they also suggest that children with ADHD are more often characterized by serious conduct problems, whereas children with ADD/WO are more likely to display anxiety, depression, and shyness.

Edelbrock et al. (1984) used DSM-III criteria to classify clinic-referred boys as ADD/H ($n = 18$) or ADD/WO ($n = 7$) based on clinical case records and then compared the groups with ADD with 62 clinic control subjects on subscales of the Teacher Rating Form of the Child Behavior Checklist (Edelbrock and Achenbach 1984). The children with diagnoses of ADD/WO obtained significantly higher ratings on social withdrawal and lower ratings on happiness, unpopularity, and aggression than the children with ADD/H.

Berry et al. (1985) similarly compared 40 children with ADD/WO and 94 children with ADD/H on a variety of behavioral characteristics. Subjects with ADD were selected from children referred to a learning disorders or pediatric neurology unit who were evaluated by one of the authors and diagnosed as ADD/H or ADD/WO according to DSM-III criteria. In addition, subjects were required to be older than 6 years and nonpsychotic and to have IQ scores greater than 70. A control group of 94 children was obtained from a sample of children who attended regular classes in a public school system and did not display attention or learning problems. Assessment measures included parent-completed historical/behavioral questionnaires, psychoeducational testing, an examination of school records, and teacher ratings on the Yale Children's Inventory (Shaywitz et al. 1986). Results indicated that subjects with ADD/H demonstrated cognitive deficits, fine motor problems, poor response to changes in routine, low self-esteem, and increased antisocial behavior. Children with ADD/WO, while also displaying cognitive deficits and low self-esteem, did not exhibit intractability, impulsivity, or increased antisocial behavior.

Lahey et al. (1987b) compared the behavioral characteristics of 41 clinic-referred children with DSM-III ADD/H and 22 clinic-referred children with ADD/WO who had been evaluated at a psychological diagnostic and referral center. A comprehensive assessment battery was administered, including structured diagnostic interviews of the child, parent, and teacher using the Schedule for Affective Disorders and Schizophrenia for School-Age Children (Puig-Antich and Chambers 1978), parent ratings on the Conners Parent Rating Scale (Conners 1989), and Revised Behavior Problem Checklist (Quay and Peterson 1983), and teacher ratings on the Conners Teacher Rating Scale (Conners 1989), the SNAP Checklist (Swanson et al., unpublished manuscript, 1981), and the Comprehensive Behavior Rating Scale for Children (CBRSC) (Neeper et al. 1990). Decisions about the presence of each DSM-III ADD symptom were made based on all sources of information, and ADD/H and ADD/WO diagnoses were then assigned based on DSM-III criteria.

Comparisons revealed markedly different behavior patterns for the two ADD groups. Children with ADD/WO were more likely to receive co-diagnoses of either anxiety or depressive disorders (43%) than children with ADD/H (10%). Although conduct disorders were more common among children with ADD/H (56%) than children with ADD/WO (36%), this latter difference was not statistically significant. In addition, teachers rated children with ADD/H significantly higher on teacher rating scale and CBRSC conduct problems scales than children with ADD/WO and rated children with ADD/H as significantly more impulsive (SNAP impulsivity) and less sluggish (CBRSC sluggish tempo) than children with ADD/WO. Finally, there were nonsignificant trends for children with ADD/WO to receive higher teacher rating scale tension anxiety ($P < .06$) and CBRSC anxiety-depression ($P < .08$) scores than children with ADD/H.

Lahey (1988) reported analyses of an extended version of the same sample described by Lahey et al. (1987b), which included 39 children with ADD/WO and 64 children with ADD/H, that confirmed the earlier findings, with two exceptions. In the larger sample, the group with ADD/H was significantly more likely to receive a co-diagnosis of conduct disorder (41%) than was the group with ADD/WO (20%), and the group with ADD/WO was significantly more likely to receive a co-diagnosis of anxiety disorder (28%–12%), but not a diagnosis of depressive disorder (9%–8%).

In this same sample, further analyses tested whether differences existed in specific patterns of conduct disorder between those children in the ADD groups who had an additional diagnosis of conduct disorder (Lahey 1988). Children with ADD/H and ADD/WO were compared on individual conduct disorder symptoms and composite indices of conduct disorder. These comparisons indicated that the ADD/H + conduct disorder group displayed a significantly greater total number of conduct disorder symptoms than the ADD/WO + conduct disorder group. In addition, the 23 children with ADD/H + conduct disorder were significantly more likely to display overt aggressive conduct disorder problems (bullying, fighting, cruelty to animals, homicidal acts, and stealing with confrontation of the victim) than children with ADD/WO + conduct disorder.

Barkley et al. (1990) reported very similar differences in the behavior problems of clinic-referred children with ADHD or ADD/WO. This study was exemplary both in the diagnostic procedures followed and in the broad range of dependent variables on which the groups were compared. Children with ADHD were again rated by their parents and teachers as more aggressive and antisocial than children with ADD/WO. Correspondingly, children with ADHD had been suspended from school more frequently and were more likely to have been placed in special education programs for children with behavior disorders.

Pliszka (1992), using a rather different strategy, also provided evidence that suggests that subgroups of children with ADD who differ in terms of level of hyperactivity/impulsivity also differ in terms of anxiety. Pliszka used a sample of 107 children who all met DSM-III-R criteria for ADHD. He compared those with comorbid overanxious disorder to those without overanxious disorder on a number of measures. The results indicated that the children with both ADHD and overanxious disorder displayed significantly less motoric behavior when observed completing an arithmetic task than children with ADHD alone. In addition, the finding that the children with ADHD and overanxious disorder made fewer commission errors on a continuous performance task can be interpreted as reflecting less impulsivity. Although all of Pliszka's subjects met DSM-III-R criteria for ADHD, these findings may be quite relevant to DSM-IV decision making about ADD/WO, because Lahey et al. (1990) reported that a sizable proportion of children with DSM-III ADD/WO meet DSM-III-R criteria for ADHD on the basis of their inattention symptoms. Considered in this light, many of the anxious children with ADHD who displayed lower levels of hyperactivity and impulsivity may well have exhibited the syndrome of ADD/WO that is under consideration for DSM-IV. It is important to note that this study (Pliszka 1992) replicated the major findings of an earlier study (Pliszka 1989) that used rating scales and observations rather than diagnostic interviews.

Peer relationships in ADD/WO and ADHD. Part of the maladjustment associated with ADD involves problems in peer relationships. Two early studies of school-based samples compared the sociometric status of children with ADHD and ADD/WO. King and Young (1982) and Lahey et al. (1984) reported that both ADD groups received significantly more "liked least" and fewer "liked most" peer nominations than control subjects. In the Lahey et al. study, however, children with ADD/H also received significantly more "liked least" ratings than children with ADD/WO. Similarly, Edelbrock et al. (1984) obtained teacher ratings of social competence on a clinic-referred sample of children with ADD/H and ADD/WO. Although both ADD groups showed social deficits, the children with ADD/H were rated as being more unpopular than the children with ADD/WO. In contrast, however, the group with ADD/WO received higher ratings of social withdrawal than the group with ADD/H.

Using a subsample of children from the Lahey et al. (1987b) clinic-referred sample, Carlson et al. (1987) examined the sociometric status of clinic-referred groups with DSM-III ADD/H and ADD/WO. When only children without co-diagnoses were compared, children with ADD/H ($n = 16$) received significantly more peer "liked least" nominations, and both children with ADD/H and children with ADD/WO ($n = 11$) received significantly fewer peer "liked most" nominations and lower social preference scores than 45 nondisabled control children. This finding is particularly important, because it suggests that clinic-referred youths with both types of ADD show impaired peer relations even when they do not exhibit other psychiatric problems. Similarly, Barkley et al. (1990) found that children with ADD/H were rated by teachers as having more problems in social competence, particularly in the areas of peer relations and peer provocation, than those with ADD/WO. However, children with ADD/WO were rated as significantly lower in social competence than both learning-disabled and nondisabled control groups.

Taken together, the results of these studies indicate that both children with ADD/H and those with ADD/WO are less popular with their peers than nonreferred children, even when these diagnoses are not accompanied by other comorbid diagnoses. There is some indication, however, that their patterns of unpopularity differ. Children with ADD/H tend to be more actively disliked than children with ADD/WO, who, in turn, appear to be more socially withdrawn.

Academic underachievement in ADD/WO and ADD/H. Academic underachievement is another problem frequently associated with ADD. Academic underachievement is typically defined as achievement in at least one academic area that is significantly below that predicted by a child's age and overall intelligence. A study of clinic-referred prepubertal boys with DSM-III-R ADHD estimated the prevalence of underachievement in either reading or mathematics to be 23% when regression artifacts and age were controlled statistically (Frick et al. 1991). It is important to note that this was a significantly higher proportion than that found in a clinic-referred control group and could not be attributed to the high degree of comorbidity of ADHD with conduct disorder. To determine whether ADD/H and

ADD/WO differ in their association with underachievement, Frick et al. divided the children with ADD into those with ADD/H ($n = 97$) and those with ADD/WO ($n = 15$) and did not find statistically significant differences. Several other studies support these findings that both children with ADD/H and children with ADD/WO are at risk for underachieving relative to their general intelligence, but that the two ADD groups do not differ from each other (Barkley et al. 1990; Carlson et al. 1986; Lahey 1988). Similarly, Lahey et al. (1984) found that both children with ADD/H and those with ADD/WO were rated by their teachers as having greater difficulties in learning than a nonimpaired control group, but the two groups with ADD did not differ significantly.

There are two notable exceptions to these findings of no differences between children with ADD/H and children with ADD/WO in terms of academic underachievement. Edelbrock et al. (1984) reported that, whereas only 16.7% of the children with ADD/H in their clinic-referred sample had failed at least one school grade, 71.4% of the group with ADD/WO had done so. Unfortunately, intelligence scores were not reported for the two groups, making it impossible to determine if the children were comparable in ability. Hynd et al. (1991) compared 10 children diagnosed with ADD/H with 10 children diagnosed with ADD/WO and found that a significantly higher proportion of children with ADD/WO (60%) had a discrepancy between their intelligence and academic achievement. In fact, none of the children with ADD/H were significant underachievers. The small sample size makes interpretation of these results difficult; firm conclusions on whether ADD/H and ADD/WO are differentially associated with academic underachievement cannot be made until these discrepant findings are clarified in future studies.

It is unfortunate that most of the existing studies of ADD have examined tested academic underachievement as their only measure of success in schooling. Clinical experience suggests that many children with ADD perform adequately on measures of academic achievement relative to their intelligence, but still cannot meet the demands of the classroom. For example, it is not uncommon for children who score well on tests of mathematics achievement to receive failing grades because of not completing homework or not finishing timed tests. It is important, therefore, that measures of both academic achievement and classroom performance be included in the DSM-IV field trials for the disruptive behavior disorders.

Patterns of inattention and cognitive style in ADD/WO and ADHD. There is some evidence that the pattern of dysfunction in attention or cognitive style is different in ADD/WO and ADHD, at least as perceived by adult raters. Two studies using teacher ratings of cognitive style found that children with ADD/WO differed from children with ADD/H and control children in showing a more sluggish and drowsy cognitive style. Lahey et al. (1985) compared nonreferred school children with ADD/H and ADD/WO on teacher ratings of the individual items on the attention problems-immaturity scale of the Revised Behavior Problem Checklist. Children with ADD/H were more likely to be rated as irresponsible, sloppy, impulsive, and distractible and likely to answer without thinking, whereas children with ADD/WO were more likely to be rated as sluggish and drowsy. Similar findings have been reported in validating the teacher-completed CBRSC rating scale (Neeper et al. 1990). Specifically, 29 clinic-referred children meeting DSM-III criteria for ADD/WO showed a significantly higher score on the CBRSC sluggish tempo scale than both a group of 148 children with ADD/H and a clinic control group of 101 children.

The behavioral descriptions of the attention problems exhibited by children with ADD/WO also seem to differ from those of children with ADD/H. In the large normative sample of 2,450 school-age children for the CBRSC, two separate scales describing attention problems were extracted through factor analyses (Neeper et al. 1990). The first scale was an inattention-disorganization scale, very similar to that found in most previous factor analyses and described earlier. However, a small three-item daydreaming scale was also found, with the symptoms of "daydreams a great deal," "stares into space," and "seems to be in a world of his or her own." When clinic-referred children with ADD/H and ADD/WO were compared on these scales, both groups differed from control children on the inattention-disorganization scale, but the two groups with ADD did not differ (Neeper et al. 1990). In contrast, children with ADD/WO showed higher scores than both children with ADD/H and control children on the daydreaming scale. Similar differences in teacher ratings of attention problems for children with ADD/H and ADD/WO were found by Barkley et al. (1990). Specifically, children with ADD/WO were found to be rated higher than children with ADD/H on the Child Behavior Checklist—Teacher Report Form (Achenbach and Edelbrock 1986) items "lost in a fog," "daydreaming or getting lost in thought," and "apathetic or unmotivated."

Cognitive/neuropsychological functioning in ADD/WO and ADD/H. Several studies have reported differences between ADD groups on laboratory measures of cognitive functioning. Sargeant and Scholton (1985a, 1985b) examined the attentional performance of eight hyperactive children (possibly equivalent to ADD/H), eight nonhyperactive children with attention problems (possibly equivalent to ADD/WO), and eight control children. On a high-speed visual search task, the performance of children with ADD/H was significantly slower and less accurate than that of control children, whereas children with ADD/WO differed from control children only in showing a slower search rate; this latter finding was accounted for by the authors as being due to children with ADD/WO being more likely than control children to trade speed for accuracy (Sargeant and Scholton 1985a).

In a second study, Sargeant and Scholton (1985b) manipulated instructional demands on the visual search task such that subjects were asked to emphasize speed, accuracy, or both. Again, children with ADD/H performed more slowly than children with ADD/WO and control children across all conditions, although accuracy of responses did not differentiate groups. In addition, only children with ADD/WO and nondisabled children were able to speed up their responses to meet task demands in the speed emphasis condition; children with ADD/H actually performed somewhat more slowly in this condition than in the "normal" instruction condition. Thus, children with ADD/H were described as showing deficits in resource allocation, because they were less able than children with ADD/WO or control children to change strategies to meet task demands. Interestingly, the performance of children with ADD/WO and control children conformed to a "fast guess" model (short latencies related to errors and long latencies related to accurate responding), whereas the performance of children with ADD/H did not, because their errors were sometimes related to fast and sometimes to slow latencies.

Frank and Ben-Nun (1988) compared 21 children with ADD/H and 11 children with ADD/WO on a neurological and neuropsychological assessment battery. Using parent and teacher ratings on Conners questionnaires, written teacher reports, and school psychological reports, children referred by school personnel to a pediatric neurology learning problem clinic were classified as ADD/H or ADD/WO based on DSM-III criteria. Comparisons between groups with ADD indicated that children with ADD/H showed significantly greater abnormality on a variety of soft neurological measures. The children with ADD/H also were more likely than children with ADD/WO to have a history of perinatal or neonatal abnormality (approximately 50% versus 12%, respectively), although no differences in likelihood of having an abnormal medical history or delayed speech or motor development emerged. Because normative data were available for cognitive measures, groups with ADD were compared with each other and with control subjects on these variables. Results indicated that, although both groups with ADD showed significantly poorer performance than control children on measures of visual perception, visual and auditory sequential memory, reading, and writing, the children with ADD/H showed significantly greater abnormalities than the children with ADD/WO in visual perception, visual sequential memory, and writing performance.

In a study of the cognitive performance of children with ADD/WO and ADD/H, Barkley et al. (1990) also found significant differences between the groups on laboratory cognitive performance tasks. Children with ADD/WO were found to have deficiencies in timed perceptual-motor tasks but did not exhibit deficits in impulsivity or sustained attention on a vigilance task. In contrast, the children with ADD/H exhibited no deficits on the timed perceptual-motor task, but did exhibit impulsive responding and difficulties in sustained attention. The group with ADD/H, but not the group with ADD/WO, exhibited difficulties with neuropsychological tasks that are thought to be sensitive to frontal lobe functioning.

Although these studies of laboratory cognitive tasks are suggestive, several controlled studies have failed to document differences between the ADD groups. Carlson et al. (1986) administered a cognitive test battery (including a test of visual-motor integration, a visual match-to-sample task, a Stroop test, a rapid naming task, and measures of language functioning, school achievement, and intelligence) to children with ADD/WO, children with ADD/H, and nondisabled control children who were identified by teacher ratings from a school population. Although both groups with ADD showed deficits compared with control children, few cognitive differences between children with ADD/H and ADD/WO emerged.

Conte et al. (1986) administered the Matching Familiar Figures Test and variously paced conditions of paired associate learning tests to eight children with ADD/H and eight children with ADD/WO. All subjects had been referred for assessment of learning problems and were classified according to teacher ratings on DSM-III symptom checklists and the Conners Teacher Rating Scale. Paired associates learning tests were administered to subjects under two conditions of presentation rate (fast or slow) and two conditions of list type (fixed rate or mixed rate). Nondisabled control children performed better than the children with ADD/H and ADD/WO in all conditions, but the groups with ADD/H and ADD/WO did not differ significantly. On the Matching Familiar Figures Test, children with ADD/WO had significantly shorter latencies than either children with ADD/H or control children and made significantly more errors than control children. Although these results would appear to indicate that children with ADD/WO were more impulsive than children with ADD/H, the authors noted that the latency scores of both groups with ADD were in the average range according to norms.

Hynd et al. (1989) examined the speed and efficiency of neurocognitive processing in 43 children with ADD/H, 22 children with ADD/WO, and 16 clinic control subjects. Subjects completed four reaction time tasks, one simple visual reaction time task, and three speeded classification tasks based on Posner's (1978) paradigm in which same-different decisions were required about stimuli involving physical match letter pairs, name match letter pairs, and letter string matches. Analyses revealed that children with ADD/H performed significantly more slowly than control subjects on letter string matches and performed significantly more variably in name match and letter string match conditions. Children with ADD/WO did not differ significantly from children with ADD/H or control children in speed or variability of response in any of the four conditions. No significant differences in speeded classification error rates among groups were obtained. When only the 16 children with ADD/H and 7 children with ADD/WO without other co-diagnoses were included in analyses, the only significant group difference was that children with ADD/H performed more variably than control subjects on the letter string match task.

Schaughency et al. (1988) compared the same clinic-referred sample on the Luria-Nebraska Neuropsychological Battery Children's Revision (Golden 1981). Both groups with ADD showed significantly more errors on the battery than a clinic control group of children without ADD. In addition, both groups with ADD were lower on Wechsler Intelligence Scale for Children—Revised full scale and verbal intelligence scores (Wechsler 1974). When full scale intelligence was covaried, however, there were no significant differences among the groups on the Luria-Nebraska battery scores, suggesting that the apparent neuropsychological deficits were merely reflective of the lower intelligence scores of children with ADD/H (96.1) and ADD/WO (96.6) compared with the clinic control group (109.0).

Effects of stimulant medication for ADD/WO and ADD/H. One of the more persuasive arguments that could be made for the validity of differentiating ADD into two types of disorders would be differential responses to treatment. Given the wide acceptance of stimulant medication and the large amount of research on its efficacy in treating ADD/H, it is not surprising that initial attempts to test the differential response to treatment of the types of ADD have focused on the response to stimulants. However, only four studies have described the use of stimulant medication with children with ADD/WO, and only one of these provided data directly comparing the response of children with ADD/H with that of children with ADD/WO.

Saul and Ashby (1986) reported that 38 of 49 subjects with ADD/WO treated at a diagnostic and developmental center were "responders" (evidently defined by "degree of response" indicated by parent ratings on the Conners Parent Questionnaire) to pemoline treatment. Subjects with ADD/WO were required to display an idiosyncratic list of characteristics (inattention, impulsive, short tempered, lack of persistence, deficient interpersonal relations, and learning problems) assessed in parent interviews or ratings on the Conners Parent Questionnaire. It is difficult to evaluate these results because of the lack of standard diagnostic criteria and because it is not clear how decisions about changing dosage were made or what specific criteria were used for defining "responders."

Ullmann and Sleator (1985) reported that a group of 86 children with ADD, including 13 with ADD/WO, showed significant improvements on .3, .5, or .8 mg/kg methylphenidate when compared with placebo. Again, it is impossible to draw conclusions from this study, because the criteria for diagnosing ADD/WO were unclear (although diagnoses were evidently based on systematic assessments) and because results from children with ADD/WO and ADD/H children were not distinguished and compared.

Famularo and Fenton (1987) examined the effects of methylphenidate on the school grades of 10 children with ADD/WO in a nonblind pre-post design study. Subjects were diagnosed as ADD/WO according to DSM-III criteria using information from parent interviews, school information, and parent and teacher ratings on a 76-item questionnaire. Dosages of methylphenidate ranged from 0.4 to 1.2 mg/kg/day administered in two dosages; the criteria used for determining dosage were not described. School grades were obtained for three consecutive grading periods representing predrug, drug treatment, and withdrawal of drug treatment periods. Results indicated that children obtained significantly higher grades during drug treatment than during either the predrug or withdrawal grading periods, with 8 of the 10 children showing improvement in at least three of five targeted subjects.

The only adequate test of possible differences in response to methylphenidate by children with ADD/WO and children with ADD/H has been provided by Barkley et al. (1991). In this study, 23 children with ADD/H and 17 with ADD/WO were given 5-, 10-, or 15-mg doses of methylphenidate in a triple-blind placebo-controlled crossover design using parent and teacher ratings, laboratory tests, and direct observations during academic tasks to assess drug effects. Although the groups did not differ significantly on any dependent measure, significantly more children with ADD/WO were found to be nonresponders or to respond best to the lowest dose in comparison with the children with ADD/H, 71% of whom responded best to the highest dose.

Taken together, these studies suggest that children with ADD/WO may respond favorably to stimulant medication in much the same manner as children with ADD/H, although perhaps at lower dosages. A potentially important cautionary note has been provided by Pliszka (1989), who found that children with clinically significant ADD with lower levels of hyperactivity/impulsivity (and higher levels of anxiety) responded to methylphenidate no better than to placebo, whereas children with ADD with higher levels of hyperactivity/impulsivity (and lower levels of anxiety) responded better to methylphenidate than to placebo. It may be, then, that at least some children with ADD/WO do not respond favorably to methylphenidate compared with placebo. This should be a topic of considerable additional research.

Discussion

The empirical literature has done much to address doubts about the validity of ADD/WO as a clinical syndrome. There is now clear evidence that substantial numbers of children are referred for mental health services who are maladjusted in some aspects of their development, most often in social and academic areas, and who have difficulties with inattention, but who are not motorically hyperactive.

Studies suggest clinically significant differences between the putative syndromes of ADD/WO and ADHD. Children with ADD/WO appear to be characterized by fewer serious conduct problems, less impulsivity, greater anxiety, and greater depressed mood. As with ADHD, children with ADD/WO are also consistently found to be unpopular with their peers. However, children with ADD/WO are often perceived as socially withdrawn and less likely to be actively rejected than children with ADHD. There is also emerging evidence that children with ADD/WO differ from those with ADHD in the behavioral descriptions of their cognitive style and types of attentional difficulties, with children with ADD/WO appearing to daydream more often, to be forgetful, and to be more sluggish and drowsy. There is also suggestive, but inconsistent, evidence that the two groups of ADD differ on laboratory measures of cognitive functioning. However, both ADD groups appear to exhibit similar deficits in school performance and academic achievement. Unfortunately, the two areas that may be of most importance in testing the validity of the subtypes of ADD—response to treatment and long-term prognosis—have been the subject of the least empirical study. Little information is currently available about the treatment of ADD/WO, and nothing is known about its long-term prognosis. Longitudinal and treatment studies of children with ADD/WO, particularly in comparison with children with ADD/H, are clearly a priority for the future.

The weight of currently available taxometric evidence appears to argue for diagnostic conceptualizations of ADD that are based on two dimensions of maladjustment: one composed primarily of symptoms of inattention and disorganization and the other composed of symptoms of motor hyperactivity and impulsive behavior. Based on cluster-analytic studies, it appears that one syndrome is characterized by dysfunction in both attention and motor hyperactivity (ADHD) and that a second syndrome is characterized by dysfunction in attention, but not in motor hyperactivity/impulsivity (ADD/WO). Because some evidence suggests that ADD/WO is also characterized by sluggishness, drowsiness, daydreaming, and forgetfulness, it is important for these additional symptoms to be considered in the DSM-IV field trials as well.

Recommendations

Since the publication of DSM-III, a useful empirical literature has emerged on the validity of a distinction between ADD/H and ADD/WO. Based on this evidence, a distinct diagnostic category of ADD/WO should be considered for DSM-IV and should be evaluated in the DSM-IV field trials for the disruptive behavior disorders.

Accordingly, possible new criteria for ADD/WO have been proposed in the *DSM-IV Options Book* based on a two-dimensional approach. Two alternatives have been proposed for ADD/WO. In the first option, ADD/WO would be defined on the basis of clinically significant dysfunction in inattention, disorganization, distractibility, and lack of completion of tasks in the absence of close supervision, but the absence of dysfunctional levels of motor hyperactivity and impulsivity. This option would employ the same list of inattention symptoms for both ADHD and ADD/WO and would distinguish the two disorders on the basis of a list of symptoms of motor hyperactivity/impulsivity. The exact symptoms in the two lists and the diagnostic thresholds (cut scores) for each list will be determined in the DSM-IV field trials and by reference to other data sets.

The second option in the *DSM-IV Options Book* is based on a different list of inattention symptoms. This list does not include the symptom of "distractibility," which, as noted, some studies have found to be more characteristic of ADHD than of ADD/WO. In addition, the list of inattention symptoms in the second option for ADD/WO includes symptoms of sluggishness, drowsiness, daydreaming, and forgetfulness. The choice between these two approaches will be made on the basis of the relative validity and reliability of the two options. It is likely that neither option will be chosen in exactly its present form; detailed analyses of the diagnostic utility of individual symptoms and other empirical and clinical considerations will likely lead to changes.

References

Achenbach JM, Edelbrock CS: Manual for the Child Behavior Checklist and Revised Child Behavior Profile. Burlington, VT, University of Vermont, Department of Psychiatry, 1986

American Psychiatric Association: Diagnostic and Statistical Manual of Mental Disorders, 2nd Edition. Washington, DC, American Psychiatric Association, 1968

American Psychiatric Association: Diagnostic and Statistical Manual of Mental Disorders, 3rd Edition. Washington, DC, American Psychiatric Association, 1980

American Psychiatric Association: Diagnostic and Statistical Manual of Mental Disorders, 3rd Edition, Revised. Washington, DC, American Psychiatric Association, 1987

American Psychiatric Association: DSM-IV Options Book: Work in Progress. Washington, DC, American Psychiatric Association, 1991

Barkley RA, DuPaul GJ, McMurray MB: Comprehensive evaluation of attention deficit disorder with and without hyperactivity as defined by research criteria. J Consult Clin Psychol 58:775–789, 1990

Barkley RA, DuPaul GJ, McMurray MB: Attention deficit disorder with and without hyperactivity: clinical response to three dose levels of methylphenidate. Pediatrics 87:519–531, 1991

Berry CA, Shaywitz SE, Shaywitz BA: Girls with attention deficit disorder: a silent majority? a report on behavioral and cognitive characteristics. Pediatrics 76:801–809, 1985

Carlson CL: Attention deficit disorder without hyperactivity: a review of preliminary experimental evidence, in Advances in Clinical Child Psychology, Vol 9. Edited by Lahey BB, Kazdin AE. New York, Plenum, 1986, pp 153–175

Carlson CL, Lahey BB, Neeper R: Direct assessment of the cognitive correlates of attention deficit disorders with and without hyperactivity. Journal of Behavioral Assessment and Psychopathology 8:69–86, 1986

Carlson CL, Lahey BB, Frame CL, et al: Sociometric status of clinic-referred children with attention deficit disorder with and without hyperactivity. J Abnorm Child Psychol 15:537–547, 1987

Clements SD, Peters J: Minimal brain dysfunctions in the school-age child. Arch Gen Psychiatry 6:185–197, 1962

Conners CK: Conners' Parent and Teacher Rating Scales. Toronto, Canada, Multi-Health Systems, 1989

Conte R, Kinsbourne M, Swanson J, et al: Presentation rate effects on paired associate learning by attention deficit disordered children. Child Dev 57:681–687, 1986

Costello AJ, Edelbrock CS, Kalas R, et al: The NIMH Diagnostic Interview Schedule for Children. Worcester, MA, University of Massachusetts Medical School, 1984

Edelbrock C, Achenbach TM: The teacher version of the Child Behavior Profile, I: boys 6–11. J Consult Clin Psychol 52:207–217, 1984

Edelbrock C, Costello AJ, Kessler MD: Empirical corroboration of the attention deficit disorder. Journal of the American Academy of Child Psychiatry 23:285–290, 1984

Famularo R, Fenton T: The effect of methylphenidate on school grades in children with attention deficit disorder without hyperactivity: a preliminary report. J Clin Psychiatry 142:112–114, 1987

Frank Y, Ben-Nun Y: Toward a clinical subgrouping of hyperactive and nonhyperactive attention deficit disorder: results of a comprehensive neurological and neuropsychological assessment. Journal of Diseases of Children 142:153–155, 1988

Frick PJ, Kamphaus RW, Lahey BB, et al: Academic underachievement and the disruptive behavior disorders. J Consult Clin Psychol 59:289–294, 1991

Golden CJ: The Luria-Nebraska Children's Battery: theory and formulation, in Neuropsychological Assessment and the School-Aged Child: Issues and Procedures. Edited by Hynd GW, Obrzut JC. New York, Grune & Stratton, 1981, pp 277–302

Healy JM, Halperin JM, Newcorn J, et al: The factor structure of ADD items in DSM-III and DSM-III-R. Paper presented at the annual meeting of the American Academy of Child and Adolescent Psychiatry, Los Angeles, CA, 1987

Hynd GW, Nieves N, Conner R, et al: Speed of neurocognitive processing in children with attention deficit disorder with and without hyperactivity. Journal of Learning Disabilities 22:573–579, 1989

Hynd GW, Lorys AR, Semrud-Clikeman M, et al: Attention deficit disorders without hyperactivity: a distinct behavioral and neurocognitive syndrome. J Child Neurol 6:35–41, 1991

King C, Young RD: Attentional deficits with and without hyperactivity: teacher and peer perceptions. J Abnorm Child Psychol 10:483–495, 1982

Lahey BB: Attention deficit disorder without hyperactivity: issues in validity. Paper presented at the annual meeting of the Bloomingdale Conference on Attention Deficit Disorder, Seattle, WA, 1988

Lahey BB, Carlson CL: Validity of the diagnostic category of attention deficit disorder without hyperactivity: a review of the literature. Journal of Learning Disabilities 24:110–120, 1991

Lahey BB, Schaughency EA, Strauss CC, et al: Are attention deficit disorders with and without hyperactivity: similar or dissimilar disorders? Journal of the American Academy of Child Psychiatry 23:302–309, 1984

Lahey BB, Schaughency EA, Frame CL, et al: Teacher ratings of attention problems in children experimentally classified as exhibiting attention deficit disorders with and without hyperactivity. Journal of the American Academy of Child Psychiatry 24:613–616, 1985

Lahey BB, McBurnett K, Piacentini JC, et al: Agreement of parent and teacher rating scales with comprehensive clinical assessments of attention deficit disorder with hyperactivity. Journal of Psychopathology and Behavioral Assessment 9:429–439, 1987a

Lahey BB, Schaughency EA, Hynd GW, et al: Attention deficit disorder with and without hyperactivity: comparison of behavioral characteristics of clinic-referred children. J Am Acad Child Adolesc Psychiatry 26:718–723, 1987b

Lahey BB, Pelham WE, Schaughency EA, et al: Dimensions and types of attention deficit disorder with hyperactivity in children: a factor and cluster analytic approach. J Am Acad Child Adolesc Psychiatry 27:330–335, 1988

Lahey BB, Loeber R, Stouthamer-Loeber M, et al: Comparison of DSM-III and DSM-III-R diagnoses of prepubertal children: changes in prevalence and validity. J Am Acad Child Adolesc Psychiatry 29:620–626, 1990

Maurer RG, Stewart MA: Attention deficit without hyperactivity in a child psychiatry clinic. J Clin Psychiatry 417:232–233, 1980

Neeper R, Lahey BB, Frick PJ: Comprehensive Behavior Rating Scale for Children. San Antonio, TX, Psychological Corporation, 1990

Pelham WE, Atkins MS, Murphy HA: Attention deficit disorder with and without hyperactivity: definitional issues and correlates. Paper presented at the annual meeting of the American Psychological Association, Los Angeles, CA, 1981a

Pelham WE, Atkins MS, Murphy HA, et al: Operationalization and validation of attention deficit disorders. Paper presented at the annual meeting of the Association for the Advancement of Behavior Therapy, Toronto, Canada, 1981b

Pelham WE, Gnagy EM, Greenslade KE, et al: Teacher ratings of DSM-III-R symptoms for the disruptive behavior disorders. J Am Acad Child Adolesc Psychiatry 31:210–218, 1992

Pliszka SR: Effect of anxiety on cognition, behavior, and stimulant response in ADHD. J Am Acad Child Adolesc Psychiatry 28:882–887, 1989

Pliszka SR: Comorbidity of attention-deficit hyperactivity disorder and overanxious disorder. J Am Acad Child Adolesc Psychiatry 31:197–203, 1992

Posner MJ: Chronometric Explorations of Mind. Hillsdale, NJ, Lawrence Erlbaum Associates, 1978

Puig-Antich J, Chambers W: The Schedule for Affective Disorders and Schizophrenia for School-Aged Children. New York, New York State Psychiatric Institute, 1978

Quay HC: Classification, in Psychopathological Disorders of Childhood. Edited by Quay HC, Werry JS. New York, Wiley, 1986, pp 1–34

Quay HC, Peterson DR: Manual for the Behavior Problem Checklist. Coral Gables, FL, University of Miami, 1975

Quay HC, Peterson DR: Interim manual for the Revised Behavior Problem Checklist. Coral Gables, FL, University of Miami, 1983

Sargeant JA, Scholton CA: On data limitations in hyperactivity. J Child Psychol Psychiatry 26:111–124, 1985a

Sargeant JA, Scholten CA: On resource strategy limitations in hyperactivity: cognitive impulsivity reconsidered. J Child Psychol Psychiatry 26:97–109, 1985b

Saul RC, Ashby CD: Measurement of whole blood serotonin as a guide for prescribing psychostimulant medication for children with attentional deficits. Clin Neuropharmacol 9:189–195, 1986

Schaughency EA, Lahey BB, Hynd GW, et al: Neuropsychological test performance and the attention deficit disorders: clinical utility of the Luria-Nebraska Neuropsychological Battery Children's Revision. J Consult Clin Psychol 57:112–116, 1988

Shaywitz SE, Schnell C, Shaywitz BA, et al: Yale Children's Inventory (YCI): an instrument to assess children with attentional deficits and learning disabilities. Journal of Child Psychology 14:347–364, 1986

Ullman RK, Sleator EK: Attention deficit disorder children with or without hyperactivity: which behaviors are helped by stimulants? Clin Pediatr (Phila) 24:547–551, 1985

Wechsler D: Manual for the Wechsler Intelligence Scale for Children—Revised. New York, Psychological Corporation, 1974

Chapter 11

Oppositional Defiant Disorder and Conduct Disorder

Benjamin B. Lahey, Ph.D., Rolf Loeber, Ph.D.,
Herbert C. Quay, Ph.D., Paul J. Frick, Ph.D., and
James Grimm, M.D.

Statement and Significance of the Issues

There are many important decisions concerning the psychiatric disorders to be defined in DSM-IV, including those disorders affecting children and adolescents. This chapter summarizes the issues that must be resolved with respect to the diagnoses of oppositional defiant disorder and conduct disorder.

The diagnoses of oppositional defiant disorder and conduct disorder are intended to distinguish patterns of disruptive behavior that "differ in severity" (American Psychiatric Association 1987, p. 56). As defined in both DSM-III (American Psychiatric Association 1980) and DSM-III-R (American Psychiatric Association 1987), oppositional defiant disorder is an enduring pattern of oppositional, irritable, and defiant behavior, whereas conduct disorder is a persistent pattern of more serious violations of the rights of others and social norms. Modifications of the DSM-III criteria for both disorders were made for DSM-III-R that increased the threshold of severity and correspondingly decreased the prevalence of both disorders (Lahey et al. 1990). Less specific and more prevalent symptoms were eliminated from the definitions of both oppositional defiant disorder (e.g., "stubborn" and "violates minor rules") and conduct disorder (e.g., "violates important rules" and "bullies"), and the minimum number of symptoms was raised to five for DSM-III-R oppositional defiant disorder and to three for DSM-III-R conduct disorder. These changes apparently resulted in improvements in the concurrent validity of the diagnosis of conduct disorder (Lahey et al. 1990).

Perhaps the most fundamental issue facing the DSM-IV Disruptive Behavior Disorders Committee is the clinical utility of the distinction between oppositional defiant disorder and conduct disorder. If one were to use published clinical research as a barometer of wider patterns of diagnostic practice, the distinction between oppositional defiant disorder and conduct disorder in DSM-III and DSM-III-R has been honored more by its nonobservance than its observance. Indeed, oppositional defiant disorder and conduct disorder have been combined in a single category in nearly all published studies since the publication of DSM-III (e.g., Anderson et al. 1987; Bird et al. 1988; Offord et al. 1987; Werry et al. 1987), except for the few studies that have specifically addressed the validity of the diagnosis of oppositional defiant disorder. This decision clearly reflects an assumption that oppositional defiant disorder and conduct disorder are similar enough to combine and still draw meaningful conclusions about the combined oppositional defiant disorder/conduct disorder group, at least in research. It is important, therefore, for the DSM-IV committee to weigh the evidence relevant to the distinction of these two diagnostic categories.

Three options for the diagnoses of oppositional defiant disorder and conduct disorder are presented in the *DSM-IV Options Book* (American Psychiatric Association 1991). The first option is to adopt DSM-III-R criteria for oppositional defiant disorder and conduct disorder without changes.

The second option is to retain the distinction between oppositional defiant disorder and conduct disorder in the same form as in DSM-III-R, but to make some changes in criteria if supported by data from the DSM-IV field trials for the disruptive behavior disorders and other sources. The specific changes proposed for consideration in this second option are adding a few new symptoms of conduct disorder that may increase diagnostic validity, especially for girls; moving some symptoms previously conceptualized as part of conduct disorder to oppositional defiant disorder (some aspects of fighting and lying); and reconsidering diagnostic thresholds.

The third option proposed for oppositional defiant disorder and conduct disorder is to eliminate much (but not all) of the distinction between oppositional defiant disorder and conduct disorder by considering them to be two developmentally staged levels of the same disorder. In this "levels of disruptive behavior disorder" option, oppositional defiant disorder would still be identified (using criteria similar to those in DSM-III-R), but it would be considered to be a milder form of conduct disorder rather than a separate disorder. This option further distinguishes two developmentally staged levels of severity of conduct disorder from within the criteria for conduct disorder. Thus, in this option, three developmental levels of a single disorder would be distinguished based on median age at onset and severity of misconduct. It is assumed that youth who progress to the most severe level of disorder will have previously met criteria for the earlier levels, but that not all youth who reach the first or second level will progress to higher levels. In this chapter, we review evidence relevant to each of the three options proposed for oppositional defiant disorder and conduct disorder.

Method

This review is based on relevant literature accessed using a combination of computer searches and reference to personal libraries. Some sections are based on recent exhaustive literature reviews by the authors and our colleagues that are cited in the text. Other sections are based on more selective reviews of literature that are believed to be relevant to the key issues to be resolved for DSM-IV in the area of oppositional behavior and conduct problems.

Results and Discussion

Statistical Covariation Among Symptoms of Oppositional Defiant Disorder and Conduct Disorder

Three papers have reviewed the large literature on the statistical covariation among the symptoms of oppositional defiant disorder and conduct disorder (Frick et al. 1991; Loeber et al. 1991; Quay 1986a). This literature consistently shows oppositional symptoms (e.g., stubborn, defiant, irritable, argumentative, and provocative behaviors) to factor together in both clinic and community samples. Similarly, a group of conduct disorder symptoms (e.g., stealing, truancy, and running away from home) also emerges consistently on a separate factor. However, several symptoms of conduct disorder (e.g., fighting, bullying, and lying) typically emerge on the same factor with the oppositional defiant disorder symptoms rather than with covert symptoms of conduct disorder.

This one type of evidence suggests that some forms of antisocial behavior designated as symptoms of conduct disorder in DSM-III and DSM-III-R might be more appropriately considered to be symptoms of oppositional defiant disorder than symptoms of conduct disorder. Because such a conclusion would result in a radical change in the way in which oppositional defiant disorder and conduct disorder are defined, the evidence relevant to such a reconceptualization should be weighed carefully. Importantly, the results of the quantitative meta-analysis of the existing factor-analytic literature conducted by Frick et al. (1993) may allow an alternative conclusion.

Multidimensional scaling was used to summarize the existing factor-analytic literature by Frick et al. (1993). This statistical procedure was used to summarize statistical patterns of co-occurrence among symptoms of oppositional defiant disorder and conduct disorder in 64 factor analyses. When one dimension of co-occurrence was extracted, the symptoms of oppositional defiant disorder and four symptoms of conduct disorder involving physical aggression clustered at one pole, and the remaining nonaggressive symptoms of conduct disorder clustered at the other pole. However, the multidimensional scaling analysis indicated that the extraction of two dimensions was more justifiable on statistical grounds. When the second dimension of co-occurrence was extracted, the symptoms of conduct disorder were separated from the symptoms of oppositional defiant disorder (Frick et al. 1993; Loeber et al. 1991).

This quantitative summary of factor analyses suggests a complex relationship between the symptoms of oppositional defiant disorder and conduct disorder. The fact that the symptoms of oppositional defiant disorder and the symptoms of conduct disorder involving mild physical aggression emerged on the same pole of the first dimension to be extracted suggests a pattern of intercorrelation among these symptoms across the 64 factor-analytic studies. The meta-analysis also suggests that the symptoms of conduct disorder that emerged at the opposite pole of the first dimension to be extracted (mostly nonaggressive symptoms) form a group of intercorrelated misbehaviors that is meaningfully distinct from the oppositional and aggressive behaviors. However, the extraction of the second dimension resulted in the separation of the symptoms of oppositional defiant disorder from all symptoms of conduct disorder, suggesting that the symptoms of oppositional defiant disorder are *partially* distinct from symptoms of conduct disorder (especially lying, fighting, and bullying) in terms of statistical covariation, although they clearly share much common variance. However, many factors other than statistical covariation must be taken into account in making decisions about the validity of the distinction between oppositional defiant disorder and conduct disorder.

Age at Onset of Symptoms of Oppositional Defiant Disorder and Conduct Disorder

Some evidence now exists on the age at onset of behavior problems that may shed light on the putative distinction between oppositional defiant disorder and conduct disorder. Loeber et al. (1991) reviewed findings on the relationship of these symptoms to age. It appears that most symptoms of oppositional defiant disorder are common by at least age 4–5 years and then decline in prevalence with increasing age in most children (Achenbach and Edelbrock 1981; Campbell 1990; MacFarlane et al. 1962). Interestingly, these same studies suggest that the symptoms of conduct disorder that were shown in the studies discussed to be most correlated with oppositional defiant disorder symptoms (lying, fighting, and bullying) are also present at early ages and decline with increasing age, at least in children without clinically significant behavioral disturbance.

In contrast, the nonaggressive symptoms of conduct disorder that were found above to factor separately (e.g., stealing, running away from home, and truancy) are uncommon before about age 10–11 years and increase in prevalence as the youth grow older. Several serious forms of aggression (e.g., rape, mugging, homicide) are also rare before age 10–11 years and increase in prevalence into early adulthood (Farrington 1986; Farrington et al. 1990; LeBlanc and Frechette 1989; Loeber 1988). These findings are consistent with the evidence on behavioral covariation cited. It appears that symptoms of oppositional defiant disorder and some symptoms of conduct disorder (e.g., fighting, bullying, and lying) are not only intercorrelated, but show similar ages at onset and developmental courses. Other symptoms of conduct disorder, however, appear to be more distinct in terms of both patterns of intercorrelation and age at onset. This latter group of conduct disorder symptoms was found to be limited to nonaggressive antisocial behaviors in the studies of statistical covariation, but this may be because symptoms of serious aggression were almost never included in these studies. The studies of age at onset, however, suggest that serious forms of aggression might be more related to the distinct cluster of nonaggressive symptoms of conduct disorder than to minor aggression (fighting and bullying) that show very different ages at onset and developmental trends.

Lahey et al. (1992) also addressed the issue of age at onset using retrospective reports of onset of symptoms of oppositional defiant disorder and conduct disorder in year 1 of the Developmental Trends Study of clinic-referred boys when they were 7–12 years old.[1] However, because the boys in the Developmental Trends Study were assessed annually for 4 years during the risk period for the onset of disruptive behaviors, the best estimate of age at onset is one that includes both the retrospective age at onset of symptoms present in year 1 and the age at onset of symptoms that were present for the first time in years 2–4. These estimates of the ages onset of symptoms of oppositional defiant disorder and conduct disorder are shown in Table 11–1, rounded to the nearest half year. Except for stubbornness and swearing, with onsets that were much earlier and much later, respectively, than other oppositional defiant disorder symptoms, the oppositional defiant disorder symptoms had median ages at onset between ages 5.0 and 8.0 years. In contrast, the conduct disorder symptoms had ages at onset between ages 8.0 and 13.0 years. It is interesting that the group of conduct disorder symptoms that were consistently found to be distinct from oppositional defiant disorder symptoms in factor-analytic studies

---

[1] In the Developmental Trends Study (described in Lahey et al. 1990), 177 clinic-referred boys from Pennsylvania and Georgia who were 7–12 years old at the time of the first evaluation have been reassessed annually for 4 years using parent, child, and teacher forms of the Diagnostic Interview for Children. The papers by Christ et al. (M. A. G. Christ, B. B. Lahey, and J. Frick: Correlates of peer rejection in clinic-referred boys, unpublished manuscript, 1991), Frick (1990), Frick et al. (1991), and Loeber et al. (1991) all report analyses based on the Developmental Trends Study sample and should not be construed as being from separate samples.

showed ages at onset that are quite distinct from the oppositional defiant disorder symptoms and rather distinct even from those symptoms of conduct disorder that tended to emerge on the same factor as the oppositional defiant disorder symptoms. Indeed, one could argue that the ages at onset of the oppositional defiant disorder symptoms and the conduct disorder symptoms that have the earliest ages at onset (up to cruelty to animals at age 10.5) form a single cluster of symptoms in terms of age at onset. DSM-III-R may have drawn a line between oppositional defiant disorder and conduct disorder in terms of age at onset and severity that is somewhat arbitrary, at least in terms of age at onset. On the other hand, the fact that all symptoms of conduct disorder emerge after the onset of 80% of the oppositional defiant disorder symptoms could be interpreted as lending developmental support to the distinction between oppositional defiant disorder and conduct disorder.

Table 11–1. Median age at onset of symptoms of oppositional defiant disorder and conduct disorder reported by parent

Median age (nearest half year)	Oppositional defiant disorder	Conduct disorder
3.0	Stubborn	
3.5		
4.0		
4.5		
5.0	Defies adults, temper tantrums	
5.5		
6.0	Irritable, argues	
6.5	Blames others	
7.0	Annoys others	
7.5	Spiteful	
8.0	Angry	Lies
8.5		Fights
9.0		Bullies, sets fires
9.5	Swears	Uses weapon
10.0		Vandalizes
10.5		Cruel to animals
11.0		
11.5		Physical cruelty
12.0		Steals, runs away from home
12.5		Truant, mugs, breaks and enters
13.0		Forces sex

Hierarchical Relation of Conduct Disorder to Oppositional Defiant Disorder

It is stated in DSM-III-R that youth who exhibit conduct disorder will also exhibit symptoms of oppositional defiant disorder, suggesting a *hierarchical relation between oppositional defiant disorder and conduct disorder.* "In Conduct Disorder all of the features of Oppositional Defiant Disorder are likely to be present; for that reason, Conduct Disorder preempts the diagnosis of Oppositional Defiant Disorder" (American Psychiatric Association 1980, p. 57). In this light, the levels of disruptive behavior disorder option for oppositional defiant disorder and conduct disorder would not represent a radical departure in the conceptualization of oppositional defiant disorder and conduct disorder from DSM-III-R. Indeed, it is understandable that many researchers have already treated conduct disorder as a more advanced form of oppositional defiant disorder rather than a distinct disorder by combining them for data analytic purposes.

Evidence from the Developmental Trends Study suggests that the assumption of a hierarchical relation between oppositional defiant disorder and conduct disorder may be defensible. Walker et al. (1991) reported that 96% of clinic-referred boys ages 7–12 years who met DSM-III-R criteria for conduct disorder also met full criteria for oppositional defiant disorder. Similarly, 84% of the clinic-referred youth with conduct disorder in the DSM-III-R field trials also met criteria for oppositional defiant disorder (Spitzer et al. 1991), and Faraone et al. (1991) reported that 96% of youth referred to an attention-deficit/hyperactivity disorder clinic who met criteria for DSM-III conduct disorder also met criteria for DSM-III oppositional disorder. These findings reinforce the view that clinic-referred children with conduct disorder exhibit the same symptoms as youth with oppositional defiant disorder and differ only by also exhibiting more serious antisocial behaviors (i.e., that conduct disorder is a more severe form of oppositional defiant disorder).

However, it needs to be demonstrated that youth with conduct disorder are more likely to exhibit oppositional defiant disorder than children with other disorders. Before the relation between oppositional defiant disorder and conduct disorder can be accurately described, it must be known whether oppositional symptoms are global indicators of malaise that are related to a variety of different diagnoses, such as depression, or are related specifically to conduct disorder.

Developmental Relation of Conduct Disorder and Oppositional Defiant Disorder

If the finding that most children with clinically significant conduct disorder exhibit substantial oppositional behavior is confirmed, the DSM-IV committees should consider the possibility that oppositional defiant disorder and conduct disorder are developmentally related. That is, as suggested in the levels of disruptive behavior disorder option for oppositional defiant disorder and conduct disorder in the *DSM-IV Options Book*, it may be that most or all youth with conduct disorder pass through a stage of oppositional symptoms before developing symptoms of conduct disorder. This would mean that some number of youth with oppositional defiant disorder at the time of first clinic referral will develop conduct disorder at a later date, whereas others will not progress beyond oppositional defiant disorder.

The possibility of a developmental progression from oppositional defiant disorder to conduct disorder can be evaluated using analyses of prospective data from the Developmental Trends Study (Hinshaw et al. 1993; Lahey et al. 1992). In year 1, 68 boys received a DSM-III-R diagnosis of conduct disorder (Lahey et al. 1990). During year 2, 15 additional boys who had not met criteria for conduct disorder in year 1 newly met conduct disorder criteria; of these 15 new cases, 13 (87%) had received a diagnosis of oppositional defiant disorder in year 1. During year 3 and year 4, 17 additional youth met criteria for conduct disorder for the first time, 14 of whom (82%) had received an oppositional defiant disorder diagnosis during at least one preceding year. In this one prospective study of boys, then, oppositional defiant disorder preceded the development of conduct disorder in the great majority of cases.

On the other hand, oppositional defiant disorder does not always portend the later development of conduct disorder. In the Developmental Trends Study, 62% of the 68 boys with oppositional defiant disorder in year 1 who did not also meet criteria for conduct disorder at that time had not progressed to conduct disorder by the end of the fourth year of the investigation. About half (47%) of these youth with only oppositional defiant disorder in year 1 received a diagnosis of oppositional defiant disorder at least one more time during years 2–4 without progressing to conduct disorder, and 15% never met criteria for oppositional defiant disorder or conduct disorder after the first year. Examining the same data in a different way, however, we see that among the total of 135 youth who met criteria for oppositional defiant disorder in year 1 (65 who also already met criteria for conduct disorder in year 1 and 68 who did not), 44 (33%) never met criteria for conduct disorder during any of the four annual assessments.

Thus, although nearly all boys with conduct disorder in year 1 also met criteria for oppositional defiant disorder in year 1, and more than 80% of boys who developed conduct disorder for the first time after year 1 had previously met criteria for oppositional defiant disorder, nearly two-thirds of boys with oppositional defiant disorder during year 1 who did not already exhibit conduct disorder did not subsequently develop conduct disorder. When considered with the differences in the age at onset of oppositional defiant disorder and conduct disorder symptoms, the data from this one study of boys suggest that there is both a developmental and hierarchical relation between oppositional defiant disorder and conduct disorder that is consistent with the levels of disruptive behavior disorder option. That is, it may be that childhood conduct disorder nearly always begins developmentally with oppositional defiant disorder in boys, but not all boys with oppositional defiant disorder progress to later conduct disorder. Confirmation of this tentative conclusion by other longitudinal studies is sorely needed, however, particularly studies including girls.

Comparison of the Correlates of Oppositional Defiant Disorder and Conduct Disorder

Given that oppositional defiant disorder and conduct disorder may be related both hierarchically and developmentally, it is important to determine if oppositional defiant disorder and conduct disorder are related to family history, impairment, persistence, and other diagnostically significant correlates in similar or different ways. If oppositional defiant disorder is related to the same correlates as conduct disorder, but to a lesser extent, a stronger argument could be made that conduct disorder should be conceptualized for DSM-IV as a more severe form of oppositional defiant disorder. On the other hand, one could argue more strongly that oppositional defiant disorder and conduct disorder should be thought of as distinct diagnostic entities if they have distinctly different correlates. Although oppositional defiant disorder has been the subject of far fewer investigations than conduct disorder, a few studies have compared the two diagnoses on a range of relevant correlates.

In considering this literature, however, it is important to keep in mind the possibility that some of the subjects who are identified as having oppositional defiant disorder in any one study may progress to conduct disorder at a later date. Thus, if some subjects with oppositional defiant disorder are similar to youth with conduct disorder (e.g., in family history of antisocial behavior), it may be the subjects with oppositional defiant disorder who will later develop conduct disorder who account for this similarity and that youth with oppositional defiant disorder who never develop conduct disorder may be more like control subjects. Indeed, an important agenda for future research will be to determine whether some of the correlates of conduct disorder can be used to predict which youth with oppositional defiant disorder will progress to conduct disorder and which will not. The results of these studies are summarized in Table 11–2.

Socioeconomic status and family psychopathology. Four studies have compared youth with oppositional defiant disorder and conduct disorder on socioeconomic status and found no differences (Faraone et al. 1991; Frick et al. 1992; Rey et al. 1988; Schachar and Wachsmuth 1990). Frick et al. (1992) found that antisocial personality disorder was significantly more prevalent in the biological parents of boys in the Developmental Trends Study with conduct disorder than oppositional defiant disorder, but that antisocial personality disorder was significantly more prevalent in the biological parents of boys with oppositional defiant disorder than in the parents of clinic-referred boys with neither oppositional defiant disorder nor conduct disorder. Parental substance abuse was significantly more common among the parents of boys with conduct disorder than in the clinic control group, but the prevalence of substance abuse among the parents of boys with oppositional defiant disorder was intermediate and did not differ significantly from either the conduct disorder or the clinic control groups.

Table 11–2. Summary of family variables, comorbidities, and impairment related to oppositional defiant disorder (ODD) and conduct disorder (CD)

Socioeconomic status			
Rey et al. 1988	CD[a]	ODD[a]	
Schachar and Wachsmuth 1990	CD[a]	ODD[a]	CC[a]
Frick et al. 1992	CD[a]	ODD[a,b]	CC[b]
Parental psychopathology			
Antisocial personality disorder			
Faraone et al. 1991	CD[a,b]	ODD[a]	CC[b]
Frick et al. 1992	CD[a]	ODD[b]	CC[c]
Substance abuse			
Faraone et al. 1991	CD[a]	ODD[b]	CC[b]
Frick et al. 1992	CD[a]	ODD[a,b]	CC[b]
General psychopathology			
Schachar and Wachsmuth 1990	CD[a]	ODD[a]	CC[b]
Impairment			
Sibling and peer problems			
Schachar and Wachsmuth 1990	CD[a]	ODD[a]	CC[b]
Social relatedness			
Schachar and Wachsmuth 1990	CD[a]	ODD[b]	CC[b]
Peer-nominated aggression			
Frick et al. 1992	CD[a]	ODD[a]	CC[b]
Peer rejection			
Christ et al. 1991	CD[a]	ODD[a]	CC[b]
School suspensions			
Frick et al. 1992	CD[a]	ODD[b]	CC[b]
Police contacts			
Frick et al. 1992	CD[a]	ODD[b]	CC[b]

Note. Diagnostic groups with different superscripts differ at the .05 level, with means or proportions labeled with *a* being significantly greater than means or proportions labeled with *b*, and means or proportions labeled with *b* being significantly greater than means or proportions labeled with *c*. CC = clinic control subjects without either CD or ODD.

Faraone et al. (1991) compared the family history of psychopathology of youth referred to an attention-deficit/hyperactivity disorder clinic who received DSM-III diagnoses of oppositional disorder, conduct disorder, or neither diagnosis. They found that the prevalence of antisocial personality disorder in the parents of children with conduct disorder did not differ significantly from the prevalence in the parents of children with oppositional disorder. However, when the frequency of either antisocial personality disorder or childhood oppositional disorder was assessed in the parents, the prevalence was highest in the conduct disorder group, intermediate in the oppositional disorder group, and lowest in the clinic control group, with all comparisons being statistically significant ($P < .05$). Similarly, the prevalence of substance abuse or dependence was found to be significantly more common among the parents of youth with conduct disorder than among the parents of youth with oppositional disorder or of youth with neither diagnosis, with the latter groups not differing significantly.

Schachar and Wachsmuth (1990) found that prepubertal clinic-referred boys with DSM-III oppositional disorder displayed rates of paternal psychopathology that were equal to rates for boys with DSM-III conduct disorder, and both groups showed greater parental psychopathology than a group of clinic-referred boys with neither oppositional disorder nor conduct disorder. Although the prevalences of specific parental diagnoses were not reported, Schachar and Wachsmuth reported that the most frequent diagnoses were substance abuse and antisocial personality disorder.

Impairment. To provide a comparison of the impairment associated with DSM-III oppositional disorder and conduct disorder, Rey et al. (1988) compared clinic-referred adolescents with these diagnoses on the norm-referenced Child Behavior Checklist (Achenbach and Edelbrock 1983). The two diagnostic groups did not differ from one another on the internalizing scale, but the conduct disorder group was rated significantly higher than the oppositional disorder group on both the externalizing and the total behavior problems scales.

Schachar and Wachsmuth (1990) reported that both DSM-III oppositional disorder and conduct disorder groups had more sibling and peer relationship difficulties than the clinic control group, but the oppositional disorder and conduct disorder groups did not differ from one another. However, the conduct disorder group was rated by clinical interviewers as demonstrating less capacity for enduring social relationships than the other two groups. Christ et al. (unpublished manuscript, 1991) compared boys in the Developmental Trends Study with DSM-III-R oppositional defiant disorder, conduct disorder, or neither diagnosis on sociometric measures and found no differences between oppositional defiant disorder and conduct disorder. The oppositional defiant disorder and conduct disorder boys received more nominations as the child who is "liked least," "meanest," and "fights most" than the clinic control group, but the oppositional defiant disorder and conduct disorder groups did not differ significantly. The three groups did not differ in terms of "liked most" nominations, but the oppositional defiant disorder and conduct disorder groups had more negative social preference scores ("liked most" minus "liked least") than the clinic control group, but did not differ from one another.

When the three diagnostic groups were compared on the number of police contacts and the number of disciplinary school suspensions, the conduct disorder group showed significantly more of both types of impairment than the clinic control group, with the oppositional defiant disorder group not differing significantly from the clinic control group on either measure. Thus, it appears that the assumption of greater severity of conduct disorder than oppositional defiant disorder is true in some areas of adjustment (police contacts and school suspensions), but not in others (peer and sibling relationships).

Continuous Versus Discontinuous Differences in Severity

Even if the view that conduct disorder is hierarchically related to oppositional defiant disorder in terms of development, family history of psychopathology, and impairment, it still may be appropriate to conceptualize oppositional defiant disorder and conduct disorder as distinct disorders in DSM-IV. If the relation between the severity of disruptive behavior and indices of impairment is *discontinuous* at approximately the point of distinction between oppositional defiant disorder and conduct disorder, a corresponding dichotomy in terms of diagnoses may also be appropriate. For example, using data from the first year of the Developmental Trends Study, Lahey et al. (1990) found curvilinear relations between the number of DSM-III-R symptoms of conduct disorder and both police contacts and disciplinary school suspensions, with both points of discontinuity (inflection) near three symptoms of conduct disorder. The risk for boys with zero, one, or two symptoms of conduct disorder was near zero, with the risk increasing dramatically past that point. This suggests that the risk of conflict with legal and school systems may be so much lower for boys with oppositional defiant disorder (who exhibit fewer than three symptoms of conduct disorder) than for boys with conduct disorder (who exhibit three or more symptoms of conduct disorder) that different diagnostic categories are indicated.

In a long-term prospective study of clinic-referred children and adolescents, Harrington et al. (1991) similarly found that individuals with fewer than three symptoms of conduct disorder at the time of referral during childhood had a 10% risk of criminal conviction through early adulthood, compared with greater than 50% for individuals with three or more symptoms of conduct disorder. Although the risk of conviction for youth with zero, one, and two symptoms was not presented separately, the risk is so low below three symptoms that it is likely that the risk function was curvilinear in these results as well.

Subtypes of Conduct Disorder

It is clear to all who study antisocial behavior in youth that conduct disorder is a heterogeneous diagnostic category (Farrington 1987; Kazdin 1987; Loeber 1988). Subtypes of conduct disorder have been proposed, therefore, in an effort to capture differences in behavior, developmental trajectories, and assumed etiology. Subclassifications from earlier editions of the DSM and the ICD, and from the field of developmental criminology, have distinguished subtypes of conduct disorder on the basis of the capacity of the youth for maintaining social relationships, the presence or absence of aggression, age at onset, and the presence or absence of comorbid diagnoses. No specific proposals concerning subtypes of conduct disorder are stated in the *DSM-IV Options Book*, but further study of alternative subtyping schema is proposed.

Group (socialized) versus solitary (undersocialized) conduct disorder. A distinction is made in DSM-III-R between group and solitary types of conduct disorder. In DSM-III, essentially the same distinction was referred to as socialized and undersocialized, respectively. The distinction is made between those youth with conduct disorder who, on the one hand, are capable of maintaining social relationships and who primarily commit antisocial behavior with other deviant peers (socialized or group type), and those youth with conduct disorder, on the other hand, who are not capable of maintaining social relationships and primarily commit antisocial acts alone (undersocialized or solitary type).

The distinction between socialized and undersocialized conduct disorder was based on a number of consistently replicated multivariate studies of psychiatric outpatients and incarcerated juvenile delinquents beginning with the pioneering studies of Jenkins (Jenkins and Glickman 1947; Jenkins and Hewitt 1944). These studies indicate that youth with undersocialized conduct disorder are more aggressive, adjust less well to juvenile detention facilities, are less successful in work-release programs, and are more likely to violate probation and be rearrested after release than youth with socialized conduct disorder (Henn et al. 1980; Quay 1986b, 1987). Furthermore, Quay (1987) suggested that socialized and undersocialized subtypes of conduct disorder differ in biological substrates that provide a predisposition to their different patterns of antisocial behavior and reviewed evidence in support of this notion. It is clear, however, that if a meaningful distinction is to be drawn between socialized and undersocialized conduct disorder in DSM-IV, it will be necessary to provide more explicit operational criteria for the distinction than in previous editions of DSM.

Aggressive versus nonaggressive conduct disorder. The socialized and undersocialized subtypes of conduct disorder distinguished in DSM-III were each subdivided into aggressive and nonaggressive subtypes. Because of the social importance of aggression and its stability over time, there is reason to believe that youth with conduct disorder who are physically aggressive should be distinguished from those who are not. For example, Henn et al. (1980) found in their 10-year follow-up of incarcerated juvenile delinquents that youth rated as physically aggressive were significantly more likely to commit violent acts including assault, murder, and rape as adults. Similarly, Stattin and Magnusson (1989) found high levels of aggression at age 10 years to be highly predictive of persistent adult male criminality, especially violent and destructive crime. Lahey et al. (1994) reviewed studies of biological correlates of aggression. They found consistent correlations between level of physical aggression, but not level of nonaggressive behaviors, and a variety of peripheral measures of sympathetic and hypothalamic-pituitary-adrenal arousal, adding credence to the possible distinction of aggressive and nonaggressive subtypes.

Childhood- versus adolescent-onset conduct disorder. Loeber (1988) proposed a distinction between childhood- and adolescent-onset forms of conduct problems and delinquency, and this distinction has been included as a subtyping schema for conduct disorder for review in the *DSM-IV Options Book*. It is important to avoid confusion between this proposal and the very different proposal to distinguish between two developmental levels of conduct disorder based on the age at onset and severity of the symptoms of conduct disorder (the levels of disruptive behavior disorder proposal). The levels of disruptive behavior disorder model suggests that some youth who develop oppositional defiant disorder early in childhood will progress to the first symptoms of conduct disorder (e.g., lying, bullying, and fighting) during childhood and will later progress to the more advanced symptoms of conduct disorder (stealing, physical cruelty, running away from home, and mugging), usually around the time of early puberty. Because the median age at onset of oppositional defiant disorder and the earliest conduct disorder symptoms are during childhood, the levels of disruptive behavior disorder proposal would seem to be relevant primarily, if not exclusively, to children whose conduct disorder has its onset during childhood. One cannot rule out the possibility that this putative developmental process could begin in adolescence, because little is known about oppositional behavior in adolescence, but the levels of disruptive behavior disorder option is intended to be relevant only to conduct disorder that begins in childhood.

In contrast, Loeber (1988) proposed that there is a form of antisocial behavior that emerges for the first time in adolescence that does not follow the developmental pathway described in the levels of disruptive behavior disorder option. His review of the developmental criminology and developmental psychopathology literatures suggested that youth with adolescent-onset antisocial behavior tend to be less severe in their offending, particularly in exhibiting markedly less aggression, and have a better prognosis for desistance in offending (Loeber 1982, 1988). Consistent with this distinction, Robins (1966) found that youth with onset of conduct disorder before age 11 years were *twice* as likely to receive a diagnosis of antisocial personality disorder (sociopathy) in adulthood as those with an onset after age 11.

More recently, Moffitt (1990) and McGee et al. (1992) provided important evidence on the question of adolescent-onset conduct disorder using the Dunedin Multidisciplinary Health and Development Study. They identified a surprisingly large group of male and female youth in a longitudinal sample who exhibited antisocial behavior for the first time after age 11. Indeed, most females who ever met criteria for conduct disorder did so for the first time after age 11. Compared with a group of childhood-onset youth who had shown persistent oppositional and antisocial behavior since age 5, the adolescent-onset antisocial youth were less likely to be aggressive; had markedly less history of oppositional defiant disorder in childhood; and exhibited higher verbal ability and reading scores, less family adversity, and higher socioeconomic status. In analyzing the results of the DSM-IV field trials for the disruptive behavior disorders, therefore, it will be important to determine whether a group of youth with conduct disorder can be identified 1) with first onset during adolescence, 2) among whom there is a higher proportion of females than for childhood-onset conduct disorder, and 3) who exhibit less aggression than is characteristic of youth with childhood onset-conduct disorder when age and sex are controlled.

Subtypes based on comorbid conditions. The draft of ICD-10 (World Health Organization 1990) distinguishes subtypes based on the comorbidity of conduct disorder with attention-deficit/hyperactivity disorder and with emotional disorders. Because of policy decisions to keep comorbid conditions separate in DSM-IV, it seems unlikely that a subtyping schema for conduct disorder based solely on comorbidity will be included.

Possible redundancy of subtyping concepts. An important goal of the DSM-IV field trials for the disruptive behavior disorders is to assess the utility of subtyping conduct disorder. The subgroups of conduct disorder created by each subtyping schema will be compared to see if they differ in terms of impairment, family history, comorbidity, and other clinically important variables. In addition, the field trials will explore the extent to which any validated approaches to subtyping conduct disorder identify the *same* groups of youth and are redundant. It may be that approaches that subtype conduct disorder on the basis of different constructs (childhood-onset, aggression, and social relatedness) actually distinguish essentially the same two subgroups. That is, because it appears that youth with adolescent-onset conduct disorder are less aggressive than youth with childhood-onset conduct disorder (Loeber 1988; McGee et al. 1992; Moffitt 1990), it is possible that the youth with conduct disorder described as solitary aggressive or undersocialized aggressive have an onset of conduct disorder during childhood for the most part, whereas youth described as group type or socialized nonaggressive generally have an onset of conduct disorder in adolescence.

Utility of Diagnostic Criteria and Possible New Criteria

A major goal of the DSM-IV field trials for the disruptive behavior disorders is to assess the utility of all potential diagnostic criteria for the disruptive behavior disorders. This will be done in three general ways. First, the conditional probability that if a youth exhibits symptom X the youth will also exhibit symptom Y may be so high that symptom Y is redundant and adds little or nothing to the diagnostic criteria. That is, it may be possible to drop one or more redundant diagnostic criteria and thus simplify the diagnostic criteria without sacrificing diagnostic precision.

Second, the power of each symptom to predict the full diagnosis will be compared. This may allow the elimination of some symptoms that are not clearly and specifically associated with the diagnosis.

Third, when symptoms are identified for possible deletion in these ways, the prevalence, reliability, and validity of the diagnosis can be assessed before and after the deletion of the symptoms to be sure that these have not changed.

Gender Differences and Age-Appropriate Criteria for Oppositional Defiant Disorder and Conduct Disorder

It is important to acknowledge that the great majority of current information about conduct disorder and oppositional defiant disorder stems from studies of males (Kazdin 1987). Based on current evidence, therefore, the extent to which one can generalize any diagnostic schema to girls is questionable. A high priority must be placed on reanalyses of existing data sets and new studies that will allow the DSM-IV Work Group to assess gender differences. It is clear, for example, that girls meet DSM-III-R criteria for conduct disorder less often than boys and have later ages at onset (Loeber 1988). This may mean that girls are less often affected by the disorder, but it is possible that a lower diagnostic cut-score would identify girls that are as impaired as boys who have higher numbers of symptoms. Similarly, possible changes in symptom lists for conduct disorder that would include more symptoms that reflect female antisocial behavior may lead to more accurate identification of girls with conduct disorder. These are important empirical questions that must be answered before appropriate criteria for oppositional defiant disorder and conduct disorder can be developed for female children and adolescents.

In addition, it is not clear to what extent the diagnostic criteria for oppositional defiant disorder are appropriate for younger and older youth. Concerns have been raised that the symptoms of this disorder are so common in unimpaired preschool children and unimpaired adolescents that DSM-III-R criteria may overidentify youth in these age ranges. It is important to consider the validity of the criteria for oppositional defiant disorder across the entire span of childhood and adolescence using a variety of sources of data.

Recommendations

In this chapter, we discussed issues that face the DSM-IV Work Group concerning possible revisions of the diagnostic criteria for oppositional defiant disorder and conduct disorder and reviewed the relevant empirical literature. The symptoms of oppositional defiant disorder emerge earlier than the symptoms of conduct disorder in most cases, but there is overlap between the ages at onset of the last oppositional defiant disorder symptoms to emerge and the first conduct disorder symptoms to emerge. In contrast, a group of conduct disorder symptoms characteristically has a later onset than the earliest group of conduct disorder symptoms.

A large and consistent literature on the statistical covariation of symptoms of oppositional defiant disorder and conduct disorder suggest both distinct patterns of covariation and overlap. That is, in factor-analytic studies, the symptoms of oppositional defiant disorder consistently load on a factor that is distinct from the factor on which many symptoms of conduct disorder load. In general, the conduct disorder symptoms that load on this latter factor are the ones that have the latest onset and are the most serious. In contrast, fighting, bullying, lying, and other symptoms of conduct disorder that have the earliest onset were found to be associated with both oppositional defiant disorder and conduct disorder in terms of statistical covariation.

The preponderance of evidence reviewed in this chapter suggests that oppositional defiant disorder and conduct disorder are related both developmentally and hierarchically. That is, although many youth with oppositional defiant disorder do not progress to conduct disorder, almost all youth with clinically significant conduct disorder whose symptoms began during childhood developed conduct disorder after oppositional defiant disorder, while retaining the symptoms of oppositional defiant disorder. Furthermore, the small existing literature comparing the two disorders suggests that oppositional defiant disorder and conduct disorder are quite similar in terms of socioeconomic status, family history of psychopathology, and impairment. When differences emerged, they almost always suggested greater impairment and stronger family history of antisocial behavior among youth with conduct disorder than oppositional defiant disorder, but with youth with oppositional defiant disorder showing more deviance on both variables than control subjects.

These tentative findings suggest that it would be reasonable to conceptualize oppositional defiant disorder and conduct disorder as two levels of severity of the same disorder and to distinguish two developmental levels of severity within conduct disorder. However, three arguments can be made against such a reconceptualization of oppositional defiant disorder and conduct disorder. First, many youth with oppositional defiant disorder do not later develop conduct disorder, indicating that oppositional defiant disorder does not always progress to conduct disorder. In oncology, the distinction between dysplasia and cancer is made on much the same basis.

Second, some recent evidence suggests that most youth who develop conduct disorder for the first time during adolescence show a more even gender ratio, show a more nonaggressive pattern of symptoms, and are less likely to have met criteria for oppositional defiant disorder. Evidence from developmental criminology suggests that these youth often come into conflict with the police, but that their prognosis is markedly better than for youth with childhood-onset conduct disorder. Thus, a simple form of the levels of disruptive behavior disorder model may be misleading because it appears that not all conduct disorder emerges on the developmental pathway described in the levels of disruptive behavior disorder model. That is, a putative adolescent-onset form of conduct disorder that does not fit the levels of disruptive behavior disorder model appears to have distinct features that are clinically and theoretically important. If the levels of disruptive behavior disorder option is adopted in DSM-IV, it may be necessary to restrict it specifically to childhood-onset conduct disorder.

Third, the point of distinction between oppositional defiant disorder and conduct disorder may be associated with a discontinuous increase in some aspects of impairment. Thus, even if the progression from oppositional defiant disorder to childhood-onset conduct disorder proves to be relatively seamless, the transition to enough symptoms of conduct disorder to meet diagnostic criteria may result in a discontinuous increase in impairment (in terms of police contacts) that is sufficient to warrant a separate diagnosis. At present, however, the evidence suggesting such a discontinuity in impairment comes from only two studies (Harrington et al. 1991; Lahey et al. 1990), and this possibility must be carefully reexamined using data from the DSM-IV field trials for the disruptive behavior disorders and other sources.

A significant body of research suggests that meaningfully distinct subtypes of conduct disorder could be distinguished. Support exists in the empirical literature for subtypes based on the capacity for social relationships, aggression, and age at onset. A major goal of the DSM-IV field trials and related studies should be to determine if some or all of these distinctions identify essentially the same subgroups of youth with conduct disorder. For example, some evidence indicates that the great majority of youth with conduct disorder that emerged during childhood are aggressive and have poor peer relationships. This suggests that subtyping on the basis of each of these dimensions may be unnecessary and that it may be possible to capture the essence of previous DSM-III and DSM-III-R subtyping schema for conduct disorder in an easily operationalized distinction based on age at onset.

The DSM-IV field trials, reanalyses of existing data sets, and other new studies will bring much new data to bear on these issues. This will give the DSM-IV Work Group a much stronger database than for any previous edition of DSM, but the fact that little research comparing oppositional defiant disorder and conduct disorder has been conducted to date will mean that the decisions will still need to be made on the basis of less information than would be optimal. The relative lack of information on girls with oppositional defiant disorder and conduct disorder is of special concern.

References

Achenbach TM, Edelbrock CS: Behavioral problems and competencies reported by parents of normal and disturbed children aged four through sixteen. Monographs of the Society for Research in Child Development 46:1–82, 1981

Achenbach TM, Edelbrock CS: Manual for the Child Behavior Checklist and Revised Child Behavior Profile. Burlington, VT, University Associates in Psychiatry, 1983

American Psychiatric Association: Diagnostic and Statistical Manual of Mental Disorders, 3rd Edition. Washington, DC, American Psychiatric Association, 1980

American Psychiatric Association: Diagnostic and Statistical Manual of Mental Disorders, 3rd Edition, Revised. Washington, DC, American Psychiatric Association, 1987

American Psychiatric Association: DSM-IV Options Book: Work in Progress. Washington, DC, American Psychiatric Association, 1991

Anderson JC, Williams S, McGee R, et al: DSM-III disorders in preadolescent children. Arch Gen Psychiatry 44:69–76, 1987

Bird HR, Canino G, Rubio-Stipec M, et al: Estimates of the prevalence of childhood maladjustment in a community survey in Puerto Rico. Arch Gen Psychiatry 45:1120–1126, 1988

Campbell SB: Behavior Problems in Preschool Children: Developmental and Clinical Issues. New York, Guilford, 1990

Faraone SV, Biederman J, Keenan K, et al: Separation of DSM-III attention deficit disorder and conduct disorder: evidence from a family genetic study of American child psychiatry patients. Psychol Med 21:109–121, 1991

Farrington DP: Age and crime. Crime and Justice: An Annual Review of Research 7:29–90, 1986

Farrington D: Epidemiology, in Handbook of Juvenile Delinquency. Edited by Quay HC. New York, John Wiley, 1987, pp 33–61

Farrington DP, Loeber R, Elliott DS, et al: Advancing knowledge about the onset of delinquency and crime, in Advances in Clinical Child Psychology, Vol 13. Edited by Lahey BB, Kazdin AE. New York, Plenum, 1990, pp 283–342

Frick PJ: Patterns of parent and family characteristics associated with oppositional defiant disorder and conduct disorder in boys. Doctoral dissertation, University of Georgia, Athens, GA, 1990

Frick PJ, Lahey BB, Loeber R, et al: Oppositional defiant disorder and conduct disorder in boys: patterns of behavioral covariation. Journal of Clinical Child Psychology 20:202–208, 1991

Frick PJ, Lahey BB, Loeber R, et al: Familial risk factors to oppositional defiant disorder: parental psychopathology and maternal parenting. J Consult Clin Psychol 60:49–55, 1992

Frick PJ, Lahey BB, Loeber R, et al: Oppositional defiant disorder and conduct disorder: a meta-analytic review of factor analyses and cross-validation in a clinic sample. Clinical Psychology Review 13:319–340, 1993

Harrington R, Fudge H, Rutter M, et al: Adult outcomes of childhood and adolescent depression, II: links with antisocial disorders. J Am Acad Child Adolesc Psychiatry 30:434–439, 1991

Henn FA, Bardwell R, Jenkins RL: Juvenile delinquents revisited: adult criminal activity. Arch Gen Psychiatry 37:1160–1163, 1980

Hinshaw SP, Lahey BB, Hart EL: Issues of taxonomy and comorbidity in the development of conduct disorder. Development and Psychopathology 5:31–50, 1993

Jenkins RL, Glickman S: Patterns of personality organization among delinquents. Nervous Children 6:329–339, 1947

Jenkins RL, Hewitt LE: Types of personality structure encountered in child guidance clinics. Am J Orthopsychiatry 14:84–89, 1944

Kazdin AE: Conduct Disorders in Childhood and Adolescence. Newbury Park, CA, Sage, 1987

Lahey BB, Loeber R, Stouthamer-Loeber M, et al: Comparison of DSM-III and DSM-III-R diagnoses for prepubertal children: changes in prevalence and validity. J Am Acad Child Adolesc Psychiatry 29:620–626, 1990

Lahey BB, Loeber R, Quay HC, et al: Oppositional defiant and conduct disorders: issues to be resolved for DSM-IV. J Am Acad Child Adolesc Psychiatry 31:539–546, 1992

Lahey BB, McBurnett K, Loeber R, et al: Psychobiology of conduct disorder, in Conduct Disorders in Children and Adolescents: Assessment and Interventions. Edited by Sholevar GP. Washington, DC, American Psychiatric Press, 1994

LeBlanc M, Frechette M: Male Criminal Activity from Childhood Through Youth: Multilevel and Developmental Perspectives. New York, Springer-Verlag, 1989

Loeber R: The stability of antisocial and delinquent child behavior: a review. Child Dev 53:1431–1446, 1982

Loeber R: Natural histories of conduct problems, delinquency, and associated substance abuse: evidence for developmental progressions, in Advances in Clinical Child Psychology, Vol 11. Edited by Lahey BB, Kazdin AE. New York, Plenum, 1988, pp 73–124

Loeber R, Lahey BB, Thomas C: The diagnostic conundrum of oppositional defiant disorder and conduct disorder. J Abnorm Psychol 100:379–390, 1991

MacFarlane JW, Allen L, Honzik MP: A Developmental Study of the Behavior Problems of Normal Children Between Twenty-One Months and Fourteen Years. Berkeley, CA, University of California Press, 1962

McGee R, Feehan M, Williams S, et al: DSM-III disorders from age 11 to age 15. J Am Acad Child Adolesc Psychiatry 31:50–59, 1992

Moffitt TE: Juvenile delinquency and attention deficit disorder: boys' developmental trajectories from age 3 to age 15. Child Dev 61:893–910, 1990

Offord DR, Boyle MH, Szatmari P, et al: Ontario Health Study, II: six-month prevalence of disorder and rates of service utilization. Arch Gen Psychiatry 44:832–836, 1987

Quay HC: Classification, in Psychopathological Disorders of Childhood, 3rd Edition. Edited by Quay HC, Werry JS. New York, John Wiley, 1986a, pp 1–34

Quay HC: Conduct disorders, in Psychopathological Disorders of Childhood, 3rd Edition. Edited by Quay HC, Werry JS. New York, John Wiley, 1986b, pp 35–72

Quay HC: Patterns of delinquent behavior, in Handbook of Juvenile Delinquency. Edited by Quay HC. New York, John Wiley, 1987, pp 118–138

Rey JM, Bashir MR, Schwartz M, et al: Oppositional disorder: fact or fiction? J Am Acad Child Adolesc Psychiatry 27:157–162, 1988

Robins L: Deviant Children Grown Up. Baltimore, MD, Williams & Wilkins, 1966

Schachar R, Wachsmuth R: Oppositional disorder in children: a validation study comparing conduct disorder, oppositional disorder, and normal control children. J Child Psychol Psychiatry 31:1089–1102, 1990

Spitzer RL, Davies M, Barkley R: The DSM-III-R field trials for the disruptive behavior disorders. J Am Acad Child Adolesc Psychiatry 29:690–697, 1991

Stattin H, Magnusson D: The role of early aggressive behavior in the frequency, seriousness, and types of crime. J Consult Clin Psychol 57:710–718, 1989

Walker JL, Lahey BB, Russo MF, et al: Anxiety, inhibition, and conduct disorder in children, I: relations to social impairment. J Am Acad Child Adolesc Psychiatry 30:187–191, 1991

Werry JS, Reeves JC, Elkind GS: Attention deficit, conduct, oppositional, and anxiety disorders in children, I: a review of research on differentiating characteristics. J Am Acad Child Adolesc Psychiatry 26:133–143, 1987

World Health Organization: ICD-10 Chapter V: Mental and Behavioral Disorders: Diagnostic Criteria for Research. Geneva, Switzerland, World Health Organization, 1990

Chapter 12

Feeding and Eating Disorders of Infancy or Early Childhood

Fred R. Volkmar, M.D., and Linda C. Mayes, M.D.

Statement and Significance of the Issues

This review is concerned with classification of eating disorders of infancy and early childhood, including pica, rumination disorder of infancy, nonorganic failure to thrive, and psychosocial dwarfism. The first two of these conditions are presently included in DSM-III-R (American Psychiatric Association 1987). ICD-10 (World Health Organization 1990) includes pica and a feeding disorder category that essentially encompasses both rumination disorder and nonorganic failure to thrive. Neither failure to thrive nor psychosocial dwarfism is accorded independent diagnostic status in DSM-III-R or ICD-10.

The considerable body of literature on eating disorders of infancy and early childhood is limited in important respects (Woolston 1986). Because the dyadic nature of eating problems of infancy and early childhood had been underemphasized in the past, more recently the term *feeding* rather than *eating* disorders has come to be used. Distinctions between "organic" and "nonorganic" pathology have commonly been made, but such distinctions can be difficult to make in practice. A medical condition may contribute to problems in feeding and in the parent-child dyad, and the latter problem can further exacerbate the child's difficulties with eating or feeding (Skuse 1985). The nature of causal mechanisms is often difficult to establish. Finally, pica and rumination disorder are observed in older individuals, especially those with significant levels of mental retardation (Accardo et al. 1988; McAlpine and Sing 1986).

An abbreviated version of this paper has appeared elsewhere: Mayes LC, Volkmar FR: "Nosology of Eating and Growth Disorders in Early Childhood." *Child and Adolescent Psychiatric Clinics of North America* 2:5–35, 1993.

Method

In preparing this review, a number of standard databases (including Medline, *Psychological Abstracts, Child Development Abstracts,* and *Index Medicus*) were reviewed, and various review articles were also examined. In addition, comments were solicited from more than 50 investigators and clinicians. Based on this review, several issues regarding the definition of the two disorders included in DSM-III-R, pica and rumination disorder of infancy, were identified. The bulk of this review focuses on failure to thrive and psychosocial dwarfism, because the inclusion of these conditions in DSM-IV would entail the addition of new categories. We considered available data regarding the natural history and treatment of failure to thrive and psychosocial dwarfism to the extent that it was relevant to issues of classification. Theoretical views (e.g., that some forms of failure to thrive represent the earliest manifestations of anorexia nervosa) were considered only to the extent that they contribute to issues of definition and classification. Because this review is essentially confined to diagnoses that are presently, or might be, included on Axis I of DSM, certain problems of eating (e.g., obesity secondary to pathological overeating) that are occasionally observed in infants and young children are not addressed.

Results and Discussion

Pica

The definition of pica is essentially the same in DSM-III (American Psychiatric Association 1980) and DSM-III-R and is characterized by the eating of nonnutritive substances for at least 1 month. The condition cannot be due to autism, schizophrenia, or Klein-Levin syndrome (a syndrome included in ICD-10 that is characterized by periodic hypersomnia and bulimia and is associated with behavioral changes during episodes but with normal functioning between episodes). No specific age at onset is required for the diagnosis. The ICD-10 definition of pica is similar to that of DSM, but requires the eating of nonnutritive substances at least twice a week for at least 1 month and excludes the presence of any other disorder except a mental handicap. The ICD-10 research diagnostic criteria further specify that the child should be at least 2 years old with a mental age of at least 18 months, thus preventing very retarded or very young children from being diagnosed with pica.

Although essentially a "monosymptomatic" condition, pica appears to deserve inclusion as a disorder because it can be an important target of effective intervention and can lead to various complications (e.g., lead encephalopathy, bowel obstruction). The exclusion of individuals with autism from the diagnosis appears to be problematic, because pica is sometimes observed in association with autism (Accardo et al. 1988). In the ICD-10 definition, the specification of lower bounds for chronological and mental age and of minimal frequencies may be useful for research purposes but may overly inhibit the clinical utility of the category, because, for example, pica may be an important clinical problem in either very young or very severely handicapped individuals (Danford and Huber 1982; McAlpine and Sing 1986).

Rumination Disorder of Infancy

This relatively rare disorder is included in DSM-III-R and ICD-10. As defined in DSM-III-R, the basic features are repeated regurgitation (without nausea or gastrointestinal illness) and weight loss or failure to gain expected weight for at least 1 month following a period of normal functioning. Although occurring predominantly in infancy, it is sometimes observed in adults, particularly those with mental retardation. Correct diagnosis and prompt treatment is important in the infantile form of the disorder given the potential fatal complications associated with it (as high as 25% in some series). Most information derives from case reports and case series (Mayes et al. 1988; Sauvage et al. 1985; Winton and Sing 1983). The literature review and comments of experts in the area suggest minor modifications of text and criteria in light of more recent research and clinical experience.

Rumination can be distinguished from ordinary vomiting by the apparently voluntary nature of the rumination (e.g., observation of characteristic preparatory movements); the voluntary nature is also important for behavioral treatment (Mayes et al. 1988; Winton and Sing 1983). Although DSM-III-R indicates that the sex ratio is equal, a male predominance has been noted (Mayes et al. 1988). The infantile form is often associated with problems in mother-child interaction. There is some suggestion that rumination in older, mentally retarded individuals occurs at a somewhat later developmental stage.

Although rumination disorder shares the general problems of monosymptomatic categories, the disorder appears to deserve its inclusion in DSM-III and DSM-III-R because 1) it is potentially life threatening and 2) effective behavioral treatments are available.

Nonorganic Failure to Thrive/
Feeding Disorder of Infancy

DSM-III included failure to thrive as a diagnostic criterion for reactive attachment disorder. Failure to thrive was not itself accorded official diagnostic status. In DSM-III-R, the failure to thrive criterion was eliminated from the reactive attachment disorder category (although the issue was discussed in the text). ICD-10, in contrast, includes a category (feeding disorder) that encompasses nonorganic failure to thrive, rumination disorder of infancy, and at least some cases of psychosocial dwarfism. The differences between these various diagnostic systems reflect various factors.

As commonly used, the unmodified term *failure to thrive* essentially defines a symptom and presenting problem rather than a disorder (i.e., similar to the term *fever of unknown origin*). This symptom may, of course, be a very legitimate and appropriate target of evaluation and treatment, regardless of its etiology. The available literature is somewhat difficult to interpret given the differences in definition and the varying theoretical assumptions of the investigators (Casey 1983; Chatoor et al. 1984; Skuse 1985; Woolston 1986). It does appear that degree of weight loss is related to caloric intake (Bell and Woolston 1985) and that the clinical course is variable. Complications can include the results of malnutrition as well as of the emotional deprivation; it is unclear whether some infants with nonorganic failure to thrive go on to develop psychosocial dwarfism. Satisfactory epidemiological data on long-term sequelae of nonorganic failure to thrive are lacking (Skuse 1985). If failure to thrive during the first year is severe and sustained, it appears that the child's subsequent growth, at least during the preschool years, is likely to be affected. Failure to thrive is more common in families that suffer from various forms of adversity. The issue of hyponutrition versus psychosocial deprivation in nonorganic failure to thrive has been somewhat controversial. The presumption in DSM-III was that psychosocial deprivation was primary, although even understimulated infants will gain weight rapidly if given enough food; usually these factors interact with each other in that starvation might produce behavioral/affective changes that in turn tend to disrupt interaction with the caregiver. Conversely, the psychosocial factors that lead parents to provide insufficient stimulation may also contribute to their inability to provide sufficient food. The dyadic and interactive nature of causal factors has been emphasized in recent research. Children with the symptom of failure to thrive are, of course, generally evaluated by pediatricians and often in inpatient settings; a host of medical conditions are included in the differential diagnosis but are infrequently identified in actual practice.

The ICD-10 feeding disorder category is defined as 1) failure to eat adequately (or persistent rumination or regurgitation of food); 2) failure to gain weight or loss of weight over a period of at least 1 month (it is suggested that, for research purposes, a 3-month duration may be indicated); 3) no syndrome meeting ICD-10 criteria for any other psychiatric disorder (other than mental handicap); and 4) no organic disease sufficient to account for the failure to eat. This definition has the disadvantage of including infants with rumination as well as with failure to thrive; it is clear that the two disturbances can be observed independently.

Psychosocial Dwarfism

Psychosocial dwarfism is an uncommon condition that has been known for many years (Green 1986; Green et al. 1987; Talbot et al. 1947). Various labels, diagnostic criteria, and guidelines have been used for the condition, thus complicating comparison of different studies. The boundaries between this condition and nonorganic failure to thrive remain controversial. DSM-III-R mentions psychosocial dwarfism in passing in the reactive attachment disorder section (i.e., as a condition to consider in the differential diagnosis of reactive attachment disorder). However, it does appear that gross and sustained abuse may be observed and that many children with psychosocial dwarfism are also likely to exhibit reactive attachment disorder. In ICD-10, some cases of psychosocial dwarfism would likely be included within the feeding disorder category; however, this diagnostic label would likely not be applicable in a majority of cases. Some (although not all) children with psychosocial dwarfism have previous histories of failure to thrive or eating problems in infancy (Borden and Hopwood 1982; Reinhard 1979).

The psychosocial dwarfism syndrome is essentially characterized by a linear deceleration in growth and characteristic behavioral features such as sleep problems and bizarre eating habits; these are reversed when the psychosocial environment is changed. Various unusual eating behaviors such as polyphagia (pica) and polydipsia may be observed (Powell et al. 1967); children may eat to the point of inducing vomiting when food is available. Food preferences may be highly unusual or markedly deviant. The polyphagia likely reflects some aspects of the child's experience and food deprivation. Children with psychosocial dwarfism may exhibit unusual patterns of relatedness, unusual behaviors, problems with impulsivity, and aggression. Other features include specific developmental delays, night roaming (in search of food), and sleep disturbance, apparently related to abnormalities in growth hormone levels (Drash et al. 1968; Wolff and Money 1973). After hospitalization, abnormal endocrine findings tend to reverse, and growth resumes. During psychotherapy, children with psychosocial dwarfism exhibit problems in forming relationships (in much the same way as is typically seen in children with reactive attachment disorder), and depression may be observed (Ferholt et al. 1985). Various medical conditions that result in growth delay or failure are included in the differential diagnosis, as is constitutional delay. Reversibility of some of the features with hospitalization is not, or course, typical in short stature caused by hypopituitarism.

The issue of overlap of psychosocial dwarfism with nonorganic failure to thrive is problematic, although various differences in phenomenology (e.g., age at onset) are apparent. Distinctions in the available literature have had to do with the absence or presence of associated malnutrition. As with failure to thrive, it is likely that some degree of interaction between the psychosocial environment and some preexisting vulnerability in the child is implicated in some cases. As Green (1986) noted, because one of the diagnostic criteria used for psychosocial dwarfism has often been stature below the third percentile, it is possible that other children exhibit growth delays as a result of psychosocial factors but are not encompassed by commonly used definitions of the disorder. Green (1986) proposed guidelines for the diagnosis; Green (1989) also argued strongly for inclusion of the disorder in DSM. Evidence in favor of its inclusion includes 1) characteristic (if highly variable) clinical findings, 2) characteristic course and response to treatment, 3) associated neuroendocrine findings, and 4) the potential morbidity associated with the syndrome. However, the validity of the condition as distinct from nonorganic failure to thrive remains controversial, as does the role of malnutrition in syndrome pathogenesis. Aspects of comorbidity are also problematic (e.g., children with psychosocial dwarfism have been noted to have a range of problems that might include reactive attachment disorder, mental retardation, specific developmental disorders, disruptive disorders, elective mutism, pica, or rumination). At present, this condition is formally included in neither DSM-III-R nor ICD-10 as a distinct diagnostic category. Children whose parents admitted to withholding food or children whose feeding or eating problems were specific to interactions with the parents would not, by definition, receive this diagnosis. The ICD-10 approach does have the merit of avoiding giving a psychiatric diagnosis to children whose problem is that they are being starved.

The issue of potential continuity with failure to thrive is unclear. Similarly, in at least some cases, actual malnutrition appears to be involved.

Recommendations

Pica

Relatively minor changes in the definition of the disorder are recommended. Given that DSM-IV is designed to be useful for both clinical work and research, it seems reasonable to allow for responsible clinical judgment regarding issues of frequency and comorbid conditions.

Criteria.

1. Change the word *repeated* (criterion A) to *persistent or recurrent*. This change more accurately captures the underlying diagnostic issue and allows for clinical judgment.

2. Include a new criterion (B) "the eating of nonnutritive substances is developmentally inappropriate." This approach appears more reasonable than assigning a precise (and arbitrary) mental age/chronological age bound as is done in ICD-10.
3. Retain an exclusionary criterion for Klein-Levin syndrome (which becomes criterion C) with a brief description of this disorder (e.g., "of periodic hypersomnia and bulimia"). This would allow individuals with disorders other than mental retardation to be accorded a diagnosis of pica. This represents a change from DSM-III-R, which excludes individuals with both autism and schizophrenia from the diagnosis; this approach also differs from that adopted in ICD-10. ICD-10 would also exclude individuals with reactive attachment disorder from the diagnosis; this seems unreasonable because pica is often observed in association with some degree of neglect.

Rumination Disorder of Infancy

The DSM-III-R definition appears, in most respects, to be satisfactory. One exception is the criterion related to the absence of nausea or associated gastrointestinal illness, because 1) it is difficult to establish this in infancy and 2) there is evidence that suggests that in infancy the disorder may be more common in infants who lack the usual physiological barrier to reflux. The phrase *of infancy* in the title may be somewhat misleading to clinicians confronted with older patients with developmental delays who exhibit rumination. If the name of the disorder is changed to reflect the reality that many individuals with mental retardation also exhibit the condition, criterion B should be eliminated; in this case, the text should indicate that failure to gain weight or weight loss may be observed in infants. If the change in name is adopted, it should be made clear that the disorder should not be used to describe more typical adolescent and adult forms of eating disorder (i.e., consistent with ICD-10, an exclusionary criterion should be included to exclude individuals with diagnoses other than mental retardation, autism/pervasive developmental disorder, and pica from the diagnosis). An alternative option would be to combine rumination disorder with nonorganic failure to thrive in a new category (feeding disorder of infancy and early childhood); this option has the advantage of being more compatible with ICD-10 but represents a major change from DSM-III-R.

Nonorganic Failure to Thrive/Feeding Disorder of Infancy

The classification of infants and young children with failure to thrive is clearly complicated. Various approaches are possible. These include 1) a separate diagnostic category; 2) a combined (rumination/nonorganic failure to thrive) category (as in ICD-10); 3) the DSM-III-R approach, which does not accord the condition official diagnostic status on Axis I or II (failure to thrive could, of course, be noted on Axis III); or 4) addition of a V code to encompass feeding problems of infancy and early childhood. Each of these approaches has advantages and disadvantages. If the DSM-III-R approach is retained in DSM-IV, it will be incompatible with ICD-10. On the other hand, if the ICD-10 approach is adopted, this would make for incompatibility with DSM-III-R and have the apparent disadvantage of combining rumination and nonorganic failure to thrive into a single category. If the disorder is accorded diagnostic status, the category would be a new one and hence incompatible with DSM-III-R. Although the use of a V code could be justified given the apparently interactive nature of the problem, the use of such a code does not sufficiently address the potential severity of the condition, the importance of treatment, and the considerable evidence in favor of the validity of the category as a diagnosis. On the basis of this review, it appears reasonable to consider inclusion of a new category in DSM-IV, *feeding disorder of infancy and early childhood*, which would essentially encompass nonorganic failure to thrive and at least some cases of psychosocial dwarfism. The name for the disorder would best reflect the interactive nature of the disturbance rather than simply reflecting the issue of an eating problem (i.e., the term *feeding disorder* would be preferable). Criteria for this condition would include

1. Feeding disturbance as manifested by persistent failure to eat adequately with significant failure to gain weight or significant loss of weight over at least 1 month.
2. The disturbance is not due to an associated gastrointestinal or other general medical condition (e.g., esophageal reflux)
3. The disturbance is not better accounted for by another mental disorder (e.g., rumination disorder) or by lack of available food.
4. The onset is before age 6 years.

This definition emphasizes the interactive nature of the problem (e.g., in the name of the disorder). The inclusion of criterion 2 reflects a desire to avoid making the diagnosis in infants who clearly exhibit feeding problems that have an organic basis. Inclusion of criterion 3 would ensure that the diagnosis could not be given concurrently with a diagnosis of anorexia nervosa or bulimia nervosa.

Psychosocial Dwarfism

Options for DSM-IV include the following: 1) inclusion of psychosocial dwarfism as a disorder; 2) elaboration of a V code to encompass feeding or growth disturbances that result from deviant patterns of parent-child interaction and/or frank parental abuse (starvation of the child); 3) elaboration of the text of the reactive attachment disorder category to discuss the issue of potential associations with problems in growth/feeding; 4) expansion of the potential new feeding disorder category to include psychosocial dwarfism; or 5) continuing with the present approach, which mentions the disorder only in passing in the differential diagnosis of reactive attachment disorder.

Inclusion of psychosocial dwarfism as a new category would entail a major shift from DSM-III-R and would also be incompatible with ICD-10. Although considerable information on psychosocial dwarfism is available, inconsistencies in the use of the term and other factors have limited our understanding of the definition and course of the disorder and its association with other conditions. Use of a V code (e.g., to indicate child abuse) would not capture the complexity of the disturbance that is often also observed in children with psychosocial dwarfism. Expansion of the potential new feeding disorder category would entail additional incompatibilities with ICD-10 and would further complicate the use of this potential new category, because the continuities of failure to thrive and psychosocial dwarfism are not clearly established. The DSM-III-R approach of including the term only in the differential diagnosis of reactive attachment disorder seems similarly unsatisfactory because it appears that many children with psychosocial dwarfism are also likely to exhibit reactive attachment disorder. On balance, additional discussion, within the reactive attachment disorder category, of children with failures of growth in association with reactive attachment disorder seems most compatible with both ICD-10 and DSM-III-R. This approach would entail addition of some text to the reactive attachment disorder category to clarify issues of associated feeding problems and disturbances of growth. It must be emphasized that the categorization of psychosocial dwarfism is likely to be controversial at least until additional data are collected. It is possible that by the time DSM-V and/or ICD-11 are prepared the category will clearly merit inclusion.

References

Accardo P, Whitman B, Caul J, et al: Autism and plumbism: a possible association. Clin Pediatr 27:41–44, 1988

American Psychiatric Association: Diagnostic and Statistical Manual of Mental Disorders, 3rd Edition. Washington, DC, American Psychiatric Association, 1980

American Psychiatric Association: Diagnostic and Statistical Manual of Mental Disorders, 3rd Edition, Revised. Washington, DC, American Psychiatric Association, 1987

Bell LS, Woolston JL: The relationship of weight gain and caloric intake in infants with organic and non-organic failure to thrive syndrome. Journal of the American Academy of Child Psychiatry 24:447–452, 1985

Borden ML, Hopwood NJ: Psychosocial dwarfism: identification, intervention, and planning. Soc Work Health Care 7:15–36, 1982

Casey PH: Failure to thrive: a reconceptualization. J Dev Behav Pediatr 4:63–66, 1983

Chatoor I, Schaefer S, Dickson L, et al: Nonorganic failure to thrive: a developmental perspective. Pediatr Ann 13:829–35, 1984

Danford DE, Huber AM: Pica among mentally retarded adults. American Journal of Mental Deficiency 87:141–146, 1982

Drash PW, Greenberg NE, Mooney J: Intelligence and personality in four syndromes of dwarfism, in Human Growth: Body Composition, Cell Growth, Energy, and Intelligence. Edited by Cheek DB. Philadelphia, PA, Lea & Febiger, 1968, pp 568–581

Ferholt JB, Rotnem DL, Genel M: A psychodynamic study of psychosomatic dwarfism: a syndrome of depression, personality disorder, and impaired growth. Journal of the American Academy of Child Psychiatry 24:49–57, 1985

Green WH: Psychosocial dwarfism: psychological and etiological considerations, in Advances in Clinical Child Psychology, Vol 9. Edited by Lahey B, Kazdin A. New York, Plenum, 1986, pp 245–278

Green WH: Reactive attachment disorder of infancy and early childhood, in Comprehensive Textbook of Psychiatry, 5th Edition, Vol 2. Edited by Kaplan HI, Sadock BJ. Baltimore, MD, Williams & Wilkins, 1989, pp 1894–1903

Green WH, Deutsch SI, Campbell M: Psychosocial dwarfism, infantile autism, and attention deficit disorder, in Handbook of Psychoneuroendocrinology. Edited by Nemeroff CB, Loosen PT. New York, Guilford, 1987, pp 109–142

Mayes SD, Hymphrey FH, Handford HA, et al: Rumination disorder: differential diagnosis. J Am Acad Child Adolesc Psychiatry 27:300–302, 1988

McAlpine C, Sing NN: Pica in institutionalized mentally retarded persons. Journal of Mental Deficiency Research 30:171–178, 1986

Powell GF, Raiti S, Blizzard RM: Emotional deprivation and growth retardation simulating idiopathic hypopituitarism, II: endocrinologic evaluation of the syndrome. N Engl J Med 276:1279–1283, 1967

Reinhard JB: Failure to thrive, in Basic Handbook of Child Psychiatry, Vol 2. Edited by Noshpitz JD. New York, Basic Books, 1979, pp 593–599

Sauvage D, Leddet L, Hameur L, et al: Infantile rumination: diagnosis and follow-up of twenty cases. Journal of the American Academy of Child Psychiatry 24:197–203, 1985

Skuse DH: Nonorganic failure to thrive: a reappraisal. Arch Dis Child 60:173–178, 1985

Talbot NB, Sobel EH, Burke BS, et al: Dwarfism in healthy children: its possible relation to emotional, nutritional, and endocrine disturbances. N Engl J Med 236:783–793, 1947

Winton ASW, Sing NN: Rumination in pediatric populations: a behavioral analysis. Journal of the American Academy of Child Psychiatry 22:269–275, 1983

Wolff G, Money J: Relationship between sleep and growth in patients with reversible somatotropin deficiency (psychosocial dwarfism). Psychol Med 3:18–27, 1973

Woolston JL: Eating disorders in childhood and adolescence, in Psychiatry, Vol 2. Edited by Michaels R. Philadelphia, PA, Lippincott, 1986, pp 1–8

World Health Organization: ICD-10 Chapter V: Mental and Behavioral Disorders: Diagnostic Criteria for Research. Geneva, Switzerland, World Health Organization, 1990

Chapter 13

Anxiety Disorders of Childhood or Adolescence

Rachel G. Klein, Ph.D., Nancy Kaplan Tancer, M.D., and John S. Werry, M.D.

Statement of the Issues

Seven issues regarding the anxiety disorders of childhood or adolescence were identified for this review:

1. Given the recent introduction of these disorders in the nomenclature, how adequately do they capture observable clinical syndromes?
2. How reliable are the diagnostic criteria?
3. Are the disorders distinct from other psychopathology with which they overlap, such as depressive disorders?
4. Are the anxiety disorders specific clinical entities, each with particular differentiating features (e.g., course)?
5. Are the childhood anxiety disorders distinct from adult anxiety disorders?
6. Do the childhood anxiety disorders describe pathological anxiety that is distinct from the normative anxiety of early life, or do these overlap too extensively?
7. What degree of compatibility with the ICD-10 (World Health Organization 1990) definitions is optimal?

Significance of the Issues

These seven issues are critical to the diagnosis of children and adolescents with anxiety disorders. Regarding the first issue, the definition of the disorders must be changed if they fail to reflect clinical presentations adequately. Regarding the second issue, a lack of diagnostic reliability would be a strong indication that the diagnostic standards are not precise enough to facilitate an understanding of the clinical criteria and need clarification. The remaining issues all address the uniqueness of the childhood anxiety disorders. To have clinical utility, the diagnoses must represent syndromes that are distinct from other similar psychopathology (e.g., depression versus childhood anxiety), from each other, and from similarly defined adult anxiety disorders. Unless these standards are met, childhood anxiety disorders will not only fail to contribute to the classification of childhood psychopathology, but will also have a negative impact by confounding other, perhaps more relevant, diagnoses (e.g., depressive disorders or adult anxiety disorders). Finally, the distinction between age-appropriate anxiety and anxiety disorders is especially relevant to young individuals, because the defining clinical features of the disorders represent quantitative exaggerations of common childhood anxiety, rather than qualitative distinctions. The purpose of the classification is to identify clinical cases. The usefulness and validity of the nomenclature depends largely on its ability to distinguish developmentally appropriate anxious features from maladaptive, pathological states.

Method

Separation anxiety, avoidant disorder, and overanxious disorder make up the anxiety disorders of childhood and adolescence. For separation anxiety disorder (key word: *separation anxiety*) Medline (1974–1990) and PsychLit (1974–1990) searches as well as examination of recent journals and bibliographies yielded 80 publications. Similar searches were conducted for avoidant disorder (key words: *avoidant, avoidant disorder*). The review of overanxious disorder relies on the article prepared for the DSM-IV Work Group on Childhood Disorders by Werry (1991) and subsequent publications (Last et al. 1991, 1992).

The goal of this chapter is to review the literature relevant to the DSM-III-R (American Psychiatric Association 1987) childhood anxiety disorders. Some studies report on anxiety disorders or "internalizing" disorders without further diagnostic refinements. Although these investigations may have important implications for an understanding of childhood psychopathology, they are not germane to the purpose of this review and are not included.

Results

Separation Anxiety Disorder

The essential features of separation anxiety disorder consist of excessive anxiety about separation from home or from parents, as well as morbid preoccupation with the parent's or the child's own death. Separation anxiety as a normal developmental phenomenon and as a pathological state has a long history (Bowlby 1969; Freud 1956). Its classification as a distinct psychiatric disorder began more recently in the DSM-III (American Psychiatric Association 1980), based on clinical presentations of children with school phobia, most of whom suffered from separation anxiety (Gittelman-Klein and Klein 1980). Similar clinical patterns have been reported using DSM-III criteria (Last et al. 1987d). Even when school phobia is not found to have a close relationship with separation anxiety, anxiety is a regular feature of school phobia (Last and Strauss 1990). In view of this clinical relationship, we decided to include key papers from the large literature on children with school phobia.

Children must have three of nine features to meet DSM-III-R criteria for the disorder. They all reflect manifestations of excessive anxiety about separation from the home, or from people to whom the child is attached. The studies that present specific clinical symptoms are summarized in Table 13–1. Among the studies before DSM-III, Hersov (1960) compared 7- to 16-year-old outpatient children with school phobia with truants and control subjects. The index cases were distinguished by a preference for staying home, multiple somatic symptoms, sleep problems, and close-knit families in which separations were rare. Based on chart reviews, Davidson (1961) found that 6- to 14-year-old outpatients with school phobia were characterized as having multiple fears, with fear of the mother dying predominating, and with nightmares, sleep problems (need to sleep with parents), clinginess, multiple somatic complaints, and high levels of anxiety when separated from the mother. In a large group of 9- to 18-year-old inpatient children with school phobia, Nichols and Berg (1970) reported excessive attachment to mothers, reduced freedom in venturing away from home, and more neuroticism. A study by Gittelman-Klein and Klein (1980) of 45 outpatient children with school phobia between ages 6 and 15 reported the presence of excessive worry about the mother dying, sleep problems, nightmares, intolerance of remaining alone, distress when separated from the mother, reduction in independent travel away from home, and multiple physical complaints. Worry about parental death is noted in several reports, but does not appear in the diagnostic criteria.

The frequency of DSM-III criteria appears well represented in both genders and at all ages except for distress on separation in late adolescence (Francis et al. 1987).

Duration. DSM-III-R stipulates a duration criterion of at least 2 weeks. Early studies of children with school phobia dealt with syndromes of months' or years' duration. Do disorders of recent onset, such as 2 weeks, reflect the same conditions? Berg et al. (1969) suggested that acute and chronic school phobia should be

Table 13–1. Studies reporting specific clinical symptoms corresponding to DSM-III-R criteria for separation anxiety disorder

Study	Subject characteristics	Worry about harm befalling attachment figure	Worry that calamitous event will separate child from attachment figure	Reluctance or refusal to go to school	Reluctance or refusal to sleep/sleep away from home	Avoidance of being home alone	Nightmares involving separation	Physical complaints on school days	Excess distress on separation	Withdrawal, apathy, sadness, or poor concentration when separated
Davidson 1961	School phobia	Yes	Yes	Yes	Yes	Yes	Yes	Yes	Yes	Yes
Francis et al. 1987	Separation anxiety	Yes	Yes	Yes	Yes	Yes	Yes	Yes	Yes	Yes
Gittelman-Klein and Klein 1980	School phobia	Yes	Yes	Yes	Yes	Yes	Yes	Yes	Yes	Yes
Hersov 1960	School phobia	?	?	Yes	?	?	Yes	Yes	?	?
Nichols and Berg 1970	School phobia	?	?	Yes	?	?	?	?	Yes	Yes

distinguished. However, the defining feature was the quality of premorbid functioning rather than the length of positive symptoms. One approach to the question is to examine outcome. This point has been addressed in two ways. First, early treatment of school phobia is reported to predict a better outcome (Eisenberg 1958a, 1958b), thus supporting the use of a brief duration to promote early identification and intervention. Second, retrospective studies of adults with anxiety disorders have obtained higher rates of separation anxiety disorder than expected when the 2-week duration criterion is applied (Ayuso et al. 1989; Breit 1982; Deltito et al. 1986; Klein 1990a; Last et al. 1987c; Perugi et al. 1988; Thyer et al. 1985; Van Der Mollen et al. 1989; Yeragani et al. 1989; Zitrin and Ross 1988). Therefore, the data lead to conflicting conclusions on this point. Finally, the ICD-10 definition requires a 4-week minimum duration, in contrast to 2 weeks in DSM-III-R. For clinical purposes, a 4-week period still allows for prompt intervention, but at the same time may eliminate the very brief, false-positive cases identified from retrospective reporting.

Differential diagnosis. The only potentially problematic differential diagnosis identified in DSM-III-R is the distinction between separation anxiety disorder and overanxious disorder. The literature does not address this. This distinction is relevant because concerns about separation are not excluded from overanxious disorder if the child does not have a pure separation anxiety disorder. This diagnostic overlap complicates the determination of whether various types of childhood anxiety represent distinct syndromes. There may be demographic differences between separation anxiety disorder and overanxious disorder (Last et al. 1987b). However, it is not clear whether these differences represent true diagnostic characteristics or epiphenomena of referral for treatment due to differences in threshold for seeking care for each condition. That separation anxiety disorder and overanxious disorder evoke different referral behaviors is suggested by longer intervals between age at onset and referral for overanxious disorder than for separation anxiety disorder (Last et al. 1992).

Comorbid major depression has been reported in 30%–50% of clinical cases (Last et al. 1987b, 1992), raising concern about distinguishing between the affects of anxiety and depression. Studies of depressed children also report high rates of anxiety disorders. In the great majority, the anxiety disorder precedes the onset of the depressive disorder (Klein 1990b; Kovacs et al. 1989). The difference in onset chronology suggests that the clinical features of each condition are distinguishable.

Distinction from adult anxiety disorders. Separation anxiety disorder has no equivalent adult diagnosis. However, there is overlap with the diagnostic item in generalized anxiety disorder, "worry about possible misfortune to one's child (who is in no danger)," because this symptom would be an adult manifestation of separation anxiety disorder. It is conceivable that some adults with separation anxiety disorder and multiple somatic symptoms may meet criteria for generalized anxiety disorder as defined in DSM-III-R.

A diagnosis of separation anxiety disorder is excluded if the symptoms always coincide with a pervasive developmental disorder, schizophrenia, or another psychotic disorder. No reports have appeared on these points. Although there is no indication that they present limitations for comprehensive clinical diagnosis, at the same time there is no obvious reason for these exclusions.

Compatibility with ICD-10. The clinical descriptions of separation anxiety disorder in DSM-III-R and ICD-10 are very similar. The two differ in duration and age at onset. Clinical reports all document extended periods of dysfunction (for sources, see Table 13–1) and point to the desirability of adopting the longer duration specified in ICD-10. ICD-10 also restricts the diagnosis to children with an onset prior to the age of 6.

Avoidant Disorder

Avoidant disorder is defined as desiring social contact with people one knows, but experiencing excessive anxiety in unfamiliar social situations and avoiding exposure to new social interactions. The key dysfunction is fear of new social contact.

Clinical samples come from two centers: a speech and hearing clinic (Cantwell and Baker 1989) and a children's anxiety disorders clinic (Last et al. 1987a, 1987b, 1992). One epidemiological study assessed 1-year rates of avoidant disorder in 7- to 11-year-old children (Benjamin et al. 1990). Because none of these reports describes the children's symptomatology, the clinical relevance of the DSM-III-R diagnostic criteria cannot be critically assessed.

Duration. The stipulated requirement for a 6-month duration has not been examined. The fact that children have been diagnosed in clinical and population studies indicates that avoidant disorder does indeed occur for 6-month periods. Whether a shorter duration would be appropriate for identifying affected children is unknown.

Differential diagnosis. According to DSM-III-R, avoidant disorder may co-occur with separation anxiety disorder and overanxious disorder, which are distinguished by a lack of fear of contact with unfamiliar people. High comorbidity with overanxious disorder (Last et al. 1987a) and social phobia has been reported (Last et al. 1992). The DSM-III-R note concerning overlap between avoidant disorder and other childhood anxiety disorders appears legitimate.

The distinction between the social withdrawal seen in avoidant disorder and in major depressive disorder noted in the DSM-III-R text relies on differences in the situations associated with social anxiety in each disorder. The fear and social withdrawal of children with avoidant disorder are restricted to unfamiliar contacts, whereas patients with major depressive disorder who fear social situations do so whether these are with familiar people or not.

In the DSM-III-R system, avoidant personality disorder supersedes avoidant disorder if symptomatic pervasiveness and severity warrant a diagnosis of the personality disorder.

Distinction from adult anxiety disorders. Social phobia is the adult equivalent of avoidant disorder. However, only generalized social anxiety is reflected in avoidant disorder; the latter does not encompass symptoms of excessive performance anxiety as social phobia does. For children with performance anxiety, but no generalized social anxiety, a diagnosis of social phobia would be considered. Children with avoidant disorder *and* performance anxiety would not receive the diagnosis of social phobia, because social phobia cannot be diagnosed in those under 18 years when criteria for avoidant disorder are met. The exclusion rules of DSM-III-R preclude the diagnosis of children with both performance and generalized social anxiety.

Avoidant disorder requires that the individual display the ability to form social relationships. The presence of this trait is implied in the description of social phobia but is not a diagnostic criterion. The only epidemiological study that included avoidant disorder and social phobia did not have enough self-reported cases of social phobia ($N = 3$) to examine the clinical distinctions or overlap between the two disorders (Benjamin et al. 1990). Clinical studies have failed to address this issue.

Compatibility with ICD-10. ICD-10 does not include a disorder equivalent to DSM-III-R avoidant disorder. ICD-10 does not provide for a childhood diagnosis unless the adult classification fails to include an appropriate disorder. Following this rule, children who meet criteria for avoidant disorder would receive the ICD-10 diagnosis of social phobias.

Overanxious Disorder

In DSM-III-R, overanxious disorder is characterized by a variety of anxious concerns: about the appropriateness of one's past performance, competence in sports or in academic or social performance, worry about future events, self-consciousness, need for reassurance, somatic complaints, and chronic tension. Unlike the other anxiety disorders, there is no common underlying anxiety construct across the diagnostic criteria.

None of the studies we located reported on the phenomenology or specific symptoms of overanxious disorder. McGee et al. (1990) noted that anxiety about academic performance and school tests was the most typical feature of overanxious disorder in a community sample of 15-year-old children. In a survey of elementary school–age children, Beidel and Turner (1988) found that overanxious disorder occurred in 25% of those with test anxiety, but in none of the children without test anxiety. In a small sample of clinic patients, overconcern about the quality of academic performance and perfectionist concerns were the only clinical features specific to overanxious disorder (Klein et al. 1992). These symptoms represent only one restricted aspect of the diagnostic criteria for overanxious disorder. These clinical observations point to a lack of syndromal specificity for several items in the overanxious disorder criteria and to their limited face validity because of their overlap with the clinical criteria of other anxiety disorders (as noted by Werry 1991). For example, several criteria (i.e., concern about past behavior, social competence, and self-consciousness) are also features of avoidant disorder and social phobia. Other criteria for overanxious disorder (e.g., worrying about future events, a need for reassurance, somatic symptoms, and chronic tension) are common in other anxiety disorders (Werry 1991). Problematically, somatic symptoms have not been found to aggregate with the other overanxious disorder symptoms. As stated by Werry, overanxious disorder should be a diagnosis whose symptoms differ from those that make up other disorders. That such is the case is not documented. The overlap in symptomatology between overanxious disorder and other anxiety disorders presents a challenge to the nomenclature, because the minimal requirement for a disorder is that it represent a phenomenologically distinct clinical syndrome. The overanxious disorder seems lacking in this key regard.

Duration. The 6-month duration required in the DSM-III-R criteria has not been studied. A longer duration of illness has been reported in clinical groups (Last et al. 1992), documenting the occurrence of the stipulated duration. Whether shorter or longer periods would enhance the validity of the diagnosis is unknown.

Differential diagnosis. DSM-III-R calls for distinguishing overanxious disorder from separation anxiety disorder, attention-deficit/hyperactivity disorder, and adjustment disorder with anxious mood. The very high comorbidity of overanxious disorder with other anxiety disorders suggests that the diagnostic criteria for overanxious disorder may be insufficiently specific or could conceivably represent complications of other anxiety disorders. If so, the onset of other anxiety disorders should precede the onset of overanxious disorder. Consistent with this notion, a small clinical study found that other anxiety disorders had earlier onsets than overanxious disorder and that overanxious disorder was never the first anxiety disorder in comorbid cases (Klein et al. 1992). However, the database on this point is very limited.

Considerable comorbidity between attention-deficit/hyperactivity disorder and anxiety disorders has been reported (Biederman et al. 1991).

Distinction from adult anxiety disorders. The adult equivalent of overanxious disorder is generalized anxiety disorder. The two disorders are characterized by nonspecific excessive worries for at least 6 months. Two features distinguish overanxious disorder from generalized anxiety disorder, and both are necessary criteria of generalized anxiety disorder but not of overanxious disorder. One is the requirement that at least six somatic symptoms be present; the second is the necessity to rule out medical disorders as initiating or maintaining the generalized anxiety disorder symptoms. It is not clear why the latter was omitted for overanxious disorder. With regard to somatic symptoms, they are one of the criteria for overanxious disorder, but are not required. In view of their lack of association with the other symptoms of overanxious disorder, there is no reason to view them as an integral part of the condition. Other than these differences, there is considerable clinical overlap between overanxious disorder and generalized anxiety disorder.

Children may receive the diagnosis of generalized anxiety disorder, but the manual does not specify the diagnostic features that differentiate it from overanxious disorder. It is possible for those younger than age 18, but not older than age 18, to receive concurrent diagnoses of overanxious disorder and generalized anxiety disorder. Among individuals older than 18, DSM-III-R restricts the diagnosis of overanxious disorder to those who do not meet criteria for generalized anxiety disorder. The rules for the co-occurrence of overanxious disorder and generalized anxiety disorder as a function of age are not based on empirical findings, nor do they appear to have clinical face validity.

Compatibility with ICD-10. ICD-9 (World Health Organization 1978) did not include a diagnosis of overanxious disorder, because such children meet criteria for the adult diagnosis of generalized anxiety disorder. However, a disorder similar to the proposed DSM-IV version will likely appear in ICD-10.

Reliability

Findings on interrater and test-retest reliability for all childhood anxiety disorders are presented in Tables 13–2 and 13–3. Five studies were based on direct interviews with child or parent. All but one used clinicians to generate diagnoses. Reliability results are satisfactory for separation anxiety disorder (kappas = .51–.91). The only report on avoidant disorder indicates reliable diagnoses (kappa = .89). The reliabil-

Table 13–2. Interrater reliability of DSM-III childhood anxiety disorders

Study	Subjects	N	Ages (years)	Raters	Method	Anxiety disorders (kappa values)				
						Avoidant disorder	Any	Separation anxiety disorder	Over-anxious disorder	Simple phobia
Ambrosini et al. 1989	Outpatient clinic, depression clinic	25	6–18	Clinicians	K-SADS videotapes	NR	NR	.85	.85	.64
Anderson et al. 1987	Community cases	792	11	Lay interviewers	DISC	NR	.70[a]	NR	NR	NR
Last et al. 1991	Relatives of children with anxiety disorders, with other disorders, without disorders (control)	1,178	Adults	Clinicians	K-SADS audiotapes	.89	.95	.91	.93	NR
Silverman et al. 1988	Offspring of anxious adults, anxiety clinic patients	51	6–18	Clinicians	ADIS with child and parent	NR	NR	NR	.54	1.0
Strober et al. 1981	Adolescent inpatients	95	12–17	Clinicians	SADS joint interviews	NR	.47	NR	NR	NR

Note. K-SADS = Schedule for Affective Disorders and Schizophrenia for School-Age Children (Chambers et al. 1985). NR = not reported. DISC = Diagnostic Interview Schedule for Children (Costello et al. 1982). ADIS = Anxiety Disorders Interview Schedule for Children (Silverman and Nelles 1988). SADS = Schedule for Affective Disorders and Schizophrenia (Endicott and Spitzer 1978).
[a] Anxiety and affective disorders combined.

Table 13–3. Test-retest reliability of DSM-III childhood anxiety disorders

Study	Subjects	N	Ages (years)	Raters	Method	Interval	Avoidant disorder	Any	Separation anxiety disorder	Over-anxious disorder	Simple phobia
Canino et al. 1987	Clinic referrals, community cases	191	4–16	Child psychiatrists	DISC current	0 days to 10 weeks	NR	NR	.51	.35	NR
Chambers et al. 1985	Outpatient clinic, depression clinic, in-patient unit	52	6–17	Clinicians and raters	K-SADS current	Up to 72 hours	NR	NR	.53	.29[a]	.38
Last et al. 1987b	Anxiety clinic patients	91	5–18	Clinicians	ISC current	A few hours	NR	NR	.81	.82	NR
Welner et al. 1987	Inpatients	27	7–17	Lay interviewers	DICA-C	1–7 days	NR	.76	NR	NR	NR
Hodges et al. 1982	Inpatients	32	6–12	Clinicians	CAS	1–10 days	NR	.72	.56	.38	NR
Fendrich et al. 1991	Offspring of depressed adults, control adults	59	6–16	Interviewers	K-SADS Lifetime	2 years	NR	.25[b] −.07[c]	NR	NR	NR

Note. The authors thank Flemming Graae, M.D., for searching the literature on avoidant disorder. DISC = Diagnostic Interview Schedule for Children (Costello et al. 1982). NR = not reported. K-SADS = Schedule for Affective Disorders and Schizophrenia for School-Age Children (Chambers et al. 1985). ISC = Interview Schedule for Children (Kovacs 1985). DICA = Diagnostic Interview for Children and Adolescents (Herjanic and Reich 1982). CAS = Child Assessment Schedule (Hodges et al. 1982).
[a] Generalized anxiety; [b] parent reliability; [c] child reliability.

ity of overanxious disorder is variable, with only some studies reporting satisfactory agreement. The study of long-term test-retest reliability of lifetime anxiety disorder indicates very poor stability of recall (Fendrich et al. 1991). Studies based on chart and clinical reviews (Rey et al. 1989; Werry et al. 1983a, 1983b) have generated good agreement for separation anxiety disorder (kappas = .80 and .72), poor reliability for avoidant disorder (.39 and .05), and inconsistent findings for overanxious disorder (.14 and .65).

Distinction From Normal Anxiety

Because manifestations of anxiety are extremely common in children, the question arises as to whether the disorders reflect pathological states associated with impairment. The fact that anxiety disorders are the most frequently diagnosed disorders in epidemiological studies but the least frequent in clinical populations suggests that the diagnostic criteria allow for the diagnosis of subclinical cases. Indeed, when epidemiological studies include an index of impairment, the rate of cases drops markedly (Bird et al. 1990; Weissman et al. 1990). The text of DSM-III-R explicitly states that each mental disorder must be accompanied by dysfunction or distress.

Discussion

Of the three childhood anxiety disorders, there is an extensive clinical descriptive literature only for separation anxiety disorder. As a result, establishing clinical criteria for avoidant and overanxious disorders remains controversial. There is ample evidence, however, that the disorders as defined in DSM-III-R are identifiable among patients as well as nonpatients (Table 13–4). Nevertheless, this feature cannot be considered to document the accuracy of the clinical diagnostic criteria. A minimum requirement is that the disorders have seemingly distinct features. The diagnostic criteria for overanxious disorder were judged not to reflect a common pathology, nor to contain mostly distinct features. Therefore, the option was considered to modify the definition of the disorder to reflect anxiety symptoms unique to it and to try to exclude features that overlapped with other anxiety disorders. Excessive concerns about the adequacy of one's performance, punctuality, and catastrophic events (such as war) are specific to overanxious disorder, whereas other criteria are not. Therefore, a purified version of overanxious disorder was formulated with less descriptive overlap with other anxiety disorders than was the case in the DSM-III-R criteria. The diagnostic hierarchies between overanxious disorder and generalized anxiety disorder are problematic, because comorbidity may occur, but only before age 18. Therefore, consideration was given to altering them.

Table 13–4. Rates of DSM-III childhood anxiety disorders in the community based on diagnostic interviews

Study	Site	N	Age (years)	Period covered	Informant	Instrument	Avoidant disorder	Anxiety disorder (percentages)				
								Any	Separation anxiety disorder	Over-anxious disorder	Simple phobia	Social phobia
Anderson et al. 1987	New Zealand	782	11	12 months	Child	DISC	NR	7.5	3.5	2.9	2.4	0.9
Benjamin et al. 1990	United States	789	7–11	12 months	Child, parent	DISC	1.6	5.4	4.1	4.6	9.1	1.0
Bird et al. 1990	Puerto Rico	777	4–16	12 months	Child, parent	DISC	NR	NR	3.5	NR	2.3	NR
Kashani and Orvaschel 1988	United States	150	14–16	6 months	Child, parent	DICA	NR	8.7	4.1	NR	9.1	NR
McGee et al. 1990	New Zealand	962	15	Present[a]	Child	DISC	NR	NR	2.0	5.9	3.6	1.1
Velez et al. 1989	United States	320	9–12	12 months	Child, parent	DISC	NR	NR	25.6	19.1	NR	NR
		456	13–18	12 months	Child, parent	DISC	NR	NR	6.8	12.7	NR	NR

Note. DISC = Diagnostic Interview Schedule for Children (Costello et al. 1982). DICA = Diagnostic Interview for Children and Adolescents (Herjanic and Reich 1982). NR = not reported.
[a] Specific time frame not indicated.

The distinctness of the childhood anxiety disorders from one another has not been demonstrated. Family history, the only correlate studied thus far, has not shown disorder-specific patterns. Related to this point is the overlap between avoidant disorder and social phobia and between overanxious disorder and generalized anxiety disorder. The option to combine the child and adult disorders was considered. Similarities between avoidant disorder and social phobia suggested that there was little reason to retain avoidant disorder as a distinct syndrome. In contrast to overanxious disorder, generalized anxiety disorder requires multiple somatic symptoms and has imprecise anxiety symptoms. The clinical distinctions between the two disorders were felt to warrant retention of overanxious disorder.

The ICD-10 principle of limiting the diagnosis of separation anxiety disorder to children with an onset prior to age 6 years is not based on empirical evidence and was felt to be problematic. How would one diagnose a child of 9 who developed separation anxiety disorder? Furthermore, if older children had had previous episodes before age 6, they could receive the diagnosis of separation anxiety disorder; if they had not, the diagnosis could not be applied. The onset rule would lead to children younger than and older than 6 years with identical symptomatology receiving different diagnoses, based on previous history. It was felt that evidence to warrant this change was lacking. ICD-10 also requires the absence of disturbance of personality development for the diagnosis of separation anxiety disorder. This criterion was viewed as relatively imprecise and difficult to establish in young children.

As noted, avoidant personality disorder and avoidant disorder are phenomenologically congruent. It seems unwise for two separate disorders to differ exclusively with respect to duration and severity.

The DSM-III-R standard of having distress as part and parcel of psychiatric diagnosis has been ignored. As a result, it is likely that, as applied, the DSM-III-R criteria for childhood anxiety disorders are too lenient.

Recommendations

Separation Anxiety Disorder

Based on the findings concerning the frequency of the DSM-III criteria (Table 13–1), the diagnostic criteria appear appropriate, and adjustments for different developmental periods or for gender do not appear indicated. Because nightmares and distress on separation were more common in younger children than in adolescents, it is possible that the criteria might be improved by specifying their likely occurrence in different developmental periods. However, this conclusion is precluded by a dearth of further studies and by the fact that only nine adolescents have been reported. On the other hand, critical perusal of the criteria revealed ambiguity in the clinical meaning of some items, such as in the reason for a child's refusal to sleep away from parents or home. Also, reported difficulties with leaving home and concerns about death are missing from the diagnostic criteria. It is recommended that the symptoms of concern about death and difficulties leaving home be added to the description of separation anxiety disorder. Furthermore, it is suggested that DSM-IV include the fact that the proximate cause of disrupted sleep in children with separation anxiety disorder is the fear of separation. Overall, the literature indicates that the essential features of separation anxiety disorder have clinical relevance. The threshold necessary for defining the disorder has not been examined. Among referred cases, it is most unusual for children to have only three diagnostic symptoms (Klein et al. 1992), but informative findings would have to come from studies of nonreferred groups. It is recommended that the ICD-10 duration criterion of 4 weeks be substituted for the 2-week duration of DSM-III-R. The limit on age at onset in ICD-10 was not recommended for adoption.

Avoidant Disorder

The clinical content of the disorder appears compatible with a diagnosis of social phobia. Therefore, it is recommended that the childhood disorder be subsumed within the adult disorder, with age-specific descriptors added to social phobia. In addition, a duration of 6 months is recommended for the diagnosis of social phobia in those younger than 18.

Overanxious Disorder

It is recommended that overanxious disorder be retained as a childhood anxiety disorder, but that it be modified to remove the considerable clinical overlap with the other anxiety disorders.

Impairment

It is recommended that the childhood anxiety disorders include a diagnostic criterion requiring the presence of impairment.

References

Ambrosini PJ, Metz C, Prabucki K, et al: Videotape reliability of the third revised edition of the K-SADS. J Am Acad Child Adolesc Psychiatry 28:723–728, 1989

American Psychiatric Association: Diagnostic and Statistical Manual of Mental Disorders, 3rd Edition. Washington, DC, American Psychiatric Association, 1980

American Psychiatric Association: Diagnostic and Statistical Manual of Mental Disorders, 3rd Edition, Revised. Washington, DC, American Psychiatric Association, 1987

Anderson JC, Williams S, McGee R, et al: DSM-III disorders in preadolescent children: prevalence in a large sample from the general population. Arch Gen Psychiatry 44:69–76, 1987

Ayuso J, Alfonso S, Rivera A: Childhood separation anxiety and panic disorder. Prog Neuropharmacol Biol Psychiatry 13:665–671, 1989

Beidel DC, Turner SM: Comorbidity of test anxiety and other anxiety disorders in children. J Abnorm Child Psychol 16:275–287, 1988

Benjamin RS, Costello EJ, Warren M: Anxiety disorders in a pediatric sample. J Anx Dis 4:293–316, 1990

Berg I, Nichols K, Pritchard C: School phobia: its classification and relationship to dependency. J Child Psychol Psychiatry 10:123–141, 1969

Biederman J, Newcorn J, Sprich S: Comorbidity of attention deficit hyperactivity disorder with conduct, depressive, anxiety, and other disorders. Am J Psychiatry 148:564–577, 1991

Bird HR, Yager TJ, Staghezza B, et al: Impairment in the epidemiological measurement of childhood psychopathology in the community. J Am Acad Child Adolesc Psychiatry 29:796–803, 1990

Bowlby J: Attachment and Loss, Vol 1. New York, Basic Books, 1969

Breit M: Separation anxiety in mothers of latency-age fearful children. J Abnorm Child Psychol 10:135–144, 1982

Canino GJ, Bird HR, Rubio-Stipec M, et al: Reliability of child diagnosis in a Hispanic sample. J Am Acad Child Adolesc Psychiatry 26:691–700, 1987

Cantwell DP, Baker L: Stability and natural history of DSM-III childhood diagnoses. J Am Acad Child Adolesc Psychiatry 28:691–700, 1989

Chambers WJ, Puig-Antich J, Hirsch M, et al: The assessment of affective disorders in children and adolescents by semi-structured interview. Arch Gen Psychiatry 42:696–702, 1985

Costello AJ, Edelbrock C, Kalas R, et al: Diagnostic Interview Schedule for Children (DISC) (Contract No RFP-DB-81-0027). Bethesda, MD, National Institute of Mental Health, 1982

Davidson S: School phobia as a manifestation of family disturbance: its structure and treatment. J Child Psychol Psychiatry 1:270–287, 1961

Deltito JA, Perugi G, Maremmani I, et al: The importance of separation anxiety in the differentiation of panic disorder from agoraphobia. Psychiatr Dev 3:227–236, 1986

Eisenberg L: School phobia: a study in the communication of anxiety. Am J Psychiatry 114:712–718, 1958a

Eisenberg L: School phobia: diagnosis, genesis and clinical management. Pediatr Clin North Am 4:645–666, 1958b

Endicott J, Spitzer RL: A diagnostic interview: the Schedule for Affective Disorders and Schizophrenia. Arch Gen Psychiatry 35:837–844, 1978

Fendrich M, Weissman MM, Warner V: Longitudinal assessment of major depression and anxiety disorders in children. J Am Acad Child Adolesc Psychiatry 30:38–42, 1991

Francis G, Last CG, Strauss C: Expression of separation anxiety disorder: the roles of age and gender. Child Psychiatry Hum Dev 18:82–89, 1987

Freud S: The Collected Papers, Vol 3. Edited by Jones E. London, England, Hogarth Press, 1956

Gittelman-Klein R, Klein DF: Separation anxiety in school refusal and its treatment with drugs, in Out of School. Edited by Hersov L, Berg I. London, England, John Wiley, 1980

Herjanic B, Reich W: Development of a structured psychiatric interview for children: agreement between child and parent on individual symptoms. J Abnorm Psychol 10:307–324, 1982

Hersov LA: Persistent non-attendance at school. Child Psychol Psychiatry 1:130–136, 1960

Hodges K, McKnew D, Cytryn L, et al: The Child Assessment Schedule (CAS) Diagnostic Interview: a report on reliability and validity. J Am Acad Child Psychiatry 21:468–473, 1982

Kashani JH, Orvaschel H: Anxiety disorder in mid-adolescence: a community sample. Am J Psychiatry 145:960–964, 1988

Klein RG: Adult consequences of separation anxiety disorder. Paper presented at the annual meeting of the American Academy of Child Psychiatry, Chicago, IL, October 25, 1990a

Klein RG: Antidepressant treatment of adolescent major depressive disorder. Paper presented at the 29th annual meeting of the American College of Neuropsychopharmacology, San Juan, Puerto Rico, December 1990b

Klein RG, Koplewicz HS, Kanner A: Imipramine treatment of children with separation anxiety disorder. J Am Acad Child Adolesc Psychiatry 31:21–28, 1992

Kovacs M: The Interview Schedule for Children (ISC). Psychopharmacol Bull 21:991–994, 1985

Kovacs M, Gatsonis C, Pauleuskas S, et al: Depressive disorders in childhood, IV: a longitudinal study of comorbidity with a risk for anxiety disorders. Arch Gen Psychiatry 46:776–782, 1989

Last CG, Strauss C: School refusal in anxiety-disordered children and adolescents. J Am Acad Child Adolesc Psychiatry 29:31–35, 1990

Last CG, Francis G, Hersen M, et al: Separation anxiety and school phobia: a comparison using DSM-III criteria. Am J Psychiatry 144:635–657, 1987a

Last CG, Hersen M, Kazdin A, et al: Comparison of DSM-III separation anxiety and overanxious disorders: demographic characteristics and patterns of comorbidity. J Am Acad Child Adolesc Psychiatry 26:527–531, 1987b

Last CG, Hersen M, Kazdin A, et al: Psychiatric illness in the mothers of anxious children. Am J Psychiatry 144:1580–1583, 1987c

Last C, Strauss C, Francis G: Comorbidity among childhood anxiety disorders. J Nerv Ment Dis 175:726–730, 1987d

Last CG, Hersen M, Kazdin A, et al: Anxiety disorders in children and their families. Arch Gen Psychiatry 48:928–934, 1991

Last CG, Perrin S, Hersen M, et al: DSM-III-R anxiety disorders in children: sociodemographic and clinical characteristics. J Am Acad Child Adolesc Psychiatry 31:1070–1076, 1992

McGee R, Feehan M, Williams S, et al: DSM-III disorders in a large sample of adolescents. J Am Acad Child Adolesc Psychiatry 29:611–619, 1990

Nichols K, Berg I: School phobia and self-examination. J Child Psychol Psychiatry 11:133–141, 1970

Perugi G, Deltito J, Soriani A, et al: Relationships between panic disorder and separation anxiety with school phobia. Compr Psychiatry 29:98–107, 1988

Rey JM, Plapp JM, Stewart GW: Reliability of psychiatric diagnosis in referred adolescents. J Child Psychol Psychiatry 30:879–888, 1989

Silverman WK, Nelles WB: The Anxiety Disorders Interview Schedule for Children. J Am Acad Child Adolesc Psychiatry 27:772–778, 1988

Silverman WK, Cerny JA, Nelles WB, et al: Behavior problems in children of parents with anxiety disorders. J Am Acad Child Adolesc Psychiatry 27:779–784, 1988

Strober M, Green J, Carlson G: Reliability of psychiatric diagnosis in hospitalized adolescents. Arch Gen Psychiatry 38:141–145, 1981

Thyer B, Nesse R, Cameron O, et al: Agoraphobia: a test of the separation anxiety hypothesis. Behav Res Ther 23:75–78, 1985

Van Der Mollen G, Van Der Hout M, Van Dieren A, et al: Child separation anxiety and adult onset panic disorders. J Anx Dis 3:97–106, 1989

Velez CN, Johnson J, Cohen P: A longitudinal analysis of selected risk factors for childhood psychopathology. J Am Acad Child Adolesc Psychiatry 28:861–864, 1989

Weissman MM, Warner V, Fendrich M: Applying impairment criteria to children's psychiatric diagnosis. J Am Acad Child Adolesc Psychiatry 29:789–795, 1990

Welner Z, Reich W, Herjanic B, et al: Reliability, validity, and parent-child agreement studies of the Diagnostic Interview for Children and Adolescents (DICA). J Am Acad Child Adolesc Psychiatry 26:649–653, 1987

Werry JS: Overanxious disorder: a review of its taxonomic properties. J Am Acad Child Adolesc Psychiatry 30:533–544, 1991

Werry JS, Methven RJ, Fitzpatrick J, et al: The DSM-III diagnoses of New Zealand children, in International Perspectives on DSM-III. Edited by Spitzer RL, Williams JBW, Skodol AE. Washington DC, American Psychiatric Press, 1983a

Werry JS, Methven RJ, Fitzpatrick J, et al: The interrater reliability of DSM-III in children. J Abnorm Child Psychol 11:341–354, 1983b

World Health Organization: ICD-9 Chapter V: Mental Disorders. Geneva, Switzerland, World Health Organization, 1978

World Health Organization: ICD-10 Chapter V: Mental and Behavioral Disorders: Diagnostic Criteria for Research. Geneva, Switzerland, World Health Organization, 1990

Yeragani VK, Meiri PC, Balon R, et al: History of separation anxiety in patients with panic disorder and depression and normal controls. Acta Psychiatr Scand 79:550–556, 1989

Zitrin C, Ross D: Early separation anxiety and adult agoraphobia. J Nerv Ment Dis 176:621–625, 1988

Further Readings

Berg I: Psychiatric illness in mothers of school-phobic adolescents. Br J Psychiatry 125:466–467, 1974

Berg I, Collins T: Willfulness in school phobic adolescents. Br J Psychiatry 125:468–469, 1974

Berg I, McGuire R: Are school phobic adolescents overdependent? Br J Psychiatry 119:167–168, 1971

Berg I, Butler A, McGuire R: Birth order and family size of school phobic adolescents. Br J Psychiatry 121:509–514, 1972

Berg I, Marks I, McGuire R, et al. School phobia and agoraphobia. Psychol Med 4:428–434, 1974

Berg I, Collins T, McGuire R, et al: Educational attainment in adolescent school phobia. Br J Psychiatry 126:435–438, 1975

Berg I, Butler A, Hall G: The outcome of adolescent school phobia. Br J Psychiatry 128:80–85, 1976

Berg I, Butler A, McGuire R: The parents of school phobia adolescents: a preliminary investigation of family life variables. Psychol Med 11:79–83, 1981

Bird HR, Canino I, Rubio-Stipec M, et al: Estimates of the prevalence of childhood maladjustment in a community survey in Puerto Rico. Arch Gen Psychiatry 45:1120–1126, 1988

Boreham J: A follow-up study of 54 persistent school refusers. Association for Child Psychology and Psychiatry News 15:8–14, 1983

Coolidge J, Brodie R, Feeney B: A ten year follow-up of 66 school phobic children. Am J Orthopsychiatry 34:675–684, 1964

Costello EJ: Developments in child psychiatric epidemiology. J Am Acad Child Adolesc Psychiatry 28:836–841, 1989

Costello EJ, Edelbrock CS, Costello AJ: Validity of the NIMH diagnostic interview schedule for children: a comparison between psychiatric referrals and pediatric referrals. J Abnorm Child Psychol 13:579–595, 1985

Costello EJ, Costello AJ, Edelbrock CS, et al: Psychiatric disorders in pediatric primary care. Arch Gen Psychiatry 45:1107–1116, 1988

Kashani JH, Orvaschel H: A community study of anxiety in children and adolescents. Am J Psychiatry 147:313–318, 1990

Klein RG: Childhood separation anxiety and adult psychopathology. (Angoisse de séparation de l'enfant et psychopathologie de l'adulte.) Actualities Medicales Internationales 79:30–35, 1988

Klein RG: Anxiety disorders, in Child and Adolescent Psychiatry, 3rd Edition. Edited by Rutter M, Hersov L. Oxford, England, Blackwell Scientific, 1994

McGee R, Feehan M, Williams S, et al: DSM-III disorders from age 11 to age 15 years. J Am Acad Child Adolesc Psychiatry 31:50–59, 1992

Rodriguez A, Rodriguez M, Eisenberg L: The outcome of school phobia: a follow-up study based on 41 cases. Am J Psychiatry 116:540–544, 1959

Smith SL: School refusal with anxiety: a review of 63 cases. Can Psychiatr Assoc J 15:257–264, 1970

Talbot M: Panic in school phobia. Am J Orthopsychiatry 27:286–295, 1957

Weiss M, Burke A: A 5 to 10 year follow-up of hospitalized school phobic children. Am J Orthopsychiatry 40:672–676, 1970

Weissman MM, Leckman JF, Merikangas KR, et al: Depression and anxiety disorders in parents and children. Arch Gen Psychiatry 41:845–852, 1984

Chapter 14

Elective Mutism

Nancy Kaplan Tancer, M.D., and Rachel G. Klein, Ph.D.

Statement of the Issues

Issues under consideration regarding elective mutism include 1) its place in the nomenclature (i.e., among the speech and language disorders, anxiety disorders, or other disorders); 2) the inclusion of mutism due to lack of language fluency (i.e., recent immigrant children); 3) the inclusion of mutism due to embarrassment about speech or language dysfunction; 4) its minimum duration (i.e., 1 month or more); and 5) whether it should be renamed *selective mutism*.

Significance of the Issues

Placement of the disorder in DSM-IV has implications for clinical care and future research. There is concern that, if elective mutism is grouped with speech and language disorders (because the primary impairment is in communication), it may mislead professionals in two ways: 1) associated symptoms and comorbid diagnoses, particularly anxiety, may be ignored; and 2) it may indicate erroneously that the disorder is one in which the language aspects of communication are impaired. Changes in diagnostic criteria, such as excluding recent immigrants, would have the important goal of making the clinical content more precise. The name elective mutism implies that children opt not to speak (i.e., are oppositional). Because the name does not reflect what is known about the disorder and may be disparaging (S. Lesczyk, personal communication, November 1991), a change of name to selective mutism has been proposed.

Method

A PsychLit computer search using the key words *mutism/language: English* generated 193 citations between 1974 and 1989. Earlier papers were considered for inclusion if they had been frequently cited.

Fifty-eight publications were examined. Most are case reports of symptoms, family pathology, and treatment strategies (Table 14–1). Because these articles contain a large number of unverifiable and anecdotal data, only papers that reported more than two cases are included (except where the paper makes a conceptual point). Articles that do not include quantitative data are excluded, as are those that do not present original data (Cantwell and Baker 1985; Hesselman 1983; Kratochwill et al. 1979; Labbe and Williamson 1984; Lowenstein 1978; Meyers 1984; Sanok and Ascione 1979). Because only a small number of appropriate studies were found, papers that did not include clearly defined diagnostic criteria were included. In addition, the usual requirements of methodological rigor, such as inclusion of appropriate comparison groups, could not be applied.

Results

Characteristics of the Studies

Using the standards described, 23 papers were identified (Table 14–2), of which 15 originated from psychiatry departments, 3 from psychology departments, and 5 from child guidance and school-based clinics. None of the reports originated from speech and language clinics, although several studies recruited subjects from such clinics. Several papers reported on prevalence (Brown and Lloyd 1975; Reed 1963), classification (Hayden 1980; Reed 1963), symptom profile (Kolvin and Fundudis 1982; Wilkins 1985; Wright 1968), and follow-up (Calhoun and Koenig 1973; Cunningham et al. 1983; Elson et al. 1965; Kolvin and Fundudis 1982; Lowenstein 1979; Paniagua and Saeed 1988; Wergeland 1980). Most define the syndrome imprecisely and lack methodological clarity. Together, however, they contribute to an understanding of elective mutism (Tancer 1991).

Two studies are of special interest as being the only systematic attempts to specify distinguishing characteristics of elective mutism (Kolvin and Fundudis 1982; Wilkins 1985). In the first, all 24 children with elective mutism, ages 6–8 years, who had been referred to a clinic for children with specific language and behavior disorders (by a variety of agencies), were compared with 84 speech-retarded children and 102 control subjects matched for age, sex, and postal zone (Kolvin and Fundudis 1982). In the second report, charts of all ($N = 24$) children with elective mutism, ages 5–17 years, diagnosed at the Maudsley Hospital in London from 1968–1980, were compared retrospectively with 24 children with other psychiatric symptoms matched for sex, age, year seen, IQ, and area of residence (Wilkins 1985). The characteristics of the comparison children are unfortunately described only vaguely, and the study by Wilkins, in particular, has been criticized for including a highly diverse comparison group (Bhide and Srinath 1985).

Elective Mutism

Table 14–1. Case reports on elective mutism

Study	N	Age (years)	M:F	Description of study
Albert and Phyllis 1986	1	13	1:0	Behavioral treatment
Ambrosino and Alessi 1979	1	10	0:1	Psychodynamic treatment
Atoynatan 1986	7	5–7	?	Family treatment
Austad et al. 1980	1	7	0:1	Behavioral treatment
Bauermeister and Jemail 1975	1	8	1:0	Behavioral treatment
Beck and Hubbard 1987	1	7	0:1	Dynamic formulation
Bozigar and Hansen 1984	4	6–9	?	Behavioral treatment
Browne et al. 1963	1	6	1:0	Psychodynamic family therapy
Carr and Afnan 1989	1	6	0:1	Behavioral treatment
Chetnick 1973	1	6	0:1	Psychodynamic treatment
Ciottone and Madonna 1984	1	11	1:0	Holistic treatment
Croghan and Craven 1982	1	8	0:1	Behavioral treatment
Cunningham et al. 1983	41	?	?	Comparisons of behavioral treatments
Eldar et al. 1985	1	16	0:1	10-year follow-up, diagnosed schizophrenic
Elson et al. 1965	4	7–10	0:4	6-month to 5-year follow-up of former hospital patients
Goll 1979	10	?	?	Family process
Goll 1980	10	?	?	Family process
Hill and Scull 1985	1	9	1:0	Behavioral treatment
Hoffman and Laub 1986	1	4	0:1	Behavioral treatment
Krolian 1988	2	7–8	1:1	Structured day hospital treatment
Kupietz and Schwartz 1982	3	4–15	3:0	Behavioral treatment
Lazarus et al. 1983	2	6–7	0:2	Individual psychotherapy
Lesser-Katz 1986	15	3	?	Behavioral treatment
Louden 1987	1	6	1:0	Evaluation with psychometric assessments
Lowenstein 1979	21	3–8	16:5	7-year follow-up of treatment outcome
Meijer 1979	5	3–10	2:3	Psychodynamic treatment

(continued)

Table 14–1. Case reports on elective mutism *(continued)*

Study	N	Age (years)	M:F	Description of study
Nash et al. 1979	3	5–9	?	Behavioral treatment
Parker et al. 1960	27	?	?	Behavioral treatment
Pigott and Gonzales 1987	1	8	1:0	Behavioral treatment
Pustrom and Speers 1964	3	8	2:1	Psychodynamic treatment
Radford 1977	1	6	1:0	Psychoanalytic treatment
Reed 1963	4	12–13	1:3	Cognitive treatment
Richards and Hansen 1978	1	8	0:1	Behavioral treatment
Rosenberg and Linblad 1978	1	?	?	Behavioral and family therapy
Sanok and Striefel 1979	1	11	0:1	Behavioral treatment
Sluckin 1977	2	5–6	1:1	Behavioral treatment
Subak et al. 1982	1	15	0:1	Discusses family psychopathology
Wassing 1973	1	?	1:0	Creative therapy
Wergeland 1980	11	6–11	4:7	8- to 18-year follow-up of treatment outcome
Williamson 1977	2	7–8	1:1	Behavioral treatment
Wright 1968	24	5–9	7:17	6-month to 7-year follow-up of treatment outcome
Wright et al. 1985	3	4–5	2:1	1-year follow-up of treatment outcome
Wulbert et al. 1973	1	6	0:1	Behavioral treatment

Essential Features of Elective Mutism

Since 1877, when elective mutism was first described, the approach for diagnosis has changed very little. The DSM-III-R (American Psychiatric Association 1987) criteria for elective mutism are: "Persistent refusal to talk in one or more major social situations (including at school)" and "Ability to comprehend spoken language and to speak" (American Psychiatric Association 1987, p. 89).

The major question concerning the first criterion is defining "persistent refusal to talk." Only five studies specify duration of speech refusal as a defining feature (Brown and Lloyd 1975; Hayden 1980; Kolvin and Fundudis 1982; Wilkins 1985; Wright et al. 1985). The minimum length of speech refusal varied from 8 weeks (Brown and Lloyd 1975; Hayden 1980) to 1 year (Kolvin and Fundudis 1982). The

Table 14–2. Study characteristics on elective mutism

Study	N	Age (years)	M:F	Source of subjects	Diagnostic criteria	Time with symptoms of elective mutism	Assessment methods	Description of study
Atoynatan 1986	7	5–7	?	Various	Refusal to speak	?	Clinical	Family treatment
Bozigar and Hansen 1984	4	6–9	?	School	Refusal to speak	?	Clinical	Behavioral treatment
Brown and Lloyd 1975	42	5	?	School	Refusal to speak	8 weeks	Parental report	Prevalence survey of 6,072 children in a Birmingham primary school
Calhoun and Koenig 1973	8	5–8	?	School	Deficient speech	?	Clinical	Controlled study behavioral treatment
Cunningham et al. 1983	41	?	?	Various	?	?	Various clinical	Comparison of behavioral treatments
Eldar et al. 1985	1	16	0:1	?	Refusal to speak	?	Clinical	10-year case follow-up; diagnosed schizophrenic
Elson et al. 1965	4	7–10	0:4	Inpatient psychiatric hospital	Refusal to speak	?	Clinical	6-month to 5-year follow-up of former hospital patients

(*continued*)

Table 14–2. Study characteristics on elective mutism *(continued)*

Study	N	Age (years)	M:F	Source of subjects	Diagnostic criteria	Time with symptoms of elective mutism	Assessment methods	Description of study
Goll 1979	10	?	?	Inpatient psychiatric hospital	Refusal or no speech	?	Clinical	Family process
Goll 1980	10	?	?	Inpatient speech	Refusal or no speech	?	Clinical	Family process
Hayden 1980	68	3–14	12:56	Various	No speech One setting	8 weeks	Clinical Wechsler Intelligence Scale for Children	Classification of cases followed for 7 years
Kolvin and Fundudis 1982	24	6–8	11:13	Various	Refusal to speak and shy	1 year	Clinical	Comparison of elective mutism with 84 speech-retarded children and 102 control subjects
Kupietz and Schwartz 1982	3	4–15	3:0	School	No speech	?	Clinical	Behavioral treatment
Lesser-Katz 1986	15	3	?	Head Start	Refusal to speak	?	Clinical	Behavioral treatment
Lowenstein 1979	21	3–8	16:5	Various	Refusal to speak	?	Clinical	7-year follow-up
Meijer 1979	5	3–10	2:3	?	Refusal to speak	?	Clinical	Psychodynamic treatment

Study	N	Age	Sex ratio	Setting	Symptom	Duration	Assessment	Treatment/Follow-up
Nash et al. 1979	3	5–9	?	School	Refusal to speak	?	Clinical	Behavioral treatment
Parker et al. 1960	27	?	?	School	Refusal to speak	?	Clinical	Behavioral treatment
Pustrom and Speers 1964	3	8	2:1	Various hospitals	Refusal to speak	?	Clinical	Psychodynamic treatment
Reed 1963	4	12–13	1:3	Various outpatients	Refusal to speak	?	Clinical	Cognitive treatment
Wergeland 1980	11	6–11	4:7	School	Refusal to speak	?	Clinical physical examination, EEG	8- to 18-year follow-up
Wilkins 1985	24	5–17	7:17	All hospital cases	Refusal to speak	6 months	Clinical	Comparison of elective mutism with 24 children with other emotional disorders
Wright 1968	24	5–9	7:17	School	Not talk in school	?	Clinical	6-month to 7-year follow-up
Wright et al. 1985	3	4–5	2:1	Various	Refusal to speak	6 months	Clinical	1-year follow-up

duration criterion is of particular importance because persistent and transient mutism may represent different disorders.

A questionnaire survey of parents of 5-year-old children, done 8 weeks after school entrance, reported a prevalence of nearly 7 per 1,000 (42/6,072) (Brown and Lloyd 1975). Of these, 20% had improved 5 months later, and 90% had improved at a 10-month follow-up. Although the children's language comprehension was not established and sampling included 42% immigrant children, the study suggests that 1) elective mutism is not common in young children at school entrance; and 2) when it occurs, it is transient, possibly representing an adjustment disorder that may be distinct from protracted elective mutism. If so, much of the current data yield ambiguous findings, because they combine transient and chronic cases.

Another issue related to the first criterion is whether elective mutism is an elective refusal to talk or an inability to communicate verbally in specific social situations as a result of anxiety, embarrassment, or shyness. This clinical distinction has not been systematically examined, and no firm conclusions can be drawn. However, the literature supports the thesis that children with elective mutism have other difficulties (i.e., communication disorders, anxious temperaments) that impair their ability to speak in certain social situations.

The critical diagnostic point in the second criterion is the exclusion of abnormality of language comprehension or production: elective mutism is defined as a motivational disorder. However, in the three studies that examined for language disorders in children with elective mutism, all found a high rate of such abnormalities. In Wright's (1968) sample, 20% of the children had a language handicap, and in Kolvin and Fundudis' (1982) sample, 50% had immaturities of speech and/or other speech abnormalities, although hearing was normal. Finally, in Wilkins' (1985) sample, 33% had language problems compared with none of the children with other emotional disorders ($P < .01$).

It remains unclear at what level of severity of comprehension and speech abnormalities the diagnosis of elective mutism should be excluded. Exclusion of any but the most impaired of these children would render most of the studies presented uninterpretable, because the reported findings do not distinguish between children with and without a history of language disorder.

Associated Features of Elective Mutism

A wide range of symptoms has been associated with the diagnosis of elective mutism. In general, these associations remain conjectural, because data collection has often been retrospective and driven by preconceptions of etiology and psychopathology. The following associated features have been reported: negativism (Hayden 1980; Kolvin and Fundudis 1982; Wilkins 1985), shyness (Elson et al. 1965; Hayden 1980; Kolvin and Fundudis 1982; Lesser-Katz 1986; Meijer 1979; Wergeland 1980; Wilkins 1985; Wright et al. 1985), controlling or oppositional behavior (Elson et al. 1965; Hayden 1980; Parker et al. 1960; Wergeland 1980), and social isolation (Elson et al. 1965; Hayden 1980; Wergeland 1980; Wright et al. 1985).

Whether elective mutism is a feature of anxiety or an anxiety disorder has never been directly examined. A number of studies report anxious temperamental features (Atoynatan 1986; Elson et al. 1965; Goll 1979; Hayden 1980; Kolvin and Fundudis 1982; Lesser-Katz 1986; Meijer 1979; Pustrom and Speers 1964; Reed 1963; Wergeland 1980; Wilkins 1985; Wright 1968; Wright et al. 1985) or anxiety symptoms (Reed 1963; Wilkins 1985; Wright 1968). In particular, Wilkins gives detailed behavioral descriptions from case notes and indicates that 88% of patients with elective mutism were described as anxious compared with 46% of psychiatric control subjects.

Kolvin and Fundudis (1982), comparing children with elective mutism with children with other psychiatric problems and with control subjects, reported enuresis (42%, 25%, and 15%, respectively) and encopresis (17%, 7%, and 2%, respectively).

Discussion

Given the large number of cases reported over the last century, it appears certain that elective mutism, a syndrome of speech refusal in children capable of speaking, exists as a clinical phenomenon. Yet it is likely to include several subgroups. Because of the paucity of relevant studies, it is not possible to suggest empirically based changes to refine the nomenclature.

Of particular interest is the relationship between elective mutism and anxiety disorders. Identifying mutism as a nonspecific symptom of anxiety, or perhaps as a manifestation of avoidance in severe forms of childhood social phobia, would direct our conceptual understanding of the disorder as well as intervention strategies. Another important area of inquiry is that of defining a minimum symptomatic period for the diagnosis of elective mutism. Further, the relationship between specific developmental disorders, particularly expressive language disorders and elective mutism, requires clarification.

The problem of how to design a study to begin to address these questions is a difficult one, particularly because of the rarity of elective mutism. One possibility would be to set up a large epidemiological sampling of children first entering school, like that by Brown and Lloyd (1975), with prospective follow-up of children with elective mutism. Careful attention should be paid to evidence of language and other developmental disorders to determine their relationship to elective mutism, as well as to assess the impact of these cognitive developmental features on the stability of the disorder. Another strategy would be to recruit children with elective mutism for systematic psychiatric evaluation. Family and twin studies would also contribute to knowledge concerning genetic contributions to the expression of elective mutism and would, in turn, clarify the diagnostic meaning of the condition.

Recommendations

The following recommendations are proposed for DSM-IV based on current findings:

1. The placement of elective mutism has implications for its conceptualization. Elective mutism is unlike any expressive language disorder in that it is not uniformly associated with functional speech abnormality; therefore, the placement of elective mutism in the language and speech disorders section would be misleading. The question of whether to place elective mutism with the anxiety disorders is of interest because there is some suggestion that mutism represents a subtype or manifestation of anxiety. However, at this time, such placement would be without scientific validation and must be viewed as premature. The recommendation is to retain elective mutism as one of the other disorders of infancy, childhood, and adolescence, unless further findings indicate that it belongs in a specific diagnostic section.
2. It is recommended that an additional criterion be introduced that excludes foreign children who do not speak the prevalent language. From the literature, it would appear wise to exclude such children for a time-limited interval, such as 6 months following immigration.
3. Although not based on research data, it is also suggested that children with severe language disorders be excluded from the diagnosis of elective mutism if the degree of language impairment can be expected, under usual circumstances, to cause embarrassment when speaking in social situations. This exclusion would eliminate many of the children with serious developmental disorders and lead to a more homogeneous clinical population of children in which to study elective mutism.
4. The data presented by Brown and Lloyd (1975) suggest that some young children exhibit only transient symptoms of mutism. Based on these reports, it seems judicious to include a minimum duration of mutism for the diagnosis of elective mutism. However, there is no empirical basis for selecting an optimal length of time that would capture true cases and exclude temporary transient states of mutism. A longer span is not recommended because it would delay professional attention for children who are functionally impaired.

5. It is recommended that the disorder be named *selective mutism*, because evidence is lacking to support the implication that children with elective mutism have a deliberate preference not to speak. The new term is more descriptive and avoids an unnecessary inferential model of psychopathology that is likely to stigmatize children with elective mutism and their families.

References

Albert S, Phyllis L: Positive reinforcement in short-term treatment of an electively mute child: a case study. Psychol Rep 58:571–576, 1986

Ambrosino S, Alessi M: Elective mutism: fixation and double bind. Am J Psychoanal 39:251–256, 1979

American Psychiatric Association: Diagnostic and Statistical Manual of Mental Disorders, 3rd Edition, Revised. Washington, DC, American Psychiatric Association, 1987

Atoynatan T: Elective mutism: involvement of the mother in the treatment of the child. Child Psychiatry Hum Dev 17:15–27, 1986

Austad C, Sininger R, Stricklin A: Successful treatment of a case of elective mutism. Behavior Therapist 3:18–19, 1980

Bauermeister J, Jemail J: Modification of "elective mutism" in the classroom setting: a case study. Behavior Therapy 6:246–250, 1975

Beck J, Hubbard M: Elective mutism in a missionary family: a case study. Journal of Psychology and Theology 15:291–299, 1987

Bhide A, Srinath S: Elective mutism (letter). Br J Psychiatry 147:731, 1985

Bozigar J, Hansen R: Group treatment of elective mute children. Social Work 29:478–480, 1984

Brown J, Lloyd H: A controlled study of not speaking in school. Journal of the Association of Workers With Maladjusted Children 3:49–63, 1975

Browne E, Wilson V, Laybourne P: Diagnosis and treatment of elective mutism in children. J Am Acad Child Adolesc Psychiatry 2:605–617, 1963

Calhoun J, Koenig K: Classroom modification of elective mutism. Behavior Therapy 4:700–702, 1973

Cantwell D, Baker L: Speech and language: development and disorders, in Child and Adolescent Psychiatry, Modern Approaches, 2nd Edition. Edited by Rutter M, Hersov L. Oxford, England, Blackwell Scientific, 1985, pp 526–544

Carr A, Afnan S: Concurrent individual and family therapy in a case of elective mutism. Journal of Family Therapy 11:29–44, 1989

Chetnick M: Amy: the intensive treatment of an elective mute. Journal of the American Academy of Child Psychiatry 12:482–498, 1973

Ciottone R, Madonna J: The treatment of elective mutism: the economics of an integrated approach. Techniques 1:23–30, 1984

Croghan L, Craven R: Elective mutism: learning from the analysis of a successful case history. J Pediatr Psychol 7:85–93, 1982

Cunningham C, Cataldo M, Mallion C: A review and controlled single case evaluation of behavioral approaches to the management of elective mutism. Child and Family Behavior Therapy 5:25–49, 1983

Eldar S, Bleich A, Apter A, et al: Elective mutism: an atypical antecedent of schizophrenia. J Adolesc 8:289–292, 1985

Elson A, Pearson C, Jones D, et al: Follow-up study of childhood elective mutism. Arch Gen Psychiatry 13:182–187, 1965

Goll K: Role structure and subculture in the families of elective mutists. Fam Process 18:55–68, 1979

Goll K: Role structure and subculture in the family of elective mutists. Advances in Family Psychiatry 2:141–161, 1980

Hayden T: Classification of elective mutism. Journal of the American Academy of Child Psychiatry 19:118–133, 1980

Hesselman S: Elective mutism in children 1877–1981. Acta Paedopsychiatrica 49:297–310, 1983

Hill L, Scull J: Elective mutism associated with selective inactivity. J Commun Dis 18:161–167, 1985

Hoffman S, Laub B: Paradoxical intervention using a polarization model of co-therapy in the treatment of elective mutism: a case study. Contemporary Family Therapy 8:136–143, 1986

Kolvin I, Fundudis T: Elective mute children: psychological, developmental and background factors, in Annual Progress in Child Psychiatry and Child Development. Edited by Chess S, Thomas A, Hertzig M. New York, Brunner/Mazel, 1982, pp 484–501

Kratochwill T, Bordy G, Piersel W: Elective mutism in children, in Advances in Clinical Child Psychology, Vol 2. Edited by Lahey B, Kazden A. New York, Plenum, 1979, pp 194–240

Krolian E: "Speech is silver, but silence is golden": day hospital treatment of two electively mute children. Clinical Social Work Journal 16:355–377, 1988

Kupietz S, Schwartz I: Elective mutism: evaluation and behavioral treatment of three cases. N Y State J Med 82:1073–1076, 1982

Labbe E, Williamson D: Behavioral treatment of elective mutism: a review of the literature. Clinical Psychology Review 4:273–292, 1984

Lazarus P, Gavil H, Moore J: The treatment of elective mutism in children within the school setting: two case studies. School Psychology Review 12:467–472, 1983

Lesser-Katz M: Stranger reaction and elective mutism in young children. Am J Orthopsychiatry 56:458–469, 1986

Louden D: Elective mutism: a case study of a disorder of childhood. J Natl Med Assoc 79:1043–1048, 1987

Lowenstein L: A summary of the research on elective mutism. Acta Paedopsychiatrica 44:17–22, 1978

Lowenstein L: The result of 21 elective mute cases. Acta Paedopsychiatrica 45:17–23, 1979

Meijer A: Elective mutism in children. Israel Annals of Psychiatry and Related Disciplines 17:93–100, 1979

Meyers S: Elective mutism in children: a family systems approach. American Journal of Family Therapy 12:39–45, 1984

Nash R, Thorpe H, Andrews M, et al: A management program of elective mutism. Psychology in the Schools 16:246–253, 1979

Paniagua F, Saeed M: A procedural distinction between elective and progressive mutism. J Behav Ther Exp Psychiatry 19:207–210, 1988

Parker E, Olson T, Throdemorton M: Social casework with elementary children who do not talk in school. Social Work 5:64–70, 1960

Pigott H, Gonzales F: Efficacy of videotape self-modeling in treating an electively mute child. Journal of Clinical Child Psychology 16:106–110, 1987

Pustrom E, Speers R: Elective mutism in children. Journal of the American Academy of Child Psychiatry 3:287–297, 1964

Radford P: A psychoanalytically-based therapy as the treatment of choice for a six year old elective mute. Journal of Child Psychotherapy 4:49–65, 1977

Reed G: Elective mutism in children: a reappraisal. J Child Psychol Psychiatry 4:99–107, 1963

Richards C, Hansen M: A further demonstration of the efficacy of stimulus fading treatment of elective mutism. J Behav Ther Exp Psychiatry 9:57–60, 1978

Rosenberg J, Linblad M: Behavior therapy in a family context: treating elective mutism. Fam Process 17:77–82, 1978

Sanok R, Ascione F: Behavioral interventions for childhood elective mutism: an evaluative review. Child Behavior Therapy 1:49–68, 1979

Sanok R, Striefel S: Elective mutism: generalization of verbal responding across people and settings. Behavior Therapy 1:357–371, 1979

Sluckin A: Children who do not talk at school. Child-Care, Health and Development 3:69–79, 1977

Subak M, West M, Carlin M: Elective mutism: an expression of family psychopathology. International Journal of Family Psychiatry 3:335–344, 1982

Tancer NK: Elective mutism: a review of the literature, in Advances in Clinical Child Psychology, Vol 14. Edited by Lahey B, Kazdin A. New York, Plenum, 1991, pp 265–288

Wassing H: A case of prolonged elective mutism in an adolescent boy: on the nature of the condition and its residential treatment. Acta Paedopsychiatrica 40:75–96, 1973

Wergeland H: Elective mutism, in Annual Progress in Child Psychiatry and Child Development. Edited by Chess S, Thomas A, Hertzig M. New York, Brunner/Mazel, 1980, pp 373–385

Wilkins R: A comparison of elective mutism and emotional disorders in children. Br J Psychiatry 146:198–203, 1985

Williamson D: The behavioral treatment of elective mutism: two case studies. J Behav Ther Exp Psychiatry 8:143–149, 1977

Wright H: A clinical study of children who refuse to talk. Journal of the American Academy of Child Psychiatry 7:603–617, 1968

Wright H, Miller M, Cook M, et al: Early to speak. Journal of the American Academy of Child Psychiatry 24:739–746, 1985

Wulbert M, Nyman B, Snow D, et al: The efficacy of stimulus fading and contingency management in the treatment of elective mutism: a case study. J Appl Behav Anal 6:435–441, 1973

Chapter 15

Reactive Attachment Disorder

Fred R. Volkmar, M.D.

Statement and Significance of the Issues

A substantial body of research suggests that some young children exhibit a particular constellation of social deficit (either lack of interest in social interaction or indiscriminate sociability) in response to sustained grossly deficient or negligent care. A specific diagnostic concept, reactive attachment disorder, was included in DSM-III (American Psychiatric Association 1980) to encompass this condition. Although various changes were made in the definition of reactive attachment disorder in DSM-III-R (American Psychiatric Association 1987), the underlying diagnostic construct remained consistent with DSM-III. The condition was not included in ICD-9 (World Health Organization 1978) but is included in ICD-10 (World Health Organization 1990), which explicitly distinguishes two forms of the condition based on the nature of the disturbance in social interaction, a distinction that is implicit in DSM-III-R. In contrast to DSM-III-R, the ICD-10 research definition does not make grossly pathological care a necessary aspect of the condition; this position makes it possible to make a diagnosis of attachment disorder on the basis of behavioral or developmental findings in the child even when gross neglect or abuse is not suspected.

This review is concerned with the following issues: 1) is continued inclusion of the category warranted in DSM-IV; 2) if the category is included, what changes in criteria or text description are justified; and 3) to what extent should the DSM-IV definition converge with that used in ICD-10? It must be noted that, although several different lines of evidence provide support for continued inclusion of the category in DSM-IV, empirical studies of reactive attachment disorder, as defined using categorical diagnostic criteria, have been extremely uncommon.

Method

As part of this review, various relevant computer databases (e.g., Medline, *Index Medicus, Psychology Abstracts, Mental Health Abstracts*) were searched for references to *attachment disorders, child neglect/abuse,* and so forth. In addition, comments from various experts in the field were solicited. A substantial body of work with general relevance to the topic was identified, although studies focused explicitly on reactive attachment disorder were few. Accordingly, a data reanalysis project was undertaken to focus specifically on aspects of the diagnosis of reactive attachment disorder in a sample of children who were presumably at risk for exhibiting the condition, because their cases had been referred for evaluation of possible termination of parental rights following suspected neglect and abuse.

Results

In one sense, the reactive attachment disorder concept has its origins in the centuries-old debate over the relative importance of biological endowment and maturation (nature) versus that of the psychosocial environment (nurture) in child development. During the first decades of this century, there was a general belief that early experience had little impact on children's development, which was thought to emerge in ways predetermined by the child's endowment. This belief was associated with the assumption of strong genetic aspects of intelligence, which was essentially viewed as fixed at birth (for a discussion, see Hunt 1961). However, several lines of evidence, notably work on children reared in institutions, suggested major influences of early experience and major untoward effects of a lack of stable and responsive caregiving early in life (Bowlby 1951; Dennis 1973; Hodges and Tizard 1989a, 1989b; Provence and Lipton 1962; Skeels and Dye 1939; Spitz 1946; Tizard 1977). Much of this literature became subsumed under the general rubric of maternal deprivation (for reviews, see Rutter 1972, 1979). It became apparent that children deprived of normally responsive caregiving often failed to form responsive affective bonds with others (Bowlby 1951) and exhibited a range of associated developmental and behavioral problems, although with a large range of individual differences (Koluchova 1971; Rutter 1972; Skuse 1984a, 1984b; Terwogt et al. 1990; Thompson 1986).

Subsequent work on this topic has extended into other areas, including both ethological and animal work on the effects of early experience. Several specific experimental paradigms have been used to assess the nature of early attachment patterns, most commonly the Ainsworth "strange situation" (Ainsworth et al. 1985). Over the past decade, a substantial body of research using the Ainsworth paradigm has emerged, and characteristic patterns of attachment have been identified (Ainsworth et al. 1985; Main and George 1985; Main and Solomon 1986). Information derived from the Ainsworth paradigm is impressive in terms of both sheer volume and general consistency, but its relevance to the definition of reactive attachment *disorder* is limited. An additional line of research has stemmed from the study of child abuse and the effects of maltreatment on children (Cicchetti and Carlson 1989). This line of research has emerged since the identification of the "battered child syndrome" (Kempe et al. 1962), and attempts to synthesize findings from both the attachment and abuse/neglect literature have been made (Crittenden and Ainsworth 1989; Zeanah and Zeanah 1989). However, the informative value of this literature for reactive attachment disorder is limited because of issues of definition, the problem of differentiating abuse and neglect, and an understandable focus on perpetrators as well as victims. The interpretation of the broader child abuse literature is also complicated because many different factors are subsumed under the general topic of abuse: marital disharmony, parental psychopathology, lack of early stimulation, and associations with other forms of psychosocial adversity. There is evidence that maltreated infants and young children are more likely to exhibit deviant attachment patterns to parents and primary caregivers, although some evidence of attachment is often observed (Egeland and Sroufe 1981), and that effects of maltreatment may be apparent in both readiness to learn and measures of social orientation (Aber and Allen 1987).

Clinically, it is clear that many children suffering from gross neglect and/or abuse have developmental and behavioral difficulties, particularly in the areas of social interaction and formation of stable relationships (Mrazek and Mrazek 1985). Other conditions that can lead to unavailability of the mother or caregiver, such as severe maternal depression, may result in similar problems. Cognitive effects of severe neglect have been noted (e.g., Dennis 1973; Hunt 1961). It has also become clear that responses to early deprivation vary considerably among individual children (Rutter 1979) and that even children who are abused may form attachments to caregivers. The inclusion of the reactive attachment disorder category in DSM-III reflected an awareness that the difficulties exhibited by some children who had suffered marked deprivation, neglect, and/or abuse were not captured by alternative diagnostic categories (Rutter and Tuma 1988). For example, an argument could be made that a diagnosis of posttraumatic stress disorder might apply in certain instances, such as after single episodes of major abuse in older children. But it is clear that this category would not necessarily, or as readily, apply to younger children whose difficulties relate more to sustained patterns of neglect/abuse rather than discrete episodes of psychic trauma. Similarly, although it is clear that the same kinds of problems that apparently lead to reactive attachment disorder might also be associated with feeding and growth disturbances (see Volkmar and Mayes, Chapter 12, this volume), such problems are not (unless made so by definition) necessarily observed with the other features of reactive attachment disorder. Finally, although reactive attachment disorder is by definition relational in nature, it differs from other relational problems and V codes in that the relational problem may have to do with the *absence* of a relationship and that the behavioral constellation observed is clearly exhibited by the child in multiple situations and contexts and over time, not just in the child-caregiver context.

Definitional Issues

As defined in DSM-III, reactive attachment disorder was a disorder of infancy with its onset before age 8 months that was observed in the context of grossly inappropriate development (e.g., as caused by gross neglect or social isolation as in institutional rearing). The apparent "reactive" nature of the condition was central so that the diagnosis could not be made in the absence of gross neglect even if the child otherwise exhibited the behavioral features of the condition. The definition was focused on infants, rather than on somewhat older preschool children, and was quite detailed. In addition to the onset and grossly pathological care criteria, other criteria included lack of developmentally appropriate signs of social responsivity (as exemplified by "several" of seven specific behavioral features); at least three of the following symptoms: weak cry, excessive sleep, lack of interest in the environment, hypomobility, poor muscle tone, and weak root and grasping in feeding attempts; and weight loss or failure to gain weight (i.e., failure to thrive). The condition could not be due to a physical disorder, mental retardation, or infantile autism. The final criterion indicated that the diagnosis was confirmed if the clinical picture reversed with adequate caretaking.

It was quickly apparent that, although the category reflected an important clinical concern, aspects of the definition were unsatisfactory (Rutter and Shaffer 1980). For example, the condition was defined as specific to infants, and criteria were provided for very young children at an age before selective attachments clearly develop. Aspects of the definition were contradictory, and the inclusion of failure to thrive as a diagnostic criterion was unfortunate. because it essentially equated reactive attachment disorder with this diagnosis. Accordingly, major revisions of the definition were undertaken in DSM-III-R.

DSM-III-R dropped failure to thrive as an essential diagnostic feature and indicated that it should be noted, when present, on Axis III. The four essential features of the condition (paraphrased from DSM-III-R) were

A. Markedly disturbed social relatedness in most contexts, beginning before the age of 5, of either of two types (an inhibited type characterized by persistent failure to initiate or respond to most social interactions, and a disinhibited type characterized by indiscriminate sociability).
B. By definition, the social disturbance could not be due to mental retardation or autism or pervasive developmental disorder not otherwise specified.
C. Grossly pathological care as evidenced by one of 1) persistent disregard of the

child's basic emotional needs, or 2) persistent disregard of the child's basic physical needs, or 3) repeated change of primary caregiver.
D. There is a presumption that the social disturbance was caused by the pathological care experience if it followed this care.

The age at onset of the condition was specified only to the extent that the disorder had to originate before age 5 (rather than by 8 months as in DSM-III). Another diagnostic concept (psychosocial dwarfism) was alluded to in the text but not included in the criteria (see Volkmar and Mayes, Chapter 12, this volume).

In contrast to DSM-III-R, ICD-10 includes two diagnostic categories (reactive attachment disorder of childhood and disinhibited attachment disorder). The distinction between the two conditions essentially parallels that encompassed by the two types of disturbed social relatedness in the DSM-III-R definition. Other points of difference from DSM-III-R include: 1) the greater emphasis in ICD-10 on associated emotional difficulties (e.g., misery, apathy, hypervigilance); 2) children with pervasive developmental disorder (but not mental retardation) are excluded from the diagnosis; 3) ICD-10 provides slightly more description of the nature of the associated attachment problem and notes that this is exhibited in a range of contexts with a wide range of individual differences; and 4) ICD-10 does not *require* that the condition always be observed in the context of inadequate care (e.g., if a child develops the behavioral features of reactive attachment disorder following brain injury, he or she would not receive the diagnosis) (Graham 1986).

Data Reanalysis

As an aspect of the review, a series of data reanalyses funded by the MacArthur Foundation were undertaken, using a previously collected data set that included criteria from the DSM-III and DSM-III-R reactive attachment disorder descriptions, as part of a broader review of nearly 120 cases of children referred for evaluation after severe neglect and/or abuse. In each instance, the child had received a comprehensive evaluation, typically including developmental and psychological testing as well as direct observation and psychiatric examination. One or more experienced raters had reviewed each case using a standard coding system. Before the results of these data reanalyses are briefly summarized, it is important to note the limitations of the study: 1) chart review material was used, and 2) although the nature of the sample made it likely that reactive attachment disorder would be exhibited, the sample was drawn from consecutive cases and was not, therefore, truly epidemiological in nature.

The reliability of DSM-III and DSM-III-R reactive attachment disorder criteria were examined. DSM-III criteria proved, generally, to be difficult to use clinically (at least in a retrospective review of this type) and had low reliability. In contrast,

DSM-III-R criteria were both clinically useful and reliable (kappas > .40). As might be expected from the nature of the sample, patterns of inhibited attachment were more common than the pattern of indiscriminate sociability, although the latter was more frequent when children had been in multiple foster homes from a very young age. Eating/feeding problems were sometimes but not always observed in association with reactive attachment disorder. Consistent with previous research, individual differences were marked. Some children with markedly deviant caretaking experiences apparently did *not* exhibit reactive attachment disorder. As might be expected, many preschool children with reactive attachment disorder also exhibited developmental delays of various types (particularly involving language and cognitive skills) that were occasionally so severe as to warrant a diagnosis of mental retardation or of a specific developmental disorder. Consistent with the DSM-III-R definition, the behavioral features of reactive attachment disorder generally appeared to remit after adequate caretaking had been instituted. Data from this reanalysis could not address the issue of whether behavioral features of reactive attachment disorder were ever observed outside the context of grossly deviant care.

The results provided evidence for the greater clinical utility of the DSM-III-R definition of reactive attachment disorder. In contrast, DSM-III criteria proved difficult to use clinically and were generally unreliable. Consistent with DSM-III-R and ICD-10, two rather different patterns of attachment problem were noted.

Discussion

Although the topic of remarkably little research, reactive attachment disorder does appear to deserve continued inclusion in DSM-IV. The particular behavioral features of children who exhibit reactive attachment disorder are not encompassed by other existing diagnostic categories, and the condition is clearly an important target both for intervention and for additional research. The rationale for excluding children with autism/pervasive developmental disorder from the category is clear, because by definition they already exhibit problems in social relatedness, presumably on a biological rather than a "reactive" basis. However, the rationale for excluding children with mental retardation from the diagnostic category seems more questionable. Relatively minor changes in criteria, such as emphasizing the developmental inappropriateness of the disturbance in social relatedness, would allow the diagnosis to be made even with children who exhibit mental retardation (Berry et al. 1980; Blacher and Meyers 1983). Both ICD-10 and DSM-III-R essentially identify two behavioral forms of reactive attachment disorder; for purposes of consistency and compatibility with ICD-10, it appears reasonable to identify two subtypes of the condition in DSM-IV, depending on the nature of the attachment problems. Relatively minor changes in criterion wording would also provide better specification of the behavioral features.

The area of greatest disagreement between ICD-10 and DSM-III-R definitions has to do with the DSM-III-R requirement of adverse care. This requirement was emphasized both in the criteria and in the name (*reactive* attachment disorder). On the one hand, it does appear quite likely that in the vast majority of instances some degree of adverse experience would likely be involved in the pathogenesis of the syndrome. On the other hand, when such adverse experience is made a necessary, etiological requirement, it becomes impossible to note that the behavioral features of the condition are present in the absence of such experience. This point probably has greater implications for research than for clinical service, but the definition does have another disadvantage because it differs from the definitions of other mental disorders by specifying an etiology.

Recommendations

Although empirical data on the reactive attachment disorder diagnostic concept, strictly defined, are rather limited, ample evidence supports its continued inclusion in DSM-IV. The pattern of disturbance exhibited by children with the condition would not be encompassed by other categories nor would it be adequately described by coding the relational disturbance as such (although such codes should, of course, be used as appropriate). Relatively minor modifications in the text and explicit adoption of the already implicit subtyping scheme would enhance compatibility with ICD-10. Unfortunately, the one substantive area of disagreement between the DSM-III-R and ICD-10 definitions—the necessity of including grossly pathological care as an essential feature of the condition—cannot be addressed on the basis of currently available data. The rationale for *not* including this as a necessary criterion for the condition is clear; it also appears quite likely that the vast majority of children with the condition would have experienced such care. Compatibility with ICD-10 would be enhanced if this criterion was not made an essential diagnostic feature (the text could then emphasize that the condition has *usually* been observed in the context of such care); alternatively, this criterion could be retained to be consistent with DSM-III-R.

References

Aber JL, Allen JP: Effects of maltreatment on young children's social emotional development: an attachment theory perspective. Developmental Psychology 23:406–414, 1987

Ainsworth MDS, Blehar MS, Waters E, et al: Patterns of Attachment: A Psychological Study of the Strange Situation. Hillsdale, NJ, Lawrence Erlbaum Associates, 1985

American Psychiatric Association: Diagnostic and Statistical Manual of Mental Disorders, 3rd Edition. Washington, DC, American Psychiatric Association, 1980

American Psychiatric Association: Diagnostic and Statistical Manual of Mental Disorders, 3rd Edition, Revised. Washington, DC, American Psychiatric Association, 1987

Berry P, Gunn P, Andrews R: Behavior of Down Syndrome infants in a strange situation. American Journal of Mental Deficiency 85:213–218, 1980

Blacher J, Meyers CE: A review of attachment formation and disorder of handicapped children. American Journal of Mental Deficiency 87:359–371, 1983

Bowlby J: Maternal Care and Mental Health. Geneva, Switzerland, World Health Organization, 1951

Cicchetti D, Carlson V (eds): Child Maltreatment: Theory and Research on the Causes and Consequences of Child Abuse and Neglect. Cambridge, MA, Cambridge University Press, 1989

Crittenden PM, Ainsworth MDS: Child maltreatment and attachment theory, in Child Maltreatment: Theory and Research on the Causes and Consequences of Child Abuse and Neglect. Edited by Cicchetti D, Carlson V. Cambridge, MA, Cambridge University Press, 1989, pp 432–463

Dennis W: Children of the Creche. New York, Appleton-Century-Crofts, 1973

Egeland B, Sroufe LA: Attachment and early maltreatment. Child Dev 52:44–52, 1981

Graham P: Child Psychiatry: A Developmental Approach. Oxford, England, Oxford University Press, 1986

Hodges J, Tizard B: IQ and behavioral adjustment of ex-institutional adolescents. J Child Psychol Psychiatry 30:53–75, 1989a

Hodges J, Tizard B: Social and family relationships of ex-institutional adolescents. J Child Psychol Psychiatry 30:77–97, 1989b

Hunt J McV: Intelligence and Experience. New York, Ronald Press, 1961

Kempe CH, Silverman FN, Steele BF: The battered-child syndrome. JAMA 181:17–24, 1962

Koluchova J: Severe deprivation in twins: a case study. J Child Psychol Psychiatry 13:107–114, 1971

Main M, George C: Responses of abused and disadvantaged toddlers to distress in age mates: a study in the day care setting. Developmental Psychology 21:407–412, 1985

Main M, Solomon J: Discovery of an insecure/disorganized attachment pattern: procedure, findings, and implications for the classification of behavior, in Affective Development in Infancy. Edited by Yogman M, Brazelton TB. Norwood, NJ, Ablex, 1986, pp 95–124

Mrazek D, Mrazek P: Child maltreatment, in Child and Adolescent Psychiatry: Modern Approaches, 2nd Edition. Edited by Rutter M, Hersov L. Oxford, England, Blackwell, 1985, pp 679–697

Provence S, Lipton R: Infants in Institutions. New York, International Universities Press, 1962

Rutter M: Maternal Deprivation Reassessed. Harmondsworth, Middlesex, England, Penguin, 1972

Rutter M: Maternal deprivation, 1972–1978: new findings, new concepts, new approaches. Child Dev 50:283–305, 1979

Rutter M, Shaffer D: DSM-III: a step forward or back in terms of classification of child psychiatric disorders? J Am Acad Child Psychiatry 19:371–394, 1980

Rutter M, Tuma AH: Diagnosis and classification: some outstanding issues, in Assessment and Diagnosis in Child Psychopathology. Edited by Rutter M, Tuma AH, Lann I. New York, Guilford, 1988, pp 437–452

Skeels HM, Dye HB: A study of the effects of differential stimulation of mentally retarded children. Proceedings of the American Association of Mental Deficiency 44:114–136, 1939

Skuse D: Extreme deprivation in early childhood, I: diverse outcomes for three siblings from an extraordinary family. J Child Psychol Psychiatry 25:523–541, 1984a

Skuse D: Extreme deprivation in early childhood, II: theoretical issues and a comparative review. J Child Psychol Psychiatry 25:543–572, 1984b

Spitz R: Anaclitic depression. Psychoanal Study Child 2:313–342, 1946

Terwogt MM, Schene J, Koops W: Concepts of emotion in institutionalized children. J Child Psychol Psychiatry 31:1131–1143, 1990

Thompson AM: Adam: a severely deprived Colombian orphan: a case report. J Child Psychol Psychiatry 27:689–695, 1986

Tizard B: Adoption: a Second Chance. New York, Free Press, 1977

World Health Organization: Mental Disorders: Glossary and Guide to Their Classification in Accordance With the Ninth Revision of the International Classification of Diseases. Geneva, Switzerland, World Health Organization, 1978

World Health Organization: ICD-10 Chapter V: Mental and Behavioral Disorders: Diagnostic Criteria for Research. Geneva, Switzerland, World Health Organization, 1990

Zeanah CH, Zeanah PD: Intergenerational transmission of maltreatment: insights from attachment theory and research. Psychiatry 52:177–196, 1989

Chapter 16

The Nosological Status of Depression in Children and Adolescents

Adrian Angold, M.B., B.S., M.R.C.Psych.

Statement of the Issues

This review addresses two central issues regarding the definition of depression in children and adolescents: 1) is there sufficient evidence to justify the use of different criteria from those applied to adults in DSM-IV, and 2) is there adequate empirical support to justify maintaining the current differences in the criteria for juvenile depressions embodied in DSM-III-R (American Psychiatric Association 1987)?

Significance of the Issues

For children younger than age 6 years, DSM-III (American Psychiatric Association 1980) introduced five modifications of the adult criteria: 1) dysphoric mood could be inferred from a persistently sad facial expression, 2) only three of the first four symptoms in part B needed to be present, 3) failure to make expected weight gains could be considered in relation to the weight loss criterion, 4) hypoactivity could stand in place of psychomotor agitation or retardation, and 5) "signs of apathy" could replace loss of interest or pleasure or loss of sexual drive. The duration criterion for dysthymia was set at 1 year for children and adolescents. At that time, there was no empirical evidence to support either the 6-year age cutoff or the specific modifications.

DSM-III-R did away with the 6-year age cutoff and all the criterion changes

---

Financial support for the preparation of this chapter was provided by the William T. Grant Foundation through their Faculty Scholar Award program.

associated with it. It also added a new modification for children and adolescents: that irritability could be the primary mood in the diagnosis of a depressive episode. Again, none of these changes was supported by empirical research.

The advent of DSM-IV provides an opportunity to examine the recent literature to determine whether further changes are justified.

Method

Robins and Guze (1970) set out five lines of investigation for the delineation of psychiatric syndromes: 1) clinical description, 2) delimitation from other disorders, 3) laboratory studies, 4) follow-up studies, and 5) family studies. This chapter is organized according to these five topics.

Results

Clinical Description

Depressed mood and irritability. There are no studies that report the frequency with which irritable mood is associated with other depressive symptoms, in the *absence* of depressed mood. Thus, the syndromic association between irritability and depression (as a diagnosis) remains to be demonstrated. The inclusion of irritability may also be partly responsible for the comorbidity that is often observed between depression and oppositional disorder, because four of the criteria symptoms for oppositional disorder would be expected to increase in the presence of irritable mood. Ryan et al. (1987) found that the symptom of anger or irritability had a loading of .68 on a "conduct" factor that included the presence of conduct disorder.

Duration of depressed mood. Poznanski (1982) distinguished between the long-lasting "downcast" mood she felt was characteristic of depression and the misery or unhappiness that may accompany a wide range of diagnoses. Her diagnostic criteria required the depressed affect to have been present for at least 1 month. She also suggested that nonverbal expressions of affect, such as a consistently sad facial expression and the absence of smiles, might be substituted for verbal self-reports of low mood, but no data have been reported in support of this position. On the other hand, Inamdar et al. (1979) found that depressed adolescents usually looked sad only when talking about their depressions and were not continuously depressed, but episodically were intensely affected and disabled. To date, no reports of the actual amount of time that children experience depressive affect have been published. However, Costello et al. (1991) reported that inpatient adolescents with mixed conduct and depressive disorders showed more mood variability than purely depressed adolescents.

Gittelman-Klein (1977) suggested that it might be best to regard the "pervasive and autonomous loss of hedonic experience" as the central feature of depression. However, some degree of anhedonia seems to be quite common in the depressions of childhood, and a marked loss of hedonic capacity might better be regarded as a marker of severity in the presence of other depressive symptoms. Once again, empirical data are lacking on this point.

Syndromic aggregation of depressive symptoms. Feinstein et al. (1984) found that dysphoric symptoms were common in all diagnostic groups but that the combination of dysphoria and self-deprecatory ideation discriminated highly between subjects who were depressed and those with conduct disorder. On the basis of this finding, they suggested that self-deprecatory ideation should be regarded as a core feature of childhood depression.

Costello and Angold (1988) found that a core group of self- and parent-reported symptoms from a depression questionnaire was a good predictor of depression scores obtained from independent interviews. This core group consisted mostly of items probing low mood, anhedonia, and self-deprecation, but it also included tiredness, restlessness, and poor concentration.

The most extensive data on the topic of the syndromic aggregation of depressive symptoms are provided by parent checklist reports collected from general population and clinical samples in a number of countries, using the Child Behavior Checklist (Achenbach et al. 1989) and similar instruments. A factor loading heavily on depressive items appears in most age groups. In general, such factors contain items relating to depressed mood, anhedonia, and depressive cognitions. However, they are never identical in content to DSM-III or DSM-III-R depression and always contain other items (particularly anxiety items) that would not usually be considered for the diagnosis of depression. Furthermore, a clearly depressive factor is often absent for teenage boys.

Age-dependent changes in depressive symptomatology. Epidemiological and clinical evidence suggests that depressive symptoms become much more common during adolescence. The female preponderance of depressive disorders is not apparent until then (Angold 1988a; Angold and Rutter 1992; Rutter 1986; Rutter et al. 1970, 1976), and suicide attempts and completions rise very rapidly in adolescence. We should recognize that if the base rates of symptoms in the population change in relation to each other with age, then their relative weights in contributing to the diagnosis of depression may also change (Digdon and Gotlib 1985). For instance, McConville et al. (1973) described three age-dependent forms of depression characterized by "affectual symptoms" (6- to 8-year-old children), guilt (adolescents), and low self-esteem (older children and adolescents), respectively. Inamdar et al. (1979) noted the absence of motor agitation or retardation, delusions of guilt, and hopelessness in their sample of 30 depressed adolescents, although these symptoms have been reported in adolescents with depression (Chambers et al. 1982; Friedman et al. 1983a, 1983b; Kazdin and Petti 1982; Strober et al. 1981).

Ryan et al. (1987) compared the symptomatology of 95 prepubertal children and 92 adolescents with major depressive disorder. The prepubertal children had more somatic complaints, psychomotor agitation, separation anxiety, phobias, and hallucinations and presented a more depressed appearance, whereas the adolescents suffered from more anhedonia, hopelessness, hypersomnia, weight change, use of illicit drugs, and lethality of suicide attempts (although not more severe suicidal ideation or intent). However, these represented only a minority of the symptoms evaluated, and the authors concluded that the similarities between the depressions of the younger and older groups were more striking than the differences. Surprisingly, psychotic depressions were more common in the prepubertal children. In contrast to the findings of Inamdar et al. (1979), psychomotor agitation and retardation and hopelessness were very common.

Mitchell et al. (1988) compared the symptoms of 45 depressed children with those of 50 depressed adolescents. They found only one significant difference in symptom rates: hypersomnia was more common in the adolescents. In a further comparison with the rates of symptoms in depressed young adults (Baker et al. 1971), the combined child and adolescent group had higher rates of guilt, somatic complaints, low self-esteem, suicidal attempts, and hallucinations, whereas the adults had higher rates of terminal insomnia, anorexia, weight loss, and delusions.

Weissman et al. (1987) found that older children with major depressive disorder reported weight loss and insomnia more often than younger depressed children. Angold et al. (1991), using a larger subset of children from the same study, found that dysphoric episodes occurring in older girls were marked by considerably more sleep and appetite disturbance and an increase in cognitive symptoms, concentration problems, and suicidality. No such age effects appeared in either the reports of the boys or the parent reports about boys or girls.

Methodological differences between these studies could be responsible for some or all of the inconsistent findings. All of the subjects in the study by Ryan et al. (1987) were highly selected for the severity of their depressions, whereas subjects in the Angold et al. (1991) study were selected on the basis of the parent's psychiatric status. Ryan et al. (1987) and Mitchell et al. (1988) also present combined analyses for boys and girls using combined parent and child reports, and this may have obscured age trends that Angold et al. found were confined to girls' self-reports.

Delimitation From Other Disorders

Numerous general population and clinical studies have indicated that childhood depressions are very frequently associated with other DSM diagnoses, in particular anxiety disorders and conduct disorders, and that only a minority of depressions are "pure" (for a review, see Angold and Costello 1993). However, because phenomenological and family-genetic studies have repeatedly demonstrated that depression in adults takes many forms and is associated with many other psychiatric diagnoses, the situation in children may not really differ very much from that in adults.

To give a single representative example, more than two-thirds of the 60 affectively disturbed children and adolescents found by Bird et al. (1988) in their general population study also met criteria for a diagnosis of conduct disorder, oppositional defiant disorder, attention-deficit disorder, or anxiety disorder. These striking findings raise the possibility that depression mostly serves as a marker for the presence of multiple disabling pathologies of other sorts and that the adult criteria are simply picking up what might better be called "misery" in the face of multiple problems.

Furthermore, these findings raise the question of whether pure, anxious, and conduct-disordered depressions all represent examples of the same depressive diathesis, or whether they should be regarded as different disorders. ICD-9 (World Health Organization 1978) has a separate grouping for mixed disorders of conduct and emotions; ICD-10 (World Health Organization 1990) includes a diagnosis of depressive conduct disorder. In both cases, these categories are regarded as being subsets of conduct disorder.

Several authors suggested that certain symptoms that are not considered in the diagnosis of depression in adults (such as school refusal, headaches, or stomachaches) are actually manifestations of depression in childhood and should be counted toward making the diagnosis, rather than being regarded simply as associated phenomena (Kazdin and Petti 1982; Kolvin et al. 1984; Ling et al. 1970; McConville et al. 1973; Pearce 1978). The danger here is that if one attempts to include all possibly associated symptoms, depression becomes just a catchall diagnosis. However, it remains quite possible that there are age-specific manifestations of these disorders.

Laboratory Studies

In the early 1970s, Cytryn et al. (1974), using urinary excretion products as markers, found evidence of abnormalities of catecholamine metabolism in affectively disturbed children. More recently, Rogeness et al. (1990), examining dopamine-beta-hydroxylase in boys who were psychiatrically hospitalized, found that those with high levels of these markers were more likely to be depressed or anxious, whereas those with low levels were more likely to manifest undersocialized conduct disorder. Increased noradrenergic activity was present in at least some forms of emotional disorders; however, these changes were associated with both depression and anxiety. Cavallo et al. (1987) found lower levels of melatonin secretion in a mixed group of depressed prepubertal and pubertal boys than in control subjects, although there was no evidence of any alteration in the melatonin secretory rhythm.

In a review of the status of the dexamethasone suppression test in children, Leckman et al. (1983) concluded that "the validity of the [dexamethasone suppression test] as a diagnostic test remains in doubt" (p. 1058). The studies that have appeared since this review have done nothing to allay such doubts (e.g., Burke and Puig-Antich 1990).

Growth hormone hyposecretion in response to insulin tolerance tests has been documented in prepubertal patients with endogenous major depression, but the same researchers found little in the way of abnormalities in the cortisol or prolactin responses to insulin-induced hypoglycemia in either endogenous or non-endogenous depressed patients (for references, see Burke and Puig-Antich 1990).

A number of studies of the sleep of depressed children and adolescents have appeared, again with conflicting results. The characteristic in-episode sleep abnormalities seen in adults with endogenous depression appear to emerge only in late adolescence. On the other hand, shortened rapid eye movement latency may characterize children with depressive diatheses between episodes (for references, see Burke and Puig-Antich 1990). Emslie et al. (1990) found differences in sleep latency and rapid eye movement latency between hospitalized depressed children and a matched group of control subjects, but other changes that have been described in depressed adults were not found.

Follow-Up Studies

Natural history. Poznanski et al. (1976) managed to follow up 10 of their original group of 14 depressed children and found that half of them still appeared to be depressed 6.5 years later. Pearce (1978) found that more than half of the children identified by an item checklist as suffering from "morbid depression" had their disorder for more than a year.

Garber et al. (1988) followed up 20 10- to 17-year-old patients an average of 8 years after hospital admission, 11 of whom, on chart review, met DSM-III criteria for major depression (whereas the remaining 9 did not). Of the depressed group, 3 were currently depressed at follow-up, and 7 had been depressed since their index episode. Only 1 of the control subjects had been depressed since the index admission.

Kovacs and colleagues (Kovacs and Gatsonis 1989; Kovacs et al. 1984a, 1984b) found that the mean duration of major depression at the time of diagnosis was 32 weeks, whereas those with dysthymic disorder had already been suffering for 3 years. The median time to recovery after diagnosis was 3.5 years for dysthymia, although the recovery rate for major depressive disorder was much faster. However, within 5 years from diagnosis, 69% of the dysthymic patients had an episode of major depression, and 72% of the major depressive patients had a second episode. The only groups to do well were those with adjustment disorder with depressive mood, who recovered relatively quickly and did not relapse, and the control group, of whom only 5% became depressed.

A study by Harrington et al. (1990) that followed children with marked depressive symptomatology into adulthood confirms and extends these findings. Strong continuity of depressive symptomatology was found in those who had adult-type depressions as adolescents. However, prepubertal depressive problems were less predictive of adult depression.

Treatment Studies

The appearance of a number of nonblind, nonplacebo-controlled trials of tricyclic antidepressants (for references, see Angold 1988b) led to a wave of enthusiasm for the use of these drugs in children. However, recent controlled, double-blind trials have so far failed to support this initial positive impression (Geller et al. 1989; Kashani et al. 1984; Klein et al. 1989; Kramer and Feiguine 1981; Puig-Antich et al. 1987; Ryan et al. 1989). The placebo response rate in children has been found to be unexpectedly high in several studies (up to more than 60%). There is also little evidence to support the presence of any significant treatment effect beyond the placebo response.

Family Studies

Numerous studies have shown that a wide range of psychiatric disorders are more common in the children of psychiatrically disturbed parents than in the children of "normal" parents (Quinton and Rutter 1985; Rutter 1966; Rutter and Quinton 1984). More recently, clear links between parental depression and child psychiatric disturbance have been established (Beardslee et al. 1983; Orvaschel 1983; Strober 1984; Weissman et al. 1984a, 1984b, 1984c, 1984d, 1986; Winokur et al. 1978). Beardslee et al. suggested that the current evidence indicates that about 40% of the children of depressed parents have a psychiatric disorder of some sort. Several studies found an increase in the risk for depressive disorders in the relatives of depressed probands, including their children, according to both parents' and children's own reports (Tsuang et al. 1980; Weissman 1984a, 1984b, 1984c, 1984d; Winokur et al. 1978). Weissman et al. (1987) found that the average age at onset for depression in children of depressed parents was 12.6 years, more than 4 years earlier than in the children of nondepressed parents. However, it should be noted that many of these children had other problems as well, particularly with anxiety and conduct disturbances.

There is overwhelming evidence that disordered family functioning is involved in the etiology of a wide range of child psychiatric problems (Rutter 1981), but the issue requires more detailed exploration, specifically in relation to childhood depression. There are also strong suggestions that depressed adults often exhibit poor parenting skills (Cox et al. 1987; Cytryn et al. 1984, 1986; Davenport et al. 1984; Gaensbauer et al. 1984; Mills et al. 1984; Parker 1979a, 1979b, 1981, 1982; Raskin et al. 1971; Weissman and Paykel 1974; Weissman et al. 1972; Zahn-Waxler et al. 1984) as well as other defects of social functioning (John and Weissman 1985). However, we are far from identifying specific links between each adult disorder and its childhood equivalent.

Discussion

1. The syndromic unity of DSM-III and DSM-III-R criteria for depressive disorders in childhood has not been adequately established. There is good evidence that rates of expression of depressive symptoms vary with age, even in children who meet current diagnostic criteria for depression. However, none of the specific modifications in the criteria for children introduced in DSM-III or DSM-III-R has empirical support. The use of depressed mood as the starting point for the diagnosis of depression is strongly indicated, but the same cannot be said of irritability. The DSM-III-R duration criterion may also be too stringent as far as selecting children with psychological impairment due to depression is concerned. It has also been well established that depressed mood, anhedonia, and depressive cognitions often appear together and thus represent a syndrome. However, it is much less clear which other "depressive" symptoms are also really part of this syndrome or whether other symptoms (such as headaches or social withdrawal) should be regarded as diagnostic criteria for depression.
2. DSM-III and DSM-III-R depressions are very frequently associated with other disorders and cannot be regarded as having been satisfactorily delimited from them.
3. Laboratory studies have suggested that there are both similarities and differences between childhood and adult depressions. These studies do not clearly

support the idea that current criteria define the same disorders in these two developmental periods.
4. Follow-up studies have indicated that syndromes associated with depressed mood in childhood greatly increase the risk of depressive disorders over the following 15 years. However, one of the most important demonstrations of this fact was based on diagnostic criteria that differed quite substantially from those in DSM-III or DSM-III-R (Harrington et al. 1990). Thus, although both DSM-III and DSM-III-R identified children at risk for continuing affective disturbance, it is not clear that their specific criteria are either necessary or sufficient for the diagnosis of long-lasting or recurrent depressive disorders in children and adolescents.
5. The evidence from family studies overwhelmingly supports the idea that parental depression is associated with psychopathology in children, but this is little evidence for a pure specific link with childhood depression as defined by DSM-III or DSM-III-R.

In view of the many outstanding questions about the nosologic status of depression in childhood, the adoption of adult criteria must still be seen as a hypothesis, rather than a statement of established fact. The clinical literature suggests that a number of other symptoms (e.g., aches and pains, school refusal, social withdrawal, poor concentration) may be central manifestations of depression in childhood, and a statement to this effect in the rubric of DSM-IV might help to prevent too literal an interpretation of criteria that have not been well validated. The same applies to changes in rates of the disorder and in individual symptoms with age.

The DSM criteria do not require any level of psychosocial impairment for the diagnosis of depression to be made (unlike the Research Diagnostic Criteria [Spitzer et al. 1978]). This makes it difficult to decide whether depressive symptoms are making an independent contribution to poor functioning or simply represent another outcome of other disorders. However, the addition of psychosocial impairment resulting directly from depressive symptomatology as a criterion for the diagnosis of depression would probably not be helpful at this stage, because the issue requires further empirical investigation.

Recommendations

The overall conclusion of this review is that it is not at all clear that adult criteria for depression define the same disorders in childhood and adolescence that they do in adulthood. However, no other set of more appropriate criteria can, as yet, be endorsed. There are very great advantages to be gained from maintaining the present DSM-III-R criteria unchanged in DSM-IV, because any redefinition of diagnostic groupings for depression will serve only to undermine an extensive ongoing research effort that is focused on these criteria.

References

Achenbach TM, Conners CK, Quay HC, et al: Replication of empirically derived syndromes as a basis for taxonomy of child/adolescent psychopathology. J Abnorm Child Psychol 17:299–323, 1989

American Psychiatric Association: Diagnostic and Statistical Manual of Mental Disorders, 3rd Edition. Washington, DC, American Psychiatric Association, 1980

American Psychiatric Association: Diagnostic and Statistical Manual of Mental Disorders, 3rd Edition, Revised. Washington, DC, American Psychiatric Association, 1987

Angold A: Childhood and adolescent depression, I: epidemiological and aetiological aspects. Br J Psychiatry 152:601–617, 1988a

Angold A: Childhood and adolescent depression, II: research in clinical populations. Br J Psychiatry 153:476–492, 1988b

Angold A, Costello EJ: Depressive comorbidity in children and adolescents: empirical, theoretical, and methodological issues. Am J Psychiatry 150:1779–1791, 1993

Angold A, Rutter M: The effects of age and pubertal status on depression in a large clinical sample. Development and Psychopathology 4:5–28, 1992

Angold A, Weissman MM, John K, et al: Parent and child reports of depressive symptoms. J Am Acad Child Adolesc Psychiatry 30:67–74, 1991

Baker M, Dorzab J, Winokur G, et al: Depressive disease: classification and clinical characteristics. Compr Psychiatry 12:354–365, 1971

Beardslee WR, Bemporad J, Keller MB, et al: Children of parents with major affective disorder: a review. Am J Psychiatry 140:825–832, 1983

Bird HR, Canino G, Rubio-Stipec M, et al: Estimates of prevalence of childhood maladjustment in a community survey in Puerto Rico. Arch Gen Psychiatry 45:1120–1126, 1988

Burke PM, Puig-Antich J: Psychobiology of childhood depression, in Handbook of Developmental Psychopathology. Edited by Lewis M, Miller SM. New York, Plenum, 1990, pp 327–339

Cavallo A, Holt KG, Hejazi MS, et al: Melatonin circadian rhythm in childhood depression. J Am Acad Child Adolesc Psychiatry 26:395–399, 1987

Chambers WJ, Puig-Antich J, Tabrizi MA, et al: Psychotic symptoms in prepubertal major depressive disorder. Arch Gen Psychiatry 39:921–927, 1982

Costello EJ, Angold A: Scales to assess child and adolescent depression: checklist, screens and nets. J Am Acad Child Adolesc Psychiatry 27:726–737, 1988

Costello EJ, Benjamin R, Angold A, et al: Mood variability in adolescents: a study of depressed, nondepressed, and comorbid patients. Paper presented at the annual meeting of the Society for Research on Child and Development Psychopathology, Zandvoort, Holland, June 1991

Cox AD, Puckering C, Pound A, et al: The impact of maternal depression in young children. J Child Psychol Psychiatry 28:917–928, 1987

Cytryn L, McKnew DH, Logue M, et al: Biochemical correlates of affective disorders in children. Arch Gen Psychiatry 31:659–661, 1974

Cytryn L, McKnew DH, Zahn-Waxler C, et al: A developmental view of affective disturbances in the children of affectively ill parents. Am J Psychiatry 141:219–222, 1984

Cytryn L, McKnew DH, Zahn-Waxler C, et al: Developmental issues in risk research: the offspring of affectively ill parents, in Depression in Young People: Issues and Perspectives. Edited by Rutter MM, Izard C, Read P. New York, Guilford, 1986, pp 163–188

Davenport YB, Zahn-Waxler C, Adland ML, et al: Early child-rearing practices in families with a manic-depressive parent. Am J Psychiatry 141:230–235, 1984

Digdon N, Gotlib IH: Developmental considerations in the study of childhood depression. Developmental Research 5:162–199, 1985

Emslie GJ, Rush AJ, Weinberg WA, et al: Children with major depression show reduced rapid eye movement latencies. Arch Gen Psychiatry 47:119–124, 1990

Feinstein C, Blouin AG, Egan J, et al: Depressive symptomatology in a child psychiatric outpatient population: correlations with diagnosis. Compr Psychiatry 25:379–391, 1984

Friedman RC, Hurt SW, Clarkin JF, et al: Primary and secondary affective disorders in adolescents and young adults. Acta Psychiatr Scand 67:226–235, 1983a

Friedman RC, Hurt SW, Clarkin JF, et al: Symptoms of depression among adolescents and young adults. J Affect Disord 5:37–43, 1983b

Gaensbauer MD, Harmon RJ, Cytryn L, et al: Social and affective development in infants with a manic depressive parent. Am J Psychiatry 141:223–229, 1984

Garber J, Kriss MR, Koch M, et al: Recurrent depression in adolescents: a follow-up study. J Am Acad Child Adolesc Psychiatry 27:49–54, 1988

Geller B, Cooper TB, Fetner H, et al: Double-blind placebo-controlled study of nortriptyline in depressed adolescents. Verbal presentation at the 36th annual meeting of the American Academy of Child and Adolescent Psychiatry, New York, October 1989

Gittelman-Klein R: Definitional and methodological issues concerning depressive illness in children, in Depression in Childhood: Diagnosis Research Treatment and Conceptual Models. Edited by Schulterbrandt JG, Raskin A. New York, Raven, 1977, pp 69–85

Harrington R, Fudge H, Rutter M, et al: Adult outcomes of childhood and adolescent depression. Arch Gen Psychiatry 47:465–473, 1990

Inamdar SC, Siomopoulos G, Osborne M, et al: Phenomenology associated with depressed moods in adolescents. Am J Psychiatry 136:150–159, 1979

John K, Weissman MM: The familial and psychosocial measurement of depression, in The Measurement of Depression: Clinical, Biological, Psychological, and Psychosocial Retrospectives. Edited by Marsella AJ, Hirschfield RMA, Katz M. New York, Guilford, 1985, pp 1–71

Kashani JH, Shekim WO, Reid JC: Amitriptyline in children with major depressive disorder: a double-blind crossover pilot study. J Am Acad Child Psychiatry 23:348–351, 1984

Kazdin AE, Petti TA: Self-report and interview measures of childhood and adolescent depression. J Child Psychol Psychiatry 23:437–457, 1982

Klein R, Klass E, Koplewitz H, et al: Tricyclic treatment of adolescent depression. Verbal presentation at the 36th annual meeting of the American Academy of Child and Adolescent Psychiatry, New York, October 1989

Kolvin I, Berney TP, Bhate SR: Classification and diagnosis of depression in school phobia. Br J Psychiatry 145:347–357, 1984

Kovacs M, Gatsonis C: Stability and change in childhood-onset depressive disorders: longitudinal course as a diagnostic validator, in The Validity of Psychiatric Diagnosis. Edited by Robins E, Barrett JE. New York, Raven, 1989, pp 57–73

Kovacs M, Feinberg TL, Crouse-Novak M, et al: Depressive disorders in childhood, I: a longitudinal prospective study of characteristics and recovery. Arch Gen Psychiatry 41:229–237, 1984a

Kovacs M, Feinberg TL, Crouse-Novak M, et al: Depressive disorders in childhood, II: a longitudinal study of the risk for a subsequent major depression. Arch Gen Psychiatry 41:643–649, 1984b

Kramer AD, Feiguine RJ: Clinical effects of amitriptyline in adolescent depression: a pilot study. J Am Acad Child Adolesc Psychiatry 20:36–44, 1981

Leckman JF, Weissman MM, Merikangas KR, et al: Panic disorder and major depression: increased risk of depression, alcoholism, panic and phobic disorders in families of depressed probands with panic disorder. Arch Gen Psychiatry 40:1055–1060, 1983

Ling W, Oftedal G, Weinberg N: Depressive illness in children presenting a severe headache. Am J Dis Child 120:122–124, 1970

McConville BJ, Boag LC, Purohit A: Three types of childhood depression. Canadian Psychiatric Association Journal 18:133–137, 1973

Mills M, Puckering C, Pound A, et al: What is it about depressed mothers that influences their children's functioning?, in Recent Research in Developmental Psychology (JCPP Monograph Supplement No 4). Edited by Stevenson J. Oxford, England, Pergamon, 1984, pp 11–17

Mitchell J, McCauley E, Burke PM, et al: Phenomenology of depression in children and adolescents. J Am Acad Child Psychiatry 27:12–20, 1988

Orvaschel H: Parental depression and child psychopathology, in Childhood Psychopathology and Development. Edited by Guze SB, Earls FJ, Barrett JE. New York, Raven, 1983, pp 53–66

Parker G: Parental characteristics in relation to depressive disorders. Br J Psychiatry 134:138–147, 1979a

Parker G: Reported parental characteristics in relation to trait depression and anxiety levels in a non-clinical group. Aust N Z J Psychiatry 13:260–264, 1979b

Parker G: Parental reports of depressives: an investigation of several explanations. J Affect Disord 3:131–140, 1981

Parker G: Parental representations and affective symptoms: examination for an hereditary link. Br J Med Psychol 55:57–61, 1982

Pearce J: The recognition of depressive disorder in children. J R Soc Med 71:494–500, 1978

Poznanski EO: The clinical phenomenology of childhood depression. Am J Orthopsychiatry 52:308–313, 1982

Poznanski EO, Krahenbull V, Zrull JP: Childhood depression: a longitudinal perspective. J Am Acad Child Psychiatry 15:491–501, 1976

Puig-Antich J, Perel JM, Lupatkin W, et al: Imipramine in prepubertal major depressive disorders. Arch Gen Psychiatry 44:81–89, 1987

Quinton D, Rutter M: Family pathology and child psychiatric disorder: a four year prospective study, in Longitudinal Studies in Child Psychology and Psychiatry: Practical Lessons from Research Experience. Edited by Nicol AR. Chichester, England, John Wiley, 1985, pp 91–134

Raskin A, Boothe HH, Reatig NA, et al: Factor analyses of normal and depressed patients' memories of parental behavior. Psychol Rep 29:871–879, 1971

Robins E, Guze SB: Establishment of diagnostic validity in psychiatric illness: its application to schizophrenia. Am J Psychiatry 126:107–111, 1970

Rogeness GA, Javors MA, Maas JW, et al: Catecholamines and diagnoses in children. J Am Acad Child Adolesc Psychiatry 29:234–241, 1990

Rutter M: Children of Sick Parents: An Environmental and Psychiatric Study (Institute of Psychiatry Maudsley Monograph No 16). London, England, Oxford University Press, 1966

Rutter M: Epidemiological longitudinal strategies and causal research in child psychiatry. J Am Acad Child Psychiatry 20:513–544, 1981

Rutter M: The developmental psychopathology of depression: issues and perspectives, in Depression in Young People: Issues and Perspectives. Edited by Rutter M, Izard C, Read P. New York, Guilford, 1986, pp 3–30

Rutter M, Quinton D: Parental psychiatric disorder: effects on children. Psychol Med 14:853–880, 1984

Rutter M, Tizard J, Whitmore K: Education, Health and Behavior. London, England, Longman, 1970

Rutter M, Graham P, Chadwick OFD, et al: Adolescent turmoil: fact or fiction? J Child Psychol Psychiatry 17:35–56, 1976

Ryan ND, Puig-Antich J, Ambrosini P, et al: The clinical picture of major depression in children and adolescents. Arch Gen Psychiatry 44:854–861, 1987

Ryan N, Puig-Antich J, Perel J: A controlled study of amitriptyline versus placebo in adolescent MDD. Verbal presentation at the 36th annual meeting of the American Academy of Child and Adolescent Psychiatry, New York, October 1989

Spitzer RL, Endicott J, Robins E: Research diagnostic criteria: rationale and reliability. Arch Gen Psychiatry 35:773–782, 1978

Strober M: Familial aspects of depressive disorder in early adolescence, in Current Perspectives on Major Depressive Disorders in Children. Edited by Weller EB, Weller RA. Washington, DC, American Psychiatric Press, 1984, pp 38–48

Strober M, Green J, Carlson G: Phenomenology and subtypes of major depressive disorder in adolescence. J Affect Disord 3:281–290, 1981

Tsuang MT, Winokur G, Crowe RR: Morbidity risk of schizophrenia and affective disorders among first degree relatives of patients with schizophrenia, mania, depression and surgical conditions. Br J Psychiatry 137:497–504, 1980

Weissman MM, Paykel ES: The Depressed Woman: A Study of Social Relationships. Chicago, IL, University of Chicago Press, 1974

Weissman MM, Paykel ES, Klerman GL: The depressed woman as a mother. Social Psychiatry 7:98–108, 1972

Weissman MM, Leckman JF, Merikangas KR, et al: Depression and anxiety disorders in parents and children. Arch Gen Psychiatry 41:845–851, 1984a

Weissman MM, Wickramaratne P, Merikangas KR, et al: Onset of major depression in early adulthood: increased familial loading and specificity. Arch Gen Psychiatry 41:1136–1143, 1984b

Weissman MM, Gershon ES, Kidd KK, et al: Psychiatric disorders in the relatives of probands with affective disorders. Arch Gen Psychiatry 41:13–21, 1984c

Weissman MM, Prusoff BA, Gammon GD, et al: Psychopathology in the children (ages 6–18) of depressed and normal parents. Journal of the American Academy of Child Psychiatry 23:78–84, 1984d

Weissman MM, John J, Merikangas KR, et al: Depressed parents and their children: general health, social, and psychiatric problems. Arch Gen Psychiatry 40:801–805, 1986

Weissman MM, Gammon GD, John K, et al: Children of depressed parents: increased psychopathology and early onset of major depression. Arch Gen Psychiatry 44:847–853, 1987

Winokur G, Behar D, Vanvalkenburg C, et al: Is a familial definition of depression both feasible and valid? J Nerv Ment Dis 166:764–768, 1978

World Health Organization: Mental Disorders: Glossary and Guide to Their Classification in Accordance With the Ninth Revision of the International Classification of Diseases. Geneva, Switzerland, World Health Organization, 1978

World Health Organization: ICD-10 Chapter V: Mental and Behavioral Disorders: Diagnostic Criteria for Research. Geneva, Switzerland, World Health Organization, 1990

Zahn-Waxler C, McKnew DH, Cummings M, et al: Problem behaviors and peer interactions of young children with a manic depressive parent. Am J Psychiatry 141:236–240, 1984

Chapter 17

Suicide in Childhood and Adolescence

Robert A. King, M.D., G. Davis Gammon, M.D.,
Cynthia R. Pfeffer, M.D., and Donald J. Cohen, M.D.

Statement of the Issues

Although the presence of suicidal ideation or acts is a frequent and compelling indication for clinical intervention, DSM-III-R (American Psychiatric Association 1987) makes no provision for the systematic classification, ascertainment, and recording of these phenomena. The purpose of this review is examine how suicidal phenomena might be most usefully classified and recorded in DSM-IV and to explore whether a new diagnostic category of suicidality of childhood and adolescence should be included in DSM-IV.

Significance of the Issues

The term *suicidality* is used in this chapter to denote the spectrum of ideation and/or behavior involving deliberate efforts to inflict death or serious physical harm to the self. Suicidality is a leading cause of morbidity and mortality in the young, and research into its causes and prevention remains a high scientific and public health priority. Despite this importance, however, suicidality is noted in DSM-III-R only as a symptom of major depressive disorder or borderline personality disorder.

The current DSM-III-R categorization of suicidality may be problematic in several important regards. First, there is the problem of inadequate coverage. A small but clinically significant number of disturbed suicidal individuals in need of clinical intervention do not meet the criteria for any DSM-III-R diagnostic category. Second, simply subsuming suicidality as a symptom of another diagnosis may be clinically uninformative or misleading; such a diagnosis may fail to capture or convey the distinctive suicidal features that may be the major determinants of the patient's clinical care or prognosis. Third, DSM-III-R's neglect of suicidality could hamper recordkeeping and clinical research about suicidal individuals by failing to provide a generally accepted framework and criteria for identifying, classifying, and recording them.

The potential problems attendant on DSM-III-R's treatment of suicidality might be remedied in several ways: 1) retain the current notion of classifying suicidality as a symptom of other, putatively "primary" diagnoses (e.g. major depression, substance abuse), perhaps treating it as a modifier in the way that psychotic features currently modify the diagnosis of major affective disorder; 2) record suicidality as a supplementary code that, while leaving open its relationship to other mental disorders (if any), would note suicidality as a "clinically significant condition" in its own right; or 3) if research data support the syndromal validity of suicidality, consider it as a mental disorder in its own right.

One crucial issue in choosing between these options is the question, as Shaffer (1982) put it, of whether "suicidal behavior can be seen as a unitary condition or 'diagnosis' arising from a limited set of antecedent circumstances with predictable consequences . . . or is it merely an epiphenomenon of a variety of different mental states each with its own and different determinants and prognoses" (p. 414).

Method

To weigh these options and to assess whether suicidality meets the desiderata for a valid diagnostic category, we have reviewed the literature on youth suicide, focusing on studies with modern research design that utilize adequate sample selection, assessment, and analytic methods. To qualify as a valid new diagnostic category, we specified that a condition should: 1) constitute a *significant mental disorder* (i.e., contribute to impaired social functioning or to personal distress); 2) be *reliably ascertainable*; and 3) have *validity* in terms of distinctive predisposing or etiological features (antecedent or postdictive validity), concomitant biological or psychological features (concurrent validity), and natural history or clinical course (predictive validity). In addition, a classification should facilitate communication, have clinical utility, and not be adequately described by existing diagnoses (Rutter and Gould 1985).

Results

Potential Limitations of the DSM-III-R Approach

Implicit in the DSM-III-R's treatment of suicidality is the notion that suicidality is "epiphenomenal"—that is, that it is primarily "a sequella or complication of various other conditions, and that the majority of suicides are secondary to such conditions. The obvious corollary is that the basic and specific treatment is of the underlying condition rather than of the suicidal inclination per se" (Miles 1977, p. 231).

Are most suicidal patients diagnosable using DSM-III-R categories, and do these diagnoses adequately convey these patients' distinctive clinical features (including natural history, prognosis, treatment needs) and salient antecedents or concomitants (e.g., family factors, genetic influences)?

Lack of adequate coverage in diagnostic studies of suicidal persons. Although most suicidal youth are clearly disturbed, a proportion of suicide attempters and completers who manifest psychopathological symptoms apparently do not meet the criteria for *any* formal DSM-III-R diagnostic category. This leads to the unsatisfactory situation of patients in clear need of clinical intervention, but who nonetheless lack a diagnosable condition. (The overuse of "adjustment disorder" as a diagnostic catchall for many such suicidal adolescents, even when they fail to meet the criteria for that condition, is a symptom of this shortcoming.)

In about 2%–20% of youthful suicides, psychological "postmortems" are unable to establish any DSM-III (American Psychiatric Association 1980) diagnoses (Clark and Horton-Deutsch 1991; Kovacs and Puig-Antich 1989). In some studies, this inability may reflect ascertainment difficulties (Brent 1989); however, even intensive interviewing of multiple informants found no Axis I diagnosis in 19% of Israeli adolescent suicides (Apter et al. 1993). Among the even more heterogeneous group of suicide ideators and attempters, many lack any categorical diagnosis. For example, Trautman et al. (1991) could establish no categorical diagnosis in 13% of female adolescent suicide attempters seen in the emergency room, and in a community sample, Kashani et al. (1989) found that 14% of children reporting suicidal ideation did not meet the criteria for any Axis I disorder. Although the proportion of undiagnosable individuals may seem relatively small, this group poses important scientific and preventive challenges, and their absence in the current nosology is problematic.

Although depression is common in suicidal youth, neither depressive symptoms nor a diagnosis of affective disorder is necessary or sufficient for suicidality. Significant numbers of suicidal individuals either do not appear depressed or do not meet the full DSM-III-R criteria for a depressive disorder. Aggression and impulsivity appear to play a role in suicide, both in combination with and independent of depression. Thus, conduct disorder, borderline personality disorder, and substance abuse are common diagnoses in suicide completers and attempters (Fowler et al. 1986; Frances and Blumenthal 1989; Marttunen et al. 1991; Shaffer et al. 1988) and may occur in the absence of a diagnosable affective disorder

(Cohen-Sandler et al. 1982; Levy and Deykin 1989; Vandivort and Locke 1979; Velez and Cohen 1988).

Failure to identify an important focus of clinical attention. Completely subsuming instances of suicidality under existing DSM-III-R diagnoses may entail other conceptual and practical difficulties as well. Although some DSM-III-R diagnoses are clearly risk factors for suicidality, the presence of a categorical diagnosis is a very nonspecific marker for suicidality. Thus, although roughly 5%–15% of patients with depression, schizophrenia, psychopathic personality, or substance abuse ultimately commit suicide (Miles 1977), this implies that 85%–95% of patients with these serious disorders do not kill themselves. Similarly, most depressed inpatients do not attempt suicide, and many do not report suicidal ideation (Mitchell et al. 1988; van Praag and Plutchik 1988).

The limited explanatory power of categorical diagnoses is further highlighted by the finding of Trautman et al. (1991) that there were no significant diagnostic differences between a group of adolescent female suicide attempters and nonattempting psychiatric outpatient control subjects.

Thus, even when a DSM-III-R diagnosis can be assigned to a suicidal patient, that diagnosis may fail to capture or convey sufficiently the clinically important aspects of the patient's condition. Rather than being a mere "epiphenomenon" of another diagnosis, the patient's suicidality (and the factors related to it) may in many cases be the crucial determinants of clinical care or prognosis.

Obstacles to recordkeeping and research. A related problem concerns clinical research and recordkeeping about suicidal patients and their care. Currently, such activities may be hampered because suicidal patients cannot readily be identified from recorded diagnoses. Instead, suicidal patients are often "submerged" under a variety of other diagnostic categories, even though their suicidality may have been the most compelling focus of clinical attention. In addition, DSM-III-R fails to provide a set of generally accepted criteria for defining such cases.

Summary. To summarize, suicidal status appears only partially linked to current diagnostic categories. Although most young suicidal individuals have psychopathological symptoms, they may meet the criteria for a wide variety of DSM-III-R diagnoses or none at all. Conversely, categorical diagnosis is a very nonspecific discriminator and descriptor of suicidal patients.

In the section that follows, we explore the hypothesis that the crucial aspects of suicidality may lie less in the area of categorical diagnosis than in several realms that cut across current diagnostic categories. Described from a psychological perspective, these appear to include deficits in the regulation of impulsivity and aggression, self-concept and perceived self-competency, quality of attachment and family experience, social adaptive skills, and sensitivity to certain cultural and experiential factors (including exposure to suicidal behavior). In turn, these psychological dimensions may reflect underlying biological, genetic, or familial factors that are also partially independent of current diagnostic categories. Beyond their importance as potential mediating variables in the causal chain leading to suicidality, these factors may have important clinical implications not fully reflected in the assigned DSM-III-R diagnoses.

Suicidality as a Potential Diagnostic Category

To qualify as a valid diagnostic category, a condition should 1) constitute a *significant source of morbidity*; 2) be the product of *mental disorder*; 3) be *reliably ascertainable*; and 4) have *content validity* in terms of possessing distinctive antecedents, concomitants, and consequences that distinguish it from other conditions. We focus on the central issue of construct and external validity (for a fuller discussion, see King et al. 1992).

Do children and adolescents who are suicidal differ from their peers (and resemble each other) in important ways other than their suicidality? This is a key distinction between a symptom and a disorder. The fact that suicidality would constitute a definitionally monosymptomatic disorder is not in itself problematic to its validity; other monosymptomatic disorders such as transient tic disorder, trichotillomania, functional encopresis, and functional enuresis occupy established places in DSM-III-R. The question at stake is whether making such a diagnosis tells one anything beyond the fact that the symptom is present. If so, assigning the diagnosis also conveys potential information about predisposing or etiologic factors, associated psychological or biological features, and/or clinical course or prognosis.

Concomitant validators

Psychological concomitants. Suicidal children and adolescents are characterized by various personality features that cut across diagnostic categories. These include aggressiveness, irritability, low frustration tolerance, resentfulness, and/or impulsivity (Cohen-Sandler et al. 1982; Frances and Blumenthal 1989; Pfeffer et al. 1983, 1989; Plutchik and van Praag 1986). Certain cognitive features are often associated with suicidality and may serve as intervening variables—for example, hopelessness (Kazdin et al. 1983), failure to generate active coping strategies (Asarnow et al. 1987), and lack of perceived competence in critical realms (Harter and Marold 1989).

Biological correlates. Neurobiological studies support the notion that suicidality may be the outcome of multiple factors that are at least partially independent of or interactive with depression and other major disorders (van Praag 1991). A possible link between suicidality and abnormal serotonin (5-hydroxytryptamine [5-HT]) regulation is suggested by postmortem and in vivo metabolite and receptor studies. The most consistent finding has been that of lowered cerebrospinal fluid concentrations of the 5-HT metabolite 5-hydroxyindoleacetic acid (5-HIAA) in suicide attempters, repeaters, and completers (Asberg 1989). However, the correlation of low cerebrospinal fluid 5-HIAA with impulsivity and aggression leaves it unclear whether abnormal 5-HT regulation is related to suicidality per se or to a broader cluster of traits, such as aggressivity and/or impulsivity, which in turn may predispose some individuals to suicidality (Brown et al. 1982; Coccaro et al. 1989; Virkkunen et al. 1989).

Antecedent or postdictive validity

Antecedents such as family and genetic factors and exposure to other suicidal individuals may predispose individuals to suicidal behavior or ideation.

Family factors. Compared with clinical control subjects, suicidal youngsters appear to have more disturbed families on a variety of measures, including abuse or neglect; lack of family warmth; and parental absence, conflict, or psychopathology (as manifested in parental depression, suicidality, or psychiatric hospitalization) (Pfeffer 1989). To what extent these familial associations represent the deleterious impact of nongenetic processes as opposed to the effects of intergenerationally shared genetic factors is unclear.

Exposure to suicidal individuals. Exposure to a peer or relative who has made a suicide attempt is significantly more common among young suicide attempters and completers than among nonsuicidal control subjects (Shafii et al. 1985). The effects of such exposure may also be responsible for the clusters of attempted and completed suicides following reports of a suicide (Brent et al. 1989) or mass media accounts of real or fictional suicides (Davidson and Gould 1989).

Genetic factors. At all stages of the life cycle, suicidal behavior appears to be associated with a family history of attempted or completed suicide. Twin, adoption, and high-risk family studies support the notion there are heritable factors predisposing individuals to suicidal behavior and suggest these factors may be to some extent independent of the major psychiatric disorders frequently associated with suicide (Egeland and Sussex 1985; Roy 1989; Roy et al. 1991; Schulsinger et al. 1979; Wender et al. 1986).

Predictive validity

Studies of suicide completers, attempters, or ideators suggest that suicidality is often a persistent form of maladaptation. Up to 45%–55% of youthful suicides are known to have made previous suicide attempts (Farberow 1989; Shaffer 1974; Shafii et al. 1985), and 10%–50% of adolescent suicide attempters repeat their attempt (Goldacre and Hawton 1985; Stanley and Barter 1970). A 6- to 8-year prospective study of preadolescents and young adolescents found that a history of a suicide attempt was an important predictor of future suicide attempts (Pfeffer et al. 1991). In a follow-up of a nonclinical school-age sample, suicidal ideation persisted in 50% of the children who had reported such ideation at baseline 2 years earlier (Pfeffer et al. 1988). Persistent suicidality was not associated with any specific DSM-III diagnosis.

Discussion and Recommendations

The Work Group on Childhood Affective Disorders considered several options. On the basis of the review, one group of correspondents suggested that, at least in children and adolescents, suicidality meets the desiderata for a new categorical diagnosis (i.e. reliability, construct and external validity, and clinical utility) and proposed model criteria for such a disorder (King et al. 1992). They argued that inclusion of a formal category for suicidality would highlight the existence of an important clinical condition with major preventive, therapeutic, and prognostic consequences that extend beyond those implied by any coexisting diagnoses. Further, it seemed inconsistent to include enuresis, transient tics, or trichotillomania as categorical disorders in DSM-IV, while potentially denying a diagnosis to a child who thinks about, plans, and perhaps then performs a lethal act.

After discussion, the Work Group rejected this proposal. Some members felt the evidence for the validity of such a disorder was not conclusive; others objected in principle, perceiving the proposal as an undesirable retreat from an approach based on syndrome to one stressing symptom.

At the same time, however, the Work Group recognized the need for improved recording of suicidal phenomena in DSM-IV. As an alternative, it was proposed to adopt a supplementary code to record and code suicidal phenomena. Unlike the V codes in DSM-III-R that denote conditions "not attributable to a mental disorder," the new supplementary codes proposed for DSM-IV would specify "clinically significant conditions," while leaving open their relationship to the categorical disorders. The *DSM-IV Options Book* (American Psychiatric Association 1991) therefore included "suicide" among its list of "newly suggested problems that might be included," while cautioning that "it is intended that these problems would be coded only when they are not better accounted for by any other condition" (American Psychiatric Association 1991, p. U:4). However, even this limited proposal for inclusion of a supplementary suicide code was opposed by some on the grounds that attempted suicide is a "single symptom . . . that cut[s] across a variety of disorders and that isolating [it] for separate attention may compromise the clinical assessment necessary to establish the full syndromal picture of which [it] may be a part" (American Psychiatric Association 1991, p. U:4).

Although the inclusion of a supplementary code for suicide may seem an appealing compromise that sidesteps the deeper nosological controversy, the *DSM-IV Options Book* proposal has several serious difficulties. First, in actual practice, supplementary codes are often omitted or used unreliably, posing problems for recordkeeping and retrieval (Sniezek et al. 1989). Second, the *DSM-IV Options Book* text refers only to "suicide attempts," whereas the proposed code simply specifies "suicide." This neglects the fact that intense suicidal ideation is also an important potential indication for clinical attention and should be included in the proposed system of supplementary codes. Third, and most serious, no clear guidelines are given for determining whether a given suicide attempt is "better accounted for by another condition." The book implies that if a suicide attempt is attributed to a categorical disorder, only that latter diagnosis is to be assigned (and the code for suicide omitted); this practice perpetuates the difficulties discussed earlier. For example, will the diagnosis of adjustment disorder preclude assignment of the supplementary code for suicide?

The assignment of other, putatively "primary" diagnoses should not preclude the simultaneous assignment of a supplementary code for suicidal behavior (or ideation). Unless the supplementary code is consistently assigned to all cases of suicidal behavior, many instances of life-threatening behavior will go unnoted in the official nosology, thereby hindering the systematic retrieval of clinical data on suicide and impeding future research.

References

American Psychiatric Association: Diagnostic and Statistical Manual of Mental Disorders, 3rd Edition. Washington, DC, American Psychiatric Association, 1980

American Psychiatric Association: Diagnostic and Statistical Manual of Mental Disorders, 3rd Edition, Revised. Washington, DC, American Psychiatric Association, 1987

American Psychiatric Association: DSM-IV Options Book: Work in Progress. Washington, DC, American Psychiatric Association, 1991

Apter A, Bleich A, King RA, et al: Death without warning? a clinical post-mortem study of 43 Israeli adolescent male suicides. Arch Gen Psychiatry 50:138–142, 1993

Asarnow J, Carlson G, Guthrie D: Coping strategies, self-perceptions, hopelessness, and perceived family environments in depressed and suicidal children. J Consult Clin Psychol 55:361–365, 1987

Asberg M: Neurotransmitter monoamine metabolites in the cerebrospinal fluid as risk factors for suicidal behavior, in Report of the Secretary's Task Force on Youth Suicide, Vol 2: Risk Factors on Youth Suicide (DHHS Publ No ADM-89-1622). Washington, DC, U.S. Government Printing Office, 1989, pp 193–212

Brent DA: The psychological autopsy: methodological considerations for the study of adolescent suicide. Suicide Life Threat Behav 19:43–57, 1989

Brent DA, Kerr MM, Goldstein C, et al: An outbreak of suicide and suicidal behavior in a high school. J Am Acad Child Adolesc Psychiatry 28:918–924, 1989

Brown GL, Ebert ME, Goyer PF, et al: Aggression, suicide, and serotonin: relationship to CSF amine metabolites. Am J Psychiatry 139:741–746, 1982

Clark DC, Horton-Deutsch SL: Assessment in absentia: the value of the psychological autopsy method for studying antecedents of suicide and predicting future suicides, in Assessment and Prediction of Suicide. Edited by Maris R, Berman A, Maltsberger J, et al. New York, Guilford, 1991, pp 144–182

Coccaro EF, Siever LJ, Klar HM, et al: Serotonergic studies in patients with affective and personality disorders. Arch Gen Psychiatry 46:587–599, 1989

Cohen-Sandler R, Berman AL, King RA: Life stress and symptomatology: determinants of suicidal behavior in children. J Am Acad Child Psychiatry 21:565–574, 1982

Davidson L, Gould M: Contagion as a risk factor for youth suicide, in Report of the Secretary's Task Force on Youth Suicide, Vol 2: Risk Factors for Youth Suicide (DHHS Publ No ADM-89-1622). Washington, DC, U.S. Government Printing Office, 1989, pp 88–106

Egeland J, Sussex J: Suicide and family loading for affective disorders. JAMA 254:915–918, 1985

Farberow NL: Preparatory and prior suicidal behavior factors, in Report of the Secretary's Task Force on Youth Suicide, Vol 2: Risk Factors for Youth Suicide (DHHS Publ No ADM-89-1622). Washington, DC, U.S. Government Printing Office, 1989, pp 34–55

Fowler FC, Rich CL, Young D: San Diego Suicide Study, II: substance abuse in young cases. Arch Gen Psychiatry 43:962–965, 1986

Frances A, Blumenthal SJ: Personality as a predictor of youthful suicide, in Report of the Secretary's Task Force on Youth Suicide, Vol 2: Risk Factors for Youth Suicide (DHHS Publ No ADM-89-1622). Washington, DC, U.S. Government Printing Office, 1989, pp 160–171

Goldacre M, Hawton K: Repetition of self-poisoning and subsequent death in adolescents who take overdoses. Br J Psychiatry 146:395–398, 1985

Harter S, Marold DB: Psychosocial risk factors contributing to adolescent suicidal ideation. New Directions for Child Development 64:71–91, 1989

Kashani JH, Goddard P, Reid JC: Correlates of suicidal ideation in a community sample of children and adolescents. J Am Acad of Child Adolesc Psychiatry 28:912–917, 1989

Kazdin AE, French NH, Unis AS, et al: Hopelessness, depression, and suicidal intent among psychiatrically disturbed inpatient children. J Consult Clin Psychol 51:504–510, 1983

King RA, Pfeffer CR, Gammon GD, et al: Suicidality of childhood and adolescence: review of the literature and proposal for establishment of a DSM-IV category, in Advances in Clinical Child Psychology, Vol 14. Edited by Lahey BB, Kazdin AE. New York, Plenum, 1992, pp 297–325

Kovacs M, Puig-Antich J: Major psychiatric disorders as risk factors in youth suicide, in Report of the Secretary's Task Force on Youth Suicide, Vol 2: Risk Factors for Youth Suicide (DHHS Publ No ADM-89-1622). Washington, DC, U.S. Government Printing Office, 1989, pp 143–159

Levy JC, Deykin EY: Suicidality, depression, and substance abuse in adolescence. Am J Psychiatry 146:1462–1467, 1989

Marttunen MJ, Aro HM, Henriksson MM, et al: Mental disorders in adolescent suicide. Arch Gen Psychiatry 48:834–839, 1991

Miles CP: Conditions predisposing to suicide: a review. J Nerv Ment Dis 164:231–246, 1977

Mitchell MD, McCauley E, Burke PM, et al: Phenomenology of depression in children and adolescents. J Am Acad Child Adolesc Psychiatry 27:12–20, 1988

Pfeffer CR: Family characteristics and support systems as risk factors for youth suicide, in Report of the Secretary's Task Force on Youth Suicide, Vol 2: Risk Factors for Youth Suicide (DHHS Publ No ADM-89-1622). Washington, DC, U.S. Government Printing Office, 1989, pp 71–87

Pfeffer CR, Plutchik R, Mizruchi MS: Suicidal and assaultive behavior in children: classification, measurement, and interrelations. Am J Psychiatry 1983; 140:154–157

Pfeffer CR, Lipkins R, Plutchik R, et al: Normal children at risk for suicidal behavior: a two-year follow-up study. J Am Acad Child Adolesc Psychiatry 27:34–41, 1988

Pfeffer CR, Newcorn J, Kaplan G, et al: Subtypes of suicidal and assaultive behaviors in adolescent psychiatric inpatients: a research note. J Child Psychol Psychiatry 30:151–163, 1989

Pfeffer CR, Klerman GL, Hurt SW, et al: Suicidal children grow up: demographic and clinical risk factors for adolescent suicide attempts. J Am Acad Child Adolesc Psychiatry 30:609–616, 1991

Plutchik R, van Praag HM: The measurement of suicidality, aggressivity, and impulsivity. Clin Neuropharmacol 9:380, 1986

Roy A: Genetics and suicidal behavior, in Report of the Secretary's Task Force on Youth Suicide, Vol 2: Risk Factors on Youth Suicide (DHHS Publ No ADM-89-1622). Washington, DC, U.S. Government Printing Office, 1989, pp 247–262

Roy A, Segal NL, Centerwall BS, et al: Suicide in twins. Arch Gen Psychiatry 48:29–32, 1991

Rutter M, Gould M: Classification, in Child and Adolescent Psychiatry, 2nd Edition. Edited by Rutter M, Hersov L. Oxford, England, Blackwell Scientific, 1985, pp 304–321

Schulsinger R, Kety S, Rosenthal D, et al: A family study of suicide, in Origins, Prevention and Treatment of Affective Disorders. Edited by Schou M, Stromgren E. New York, Academic Press, 1979, pp 277–287

Shaffer D: Suicide in childhood and early adolescence. J Child Psychol Psychiatry 15:275–291, 1974

Shaffer D: Diagnostic considerations in suicidal behavior in children and adolescents. J Am Acad Child Psychiatry 21:414–415, 1982

Shaffer D, Garland A, Gould M, et al: Preventing teenage suicide: a critical review. J Am Acad Child Adolesc Psychiatry 27:675–687, 1988

Shafii M, Carrigan S, Whittinghill JR, et al: Psychological autopsy of completed suicide in children and adolescents. Am J Psychiatry 142:1061–1064, 1985

Sniezek JE, Finklea JF, Graitcer PL: Injury coding and hospital discharge data. JAMA 262:2270–2272, 1989

Stanley EJ, Barter JT: Adolescent suicidal behavior. Am J Orthopsychiatry 40:87–96, 1970

Trautman PD, Rotheram-Borus MJ, Dopkins S, et al: Psychiatric diagnoses in minority female adolescent suicide attempters. J Am Acad Child Adolesc Psychiatry 30:617–622, 1991

Vandivort DS, Locke BZ: Suicide ideation; its relation to depression, suicide and suicide attempt. Suicide Life Threat Behav 9:205–218, 1979

van Praag HM: Serotonergic dysfunction and aggression control. Psychol Med 21:15–19, 1991

van Praag HM, Plutchik R: Increased suicidality in depression: group or subgroup characteristic? Psychiatry Res 26:273–278, 1988

Velez C, Cohen P: Suicidal behavior and ideation in a community sample of children. J Am Acad Child Adolesc Psychiatry 27:349–356, 1988

Virkkunen M, DeJong J, Bartko J, et al: Relationship of psychobiological variables to recidivism in violent offenders and impulsive fire setters. Arch Gen Psychiatry 46:600–603, 1989

Wender PH, Kety SS, Rosenthal D, et al: Psychiatric disorders in the biological and adoptive families of adopted individuals with affective disorders. Arch Gen Psychiatry 43:923–992, 1986

Chapter 18

Adjustment Disorder in Children and Adolescents

Jeffrey H. Newcorn, M.D., and James Strain, M.D.

Statement of the Issues

Two principal issues are considered in this review: 1) does the DSM-III-R (American Psychiatric Association 1987) definition of adjustment disorder accurately reflect the clinical presentation seen in children and adolescents, and 2) are there differences between adjustment disorder in youth and adults that should be reflected in the DSM-IV criteria?

Significance of the Issues

The DSM-III-R definition of adjustment disorder consists of three essential components. There must be a maladaptive reaction to an identified psychosocial stressor that involves impairment in either social, occupational, or school functioning, or is in excess of a normal and expectable reaction to the stressor. The maladaptive reaction must occur within 3 months of the occurrence of the stressor and must not persist for longer than 6 months. The disturbance must not fulfill the diagnostic criteria for another major psychiatric disorder or the V code "uncomplicated bereavement." A variety of symptomatic presentations of adjustment disorder are identified, which are categorized as subtypes.

The combination of subsyndromal symptomatology and the presence of an identified psychosocial stressor serves to distinguish adjustment disorder from all other Axis I and Axis II disorders. Adjustment disorder and posttraumatic stress disorder both require the presence of a psychosocial stressor. However, posttraumatic stress disorder is characterized by severe psychosocial stress and a specific constellation of affective and autonomic symptoms, whereas adjustment disorder can be triggered by a stressor of any severity and may present with a wide range of symptomatology. Similarly, although the individual subtypes of adjustment disorder resemble atypical or subthreshold presentations of many other disorders, the latter need not be stress-related and are therefore classified under the appropriate symptom domain using the designation "not otherwise specified."

Historically, adjustment disorder has been a frequently used diagnosis in children and adolescents. However, it has also been problematic. The complex and uncertain relationship between stress and psychiatric disorder (Rutter 1981; Woolston 1988) raises questions regarding the suitability of the concepts that have formed the basis of adjustment disorder in DSM-III (American Psychiatric Association 1980) and DSM-III-R. Furthermore, the lack of specificity of adjustment disorder and the ease with which it may be assigned offer considerable potential for overuse as a means of "protecting" patients from receiving other diagnostic labels that may be perceived as more "stigmatizing" (Wynne 1975). This may result in the incorrect classification of children with more severe psychiatric disorders (Looney and Gunderson 1978) and thereby contribute to delays in treatment planning (Weiner and Del Gaudio 1976).

Method

A Medline search was conducted to identify all refereed publications from approximately 1980–1990 concerning adjustment disorder or the relationship of life events to the development of psychiatric disorders in youth. Selected journal articles published prior to DSM-III and relevant textbook chapters were also reviewed.

Results

Prevalence

Prevalence estimates of adjustment disorder are characterized by considerable variability, with generally high rates (Table 18–1). However, the inconsistent use of structured diagnostic instruments in case identification limits the utility of some of these reports. Only one study examined the prevalence of adjustment disorder in the general population (Bird et al. 1988). Using a Children's Global Assessment Scale (Shaffer et al. 1983) score ≤70 as the cutoff for caseness, the prevalence of adjustment disorder was determined to be 7.6%. However, if children with scores between 61 and 70 were excluded, the prevalence of adjustment disorder dropped to 4.2%, suggesting a low level of impairment in about 40% of the cases.

Nature of Symptomatology

In all age groups, depressive symptoms are prominently represented (Table 18–2). However, studies in child and adolescent populations point to the importance of

Table 18–1. Prevalence of adjustment disorder

Study	Sample type	Sample size	Assessment method	Prevalence
Bird et al. 1988	Epidemiological general population	Probability estimate of 2,036 households	Structured rating scales, clinical interview	7.6% (CGAS ≤ 70), 4.2% (CGAS ≤ 60)
Weiner and Del Gaudio 1976	Epidemiological clinical services	1,344	Clinical diagnosis	27% of all cases
J. E. Mezzich et al. 1989	Clinical screening evaluation (all services)	11,292	Semistructured assessment instrument	10% (all ages) 16% (< 18 years old)
Faulstich et al. 1986	Clinical (adolescent inpatient)	392	Chart review, clinical diagnosis	12.5%
Hillard et al. 1987	Clinical (emergency room)	100 adolescents, 100 adults (random)	Chart review, clinical diagnosis	42% of adolescents, 13% of adults
Doan and Petti 1988	Clinical (partial hospital)	796	Chart review, clinical diagnosis	7%
Jacobson et al. 1980	Clinical (4 outpatient pediatric clinics)	20,000 pediatric patients	Clinical diagnosis	25%–65% of cases with psychiatric diagnosis

Note. CGAS = Children's Global Assessment Scale.

Table 18–2. Nature of symptomatology in adjustment disorder

Study	Sample/design	N	Age	Finding
J. E. Mezzich et al. 1989	Clinical population, semi-structured evaluation instrument	11,292 (10% with adjustment disorder)	All ages (1,868 < 18 years old)	Half of adjustment disorder group had adjustment disorder with depressed mood
Cantwell and Baker 1989	Outpatient speech and language clinic, follow-up design	151 cases (19 with adjustment disorder)	3.0–15.8 years (mean, 6.4 years)	13/19 cases (68%) mixed types: 42% mixed emotions, 26% mixed emotions/conduct
Faulstich et al. 1986	Chart review (inpatients)	392 (49 with adjustment disorder)	Adolescent	Adjustment disorder subtypes: mixed 35%, depressed 27%, atypical 22%, conduct 12%
Andreasen and Wasek 1980	Chart review (outpatients)	199, 303	Adolescent, adult	Behavioral symptoms: 77% adolescents, 25% adults; depressive symptoms: 87% adults, 50% adolescents
Fabrega et al. 1987	Mixed clinical sample (subset of Mezzich et al. 1989 data set)	5,569 (127 with adjustment disorder only)	All ages	Symptoms of adjustment disorder group: 76% depressed mood, 58% insomnia, 29% social withdrawal, 29% suicidal indicators

behavioral symptoms and the frequency of mixed clinical presentations. There is also a significant association with suicidal behavior. Minnaar et al. (1980) found that 56% of all patients hospitalized for suicidal behavior (studied prospectively) met DSM-II (American Psychiatric Association 1968) criteria for transient situational disturbance. McGrath (1989) reported that 58% of 325 consecutive admissions for deliberate self-poisoning met criteria for adjustment disorder with depressed mood, the majority of whom were ages 15–24 years and female. Psychological autopsy studies have yielded similar results. Runeson (1989) reported that 14% of 58 consecutive suicide victims ages 15–29 years were best classified as adjustment disorder with depressed mood. Similarly, Fowler et al. (1986) reported that 9% of 133 suicide victims ages 10–29 years met criteria for adjustment disorder.

Reliability

A. C. Mezzich et al. (1985) determined the interrater agreement (kappa) for adjustment disorder to be .05 (not significant) in a study in which psychiatrists and psychologists evaluated 27 child and adolescent case histories; agreement regarding DSM-II transient situational disturbance was higher (kappa = .28, $P < .05$). Similarly, Werry et al. (1983) found low reliability for adjustment disorder (kappa = .23).

Results of the United Kingdom–World Health Organization study of the reliability of ICD-9 (World Health Organization 1978) categories (Gould et al. 1988) are consistent with the findings from studies of DSM-III. The kappa for adjustment disorder was .23, considerably lower than for other categories studied. However, use of a psychiatric glossary improved reliability (kappa = .33). Rey et al. (1988) reported a kappa of .46 for adjustment disorder in adolescent patients using a combination of structured ratings and unstructured clinical interviews, lending further support to the conclusion that structured methods can improve the reliability of adjustment disorder.

Stability and Outcome

Weiner and Del Gaudio (1976) found a 15% stability rate for adolescents originally diagnosed with transient situational disturbance on 10-year follow-up. Cantwell and Baker (1989) found that none of a group of 19 children and adolescents with adjustment disorder retained the diagnosis after 4 years, noting movement toward both improved health and more serious illness. Individuals with mild symptomatology generally recover (Thomas and Chess 1984). However, many cases progress to more severe forms of psychopathology (Fard et al. 1978; Weiner and Del Gaudio 1976). Andreasen and Hoenk (1982) reported that only 44% of a group of 52 adolescents originally diagnosed with adjustment disorder were well at 5-year follow-up. An additional 13% were well at follow-up but had intervening difficulties.

However, the adjustment disorder subtype in adolescence did not predict the follow-up diagnosis. Similarly, Cantwell and Baker (1989) found that the recovery rate from adjustment disorder was 26%, the most common follow-up diagnoses being disruptive behavior and anxiety disorders.

Comorbidity

Fabrega et al. (1987) reported that in only 2.3% of a large cohort of child and adult patients with adjustment disorder was this the only Axis I or Axis II diagnosis. Kovacs et al. (1984) found that 45% of 11 children with adjustment disorder with depressed mood had a comorbid psychiatric diagnosis. A subsequent publication that included 8 additional children with adjustment disorder with depressed mood reported the incidence of comorbidity to be 58% (Kovacs et al. 1988). Comorbidity in adjustment disorder was lower than in either dysthymic disorder or major depressive disorder.

Temporal Characteristics

There are no data regarding the suitability of the onset criterion in adjustment disorder. However, several studies have evaluated duration. Andreasen and Wasek (1980) reported that persistent symptomatology was more characteristic of adolescents than adults; 66% of adolescents and 35% of adults were symptomatic for more than 6 months, whereas 47% of adolescents and 23% of adults were ill for longer than 1 year.

Kovacs et al. (1984) studied the correlates of depressive disorders in children and found the mean duration of adjustment disorder with depressed mood to be 25 weeks (SD = 18 weeks). The peak interval-specific probability of recovery was determined to be 6–9 months, and, by 9 months, 90% of the children had recovered. Similarly, recovery from adjustment disorder in a group of newly diagnosed diabetic children was 50% by 2.5 months and 93% by 9 months (Kovacs et al. 1985).

Goodyear et al. (1987) more broadly examined the temporal relationship between the occurrence of undesirable life events and the development of psychiatric disorders in child psychiatric outpatients and community control subjects. The occurrence of negative life events increased the risk of disorder by three to six times, although the temporal relationship of stressor to disorder varied. The onset of symptoms was within 16 weeks of an event in 49% of the cases and within 6 months in 70% of the cases. However, 30% of the cases did not develop symptoms until 6 months to 1 year following the undesirable event.

Stressor Criterion

Andreasen and Wasek (1980) found that stressors were more likely to be chronic (>1 year) in adolescents than in adults (59% versus 36%). School problems were the most frequently identified precipitant for symptomatology in the adolescent population (> 60%), although a variety of family, boyfriend-girlfriend, and substance abuse problems were also common. In contrast, marital problems, including separation and divorce, were the most common stressors in adults.

Additional data regarding the stressor criterion in adjustment disorder may be extrapolated from studies that have examined the relationship between life events and psychiatric disturbance more broadly. Monroe (1982) found that individuals with and without preexisting psychiatric symptoms responded differently to the presence of stressful events. Brown and Siegel (1988) reported that internal, global attributions for negative life events were positively correlated with depression in adolescents only when the causes were uncontrollable. Hammen (1988) found that children's cognitions about self-worth and self-efficacy were mediating factors in determining the likelihood of developing depression in response to stressful life events. In other words, it is not the exposure to stress per se that leads to psychopathology, but rather an interaction between certain key features of the stressor and the individual's psychological and cognitive makeup. These findings challenge the notion that stress is universally related to psychopathology and argue for increased specificity of the stressor criterion in adjustment disorder. However, they do not provide clear direction as to how this criterion might be reformulated.

Discussion

There have been few systematic studies of adjustment disorder. Some of these were begun prior to 1980 and did not use current diagnostic criteria. Because other studies of adjustment to stressful life events have not been linked to clinical diagnosis, conclusions about specific categories such as adjustment disorder are at best inferential. The lack of algorithms for adjustment disorder on many structured diagnostic interviews has compounded this problem, because data on adjustment disorder were not collected in a number of recent surveys of child and adolescent psychopathology.

Nevertheless, the available data indicate that adjustment disorder is a serious condition in children and adolescents, as evidenced by the following: 1) adjustment disorder accounts for a significant number of cases in all treatment settings; 2) although the severity of impairment is not uniformly high, adjustment disorder is associated with considerable morbidity (emergency room visits and hospital admissions) and even mortality (completed suicide) in a significant number of individuals; and 3) a substantial number of children and adolescents with this condition go on to develop other, more severe disorders. In this respect, adjustment disorder appears to be different in children and adolescents than in adults: the course in adults is more often benign. However, the adjustment disorder subtype has not been shown to predict follow-up diagnosis. The large number of youth with adjustment disorder who present with mixed syndromes provides further evidence that subtyping according to symptom domain may be of limited utility.

Another serious problem is low reliability. Some authors have speculated that the interpretation of descriptors such as "maladaptive" and "symptoms in excess of a normal and expectable reaction" may contribute to low reliability, because these terms are culturally bound, and their meaning may vary greatly among physicians and patients alike (Fabrega and Mezzich 1987; Malt 1986). Lack of clarity as to whether comorbidity of adjustment disorder and other psychiatric disorders is permitted may further contribute to low reliability. However, the absence of a specific symptom profile and lack of clarity regarding what should constitute a stressor represent other formidable obstacles to achieving reliability.

Studies of temporal characteristics of stress-related conditions highlight further difficulties. Although children's reactions to stress are frequently brief, chronic maladjustment may also occur, most often in the context of enduring stress such as chronic medical illness, parental death, or separation (Newcorn and Strain 1992). Over time, those conditions that persist generally progress to meet criteria for another mental disorder. However, this does not necessarily occur within 6 months.

Other important questions also remain unanswered. There are little published data available to assess the discriminant validity of adjustment disorder in youth. Such information would be useful in determining whether adjustment disorder should be viewed as representing a subthreshold presentation of posttraumatic stress disorder; a variant of the "minor" mood, anxiety, and behavioral disorders; or a separate disorder independent of any of these conditions.

Recommendations and Proposed Revisions

It is proposed that adjustment disorder remain a separate diagnostic category in DSM-IV, much as it has been in DSM-III and DSM-III-R. There are insufficient data to recommend any of the other possibilities at present. The creation of a separate adjustment disorder category for children and adolescents is not indicated, despite differences in outcome and prevalence of adjustment disorder subtypes, because similar symptomatic profiles can be identified across the life span. Inclusion of adjustment disorder in a new class of stress-related disorders (including posttraumatic stress disorder) remains an option, provided that data can demonstrate a similarity between these conditions.

The following revisions are recommended

1. The criteria should attempt to minimize the use of terms laden with value judgments (e.g., *maladaptive*) and clarify that the existence of another mental disorder is exclusionary only if it better accounts for the stress-related symptoms. This would help to improve reliability.
2. The duration criterion should be altered to better account for the persistence of adjustment disorder symptoms beyond 6 months, provided the stressor is ongoing and the disorder does not fulfill criteria for another mental disorder.
3. The text should be specific, to the extent this is possible, regarding which types of life events are likely to result in adjustment disorder.
4. Differences between adjustment disorder and other subthreshold disorders that are not stress-related (i.e., the "not otherwise specified" categories) should be highlighted.

The feasibility of deleting little-used or unsubstantiated subtypes will be assessed in analyses of existing data sets from Western Psychiatric Institute and Clinic (Mezzich et al. 1989) and the National Institute of Mental Health.

References

American Psychiatric Association: Diagnostic and Statistical Manual of Mental Disorders, 2nd Edition. Washington, DC, American Psychiatric Association, 1968

American Psychiatric Association: Diagnostic and Statistical Manual of Mental Disorders, 3rd Edition. Washington, DC, American Psychiatric Association, 1980

American Psychiatric Association: Diagnostic and Statistical Manual of Mental Disorders, 3rd Edition, Revised. Washington, DC, American Psychiatric Association, 1987

Andreasen NC, Hoenk PR: The predictive value of adjustment disorders: a follow-up study. Am J Psychiatry 139:584–590, 1982

Andreasen NC, Wasek P: Adjustment disorders in adolescents and adults. Arch Gen Psychiatry 37:1166–1170, 1980

Bird HR, Canino G, Rubio-Stipec M, et al: Estimates of the prevalence of childhood maladjustment in a community survey in Puerto Rico: the use of combined measures. Arch Gen Psychiatry 45:1120–1126, 1988

Brown JD, Siegel JM: Attributions for negative life events and depression: the role of perceived control. J Pers Soc Psychol 54:316–322, 1988

Cantwell DP, Baker L: Stability and natural history of DSM-III childhood diagnoses. J Am Acad Child Adolesc Psychiatry 28:691–700, 1989

Doan RJ, Petti TA: Clinical and demographic characteristics of child and adolescent partial hospital patients. J Am Acad Child Adolesc Psychiatry 28:66–69, 1988

Fabrega H Jr, Mezzich J: Adjustment disorder and psychiatric practice: cultural and historical aspects. Psychiatry 50:31–49, 1987

Fabrega H Jr, Mezzich JE, Mezzich AC: Adjustment disorder as a marginal or transitional illness category in DSM-III. Arch Gen Psychiatry 44:567–572, 1987

Fard K, Hudgens RW, Welner A: Undiagnosed psychiatric illness in adolescents: a prospective study and seven-year follow-up. Arch Gen Psychiatry 35:279–282, 1978

Faulstich ME, Moore JR, Carey MP, et al: Prevalence of DSM-III conduct and adjustment disorders for adolescent psychiatric inpatients. Adolescence 21:333–337, 1986

Fowler RC, Rich CL, Young D: San Diego suicide study, II: substance abuse in young cases. Arch Gen Psychiatry 43:962–965, 1986

Goodyear IM, Kolvin I, Gatzanis S: The impact of recent undesirable life events on psychiatric disorders in childhood and adolescence. Br J Psychiatry 151:179–184, 1987

Gould M, Rutter M, Shaffer D, et al: UK/WHO study of ICD-9, in Assessment and Diagnosis in Child Psychopathology. Edited by Rutter M, Tuma AH, Lann IS. New York, Guilford, 1988, pp 37–65

Hammen C: Self-cognitions, stressful events, and the prediction of depression in children of depressed mothers. J Abnorm Child Psychol 16:347–360, 1988

Hillard JR, Slomowitz M, Levi LS: A retrospective study of adolescents' visits to a general hospital psychiatric emergency service. Am J Psychiatry 144:432–436, 1987

Jacobson AM, Goldberg ID, Burns BJ, et al: Diagnosed mental disorder in children and use of health services in four organized health care settings. Am J Psychiatry 137:559–565, 1980

Kovacs M, Feinberg TL, Crouse-Novak MA, et al: Depressive disorders in childhood, I: a longitudinal prospective study of characteristics and recovery. Arch Gen Psychiatry 41:229–237, 1984

Kovacs M, Feinberg TL, Paulauskas S, et al: Initial coping responses and psychosocial characteristics of children with insulin-dependent diabetes mellitus. J Pediatr 106:827–834, 1985

Kovacs M, Paulauskas S, Gatsonis C, et al: Depressive disorders in childhood, III: a longitudinal study of comorbidity with and risk for conduct disorders. J Affect Disord 15:205–217, 1988

Looney JG, Gunderson EKE: Transient situational disturbances: course and outcome. Am J Psychiatry 135:660–663, 1978

Malt U: Five years of experience with the DSM-III system in clinical work and research: some concluding remarks. Acta Psychiatr Scand Suppl 328:76–84, 1986

McGrath J: A survey of deliberate self-poisoning. Med J Aust 150:317–324, 1989

Mezzich AC, Mezzich JE, Coffman GA: Reliability of DSM-III and DSM-II in child psychopathology. J Am Acad Child Psychiatry 24:273–280, 1985

Mezzich JE, Fabrega H Jr, Coffman GA, et al: DSM-III disorders in a large sample of psychiatric patients: frequency and specificity of diagnoses. Am J Psychiatry 146:212–219, 1989

Minnaar GK, Schlebusch L, Levin A: A current study of parasuicide in Durban. S Afr Med J 57:204–207, 1980

Monroe SM: Life events and disorder: event-symptom associations and the course of disorder. J Abnorm Psychol 91:14–24, 1982

Newcorn JH, Strain J: Adjustment disorders in children and adolescents. J Am Acad Child Adolesc Psychiatry 31(2):318–327, 1992

Rey JM, Bashir MR, Schwarz M, et al: Oppositional disorder: fact or fiction? J Am Acad Child Adolesc Psychiatry 27:157–162, 1988

Runeson B: Mental disorder in youth suicide: DSM-III-R Axes I and II. Acta Psychiatr Scand 79:490–497, 1989

Rutter M: Stress, coping and development: some issues and some questions. J Child Psychol Psychiatry 22:323–356, 1981
Shaffer D, Brassic J, Ambrosini P, et al: A Children's Global Assessment Scale (CGAS). Arch Gen Psychiatry 40:1228–1231, 1983
Thomas A, Chess S: Genesis and evolution of behavioral disorders: from infancy to early adult life. Am J Psychiatry 141:1–9, 1984
Weiner IB, Del Gaudio AC: Psychopathology in adolescence: an epidemiological study. Arch Gen Psychiatry 33:187–193, 1976
Werry JS, Methven RJ, Fitzpatrick J, et al: The interrater reliability of DSM-III in children. J Abnorm Child Psychol 11:341–354, 1983
Woolston JL: Theoretical considerations of the adjustment disorders. J Am Acad Child Adolesc Psychiatry 27:280–287, 1988
World Health Organization: ICD-9 Chapter V: Mental and Behavioural Disorders. Geneva, Switzerland, World Health Organization, 1978
Wynne LC: Adjustment reaction of adult life, in Comprehensive Textbook of Psychiatry, 2nd Edition. Edited by Freedman AM, Kaplan HJ, Sadock BJ. Baltimore, MD, Williams & Wilkins, 1975, pp 1609–1618

Chapter 19

Trichotillomania

Ronald M. Winchel, M.D.

Introduction

Conclusions about trichotillomania are severely limited by the unavailability of well-designed studies. Except for several recent treatment studies, the available literature on trichotillomania consists almost entirely of case reports or retrospective reviews of open clinical experience. No studies of this condition have examined randomly selected samples.

In addition, it is impossible to restrict this review to reports in which trichotillomania is defined by a conventional diagnostic standard. Even the few studies that have appeared since the publication of the DSM-III-R (American Psychiatric Association 1987) have not restricted subjects to DSM-III-R criteria. Consequently, for the purpose of this review, trichotillomania was considered to be present if unwanted hair-pulling occurred in the absence of a primary dermatological condition that could account for the behavior.

Statement of the Issues

1. Does trichotillomania deserve a separate diagnosis in DSM-IV? Is trichotillomania merely a monosymptomatic form of obsessive-compulsive disorder? Should trichotillomania be viewed only as a symptom of other conditions (such as mood and anxiety disorders?)
2. Is there a difference between early childhood onset and adolescent/adult onset trichotillomania?
3. Where should trichotillomania be placed in DSM-IV? In DSM-III-R, the diagnosis can be made under either of two categories: impulse control disorders not elsewhere classified or stereotypy/habit. Should it be placed in the childhood onset section? Should trichotillomania be categorized as an anxiety disorder? Should the current classification be maintained? (i.e., under impulse control disorders not elsewhere classified.)

Significance of the Issues

Does Trichotillomania Deserve a Separate Diagnosis?

There are several reasons for questioning the appropriateness of maintaining a separate classification for trichotillomania:

1. Trichotillomania can already be diagnosed under other existing categories: stereotypy/habit disorder and obsessive-compulsive disorder.
2. Trichotillomania in childhood may be a normative, phase-specific experience, such as thumb-sucking, and, as such, should not be "pathologized" with a diagnosis.
3. Trichotillomania may be a symptom of other, primary, conditions.

Is There a Difference Between Early Childhood Onset and Adolescent/Adult Onset Trichotillomania?

Both the course and epidemiological characteristics of trichotillomania may differ between childhood and later-onset presentations. It may be reasonable to view early childhood onset trichotillomania as a benign habit of self-limited course. Therefore, if trichotillomania is maintained as a diagnosable entity, it is important to determine if it fits conventionally accepted criteria for a "condition" in childhood. Otherwise, it may be appropriate to restrict the diagnosis of the condition to cases with later onset. To address this question, it is important to determine if the pattern of childhood trichotillomania differs from that of later-onset trichotillomania, both as an aid to developing appropriate diagnostic criteria for childhood presentations and also to determine if the appearance of trichotillomania in childhood can be said to represent a "disorder."

Where Should Trichotillomania Be Placed?

In DSM-III-R, trichotillomania can be diagnosed under either of two categories: impulse control disorders not elsewhere classified or stereotypy/habit. It may be argued that trichotillomania fits the DSM-III-R designation of a "disorder usually first evident in infancy, childhood, or adolescence" and should be placed in the childhood onset section. Alternatively, one might consider that a primary component of trichotillomania is the anxiety associated with attempts to resist hair-pulling. In addition, trichotillomania has been referred to as an obsessive-compulsive disorder spectrum disorder. Given the prominence of anxiety in this condition, and the precedent that obsessive-compulsive disorder itself is considered an anxiety disorder, it is reasonable to suggest that trichotillomania be placed in the anxiety disorders section of DSM-IV.

Method

Two computer databases were searched for this review: Medline from January 1973 to February 1991 and *Excerpta Medica* Psychiatry from 1980 through 1990. Index terms used for both database searches were *trichotillomania or hair-pull* or *alopecia*. The number of references generated by each search using these index terms was 88 and 126, respectively.

Several published reviews of trichotillomania were also used to find pertinent references (Christenson et al. 1991; Krishnan et al. 1985; Mannino and Delgado 1969; Muller 1990; Sorosky and Sticher 1980; Swedo and Rapoport 1991). References cited in these reviews (including references from publication dates prior to the span of the computer database search), as well as references cited in the papers found in the database search, were reviewed if they appeared to provide useful data regarding incidence, prevalence, associated features, sex ratio, or any other information that might be relevant to this review. A total of 96 publications were reviewed.

Results

Does Trichotillomania Deserve a Separate Diagnosis?

Trichotillomania and obsessive-compulsive disorder

The suggestion that trichotillomania may be viewed as a subtype of obsessive-compulsive disorder is based on three observations: 1) the phenomenological similarity between obsessive-compulsive disorder and trichotillomania, 2) the apparent increased incidence of obsessive-compulsive disorder in family members of trichotillomania patients (an incidence of 11.9% of obsessive-compulsive disorder among 65 first-degree relatives of 16 probands with trichotillomania versus an incidence of 2% in the general population) (Swedo and Rapoport 1991), and 3) apparently similar patterns of pharmacological response (i.e., response to serotonin reuptake inhibition) (Swedo et al. 1989; Winchel et al. 1989, 1992).

However, several sources of data suggest that trichotillomania should not be viewed merely as a specific type of obsessive-compulsive disorder.

Symptom specificity. Goodman et al. (1990) demonstrated that 84% of a sample of 544 patients with standard presentations of obsessive-compulsive disorder had more than one form of obsession and that 87% had more than one form of compulsion. In contrast, patients with trichotillomania did not typically have other symptoms that fulfill criteria for obsessive-compulsive disorder. Winchel et al. (1992) found that only 1 of 20 patients (5%) who presented for treatment of trichotillomania had other behaviors that fulfilled criteria for obsessive-compulsive disorder. Christenson et al. (1991) found 9 of 60 patients (15%) with trichotillomania had other features consistent with obsessive-compulsive disorder (past or present). This range of incidence (5%–15%) is greater than that for the general population, but it is markedly different from the approximately 85% rate of multiple symptoms among patients with obsessive-compulsive disorder as described by Goodman et al.

Evidence of divergent biological characteristics. Swedo et al. (1991) used a positron-emission tomography scanner to study regional brain metabolism in 10 female patients with trichotillomania. Although regional glucose metabolism among the trichotillomania patients was clearly different from that of control subjects, it was also different from that previously demonstrated among patients with obsessive-compulsive disorder.

Evidence of divergent character and personality traits. Winchel et al. (1989, 1992) found that patients with trichotillomania could be distinguished from patients with obsessive-compulsive disorder by their scores on the Leyton Obsessional Inventory (Cooper 1970). This instrument does not specifically gauge the presence or severity of DSM-III-R obsessive-compulsive disorder. Rather, it combines ratings of many "obsessional traits" with scores for interference with functioning. Patients with obsessive-compulsive disorder consistently have high scores on this instrument. Winchel et al. (1989, 1992) found that patients with trichotillomania had dramatically lower scores and could not be distinguished from control subjects.

Gender ratio. In contrast with obsessive-compulsive disorder, most authors suggest trichotillomania (at least among adults) is far more common among females than males (Greenberg and Sarner 1965; Mannino and Delgado 1969; Oguchi and Miura 1977). The male:female ratio in the adult samples reported by Christenson et al. (1991) and Winchel et al. (1992) are 4:56 and 3:17, respectively. In Muller's (1990) sample of 174 patients with trichotillomania who presented to the Mayo Clinic, Rochester, Minnesota, 76% were female. Ages ranged from early childhood to older than age 70 years. Among children with early-onset trichotillomania, the disparity between the number of males and females may be smaller. Several authors suggested that in childhood trichotillomania, the number of boys may be no different from the number of girls (Bartsch 1956; Buttwerworth and Strean 1963; Mannino and Delgado 1969; Muller 1990).

Should trichotillomania be considered as a symptom of other primary conditions rather than an independent diagnosis?

Three reports (Christenson et al. 1991; Swedo et al. 1989; Winchel et al. 1992) provide data on the presence of other conditions in adult patients with trichotillomania. Data were collected from nonrandom groups of self-identified hair-pullers who responded to advertisements or were seeking treatment. As may be seen from Table 19–1, both Winchel et al. (1992) and Christenson et al. (1991) found that a significant portion of their samples had no other lifetime Axis I diagnosis. It is not clear from the report of Swedo et al. (1989) whether any of their subjects had only trichotillomania as a diagnosis. The data from these three studies are fairly consistent, except for the low frequency of anxiety disorders in Winchel et al.'s sample. Although anxiety *disorders* were not frequently diagnosed in Winchel et al.'s sample, they found a high incidence of anxiety *symptoms* as demonstrated by a mean score of 21 on the Hamilton Anxiety Scale. In Swedo et al.'s sample, 5 of the 6 patients with anxiety disorder diagnoses had generalized anxiety disorder. Because the criteria for generalized anxiety disorder in the instrument used by Swedo et al. (Schedule for Affective Disorders and Schizophrenia [Endicott and Spitzer 1978]) are less restrictive than the DSM-III-R criteria employed by Winchel et al., this group may be symptomatically similar to the patients in Winchel et al.'s group, despite the difference in anxiety diagnoses.

The data in Table 19–1 represent lifetime incidence. Some of these were past diagnoses and were not present at the time of evaluation, further decreasing the frequencies of concurrent conditions that it might be preferable to diagnose instead

Table 19–1. Lifetime comorbidity (in percent) for adults with trichotillomania

Study	N	No Axis I disorders	Anxiety disorders	Mood disorders	Psychoactive substance use disorders	Obsessive-compulsive disorder	Eating disorders
Christenson et al. 1991	60	18	57	65	22	15	20
Winchel et al. 1992	20	45	5	45	15	5	0
Swedo et al. 1989	14	—[a]	43	57	29	—[b]	0

[a] Data not available.
[b] Patients with obsessive-compulsive disorder were excluded from this sample.

Table 19–2. Concurrent comorbidity (in percent) at time of presentation with trichotillomania (adults)

Study	N	No Axis I disorders	Anxiety disorders	Mood disorders	Psychoactive substance use disorders	Obsessive-compulsive disorder	Eating disorders
Christenson et al. 1991[a]	60			23		10	
Winchel et al. 1992	20	70	5	25	5	5	0

[a]Distinguished past/present diagnoses only for mood disorders and obsessive-compulsive disorder.

of trichotillomania. Table 19–2 demonstrates that the number of comorbid conditions drops significantly when current diagnoses alone are considered. Although Christenson et al. (1991) distinguished past and present diagnoses only for mood disorders and obsessive-compulsive disorder, note in particular that the presence of mood disorders dropped from 65% lifetime to 23% comorbid. Past and current diagnoses cannot be clearly distinguished in the data reported by Swedo et al. (1989).

Our ability to generalize from these data is limited. As noted, none of these samples was random, and in only one of these studies (Swedo et al. 1989) was a structured diagnostic instrument used. Although DSM-III-R criteria were employed in the other two reports, in neither study was a standard diagnostic instrument used. However, despite the limitations, and despite a high incidence of lifetime mood and anxiety disorders among these patients, no pattern emerges in support of the contention that trichotillomania represents only a symptom of other conditions.

Is There a Difference Between Early Childhood Onset and Later-Onset Trichotillomania?

Several studies (Bartsch 1956; Buttwerworth and Strean 1963; Friman and Hove 1987; Mannino and Delgado 1969; Mehregan 1970; Sorosky and Sticher 1980) noted differences between children and adults who present with trichotillomania. Individuals with trichotillomania may be divided into two populations: early onset (toddler to early childhood) and later onset (school age and later). The basis for this distinction would be apparent differences on the following dimensions: gender ratio, severity and duration of symptoms, and association with other forms of psychopathology (Table 19–3).

Table 19–3. A model for distinguishing early versus later onset trichotillomania

Dimension	Early onset	Later onset
Age at onset	Infant, toddler to about age 6	Approximately 6 years and up; may peak around age 13
Gender ratio	Frequency among boys and girls similar	Females seem to greatly outnumber males
Duration	Often brief (weeks to several months)	May last up to decades
Prognosis	Often responds to simple interventions	Unclear, but for some, refractory to all treatments
Association with other pathology	Increased developmental pathology has been suggested, but no convincing evidence available; may be associated with other (benign) habits (e.g., thumb-sucking)	Apparent high lifetime incidence of mood and anxiety disorders

Gender ratio. There is general agreement, as noted, that among patients with trichotillomania who present in later childhood and after, females seem to greatly outnumber males. In contrast, several authors suggested that in childhood trichotillomania, the number of boys may differ little from the number of girls (Bartsch 1956; Buttwerworth and Strean 1963; Mannino and Delgado 1969). In Muller's (1990) large sample of adult and child patients, there was no difference between the number of boys and the number of girls in the preschool age group.

Severity, duration, and prognosis. Sorosky and Sticher (1980) discussed the possible relationship between age at onset and severity and prognosis, citing several authors who suggest that childhood and preadolescent onset is frequently more benign, whereas adolescent and adult onset tends to be more severe with a more protracted course. Oranje et al. (1986) also concluded that adult trichotillomania is likely to be more severe. Friman and Rostain (1990) stated that hair-pulling in children rarely creates the same kind of problems that it does in adults and noted that milder forms in childhood seem to respond more easily to behavioral interventions.

In the dermatology literature, clinicians often state that it is relatively easy to treat childhood trichotillomania with minor interventions (e.g., applying a placebo salve, drawing the child's attention to the behavior and indicating that it is undesirable). Several authors noted that when trichotillomania is accompanied by thumb-sucking, treatment of the thumb-sucking often is followed by disappearance of the trichotillomania (Friman and Hove 1987; Knell and Moore 1988).

Associated pathology. Childhood trichotillomania may be associated with other habits, usually benign and self-limited, such as thumb-sucking, nail-biting, and nose-picking (Oranje et al. 1986). A number of authors suggested that childhood trichotillomania is associated with disturbances in psychosexual development or disturbed family dynamics, but the clinical case reports invoked in support of this contention are not sufficient to support this thesis in general. The association with adult psychopathology has been discussed earlier.

Summary. If the distinction between ages at onset is valid, it may support the assertion that childhood trichotillomania represents a normative, stereotypic behavior of childhood and should not be classified as an illness. Later-onset trichotillomania may be more clearly labeled as pathological.

In the absence of a longitudinal or controlled, random-sample study of the general population, it is not possible to assert with any certainty that this distinction is valid. It may be more conservative to view adults with chronic trichotillomania as representing the more severe and tenacious end of a spectrum rather than suggesting that early-onset and later-onset trichotillomania may represent qualitatively different conditions. Because all literature about adult trichotillomania is based on the reports of individuals with ongoing symptoms, there is no means of testing the validity of the distinction between early- and later-onset trichotillomania. Later-onset trichotillomania that is relatively short-lived and benign may never be seen by treating clinicians, whereas parents of small children may have a low threshold for seeking the advice of a clinician when trichotillomania is first noted.

Where Should Trichotillomania Be Placed?

In DSM-III-R, trichotillomania can be diagnosed either as trichotillomania, under impulse control disorders not elsewhere classified or under stereotypy/habit, if significant morbidity accompanies the condition.

Disorders usually first evident in infancy, childhood, or adolescence. Usual age at onset is the only factor regarding trichotillomania about which there is general agreement in the literature. The mean ages at onset of the three adult samples (Christenson et al. 1991; Swedo et al. 1989; Winchel et al. 1992) were 13.0 ± 8, 13.8 ± 7.2, and 12.7 ± 6.2 years, respectively. Mean ages at presentation to the investigators were 34 ± 8 (range, 18–61), 31.6 ± 7.6 (range, 16–44), and 34.1 ± 8.2 (range, 22–60) years, respectively. There have been reports of onset as early as age 14 months (Delgado and Mannino 1969), and there are many reports in the literature of trichotillomania presenting in early childhood (ages 4–8).

Should trichotillomania be categorized as an anxiety disorder? In DSM-III-R, the characteristic features of anxiety disorders are listed as symptoms of anxiety and/or avoidance. Individuals with trichotillomania occasionally demonstrate avoidant behavior in situations where they cannot hide embarrassing hair loss (e.g., certain athletic activities such as swimming, going to a professional hair dresser, or even intimate relationships). Nevertheless, significant behavioral avoidance does not appear to be a common or characteristic feature of these patients.

The ubiquitous presence of anxiety among these patients is generally assumed and is present as a necessary criterion (criterion B) for the diagnosis in DSM-III-R. Yet, although anxiety is often present before an episode of hair-pulling or manifests itself when attempts are made to interrupt the behavior, it may not inevitably precede hair-pulling. Christenson et al. (1991) found that 57/60 (95%) of their sample experienced tension preceding hair-pulling behavior at least some of the time. Of the same sample, 88% described a relief of tension after the act at least some of the time. In my clinical experience, anxiety is not inevitably associated with hair-pulling. Some patients note they "find themselves" pulling hair when the episode has already been going on "unconsciously." In such circumstances, there is no preceding awareness of anxiety. Tension will often occur if they then seek to stop, but because some patients allow the hair-pulling to continue until the episode spontaneously abates, there may be no anxiety associated with a particular episode at all. Although this is not the usual experience, it is not particularly uncommon. Many individuals with trichotillomania note that episodes of hair-pulling are facilitated by two conditions: states of anxiety and, paradoxically, states of relaxation and distraction (such as when absorbed in a book or watching television). These observations highlight the fact that conscious awareness of anxiety is not inevitably associated with hair-pulling.

Impulse control disorders not elsewhere classified. Swedo and Rapoport (1991) discussed data collected by Winchel et al. (1992) and Lenane et al. (1992) suggesting that patients with trichotillomania do not demonstrate unusual levels of generalized impulsivity. This observation is rooted in an apparent lack of significant association with other impulsive behaviors (such as self-injury) and unremarkable results on personality inventories that seek to measure "impulsivity."

Discussion and Recommendations

Subtype of Obsessive-Compulsive Disorder?

The phenomenological similarity between trichotillomania and obsessive-compulsive disorder and the incidence of obsessive-compulsive disorder in relatives of individuals with trichotillomania suggest that trichotillomania may be a variant of obsessive-compulsive disorder. But metabolic studies of brain glucose utilization, the infrequency of other obsessive-compulsive disorder symptoms, dissimilar patterns on personality inventories, and gender differences suggest that trichotillomania may be sufficiently distinguished from obsessive-compulsive disorder to argue against viewing is as a specific subtype.

Symptom of Other Conditions?

Comorbidity data suggest that trichotillomania is associated with a high lifetime incidence of mood and anxiety disorders. But trichotillomania appears to persist, even in the absence or after the resolution of these other conditions. Many patients have no other diagnosis at the time of presentation for treatment. Despite the frequency of mood and anxiety syndromes in patients with trichotillomania, the data do not present a compelling argument for viewing trichotillomania as merely a component of other conditions.

Difference Between Adult and Childhood Trichotillomania?

Although no data from controlled studies are currently available to support such a view, many authors agree that early-onset trichotillomania is less severe, more responsive to treatment, and more equally distributed between boys and girls than later-onset trichotillomania. In general, the clinical literature is consistent with such a view.

DSM Location

Trichotillomania can clearly be described as a "disorder usually first evident in infancy, childhood, or adolescence." Its classification as an anxiety disorder is somewhat problematic. Although behavioral avoidance occurs, it is often not present or not severe, and it may be difficult to view it as a characteristic feature. In addition, although anxiety is a frequent concomitant of trichotillomania, it is not inevitable. It is perhaps more accurate to state that anxiety is associated with attempts to resist the behavior (which may already be occurring) rather than to say it precedes the behavior. It is reasonable to consider trichotillomania as a disorder of impulse control, although there are no data to suggest that these patients are generally impulsive.

Should Trichotillomania Be Maintained as a Psychiatric Diagnosis?

Trichotillomania is apparently a real phenomenon. Although it may be mild and transient, it may also be severe, leading to significant distress, social avoidance, stigma, economic costs, and, occasionally, medical complications. Although no data are available to support such a conclusion, there is an emerging opinion that the condition may be very common. The absence of dermatological pathology and the inability to control an undesirable behavior support the classification of trichotillomania as a psychiatric (rather than a dermatological) illness.

As has been discussed, despite its shared features with obsessive-compulsive disorder, at this time an argument can be made for distinguishing trichotillomania from obsessive-compulsive disorder and not viewing it merely as a specific variant of obsessive-compulsive disorder.

Similarly, despite the apparent prevalence of mood and anxiety disorders among patients with trichotillomania, it does not seem to be only a symptom of other conditions. Trichotillomania may appear independently, and often does.

Where Should Trichotillomania Be Placed?

The main problem with the current classification is that trichotillomania is a condition that is usually first evident in childhood, and it is reasonable to argue that it should go into that section. In the entire literature about trichotillomania, the one factor that can probably be asserted with the greatest confidence is that most patients present in childhood or adolescence. If the guiding principles of the DSM indicate strict adherence to the issue of when symptoms first present, then there would seem to be little choice about where it should be located. It should be noted, however, that a significant number of patients present to clinicians in adulthood.

Otherwise, if strict adherence to the principle of symptom onset is not required, I favor continuing the current classification as an impulse control disorder not elsewhere classified. Calling trichotillomania an impulse control disorder is probably the most apt way to describe it.

An argument can be made for associating trichotillomania with obsessive-compulsive disorder. But, as stated, it does not seem to be just a specific form of obsessive-compulsive disorder, and the same features of irresistible urge are also shared by other conditions that are not classified as obsessive-compulsive disorder variants (e.g., kleptomania or bulimia).

Consequently, I recommend that there are insufficient data to redesignate trichotillomania as a subtype of obsessive-compulsive disorder or to move it to the anxiety disorders section. Compelling data do exist to support the contention that trichotillomania is *not* merely a single symptom of other syndromes. Further research may yield evidence of a bimodal (early- versus late-onset) presentation with variant patterns, but insufficient data are currently available to suggest the occurrence of two separate and distinguishable syndromes.

References

American Psychiatric Association: Diagnostic and Statistical Manual of Mental Disorders, 3rd Edition, Revised. Washington, DC, American Psychiatric Association, 1987

Bartsch VE: Contributions toward the aetiology of trichotillomania in infancy (abstract). Psychiatrie Neurologie und Medicalnische Psychologie 8:173–182, 1956

Buttwerworth T, Strean LP: Behavior disorders of interest to dermatologists (abstract). Archives of Dermatology 88:859–867, 1963

Christenson GA, Mackenzie TB, Mitchell JE: Characteristics of 60 adult chronic hair pullers. Am J Psychiatry 148:365–370, 1991

Cooper J: The Leyton Obsessional Inventory. Psychol Med 1:48–64, 1970

Delgado RA, Mannino FV: Some observations of trichotillomania in children. Journal of the American Academy of Child Psychiatry 8:229–246, 1969

Endicott J, Spitzer RL: A diagnostic interview: the Schedule for Affective Disorders and Schizophrenia. Arch Gen Psychiatry 35:837–844, 1978

Friman PC, Hove G: Apparent covariation between child habit disorders: effects of successful treatment for thumb sucking on untargeted chronic hair pulling. J Appl Behav Anal 20:421–425, 1987

Friman PC, Rostain A: Trichotillomania (hair pulling), II. N Engl J Med 322:471, 1990

Goodman KW, Rasmussen AS, Price HL: Types of symptoms and response to clomipramine in obsessive-compulsive disorder (abstract) (annual meeting of the American Psychiatric Association). New Research, Vol 112, 1990

Greenberg HR, Sarner CA: Trichotillomania, symptom and syndrome. Arch Gen Psychiatry 12:482–489, 1965

Knell SM, Moore DJ: Childhood trichotillomania treated indirectly by punishing thumb sucking (abstract). J Behav Ther Exp Psychiatry 19:305–310, 1988

Krishnan KRR, Davidson JRT, Guajardo C: Trichotillomania: a review. Compr Psychiatry 26:123–128, 1985

Lenane MC, Swedo SE, Rapoport JL, et al: Increased rates of OCD in first degree relatives of patients with trichotillomania. J Child Psychol Psychiatry 33(5):925–933, 1992

Mannino FV, Delgado RA: Trichotillomania in children: a review. Am J Psychiatry 126:505–511, 1969

Mehregan AH: Trichotillomania: a clinicopathologic study (abstract). Archives of Dermatology 102:129–133, 1970

Muller SA: Trichotillomania: a histopathologic study in sixty-six patients. Journal of the American Academy of Dermatology 23:56–62, 1990

Oguchi T, Miura S: Trichotillomania: its psychopathological aspect. Compr Psychiatry 18:177–182, 1977

Oranje AP, Peereboom-Wynia JD, De-Raeymaecker DM: Trichotillomania in childhood. Journal of the American Academy of Dermatology 15:614–619, 1986

Sorosky AD, Sticher MB: Trichotillomania in adolescence. Adolesc Psychiatry 8:437–454, 1980

Swedo SE, Rapoport JL: Annotation: trichotillomania. J Child Psychol Psychiatry 32:401–409, 1991

Swedo SE, Leonard HL, Rapoport JL, et al: A double-blind comparison of clomipramine and desipramine in the treatment of trichotillomania (hair pulling). N Engl J Med 321:497–501, 1989

Swedo SE, Rapoport JL, Leonard HL, et al: Regional cerebral glucose metabolism in women with trichotillomania. Arch Gen Psychiatry 48:828–833, 1991

Winchel RM, Stanley B, Guido J, et al: An open trial of fluoxetine for trichotillomania (abstract). Paper presented at the 28th annual meeting of the American College of Neuropsychopharmacology, Maui, HI, December 1989

Winchel RM, Jones JS, Stanley B, et al: Clinical characteristics of trichotillomania and its response to fluoxetine. J Clin Psychiatry 53:304–308, 1992

Chapter 20

Gender Identity Disorder

Susan J. Bradley, M.D., Ray Blanchard, Ph.D., Susan Coates, Ph.D.,
Richard Green, M.D., J.D., Stephen B. Levine, M.D.,
Heino F. L. Meyer-Bahlburg, Dr. rer. nat., Ira B. Pauly, M.D., and
Kenneth J. Zucker, Ph.D.

Statement of the Issues

The issues reviewed in this chapter include

1. Is it more appropriate to employ the concept of a spectrum of gender dysphoria rather than discrete diagnostic categories?
2. How valid are criticisms of the current diagnostic criteria?
3. Is there support for different criteria for boys and girls?
4. Of what importance in children is a stated wish to be the opposite sex?
5. Should subtyping by sexual orientation be included?
6. Should fetishistic cross-dressers be excluded from the category of gender identity disorder?
7. Should individuals with physical intersex conditions be excluded from the disorder?

Method

Because the members of the DSM-IV Work Group are responsible for most of the recent literature in the area of gender identity disorder and particularly for those studies that are methodologically adequate, the authors relied on their knowledge of and experience with the issue of a spectrum of gender dysphorias and placement

---

The authors thank the following individuals who have offered comments and suggestions: Neil Buhrich, Charles W. Davenport, Michael B. First, Richard C. Friedman, Leslie M. Lothstein, John Money, Richard R. Pleak, Thomas N. Wise, and Bernard Zuger.

in the nomenclature. K. J. Zucker (Gender identity disorder of childhood: diagnostic issues: discussion paper for the DSM-IV Subcommittee on Gender Identity Disorders, unpublished manuscript, 1990) reviewed the child literature on differences in criteria and the importance of the stated wish to be the opposite sex. R. Blanchard and P. M. Sheridan (In consideration of specifying a bisexual subtype of gender identity disorder in the DSM-IV: literature review for the DSM-IV subcommittee on gender identity disorder, unpublished manuscript, 1990) reviewed the literature on adults with respect to subtyping and exclusion of fetishistic cross-dressers. Meyer-Bahlburg (1994) reviewed the intersex literature regarding the issue of whether intersex patients differ sufficiently from non-intersex patients to be excluded from the diagnosis.

Results and Discussion

Spectrum of Gender Dysphoria Versus Discrete Categories

Concern for adequate diagnosis of individuals with gender identity disorders developed as these patients began presenting themselves in the early 1960s requesting sex reassignment surgery. Earlier work naturally focused on formulating diagnostic criteria that would permit clinicians to safely judge who should have surgery. DSM-III-R (American Psychiatric Association 1987) clearly reflects this tradition by dividing disorders into transsexualism and gender identity disorder of adolescence or adulthood, nontranssexual type (GIDAANT).

As clinicians were exposed to a broad range of children, adolescents, and adults with gender identity disorders, it became apparent that patients vary greatly in the severity, constancy, and natural history of their gender dysphoria. For example, when followed prospectively, only a small minority of children identified with cross-gender concerns go on to develop transsexualism (Green 1987); in contrast, a much larger percentage of persons who first present in adolescence with cross-gender concerns will remain gender dysphoric or eventually receive a diagnosis of transsexualism (McCauley and Ehrhardt 1984). It is also clear from referrals to adult gender identity clinics that differences between individuals who proceed toward sex reassignment surgery and those who do not may be more quantitative than qualitative.

The DSM-III-R transsexualism and GIDAANT categories are similar except that transsexualism appears to describe gender-dysphoric individuals who have decided on surgical sex reassignment as the solution to their inner distress (Levine 1989). The desire to uncouple the clinical diagnosis of gender dysphoria from criteria for approving patients for sex reassignment surgery was one factor in the subcommittee's recommendation that these categories be merged under the heading of gender identity disorder. It is also the perception of many clinicians that there are no distinct boundaries between patients with gender dysphoria who request sex reassignment surgery and those whose cross-gender wishes are of lesser intensity or constancy (Benjamin 1966; Fisk 1973; Freund et al. 1982; Person and Ovesey 1974a, 1974b). This viewpoint, which reflects clinical experience over a number of years, has led to the belief that there is no longer a justification for maintaining discrete categories within the broad category of gender identity disorder.

Placement in the Nomenclature

In DSM-III (American Psychiatric Association 1980), transsexualism and gender identity disorder of childhood were placed under the larger category entitled *psychosexual disorders*. In DSM-III-R, the category psychosexual disorders was eliminated, with many of the former diagnoses placed under a new category termed *sexual disorders*. Transsexualism and gender identity disorder of childhood were placed under the larger category entitled *disorders usually first evident in infancy, childhood, or adolescence*. The DSM-III-R placement had the advantage of ensuring that clinicians treating child and adolescent patients would recognize and give more attention to gender identity disorders. On the other hand, clinicians treating adult patients felt that such placement was inappropriate for transsexualism, particularly given that behavioral precursors of some cases of adult transsexualism are not evident in childhood.

Child Issues

Diagnostic criteria for boys and girls. In DSM-III-R, a girl is required not only to have "persistent and intense distress" about being a girl but also to have a "stated desire" to be a boy. Boys must also have a "persistent and intense distress" about being a boy, but need to have only an "intense desire" to be a girl. In other words, girls must state their desire to be a boy, whereas boys need not verbalize such wishes. Moreover, for boys, the desire must be "intense" whereas for girls no specification regarding intensity is made with regard to the verbalized wish to be a boy.

Another issue involving girls concerns the statement in criterion A that the desire to be a boy is not due to "perceived cultural advantages from being a boy."

Should the desire to be of the opposite sex be a distinct criterion? Clinical experience suggests that children may manifest significant cross-gender identification without verbalizing the wish to be of the opposite sex. This appears particularly true of children over the age of 6 or 7 years, perhaps because of the social opprobrium that ensues (Zucker 1991). Currently, the authors are analyzing data sets from

Green's (1987) study and from the database of the Child and Adolescent Gender Identity Clinic at the Clarke Institute of Psychiatry, Toronto, Canada, to examine the similarities and differences between children referred for gender identity concerns who do and do not verbalize the wish to be of the opposite sex. Analyses of the Clarke Institute and Green data sets identified one common factor of cross-gender identification, which included the verbal wish to be of the opposite sex.. Further, reliance on a stated wish as a separate and necessary criterion appears to exclude older children disproportionately (Zucker et al., in press).

Adult Issues

Exclusion of fetishistic cross-dressers from the present transsexual and GIDAANT categories. In DSM-III-R, any individual who reported being currently gender dysphoric and currently aroused by cross-dressing would necessarily be diagnosed with gender identity disorder not otherwise specified. The "not otherwise specified" label is the only one applicable because gender dysphoria precludes the diagnosis of transvestic fetishism, whereas fetishistic arousal precludes the diagnoses of transsexualism and GIDAANT. The diagnostic rule is discordant with both clinical experience and the available research literature, which suggests that about half of even the most strongly gender-dysphoric nonhomosexual men acknowledge that they still become sexually aroused or masturbate at least occasionally when cross-dressing (Blanchard and Clemmensen 1988).

The Sexual Disorders Work Group proposed that the diagnosis of transvestic fetishism be subtyped as with or without gender dysphoria (T. N. Wise: Transvestitic fetishism: DSM-IV Work Group on Sexual Disorders, unpublished manuscript, 1989). The authors found that proposal problematic because many such individuals appear to lose the fetishistic arousal as the gender dysphoria develops (Benjamin 1966; Buhrich and Beaumont 1981; Buhrich and McConaghy 1977; Person and Ovesey 1978; Wise and Meyer 1980). Subtyping such individuals according to the presence of gender dysphoria could then require changing the diagnosis from transvestic fetishism to gender identity disorder in individuals whose fetishistic arousal has diminished. This would appear to be unduly cumbersome.

Subtypes of gender identity disorder. After reviewing Blanchard's (1985, 1988, 1989a, 1989b) analyses of the various subtypes presenting to the (adult) Gender Identity Clinic of the Clarke Institute of Psychiatry, the authors agreed that there are two common routes leading to a gender identity disorder in adolescence or adulthood. The first group of cases progresses from gender identity disorder of childhood and are sexually oriented toward members of their own biological sex; the second appears to progress from transvestitic fetishism over time to a full-blown gender identity disorder. The latter group may have had, or may still have, erotic attraction to members of the opposite biological sex; mixed within this group are others who might be described as bisexual or asexual.

A great deal of discussion was devoted to the question of subtype labels. Many patients object to being labeled "homosexual" or "heterosexual," and many professionals appear confused about whether to apply such terminology from the point of view of the patient's anatomic sex or subjective gender identity (Pauly 1990).

Intersexuality and gender dysphoria. The authors considered whether individuals who appear to be identified as having marked cross-gender behavior and who have a history of ambiguous genitalia or some significant chromosomal anomaly should be given a psychiatric diagnosis. In DSM-III, individuals with intersex conditions were excluded.

DSM-III-R changed this to permit assigning a diagnosis with notation of the intersex condition on Axis III. The review by Meyer-Bahlburg (1994) recommended a return to the DSM-III exclusion of intersex conditions based on etiological differences, some phenomenological differences, and concern regarding the stigma of a psychiatric diagnosis in a poorly managed medical intersex patient. The majority of the current authors, therefore, endorsed the exclusion of intersex conditions from the gender identity disorder diagnosis. However, several authors expressed concern that, although there may be etiological and phenomenological differences, the evidence that such disorders differ from gender identity disorders presenting in physically normal individuals is questionable enough that a change from DSM-III-R at this time may be premature. It was suggested that there is a need for further research in this area to clarify whether the factors thought to be relevant in the development of gender disorders in physically normal individuals are essentially the same as those in individuals with clear-cut physical or biochemical abnormalities.

Recommendations

1. The authors recommended the adoption of one category of gender identity disorder with elaboration within the criteria for the differences between children and adults.
2. The authors agreed that a distinct diagnostic category, gender identity disorders, should be created in DSM-IV. Such a category would have the same status as, for example, anxiety disorders and mood disorders, in which there may be childhood precursors, if not identical symptoms, to what is observed in adults (see Shaffer et al. 1989).

3. The authors have taken the position that the reasons for the distinctions in criteria for boys and girls are not clear. It was felt that whatever criterion was adopted regarding the verbalized wish to be of the opposite sex should be the same for boys and girls. The authors also felt that the desire to be of the opposite sex would be difficult to infer independently of other aspects of the criteria as they stood in DSM-III-R.
4. The authors took the position that it was inappropriate to place an exclusion rule regarding cultural advantage in the criteria themselves, because there may be many reasons why a child adopts a cross-gender identity, and that these issues should be dealt with in the text (for further discussion of these points, see Zucker 1991). Further discussion at the level of the Work Group led to the proposal to place this qualifier in the criteria for both boys and girls.
5. The authors recommended that the explicit wish to be of the opposite sex be combined with other behavioral markers of gender identity disorder in one criterion. This would eliminate the pivotal role that the verbalized wish to change sex plays in the DSM-III-R criteria.
6. The authors recommend that fetishistic arousal should not be an exclusion criterion for gender identity disorder. Individuals who currently experience erotic arousal in association with cross-dressing as well as gender dysphoria would receive two diagnoses: gender identity disorder and transvestic fetishism.
7. The authors debated the utility of subtyping, various methods of subtyping, and the diagnostic labels to apply to subtypes. There was consensus that it is important for clinical management as well as research purposes to note the sexual preference of mature individuals with gender identity disorder (e.g., Blanchard et al. 1989). With regard to the method of subtyping, notwithstanding the above-mentioned evidence that there may be only two fundamentally different types of gender identity disorder, the authors felt that it was better to anchor subtyping at the descriptive level and to distinguish four different subtypes.
8. The authors' recommendations were intended to make the principles of subtyping clear to professionals and the language inoffensive to the patients themselves. The recommended system of subtyping is as follows: sexually attracted to males, sexually attracted to females, sexually attracted to both, sexually attracted to neither, and unspecified.
9. The authors further agreed that, because the rationale for subtyping is not entirely clear to those not working in this area, explanation of the need for this will be provided in the text.
10. The authors recommended exclusion of intersex patients.

Table 20–1. Proposed DSM-IV criteria for gender identity disorder

A. A strong and persistent cross-gender identification (not merely a desire for any perceived cultural advantage of being the opposite sex)
  In children, as manifested by at least 4 of the following:
  1) repeatedly stated desire to be, or insistence that he or she is, the opposite sex
  2) in boys, preference for cross-dressing or simulating female attire; in girls, insistence on wearing stereotypical masculine clothing
  3) strong and persistent preferences for cross-sex roles in fantasy play or persistent fantasies of being the opposite sex
  4) intense desire to participate in the games and pastimes of the opposite sex
  5) strong preference for playmates of the opposite sex

  In adolescents and adults, as manifested by symptoms such as a stated desire to be the opposite sex, frequent passing as the opposite sex, desire to live or be treated as the opposite sex, or the conviction that one has the typical feelings and reactions of the opposite sex.

B. Persistent discomfort with one's assigned sex or sense of inappropriateness in that gender role.
  In children, manifested by any of the following:

  in boys, assertion that his penis or testes are disgusting or will disappear or assertion that it would be better not to have a penis, or aversion toward rough-and-tumble play and rejection of male stereotypical toys, games, and activities;

  in girls, rejection of urinating in a sitting position or assertion that she does not want to grow breasts or menstruate, or marked aversion toward normative feminine clothing.

  In adolescents and adults, manifested by symptoms such as preoccupation with getting rid of one's primary and secondary sex characteristics (e.g., request for hormones, surgery, or other procedures to alter sexual characteristics physically to simulate the opposite sex), or belief that one was born the wrong sex.

C. Not due to a nonpsychiatric medical condition (e.g., hermaphroditism).

D. The disturbance causes significant impairment in social or occupational functioning, or causes marked distress.
  Specific history of sexual attraction (for sexually mature individuals):

  Sexually attracted to males
  Sexually attracted to females
  Sexually attracted to both
  Sexually attracted to neither
  Unspecified

Proposed Diagnostic Criteria

As a result of the extensive discussions within the Child Psychiatry Work Group, presentations at the American Academy of Child Psychiatry, and consultation with advisers, the authors recommended one set of criteria for gender identity disorder (Table 20–1). The authors felt that a statement of the essential, common elements of gender identity disorder could be applied to patients at different phases of the life cycle (i.e., childhood, adolescence, and adulthood), thus obviating the necessity for arbitrary age-related delineations (e.g., puberty). The criteria have been separated for children and adults to reflect developmental differences.

For children, it is proposed that a repeatedly stated desire to be of the opposite sex be one of five behavioral signs, of which four must be present for this criterion to be met. Conceptually, this criterion is intended to reflect the child's marked cross-gender identification. At present, the empirical basis for a cutoff of four signs or symptoms is debatable, although this was the consensus of the authors. The authors are currently analyzing available databases to evaluate further the legitimacy of this recommendation.

It can also be seen in Table 20–1 that the proposed B criterion is intended to reflect the child's severe discomfort with characteristics of his or her own assigned sex, including expressions of anatomic dysphoria and the intense rejection of certain normative behavioral attributes.

It should be noted that polythetic criteria are not proposed for adults and that the specific symptoms listed are intended only as examples.

References

American Psychiatric Association: Diagnostic and Statistical Manual of Mental Disorders, 3rd Edition. Washington, DC, American Psychiatric Association, 1980

American Psychiatric Association: Diagnostic and Statistical Manual of Mental Disorders, 3rd Edition, Revised. Washington, DC, American Psychiatric Association, 1987

Benjamin H: The Transsexual Phenomenon. New York, Julian Press, 1966

Blanchard R: Typology of male-to-female transsexualism. Arch Sex Behav 14:247–261, 1985

Blanchard R: Nonhomosexual gender dysphoria. Journal of Sex Research 24:188–193, 1988

Blanchard R: The classification and labeling of nonhomosexual gender dysphorias. Arch Sex Behav 18:315–334, 1989a

Blanchard R: The concept of autogynephilia and the typology of male gender dysphoria. J Nerv Ment Dis 177:616–623, 1989b

Blanchard R, Clemmensen LH: A test of the DSM-III-R's implicit assumption that fetishistic arousal and gender dysphoria are mutually exclusive. Journal of Sex Research 25:426–432, 1988

Blanchard R, Steiner BW, Clemmensen LH, et al: Prediction of regrets in postoperative transsexuals. Can J Psychiatry 34:43–45, 1989

Buhrich N, Beaumont T: Comparison of transvestism in Australia and America. Arch Sex Behav 10:269–279, 1981

Buhrich N, McConaghy N: The clinical syndromes of femmiphilic transvestism. Arch Sex Behav 6:397–412, 1977

Fisk N: Gender dysphoria syndrome (the how, what and why of a disease), in Proceedings of the Second Interdisciplinary Symposium on Gender Dysphoria Syndrome. Edited by Laub DR, Gandy P. Stanford, CA, Stanford University Medical Center, 1973, pp 7–14

Freund K, Steiner BW, Chan S: Two types of cross-gender identity. Arch Sex Behav 11:49–63, 1982

Green R: The "Sissy Boy Syndrome" and the Development of Homosexuality. New Haven, CT, Yale University Press, 1987

Levine SB: Gender identity disorders of childhood, adolescence, and adulthood, in Comprehensive Textbook of Psychiatry, 5th Edition, Vol 1. Edited by Kaplan HI, Sadock BJ. Baltimore, MD, William & Wilkins, 1989, pp 1061–1069

McCauley E, Ehrhardt AA: Follow-up of females with gender identity disorder. J Nerv Ment Dis 172:353–358, 1984

Meyer-Bahlburg HFL: Intersexuality and the diagnosis of gender identity disorder. Arch Sex Behav 23:21–40, 1994

Pauly IB: Gender identity disorders: evaluation and treatment. Journal of Sex Education and Therapy 16:2–24, 1990

Person E, Ovesey L: The transsexual syndrome in males, I: primary transsexualism. Am J Psychother 28:4–20, 1974a

Person E, Ovesey L: The transsexual syndrome in males, II: secondary transsexualism. Am J Psychother 28:174–193, 1974b

Person E, Ovesey L: Transvestism: new perspectives. J Am Acad Psychoanal 6:301–323, 1978

Shaffer D, Campbell M, Cantwell D, et al: Child and adolescent psychiatric disorders in DSM-IV: issues facing the Child Psychiatry Work Group. J Am Acad Child Adolesc Psychiatry 28:830–835, 1989

Wise TN, Meyer JK: The border area between transvestism and gender dysphoria: transvestitic applicants for sex reassignment. Arch Sex Behav 9:327–342, 1980

Zucker KJ: Gender identity disorder, in Child Psychopathology: Diagnostic Criteria and Clinical Assessment. Edited by Hooper SR, Hynd GW, Mattison RE. Hillsdale, NJ, Lawrence Erlbaum Associates, 1991, pp 305–342

Zucker KJ, Green R, Bradley SJ, et al: Gender identity disorder of childhood: diagnostic issues, in DSM-IV Sourcebook, Vol 4. Edited by Widiger TA, Frances AJ, Pincus HA, et al. Washington, DC, American Psychiatric Association, in press

Chapter 21

Sibling Rivalry: Diagnostic Category or Focus of Treatment?

Fred R. Volkmar, M.D., and Alice S. Carter, Ph.D.

Statement and Significance of the Issues

Sibling rivalry refers to a marked change in a child's affect and/or behavior that occurs in response to the birth of a sibling. The feelings and behaviors that characterize sibling rivalry include increased negative affect with predominant feelings of jealousy, anger, and rejection; lack of positive regard for the sibling; increased oppositionality; overt or covert aggression toward the sibling; marked competition for parental affection and attention; and regression to earlier stages of development. Although sibling rivalry is sometimes reported by parents, there are few empirical data about the prevalence, incidence, or stability of the phenomenon, nor are there data suggesting external validity (e.g., is the condition related to other aspects of intrapersonal or interpersonal dysfunction?).

Sibling rivalry disorder has been included as an official childhood emotional disorder in ICD-10 (World Health Organization 1990); a similar category does not exist in DSM-III-R (American Psychiatric Association 1987). The ICD-10 clinical description recognizes that sibling rivalry occurs in the context of normal child development and notes that a large proportion of young children show some degree of emotional disturbance following the birth of a sibling and that usually such a disturbance is mild and transient. A diagnosis of sibling rivalry is reserved only for those cases in which

---

A more detailed version of this paper has appeared in Lahey BB, Kazdin AE (eds): *Advances in Clinical Child Psychology,* Vol. 14. New York, Plenum, 1992, pp. 289–296.

1. The disturbance is persistent.
2. There is a change in a child's behavior following the birth of an immediately younger sibling.
3. Rivalry with or jealousy of the younger sibling is unambiguously present.
4. The degree and/or persistence of the disturbance is both statistically unusual and associated with social impairment.

Research criteria for the disorder in ICD-10 include

1. Abnormally negative feelings including jealousy toward an immediately younger sibling.
2. Emotional disturbance as evidenced by at least two of: regression, tantrums, dysphoria, sleep disturbance, oppositional behavior, or attention seeking with one or both parents.
3. Onset within 6 months of the birth of the younger sibling.
4. Duration of at least 4 weeks.

In ICD-10, the diagnosis of a sibling rivalry disorder must reflect a pattern of *extreme* behaviors that interfere with the child's developmental progress and take into account the developmental stage of the child and recent events within the family besides the birth of a sibling.

This review summarizes available research relevant to including sibling rivalry in DSM-IV either as a diagnostic category for children or as a relational problem that can be noted as an appropriate focus of treatment. Conceptualizing sibling rivalry in the latter way would lead to inclusion as a V code as opposed to an Axis I diagnosis.

Method

In preparing this review, we conducted a number of literature searches (including Medline, *Psychological Abstracts, Child Development Abstracts,* and *Index Medicus*) and examined various review articles. Although occasional case reports of sibling rivalry or sibling-related mental health problems were noted, most of the relevant literature is focused more generally on aspects of the role of siblings in child and family development. Empirical studies of sibling rivalry as a disorder were uncommon.

Results

The available literature clearly suggests that it is essential to frame the issue of sibling rivalry within the context of normal development. Further, it is critical that diagnostic criteria for this, or any, condition define deviant behavior in ways that are sensitive to the developmental, familial, and sociocultural conditions in which sibling rivalry emerges. Sibling experiences are always shaped by several interacting, dynamic influences: the nature of the relationships between the parents and the children, the developmental capacities and individual characteristics of the children (e.g., temperament) (Brody et al. 1987; Solnit 1983), and the relationships of the siblings to each other as peers (Kris and Ritvo 1983). In addition, the sociocultural environmental context provides a background that further guides the unfolding of sibling relationships (Zukow 1989). Only recently have studies begun to examine social and affective aspects of sibling relationships within the family (Furman and Buhrmester 1985). In terms of the taxonomic validity of sibling rivalry (i.e., the utility of an independent diagnostic category), it is important to note that no information of an epidemiological nature currently exists.

In many families, arguments between young siblings are customary and a cause for much parental concern and consternation (Abramovitch et al. 1982; Baskett and Johnson 1982; Dunn 1983; Newson and Newson 1970); physical aggression between siblings is not uncommon (Newson and Newson 1978). Thus, if a diagnostic category is warranted, it is important to develop assessment strategies that can distinguish severe or extreme cases of sibling rivalry from those expressions of aggression and hostility that are commonly found in sibling relationships. The adaptive or growth-promoting aspects of some features associated with sibling rivalry must be acknowledged (Howe and Ross 1990; Stewart and Marvin 1984). It is also possible that advances in general cognitive and social abilities facilitate sibling relationships (Dunn 1988).

Both prosocial and contentious aspects of sibling relationships are influenced by patterns of interaction in other family relationships (e.g., interparental conflict) and the emotional climate in the family (Brody et al. 1987; Dunn 1988). Prosocial behaviors such as friendliness, cooperation, and affection appear to be independent of antagonistic behaviors such as conflict and rivalry (cf., Dunn 1988). Parental response to aggression is of major importance in shaping children's antagonistic behavior (Dunn and Munn 1986) as well as their altruistic and empathic responses (Zahn-Waxler et al. 1979). It appears that mothers who talk about newborns as persons with needs and feelings foster positive sibling relationships (Dunn and Kendrick 1982).

Two models have been applied to understand the impact of parental intervention in sibling conflicts. First, parental intervention may unwittingly serve to reinforce conflicts (Brody and Stoneman 1983). Parental involvement with a new infant may minimize the opportunities for developing a sibling relationship, thus reducing the likelihood of both positive and negative interactions (Howe and Ross 1990). The second model views parental intervention as decreasing the likelihood of future aggressive actions (Zahn-Waxler et al. 1979). Both models may contribute to the constellation of sibling behaviors that emerges in any given sibling pair. Howe and Ross (1990) reported that, although maternal references to the infant's internal experience were positively associated with friendly sibling relationships, intense maternal interaction with children was negatively associated with friendly sibling relations. In addition, differential maternal behavior is clearly associated with increased negativity in sibling relationships (Brody et al. 1987). Although these patterns of mutual influence within the family are complex, it is clear that sibling rivalry must be assessed and treated within the broader context of family functioning.

Siblings appear to play a role in shaping children's aggressive and coercive behaviors, as well as cooperative and social fantasy play, independent of the contribution of parental behavior (Dunn 1983; Dunn and Munn 1986; Patterson 1986; Patterson and Cobb 1971). Further, Patterson (1986) reported that coercive behavior by a sibling toward a target child is associated with the target child having problems with peers outside of the family. Although there is no evidence of a causal link, this association suggests that when coercion is part of a larger constellation of behaviors associated with sibling rivalry, identification and intervention should impact not only the child who is experiencing the sibling rivalry, but also the child who is the target of coercive or aggressive actions.

Discussion

In the absence of any epidemiological information regarding the incidence, prevalence, stability, or range of severity of children's typical responses to the birth of a sibling, it is not possible to determine statistical criteria for making a diagnosis of sibling rivalry. For example, ICD-10 criteria for sibling rivalry disorder note that the negative feelings of the child toward the younger child must be abnormally intense. However, the absence of epidemiological and other data make it unclear how this criterion would be operationalized in actual use. There is a similar dearth of descriptive information about children referred for mental health services who present with a primary complaint of "sibling rivalry."

Recommendations

To date, there is insufficient evidence to argue that a constellation of behaviors associated with sibling rivalry constitutes a *syndrome* of mental disorder. These behaviors can be more conservatively viewed as evidence of a condition that is not attributed to a mental disorder but that may be the focus of individual child or family therapy. Given the evidence that many of the behaviors that compose sibling rivalry appear to be strongly related to patterns of family interaction and the emotional climate within the family, sibling rivalry may be best conceptualized within the larger rubric of family functioning. From this point of view, a V code may be the most appropriate mechanism for identifying sibling rivalry in DSM-IV. Coding it in this way would indicate that the condition may be an important focus of treatment and would facilitate both future research and clinical service.

References

Abramovitch R, Pepler D, Corter C: Pattern of sibling interaction among pre-school age children, in Sibling Relationships: Their Nature and Significance Across the Lifespan. Edited by Lamb ME, Sutton-Smith B. Hillsdale, NJ, Lawrence Erlbaum Associates, 1982, pp 61–86

American Psychiatric Association: Diagnostic and Statistical Manual of Mental Disorders, 3rd Edition, Revised. Washington, DC, American Psychiatric Association, 1987

Baskett LM, Johnson SM: The young child's interactions with parents versus siblings: a behavioral analysis. Child Dev 53:643–650, 1982

Brody GH, Stoneman Z: Children with atypical siblings, in Advances in Clinical Child Psychology, Vol 6. Edited by Lahey BB, Kadzin AE. New York, Plenum, 1983, pp 285–386

Brody GH, Stoneman Z, Burke M: Family system and individual child correlates of sibling behavior. Am J Orthopsychiatry 57:561–569, 1987

Dunn J: Sibling relationships in early childhood. Child Dev 54:787–811, 1983

Dunn J: Sibling influences on childhood development. Journal of Child and Adolescent Psychiatry 29:119–127, 1988

Dunn J, Kendrick C: Siblings. Cambridge, MA, Harvard University Press, 1982

Dunn J, Munn P: Sibling quarrels and maternal intervention: individual differences in understanding and aggression. J Child Psychol Psychiatry 27:583–595, 1986

Furman W, Buhrmester D: Children's perception of the qualities of sibling relationships. Child Dev 56:448–461, 1985

Howe N, Ross HS: Socialization, perspective-taking, and the sibling relationship. Developmental Psychology 26:160–165, 1990

Kris M, Ritvo S: Parent and siblings: their mutual influence. Psychoanal Study Child 38:311–324, 1983

Newson J, Newson E: Four Years Old in an Urban Community. Harmondsworth, United Kingdom, Penguin Books, 1970

Newson J, Newson E: Seven Years Old in the Home Environment. Harmondsworth, United Kingdom, Penguin Books, 1978

Patterson GR: The contribution of siblings to training for fighting: a microsocial analysis, in Development of Antisocial and Prosocial Behavior: Research, Theories and Issues. Edited by Olweus D, Block J, Radke-Yarrow M. New York, Academic Press, 1986, pp 263–284

Patterson GR, Cobb JA: A dyadic analysis of "aggressive" behaviors, in Minnesota Symposia on Child Psychology, Vol 5. Edited by Hill JP. Minneapolis, MN, University of Minnesota Press, 1971, pp 235–261

Solnit AJ: The sibling experience. Psychoanal Study Child 38:281–284, 1983

Stewart R, Marvin RS: Sibling relations: the role of conceptual perspective-taking in the ontogeny of sibling caregiving. Child Dev 55:1322–1332, 1984

World Health Organization: ICD-10 Chapter V: Mental and Behavioral Disorders: Diagnostic Criteria for Research. Geneva, Switzerland, World Health Organization, 1990

Zahn-Waxler C, Radke-Yarrow M, King RC: Child rearing and children's prosocial initiations towards victims of distress. Child Dev 50:319–330, 1979

Zukow PG (ed): Sibling Interaction Across Cultures: Theoretical and Methodological Issues. New York, Springer, 1989

Section III

Eating Disorders

Introduction to Section III

Eating Disorders

B. Timothy Walsh, M.D.

Introduction

The purpose of this section is to provide a synopsis of the considerations of the Work Group on Eating Disorders. The initial focus of the Work Group was on the two diagnostic categories for eating disorders in DSM-III-R (American Psychiatric Association 1987): anorexia nervosa and bulimia nervosa. (Categories for pica and rumination disorder of infancy were also included in the eating disorders section of DSM-III-R, but were under the purview of the Work Group on Child and Adolescent disorders for DSM-IV.) In addition, the Work Group reviewed information suggesting a need for an additional eating disorder in DSM-IV.

Anorexia Nervosa

Anorexia nervosa is a syndrome that has been recognized for more than a century, and its essential features are generally well accepted. In the discussions and correspondence that preceded the literature reviews that are presented in this *Sourcebook*, only one major question concerning anorexia nervosa consistently arose: whether it was useful to subdivide patients with anorexia nervosa into a group of patients who binged and purged and a group of patients who did not.

In their review on subtyping anorexia nervosa, DaCosta and Halmi (Chapter 22) found a substantial body of data suggesting that the distinction between bulimic and nonbulimic subtypes of anorexia nervosa is a useful one, and a proposal that individuals with anorexia nervosa be subtyped based on the presence or absence of binge eating is included in the *DSM-IV Options Book* (American Psychiatric Asso-

---

Some of the material presented here was previously published in Walsh BT: "Diagnostic Criteria for Eating Disorders in DSM-IV: Work in Progress." *International Journal of Eating Disorders* 11:301–304, 1992.

ciation 1991). If anorexia nervosa is subtyped, patients with anorexia nervosa who have bulimia will be diagnosed as having "anorexia nervosa, bulimic type" rather than being given simultaneous diagnoses of anorexia nervosa and bulimia nervosa, as was the case in DSM-III-R.

One other change in the criteria for anorexia nervosa is being considered: a revision of the wording of criterion C, which requires the presence of a disturbance in the person's perception of weight or shape. The rewording is not suggested on the basis of a formal literature review and is intended primarily to clarify the concept described in this criterion. The Work Group felt that the examples in criterion C in DSM-III-R were not typical of many individuals with this illness and therefore suggested that the criterion be broadened to identify additional manifestations of a disturbance of body shape and weight.

Bulimia Nervosa

Although the phenomenon of episodic "binge eating" has been noted for centuries, the syndrome of bulimia nervosa was described only in 1979 by Russell. Perhaps because this category was recently introduced, a number of questions were raised about the criteria used for its recognition in DSM-III-R, and three of the reviews conducted by the Work Group focused on diagnostic criteria for this disorder.

In his review of bulimia diagnostic criteria, Wilson (Chapter 23) attempted to obtain information to clarify several of the terms used in DSM-III-R to describe a binge, such as its being "rapid" and "large." Unfortunately, relatively little relevant information was uncovered. Because limited empirical data are available documenting that "rapid" food consumption is a critical feature of bulimia nervosa and because a number of advisers to the Work Group expressed concern about the necessity of this feature, the Work Group is recommending that this term be eliminated from the definition of a binge in DSM-IV. Although the available data do suggest that many individuals with bulimia nervosa sometimes use the term *binge* to describe the consumption of amounts of food that are *not* unusually large, data from eating diaries and from laboratory studies indicate that patients with this syndrome do, indeed, consume large amounts of food when binge eating. For this reason, and because the consumption of a large amount of food has been a required characteristic of a binge since the recognition of bulimia as a diagnostic category in DSM-III (American Psychiatric Association 1980), the Work Group is recommending that "large" be retained in DSM-IV.

In reviewing these issues, the Work Group concluded that it would be useful to define more clearly what is meant by the term *binge eating*. The proposed definition in DSM-IV would include in a single criterion two elements that, in

DSM-III-R, were in separate criteria: excessive eating (criterion A in DSM-III-R) and a sense of loss of control (criterion C in DSM-III-R). In addition, the Work Group believed that, although quantitative guidelines could not be provided regarding, for example, a minimum number of calories to be considered "large," a binge could be described in more operational terms. In doing so, the Work Group used terminology that was initially developed by Cooper and Fairburn (1987) and modified slightly by the consortium of investigators studying binge eating disorder (Spitzer et al. 1992).

Wilson's (Chapter 23) review also examined information on the validity of the DSM-III-R criterion that required that binges occur twice a week for 3 months. A few data were uncovered suggesting that a criterion frequency of once a week might be as or more appropriate, but the Work Group did not believe that the data presently available were sufficiently compelling to justify a recommendation for a change in the diagnostic criteria.

Mitchell (Chapter 24) reviewed information regarding whether it might be advantageous to subdivide the syndrome of bulimia nervosa on the basis of various clinical characteristics (e.g., the regular use of purging behavior). Although the data reviewed by Mitchell are not definitive, they suggest the existence of important differences between purging and nonpurging individuals with bulimia nervosa. Two possible options for change are therefore proposed in the *DSM-IV Options Book*. One option would retain the DSM-III-R criterion requiring that the person regularly engage in behaviors to prevent weight gain, but add a subtyping scheme to allow the clinician to distinguish those individuals who purge from those who do not. A second, more radical option is to narrow the definition of bulimia nervosa by restricting the diagnosis to those individuals who regularly purge after binge eating.

Finally, in DSM-III-R, a criterion was added to require that individuals with bulimia nervosa manifest a "persistent overconcern with shape and weight." Garfinkel's (Chapter 25) review clearly documented that this is a relatively specific and highly characteristic feature of patients with this disorder. The Work Group therefore recommends that this criterion be retained in DSM-IV. However, to describe the concept more clearly, the Work Group suggests that it be reworded.

Other Forms of Overeating

Since the recognition of bulimia nervosa as a distinct syndrome, increased attention has been focused on the presence of overeating among individuals who do not meet criteria for any DSM-III-R eating disorder (Devlin and Walsh, Chapter 26). A review of the literature was therefore undertaken to examine information about syndromes of overeating other than bulimia nervosa. This review concluded that there may be a significant number of individuals who report binge eating but who fail to meet DSM-III-R criteria for bulimia nervosa because they do not regularly engage in compensatory behaviors to avoid weight gain. However, the available literature did not permit such a syndrome to be clearly defined.

Since this literature review was completed, a consortium of investigators developed criteria for the recognition of a disorder named "binge eating disorder" and conducted preliminary studies using these criteria (Spitzer et al. 1992). On the basis of this work, the Work Group believed that there were sufficient indications of the clinical utility of binge eating disorder to justify its inclusion in the *DSM-IV Options Book*.

References

American Psychiatric Association: Diagnostic and Statistical Manual of Mental Disorders, 3rd Edition. Washington, DC, American Psychiatric Association, 1980

American Psychiatric Association: Diagnostic and Statistical Manual of Mental Disorders, 3rd Edition, Revised. Washington, DC, American Psychiatric Association, 1987

American Psychiatric Association: DSM-IV Options Book: Work in Progress. Washington, DC, American Psychiatric Association, 1991

Cooper Z, Fairburn CG: The Eating Disorder Examination: a semi-structured interview for the assessment of the specific psychopathology of eating disorders. International Journal of Eating Disorders 6:1–8, 1987

Russell G: Bulimia nervosa: an ominous variant of anorexia nervosa. Psychol Med 9:429–448, 1979

Spitzer RL, Devlin MJ, Walsh BT, et al: Binge eating disorder: a multisite field trial for the diagnostic criteria. International Journal of Eating Disorders 11:191–203, 1992

Chapter 22

Subtyping Anorexia Nervosa

Maria DaCosta, M.D., and Katherine A. Halmi, M.D.

Statement of the Issues

The issue considered in this review is whether the classification system as it exists in DSM-III-R (American Psychiatric Association 1987) should be maintained so that patients who have anorexia nervosa and experience episodes of binge eating receive a dual diagnosis of anorexia nervosa and bulimia nervosa, or whether there should be a subtyping of anorexia nervosa for patients who binge versus those who solely restrict food intake severely.

Significance of the Issues

The existence of subtypes within the spectrum of anorexia nervosa has been described by numerous clinicians dating back to Janet in 1903. He subdivided anorectic patients into an "obsessional" group and a "hysterical" group. Dally (1969) also acknowledged these two subtypes as well as a third, which consisted of patients with "mixed" features. Beumont (1977) described his collected data on a group of 31 patients with anorexia nervosa. He subtyped his group based on contrasting patterns of food consumption: 17 were restrictors who maintained very rigid eating rituals, and 14 were vomiters who experienced episodes of disinhibition and engaged in eating binges. Garfinkel et al. (1980) described 141 patients with anorexia nervosa, 68 of whom had bulimia, 73 of who did not. Casper et al. (1980) compared 48 anorectic-bulimics with 56 anorectic-restrictors. Although both groups shared features in common, the anorectic-bulimics appeared to be a distinct subgroup that carried a worse prognosis in both studies.

Method

To locate clinical data substantiating either position, Medline was searched using the key words *anorexia, binge, bulimia,* and *amenorrhea*. Potentially relevant articles were identified in the bibliographies of articles obtained via the Medline search, and review bibliographies from the *International Journal of Eating Disorders* were scanned. The main focus of this review was to determine whether there is any validity and/or utility in subclassifying anorexia nervosa into bulimic or restrictor types. We also included studies that examined parental personality traits and family psychiatric morbidity in both groups.

Results

Fourteen studies were reviewed in detail. Table 22–1 summarizes the methodology for 12 studies that are to be discussed in detail. Table 22–2 provides the demographic data. Reliability of diagnosis was determined in only eight studies. All of the studies except two limited their investigation to female subjects; one of the studies included 6 males (4 anorectic-restrictors and 2 anorectic-bulimics) and the other included 2 males (1 anorectic-restrictor and 1 anorectic-bulimic). The number of subjects among the anorectic-restrictors varied from 16 to 73, and the anorectic-bulimics varied from 7 to 76. The anorectic-bulimics were consistently older at the time of diagnosis in all the studies. The results were inconsistent in terms of mean age at onset: in four of the studies, the anorectic-bulimics were older than the anorectic-restrictors at time of onset, whereas, in three others, they were younger. The duration of illness was consistently longer for the anorectic-bulimics than for the anorectic-restrictors. Both premorbid weight and admission weight were consistently greater for the anorectic-bulimics than for the anorectic-restrictors.

Table 22–3 summarizes data from articles that reported a significant increase in impulsive behavior among anorectic-bulimics in comparison with anorectic-restrictors. The prevalence of stealing was much greater in the anorectic-bulimics than in the anorectic-restrictors. The prevalence of drug and alcohol use was also consistently greater in the anorectic-bulimic population. Other types of impulsivity were also higher in the anorectic-bulimics compared with the restrictors.

Table 22–4 summarizes data from articles that studied personality traits in an attempt to differentiate between the two groups. There was no consistent difference in the extent of depression between the two groups, nor was there a difference between obsessive-compulsive disorder symptoms unrelated to eating. Anxiety was higher in two studies, but no differences were found in another. The prevalence of anorectic complaints was higher in the anorectic-bulimics in two studies compared with anorectic-restrictors. Mood lability was higher in two studies in the anorectic-bulimics compared with anorectic-restrictors. Factors in the Hopkins Symptom Check List were used to assess the personality traits presented in the Casper et al.

Table 22–1. Methodological and design features

Study	Diagnostic criteria[a]	Method of data collection	Source of information	Setting	Subject selection procedure
Anderson 1985	DSM-III	Structured interview, self-report inventory	Patient	Inpatient university medical center	Sequential admissions
Casper et al. 1980	Feighner	Structured interview, self-report inventory	Patient	University medical center	Sequential admissions
Eckert et al. 1987	DSM-III	Clinical interview, self-report inventory	Patient	Inpatient university medical center	Not specified
Garfinkel et al. 1980	Feighner	Semistructured interview	Patient	Clark Institute inpatient/outpatient	Not specified
Garner et al. 1985	DSM-III	Clinical interview, self-report inventory	Patient	University medical center	Sequential admissions
Holmgren et al. 1983	DSM-III	Clinical interview, self-report inventory	Patient	Specialty clinic	Sequential admissions
Kassett et al. 1988	Feighner	Semistructured interview	Chart	Specialty clinic	Not specified
Laessle et al. 1989	DSM-III	Clinical interview, semistructured interview	Patient	Max Planck Institute of Psychiatry	Sequential consultation

(continued)

Table 22–1. Methodological and design features *(continued)*

Study	Diagnostic criteria[a]	Method of data collection	Source of information	Setting	Subject selection procedure
Mickalide and Anderson 1985	DSM-III	Clinical interview, self-report inventory	Chart	Specialty clinic	Sequential consultation
Strober 1981	Feighner	Structured interview, self-report inventory	Patient	University medical center	Not specified
Vandereycken and Pierloot 1983	Feighner	Clinical interview	Chart	University medical center	Sequential admissions
Yellowlees 1985	DSM-III	Clinical interview	Patient	Inpatient/outpatient	Not specified

[a] Feighner = Feighner's criteria (Feighner et al. 1972).

Table 22–2. Clinical demographic data and weight-related features: anorexia nervosa restricting patients and anorexia nervosa bulimic patients

Study	Number of subjects	Reliability of diagnosis	Sex	Mean age at time of diagnosis	Mean age at onset	Duration of disorder (months)	Premorbid weight (kg)	Admission weight (kg)
Restricting								
Anderson 1985	48		F	20.5	17.5	37.2		
Casper et al. 1980	56	Yes	F	19.7	50% 12–17			
Eckert et al. 1987	39	Yes	F					
Garfinkel et al. 1980	73		4M	21.2		38.8	56.4	39.6
Garner et al. 1985	59	Yes	F	22.1	18.7	37.3		40.9
Holmgren et al. 1983	16	Yes	F		19.7	62.1	54.5	35.7
Kassett et al. 1988	43	Yes	F	22.9	17.9			
Laessle et al. 1989	21	Yes	F	20.9		55.8	49.9	34.1

(continued)

Table 22–2. Clinical demographic data and weight-related features: anorexia nervosa restricting patients and anorexia nervosa bulimic patients *(continued)*

Study	Number of subjects	Reliability of diagnosis	Sex	Mean age at time of diagnosis	Mean age at onset	Duration of disorder (months)	Premorbid weight (kg)	Admission weight (kg)
Mickalide and Anderson 1985	54	Yes	F	22.13				
Strober 1981	22	Yes	F					35.4
Vandereycken and Pierloot 1983	65		F	18.36	16.48	23.52		
Yellowlees 1985	16		1M	20.4	16.7		50.2	44.6
Bulimic								
Anderson 1985	28		F	24.4	18.5	70.8		
Casper et al. 1980	49	Yes	F	20.2	≥18			
Garfinkel et al. 1980	68		2M	21.5		49.6	62.0	44.8
Garner et al. 1985	59	Yes	F	22.5	18.4	52.3		47.9
Holmgren et al. 1983	7	Yes	F		17.3	74.9	57.3	38.4

Kassett et al. 1988	31	Yes	F	23.5	19.4			
Laessle et al. 1989	20	Yes	F	22.1		55.2	43.8	33.0
Mickalide and Anderson 1985	54	Yes	F	23.56				
Strober 1981	22	Yes	F					35.9
Vandereycken and Pierloot 1983	76		F	22.24	18.18	48.72		
Yellowlees 1985	15		1M	25.9	17.8		60.3	52.1

Table 22–3. Impulsivity measures, in percent

Study	Stealing	Drug use/alcohol use	Suicidality	Self-mutilation	Other impulsivity
Anorexia nervosa restrictors					
Casper et al. 1980	4				
Garfinkel et al. 1980	0	11.6/4.8	7.1	1.5	
Garner et al. 1985	9	19/34	12	10	19
Laessle et al. 1989		4.8/0			
Strober 1981	0				
Vandereycken and Pierloot 1983		0/0	0		5
Anorexia nervosa bulimics					
Casper et al. 1980	24		23.1		
Garfinkel et al. 1980	12.1	28.6/20.4	25	9.2	
Garner et al. 1985	26	40/45		19	39
Laessle et al. 1989		0/20			
Strober 1981	9				
Vandereycken and Pierloot 1983		11	9		33.3

Table 22–4. Personality traits, in percent

Study	Depression	Obsessive-compulsive disorder	Anxiety	Somatic complaints	Mood lability
Anorexia nervosa restrictors					
Eckert et al. 1987	20.2			6.5	
Garfinkel et al. 1980					1.2
Garner et al. 1985					43
Laessle et al. 1989	9.5	9.5	33.3		
Strober 1981	9	9	32	9	
Yellowlees 1985	94	59	88	18	
Anorexia nervosa bulimics					
Eckert et al. 1987	21.1			7.9	
Garfinkel et al. 1980					1.7
Garner et al. 1985					60
Laessle et al. 1989	50	10	55		
Strober 1981	41	36	41	32	
Yellowlees 1985	100	67	87	27	

(1980) study. Only mean scores and no frequency data were presented. In this study, anorectic-restrictors compared with anorectic-bulimics had the following mean scores for depression (27.0 ± 5.4 versus 30.0 ± 5.9), obsession (17.2 ± 3.9 versus 18.8 ± 3.3), somatization (14.0 ± 3.6 versus 15.7 ± 5.2), and anxiety (10.4 ± 3.4 versus 11.5 ± 3.4).

Table 22–5 summarizes data available on developmental history, sexual history, and menarche. In three studies, there were no significant differences with regard to prevalence of amenorrhea at time of diagnosis or age at menarche. There was no consistent difference with regard to marital status or disinterest in sex.

Table 22–6 summarizes data from studies comparing familial, physical, and psychological traits as well as premorbid obesity among anorectic-restrictors and anorectic-bulimics. Three studies reported a higher prevalence of maternal obesity, and two studies reported a higher prevalence of premorbid obesity in anorectic-bulimics than in anorectic-restrictors. One of the articles did not find a difference in paternal obesity between the two groups. There was a higher prevalence of psychiatric illness in the mothers of anorectic-bulimics than in those of anorectic-restrictors in two articles. One of the articles reported an increase in prevalence of psychiatric illness in the fathers as well.

In their study involving 165 females, Mickalide and Anderson (1985) found evidence supporting a distinct and separate diagnosis for anorexia nervosa and normal-weight bulimia. Of the anorectic-restrictors and anorectic-bulimics, only 9% had regular menses in comparison with 60% of the normal-weight bulimics. There was a lack of statistical significance on the total and subscale General Health Questionnaire scores (somatic symptoms, anxiety, social dysfunction, and depression) when comparing anorectic-bulimics, anorectic-restrictors, and normal-weight bulimics. On the Eating Disorders Inventory, there were no statistically significant differences among the subgroups on the ineffectiveness, perfectionism, interpersonal distrust, and maturity fears subscales. However, the anorectic-restrictors attained the lowest scores on all Eating Disorders Inventory subscales with the exception of maturity fears, for which scores were equivalent. This research supported clinical observations that anorectic-bulimics exhibit more psychopathology than do anorectic-restrictors.

Strober (1983) assigned 106 females into one of three subtypes according to Minnesota Multiphasic Personality Inventory profiles. Type I was the largest and was characterized by the presence of hypomania. Type II was characterized by obsessional features and rigidity. Type III was the smallest and consisted of patients with low frustration tolerance, high impulsivity, binge eating, purgation, and addictive behaviors. Strober concluded that there was validity in developing a taxonomy of anorectic patients.

Table 22-5. Developmental history, sexual history, and menarche, in percent

Study	Amenorrhea	Age at menarche (years)	Single	Uninterested in sex	Decreased sexual interest since onset	Sexual interference
Anorexia nervosa restrictors						
Anderson 1985		13.0	85.5	42.6		
Casper et al. 1980	100	12.9	84	51	52	
Garfinkel et al. 1980		12.8	86.3			
Garner et al. 1985	98					
Holmgren et al. 1983	100					
Yellowlees 1985						0
Anorexia nervosa bulimics						
Anderson 1985		13.0	57.1	18.5		
Casper et al. 1980	100	13.0	82	80	73	
Garfinkel et al. 1980		12.9	82.4			
Garner et al. 1985	93					
Holmgren et al. 1983	100					
Yellowlees 1985						0

Table 22–6. Parental psychopathology, parental obesity, and premorbid obesity in anorexia nervosa, in percent

Study	Maternal obesity	Paternal obesity	Premorbid obesity	Mother with history of psychiatric illness	Father with history of psychiatric illness
Anorexia nervosa restrictors					
Garfinkel et al. 1980	28	18	10	9.5	
Garner et al. 1985	28	12	17		
Strober 1981	18	14		18	14
Anorexia nervosa bulimics					
Garfinkel et al. 1980	48	18.4	32	18.2	
Garner et al. 1985	30	25	20		
Strober 1981	41	32		50	50

Discussion

The research has consistently demonstrated that impulsive behaviors, including stealing, drug abuse, suicide attempts, self-mutilations, and other "unstable" traits such as mood lability, are more prevalent in anorectic-bulimics than in anorectic-restrictors. The former also have a higher prevalence of premorbid obesity, familial obesity, debilitating personality traits, and familial psychopathology.

Therefore, it seems warranted to subclassify the diagnosis of anorexia nervosa into anorexia nervosa, nonbulimic type and anorexia nervosa, bulimic type. The predominant features of anorexia nervosa are an irrational pursuit of thinness regardless of weight, an intense fear of becoming fat, a distorted perception of one's appearance, and amenorrhea. These issues are of major concern to anorectic-restrictors and anorectic-bulimics alike. Binge eating represents a loss of control in reaction to severe and effective starvation. The vomiting and purging represent attempts to regain control and maintain the thin body ideal.

The alternative to subtyping is to maintain the system of classification as it exists in DSM-III-R. Anorectic patients who binge eat would receive a dual diagnosis of anorexia nervosa and bulimia nervosa. It seems cumbersome and inconsistent with the rest of the DSM classifications to give two Axis I diagnoses within the same restricted category (in this case, the "Eating Disorder" category). All underweight patients who binge and purge have anorexia nervosa. The converse is not true; that is, not all patients who have anorexia nervosa binge and purge. A primary diagnosis of bulimia nervosa implies to most clinicians that the patient is within the normal-weight range. It may be confusing to apply this diagnostic label to emaciated anorexia nervosa patients to denote bingeing behavior. The emaciation inherent in anorexia nervosa also has specific medical complications as well as specific treatment requirements. The necessity of hospitalization for adequate treatment is far more frequent in the anorectic-bulimic compared with the normal-weight bulimia nervosa patient. These are reasons to support a subclassification of anorexia nervosa into restrictor and bulimic types and to confine the diagnosis of bulimia nervosa to individuals who are not underweight.

On the other hand, there are many personality characteristics and behaviors that bulimia nervosa patients and anorectic-bulimics have in common. Further, a major purpose of diagnostic classification systems is to facilitate communication. The DSM-III-R system of diagnosis has been in effect for several years, and it is only recently that it has become well understood and accurately used for eating disorder diagnoses. This would be a strong argument for keeping the DSM-III-R eating disorder classification schema.

Recommendations

Assessments of the accuracy of eating disorder diagnoses using the DSM-III-R classification would be useful to determine if this schema should be changed. Chart studies could be conducted in centers with high-quality records. Prospective studies with general psychiatric practitioners diagnosing eating disorders using either the present DSM-III-R classification or a newly proposed scheme, with anorexia nervosa divided into subtypes and a separate bulimia nervosa category, would provide the best evidence for determining which diagnostic system promotes the greatest accuracy of diagnoses.

Although the studies recommended have not been conducted, the Eating Disorders Work Group recommended that enough evidence was present in the literature to warrant the classification of anorexia nervosa into the subtypes of anorexia nervosa, nonbulimic type and anorexia nervosa, bulimic type. The proposed criteria for subtyping are

- *Bulimic type:* During the episode of anorexia nervosa, the person engages in recurrent episodes of binge eating.
- *Nonbulimic type:* During the episode of anorexia nervosa, the person does not engage in recurrent episodes of binge eating.

References

American Psychiatric Association: Diagnostic and Statistical Manual of Mental Disorders, 3rd Edition, Revised. Washington, DC, American Psychiatric Association, 1987

Anderson AE: Practical comprehensive treatment of Anorexia Nervosa and Bulimia. Baltimore, MD, Johns Hopkins University Press, 1985

Beumont PJV: Further categorization of patients with anorexia nervosa. Aust N Z J Psychiatry 11:223–226, 1977

Casper RC, Eckert ED, Halmi KA: Bulimia: its incidence and clinical importance in patients with anorexia nervosa. Arch Gen Psychiatry 37:1030–1035, 1980

Dally P: Anorexia Nervosa. London, England, William Heineman Medical Books, 1969

Eckert E, Halmi KA, Marchi P, et al: Comparison of bulimic and non-bulimic anorexia nervosa patients during treatment. Psychol Med 17:891–898, 1987

Feighner JP, Robins E, Guze S, et al: Diagnostic criteria for use in psychiatric research. Arch Gen Psychiatry 26:57–63, 1972

Garfinkel PE, Moldofsky H, Garner DM: The heterogeneity of anorexia nervosa. Arch Gen Psychiatry 37:1036–1040, 1980

Garner DM, Garfinkel PE, O'Shaughnessy M: The validity of the distinction between bulimia with and without anorexia nervosa. Am J Psychiatry 142:581–582, 1985

Holmgren S, Humble K, Norring C, et al: The anorectic bulimic conflict: an alternative diagnostic approach to anorexia nervosa and bulimia. Int J Eating Disord 2:3–14, 1983

Janet P: Les Obsessions et La Psychiasthenie. Paris, France, Felix Alean, 1903

Kassett JA, Gwirtsman HE, Kaye W, et al: Pattern of onset of bulimic symptoms in anorexia nervosa. Am J Psychiatry 145:1287–1288, 1988

Laessle RG, Wittchen HV, Fichter M et al: The validity of subgroups of bulimia and anorexia nervosa: lifetime history of psychiatry disorders. Int J Eating Disord 8:569–574, 1989

Mickalide A, Anderson A: Subgroups of anorexia nervosa and bulimia: validity and utility. J Psychiatr Res 19:121–128, 1985

Strober M: The significance of bulimia in juvenile anorexia nervosa: an exploration of possible etiologic factors. Int J Eating Disord 1:28–43, 1981

Strober M: An empirically derived typology of anorexia nervosa, in Anorexia Nervosa: Recent Developments in Research. Edited by Darby PL, Garfinkel PE, Garner DM, et al. New York, Alan R Liss, 1983, pp 185–198

Vandereycken W, Pierloot R: The significance of subclassification in anorexia nervosa: a comparative study of clinical features in 141 patients. Psychol Med 13:543–549, 1983

Yellowlees AJ: Anorexia and bulimia in anorexia nervosa: a study of psychosocial functioning and associated psychiatric symptomatology. Br J Psychiatry 146:648–652, 1985

Chapter 23

Diagnostic Criteria for Bulimia Nervosa

G. Terence Wilson, Ph.D.

Statement of the Issues

The DSM-III-R (American Psychiatric Association 1987) criteria for bulimia nervosa include the following two items: "Recurrent episodes of binge eating (rapid consumption of a large amount of food in a discrete period of time)" (p. 68) and "A minimum average of two binge eating episodes a week for at least three months" (p. 69). The issue for this review is whether these thresholds are optimal, valid, or useful.

Significance of the Issues

The threshold for determining when a person is given the diagnosis of a mental disorder has substantial social, theoretical, and clinical significance. DSM-III-R contained specific criteria for this judgment for many of the mental disorders, but there was often little empirical justification for the criteria. The criteria for bulimia nervosa are quite specific with respect to the frequency of binge eating that is necessary to diagnose the disorder (i.e., two episodes a week for at least 3 months), but not with respect to what constitutes a binge-eating episode (i.e., it is not clear what constitutes a "large" amount of food or "rapid" consumption). The purpose of this review is to determine whether there is empirical justification for more specific criteria and whether the existing criteria are necessary.

Method

A review of relevant articles and book chapters on eating disorders was conducted, including a systematic review of all articles from 1981 to 1990 from the *International Journal of Eating Disorders* and a printout of articles on eating disorders from the database for the 1988–1989 *Current Opinion in Psychiatry*. In addition, Dr. B. T. Walsh solicited comments on diagnostic criteria from authorities on eating disorders.

Results

Binge-Eating Threshold

There appears to be no empirical evidence that addresses the diagnostic significance of the rapidity of eating. There is little empirical evidence that addresses the diagnostic significance of specifying that a binge be defined in terms of the consumption of a "large" amount of food. Studies in which the eating behavior of bulimic patients has been monitored in the laboratory consistently indicate mean consumption in binges ranging from 3,500 kcal to 4,476 kcal (Kaye et al. 1986; Kissileff et al. 1986; Mitchell and Laine 1985). Nevertheless, two published reports argue that patients who otherwise meet the DSM-III-R criteria for bulimia nervosa often consume relatively "small" amounts of food. Rossiter et al. (1988) noted that one-third of their bulimic patients reported consuming less than 100 kcal per binge. Rosen et al. (1986) observed that one-third of their patients reported binges of less than 600 kcal and that roughly 50% of all reported binges were less than 100 kcal.

An inevitable problem with self-reported binge eating is its accuracy, even when guided self-monitoring is used. Self-reports may under- or overestimate actual caloric intake during binges (Ortega et al. 1987; Wilson 1987). Rosen et al. (1986) defended the accuracy of their measures, pointing out that their subjects had been trained in and had practiced recording food consumption in standard units of measurement.

The most explicit attempt to develop an operational definition of "large amount" comes from Fairburn (1987). His Eating Disorders Examination distinguishes between "objective" and "subjective" binges. The former is defined by the consumption of a large amount of food and loss of control.

> To reach this decision, the interviewer should take into account what might be the usual amount eaten under such circumstances. This requires some knowledge of the eating habits of the subject's social group. The episode of eating should involve the consumption of more than 1,000 kcal of food. (Fairburn 1987, p. 4)

It should be noted that Fairburn no longer adheres to the 1,000 kcal cutoff, claiming that these guidelines reliably yield episodes of eating in excess of 1,000 kcal (C. G. Fairburn, personal communication, 1989).

The consensus of the experts whose opinions were polled is that the requirement of a "large" amount of food should be retained.

Frequency of Binge Eating

One way of assessing the validity of the frequency criterion is to examine the association between frequency of binge eating and concurrent psychopathology. The data are mixed. In their community study, Fairburn and Cooper (1984) found no clinical differences among probable cases of bulimia nervosa who vomited once a week or less, two to six times a week, or at least once a day. They concluded that "behavioral indices of bulimia nervosa, such as frequency of binge-eating or self-induced vomiting, may be a poor measure of clinical severity" (p. 409). Wilson and Eldredge (1991) obtained comparable results. They divided a series of 30 patients into the following weekly binge-eating frequencies: once a week, 2–3 times, 4–5 times, and more than 5 times. These frequencies were unrelated to various measures of psychopathology. Binge eating was highly correlated ($r = .75$) with purging (vomiting). The more frequent the purging, the greater the concern with weight and the greater the degree of psychopathology.

Other studies have found a relationship between frequency of binge eating and psychopathology. Williamson et al. (1987), using a median split, divided 35 bulimic patients into those who purged fewer or more than three times a week. The means were 1.7 and 9.9, respectively. The two groups did not differ on a range of measures of psychopathology, including depression. Subsequent correlational analysis showed that frequency of binge eating was significantly associated with depression, anxiety, and a general index of psychopathology. Frequency of binge eating was also correlated with measures of psychopathology in studies by Hatsukami et al. (1982) and Johnson et al. (1982).

Another, more powerful, approach to determining the diagnostic significance of frequency of binge eating is to examine its predictive value. In their small sample, Wilson and Eldredge (1991) found that neither pretreatment frequencies of binge eating nor purging predicted posttreatment outcome defined in terms of binge-purge frequency. However, in their study of 40 patients, Garner et al. (1990) found that pretreatment binge-eating frequency (but not purge frequency) was related to posttreatment outcome. The higher the frequency, the worse the prognosis. (The problem here is that their "low frequency" patients binged an average of 4 times a week and their "high frequency" patients binged an average of 8.6 times a week.) Neither of these two reports distinguishes between "subjective" and "objective" binges, although both used the Eating Disorders Examination.

Discussion

There is scant empirical basis for requiring that binges be "large," and no accepted cutoff or guidelines for determining what constitutes a large binge. There is no documented justification for requiring that binge eating be "rapid." Although the evidence is mixed, some studies have found a significant association between frequency of binge eating and other forms of psychopathology. Even if it is concluded that greater frequency of binge eating is reliably correlated with increased psychopathology, the present cutoff of twice a week remains arbitrary. Frequency of binge eating may be related to treatment outcome. There is a body of opinion that favors changing the frequency criterion to once a week for the past 3 or 6 months.

Recommendations

1. Retain the requirement that a binge be "large" but undertake secondary analyses of existing and future data sets to evaluate the validity and utility of this criterion. In particular, future research must identify guidelines to help the clinician make a reliable determination of "large."
2. For the time being, retain the requirement that binge eating occur at least twice a week despite the absence of any supportive empirical evidence. Review this interim conclusion in the light of the reanalyses of existing data sets.

References

American Psychiatric Association: Diagnostic and Statistical Manual of Mental Disorders, 3rd Edition, Revised. Washington, DC, American Psychiatric Association, 1987

Fairburn CG: The definition of bulimia nervosa: guidelines for clinicians and research workers. Annals of Behavioral Medicine 9:3–7, 1987

Fairburn DG, Cooper PJ: Binge-eating, self-induced vomiting, and laxative abuse: a community study. Psychol Med 14:401–410, 1984

Garner DM, Olmsted MP, Davis R, et al: The association between bulimic symptoms and reported psychopathology. International Journal of Eating Disorders 9:1–15, 1990

Hatsukami D, Owen P, Pyle R, et al: Similarities and differences on the MMPI between women with bulimia and women with alcohol and drug abuse problems. Addict Behav 7:435–439, 1982

Johnson CL, Stuckey M, Lewis LD, et al: Bulimia: a descriptive study of 316 patients. International Journal of Eating Disorders 2:1–15, 1982

Kaye WH, Gwirtsman HE, George DT, et al: Relationship of mood alterations to bingeing behaviour in bulimia. Br J Psychiatry 149:479–485, 1986

Kissileff HR, Walsh BT, Kral JG, et al: Laboratory studies of eating behavior in women with bulimia. Physiol Behav 38:563–570, 1986

Mitchell JE, Laine DC: Monitored binge-eating behavior in patients with bulimia. International Journal of Eating Disorders 4:177–183, 1985

Ortega DF, Waranch HR, Maldonado AJ, et al: A comparative analysis of self-report measures of bulimia. International Journal of Eating Disorders 6:301–311, 1987

Rosen JC, Leitenberg H, Fisher C, et al: Binge-eating episodes in bulimia nervosa: the amount and type of food consumed. International Journal of Eating Disorders 5:255–267, 1986

Rossiter EM, Agras WS, Losch M: Changes in self-reported food intake in bulimics as a consequence of antidepressant treatment. International Journal of Eating Disorders 7:779–783, 1988

Williamson DA, Prather RC, Upton L, et al: Severity of bulimia: relationship with depression and other psychopathology. International Journal of Eating Disorders 6:39–47, 1987

Wilson GT: Assessing treatment outcome in bulimia nervosa: a methodological note. International Journal of Eating Disorders 6:339–348, 1987

Wilson GT, Eldredge K: Frequency of binge eating in bulimic patients: diagnostic validity. International Journal of Eating Disorders 10:557–561, 1991

Chapter 24

Subtyping of Bulimia Nervosa

James E. Mitchell, M.D.

Statement of the Issues

Should the DSM-IV diagnosis of bulimia nervosa be restricted to individuals who purge, or should it be subtyped in some other way? Four possible subtyping options are explored.

1. Bulimia nervosa with and without accompanying purging behavior
2. Bulimia nervosa with and without history of anorexia nervosa
3. Bulimia nervosa with and without a history of obesity
4. Bulimia nervosa in normal-weight versus overweight individuals

Significance of the Issues

Many clinicians and investigators working in the area of eating disorders think that the DSM-III-R (American Psychiatric Association 1987) criteria for bulimia nervosa are too broad and vague and that they should be "tightened up" to describe a more homogeneous group of individuals, whereas others are quite satisfied with the DSM-III-R criteria. Researchers frequently use more stringent criteria than DSM-III-R, such as requiring binge eating coupled with self-induced vomiting or laxative abuse at a frequency of three times a week to identify subjects who have a similar level of severity of symptoms. However, using such strict criteria might pose problems for clinicians in that many of their patients who may have clinically significant eating problems do not meet such criteria. Therefore, the advisability of subtyping and/or requiring purging as a criterion needs to be explored further.

Method

The four topics listed were searched using Minnesota Medline (1984–1991, 316 citations) and PsychLit (1985–1991, 160 citations). Additional data relative to several of the possible subtyping systems were obtained from the University of Toronto (Paul Garfinkel, M.D.), the University of North Dakota (Steve Wonderlich, Ph.D.), the unpublished thesis of Valerie McClain at the Florida Institute of Technology, and the University of Minnesota (James Mitchell, M.D.).

Results

Purging Versus Nonpurging Bulimia Nervosa

Very little has been published concerning bulimia nervosa patients who do not purge; in most reported series, the vast majority of patients with bulimia nervosa engage in one or more purging behaviors. As pointed out by Willmuth et al. (1988), one of the issues in evaluating the literature on purging versus nonpurging bulimic patients concerns weight. In their observation, the authors noted that nonpurging bulimic patients tend to be overweight, and therefore it is difficult to know whether any differences between the two groups are attributable to weight differences rather than to purging. In two studies (Davis et al. 1986; Duchman et al. 1986), nonpurging bulimic patients reported less body image disturbance and less anxiety concerning eating compared with purging bulimic patients. However, the mean weight of those in the nonpurging group was in the obese range, whereas the mean weight of the purging group was in the normal-weight range. Viesselman and Roig (1985) reported that nonpurging bulimic patients reported fewer problems with concentration, fewer feelings of guilt or worthlessness, and less suicidal ideation compared with purging bulimic patients. V. McClain (unpublished data, 1990) found that purging bulimic patients evidence a greater degree of depression and body dissatisfaction compared with nonpurging patients, and they report more severe personality disorder traits.

A few studies have examined these two subgroups controlling for weight. Grace et al. (1985) studied control subjects, nonpurging bulimic patients, and purging bulimic patients selected from a university undergraduate population. They found that the two bulimic subtypes reported more anxiety and lower self-esteem than control subjects, but the two bulimic subgroups did not differ on these measures. Post and Crowther (1987) found that purging bulimic patients had a more negative body image than nonpurging bulimic patients; however, the frequency of bulimic behaviors in both samples was low. Willmuth et al. (1988) compared 20 normal-weight purging bulimic patients with 20 normal-weight nonpurging bulimic patients and 20 normal-weight control subjects. Compared with the nonpurging bulimic patients, the purging bulimic patients showed greater anxiety about eating and more disturbance on measures of eating attitudes and associated psychopathology as measured by Eating Attitudes Test (Garner et al. 1982) and Eating

Disorders Inventory (Garner et al. 1983) scores. The nonpurging bulimic patients were never more significantly maladjusted than the purging bulimic patients on any of the measures employed, although they did exhibit more anxiety about eating, more disturbance on the eating disorder questionnaires, and more depressive symptoms than the control subjects. Willmuth et al. also noted that they had difficulty recruiting normal-weight nonpurging bulimic patients, because most nonpurging applicants for the study tended to be overweight.

We reviewed the records of 200 consecutive patients evaluated at the University of Minnesota who satisfied DSM-III-R criteria for bulimia nervosa (Mitchell et al. 1985a). Of these patients, 17 (8%) did not self-induce vomiting or engage in laxative abuse. They were considerably older than our typical patients at the time of presentation (mean age 33.4 ± 9.6 years). Only 3 were younger than 25, and 11 were older than 30. Most were overweight. Of the 17 patients, 15 were greater than 110% ideal body weight, 12 were greater than 120% of ideal body weight, and 8 were greater than 160% ideal body weight (Metropolitan Life Insurance 1964); 13 engaged in fasting and restrictive dieting, 3 exercised excessively, and 1 abused diuretics.

To address the purging versus nonpurging dichotomy further, we examined 275 additional charts of patients who satisfied DSM-III-R criteria for bulimia nervosa. Of these, 16 (6%) were nonpurgers. Summary data are shown in Table 24–1. Of interest is the finding that nonpurging bulimic patients tended to binge eat less often and were also less likely to engage in self-injurious behavior. Paul Garfinkel, M.D., contributed a data set from the eating disorders program at Toronto General Hospital. These data are based on a sample of 54 nonpurging subjects and a sample of 235 purging subjects. In this series, the mean weights did not differ between the nonpurging bulimic patients and laxative-abusing bulimic patients; however, those who vomited but did not use laxatives tended to have a lower body weight. The nonpurging bulimic patients had lower total scores on the Eating Attitudes Test but very similar scores on Eating Disorders Inventory symptom and personality subscales compared with the purging groups.

Steve Wonderlich, Ph.D., also contributed a data set, summarized in Table 24–2, from the University of North Dakota eating disorders clinic. These data are based on a sample of 16 nonpurging subjects and a sample of 24 purging subjects. In this data set, purging bulimic patients tended to be younger and were more likely to have never married. There were no significant differences overall in weight. The nonpurging bulimic patients had been ill for a longer mean period of time, whereas the purging bulimic patients were more likely to engage in self-injurious behavior and suicide attempts. It is of note that 37.5% of the nonpurging bulimic patients had a history of vomiting or spitting out food, and 18.8% had used laxatives for weight control.

Table 24–1. Comparison of purging and nonpurging bulimic subjects, Minnesota data

	Purging ($n = 259$)	Nonpurging ($n = 16$)	χ^2	t	P
Age	26.1 ± 5.4	26.4 ± 4.1		.222	.825
Age at onset	16.0 ± 2.8	16.2 ± 5.2		.102	.920
History of					
vomiting	87.5%	57.1%	3.519		.061
laxatives	75.0%	37.2%	4.571		.033
diet pills	68.8%	31.3%	.155		.694
chew and spit	68.8%	68.8%	.000		1.000
Self-injury	53.3%	18.8%	4.045		.044
Suicide attempt(s)	31.3%	18.8%	.667		.414
Stealing	75.0%	56.3%	.554		.457
Frequency of binge eating last month			7.759		.021
> 1/day	37.5%	0 (0%)			
1/day	12.5%	5 (31.3%)			
< 1/day	50.0%	11 (68.8%)			
Frequency of vomiting last month			24.889		.000
> 1/day	31.3%	—			
1/day	12.5%	—			
< 1/day	43.8%	—			
None	12.5%	100%			
Frequency of laxatives last month			17.143		.002
> 1/day	—	—			
1/day	—	—			
< 1/day	71.4%	—			
None	28.6%	100%			
Max frequency of binge eating			1.591		.451
> 1/day	81.3%	62.5%			
1/day	6.3%	18.8%			
< 1/day	12.5%	18.8%			
Max frequency of vomiting			23.720		.000
> 1/day	62.5%	6.7%			
1/day	18.8%	0.0%			
< 1/day	12.5%	26.7%			
None	6.3%	66.7%			

(continued)

Table 24–1. Comparison of purging and nonpurging bulimic subjects, Minnesota data (*continued*)

	Purging ($n = 259$)	Nonpurging ($n = 16$)	χ^2	t	P
Max frequency of laxatives			13.402		.020
> 1/day	14.3%	6.3%			
1/day	21.4%	6.3%			
< 1/day	50.0%	12.5%			
None	14.3%	75.0%			

Overall, the data derived from these different samples are not entirely consistent, probably owing to differences in referral patterns and the presence or absence of obese/overweight subjects in various studies. However, the data suggest that nonpurging bulimic patients in some studies are older and heavier, have less associated psychopathology, and binge eat less often than purging bulimic patients.

Bulimia Nervosa With and Without a History of Anorexia Nervosa

It is clear that bulimia nervosa or bulimic symptoms develop in a subgroup of individuals with anorexia nervosa (Beumont et al. 1976; Casper et al. 1980; Garfinkel et al. 1980), and, more rarely, bulimia nervosa can also precede anorexia nervosa (Kasset et al. 1988).

Russell (1979), in his original description of bulimia nervosa, stressed that most of his patients had a history of actual or "cryptic" anorexia nervosa; however, treatment centers working with these disorders encounter patients without such symptoms or history.

Research at the University of Minnesota identified two subgroups of patients with bulimia nervosa (Mitchell et al. 1990b). The first subgroup was composed of 50 individuals with a history of anorexia nervosa (HAN) prior to the onset or during the course of their bulimia nervosa, but who had maintained a normal adult weight for at least 6 months. The other subgroup was composed of 50 individuals with bulimia nervosa who had never had a period of significant weight loss sufficient to qualify for a diagnosis of anorexia nervosa (NHAN). All subjects were female, all satisfied DSM-III-R criteria for bulimia nervosa, and all were within 10% of ideal body weight at the time of evaluation. Whenever possible, a prior history of anorexia nervosa was confirmed through obtaining old records. Data were extracted from the Eating Disorders Questionnaire (Mitchell et al. 1985b), from the psychiatric database used in the Minnesota clinic, and from the evaluation summaries dictated by the evaluating staff member.

Table 24–2. Comparison of purging and nonpurging bulimic subjects, North Dakota data

	Purging ($n = 24$)	Non-purging ($n = 16$)	χ^2	t	P
Mean age (years)	22.6	33.9		−4.4	.0003
Marital status (%)			14.02		.001
Married	4.2	56.2			
Divorced	8.3	6.2			
Never married	87.5	37.5			
Weight history					
Current weight (% ideal)	104.6	110.4		−1.19	.24
Desired weight (% ideal)	92.5	92.6		−0.04	.96
Highest adult weight (% ideal)	117.7	125.7		−1.22	.21
Lowest adult weight (% ideal)	91.0	96.3		−1.10	.27
Age binge eating began (years)	16.7	20.3		−1.19	.25
Mean duration of binge eating problem (months)	76.6	185.3		−2.49	.03
Binges/week (last month only)	10.2	5.9		1.5	.14
Frequency of the following behaviors in last month (1 = never, 7 = more than once a day)					
Binge eating	5.0	4.8		.32	.75
Vomiting	5.4	1.0		9.06	.0001
Laxatives	2.3	1.1		2.91	.008
Diet pills	2.0	1.5		.93	.36
Water pills	2.0	1.3		1.49	.14
Enemas	1.2	1.0		1.01	.31
Exercise for weight control	4.1	4.9		−1.19	.24
Fasting	2.0	2.7		−1.31	.19
Ever made suicide attempt (%)			6.13		.01
Yes	45.8	7.1			
No	54.2	92.9			
Ever tried to hurt self (%)			7.04		.008
Yes	58.3	14.3			
No	41.7	85.7			
Ever been involved in stealing (%)			6.13		.013
Yes	62.5	20.0			
No	37.5	80.0			

All subjects were Caucasian, with the exception of one subject in the NHAN group who was Native American. Although the majority in both groups were single (HAN = 43, 86%; NHAN = 32, 64%), there was a trend suggesting a higher marriage rate in the NHAN group (HAN divorced = 3, 6%; HAN married = 4, 8%; NHAN divorced = 5, 10%; NHAN divorced/remarried = 1, 2%; NHAN married = 12, 24%; $P = .068$). Social class distribution using the Hollingshead and Redlich (1958) two-factor index of social position was similar between the two groups.

The two groups were essentially identical as to the age of presentation for bulimia nervosa (HAN = 24.7 ± 6.0; NHAN = 24.7 ± 5.0; $P = 1.00$) and as to age at onset of binge eating (HAN = 17.5 ± 3.9; NHAN = 18.3 ± 4.8; $P = .324$). There were no significant differences between the two groups in terms of percentage of ideal body weight at evaluation (HAN = 100.4 ± 14.5; NHAN = 103.1 ± 11.2; $P = .285$); however, those in the HAN group desired a lower body weight when they were asked what they would prefer to weigh (HAN = 90.8 ± 8.7; NHAN = 94.7 ± 6.7; $P = .016$).

Abnormal eating-related behaviors were also examined. Those in the HAN group were less likely to report self-induced vomiting as a weight-control technique (HAN = 44, 88%; NHAN = 50, 100%; $P = .035$), whereas those in the NHAN group were more likely to report laxative abuse (HAN = 35, 70%; NHAN = 20, 40%; $P = .007$). Prevalence and frequencies of use of diuretics and diet pills were similar in the two groups. Binge-eating frequencies were also similar.

In both groups, 88% indicated they felt "fat" ($P = .507$). There were no significant differences between the two groups as to history of alcohol or drug abuse (HAN = 14, 28.6%; NHAN = 12, 24%; $P = .773$); stealing behavior (HAN = 26, 54.0%; NHAN = 22, 44.0%; $P = .424$); self-injurious behavior, including cutting, burning, or hitting themselves (HAN = 12, 24.5%; NHAN = 7, 14%; $P = .282$); or suicide attempts (HAN = 13, 26.5%; NHAN = 6, 12.5%; $P = .137$). As would be expected, those in the HAN group reported a longer mean period of amenorrhea (HAN = 18.5 ± 20.9 months; NHAN = 6.8 ± 9.5 months; $P = .001$) associated with their eating disorder.

Bulimia Nervosa With and Without a History of Obesity

Several researchers reported that a subgroup of patients of normal weight with bulimia nervosa have a history of having been overweight, and it is reasonable to discuss whether the presence or absence of such a history would be an appropriate way to subclassify bulimia nervosa.

Only one study systematically examined this dichotomy (Mitchell et al. 1990c). In this study, the authors identified 87 individuals who were currently of normal body weight (±20% ideal body weight), but who reported a history of having weighed in excess of 130% of ideal body weight during adolescence or adulthood

(HOW). A comparison group of 87 subjects who denied a history of anorexia nervosa or being overweight (NHOW) was randomly selected. Summary data on the two groups of patients are shown in Table 24–3. As can be seen, those in the HOW group reported a later age at onset of bulimic symptoms and were older when they presented for treatment. They also weighed significantly more at the time of evaluation and were more likely to be married or divorced. Although of normal weight, they were more likely to report feeling moderately or extremely overweight (HOW = 65, 74.7%; NHOW = 50, 57.4%; P = .037) and were more likely to report "extreme" fear of becoming "fat" (HOW = 64, 73.6%; NHOW = 41, 47.1%; P = .003). However, the two groups did not differ in terms of the methods of dieting they had tried, such as skipping meals (HOW = 56, 66.7%; NHOW = 57, 66.3%;

Table 24–3. Characteristics of bulimia nervosa subjects with and without a history of being overweight

	History (n = 87)	No history (n = 87)	χ^2	P
Age at evaluation (years)	27.4 ± 6.5	22.1 ± 4.1		.000
Weight (% ideal body weight)	111.3 ± 14.9	99.7 ± 6.1		.000
Max weight > age 18 (% ideal body weight)	144.4 ± 20.8	106.3 ± 5.0		.000
Min weight > age 18 (% ideal body weight)	98.2 ± 11.0	91.8 ± 5.0		.000
Age at onset of binge eating	18.2 ± 5.4	16.5 ± 3.3		.013
Age at onset of vomiting	20.5 ± 4.9	16.8 ± 3.2		.000
Age at onset of laxatives	21.9 ± 5.4	19.0 ± 4.0		.009
Age at onset of diet pills	20.0 ± 5.3	17.9 ± 5.7		.181
Social class			8.95	.062
I	15 (17.6%)	31 (36.5%)		
II	28 (32.9%)	35 (41.2%)		
III	35 (41.7%)	24 (28.6%)		
IV	24 (28.6%)	20 (23.8%)		
V	2 (3.6%)	1 (1.2%)		
Living situation			15.11	.002
Parents/relative	15 (17.6%)	31 (36.5%)		
Friends	28 (32.9%)	35 (41.1%)		
Conjugal	24 (28.6%)	10 (11.8%)		
Alone	18 (21.2%)	9 (10.6%)		

$P = .100$), fasting (HOW = 22, 31.9%; NHOW = 35, 40.7%; $P = .335$), restricting carbohydrate intake (HOW = 24, 35.3%; NHOW = 27, 31.4%; $P = .735$), restricting fat intake (HOW = 41, 59.4%; NHOW = 56, 65.1%; $P = .575$), or going on "fad" diets (HOW = 14, 20.3%; NHOW = 16, 18.6%; $P = .953$).

Their descriptions of their binge-eating behaviors were quite similar, as were their choices of binge foods. The majority in both groups had used self-induced vomiting as a weight-control technique (HOW = 84, 96.6%; NHOW = 85, 97.7%; $P = 1.00$). The number of patients in both groups who reported laxative abuse (HOW = 48, 57.1%; NHOW = 43, 49.4%; $P = .391$) and diet pill use (HOW = 41, 58.6%; NHOW = 29, 33.3%; $P = .886$) were not significantly different. They did not differ in their reported prevalences of alcohol or drug abuse problems, suicide attempts, or self-injurious behavior. Not unexpectedly, those in the HOW group were much more likely to report obesity in at least one first-degree family member (HOW = 39, 46.4%; NHOW = 15, 17.2%; $P = .001$), but family histories of affective disorders, alcohol or drug abuse problems, and eating disorders were similar.

Obese Versus Normal-Weight Bulimia Nervosa

A subgroup of patients with bulimia or bulimia nervosa are overweight, although most individuals with this condition are of relatively normal body weight. This overweight subgroup has received very little attention in the eating disorders literature; however, a larger literature has discussed binge eating among obese persons.

In 1959, Stunkard first described an eating pattern displayed by a subgroup of his obese patients in which enormous quantities of food were consumed in a relatively short period of time. Such "binge eating" was described as having an "orgiastic quality" and was followed by self-condemnation. More recent evidence suggests that between 25% to 50% of obese patients engage in binge eating on a regular basis (Hudson et al. 1988; Kolotkin and Revis 1987; Loro and Orleans 1981; Marcus and Wing 1987; Marcus et al. 1985, 1988; Smith 1981; Wilson 1976). Given that approximately 25% of the adult American population can be classified as obese, the number of binge eaters is substantial.

In addition to binge-eating behavior, many of the binge-eating obese also experience other symptoms (e.g., concern about weight, self-deprecating thoughts, stringent attempts at dieting), and therefore a subgroup meet DSM-III-R criteria for bulimia nervosa (Hudson et al. 1988). Unfortunately, these individuals do not appear to fare as well in conventional behavioral weight-loss treatment as do their nonbinge-eating counterparts. As of this writing, four studies have systematically examined the treatment of obese binge eaters. Using a retrospective design, Keefe et al. (1984) found that women binge eaters lost significantly less weight than did nonbinge eaters, both at the end of a 9-week behavioral treatment program

(4.2 ± 5.3 lb and 6.9 ± 8.8 lb, respectively) and at 6 months follow-up (6.7 ± 8.8 lb and 12.1 ± 8.1 lb, respectively).

In a more comprehensive prospective investigation, Marcus et al. (1988) found that women binge eaters tended to drop out of behavioral treatment more than nonbinge eaters, including behavioral treatment specifically geared to address binge eating, and that dropouts had significantly higher scores on a pretreatment measure of binge-eating severity. Although no differences in weight loss were found between binge and nonbinge groups after 10 weeks, significant differences were found after 36 weeks, with binge eaters having lost significantly less weight.

In a study comparing the response to fluoxetine, nonbinge eaters lost significantly more weight (23.8 lb) than did binge eaters (8.5 lb) after 1 year (Marcus et al. 1990).

LaPorte et al. (personal communication, 1990) used a very low calorie diet approach and found that binge-eating females reported elevated pretreatment and within-treatment levels of anxiety and depression; however, they did not differ from nonbinge-eating control subjects in the amount of weight lost, adherence to the diet, or dropout rate. These results suggest that a very low calorie diet and concurrent behavior therapy may be an effective method of weight loss for this refractory portion of the obese population.

Hudson et al. (1988) compared 23 obese bulimic subjects diagnosed by DSM-III (American Psychiatric Association 1980) criteria with 47 obese nonbulimic subjects and 47 normal-weight bulimic control subjects. The obese bulimic subjects were similar to normal-weight bulimic subjects in exhibiting a higher lifetime prevalence of major affective disorder compared with the nonbulimic obese sample, and the obese bulimic subjects were less likely than normal-weight bulimic patients to self-induce vomiting as a method of weight control.

Mitchell et al. (1990a) screened records of 591 patients evaluated in the Minnesota clinic who satisfied criteria for bulimia nervosa. Twenty-five (4%) weighed more than 130% of ideal body weight. These 25 patients were compared with 25 randomly selected control bulimic subjects who were between 90% and 110% of ideal body weight. The characteristics of the two subgroups are summarized in Table 24–4. The overweight bulimia nervosa subjects were significantly older at time of presentation and older at the onset of self-inducing vomiting. However, they did not differ significantly from the normal-weight bulimic patients in terms of age at onset of binge eating. They tended to come from lower socioeconomic strata; were more likely to be living alone; and were less likely to be living with parents, relatives, or friends.

Binge eating was more frequent among normal-weight bulimia nervosa subjects (NWBN) than among overweight bulimia nervosa subjects (OBN) (OBN: several times/day = 15, 67.5%; once/day = 5, 20.8%; several times/week = 4,

16.7%; NWBN: several times/day = 24, 96%; once/day = 1, 4%; $\chi^2 = 8.73$, $P = .013$). More laxative abuse was seen in the OBN group (OBN: several times/day = 3, 12.5%; once/day = 4, 16.7%; several times/week = 8, 33.3%; once/week = 3, 12.5%; < once/week = 3, 12.5%; never = 3, 12.5%; NWBN: several times/day = 6, 24.0%; once/day = 4, 16.0%; several times/week = 1, 4.0%; never = 14, 56.0%; $\chi^2 = 19.55$, $P = .002$). The prevalence of other associated problems was also examined. The OBN were twice as likely to report a history of self-injurious behavior (includ-

Table 24–4. Characteristics of overweight bulimia nervosa and normal-weight bulimia nervosa subjects

	Overweight bulimia nervosa ($n = 25$)	Normal-weight bulimia nervosa ($n = 25$)	χ^2	t	P
Age (years)	27.8 ± 4.8	21.8 ± 4.2		21.19	.000
Age at onset of binge eating	15.1 ± 4.9	16.7 ± 4.6		1.43	.237
Age at onset of vomiting	20.4 ± 4.5	17.4 ± 4.4		4.74	.035
Ideal body weight (%)	159.7 ± 27.8	101.9 ± 8.8		98.46	.000
High weight since 18 years (kg)	105.9 ± 24.7	62.7 ± 7.0		64.60	.000
Low weight since 18 years (kg)	64.5 ± 12.4	52.3 ± 5.1		16.92	.000
High weight 12–18 years (kg)	74.1 ± 17.3	59.7 ± 7.0		12.63	.001
Low weight 12–18 years (kg)	56.5 ± 20.1	46.1 ± 4.8		5.17	.030
Social class			10.24		.017
I	1 (4.5%)	5 (20.0%)			
II	0 (0.0%)	3 (12.0%)			
III	9 (40.9%)	13 (52.0%)			
IV	12 (54.5%)	4 (16.0%)			
V	0 (0.0%)	0 (0.0%)			
Living situation			16.60		.001
Parents/relatives	1 (4.0%)	7 (28.0%)			
Friends	8 (32.0%)	15 (60.0%)			
Conjugal	4 (16.0%)	2 (8.0%)			
Alone	12 (48.0%)	1 (4.0%)			

ing cutting, burning, or hitting themselves) (OBN = 15, 62.5%; NWBN = 5, 30.8%; $\chi^2 = 6.94$, $P = .088$) and more than three times as likely to report a history of a suicide attempt (OBN = 14, 56.0%; NWBN = 4, 18.2%; $\chi^2 = 5.57$, $P = .018$).

These data suggest many similarities and some differences between the OBN and NWBN groups.

Discussion

A minority of patients who present for treatment with bulimia nervosa do not engage in self-induced vomiting or laxative abuse for weight-control purposes. A significant subgroup of these patients have purged in the past. It is not clear how nonpurging bulimia nervosa differs from compulsive overeating or obese binge eating. The available data suggest that nonpurging bulimic patients tend to be somewhat older and, in some of those data, to weigh more than purging bulimic patients. It is of particular importance to note that much of the literature on bulimia nervosa, particularly the controlled treatment studies, have specifically selected purging bulimic subjects, and it is clear that many clinicians and researchers favor the use of purging as a criterion. For example, in a review by B. T. Walsh (personal communication, 1990) that examined the purging versus nonpurging status of subjects in 23 controlled psychotherapy and pharmacotherapy studies of bulimia nervosa, only 36 (3%) of 1,197 subjects did not purge.

The data suggest that bulimia nervosa patients with and without a history of anorexia nervosa are similar in terms of their current weight, associated pathological behaviors, and other associated problems. However, those with a history of anorexia nervosa appear to desire lower body weight. Overall, the two groups were similar on most variables examined. The database in this area is clearly inadequate.

Normal-weight individuals with bulimia nervosa who have a history of having been overweight tend to have a later age at onset for their bulimic symptoms and tend to be heavier at the time of evaluation. They are fairly similar to other bulimic patients in terms of their eating behavior and purging techniques.

The available data suggest that overweight subjects with bulimia nervosa are less likely to report frequent vomiting and more likely to report laxative abuse for weight-control purposes. Their binge-eating frequency is high but not as high as the frequency of normal-weight bulimia subjects. The database in this area is inadequate.

Recommendations

There does not appear to be any compelling evidence for subtyping bulimia nervosa on most of the variables examined, given the inadequate database. Many clinicians and researchers, however, are already using the presence of purging as a criterion for the diagnosis. Further, the growing body of treatment literature on bulimia nervosa has focused almost exclusively on purging bulimic subjects. Therefore, to reflect what is already common practice in many clinical and research settings, and to stimulate interest in research concerning nonpurging individuals, it seems prudent to consider either subtyping bulimia nervosa on the basis of purging behavior or restricting the diagnosis to those who purge.

References

American Psychiatric Association: Diagnostic and Statistical Manual of Mental Disorders, 3rd Edition. Washington, DC, American Psychiatric Association, 1980

American Psychiatric Association: Diagnostic and Statistical Manual of Mental Disorders, 3rd Edition, Revised. Washington, DC, American Psychiatric Association, 1987

Beumont PJV, George GCW, Smart DE: "Dieters" and "vomiters and purgers" in anorexia nervosa. Psychol Med 6:617–622, 1976

Casper RC, Eckert ED, Halmi KA, et al: Bulimia: its incidence and clinical importance in patients with anorexia nervosa. Arch Gen Psychiatry 37:1030–1035, 1980

Davis CJ, Williamson DA, Goreczny T: Body image distortion in bulimia: an important distinction between binge-purgers and binge eaters. Paper presented at the annual convention of the Association for the Advancement of Behavior Therapy, Chicago, IL, 1986

Duchman EG, Williamson DA, Strickler PM: Dietary restraint and bulimia. Paper presented at the annual convention of the Association for the Advancement of Behavior Therapy, Chicago, IL, 1986

Garner DM, Olmsted MP, Bohn Y, et al: The Eating Attitudes Test: psychometric features and clinical correlates. Psychosom Med 12:877–878, 1982

Garner DM, Olmsted MP, Polivy S: Development and validation of a multidimensional eating disorder inventory for anorexia nervosa and bulimia. International Journal of Eating Disorders 2:15–24, 1983

Garfinkel PE, Moldofsky H, Garner DM: The heterogeneity of anorexia nervosa: bulimia as a distinct subgroup. Arch Gen Psychiatry 37:1036–1040, 1980

Grace PS, Jacobson RS, Fullager CJ: A pilot comparison of purging and non-purging bulimics. J Clin Psychol 41:173–180, 1985

Hollingshead AB, Redlich FC: Social Class and Mental Illness. New York, John Wiley, 1958

Hudson JI, Pope HG, Wurtman J, et al: Bulimia in obese individuals: relationship to normal-weight bulimia. J Nerv Ment Dis 176:144–152, 1988

Kasset JA, Gwirtsman HE, Kaye WH, et al: Pattern of onset of bulimic symptoms in anorexia nervosa. Am J Psychiatry 145:1287–1288, 1988

Keefe PH, Wyshogrod D, Weinberger E, et al: Binge eating and outcome of behavioral treatment in obesity: a preliminary report. Behav Res Ther 3:319–321, 1984

Kolotkin RL, Revis ES: Binge-eating in obesity: associated MMPI characteristics. J Consult Clin Psychol 55:872–876, 1987

Loro AD, Orleans CS: Binge eating in obesity: preliminary findings and guidelines for behavioral analysis and treatment. Addict Behav 6:155–166, 1981

Marcus MD, Wing RR: Binge eating among the obese. Society of Behav Med 9:23–27, 1987

Marcus MD, Wing RR, Lamparski DM: Binge eating and dietary restraint in obese patients. Addict Behav 10:163–168, 1985

Marcus MD, Wing RR, Hopkins J: Obese binge eaters: affect, cognitions, and response to behavioral weight control. J Consult Clin Psychol 56:433–439, 1988

Marcus MD, Wing RR, Ewing L, et al: Double blind, placebo controlled trial of fluoxetine plus behavior modification in the treatment of obese binge eaters and non-binge eaters. Am J Psychiatry 147:876–881, 1990

Metropolitan Life Insurance Company: New height standards for men and women. Stat Bull 40:1–4, 1964

Mitchell JE, Hatsukami D, Eckert E, et al: Characteristics of 275 patients with bulimia. Am J Psychiatry 142:482–485, 1985a

Mitchell JE, Hatsukami D, Eckert E, et al: Eating disorders questionnaire. International Journal of Eating Disorders 6:757–761, 1985b

Mitchell JE, Pyle RL, Eckert ED, et al: Bulimia nervosa in overweight individuals. J Nerv Ment Dis 178:324–327, 1990a

Mitchell JE, Pyle RL, Eckert ED, et al: Bulimia nervosa with and without a history of anorexia nervosa. Compr Psychiatry 31:171–175, 1990b

Mitchell JE, Pyle RL, Eckert ED, et al: Bulimia nervosa with and without a history of overweight. Journal of Substance Abuse 2:369–374, 1990c

Post G, Crowther JH: Restricter-purger differences in bulimic adolescent females. International Journal of Eating Disorders 6:757–761, 1987

Russell G: Bulimia nervosa: an ominous variant of anorexia nervosa. Psychol Med 9:429–499, 1979

Smith GR: Modification of binge eating in obesity. J Behav Ther Exp Psychiatry 12:333–336, 1981

Stunkard AJ: Eating patterns and obesity. Psychiatr Q 33:284–295, 1959

Viesselman JO, Roig M: Depression and suicidality in eating disorders. J Clin Psychiatry 46:118–124, 1985

Willmuth ME, Leitenberg H, Rosen JC, et al: A comparison of purging and non-purging normal weight bulimics. International Journal of Eating Disorders 7:825–835, 1988

Wilson GT: Obesity, binge eating, and behavior therapy: some clinical observations. Behavior Therapy 7:700–701, 1976

Chapter 25

Importance of Attitudes Regarding Shape and Weight to the Diagnosis of Bulimia Nervosa

Paul E. Garfinkel, M.D.

Statement of the Issues

DSM-III-R (American Psychiatric Association 1987) specifies a persistent overconcern with body shape and weight as a necessary criterion for the diagnosis of bulimia nervosa. The issue for this review was whether this criterion should be retained in DSM-IV.

Significance of the Issues

A concern regarding shape and weight was not included in DSM-III (American Psychiatric Association 1980). The requirement for abnormal attitudes regarding shape and weight may not be supported by empirical research. This review considers in particular the following questions: Are weight and shape concerns regularly seen in bulimia nervosa? Do the concerns with weight and shape differ between a bulimic sample and women without an eating disorder? Do the concerns differ between a sample of women with bulimia nervosa and women who are restrained eaters?

Method

The results from an unpublished data set and from the findings reported by Cooper et al. (1989) and Wilson and Smith (1989) are considered. Additional research is provided in Fairburn and Garner (1988).

Results

Prevalence of Weight and Shape Concerns in Bulimia Nervosa

We obtained the prevalence of weight and shape concerns from 104 consecutive patients presenting to the Toronto General Hospital with eating problems. Their weight was 85%–125% of the average for their age and height. Each had reported an objective episode of binge eating in the month prior to their assessment according to the Eating Disorders Examination (Cooper et al. 1989); 77% met DSM-III-R criteria for bulimia nervosa, with more than eight binge episodes in the preceding 4 weeks. Only 7% did not evidence an overconcern for weight (item 56 of the Eating Disorders Examination); only 5% did not evidence overconcern for shape (item 63); only 3% did not evidence overconcern for shape or weight. The importance of weight and shape were both unrelated to the frequency of binge eating ($r = .17$ and .08, respectively) and frequency of vomiting ($r = .06$ and $-.05$, respectively). We concluded that most bulimia nervosa patients at the Toronto General Hospital are overly concerned with weight and shape.

Normal Women With No History of an Eating Disorder

Cooper et al. (1989) described the results from the Eating Disorders Examination administered to three groups of women: 1) 53 patients with bulimia nervosa diagnosed by the DSM-III-R (outpatients at clinics in Oxford and Cambridge); 2) 47 patients with anorexia nervosa diagnosed by DSM-III-R at outpatient clinics in Oxford, Cambridge, and the Toronto General Hospital; and 3) 42 control subjects recruited using a general practice register in Cambridge to identify healthy young women ages 18–35 years. The three groups obtained mean (±SD) weight concern scores of 3.14 ± 1.4, 2.4 ± 1.5, and $.52 \pm .6$, respectively; and shape concern scores of 3.6 ± 1.4, 2.8 ± 1.2, and $.64 \pm .8$, respectively. The patients with anorexia and bulimia nervosa obtained significantly higher levels of weight and shape concerns than did the control women.

Restrained Eaters

A problem with the previous study is that the control subjects were selected for an absence of any history of eating disorders. Dietary restraint is common among women, and a concern for weight and shape may be related to dietary restraint rather than to an eating disorder per se. Wilson and Smith (1989) addressed this issue by administering the Eating Disorders Examination to patients with bulimia nervosa (according to Russell's [1979] criteria and DSM-III) and to psychology students who scored as restrained eaters on the revised Restrained Scale. The bulimia and restrained subjects obtained Eating Disorders Examination scores for concern about shape of $3.8 \pm .31$) and $2.6 \pm .20$, respectively ($P < .002$); and scores for concern about weight of $4.0 \pm .34$ and $2.1 \pm .19$, respectively ($P < .001$). These results support the idea of elevated weight and shape concerns among bulimic subjects.

Discussion

The empirical data support the inclusion of the shape and weight criterion. There are also a number of advantages to retaining this criterion (Fairburn and Garner 1988). A morbid fear of becoming fat was one of Russell's (1979) original three criteria for diagnosing bulimia nervosa. Many consider a concern regarding shape and weight (i.e., a morbid fear of becoming fat) to be the central psychopathology leading to behavior to control body weight. The criterion also distinguishes bulimia nervosa from binge eating, which may occur independently of weight concerns. The shape and weight criterion also makes the diagnosis more restrictive. The DSM-III criteria were little more than a description of "binge eating." For example, DSM-III did not distinguish bulimic behavior in the context of a depressive disorder from bulimia that specifically involves a concern regarding shape and weight and an effort to control weight. The inclusion of the shape and weight criterion also brings the syndrome closer to its related disorder, anorexia nervosa. Finally, the shape and weight criterion draws the DSM closer to ICD-10 (World Health Organization 1990), where bulimia nervosa is characterized by a morbid fear of being fat, with patients setting a sharply defined weight threshold for themselves that is well below their premorbid weight.

Recommendations

A persistent overconcern with shape and weight should be retained in the DSM-IV diagnosis of bulimia nervosa.

However, a related question is whether body dissatisfaction should be linked to these weight and shape concerns. To answer this question, one could examine 1) the frequency of body dissatisfaction in women with bulimia nervosa, 2) the intensity of this dissatisfaction in bulimic women versus those with no history of an eating disorder, 3) the intensity in bulimic women versus those who are restrained eaters, and 4) the correlates of body dissatisfaction in women without an eating disorder and in those with bulimia nervosa.

References

American Psychiatric Association: Diagnostic and Statistical Manual of Mental Disorders, 3rd Edition. Washington, DC, American Psychiatric Association, 1980

American Psychiatric Association: Diagnostic and Statistical Manual of Mental Disorders, 3rd Edition, Revised. Washington, DC, American Psychiatric Association, 1987

Cooper Z, Cooper PJ, Fairburn CG: The validity of the Eating Disorders Examination. Br J Psychiatry 154:807–812, 1989

Fairburn L, Garner D: Diagnostic criteria for anorexia nervosa and bulimia nervosa: the importance of attitudes to weight and shape, in Diagnostic Issues in Anorexia Nervosa and Bulimia Nervosa. Edited by Garner DM, Garfinkel PE. New York, Brunner/Mazel, 1988

Russell GFM: Bulimia nervosa: an ominous variant of anorexia nervosa. Psychol Med 9:428–449, 1979

Wilson G, Smith D: Assessment of bulimia nervosa: an evaluation of the Eating Disorders Examination. International Journal of Eating Disorders 8:173–179, 1989

World Health Organization: ICD-10 Chapter V: Mental and Behavioral Disorders: Diagnostic Criteria for Research. Geneva, Switzerland, World Health Organization, 1990

Chapter 26

Forms of Overeating Not Meeting DSM-III-R Behavioral Criteria: Pathological Overeating

Michael J. Devlin, M.D., and B. Timothy Walsh, M.D.

Statement of the Issues

The purpose of this review is to determine whether there are syndromes of "pathological overeating" that can be distinguished from bulimia nervosa, either because they do not involve binge eating or because of failure to meet the bulimia nervosa criteria of self-induced vomiting, use of laxatives or diuretics, strict dieting, or vigorous exercise. In addition, a potential new syndrome should occur in a significant number of individuals and should be associated with significant psychological distress or impairment.

Significance of the Issues

Epidemiological studies suggest that the point prevalence of bulimia nervosa, as defined by DSM-III-R (American Psychiatric Association 1987) criteria, is 1%–4% among groups of young women, primarily college students. There are suggestions that an additional and possibly sizable number of individuals have a significant problem with overeating but do not meet DSM-III-R criteria for bulimia nervosa. For example, Overeaters Anonymous is a large national organization of people who are distressed and seeking help for a self-perceived eating problem, but who may not engage in self-induced vomiting, use of laxatives or diuretics, strict dieting or fasting, or vigorous exercise.

Method

To determine if such syndromes had been described, the medical literature was reviewed via Medline (as available via Silver Platter for the period 1983 to February 1989) using the key words *binge* and *overeating*. In addition, the titles of all articles in the *International Journal of Eating Disorders* (1981–1988) and the *International Journal of Obesity* (1984–1988) were scanned. Potentially relevant articles were also identified in the bibliographies of articles obtained by the two methods described. All articles in English presenting original data describing the frequencies of abnormal human eating behaviors were examined. We excluded single case reports and reports of changes in eating behavior following surgical and medical intervention.

A major focus of this review was to determine if there were individuals who met criteria for binge eating but did not meet the DSM-III-R criterion C for bulimia nervosa ("The person regularly engages in either self-induced vomiting, use of laxatives or diuretics, strict dieting or fasting, or vigorous exercise in order to prevent weight gain" [p. 69]). We therefore included for further review: 1) articles meeting the above criteria that described the presence of binge eating in an obese population (who theoretically could be obese because of binge eating without use of the "compensatory" techniques described in criterion C); and 2) articles meeting the above criteria that described the prevalence of binge eating in a nonobese population and also provided sufficient information to estimate how many individuals did *not* meet criterion C for DSM-III-R bulimia nervosa. We also included articles describing patterns of eating behavior other than binge eating.

Results

Table 26–1 summarizes data from articles focusing on binge eating among obese populations. The nature of the samples and the definitions of binge eating employed varied considerably from study to study. However, a large proportion of obese individuals in most studies reported binge eating. What is not clear is what proportion of obese binge eaters met criteria for bulimia nervosa. In one study (Telch et al. 1988), none of the obese binge eaters was using laxatives, diuretics, or self-induced vomiting, but the number using exercise, strict dieting, or fasting was not available. In the study by Hudson et al. (1988), 26% of the binge eaters reported no specific method other than dieting (of unspecified strictness) for weight control. If one makes the plausible but unproven assumption that most of these patients would fail to meet criterion C for bulimia nervosa, these data suggest that there may be a significant number of obese individuals who binge eat (at some unspecified frequency) without meeting criteria for DSM-III-R bulimia nervosa.

Table 26–1. Binge eating in obese persons

Study	Sample source and N	Sex and age	Binge definition (method of diagnosis)	Binge frequency	Prevalence of binge eating (%)	Proportion not meeting DSM-III-R criterion C (%)	Prevalence of binge eating in the absence of bulimia nervosa (%)	Comments
Stunkard 1959	Obesity clinic: 40	?	"Enormous amount of food in a short period of time" (interview)	?	7.5	?	7.5 or less	No information on purging, fasting, or exercise
Loro and Orleans 1981	Obesity clinic: 280	56% F, mean age 42.7	"Large amount of food in a short period of time" (questionnaire, records)	≥1 time/week (majority ≥2 times/week)	50.7	?	50.7 or less	No information on purging, fasting, or exercise
Gormally et al. 1982	Obesity clinic: 65	100% F, mean age 39.3	"Behavior, emotion, control" (interview)	?	21.5	?	21.5 or less	No information on purging, fasting, or exercise

(*continued*)

Table 26–1. Binge eating in obese persons (continued)

Study	Sample source and N	Sex and age	Binge definition (method of diagnosis)	Binge frequency	Prevalence of binge eating (%)	Proportion not meeting DSM-III-R criterion C (%)	Prevalence of binge eating in the absence of bulimia nervosa (%)	Comments
Gormally et al. 1982	Obesity clinic: 47	68% F, mean age 41.2	"Behavior, emotion, control" (interview)	?	25.5	?	25.5 or less	No information on purging, fasting, or exercise
Keefe et al. 1984	Obesity clinic: 44	86% F, mean age 45.4	DSM-III (telephone interview)	?	52.3 (22.7 definite, 29.6 probable DSM-III bulimia)	?	52.3 or less	No information on purging, fasting, or exercise
Marcus et al. 1985	Obesity clinic: 432	100% F, mean age 39.3	BES > 27 (questionnaire)	?	46	?	46 or less	No information on purging, fasting, or exercise
Telch et al. 1988	Obesity clinic: 81	95% F, mean age 42.9	DSM-III (interview)	?	45 (17 definite, 28 probable DSM-III bulimia	All were "non-purging" (i.e., no vomiting, cathartics, or diuretics)	45 or less	No information on fasting or exercise

Hudson et al. 1988	Paid responders: 29; obesity clinic: 41	100% F, mean age 33	DSM-III (interview)	≥1 time/week (majority daily or more)	33 lifetime prevalence of modified DSM-III bulimia	26 "dieting" only (severity of dieting not specified)	8.6 or less (lifetime)	Of obese bulimics: 9 vomiting, 17 laxatives, 39 diuretics, 61 diet pills
Marcus et al. 1988	Obesity clinic: 68	100% F, mean age 38.6	DSM-III and BES > 27 (interview)	63% weekly, 34% daily	Not available (study specifically selected binge eaters)	0–32	Not available	5.7 occasional vomiting, 8.5 usual vomiting, 26 laxatives or diuretics, 68 frequent strict diets

[a] BES = Binge Eating Severity (Gormally et al. 1982).

Table 26–2 summarizes data from articles that report the prevalence of binge eating and also provide sufficient information to estimate the number of individuals who probably would not meet criterion C for bulimia nervosa. Although the prevalence of binge eating that does not meet criteria for bulimia nervosa varies considerably across studies, most studies suggest the existence of a significant proportion of individuals with such a problem. However, there are several problems in drawing firm conclusions from these studies. First, most of the studies were based on self-report. Second, the criteria for the size and frequency of binge meals were rarely specified. Third, there are few data to indicate if nonbulimic individuals who binge eat experience distress or impairment. Finally, there is no descriptive information on the characteristics of this behavior and how it may compare and contrast with the binge eating associated with bulimia nervosa.

Table 26–3 summarizes data from articles reporting the prevalence of other well-defined forms of overeating behavior. Most such articles dealt with the "night eating syndrome" originally described by Stunkard et al. (1955) characterized by morning anorexia, evening hyperphagia, and insomnia. The data suggest that a significant proportion of obese individuals but relatively few normal-weight individuals display this pattern. The current review uncovered virtually no articles that attempted to define and study other forms of overeating (such as overeating spread out over several hours) in either obese or normal-weight populations.

Discussion

The results of the studies reviewed are consistent in suggesting that there may exist a significant number of individuals who report binge eating but who do not meet DSM-III-R criteria for bulimia nervosa because they fail to meet criterion C. The studies suggest that the prevalence of this problem may even be higher than that of bulimia nervosa. However, the available studies are not sufficiently detailed to permit definitive conclusions about the existence of such a syndrome or its characteristics.

Recommendations

The evidence reviewed is not sufficient to warrant the addition of a new category (e.g., pathological overeating). However, the available studies clearly raise the possibility that there are individuals who suffer from a nonbulimic overeating syndrome that is not covered by our current classification system. Further research is needed to identify the features of this putative syndrome as well as to establish

Table 26–2. Binge eating without weight control

Study	Sample source and N	Sex and age	Binge definition (method of diagnosis)	Binge frequency	Prevalence of binge eating (%)	Proportion not meeting DSM-III-R criterion C (%)	Prevalence of binge eating in the absence of bulimia nervosa (%)	DSM-III-R criterion C weight-control methods covered by study
Halmi et al. 1981	College students: 355	59.8% F, mean age 25.6	"Consider self a binge eater" (questionnaire)	?	25.2	≥32.6	≥8.2	Vomiting, laxatives, diuretics, diet pills (all ≥1 time/week), exercise, diet
Pyle et al. 1983	College students: 1,355	42.4% F, ? age	DSM-III criterion A (questionnaire)	?	49.8 (lifetime)	25.6 (lifetime)	12.7 (lifetime)	Vomiting, laxatives, diuretics, enemas, fasting
Katzman et al. 1984	College students: 485	100% F, ? age	"≥1,200 kcal in < 2 hours" (questionnaire)	≥8 times/month	7.4	22.2	1.6	Vomiting, cathartics, diuretics, severe dieting (≥2 times/month)
Healy et al. 1985	College students: 1,063	65.9% F, 17–25	DSM-III criterion A (questionnaire)	≥1 time/week	10.2	44.4	4.5	Laxatives, diet pills, diuretics, all ≥1 time/week, harsh diet, ? vomiting

(continued)

Table 26–2. Binge eating without weight control (continued)

Study	Sample source and N	Sex and age	Binge definition (method of diagnosis)	Binge frequency	Prevalence of binge eating (%)	Proportion not meeting DSM-III-R criterion C (%)	Prevalence of binge eating in the absence of bulimia nervosa (%)	DSM-III-R criterion C weight-control methods covered by study
Pyle et al. 1986	College students: 1,382	55.9% F, ? age	DSM-III criterion A (questionnaire)	?	13.7 (lifetime)	1.6 (lifetime)	0.2 (lifetime)	Vomiting, laxatives, diuretics, enemas, fasting
Pertschuk et al. 1986	College students: 957	100% F, ? age	"Abnormally large quantities of food over 1/2–3 hours" (questionnaire)	≥1 time/ month	7.1	45	3.2	Vomiting, laxatives, diuretics, fasting
Zuckerman et al. 1986	College students: 907	70% F, ? age	DSM-III criterion A (questionnaire)	≥1 time/ week	20.5	≥7.5	≥1.5	Vomiting, laxatives, diuretics, fasting
Meadows et al. 1986	General practice: 411	100% F, 18–22	"Have binges where I eat lots of fattening foods"	"always," "usually," or "often"	11.6	≥79.3	≥9.2	Vomiting, laxatives, strict dieting ("weight varies by over a stone in a few days")

Study	Sample	Criteria	Frequency	% binge	% purge	%	Methods
Gray et al. 1987	Black college students: 507	67.3% F, ? age	DSM-III criterion A (questionnaire)	?	74	30	22.2	Vomiting, laxatives, diuretics, dieting, fasting
Drewnowski et al. 1988	College students: 1,007	50.3% F, mean age 22.3	DSM-III criterion A (telephone interview)	≥2 times/week	8	≥77.8	≥6.3	Vomiting, laxatives, fasting
Lachenmeyer and Muni-Brander 1988	High school students: 712	46.1% F, age 13–19	DSM-III criterion A (questionnaire)	?	50	≥37.6	≥18.8	Vomiting, laxatives, diuretics, diet pills, restricting
Lachenmeyer and Muni-Brander 1988	High school students: 549	55.7% F, age 13–19	DSM-III criterion A (questionnaire)	?	62.3	≥25	≥15.6	Vomiting, laxatives, diuretics, diet pills, restricting

Table 26–3. Other abnormal eating patterns

Study	Sample source and N	Sex and age	Eating pattern (method of diagnosis)	Prevalence (%)	Comments
Stunkard et al. 1955	Obesity clinic: 25	92% F, mean age 36.8	Night eating syndrome (morning anorexia, evening hyperphagia, insomnia) (interview)	64	Predicts poor response to weight reduction treatment
Stunkard 1959	Obesity clinic: 40	?	Night eating syndrome (interview)	65	Special Study Clinic (refractory patients)
Stunkard 1959	Obesity clinic: 100	?	Night eating syndrome (interview)	12	General Nutrition Clinic
Rand and Kuldau 1986	Normal-weight volunteers: 232	62% F, mean age 35.3	Night eating syndrome (interview)	0.4	
Kuldau and Rand 1986	Morbidly obese patients admitted for surgery: 25	84% F, mean age 36	Night eating syndrome (interview)	15	Correlated with psychoneuroticism (health opinion survey)
Nevo 1985	College students ≥15% overweight: 43	100% F, ? age	Overweight snackers ("snacking much or extremely characteristic of your eating," bulimics excluded) (interview)	44	9/43 overweight women had DSM-III bulimia; 5 additional overweight women declined interview

its prevalence, its diagnostic reliability and stability over time, and external validating features. The existence of data to address these issues is a necessary prerequisite for an informed decision about whether and how an additional overeating syndrome should be included in our diagnostic system.

A group of interested investigators, including the authors, has begun to conduct, in consultation with the Eating Disorders Work Group, studies of overeating syndromes distinct from bulimia nervosa (Spitzer et al. 1992). In particular, this group has studied a syndrome characterized by 1) binge eating at least twice a week for 6 months, 2) a feeling of loss of control during the eating binge, 3) associated behavioral indicators of loss of control, and 4) significant distress. This syndrome has been referred to as binge eating disorder. Preliminary evidence stemming from a multisite survey indicates that the hypothesized disorder is common among subjects attending hospital-affiliated weight-control programs but is relatively rare in the community. Further studies are needed to provide validation of the survey results by clinical interview, longitudinal information on the stability of the syndrome over time, and further data on potential external validators (such as response to treatment).

References

American Psychiatric Association: Diagnostic and Statistical Manual of Mental Disorders, 3rd Edition, Revised. Washington, DC, American Psychiatric Association, 1987
Drewnowski A, Hopkins SA, Kessler RC: The prevalence of bulimia nervosa in the US college student population. Am J Public Health 78:1322–1325, 1988
Gormally J, Black S, Daston S, et al: The assessment of binge eating severity among obese persons. Addict Behav 7:47–55, 1982
Gray JJ, Ford K, Kelly LM: The prevalence of bulimia in a black college population. International Journal of Eating Disorders 6:733–740, 1987
Halmi KA, Flak JR, Schwartz E: Binge-eating and vomiting: a survey of a college population. Psychol Med 11:697–706, 1981
Healy K, Conroy R, Walsh N: The prevalence of binge-eating and bulimia in 1063 college students. J Psychiatr Res 19:161–166, 1985
Hudson JI, Pope HG, Wurtman J, et al: Bulimia in obese individuals: relationship to normal-weight bulimia. J Nerv Ment Dis 176:144–152, 1988
Katzman MA, Wolchik SA, Braver SL: The prevalence of frequent binge eating and bulimia in a nonclinical college sample. International Journal of Eating Disorders 3:53–62, 1984
Keefe PH, Wyshogrod D, Weinberger E, et al: Binge eating and outcome of behavioral treatment of obesity: a preliminary report. Behav Res Ther 22:319–321, 1984
Kuldau JM, Rand CSW: The night eating syndrome and bulimia in the morbidly obese. International Journal of Eating Disorders 5:143–148, 1986
Lachenmeyer JR, Muni-Brander P: Eating disorders in a nonclinical adolescent population: implications for treatment. Adolescence 23:303–312, 1988

Loro AD, Orleans CS: Binge eating in obesity: preliminary findings and guidelines. Addict Behav 6:155–166, 1981

Marcus MD, Wing RR, Lamparski DM: Binge eating and dietary restraint in obese patients. Addict Behav 10:163–168, 1985

Marcus MD, Wing RR, Hopkins J: Obese binge eaters: affect, cognitions, and response to behavioral weight control. J Consult Clin Psychol 3:433–439, 1988

Meadows GN, Palmer RL, Newball EUM, et al: Eating attitudes and disorder in young women: a general practice based survey. Psychol Med 16:351–357, 1986

Nevo S: Bulimia symptoms: prevalence and ethnic differences among college women. International Journal of Eating Disorders 4:151–168, 1985

Pertschuk MJ, Collins M, Kreisber J, et al: Psychiatric symptoms associated with eating disorders in a college population. International Journal of Eating Disorders 5:563–568, 1986

Pyle RL, Mitchell JE, Eckert EE, et al: The incidence of bulimia in freshman college students. International Journal of Eating Disorders 2:75–85, 1983

Pyle RL, Halvorson PA, Neuman PA, et al: The increasing prevalence of bulimia in freshman college students. International Journal of Eating Disorders 5:631–647, 1986

Rand CSW, Kuldau JM: Eating patterns in normal weight individuals: bulimia, restrained eating, and the night eating syndrome. International Journal of Eating Disorders 5:75–84, 1986

Spitzer RL, Devlin MJ, Walsh BT, et al: Binge eating disorder: a multisite field trial of diagnostic criteria. International Journal of Eating Disorders 11:191–203, 1992

Stunkard AJ: Eating patterns and obesity. Psychiatr Q 33:284–295, 1959

Stunkard AJ, Grace WJ, Wolff HG: The night-eating syndrome. Am J Med 19:78–86, 1955

Telch CF, Agras WS, Rossiter EM: Binge eating increases with increasing adiposity. International Journal of Eating Disorders 7:115–119, 1988

Zuckerman DM, Colby A, Lazerson JS: The prevalence of bulimia among college students. Am J Public Health 76:1135–1137, 1986

Section IV

The DSM-IV Multiaxial System

Introduction to Section IV

The DSM-IV Multiaxial System

Janet B. W. Williams, D.S.W.

The multiaxial system for evaluation in DSM-III (American Psychiatric Association 1980) and DSM-III-R (American Psychiatric Association 1987) has been widely regarded as one of the major innovations of DSM-III (Williams 1985). This system encourages clinicians to evaluate an individual in terms of several different domains of information that are related to planning treatment and predicting outcome. It provides a scheme for organizing and communicating clinical information and helps ensure that a comprehensive evaluation is conducted. Nonetheless, after 10 years of experience and one revision, there is disappointment about the relatively infrequent use of the multiaxial system in clinical and research settings.

The Multiaxial Issues Work Group began its deliberations by considering possible reasons for this lack of use. We determined that there were three: 1) the multiaxial system was not useful in facilitating a comprehensive evaluation, 2) no prototypic recording form had been provided for agencies to adopt that would facilitate their systematic inclusion of all five axes in their regular clinical evaluations, and 3) clinicians had not received adequate training in how to make ratings on Axes IV and V (the multiaxial system was not universally taught in training programs).

Throughout the first years of work, the Multiaxial Issues Work Group also considered proposals that had been made for the elimination or revision of the multiaxial system. These were based on the following notions: 1) the ICD-10 (World Health Organization 1989) will not include a multiaxial system (although an optional one may be available in a separate manual); 2) placing personality disorders on a separate axis (Axis II) incorrectly implies that they are less important than the Axis I disorders; 3) having a separate axis (Axis III) for nonpsychiatric medical disorders implies a false separation between mental disorder and these other medical disorders; and 4) nondiagnostic axes, such as Axes IV and V, should not be included in a diagnostic manual and are not commonly used anyway.

All of these issues guided the Work Group's initial proceedings. What follows is a summary of specific proposals that were made for changes in each axis and the Work Group's summary of the advantages and disadvantages of each proposal. In addition to considering these specific proposals, the Work Group continued to discuss the proposal to eliminate the multiaxial system altogether.

Proposals for Axes I and II

Axis II of DSM-III-R included both personality disorders and developmental disorders; therefore, the distinction between Axis I and Axis II was considered not only by the Multiaxial Issues Work Group but also by the Personality Disorders Work Group and the Childhood Disorders Work Group. The original inclusion (in DSM-III) of certain disorders on Axis II was to ensure that consideration be given to these relatively stable conditions that might otherwise be overlooked when attention is paid to a usually more-florid Axis I condition. The value of placing personality disorders on Axis II has been evidenced in part by its wide clinical acceptance and its contribution to stimulating research in this area.

Despite this reasoning, there are several conditions that the various Work Groups are considering moving back to Axis I. For example, the Personality Disorder Work Group and the Psychotic Disorders Work Group have considered moving schizotypal personality (Siever et al. 1996) disorder to the schizophrenia section on Axis I. It has also been suggested that pervasive developmental disorders belong more logically on Axis I (see Campbell, Introduction to Section I, this volume).

Axis III

In DSM-III-R, Axis III was named "Physical Disorders and Conditions," with the unfortunate implication that disorders listed on Axes I and II do not also have a physical component. Although no truly satisfactory solution exists to this terminology problem, the term *nonpsychiatric medical condition* has been proposed as a replacement.

There is some evidence that Axis III is underutilized in many clinical settings, and the Multiaxial Issues Work Group has considered proposals to enhance the usefulness of this axis. One proposal for DSM-IV, as described by Gruenberg et al. in Chapter 27, is to include those Axis III disorders that are etiological to the Axis I disorders (e.g., secondary mood disorder due to hypothyroidism) as part of the Axis I diagnosis. Other clinically relevant relationships between Axis I disorders and

Axis III disorders could then be indicated by the use of modifiers applied to the Axis III disorders. This convention would allow a clinician to indicate for each Axis III disorder whether it is "exacerbating," "treatment relevant," or "coexisting" with the Axis I disorders. Although the inclusion of these proposed modifiers may have clinical and educational value, their reliability is unknown, and they may instead add unwanted complexity to the multiaxial system. In addition, in the majority of clinical cases, there may be uncertainty about the relationship between the mental disorder(s) and any coexisting nonpsychiatric medical conditions. If the proposal to list on Axis I those nonpsychiatric medical conditions that have an etiological relationship is not adopted, the indication of such relationships could instead be made on Axis III, in addition to the other modifiers described.

Axis IV

DSM-III-R Axis IV provides a rating scale for indicating the severity of psychosocial stressors that have contributed to the onset or exacerbation of the mental disorders listed on Axes I and II. There is an extensive literature supporting the importance of stress in the pathogenesis and exacerbation of a variety of mental disorders. The inclusion of an Axis IV rating of stressors was intended to be useful for treatment planning and outcome prediction. Axis IV was modestly revised in DSM-III-R to include separate sets of examples for rating acute events and enduring circumstances, both in children and adolescents and in adults. In addition, the severity rating scale was truncated by one point, so that the DSM-III-R scale ranges from 0 to 6. Finally, clinicians were asked to make a distinction between "predominantly acute events" and "predominantly enduring circumstances," based on evidence that these may exert different effects.

As summarized by Skodol in Chapter 28, several problems have been identified in the DSM-III-R approach to rating stress on Axis IV: 1) DSM-III-R Axis IV is not commonly used in clinical practice and research, 2) its reliability is only modest, and 3) the validity of Axis IV with respect to predicting outcome is uncertain. The disappointing underuse of Axis IV has been documented in several surveys, although the reasons for this lack of use are less clear. It may be due to a flaw in the basic assumption that such a rating is helpful for treatment planning, or because the guidelines for use are too complicated to incorporate into routine clinical practice, or because clinicians have not received adequate training in its use. The lack of adequate training may also have affected the few studies on the reliability of Axis IV that have been conducted. Thus, the very modest agreement that has been measured may represent an underestimate of what the reliability would be if such studies had been carried out following rigorous training, as would be done for a test of a research instrument.

The validity of the various conventions governing Axis IV has been questioned, such as the guideline to rate the stressor severity according to how stressful it would be to an "average" person, and the emphasis on a single global rating of stress severity. However, life events research has not provided clear evidence that these conventions do not represent the most useful compromise, nor have feasible alternative ways to quantify life events been proposed. In fact, most studies of the validity of Axis IV have demonstrated some measure of concurrent and construct validity.

In summary, despite some indications of adequate reliability and validity, Axis IV remains underutilized. Thus, the Multiaxial Issues Work Group is considering options that include the following: 1) retain Axis IV as is but promote more rigorous training; 2) clarify and/or modify the instructions to make them easier to apply; 3) eliminate the severity scale and provide a checklist on which clinicians can indicate the presence of certain psychosocial stressors, because clinicians may find problem lists more useful than dimensional ratings; or 4) include a different domain of information on Axis IV (e.g., social supports, environmental resources) that may be more clinically useful than a rating of stress.

Several specific proposals have been suggested for replacing the DSM-III-R rating of stressors. In one, Axis IV would consist of a rating of the adequacy of an individual's resources, a variable that could help guide treatment and predict outcome. Two Personal Resource Scales (for social supports and environmental resources) were developed after reviewing the literature and determining that existing scales were too cumbersome for general clinical use. Although these proposed scales are now being tried out on a pilot basis, their reliability and validity have not yet been systematically studied. This proposal has been criticized as being user-unfriendly because it requires two separate dimensional ratings. An alternative that would meet this concern would be to restrict Axis IV to a scale for rating the adequacy of social supports, as described in Chapter 29 by Cohen et al. Moreover, it seems likely that the Axis IV rating of stress (as in DSM-III-R) and the Axis IV rating of personal resources (as suggested for DSM-IV) are both important factors in clinical assessment, so that choosing between them may be difficult.

An alternative proposal provides a psychosocial problem checklist for clinicians to indicate those life areas in which problems exist and to specify, in their own words, the nature of the problems. This proposal differs from the current Axis IV rating of stressors, in which one overall severity rating is made. The main advantages of the psychosocial problem checklist are simplicity and the fact that it allows the clinician to note the specific problem of concern. Its disadvantages are that it does not include a method to indicate the severity of problems (other than counting the number of problems listed) and that this method may be less useful for research. Its reliability and validity have also not yet been systematically studied.

Axis V

In DSM-III-R, Axis V consists of the Global Assessment of Functioning Scale, derived from the Global Assessment Scale (Endicott et al. 1976). The Global Assessment Scale has been widely used for many years and has proven to be both reliable and valid for many purposes. DSM-III-R instructs the user to make ratings for two time periods, current and highest level for the past year, to increase the prognostic significance of the Global Assessment of Functioning Scale ratings. The scale also includes an instruction to "not include impairment in functioning due to physical (or environmental) limitations" (American Psychiatric Association 1987, p. 12).

Three problems have been identified with the utility of the Global Assessment of Functioning Scale, as reviewed by Goldman et al. in Chapter 30. First, requiring two ratings introduces additional complexity to the system. Second, this scale combines measures of social and occupational functioning and measures of psychological symptom severity into one single rating scale. This has been criticized both because these dimensions may vary independently and because the scale in this form provides information that may be somewhat redundant with the Axis I and Axis II diagnoses and their severity modifiers. Finally, the instruction to exclude physical impairment from the assessment of functioning sometimes calls for extremely difficult clinical judgments and may reduce the utility of the Global Assessment of Functioning Scale in some settings, such as primary care and geriatric settings.

The Work Group is considering several types of changes in Axis V. First, it may facilitate the use of this axis if the rating is restricted to the current time period alone. Second, perhaps the three different areas of functioning that are summarized into a single rating (psychological, social, and occupational) should be disaggregated. Ideally, three separate scales could be presented, although in reality this would clearly overload the system. An alternative might be to remove one of the three areas for separate evaluation. Finally, since in many settings it is too difficult to discount impairment due to physical disability, perhaps this area of functioning should be added back for consideration of overall functioning.

Proposals for Additional Axes

In the course of our work, several proposals have been made for additional axes. The Work Group advised that it might not be feasible to include more than five axes in the "official" multiaxial system; however, it would be possible to include some optional axes in the appendix of DSM-IV.

Relational Functioning

It has been well recognized that DSM-III and DSM-III-R have been of little use to family therapists, primarily because of the traditional focus in the DSM on individual psychopathology. Some clinicians and clinical researchers dealing with couples, families, and relational networks have suggested the utility of an independent assessment of the degree to which a family or other relational unit meets the needs of its members. A Coalition on Family Diagnosis was formed during the development of DSM-IV to address such issues. The coalition is an interorganizational group that includes representatives from a wide array of professional associations involved with families and interested in the process of revising the DSM (e.g., American Family Therapy Association, American Psychological Association, American Psychiatric Nurses Association, Group for the Advancement of Psychiatry, National Association of Social Workers). Originally convened by a Task Force of the American Association for Marriage and Family Therapy, the coalition eventually developed a Global Assessment of Relational Functioning Scale. This dimensional scale resembles the Global Assessment of Functioning Scale in overall format, and has been proposed as a possible optional axis. The Global Assessment of Relational Functioning Scale is in the process of being pilot-tested to determine its reliability and clinical utility. However, major concerns about providing this scale as an optional axis are that it may be too cumbersome and specialized and that the terminology may be too unfamiliar for use by nonfamily clinicians.

Defense or Coping Axis

The reliance on descriptive psychopathology in DSM-III was criticized by psychodynamically oriented clinicians. This led to the inclusion in the DSM-III-R glossary of an extensive list of defense mechanisms, with the recommendation that particular defense mechanisms might be indicated on Axis II. As summarized in Chapter 33 by Skodol and Perry, research suggests the possible reliability, prognostic value, and clinical utility of methods for specifying and rating defense mechanisms. Therefore, it has been proposed that a scale for defense or coping styles be included in the DSM-IV appendix. The optimal organization of the scale and instructions for using it are being refined in an ongoing pilot study. Major concerns about including this scale are that it may be too cumbersome and specialized and that the terminology may be too unfamiliar for use by clinicians who do not employ psychodynamic methods.

Proposals for Qualifying Severity and Course of Axis I and II Disorders

Proposals for Classification of Course of Illness

The DSM-III-R classification primarily focuses on symptomatic descriptions of disorders. Course features are characterized in two ways: 1) by the use of the "in full remission" or "in partial remission" severity modifiers, and 2) by the use of disorder-specific course modifiers (e.g., "recurrent" in major depressive disorder, "chronic with acute exacerbation" in schizophrenia). The literature review by Mezzich and Jorge in Chapter 31 identified five course variables as being most important: 1) age at onset, 2) mode of onset (e.g., abrupt or insidious), 3) duration or chronicity, 4) episodicity, and 5) progression of illness. To emphasize the importance of the course of illness, the text section on course for each disorder will systematically consider each of these course variables. The possible use of more specific course modifiers for mood disorders is being tested in a field trial.

Proposals for Severity

In DSM-III-R, guidelines are provided for noting the severity of the mental disorders as "mild," "moderate," or "severe." In addition, if criteria for the disorder are not currently met, the modifiers "in partial remission" or "in full remission" can be used. After an unspecified duration of being in full remission, the clinician can consider the individual "recovered" (i.e., with no current mental disorder).

An alternative approach, described by Mezzich and Sullivan in Chapter 32, would be to note severity in a purely cross-sectional manner to separate ratings of severity from ratings of course. With this proposal, a disorder would be rated as "asymptomatic," "subthreshold," "mild," "moderate," or "severe." The major problem with this proposal is its novelty, and potential confusion about its use of the term *subthreshold*. A less radical alternative that refines the DSM-III-R convention would allow the clinician to differentiate three types of subthreshold cases: 1) individuals whose disorder is in "partial remission" (a term already included in DSM-III-R); 2) individuals whose disorder is in "partial relapse" (a suggested new term for DSM-IV) whose symptoms have met full criteria for a disorder in the past but who, after a period of full remission, have developed symptoms at a subthreshold level; and 3) for individuals whose symptoms have never met full diagnostic criteria for a condition, "subthreshold" could be used as a modifier of a not otherwise specified category (e.g., depressive disorder not otherwise specified [subthreshold major depressive disorder]).

References

American Psychiatric Association: Diagnostic and Statistical Manual of Mental Disorders, 3rd Edition. Washington, DC, American Psychiatric Association, 1980

American Psychiatric Association: Diagnostic and Statistical Manual of Mental Disorders, 3rd Edition, Revised. Washington, DC, American Psychiatric Association, 1987

Endicott J, Spitzer RL, Fleiss J, et al: The Global Assessment Scale: a procedure for measuring overall severity of psychiatric disturbance. Arch Gen Psychiatry 33:766–771, 1976

Siever LJ, Bernstein DP, Silverman JM: Schizotypal personality disorder, in DSM-IV Sourcebook, Vol 2. Edited by Widiger TA, Frances AJ, Pincus HA, et al. Washington, DC, American Psychiatric Association, 1996, pp 685–702

Williams JBW: The multiaxial system of DSM-III: where did it come from and where should it go? I: its origins and critiques. Arch Gen Psychiatry 42:175–180, 1985

World Health Organization: International Classification of Diseases, 10th Edition Draft. Geneva, Switzerland, World Health Organization, 1989

Chapter 27

Axis III: Relationship Between Psychiatric Syndromes and Medical Disorders

Alan M. Gruenberg, M.D., Martin Rosenzweig, M.D., and
Reed Goldstein, Ph.D.

Statement of the Issues

Investigation of individuals with psychiatric disorders in a variety of treatment settings suggests that having a psychiatric illness places one at substantial risk for coexisting medical illness (Black et al. 1985; Winoker and Black 1987). The reported incidence of medical disorders in psychiatric patients is quite variable, ranging from 10% to 80% depending on the setting. Studies have highlighted the importance of carefully screening psychiatric patients for medical disorders (Hoffman and Koran 1984). This literature review reveals general inconsistency in the documentation of the relationship between psychiatric and general medical disorders in a screened psychiatric population. Further, the current multiaxial system developed for DSM-III (American Psychiatric Association 1980) and revised in DSM-III-R (American Psychiatric Association 1987) offers minimal guidelines for specifying the relationship between Axis I and Axis III disorders. In this chapter, we review the pertinent literature and propose a method for denoting the relationship between a specific psychiatric disorder and a coexisting general medical disorder.

Significance of the Issues

In considering diagnoses, psychiatrists assume that significant medical disorders may influence the onset or course of a major psychiatric disorder. The introduction of DSM-III in 1980 encouraged the use of a multiaxial format to communicate the presence of several concurrent psychiatric and medical diagnoses. This was important from a heuristic perspective. On Axis III, the psychiatrist is encouraged to indicate any physical condition that is potentially relevant to the understanding and management of the clinical psychiatric syndrome. The clinician is also expected to note any significant medical findings such as soft neurological signs that might affect the response to specific psychiatric treatments. Many psychiatrists have urged that a heightened awareness of the relationship between medical and psychiatric conditions is essential. This includes a broader conceptual focus both on the effects of medical conditions on psychiatric diagnosis and treatment and on the effect of psychiatric disorders on general medical conditions.

Several authors (e.g., Mezzich et al. 1982) have suggested procedures for using Axis III to delineate the nature of these relationships more fully. The development of a taxonomy for assessing relationships would allow a clinician to denote more precisely and reliably the impact of a major medical disorder on the psychiatric presentation. In this way, a broader conceptualization of diagnosis would be incorporated into the multiaxial assessment and would allow for more specific treatment.

Method

In this review, we conducted a Medline search for studies that examine the co-occurrence of psychiatric and medical disorders. We also examined references that documented the actual use of Axis III in clinical practice. We excluded articles and individual case reports that discussed a specific association between particular medical disorders and a distinct psychiatric presentation (Popkin and Tucker 1994).

Results

The development of our understanding of the association between medical and psychiatric illness parallels the evolution of more general psychiatric diagnostic procedures. Camroe (1936) suggested that significant organic disease may account for nonspecific neurotic symptomatology within an 8-month follow-up period. Of 100 "neurotic" patients, 24 developed a specific medical illness within an 8-month follow-up period that accounted for psychiatric and behavioral symptomatology. He highlighted the significance of the psychiatric presentation as heralding the subsequent occurrence of a diagnosable medical illness. Between 1940 and 1960, little attention was devoted to the issue of classifying comorbid medical and psychiatric conditions. Herridge (1960) evaluated the impact that a medical disorder had on the psychiatric presentation. This study reported that 50% of 209 patients had demonstrable comorbid medical disorders. He reported that 5% of the medical disorders were "causal" of the psychiatric symptoms and 21% were "apparently contributing." The assumption is that the others were "concomitant." In his study of psychiatric outpatients, Wynne-Davies (1965) found a 42% incidence of medical disorders that were considered "causative" of the initial psychiatric disturbance. Maguire and Granville-Grossman (1968) found a 33% incidence of comorbid medical illness in 200 consecutive psychiatric inpatients, but did not describe a causal link. Of the 33% of the patients with a medical illness, half were diagnosed for the first time. The findings of these 1960s studies increased the psychiatric community's awareness of the need for medical assessment in psychiatric patients.

Hall et al. (1978) reported a 46% incidence of previously undiagnosed physical illness in 658 consecutive outpatients. In 9.1% of the medical disorders, the physical illness was considered "productive of the psychiatric symptoms." Most of the patients had no prior knowledge of the "causal" effect of their physical illness on their psychiatric presentation. In this study, certain threshold criteria were established to prove causality: 1) psychiatric symptomatology abated with medical treatment; 2) medical symptomatology was related to the onset of the psychiatric disorder; and 3) the medical disorder, if untreated, explained the patient's behavioral symptom pattern. In a similar study, Hall et al. (1980) demonstrated a 46% incidence of causal or exacerbating medical problems in 100 state hospital inpatients. Koranyi (1979) noted that 43% of 2,090 psychiatric clinic patients had one or more physical disorders. Almost half of these physical disorders had not been detected by the referring source, and general medical physicians had overlooked the physical disorder in one-third of the referrals. Muecke and Krueger (1981) found that 20.4% of 910 consecutively admitted psychiatric inpatients had a previously undiagnosed medical disorder. In contrast, a study by Glass et al. (1985) did not demonstrate a significant coexistence of medical disorders in a private hospital psychiatric population.

Koran et al. (1989) assessed 529 patients in California's public mental health system, 200 of whom were found to have significant physical symptoms. The mental health care system had recognized 47% of the patients' physical conditions. These authors assigned an estimate to the relationship between medical disorders and psychiatric syndromes based on similar cases in the literature, the temporal relationship between the onset of the general medical condition and the psychiatric disorder, and the degree of response to medical treatment. Bartsch et al. (1990) found that 46% of 175 outpatients had medical conditions or laboratory test findings that required further medical evaluation. Previously undiagnosed physical problems were present in 20% of the patients, and 16% had medical conditions that might "cause or exacerbate" the psychiatric disorder on the basis of an evaluation of the patient by an independent physician. No specific criteria were applied in making this judgment. As of this writing, there is no study in the literature examining reliability in the attribution of a causal relationship between physical and psychiatric disorders.

There is limited literature on the use of Axis III since its introduction in DSM-III. Maricle et al. (1987) examined the application of Axis III in the diagnosis of 50 discharged psychiatric inpatients and found that psychiatrists underused Axis III. Few psychiatrists noted physical findings that might affect the psychiatric disorder or its management, and none noted conditions considered to be of etiological significance. This may reflect the lack of more specific criteria for making such a judgment or the lack of attention to general medical disorders in regular clinical assessment.

Mezzich et al. (1982) proposed a format to organize DSM-III diagnoses according to a multiaxial system and tested their formulation on 1,011 consecutive patients. A systematized program facilitated the use of the multiaxial system and allowed the clinician to consider the Axis III disorder as primary, secondary, or tertiary and comment on its importance in the overall clinical picture. The multiaxial format of Mezzich et al. helped to prevent the omission of important physical disorders in the overall diagnostic formulation. However, the format did not provide for any classification of a causal, contributory, or exacerbating relationship between medical and psychiatric disorders.

There are many examples in clinical practice in which the assessment of the relationship between medical and psychiatric disorders is highly relevant. It is impossible to assess the diagnosis of depression without considering pertinent medical conditions. These include the presence of hyperthyroidism or hypothyroidism as examples of neuroendocrine abnormalities that may be considered causative in the psychiatric diagnosis. Similarly, the presence of a recent stroke may cause subsequent depression. In the diagnosis of psychotic illness, one may see coexisting schizophrenia and systemic lupus erythematosus, and the use of steroids to treat lupus may either exacerbate or improve the psychiatric manifestations. This is a situation in which the psychiatric syndrome may be exacerbated by the treatment of the associated medical condition.

Discussion

According to DSM-III-R, Axis III is to be used to indicate any current physical disorder or condition that is relevant to the understanding and management of the case. It is also currently used to indicate etiological medical conditions. Spitzer et al. (1989) proposed that the problem of organic versus nonorganic psychiatric syndromes could be solved by introducing the concept of "secondary" disorders. In this system, the clinician would indicate a secondary mental disorder "due to" a specific organic syndrome on Axis I. Popkin and Tucker (1994) reviewed the literature on the organic syndromes and concluded that only in cases in which there was clear structural injury to the central nervous system could a strong case be made for definite secondary syndromes.

The concept of secondary syndromes may be a categorical solution to the organic versus nonorganic problem. However, no clear threshold is offered by which the clinician can determine whether the psychiatric disorder is due to a medical disorder. Nevertheless, the organic affective, organic delusional, organic personality, and organic anxiety disorder categories in DSM-III and DSM-III-R are based on the concept of an etiological syndrome. Thus, in making a diagnosis of a secondary syndrome, one is simply shifting the emphasis from organic syndromes in general to the more specific diagnosis in which the psychiatric presentation occurs. The clinician is not provided with clear guidelines for making the diagnosis of the secondary syndrome. This lack of guidelines may imply a level of understanding of causation that is beyond the current state of medical knowledge.

The alternative solution is to offer a continuum through which the relationship between psychiatric and medical disorders can be assessed. On one end of the continuum are those disorders in which a causative agent can be identified that clearly explains the medical and psychiatric presentation. At the other end of the continuum are those disorders that coexist independently without affecting one another. In the middle of the continuum lie those disorders in which the medical syndrome may exacerbate the psychiatric symptoms or may potentially influence the treatment and management of the patient.

Given the nonspecificity of criteria for assessing the role of medical disorders in general psychiatric conditions, clinicians may fail to make the judgment on Axis III that is recommended in DSM-III-R. Prior investigations have suggested that individual researchers each define their own classification system for determining the impact of medical conditions on psychiatric presentations. This leads to inconsistent reporting of results and difficulty in generalizing from one study to another. One of the aims of a diagnostic system is to improve communication among researchers and clinicians. It seems appropriate, therefore, to offer a taxonomy in which the relationship of Axis I and Axis III disorders can be classified.

Recommendations

Within Axis III, four possible relationships between the general medical disorder and the psychiatric condition are suggested: 1) causative (due to), 2) exacerbating,

3) treatment relevant (clinically significant for management and treatment), and 4) coexisting.

Causative

In this case, the Axis III disorder directly causes the Axis I or Axis II syndrome. A strong association between the two disorders can be demonstrated in terms of onset of symptoms, somewhat parallel course, and the alleviation of symptoms with appropriate treatment. Both disorders can be explained by a physiological or pathological mechanism if present.

Exacerbating

In this case, the Axis III disorder should promote pathological or physiological mechanisms that exacerbate the underlying and persistent psychiatric syndrome. Within this relationship, there are independent disorders that are well established. The evolution of the general medical disorder may contribute to greater complications in the overall psychiatric presentation. An example of this relationship may be seen in an individual with schizophrenia and systemic lupus, when the autoimmune disease progresses.

Treatment Relevant

The Axis III disorder should affect the choice of treatment provided for the psychiatric illness. An example might involve a patient with first-degree heart block and major depression. The medical disorder may interfere with compliance with treatment of a specific psychiatric disorder. The medical disorder could also have such significant psychosocial impact on the patient that the patient's ability to obtain treatment for both the medical and psychiatric disorder becomes compromised.

Coexisting

To identify a psychiatric disorder that merely coexists with a medical disorder, there must be no clear etiological, temporal, or treatment relevant relationship between the two disorders. The disorders should respond independently to treatment, and no common pathophysiological relationship should occur. An example would be a patient with coexisting pneumonia and panic disorder.

The proposed classification may provide important guidelines for improved communication regarding the impact of Axis III disorders within general psychiatry. The DSM-IV Task Force is considering the proposal to include "secondary" syndromes on Axis I and Axis II with specified medical disorders as "causative or due to." The DSM-IV Organic Disorders Work Group has supported this proposal. The proposed system outlined in this review could serve to clarify the complex relationship between general medical disorders and psychiatric syndromes. We recommend studies to assess the reliability of these categories and further research on the validity of such a classification system.

References

American Psychiatric Association: Diagnostic and Statistical Manual of Mental Disorders, 3rd Edition. Washington, DC, American Psychiatric Association, 1980

American Psychiatric Association: Diagnostic and Statistical Manual of Mental Disorders, 3rd Edition, Revised. Washington, DC, American Psychiatric Association, 1987

Bartsch DA, Shern DL, Feinberg LE, et al: Screening CMHC outpatients for physical illness. Hosp Community Psychiatry 41:786–790, 1990

Black DW, Warrack G, Winoker G: Excess mortality among psychiatric patients. JAMA 253:58–61, 1985

Camroe BI: Follow up study of 100 patients diagnosed as neurotic. J Nerv Ment Dis 83:679–684, 1936

Glass J, Gossett JT, Barnhart FD, et al: Chest x-ray and laboratory findings in a private psychiatric hospital population. Am J Psychiatry 142:664–665, 1985

Hall RCW, Popkin MK, Devaul RA, et al: Physical illness presenting as psychiatric disease. Arch Gen Psychiatry 35:1315–1320, 1978

Hall RCW, Gardner ER, Stickney SK, et al: Physical illness manifesting as psychiatric disease. Arch Gen Psychiatry 37:989–995, 1980

Herridge CF: Physical disorders in psychiatric illness. Lancet 2:949–951, 1960

Hoffman SK, Koran LM: Detecting physical illness in patients with mental disorders. Psychosomatics 25:654–660, 1984

Koran LM, Sox HC, Marton KI, et al: Medical evaluation of psychiatric patients. Arch Gen Psychiatry 46:733–740, 1989

Koranyi EK: Morbidity and rate of undiagnosed physical illness in a psychiatric clinic population. Arch Gen Psychiatry 36:414–419, 1979

Maguire GP, Granville-Grossman KL: Physical illness in psychiatric patients. Br J Psychiatry 111:18–26, 1968

Maricle R, Leung P, Bloom JD: The use of DSM-III Axis III in recording physical illness in psychiatric patients. Am J Psychiatry 144:1484–1486, 1987

Mezzich JE, Coffman GA, Goodpastor SM: A format for DSM-III diagnostic formulation: experience with 1,111 consecutive patients. Am J Psychiatry 139:591–596, 1982

Muecke LN, Krueger DW: Physical findings in a psychiatric outpatient clinic. Am J Psychiatry 138:1241–1242, 1981

Popkin MK, Tucker GJ: Mental disorders due to a general medical condition and substance-induced disorders: mood, anxiety, psychotic, catatonic, and personality disorders, in DSM-IV Sourcebook, Vol 1. Edited by Widiger TA, Frances AJ, Pincus HA, et al. Washington, DC, American Psychiatric Association, 1994, pp 243–276

Spitzer RL, Williams JBW, First M, et al: A proposal for DSM-IV: solving the organic-non-organic problem. Journal of Neuropsychiatry 1:126–127, 1989

Winoker G, Black DW: Psychiatric and medical diagnosis as risk factors for mortality in psychiatric patients: a case control study. Am J Psychiatry 144:208–211, 1987

Wynne-Davies D: Physical illness in psychiatric out-patients. Br J Psychiatry 111:27–33, 1965

Chapter 28

Axis IV

Andrew E. Skodol, M.D.

Statement of the Issues

It is generally believed that Axis IV, "Severity of Psychosocial Stressors," in DSM-III (American Psychiatric Association 1980) and DSM-III-R (American Psychiatric Association 1987) is used infrequently in clinical settings and research studies. The purpose of this chapter is to review evidence regarding the use and usefulness of Axis IV. I summarize surveys of the clinical use of Axis IV, results concerning the reliability of severity ratings, and data on the usefulness of the axis as assessed in theoretical papers and empirical studies that are relevant to the construct validity of the scale or address its predictive validity.

Significance of the Issues

The inclusion of a multiaxial evaluation system was widely heralded as one of the major achievements of DSM-III (Williams 1985). Multiaxial evaluation acknowledges that the salient clinical features of mental disorders can be complex and, consequently, difficult to capture with single diagnostic concepts (Strauss 1975).

A version of this chapter titled "Axis IV: A Reliable and Valid Measure of Psychosocial Stressors?" by A. E. Skodol has previously been published in *Comprehensive Psychiatry* 32:503–515, 1991. Used with permission.

The author gratefully acknowledges the comments of the other members of the DSM-IV Multiaxial Issues Work Group (Co-chair, Howard H. Goldman, M.D., Ph.D.; Alan M. Gruenberg, M.D.; Juan E. Mezzich, M.D., Ph.D.; and Chair, Janet B.W. Williams, D.S.W.) and advisers to the Work Group (Richard E. Gordon, M.D., Ph.D.; Dr. Geoff Schrader; John S. Strauss, M.D.; Professor Christopher Tennant; Mary Durand Thomas, Ph.D., R.N., C.S.; and Holly Skodol Wilson, R.N., Ph.D., F.A.A.N.) on an earlier draft of this work.

Axis IV was included in the DSM-III multiaxial system because it was thought to be important for treatment planning to identify psychosocial stressors that may have contributed to the onset or exacerbation of a current mental disorder and also because rating the severity of the stressors was expected to have prognostic value.

Axis IV was modestly revised in DSM-III-R. DSM-III-R Axis IV differs from its DSM-III counterpart by providing separate sets of examples for rating acute events and enduring circumstances. DSM-III-R severity ratings are made on a 6-point scale; DSM-III's "minimal" stress rating was eliminated. Certain of the stressor examples were changed to make them more consistent with other lists of psychosocial stressors that are used in research.

For those charged with the development of DSM-IV, the underutilization of Axis IV has been a disappointment. It is not clear whether the architects of DSM-III were mistaken in assuming that psychosocial stressors should be accorded a separate axis, or whether the implementation of Axis IV has been conceptually or practically flawed. Because many believe that Axis IV requires drastic revision for DSM-IV, it has been necessary to consider the existing published literature to determine the extent and nature of the problems associated with Axis IV to guide a revision, if one is justified.

Method

The point of departure for this review was the index and complete bibliographic listing of *An Annotated Bibliography of DSM-III* (Skodol and Spitzer 1987). The bibliography was based on four computer searches that used terms relevant to diagnosis, including multiaxial diagnosis, and hand searches of 10 of the most popular psychiatric journals from 1980 through June 1986 for articles on topics related to DSM-III. The Medline computer search was continued monthly through November 1990 and yielded additional articles. Finally, a preliminary draft of this chapter was circulated to the members of the Multiaxial Issues Work Group and to 20 advisers who were selected on the basis of their publications or expressed interest in multiaxial diagnosis or psychosocial stress. In this way, several recently published studies and prepublication manuscripts were identified. No attempt was made to review systematically the vast research literature on psychosocial stress.

After excluding surveys of patterns of use and educational practices as well as theoretical critiques, as of November 30, 1990, I had found 22 published papers that empirically evaluated some aspect of DSM-III Axis IV. This compares with 24 papers that focused on Axis V and 12 papers dealing with Axis III.

Results

Clinical Use of Axis IV

In the DSM-III field trials (Spitzer and Forman 1979), reaction to Axis IV was mixed. Almost half of the field trial participants favored some major change in the conventions for identifying stressors or making the severity rating or elimination of the axis altogether. Only 38% believed that Axis IV was likely to be clinically useful and said that they would use it regularly in their diagnostic evaluations. Spitzer and Forman concluded that future studies were necessary to determine the extent to which Axis IV would be used in clinical practice and its impact on patient care.

Jampala et al. (1986) surveyed practicing psychiatrists and 1984 graduates of residency training and found considerable resistance to the use of the DSM-III multiaxial system because of its complexity and their incomplete knowledge of how to use it. Similar resistance for the same reasons was reported for Axis I and II diagnoses as well as for Axes IV and V. In contrast, DSM-III became the preferred system of classification in Canada shortly after its publication. In a survey by Junek (1983), two-thirds of responding Canadian practitioners recommended that a multiaxial system similar to that in DSM-III be included in ICD-10 (World Health Organization 1992). Junek and Leichner (1986) later found that psychiatric residents who had trained since publication of DSM-III preferred the DSM-III system to ICD-9 (World Health Organization 1978) more than twice as often as members of the Canadian Psychiatric Association, most of whom were trained in the pre-DSM-III era. More than 90% of residents recommended a multiaxial system for ICD-10. A multinational panel of experts in psychiatric diagnosis, many of whom were clinicians (J. E. Mezzich et al. 1985a), used the DSM-III multiaxial system more than any other. Identification of psychosocial stressors was rated less valuable in a multiaxial schema than psychiatric syndromes, personality disorders, physical disorders with brain dysfunction, and course or duration of illness, but more valuable than physical disorders without brain dysfunction and either highest or current level of adaptive functioning. Rating the overall severity of psychosocial stressors was deemed less useful than their specific identification, and "unclear principles" guiding Axis IV was occasionally mentioned as a specific problem (J. E. Mezzich et al. 1985b).

The studies in the United States and Canada suffer from modest completion rates and the lack of assessment of potential differences between responders and nonresponders. They also point to limited knowledge as a result of inadequate training as a potential source of reluctance to use the multiaxial system, making the causes, and thus the cure, ambiguous. Among practicing psychiatrists who responded to the survey of Jampala et al. (1986), the perception that Axis IV was not useful was only slightly more pronounced than a similar perception of Axis V. Similar proportions of all respondents to the survey did not believe that the Axis I/Axis II distinction was valid. All surveys have relied on reported use and usefulness rather than on systematic reviews of actual practice patterns (e.g., through records).

Two surveys of psychiatric residency training directors (Williams et al. 1985) and of directors of medical student education in psychiatry (Williams et al. 1986) indicated that, by 1983, fewer than half of the training programs in psychiatry in the United States had integrated the complete multiaxial system into their curricula or required its use by trainees. In contrast, nearly 75% taught and used the first three axes. At about the same time, 45% of Canadian academic psychiatrists taught Axis IV to trainees and 40% taught Axis V (Engles et al. 1985). In a subsequent survey, only 18% of directors of residency training programs in Canada expected residents to use Axes IV and V most or all of the time (Velamoor et al. 1989).

Thus, although use of Axis IV has lagged behind the use of Axes I through III, the limited surveys available suggest that there are no significant differences between the use of Axis IV and of Axis V and point to incomplete understanding as the reason for nonuse. The findings that few training programs emphasize Axes IV and V, but that, when trained, clinicians more readily accept the multiaxial system, suggest that changes to the system that are not accompanied by rigorous training will be unlikely to increase the use of additional axes.

Reliability

Only three studies reported on the reliability of Axis IV severity ratings. The best figures were obtained during the DSM-III field trials (Spitzer and Forman 1979): joint interviews yielded an intraclass correlation coefficient of .62 and test-retest evaluations of .58. This is the only study that reported reliability figures for Axis IV ratings on adult patients. Two studies reported poor reliability for Axis IV ratings on adolescents (intraclass correlation coefficient = .44) (Rey et al. 1987) and on children (intraclass correlation coefficient = .25) (A. C. Mezzich et al. 1985). One additional study of children reported modest agreement on the listing of psychosocial stressors on Axis IV (Russell et al. 1979). The latter two studies used written case vignettes rather than live interviews for the ratings.

Sources of error. In a study that employed diagnostic supervision to identify common errors in the use of DSM-III, Skodol et al. (1984) found an error rate of 22.5% on Axis IV, with 10% of cases requiring a change of 2 scale points or more. Errors were due to the complicated conventions for making ratings that are described in the brief instructions for the use of Axis IV included in DSM-III.

Skodol and Shrout (1989b) have demonstrated, for example, that the instruction that the rating should reflect the summed effect of all stressors listed was too complex to be incorporated into routine clinical practice, even by relatively well-trained evaluators with expert supervision. Rey et al. (1987) also cited the complex instructions for making severity ratings as sources of unreliability. In contrast, despite low reliability in their ratings, more than three-quarters of the respondents in the A. C. Mezzich et al. (1985) study judged the clarity of the Axis IV scale to be "more clear than unclear" or "very clear." No reliability study appears to have been done following intensive training, such as commonly precedes a formal study of the reliability of a semistructured diagnostic interview (Skodol and Shrout 1988).

Validity

Much has been written about how well (or poorly) Axis IV with its scale and rating conventions fulfills its functions. Most critics have been negative, although their views were not based on empirical studies. One of the most commonly cited criticisms has been of the convention to rate severity on the basis of an average person's reaction rather than on the basis of the patient's possibly idiosyncratic reaction (Frances and Cooper 1981; Roth 1983); a patient's peculiar vulnerability to particular stressors might be more clinically meaningful. Also criticized was the decision to combine all stressors, including chronic and acute, into a single global rating implying a single mechanism of effect (Kendell 1984; Rutter and Shaffer 1980).

Stressor theory and Axis IV severity ratings. Rey et al. (1988) commented on the Axis IV conventions that bear on the DSM-III operationalization of the rating of stress: 1) assessing the impact of individual stressors, 2) assessing the impact of multiple stressors, and 3) assessing the relevance of the stressors. The authors noted that numerous models and methods exist for qualitatively describing and quantitatively estimating the impact of individual psychosocial stressors on a person. DSM-III Axis IV requires a composite impact rating that includes consideration of the amount of change in the person's life caused by the stressor and the degree to which the event is desired and under the person's control. Change or adjustment resulting from a stressor is considered in many attempts to quantify stressor impact in the life events literature (Henderson et al. 1982; Holmes and Rahe 1967; Isherwood et al. 1982), and undesirability or other indications of negative impact (threat, loss, or exit) frequently characterize descriptions of important life events (Paykel et al. 1969). The fact that such theoretically independent dimensions of impact are often highly correlated (Isherwood et al. 1982) makes the DSM-III approach of an overall rating reasonable.

Approaches to assigning a specific severity rating to a particular event also vary.

The original approach of Holmes and Rahe (1967) used objective raters to assign severity scores. They viewed subjective ratings by affected individuals as biased because someone with a negative health outcome would view events retrospectively as more severe (Grant et al. 1976; Schless et al. 1974). This bias became known as "effort after meaning" (Brown 1974). A single scale for rating severity of specific events does not, however, take into account intra-event variability (i.e., not all equivalent events have the same impact on all people in all situations) (Dohrenwend et al. 1990). This led Brown and Harris (1978) to include a measure of "contextual threat" in determining severity. Brown and Harris' approach has in turn been criticized by Tennant et al. (1981) for producing an artificial association between life events and other antecedent conditions, such as an individual's social situation and personality attributes, that results in an overestimate of the causal role of life events in illness. The Axis IV approach, in which the severity rating is made by the presumably more objective clinician taking into account some of the particulars of each patient's situation, again appears to be reasonably justifiable.

DSM-III stated that the Axis IV severity rating should reflect the summed effect of all stressors judged relevant, but no guidelines were given on which to base these combined ratings. There is controversy in the life events literature over whether multiple but less severe events are as stressful as a single major event, or whether an accumulation of mild stressors might not also be pathogenic. As Rey et al. (1988) pointed out, the lack of explicit guidelines in DSM-III may again be a compromise justified by ambiguity in life events research.

Finally, given the controversy surrounding the role of stressful life events in the development and continuation of mental disorders (Depue and Monroe 1986; Lloyd 1980; Tennant 1983), the DSM-III convention that only stressors judged relevant to the onset or exacerbation of a current disorder be rated appears to Rey et al. (1988) to require judgments on etiological significance that are beyond the ability of the clinician.

Evaluation of Axis IV severity ratings. Skodol and Shrout (1989b), studying a combined sample of inpatients and outpatients, found that Axis I diagnoses of V codes, adjustment disorder, anxiety disorders, and major depression were associated with more severe stressors than was schizophrenia. Axis IV ratings were not redundant, however, because considerable variability existed within the Axis I diagnostic categories. Schrader et al. (1986) reported higher Axis IV ratings for nonpsychotic than for psychotic inpatients and for affective psychotic than for nonaffective psychotic inpatients. In a sample of more than 10,000 psychiatric patients, J. E. Mezzich et al. (1987) found that patients with depressive disorders had higher Axis IV ratings than patients with other mental disorders. Bronheim et al. (1989) found that more severe Axis IV ratings distinguished patients hospitalized on ear, nose, and throat services from other hospitalized patients for whom psychiatric consultation was sought, despite higher levels of premorbid adaptive functioning and lower rates of severe mental disorder in the ear, nose, and throat group. More severe stressors also appear to be associated with first episodes of any mental disorder than with repeat episodes (Skodol and Shrout 1989b). In contrast, Westermeyer (1988) found no correlation between Axis I diagnoses and the severity of psychosocial stressor ratings in a group of Asian refugees. Trzepacz et al. (1989) found no difference on Axis IV between delirious and nondelirious patients awaiting liver transplants.

Plapp et al. (1987) reported that raters had difficulty assigning Axis IV severity ratings to a list of psychosocial stressors, even using simpler 5-point or 3-point severity scales. This was interpreted as a demonstration of the difficulty of applying DSM-III's complicated definition of impact. Skodol and Shrout (1989b), however, found that residents and psychology intern raters could assign severity ratings that corresponded well ($r = .72$) with a standardized severity rating system used in life events research (Dohrenwend et al. 1978).

Neither Rey et al. (1987) nor Skodol and Shrout (1989b) found that multiple stressors materially changed a severity rating. In both studies the severity rating was predominantly determined by the first-listed, most severe stressor.

Zimmerman et al. (1985) found that Axis IV severity ratings in a sample of depressed patients were more highly correlated with undesirable than with desirable events; with exits (i.e., losses) than with entrances; and with discrete, short-term events than with ongoing circumstances. Higher Axis IV ratings were also associated with a lower rate of abnormal dexamethasone suppression test results, a higher rate of risk for alcoholism, a greater likelihood of comorbid personality disorders, and a greater frequency of attempted suicide during the index depressive episode. These results support the construct validity of Axis IV for depressed patients, but similar studies have not been reported for other diagnostic groups. It should be noted that the ratings were made following administration of a systematic life-events interview, rather than on the basis of a routine clinical evaluation of stressors.

Identifying psychosocial stressors using Axis IV. Brugha et al. (1985), using the methods of Brown and Harris (1978), found that most etiologically significant life events fall into a relatively small group of more severely stressful experiences. Skodol and Shrout (1989a) found that Axis IV functions well in practice as a shorthand method for identifying severe psychosocial stressors compared with the use of a lengthy, comprehensive assessment of life events. Discrepancies were found between the methods, however, for less severe events and for events that clinicians judged either were the result of a patient's mental disorder or produced no change in a patient's condition. Some etiologically significant stressors were not acute, discrete events, but rather chronic strains such as poverty. DSM-III-R Axis IV may be an improvement over DSM-III because it includes separate examples of rating scale points for acute events and for enduring circumstances.

Relationship to treatment planning and predictive validity. J. E. Mezzich et al. (1984) studied the relationship of Axis IV ratings to treatment decisions. They found a modest but significant correlation between Axis IV ratings and the decision to admit a patient from a walk-in clinic to inpatient hospital care. The relationship was weaker than that found for Axis V ratings of highest level of adaptive functioning, which was in turn weaker than that found for a rating of current adaptive functioning.

The ability of Axis IV severity ratings to predict outcome remains an open question. Gordon et al. (1985a, 1985b) found that a measure they call the "strain ratio," derived by dividing Axis IV ratings by inverted Axis V ratings (8 minus the Axis V score), is related to the length of hospital stay. The higher the strain ratio (i.e., the greater the degree of psychosocial stress associated with the disorder compared with the level of adaptive functioning), the longer patients needed to be hospitalized. Gordon and Gordon (1987) also found in subsequent analyses that high Axis IV ratings alone appeared to be related to longer inpatient stays. A study comparing outcomes after 6 months between two groups of patients with depressive disorders, one of which rated high on the Axis IV scale and the other low, failed to find the predicted relationship between high severity of stressor ratings and good prognosis (Zimmerman et al. 1987).

Discussion

It seems reasonable to conclude that a thorough evaluation of Axis IV has yet to be done. There are, for example, no published studies using the DSM-III-R version of Axis IV and thus no way to evaluate whether the revisions made in DSM-III-R are improvements or address the problems of underuse found for the DSM-III version of Axis IV. The preceding review, however, suggests a number of different options for Axis IV in DSM-IV.

One option is to make no changes in the current DSM-III-R Axis IV, to try to promote its use through better training, and to study the impact of the changes already made. This option has the advantages of allowing continuity in clinical practice and research and resisting the temptation to make changes despite limited data on which to base them. Reliability should be studied using live patients following focused training of clinicians such as would precede reliability testing of a structured interview. Reliability might be improved by changing instructions for use so that the rating is based solely on the most severe stressor or is made on any significant stressor whether clearly etiological or not. Pending the outcome of validity studies, statements in the text describing Axis IV could continue (as in DSM-III-R) to describe its usefulness in terms of planning or focusing treatment, but not in terms of its prognostic significance. Making minimal changes would be a mistake, however, if dissatisfaction with the axis is so widespread and so deep that few will work with it.

Another option is to eliminate the Axis IV severity rating scale, but to continue to note acute or enduring psychosocial stressors that are valuable in planning clinical interventions (J. E. Mezzich 1988; J. E. Mezzich et al. 1989). Identification could be limited only to those stressors associated with ratings of severe or greater, the stressors that are both most readily apparent and most likely to be pathogenic. A list of severe stressors could also be conceptualized within a broad context of psychosocial problems, maintaining discrimination between discrete life event stress and ongoing stressful life circumstances. Support for the content of such a list comes from at least three sources. First, ICD-10 includes a chapter (Chapter XXI) for codes referring to "Factors Influencing Health Status and Contact With Health Services" (Z codes). Second, primary care physicians have developed their own classification, the International Classification of Health Problems in Primary Care, which includes a Chapter Z, "Social Problems" (Jenkins et al. 1988). Finally, Karls and Wandrei (1992) proposed a system for classifying the problems that clients of social workers may present. Their Person in Environment System lists "environmental problems" as its factor II. Table 28–1 compares these three systems.

Recommendations

Three alternative options have been proposed for Axis IV in the *DSM-IV Options Book* (American Psychiatric Association 1991). The first is to retain the current DSM-III-R Axis IV. The second is to adopt a revised Axis IV consisting of two brief personal resource scales that would be used to indicate the adequacy of a person's social supports and environmental resources. The third option is to replace Axis IV with a simple checklist of psychosocial problems. The rater would check problem areas judged adversely to affect the individual and associated, either causally or in a contributory fashion, with mental disorders, nonpsychiatric medical conditions, or other clinically significant problems coded on Axes I, II, or III. The rater would have the opportunity to list specific problems. The proposed formats for options 2 and 3 may be found in the *DSM-IV Options Book*.

Although desired, no funding was available for a field test comparing the three options for Axis IV with regard to reliability, feasibility, and usefulness in aiding

Table 28–1. Comparison of three coding systems related to Axis IV: ICD-10 draft Chapter XXI Z codes, ICHPPC Chapter Z social problems, and factor II of the PIE[a]

ICD-10 term	Code	ICHPPC term	Code	PIE term	Code
Education and literacy	Z55	Education	Z07	Education and training	610X
				Discrimination in education/training system	62XX
Employment and unemployment	Z56	Working conditions	Z05	Employment	530X
		Unemployment	Z06		
Exposure to occupational risk factors	Z57	Working conditions	Z05		
Social environment	Z58	Migration	Z04	Religious groups	910X
		Social/cultural system	Z11	Community groups	920X
		Friends	Z24	Discrimination in voluntary association system	930X
		Fear of social problem	Z27		
		Social handicap	Z28		
Housing and economic circumstances	Z59	Financial	Z01	Food/nutrition	510X
		Food and water	Z02	Shelter	520X
		Housing	Z03	Economic resources	540X
		Welfare	Z08	Transportation	550X
				Discrimination	560X
Physical environment	Z60	Food and water	Z02	—	
Negative events in childhood	Z61	Child abuse	Z16	—	
Upbringing of child	Z62	—		—	

Category	Z code	Subcategory	Z code	Subcategory	Code
Primary support group/family	Z63	Partner/parent	Z12 Z20	Affectional support Discrimination in affectional support system	1010X 102XX
		Partner/child/parent behavior	Z13 Z17 Z21		
		Ill partner/child/parent	Z14 Z18 Z22		
		Death of partner/child/parent	Z15 Z19 Z23		
Other psychosocial circumstances	Z64	—		—	
	Z65	Legal	Z09	Safety	820X
				Justice/legal	710X
				Discrimination in justice/legal system	72XX
		Assault	Z25		
Health care	Z75	Health care	Z10	Health/mental health	810X
				Social services	830X
				Discrimination in health/safety/social service system	84XX
Life style	Z72	—		—	
Life management difficulty	Z73	—		—	
Care provider dependency	Z74	—		—	
Family history of mental disorder	Z81	—		—	

[a]ICD-10 Chapter XXI refers to "Factors Influencing Health Status and Contact With Health Services" (Z codes); International Classification of Health Problems in Primary Care (ICHPPC) includes Chapter Z ("Social Problems") (Jenkins et al. 1988); Person in Environment (PIE) system lists "environmental problems" as its factor II (Karls and Wandrei 1992).

clinicians to make decisions regarding treatment and management. A questionnaire has been mailed to 1,000 randomly selected members of the American Psychiatric Association to solicit views about the relative importance of identifying stressors, rating their severity, and rating the adequacy of social supports and environmental resources, as well as other multiaxial issues. The results of this questionnaire and data from a few settings, such as the HIV Center at Columbia in New York where one or another of the options have been tested, will help determine which Axis IV option should be recommended to the DSM-IV Task Force.

References

American Psychiatric Association: Diagnostic and Statistical Manual of Mental Disorders, 3rd Edition. Washington, DC, American Psychiatric Association, 1980

American Psychiatric Association: Diagnostic and Statistical Manual of Mental Disorders, 3rd Edition, Revised. Washington, DC, American Psychiatric Association, 1987

American Psychiatric Association: DSM-IV Options Book. Washington, DC, American Psychiatric Association, 1991

Bronheim H, Strain JJ, Biller HF, et al: Psychiatric consultation on an otolaryngology service. Gen Hosp Psychiatry 11:95–102, 1989

Brown GW: Meaning, measurement, and stress of life events, in Stressful Life Events: Their Nature and Effects. Edited by Dohrenwend BS, Dohrenwend BP. New York, John Wiley, 1974, pp 217–243

Brown G, Harris T: Social Origins of Depression: A Study of Psychiatric Disorder in Women. New York, Free Press, 1978

Brugha T, Bebbington P, Tennant C, et al: The list of threatening experiences: a subset of 12 life event categories with considerable long-term contextual threat. Psychol Med 15:189–194, 1985

Depue RA, Monroe SM: Conceptualization and measurement of human disorder in life stress research: the problem of chronic disturbance. Psychol Bull 99:36–51, 1986

Dohrenwend BS, Krasnoff L, Askenasy A, et al: Exemplification of a method for scaling life events: the PERI life events scale. J Health Soc Behav 19:205–229, 1978

Dohrenwend BP, Link B, Kern R, et al: Measuring life events: the problem of variability within event categories. Stress Medicine 6:179–187, 1990

Engles ML, Ghadirian AM, Dongier M: DSM-III: the view from the Canadian academe. Psychiatr J Univ Ottawa 10:37–40, 1985

Frances A, Cooper AM: Descriptive and dynamic psychiatry: a perspective on DSM-III. Am J Psychiatry 138:1198–1202, 1981

Gordon RE, Gordon KK: Relating Axes IV and V of DSM-III to clinical severity of psychiatric disorders. Can J Psychiatry 32:423–424, 1987

Gordon RE, Vijay J, Sloate SG, et al: Aggravating stress and functional level as predictors of length of psychiatric hospitalization. Hosp Community Psychiatry 36:773–774, 1985a

Gordon RE, Jardiolin P, Gordon KK: Predicting length of hospital stay of psychiatric patients. Am J Psychiatry 142:235–237, 1985b

Grant I, Gerst M, Yager J: Scaling of life events by psychiatric patients and normals. J Psychosom Res 20:141–149, 1976

Henderson S, Byrne DG, Duncan-Jones P: Neurosis and the Social Environment. London, England, Academic Press, 1982

Holmes TH, Rahe RH: The social readjustment rating scale. J Psychosom Res 11:213–218, 1967

Isherwood J, Adam KS, Hornblow AR: Readjustment, desirability, expectedness, mastery and outcome dimensions of life stress, suicide and auto-accident. J Human Stress 8:11–18, 1982

Jampala VC, Sierles FS, Taylor MA: Consumers' views of DSM-III: attitudes and practices of U.S. psychiatrists and 1984 graduating psychiatric residents. Am J Psychiatry 143:148–153, 1986

Jenkins R, Smeeton N, Shepherd M: Classification of mental disorders in primary care. Psychol Med Suppl 12:1–59, 1988

Junek RW: The DSM-III in Canada: a survey. Can J Psychiatry 28:182–187, 1983

Junek W, Leichner PP: Opinions of Canadian residents regarding DSM-III. Journal of Psychiatric Education 10:87–91, 1986

Karls JM, Wandrei K: PIE: a new language for social work. Social Work 37:80–85, 1992

Kendell RE: Reflections on psychiatric classification for the architects of DSM-III and ICD-10. Integrative Psychiatry 2:43–47, 1984

Lloyd C: Life events and depressive disorder revisited, II: events as precipitating factors. Arch Gen Psychiatry 37:541–548, 1980

Mezzich AC, Mezzich JE, Coffman GA: Reliability of DSM-III vs DSM-II in child psychopathology. Journal of the American Academy of Child Psychiatry 24:273–280, 1985

Mezzich JE: On developing a psychiatric multiaxial schema for ICD-10. Br J Psychiatry Suppl 1:38–43, 1988

Mezzich JE, Evanczuk KJ, Mathias RJ, et al: Admission decisions and multiaxial diagnosis. Arch Gen Psychiatry 41:1001–1004, 1984

Mezzich JE, Fabrega H Jr, Mezzich AC: An international consultation on multiaxial diagnosis, in Psychiatry, Vol 1. Edited by Pichot P, Berner P, Wolf R, et al. London, England, Plenum, 1985a, pp 51–56

Mezzich JE, Fabrega H Jr, Mezzich AC, et al: International experience with DSM-III. J Nerv Ment Dis 173:738–741, 1985b

Mezzich JE, Fabrega H Jr, Coffman GA: Multiaxial characterization of depressive patients. J Nerv Ment Dis 175:339–345, 1987

Mezzich JE, Fabrega H Jr, Coffman GA, et al: DSM-III disorders in a large sample of psychiatric patients: frequency and specificity of diagnoses. Am J Psychiatry 146:212–219, 1989

Paykel ES, Myers JK, Dienelt MN, et al: Life events and depression: a controlled study. Arch Gen Psychiatry 21:753–760, 1969

Plapp JM, Rey JM, Stewart GM, et al: Ratings of psychosocial stressors in adolescence using DSM-III Axis IV criteria. Journal of the American Academy of Child Psychiatry 26:80–86, 1987

Rey JM, Plapp JM, Stewart GW, et al: Reliability of the psychosocial axes of the DSM-III in an adolescent population. Br J Psychiatry 150:228–234, 1987

Rey JM, Stewart GW, Plapp JM, et al: DSM-III Axis IV revisited. Am J Psychiatry 145:286–292, 1988

Roth Sir M: The achievements and limitations of DSM-III, in International Perspectives on DSM-III. Edited by Spitzer RL, Williams JBW, Skodol AE. Washington, DC, American Psychiatric Press, 1983, pp 91–105

Russell AT, Cantwell DP, Mattison R, et al: A comparison of DSM-II and DSM-III in the diagnosis of childhood psychiatric disorders, III: multiaxial features. Arch Gen Psychiatry 36:1223–1226, 1979

Rutter M, Shaffer D: DSM-III: a step forward or back in terms of the classification of child psychiatric disorders? Journal of the American Academy of Child Psychiatry 19:371–394, 1980

Schless AP, Schwartz L, Goetz C, et al: How depressives view the significance of life events. Br J Psychiatry 125:406–410, 1974

Schrader G, Gordon M, Harcourt R: The usefulness of DSM-III Axis IV and Axis V assessments. Am J Psychiatry 143:904–907, 1986

Skodol AE, Shrout PE: Axis IV of DSM-III (letter). Am J Psychiatry 145:1046, 1988

Skodol AE, Shrout PE: Use of DSM-III Axis IV in clinical practice: rating etiologically significant stressors. Am J Psychiatry 146:61–66, 1989a

Skodol AE, Shrout PE: Use of DSM-III Axis IV in clinical practice: rating the severity of psychosocial stressors. Psychiatry Res 30:201–211, 1989b

Skodol AE, Spitzer RL: An Annotated Bibliography of DSM-III. Washington, DC, American Psychiatric Press, 1987

Skodol AE, Williams JBW, Spitzer RL, et al: Identifying common errors in the use of DSM-III through diagnostic supervision. Hosp Community Psychiatry 35:251–255, 1984

Spitzer RL, Forman JB: DSM-III field trials, II: initial experience with the multiaxial system. Am J Psychiatry 136:818–820, 1979

Strauss JS: A comprehensive approach to psychiatric diagnosis. Am J Psychiatry 132:1193–1197, 1975

Tennant C: Life events and psychological morbidity: the evidence from prospective studies. Psychol Med 13:483–486, 1983

Tennant C, Bebbington P, Hurry J: The role of life events in depressive illness: is there a substantial causal relation? Psychol Med 11:379–389, 1981

Trzepacz PT, Brenner R, Van Thiel DH: A psychiatric study of 247 liver transplantation candidates. Psychosomatics 30:147–153, 1989

Velamoor VR, Waring EM, Fisman S, et al: DSM-III in residency training: results of a Canadian Survey. Can J Psychiatry 34:103–106, 1989

Westermeyer J: DSM-III psychiatric disorders among Hmong refugees in the United States: a point prevalence study. Am J Psychiatry 145:197–202, 1988

Williams JBW: The multiaxial system of DSM-III: where did it come from and where should it go? I: its origins and critiques. Arch Gen Psychiatry 42:175–180, 1985

Williams JBW, Spitzer RL, Skodol AE: DSM-III in residency training: results of a national survey. Am J Psychiatry 142:755–758, 1985

Williams JBW, Spitzer RL, Skodol AE: DSM-III in the training of psychiatric residents and medical students: a national survey. Journal of Psychiatric Education 10:75–86, 1986

World Health Organization: International Classification of Diseases, 9th Edition. Geneva, Switzerland, World Health Organization, 1978

World Health Organization: Chapter XXI, Factors Influencing Health Status and Contact With Health Services. Geneva, Switzerland, World Health Organization, 1992

Zimmerman M, Pfohl B, Stangl D, et al: The validity of DSM-III Axis IV (severity of psychosocial stressors). Am J Psychiatry 142:1437–1441, 1985

Zimmerman M, Pfohl B, Coryell W, et al: The prognostic validity of DSM-III Axis IV in depressed inpatients. Am J Psychiatry 144:102–106, 1987

Chapter 29

A Proposed Axis for Social Supports

Cheryl S. Cohen, M.S., Janet B. W. Williams, D.S.W., and Judith G. Rabkin, Ph.D., M.P.H.

Statement of the Issues

The multiaxial system of DSM-III (American Psychiatric Association 1980 and DSM-III-R (American Psychiatric Association 1987) was hailed as a major innovation and signaled official recognition of the importance of social and environmental factors in planning treatment and predicting outcome (Kendell 1983; Williams 1985a, 1985b, 1987). Axis IV presented rating scales for indicating the severity of psychosocial stressors that were judged to be related to the initiation or exacerbation of the mental disorders listed on Axes I and II. Axis V in DSM-III provided a rating scale for measuring adaptive (social and occupational) functioning, and in DSM-III-R the Global Assessment of Functioning Scale was adopted as an expanded measure of overall functioning (i.e., social, occupational, and psychological). In this chapter, we focus on Axis IV; a separate review of issues regarding Axis V is provided by Goldman et al. (Chapter 30, this volume).

Although the multiaxial system has been widely regarded as an important innovative feature of DSM-III and DSM-III-R, the relative infrequency of use of Axis IV has been disappointing (Bassett and Beiser 1991; Skodol, Chapter 28, this volume; Williams et al. 1985). An alternative to Axis IV has been proposed that would consist of a clinician-rated scale for determining the adequacy of an adult's or child's social supports. The purpose of this literature review is to examine the empirical basis for refocusing Axis IV on the assessment of social supports and to assess the extent to which this would fulfill the purpose of the Axis.

Significance of the Issues

Axis IV has not been used as widely as was hoped: a survey polling 10% of America's child psychiatrists found that only 39% often used Axes IV or V (Setterberg et al. 1991). There are several possible reasons for this low rate of use. Clinicians may find that noting the severity of psychosocial stressors is not as helpful as hoped for planning treatment and predicting outcome, the major purposes for which the multiaxial system was intended. Another possibility is that neither DSM-III nor DSM-III-R included a sample format indicating how the results of a multiaxial evaluation should be recorded. Bassett and Beiser (1991) demonstrated that the use of the multiaxial system greatly increased when a standardized form for recording multiple axes ("compact visual reminder summarizing [its] intricacies," p. 273) was put into place. Finally, it is possible that many clinicians never received proper training in the use of the five axes, and their lack of understanding of the system has hindered their use of it. Other critiques of the multiaxial system, and Axis IV in particular, are summarized by Skodol (Chapter 28, this volume).

Because of the shortcomings of Axis IV in its present form, we felt it prudent to reevaluate the degree to which it furthers the larger objectives of the multiaxial system—facilitating treatment planning and predicting outcome—and to consider whether another approach might better serve those goals. A preliminary review of the literature identified social support as an environmental factor likely to play an important role in the prevention, course, and outcome of mental disorders.

The construct of social support has been the focus of wide attention for the past two decades, and an extensive literature on the subject has evolved. The possible role of social support or its absence in disease etiology, progression, and treatment has prompted researchers from a variety of disciplines to continue trying to refine the concept's definition and to delineate the mechanisms by which it may be linked to well-being. Although no single conceptualization has been agreed on, and although the precise process by which social support influences health remains elusive, the consistency of findings across populations and study conditions is striking.

This being so, the inclusion of a brief, easy-to-use, quantitative measure of the adequacy of social supports would provide recognition of the important relationship between this factor and morbidity. Attention to deficiencies in this area should be part of any treatment plan, given the relevance of social support to disease progression. Likewise, because of the strong association between social support and long-term outcome, formal acknowledgment of this variable helps fulfill one of the major goals of a multiaxial system, prediction of outcome. Focusing on social support should help promote a greater understanding of the patient's total life circumstances. To ignore the likely effect of inadequate social support would be to deprive our patients of a more integrated biopsychosocial approach to their problems.

Method

This review is selective rather than exhaustive; it focuses on those areas that clearly appear to be most significant for understanding and interpreting the construct of social support. All articles reporting research in the area of social support for the period 1974–1990 were accessed using the PsychLit computer database. These references then led to collections of articles in book form, to texts devoted to the topic, and to early works not included in the database.

Results

In this review, we focus on specific research relating social support to mental health, physical morbidity, and mortality and include a brief discussion of measurement issues.

Conceptualizations of Social Support

Social support is a multidimensional construct and can be thought of as having both quantitative properties (e.g., the number of people in whom one can confide, the frequency of contact with them) and qualitative or emotional properties (e.g., empathy or affection). Leavy (1983) viewed support as having both structure (e.g., availability and nature of linkages) and content (e.g., form in which help takes place). According to some researchers, content and quality of relationships are more significant than the quantity and composition of relationships (Kessler and McLeod 1985). Other researchers discuss the difference between perceived and enacted social support. Perceived support can be thought of as appraisal of being reliably connected (Barrerra 1986), whereas enacted support is what people actually do when they provide support. Sarason et al. (1987) concluded that the perception of social support is more important than actually receiving it. Other conceptualizations of social support abound. House (1981) defined social support as an interpersonal transaction involving emotional concern, instrumental aid, information, and appraisal. Kahn and Antonucci (1980) defined social support as a combination of affect, affirmation, and aid. All these definitions illustrate what Barrerra and Ainlay (1983) referred to as the "elasticity of the social support concept."

Two main hypotheses address the question of how social support contributes to well-being. The direct or main effects hypothesis suggests that social support directly enhances health (Andrews et al. 1978; Turner 1981). The buffering hypothesis suggests that social support has an effect only in the presence of stress, acting to lessen or mediate its negative consequences (House et al. 1988a; Patrick et al. 1986). The direct effects hypothesis views support as promoting normal growth and development while reducing social isolation (Litwin and Auslander 1990) or as providing a sense of identity, belonging, self-esteem, and mastery (Thoits 1985). Advocates of the buffering hypothesis believe that social support reduces the harmful impact of negative life events, perhaps by serving as a "resistance resource" (Antonovsky 1974). Some studies have found both direct and indirect effects of social support (Dean and Ensel 1982; Henderson et al. 1978), concluding that support reduces symptoms directly while also reducing negative consequences of stressful events. It should be noted that a minority of studies have found that social support can increase the effects of some stressors (Kaufmann and Beehr 1986).

Social Support and Psychiatric Morbidity

Studies investigating the relationship between social support and mental health approach the issue in a number of ways, comparing clinical and normal populations, focusing on normal population surveys or case control studies, looking at purely clinical populations, and assessing the role of social support in adjustment to life crises.

Much research in the area of social support was prompted by findings of consistent differences in the social networks of psychiatric patients and others. The evidence includes Garrison's (1978) study comparing Puerto Rican-born women with and without schizophrenia. Diminished support networks were found among the most severely disturbed, whereas the comparison group had multiple sources of support. Henderson et al. (1978) compared nonpsychotic psychiatric outpatients with healthy control subjects matched for age and sex. The patients had smaller support systems and lower levels of perceived support. Froland et al. (1979) looked at several components of social support, including size of system, perceived supportiveness, nature of relationships, and density of support. Subjects from the general population were compared with psychiatric inpatients, day-treatment patients, and outpatients. Those with more severe psychopathology were found to have less available support. In general, it appears that clinical populations have support systems that are smaller and less reciprocal than those of general populations (Leavy 1983). It remains unclear, however, whether deficient support is causally related to mental disorder or whether the diminished support is a result of the disorder.

In general population samples, there is clear evidence that social support serves as a buffer against psychological distress and is associated with well-being. In a sample of women who had experienced life stress, Brown and Harris (1978) found that the presence of a confiding relationship with a boyfriend or husband protected them from depression. This result has been replicated by Miller and Ingham (1976) and by Slater and Depue (1981). In a study of urban women, Caspi et al. (1987) found that perceived available support helped lessen the effects of the previous day's stressful events on mood. In a review of panel studies (in which a control population sample is interviewed at two or more points in time), Kessler and McLeod (1985) found that emotional support and the perception of available support could buffer the impact of stress on mental discomfort. The same review concluded that emotional support is more effective in protecting people from the negative effects of stress than structural measures of support, such as size of network or frequency of contact. Holahan and Moos (1981) found that decreased support in work and family environments was significantly related to increased psychological maladjustment.

Most studies assessing the effect of social support on adjustment to crises have found it to be related to later emotional adjustment. Vachon et al. (1982) found that, among those who had lost a spouse, satisfaction with social support at 1 month predicted the level of distress 2 years later. In a longitudinal study of the effects of job loss on factory workers, Gore (1978) found depression to remain high over a 2-year follow-up period among those with low support; depressive symptoms declined or remained stable in the higher support group. One problem in trying to assess adjustment is how to gauge appropriately what is successful. As Kessler et al. (1985) pointed out, emotional distress is not always a sign of poor adjustment. It may, in certain circumstances, serve to motivate effective coping (Goldsmith 1955). Intervention studies in which a group receiving a particular type of support is compared with a group not receiving the support strongly suggest that social support has a protective effect against psychological distress. Raphael (1977) studied the effect of preventive intervention on recently bereaved widows. Subjects considered at risk for morbidity were selected from a sample of 200 widows and randomly assigned to treatment and control groups. The treatment group received individual psychotherapy, including support for grieving, for approximately 3 months following their loss. The control group received no intervention. Follow-up at 13-months posttreatment showed significantly greater morbidity in the control group, including more physical symptoms and more severe depressive symptoms. Porritt (1979) found that, among men hospitalized for injuries, those who were randomly assigned to receive practical and emotional support did better on measures of emotional distress than did the control group. Results from similar intervention studies are consistent. However, it is difficult to ascertain just what aspect of support is most salient because the interventions are so varied, consisting of differing combinations of emotional and instrumental support.

Data from numerous other studies, involving both clinical and control populations, continue to point to the strong relationship between social support and positive outcome. Flaherty et al. (1983) found social support to have a positive effect in patients with unipolar depression. George et al. (1989) assessed 150 adult inpatients who were diagnosed with major depression. Perceptions of inadequate support at baseline predicted higher levels of depression at follow-up, 6 to 32 months later. In a study of homosexual males with AIDS (Namir et al. 1989), inverse relationships were found between measures of emotional support and depression, anxiety, and anger, and between measures of satisfaction with support and the same three outcomes. O'Connell et al. (1985) found social support to be related to positive outcome in a bipolar population treated with lithium. Data from a large random sample of people older than age 65, taken in 1975 and followed up in 1984, indicate that social support can serve as an important coping resource for the elderly, helping to delay decline of mental health over time (Haug et al. 1989).

Adaptation to illness is another area in which social support appears to be of considerable benefit. Funch and Mettlin (1982) found that the degree of perceived social support was positively related to psychological adjustment in women recovering from surgery for breast cancer. Bloom and Spiegel (1984) found emotional support from the family to be positively related to psychological adjustment in women with advanced breast cancer. In a study of male and female patients with breast, colorectal, or lung cancer, Ell et al. (1989) similarly determined availability and adequacy of social support to be a significant predictor of psychological adaptation to the disease.

Social Support and Physical Health

The literature suggests that the relationship between social support and physical health is somewhat tenuous (Cohen 1988; Ganster and Victor 1988). It is not clear at what point in the disease process—onset, progression, or recovery—social support may exert its influence. Results of research are equivocal. Two studies of Japanese-American men looked at the relationship between measures of social affiliation and coronary heart disease (Joseph 1980; Reed et al. 1983). In the first study, social affiliation, as assessed by marital status, attendance at religious services, and organizational membership, was independently associated with prevalence of coronary heart disease. The latter study assessed social interactions with both intimate and casual contacts. Prevalence rates for myocardial infarction, angina, and "total coronary disease" were inversely related to subjects' social network scores. The Israeli Ischemic Heart Disease Study looked at predictors of angina pectoris in adult males over a 5-year period (Medalie and Goldbourt 1976) and found the perceived love and support of a wife to be inversely predictive of the incidence of angina.

In the workplace, it has been found that female clerical workers with nonsupportive supervisors are more likely to develop coronary heart disease (Haynes and Feinlieb 1980). Matthews et al. (1987) found the presence of supportive coworkers and supervisors to be negatively associated with level of blood pressure. Sosa et al. (1980) experimentally studied pregnant women for effects of a supportive companion on labor and mother-infant interactions. Women who were assigned a companion had shorter labors and engaged in more interaction with their infants after delivery.

There appears to be a relationship between social support and adherence to medical treatment. In a study of compliance with taking medication, Porter (1969) found support directly related. In a study of treatment for hypertension, Caldwell et al. (1970) again found support directly related to compliance. These studies were correlational in design; among intervention studies, group support has appeared to help in controlling asthma (Green et al. 1977); patients with hypertension who received both information on the disease in the form of lectures as well as support and encouragement did better at controlling their pressure than did patients who received only lectures (Caplan et al. 1976).

Evidence also exists for a relationship between social support and recovery from physical illness (Wortman and Conway 1985). An intervention study of heart attack patients by Gruen (1975) found that those given support in the form of reassurance, encouragement, and positive feedback spent less time in the hospital and were less anxious and more active at a follow-up visit.

Social Support and Mortality

As early as the 1950s, investigators were taking note of the higher death rate among the unmarried, which held across gender, race, and age groups (Krauss and Lilienfeld 1959). In an early follow-up study, widowed men were found to have a 40% greater rate of mortality in the first 6 months after bereavement than married men of the same age (Young et al. 1963). In a later study of this same widowed group, memorable for its title "Broken Heart," Parkes et al. (1969) documented that diseases of the heart and circulatory system accounted for two-thirds of the increased mortality rate. In an extensive review of past research, Lynch et al. (1977) looked into epidemiological data, bereavement studies, and animal experiments and discovered a relationship between social support and mortality from heart disease. He concluded that unmarried men and women, of all ages and races, had a higher rate of premature cardiac death.

In one of the first major prospective studies of social relationships and mortality, Berkman and Syme (1979) analyzed data from a large general population sample of 4,725 residents of Alameda County, California. The presence or absence of four types of social ties—marriage, contacts with family and friends, church membership, and other group associations—each independently predicted mortality rate over the following 9 years. In every age group, and for both genders, people with the fewest social contacts had the highest mortality rate. The relationship held when self-reported baseline health status and several risk factors (including smoking and alcohol consumption) were controlled for.

House et al. (1982) extended and partly replicated these results with the Tecumseh, Michigan, Community Health Study of 2,754 men and women. Three types of social contacts were included: intimate social relationships, formal organizational involvements, and active leisure pursuits involving social contact. Again, those individuals with the lowest levels of social relationships and activities had the highest mortality rates over a 12-year follow-up period.

Prospective studies by Blazer (1982) and Schoenbach et al. (1986) each found deficient social support to be strongly predictive of mortality. Blazer assessed mortality status 30 months after first assessment in a community sample of 331 adults older than age 65. He found that three indices of social support—available attachments, perceived social support, and frequency of social interaction—each independently predicted mortality. Schoenbach et al. looked at the relationship between social networks and mortality in a cohort of 2,059 men and women. Results supported the hypothesis that those with fewest social ties have increased mortality risk. The relationship was strongest for older white males. House et al. (1988b), in their review of studies of social relationships, speak of the "remarkable consistency" with which they predict mortality. In a 1985 study, Cassileth et al. found that psychosocial variables, including measures of social ties, failed to predict survival time in patients with advanced cancer. However, in a follow-up of an intervention study of women with metastatic breast cancer conducted 10 years earlier, Spiegel et al. (1989) found a dramatic difference in survival time between women randomly assigned to intervention (weekly group meetings at which discussion of problems, feelings, and so on was encouraged) and those in the control group. Both groups received regular oncological treatment. Originally, the researchers had hoped to improve the subjects' quality of life; they had not predicted that survival time would be affected. The researchers speculated that the social support provided by group members may have been a key factor in accounting for the difference in mortality. Studies are currently under way to attempt to replicate these results.

Measurement

Instruments used to assess social support vary widely across studies. They include measures of social support satisfaction (Blaik and Genser 1980) as well as instruments for measuring the perceived availability of social support (Procidano and

Heller 1983). Some scales focus on specific relationships, such as those in the workplace (Billings and Moos 1981; Holahan and Moos 1982). There are global measures using just two or three items, such as Lowenthal and Haven's (1968) assessment of presence or absence of a confidante, as well as lengthy questionnaires of 100 items or more, such as the Norbeck Social Support Questionnaire (Norbeck et al. 1981).

Failure to establish the reliability and validity of instruments before collecting data is a common problem. In his review of social support instruments, O'Reilly (1988) found that 7 of 24 failed even to mention reliability. Only 9 of the 24 actually tested reliability. Validation studies often turned out to provide poor support for the instruments' validity.

Discussion

There is overwhelming evidence demonstrating a relationship between social support and both morbidity and mortality. Because of the strong relationship between social support and mental health, a scale for the measurement of social support deserves serious consideration for inclusion in the multiaxial system of DSM-IV. Such a scale would focus attention on an area of functioning that is clearly related to treatment compliance and outcome. For patients, it would ensure that this very significant aspect of their lives is not overlooked; for clinicians, focus on social supports may reveal additional resources that can aid in the treatment plan, or deficiencies that need to be addressed in the treatment plan. It is possible that development of adequate support could be a specific goal of treatment.

Recommendations

Because DSM-IV is a manual for general clinical use, it is likely that only a simple scheme will be successful as an axis. Therefore, a new, global 5-point scale to measure social supports has been proposed (see Table 29–1). This scale would address clinicians' need for simplicity and brevity when making a multiaxial assessment. The construct of "overall adequacy of social supports" is assessed to consider both its quantity and quality, from both familial and nonfamilial sources. Although two scales were initially developed, one for children and adolescents and one for adults, they were finally combined so that a clinician need learn only one scale. At the time of the evaluation, the adequacy of social supports is assessed for the current time period. Ratings are made regardless of cause of inadequacy (e.g., even if inadequacy is due to psychopathology). Scale points include "optimal,"

Table 29–1. Personal resources scales

These scales are for coding the adequacy of two areas of personal resources in children and adults: social supports and environmental resources. The adequacy of each of these areas should be rated for the current time period at the time of evaluation.

The following descriptors are to be used as *general* guidelines. Ratings should be made regardless of cause of inadequacy (e.g., rate "1" in Environmental Resources Scale even if lack of finances and housing is related to psychopathology).

Social Supports Scale

Consider the quantity and quality of social relationships and contact; include familial and nonfamilial resources. For children and adolescents, include the supervision, guidance, warmth, and security provided by important caretakers.

5—Optimal: Relationships provide extensive social support with little or no social conflict—for example, frequent contact with several close friends, and excellent relations with family, including consistent and appropriate supervision and guidance for children.

4—Adequate: Relationships provide an average amount of social support, with occasional social conflict.

3—Somewhat inadequate: Relationships provide less than adequate social support, with frequent social conflict—for example, some contact with a small number of friends, no close friends, and a minimal frequency of contact with family and/or somewhat strained relations with family. For children, inadequacies of supervision or caretakers' sensitivity to developmental needs fall short of neglect or abuse.

2—Clearly deficient: Social relationships provide little nurturance or support. Family contacts, if any, are insensitive and unsupportive. For children, neglect or abuse *may* be present due to inadequate supervision or hostility.

1—Markedly deficient: Social relationships are nonexistent or, if present, are generally unsupportive or abusive. No contact with family, or family relations are extremely strained or hostile. Overt child neglect or abuse is present at this level.

Environmental Resources Scale

Consider the adequacy of housing, finances, safety of the environment, access to health and other services, and so on.

5—Optimal: No significant financial problems, comfortable housing in a safe neighborhood, easy access to health and other services.

4—Adequate: Adequate finances to meet basic needs (including entertainment), housing is adequate in size and location, health and other services may be accessed with minimal effort.

3—Somewhat inadequate: Finances adequate for necessities only, somewhat cramped or decrepit housing in neighborhood of questionable safety, limited access to health and other services.

(continued)

Table 29–1. Personal resources scales *(continued)*

2—Clearly deficient: Income regularly inadequate for meeting basic needs, housing extremely decrepit in an unsafe neighborhood, health and other services not available without extreme effort (e.g., traveling great distances).

1—Markedly deficient: No sources of income, homeless.

"adequate," "somewhat inadequate," "clearly deficient," and "markedly deficient." With this range, the scale significantly indicates both strengths or resources as well as difficulties or deficiencies, and a greater range is provided for the latter. Descriptors are provided for each scale point to serve as general guidelines. For example, social supports are "clearly deficient" in the following case: "Social relationships provide little nurturance or support. Family contacts, if any, are insensitive and unsupportive. For children, neglect or abuse *may* be present due to inadequate supervision or hostility." The scale point descriptors were arrived at after considering a number of alternatives. Clinicians found these final choices useful during pilot testing. The scale points were easily memorized in actual use.

This scale is proposed for Axis IV in combination with a similar scale for measuring the adequacy of environmental resources, another major source of difficulty outside the organism that might affect its internal functioning (see Table 29–1). Environmental resources reflect the state of finances, housing, access to health care, and so on. Initially, a third scale for measuring occupational resources had been proposed to accompany these two. This scale would have ascertained whether one's job was a challenge and a source of satisfaction and support or whether the patient was unemployed and had a serious deficiency in that area. However, when this scale was pilot-tested, clinicians found it too difficult to apply to the vast range of occupational situations and did not find that it was useful in discriminating optimal occupational situations from those that were clearly deficient. Similar problems were noted in discussions of a proposed scale to rate the educational situations of children and adolescents.

In practice, clinicians find that most of the time they can easily rate the social supports and environmental resource scales following a thorough routine evaluation. It is good practice to evaluate the features of a patient's social and physical environment. Many treatment plans include the involvement of "significant others," recognizing that they may be part of the problem, or may be helpful in ensuring compliance with a treatment regimen. At hospital discharge, relevant others, if they are available, must be involved to facilitate readjustment to the nonhospital world and to ensure cooperation with follow-up plans. Likewise, a patient who lacks adequate financial resources may not be able to maintain a medication regimen or travel to a clinic for follow-up care. It may be difficult to maintain contact with a homeless patient. The requirement for completing these two rating scales would serve as a reminder to the clinician of the importance of assessing these factors.

The addition of the social supports and environmental resource scales to the multiaxial system would help ensure that a clinician obtains a complete picture of the individual being evaluated—a picture of both internal states (i.e., psychopathology and physical condition) and external difficulties or resources (i.e., social support and environment). It should be noted that these ideas were derived in part from a new classification of social role and environmental problems developed by social workers (Williams et al. 1989). Of course, studies of the scales' reliability and validity must be completed before they can be given full consideration as an alternative to DSM-III-R's Axis IV, and appropriate field trials are currently under way.

References

American Psychiatric Association: Diagnostic and Statistical Manual of Mental Disorders, 3rd Edition. Washington, DC, American Psychiatric Association, 1980
American Psychiatric Association: Diagnostic and Statistical Manual of Mental Disorders, 3rd Edition, Revised. Washington, DC, American Psychiatric Association, 1987
Andrews G, Tennant C, Hewson DM, et al: Life event stress, social support, coping style, and risk of psychological impairment. J Nerv Ment Dis 166:307–316, 1978
Antonovsky A: Conceptual and methodological problems in the study of resistance resources and stressful life events, in Stressful Life Events: Their Nature and Effects. Edited by Dohrenwend BS, Dohrenwend BP. New York, Wiley, 1974, pp 245–258
Barrera M Jr: Distinctions between social support concepts, measures, and models. Am J Community Psychol 14:413–445, 1986
Barrera M Jr, Ainlay SL: The structure of social support: a conceptual and empirical analysis. Journal of Community Psychology 11:133–143, 1983
Bassett AS, Beiser M: DSM-III: use of the multiaxial diagnostic system in clinical practice. Can J Psychiatry 36:270-274, 1991
Berkman LF, Syme SL: Social networks, host resistance, and mortality: a nine-year follow-up study of Alameda County residents. Am J Epidemiol 109:186–204, 1979
Billings AG, Moos RH: The role of coping responses and social resources in attenuating the stress of life events. J Behav Med 4:139–157, 1981
Blaik R, Genser SG: Perception of social support satisfaction: scale development. Personality and Social Psychology Bulletin 6:172, 1980
Blazer DG: Social support and mortality in an elderly community population. Am J Epidemiol 115:684–694, 1982
Bloom JR, Spiegel D: The relationship of two dimensions of social support to the psychological well-being and social functioning of women with advanced breast cancer. Soc Sci Med 19:831–837, 1984
Brown GW, Harris T: The Social Origins of Depression. London, England, Tavistock, 1978

Caldwell JR, Cobb S, Dowling MD, et al: The dropout problem in antihypertensive treatment: a pilot study of social and emotional factors influencing a patient's ability to follow antihypertensive treatment. Journal of Chronic Disease 22:579–592, 1970

Caplan RD, Robinson EAR, French JRP Jr, et al: Adherence to Medical Regimens: Pilot Experiments in Patient Education and Social Support. Ann Arbor, MI, University of Michigan Research Center for Group Dynamics, Institute for Social Research, 1976

Caspi A, Bolger N, Eckenrode J: Linking person and context in the daily stress process. J Pers Soc Psychol 52:184–195, 1987

Cassileth BR, Lusk EJ, Miller DS, et al: Psychosocial correlates of survival in advanced malignant disease. N Engl J Med 312:1551–1555, 1985

Cohen S: Psychosocial models of the role of social support in the etiology of physical disease. Health Psychology 7:269–297, 1988

Dean A, Ensel WM: Modeling social support, life events, competence, and depression in the context of age and sex. Journal of Community Psychology 10:392–408, 1982

Ell K, Mantell JE, Hamovitch MB, et al: Social support, sense of control, and coping among patients with breast, lung, or colorectal cancer. Journal of Psychosocial Oncology 7:63–89, 1989

Flaherty JA, Gaviria FM, Black EM, et al: The role of social support in the functioning of patients with unipolar depression. Am J Psychiatry 140:473–476, 1983

Froland C, Brodsky G, Olson M, et al: Social support and social adjustment: implications for mental health professionals. Community Ment Health J 15:82–93, 1979

Funch DP, Mettlin C: The role of support in relation to recovery from breast surgery. Soc Sci Med 16:91–98, 1982

Ganster DC, Victor B: The impact of social support on mental and physical health. Br J Med Psychol 61:17–36, 1988

Garrison V: Support systems of schizophrenic and non-schizophrenic Puerto Rican migrant women in New York City. Schizophr Bull 39:561–596, 1978

George LK, Blazer DG, Hughes DC, et al: Social support and the outcome of major depression. Br J Psychiatry 154:478–485, 1989

Goldsmith HH: A contribution of certain personality characteristics of male paraplegics to the degree of improvement in rehabilitation (thesis). New York, New York University; 1955

Gore S: The effect of social support in moderating the health consequences of unemployment. J Health Soc Behav 19:157–165, 1978

Green LW, Werlin SH, Schauffler HH, et al: Research and demonstration issues in self-care: measuring the decline of mediocentrism. Health Education Monographs 5:161–189, 1977

Gruen W: Effects of brief psychotherapy during the hospitalization period on the recovery process in heart attacks. J Consult Clin Psychol 43:223–232, 1975

Haug MR, Breslau N, Folmar SJ: Coping resources and selective survival in mental health of the elderly. Res Aging 11:468–491, 1989

Haynes SG, Feinleib M: Women, work, and coronary heart disease: prospective findings from the Framingham Heart Study. Am J Public Health 70:133–141, 1980

Henderson S, Byrne DG, Duncan-Jones P, et al: Social bonds in the epidemiology of neurosis: a preliminary communication. Br J Psychiatry 132:463–466, 1978

Holahan CJ, Moos RH: Social support and psychological distress: a longitudinal analysis. J Abnorm Psychol 90:365–370, 1981

Holahan CJ, Moos RH: Social support and adjustment: predictive benefits of social climate indices. Am J Community Psychol 10:403–413, 1982

House JS: Work Stress and Social Support. Reading, PA, Addison-Wesley, 1981

House JS, Robbins C, Metzner HL: The association of social relationships and activities with mortality: prospective evidence from the Tecumseh Community Health Study. Am J Epidemiol 116:123–140, 1982

House JS, Umberson D, Landis KR: Structures and processes of social support. Annu Rev Sociol 14:293–318, 1988a

House JS, Landis KR, Umberson D: Social relationships and health. Science 24:540–545, 1988b

Joseph JV: Social affiliation, risk factor status, and coronary heart disease: a cross-sectional study of Japanese-American men (thesis). Berkeley, CA, University of California, 1980

Kahn RL, Antonucci TC: Convoys over the life course: attachment, roles, and social support. Lifespan Development and Behavior 3:253–286, 1980

Kaufmann GM, Beehr TA: Interactions between job stressors and social support: some counterintuitive results. J Appl Psychol 71:522–526, 1986

Kendell RE: DSM-III: a major advance in psychiatric nosology, in International Perspectives on DSM-III. Edited by Spitzer RL, Williams JBW, Skodol AE. Washington, DC, American Psychiatric Press, 1983, pp 55–68

Kessler RC, McLeod JD: Social support and mental health in community samples, in Social Support and Health. Edited by Cohen S, Syme SL. Orlando, FL, Academic Press, 1985, pp 219–240

Kessler RC, Price RH, Wortman CB: Social factors in psychopathology: stress, social support, and coping processes. Annu Rev Psychol 36:531–572, 1985

Krauss AS, Lilienfeld AM: Some epidemic aspects of the high mortality rate in the young widowed group. Journal of Chronic Disease 10:207–217, 1959

Leavy RL: Social support and psychological disorder: a review. Journal of Community Psychology 11:3–21, 1983

Litwin H, Auslander GK: Evaluating informal support. Evaluation Review 14:42–56, 1990

Lowenthal MF, Haven C: Interaction and adaptation: intimacy as critical variable. American Sociological Review 33:20–30, 1968

Lynch JJ, Thomas SA, Paskewitz DA, et al. Human contact and cardiac arrhythmia in a coronary care unit. Psychosom Med 39:188–192, 1977

Matthews KA, Cottington EM, Talbott E, et al: Stressful work conditions and diastolic blood pressure among blue collar factory workers. Am J Epidemiol 126:280–291, 1987

Medalie JH, Goldbourt U: Angina pectoris among 10,000 men, II: psychosocial and other risk factors as evidenced by a multivariate analysis of a five-year incidence study. Am J Med 60:910–921, 1976

Miller PM, Ingham JG: Friends, confidants and symptoms. Social Psychiatry 11:51–58, 1976

Namir S, Alumbaugh MJ, Fawzy FI, et al: The relationship of social support to physical and psychological aspects of AIDS. Psychology and Health 3:77–86, 1989

Norbeck JS, Lindsey AM, Carrieri VL: The development of an instrument to measure social support. Nursing Research 30:264–269, 1981

O'Connell RA, Mayo JA, Eng LK, et al: Social support and long-term lithium outcome. Br J Psychiatry 147:272–275, 1985

O'Reilly P: Methodological issues in social support and social network research. Soc Sci Med 26:863–873, 1988

Parkes CM, Benjamin B, Fitzgerald RG: Broken heart: a statistical study of increased mortality among widowers. BMJ 1:740–743, 1969
Patrick DL, Morgan F, Charlton JRH: Psychosocial support and change in the health status of physically disabled people. Soc Sci Med 22:1347–1354, 1986
Porritt D: Social support in crisis: quantity or quality. Soc Sci Med 13:715–721, 1979
Porter AMW: Drug defaulting in a general practice. BMJ 1:218–222, 1969
Procidano ME, Heller K: Measures of perceived social support from friends and from family: three validation studies. Am J Community Psychol 11:1–24, 1983
Raphael B: Preventive intervention with the recently bereaved. Arch Gen Psychiatry 34:1450–1454, 1977
Reed D, McGee D, Yano K: Social networks and coronary heart disease among Japanese men in Hawaii. Am J Epidemiol 117:384–396, 1983
Sarason BR, Shearin EN, Pierce GR, et al: Interrelations of social support measures: theoretical and practical implications. J Pers Soc Psychol 52:813–832, 1987
Schoenbach VJ, Kaplan BH, Fredman L, et al: Social ties and mortality in Evans County, Georgia. Am J Epidemiol 123:577–591, 1986
Setterberg SR, Ernst M, Rao U, et al: Child psychiatrist's views of DSM-III-R: a survey of usage and opinions. J Am Acad Child Adolesc Psychiatry 30:652–658, 1991
Slater J, Depue RA: The contributions of environmental events and social support to serious suicide attempts in primary depressive disorder. J Abnorm Psychol 90:275–285, 1981
Sosa R, Kennell J, Klaus M, et al: The effect of a supportive companion on perinatal problems, length of labor, and mother-infant interaction. N Engl J Med 303:597–600, 1980
Spiegel D, Bloom JR, Kraemer HC, et al: Effect of psychosocial treatment on survival of patients with metastatic breast cancer. Lancet 2:888–891, 1989
Thoits PA: Social support and psychological well-being: theoretical possibilities, in Social Support: Theory, Research and Applications. Edited by Sarason IG, Sarason B. The Hague, Netherlands, Martinus Nijhoff, 1985, pp 51–72
Turner RJ: Social support as a contingency in psychological well-being. J Health Soc Behav 22:357–367, 1981
Vachon MLS, Rogers J, Lyall WAL, et al: Predictors and correlates of adaptation to conjugal bereavement. Am J Psychiatry 139:998–1002, 1982
Williams JBW: The multiaxial system of DSM-III: where did it come from and where should it go? I: its origins and critiques. Arch Gen Psychiatry 42:175–180, 1985a
Williams JBW: The multiaxial system of DSM-III: where did it come from and where should it go? II: empirical studies, innovations, recommendations. Arch Gen Psychiatry 42:181–186, 1985b
Williams JBW: Multiaxial diagnosis, in An Annotated Bibliography of DSM-III. Edited by Skodol AE, Spitzer RL. Washington, DC, American Psychiatric Press, 1987, pp 31–36
Williams JBW, Spitzer RL, Skodol AE: DSM-III in residency training: results of a national survey. Am J Psychiatry 142:755–758, 1985
Williams JBW, Karls JM, Wandrei K: The Person-in-Environment (PIE) system for describing problems of social functioning. Hosp Community Psychiatry 40:1125–1127, 1989
Wortman CB, Conway TL: The role of social support in adaptation and recovery from physical illness, in Social Support and Health. Edited by Cohen S, Syme SL. New York, Academic Press, 1985, pp 281–302
Young M, Benjamin B, Wallis C: The mortality of widowers. Lancet 2:454–456, 1963

Chapter 30

Revising Axis V for DSM-IV: A Review of Measures of Social Functioning

Howard H. Goldman, M.D., Ph.D., Andrew E. Skodol, M.D., and Tamara R. Lave, B.A.

Statement and Significance of the Issues

Axis V was introduced in DSM-III (American Psychiatric Association 1980) as a measure of "adaptive functioning" on a 7-point scale, ranging from "superior" to "grossly impaired." Axis V was modified for DSM-III-R (American Psychiatric Association 1987) in an effort to increase its utility. According to DSM-III-R, Axis V, the Global Assessment of Functioning Scale (GAFS), is to be used to assess "psychological, social, and occupational functioning" (p. 20). It is "available for use in special clinical and research settings" (p. 16). It is not a required element of patient evaluation and is regarded as a supplement to the "official" diagnoses (on Axes I, II, III). There is little evidence (Schrader et al. 1986) concerning how frequently Axis V is used for "planning treatment and predicting outcome."

As a result of the revision of Axis V in DSM-III-R, a simple measure of adaptive functioning was replaced by a 90-point scale that combines assessments of psychological, social, and occupational functioning, based on the widely used Global

---

A version of this chapter titled "Revising Axis V for DSM-IV: A Review of Measures of Social Functioning" by H. H. Goldman, A. E. Skodol, and T. R. Lave has previously been published in *American Journal of Psychiatry* 149:1148–1156, 1992. Used with permission.

The authors thank S. B. Fine, R. E. Gordon, J. S. Strauss, M. D. Thomas, and H. S. Wilson for comments on earlier drafts of this chapter. We acknowledge the contributions of the other members of the Work Group on Multiaxial Issues, J. B. Williams (chair), A. Gruenberg, and J. Mezzich, as well as its consultants and liaisons (A. Frances, H. A. Pincus, D. Shaffer, S. Sotterberg, R. Spitzer, and T. Widiger).

Assessment Scale (Spitzer et al. 1973). It was thought that the GAFS would be a more useful element of the multiaxial evaluation system than DSM-III Axis V because the Global Assessment Scale has been employed in hundreds of studies and clinical settings. There is little or no information, however, on the impact of the changes made for DSM-III-R on the utility or acceptability of this supplementary axis.

In this chapter, we review what is known about Axis V of DSM-III and DSM-III-R, review other measures of social functioning, and discuss several proposals for further revision of Axis V for DSM-IV.

Method

Two comprehensive reviews of the literature on measures of social and occupational functioning (Wallace 1986; Weissmann et al. 1981) served as the basis for our work. Several newer papers in the literature were added as well. In addition, we searched the entire published literature for material on the reliability and validity of Axis V. Our initial review was circulated within the Work Group on Multiaxial Issues and to a list of outside experts for comments and additions. This process yielded several additional instruments and references.

Results

Reliability

In the DSM-III field trials, intraclass reliability coefficients for Axis V ratings on adult patients were .80 using the joint interview method and .69 for test-retest evaluations (Spitzer and Forman 1986). Fernando et al. (1986) reported a lower figure of .49 from the ratings of a multidisciplinary group of clinical workers on an inpatient service.

Russell et al. (1979) give a figure of 64% agreement between raters using a preliminary version of Axis V, consisting of a 4-point scale of current impairment in adaptive functioning in cases of child psychopathology. Using DSM-III Axis V, A. C. Mezzich et al. (1985) found an intraclass correlation coefficient of .61 for ratings of a mixed group of child and adolescent cases. Rey et al. (1988) reported an intraclass correlation coefficient of .57 for a group of adolescents. All three of these studies had clinicians rate written case summaries rather than live patients.

Overall, the reliability of Axis V has been found to be higher than that of Axis IV. Given the relatively restricted diversity of clinicians, patients, information, and time frames in the published studies, however, the demonstrated reliability of Axis V has not been especially good (Rey et al. 1987). Although special training in the use of the measures of functioning for Axis V may improve reliability, we are not aware of any studies of the impact of training.

Validity

Most validity studies have compared adaptive functioning as measured by Axis V for different patient groups identified by diagnosis or referral status. A few have approached concurrent or construct validity by comparing Axis V ratings with other measures of adaptive functioning. The relationship of Axis V to disposition or treatment status has been studied, mostly retrospectively. Two studies have examined the predictive validity of Axis V using prospective designs.

Five studies reported predictable diagnostic group differences on Axis V in diverse patient populations. In a mixed group of inpatients and outpatients, Skodol et al. (1988a) found significant variation in Axis V ratings across 10 diagnostic groups. Patients with schizophrenia received ratings of the poorest adaptive functioning; patients with V codes, no Axis I diagnosis, anxiety disorders, adjustment disorder, and major depression (single episode) received the best. In a sample of more than 10,000 patients, J. E. Mezzich et al. (1987) found that depressed patients had higher Axis V ratings than nondepressed patients. Trzepacz et al. (1989) found that liver transplant candidates who were delirious and were seen by a consultation-liaison service had lower Axis V ratings than nondelirious cases. Westermeyer (1986) reported lower levels of adaptive functioning among Asian refugees to the United States who had any Axis I diagnosis compared with those who had none, and Fabrega et al. (1990) showed a trend toward greater Axis V impairment in patients who had more complex Axis I diagnoses at intake. A highly significant relationship was found between Axis I complexity and deficits in current functioning. A sixth study (Schrader et al. 1986) had mixed results. No difference on Axis V was found between psychotic and nonpsychotic, psychotic and organic, or nonpsychotic and organic patient groups. When psychotic patients were divided into those with affective psychoses and those with nonaffective psychoses, the former had higher levels of functioning than the latter, who also had lower levels than patients with nonpsychotic disorder. Bronheim et al. (1989) reported that patients referred for psychiatric consultation from an ear, nose, and throat service had better functioning on Axis V than other referrals.

Three studies examined the relationship of Axis V to other measures. Skodol et al. (1988a) compared Axis V with those measures of social and occupational functioning included in the Psychiatric Epidemiology Research Interview and with other social network variables assessed independently. They found significant correlations between Axis V adaptive functioning and both social and occupational variables, with occupational factors predominating. Among patients with substance abuse, Westermeyer and Neider (1988) found highly significant negative correlations between Axis V ratings and two separate components of social networks: number of people and number of separate social groups. Finally, Rey et al. (1988) reported that Axis V functioned similarly to independent ratings of premorbid functioning and less like measures of social competence or present functioning in their samples of adolescents.

In a series of analyses, Gordon and associates have examined the relationship of Axis V to treatment status. Initially, Gordon et al. (1985a, 1985b) developed a measure called the "strain ratio," which is the ratio of Axis IV ratings of severity of psychosocial stressors to Axis V ratings, transformed so that higher ratings indicated better adaptive functioning. They found that length of inpatient hospitalization was correlated with higher strain ratios: when patients' rescaled level of functioning exceeded their scores on Axis IV, they tended to remain in the hospital for a shorter period. Subsequently, Gordon and Gordon (1987) reported predictable differences on Axis V between chronically ill state hospital patients, long-term inpatients, short-term inpatients, and outpatients.

J. E. Mezzich et al. (1984) found that ratings of highest level of adaptive functioning in the past year had a correlation of .27 with the decision to admit a patient for inpatient treatment from a walk-in clinic. These investigators found an even greater relationship ($r = .45$) between impairment in current adaptive functioning measured over the preceding month and inpatient disposition.

In the first of two prospective studies of the ability of Axis V ratings to predict outcome, Mellsop et al. (1987) found a significant relationship for inpatients between preadmission adaptive functioning as measured by Axis V and symptomatic outcome at 6 months. They also found, however, an even greater relationship between outcome and functioning as measured by the self-report Social Adjustment Scale (Schooler et al. 1979). In the second study of predictive validity, Beiser et al. (1988) found that Axis V was a powerful predictor of which patients receiving a schizophreniform disorder diagnosis early in a psychotic episode would, in fact, recover within the 6-month time frame stipulated by DSM-III and which would not recover and need a change in diagnosis to schizophrenia.

DSM-III-R Axis V

As of this writing, there are no published studies on the GAFS of DSM-III-R, but a number of the reports mentioned earlier and two additional studies have some bearing on the changes in the adaptive functioning construct in DSM-III-R. The two major changes in concept are 1) the provision for rating both the highest level of adaptive functioning in the past year and current functioning and 2) the inclusion of symptom severity, as well as indicators of social and occupational functioning, in the ratings.

On the first change, Skodol et al. (1988a) found few differences on social and occupational functioning when measured over the past year and measured over the past month when these were correlated with Axis V ratings of highest level of functioning in the past year. Rey et al. (1988) also found a greater relationship between Axis V and independent ratings of premorbid rather than present functioning. The analyses of Fabrega et al. (1990) and A. C. Mezzich et al. (1985), however, both point to the potential importance of current functional impairment as a consideration in diagnosis and treatment planning.

On the second change, several different groups have attempted to divide Axis V into its component parts and examine each component separately. In the study by Trzepacz et al. (1989), separate ratings of current occupational, family, and social functioning all bore the same relationship to delirious versus nondelirious diagnostic status as did the overall Axis V rating. On the other hand, Mellsop et al. (1987) observed some variations in the relationship of three similar factors and outcome prediction and suspected that global ratings of adaptive functioning masked significant variability. Beiser et al. (1988) believed that the inclusion of symptoms in DSM-III-R Axis V would undermine its ability to discriminate schizophreniform from schizophrenic patients. Gordon et al. (1988) showed that symptom improvement and functional improvement as measured by Axis V did not go hand in hand in discharged patients followed in outpatient treatment over time. Finally, Skodol et al. (1988b) demonstrated that symptoms had a larger effect on Axis V ratings, in terms of explained variance, than adaptive functioning variables and tended to detract from the latter's significance. Although the effect of symptom measures on explained variance may be taken as support for changing Axis V into the GAFS, the change may also make Axis V more redundant with Axis I diagnosis. If a major objective of a multiaxial approach is the quasi-independent assessment of different domains relevant to a comprehensive psychiatric diagnosis, then explicit inclusion of symptoms in the Axis V ratings would seem to defeat this purpose.

Strengths and Weaknesses of Axis V

This review suggests that Axis V is a reasonably valid measure of adaptive functioning, limited in part by its modest reliability. In addition, some problems have been identified with the changes introduced when DSM-III was revised. For example, the evidence is mixed on the value of obtaining measures of functioning during two time periods (i.e., past month and past year). As might be expected, the value seems to depend on the nature of the question being asked, suggesting that assessments in both time periods have merit. Consequently, there is no great pressure to change Axis V again, to a rating of a single period. Two other problems, however, are believed by some to limit the utility of Axis V in DSM-III-R. In particular, there is concern that 1) the assessment of functioning is attributed to mental impairment alone, and 2) one axis combines measures of psychological, social, and occupational functioning. In the first instance, it may be impossible to disentangle the combined limitations imposed by mental and physical impairments; in the latter, it may be too difficult to assess these distinct domains of functioning with a global measure.

These problems may be related. The progenitor of the GAFS, the Global Assessment Scale, was designed as a global measure of psychopathology and focused heavily on current psychological functioning. As such, it was logical to focus on functioning related to mental disorders alone. When used more broadly, emphasizing social and occupational functioning over the past year, it may be much more problematic to attribute functioning to a mental disorder alone. Furthermore, when used in general medical settings or with elderly patients with multiple impairments, such attribution is even more difficult to make reliably (E. Caine, personal communication, September 1990).

The combination on a single axis of measures of psychological, occupational, and social functioning is problematic for two reasons. First, it violates the principle of a multiaxial system that each axis "refers to a different class of information." Second, it may also confuse raters because of the complexity of making a single rating integrating three different dimensions that do not always vary together. As noted, there is evidence from Skodol et al. (1988a, 1988b), supported by the findings of other studies (Beiser et al. 1988; Gordon et al. 1988; Mellsop et al. 1987), that ratings on Axis V are highly correlated with Axis I, indicating that Axis V does not provide a sufficiently independent class of information. In addition, other investigators (Anthony and Cohen 1984; Strauss and Carpenter 1974, 1977) have indicated that psychological functioning often does not correlate well with social and occupational functioning. Although a set of studies by Liberman (1990) suggest a significant relationship between symptom measures and occupational functioning, it is a relationship mediated by functional impairments in the capacity to work (such as limitations in social interaction and activities of daily living).

Before deciding to recommend retaining the GAFS for Axis V or changing to another measure, we turned again to the literature.

Measures of Social Functioning

We reviewed the literature on measures of social functioning in an effort to find out what other measures of functioning might be used as models for Axis V. Our review relies heavily on two existing articles in the literature: Weissman et al. (1981) and Wallace (1986). Promising instruments were viewed in more detail from their original sources. Although each of the instruments was reviewed for depth and breadth of measures, appropriate target population, and psychometric properties, the special criteria used to evaluate these scales for use in Axis V focused additionally on simplicity ("user-friendliness") and unidimensionality (i.e., involving a single class of information).

The instruments reviewed by Weissman et al. (1981) and Wallace (1986) are shown in Table 30–1. Original references are provided. Table 30–2 summarizes the reviews of each of these instruments along several dimensions, including psychometric properties and method of scoring. Each is placed into one of seven groups, based on inclusion of symptoms in the instrument or schedule, depth and breadth of dimensions of functioning, and applicability to the general population (rather than to a specific clinical group).

As shown in Table 30–2, Group 1 includes the Denver Community Mental Health Questionnaire (DCMHQ) and the KDS-15 Marital Questionnaire (KDS-

Table 30–1. Measures of social adjustment and functioning

DCMHQ: Denver Community Mental Health Questionnaire (Ciarlo and Reihman 1975, 1977)

KDS-15: KDS-15 Marital Questionnaire (Kupfer and Frank 1974)

KAS: Katz Adjustment Scale (Katz and Lyerly 1963)

PARS: Personal Adjustment and Role Skills Scale (Ellsworth et al. 1968)

PSS: Psychiatric Status Schedule (Spitzer et al. 1970)

PEF: Psychiatric Evaluation Form (Endicott and Spitzer 1972b)

CAPPS: Current and Past Psychopathology Scale (Endicott and Spitzer 1972a)

REHAB: Rehabilitation Evaluation of Baker and Hall (Baker and Hall 1983)

CLAS: Community Living Assessment Scale (Willer and Gustafero 1974, 1985)

PRI: Personal Resources Inventory (Clayton and Hirschfeld 1977)

ISSI: Interview Schedule for Social Interaction (Duncan-Jones and Henderson 1978; Henderson et al. 1980)

SBAS: Social Behavior and Adjustment Scale (Platt et al. 1980)

SAG: Self-Assessment Guide (Willer and Biggen 1976)

CAS: Community Adaptation Schedule (Burnes and Rosen 1967)

SSIAM: Structured and Scaled Interview to Assess Maladjustment (Gurland et al. 1962a, 1962b)

SIASM: Standardized Interview to Assess Social Maladjustment (Clare and Cairns 1978, 1979)

CAPS: Community Adjustment Profile System (Evanson et al. 1974)

SSFIPD: Social Stress and Functioning Inventory for Psychotic Disorders (Serban 1978)

SFS: Social Functioning Schedule (Remington and Tyrer 1979)

SAS: Social Adjustment Scale (Self Report-SR) (Version II) (Schooler et al. 1979; Weissman and Bothwell 1976)

15), which include symptom measures; do not include role performance measures (especially the DCMHQ); and focus on specific clinical groups (i.e., community mental health clinic clients and married couples, in the case of the KDS-15). Group 2 includes the Katz Adjustment Scale, Personal Adjustment and Role Skills Scale, Psychiatric Status Schedule, Psychiatric Evaluation Form, and Current and Past Psychopathology Scale. This distinguished group also includes symptoms, is somewhat more inclusive of areas of functioning than Group 1, and is broadly applicable to the entire clinical population. It is similar to Group 5, which includes the Social Behavior and Adjustment Scale and the Self-Assessment Guide, both of which are more detailed measures of functioning than the instruments in Group 2. Group 3 includes Rehabilitation Evaluation of Baker and Hall and Community Living Assessment Scale, which do not include symptom measures, focus on a narrow domain of functioning, and principally apply to a limited population in 24-hour care. The Personal Resources Inventory and Interview Schedule for Social Interaction are in Group 4. They do not include symptom measures and focus on a narrow range of functioning, but are more broadly applicable than the instruments in Group 3.

Groups 6 and 7 are similar. All of the instruments (Community Adaptation Schedule [CAS], Structured and Scaled Interview to Assess Maladjustment, Standardized Interview to Assess Social Maladjustment, Community Adjustment Profile System, Social Stress and Functioning Inventory for Psychotic Disorders, Social Functioning Schedule, and the various versions of the Social Adjustment Scale) measure a broad range of functioning without assessing symptoms. The social functioning scales from the Psychiatric Epidemiology Research Interview (Dohrenwend et al. 1983) and the Longitudinal Interval Follow-up Evaluation (Keller et al. 1987) were not included in either review and should be added to Group 7. The same is true for the Role Activity Performance Scale (Good-Ellis et al. 1987). All are applicable to a broad population. Almost all of them give global ratings, but, according to Wallace (1986), there is limited information on the psychometric properties of the CAS.

The interested reader is referred to the review articles and the original material in the literature for a more comprehensive assessment of these instruments. Our brief review focuses on the suitability of alternatives to the GAFS for inclusion in DSM-IV.

Given our criteria of unidimensionality, the instruments in Groups 3, 4, 6, and 7 should be considered as alternatives to the GAFS. Groups 3 and 4, however, cover too limited a domain of functioning, and Group 3 is also limited in its applicability. The CAS in Group 6 might also be eliminated because of limited psychometric data, leaving the instruments in Group 7. If the criterion of unidimensionality is de-emphasized, then Groups 1, 2, and 5 must also be considered. Group 1 is a weaker

Table 30–2. Assessing the measures of social adjustment and functioning

Group	Instruments	Inclusion of symptoms	Depth	Scoring	Applicable group	Psychometric characteristics	Other characteristics
1	DCMHQ, KDS-15	Yes	Not much depth DCMHO: gives little attention to role performance KDS-15: looks only at marriage	Give specific and more general scores	Highly specific DCMHG: designed only for mental health patients KDS-15: designed only for married couples	Reliable and valid	
2	KAS, PARS, PSS, PEF, CAPPS	Yes	Not much depth KSA: ignores many roles and does not discuss cause of problems PSS, PEF, CAPPS: does not discuss cause of problems	Give specific and more general scores PARS, PSS, PEF, CAPPS: give global rating	Generally applicable	Reliable and valid	KAS: short and simple, can be used with significant other PSS: flexible, includes probes, can be used with significant other

(continued)

Table 30–2. Assessing the measures of social adjustment and functioning (continued)

Group	Instruments	Inclusion of symptoms	Depth	Scoring	Applicable group	Psychometric characteristics	Other characteristics
3	REHAB, CLAS	No	Not much depth	Give specific and more general scores. REHAB: gives global rating	Highly specific. REHAB: designed only for institutionalized patients. CLAS: designed for individuals in residential care facility	Reliable and valid (CLAS should be further investigated)	REHAB: well explained, simple to use, easy to interpret
4	PRI, ISSI	No	Not much detail, look only at individual's support network	Give specific and more general scores	Generally applicable	Reliable and valid (PRI should be further investigated)	
5	SBAS, SAG	Yes	Very detailed	Give specific and more general scores	Generally applicable	Reliable and valid	SAG: self-report, short
6	CAS	No	Very detailed	Gives specific and more general scores; also gives a global rating	Generally applicable	Further investigation needed of reliability and validity	Self-report

| 7 | SSIAM, SIASM, CAPS, SSIFPD, SFS, SAS, SAS-SR, SAS-II, PERI, LIFE | No (except SSIAM) | Very detailed | Give specific and more general scores SSIAM: gives global rating SAS: gives global rating | Generally applicable | Reliable and valid | SSIAM: careful about interview bias, can be used with significant other SIASM, SSIFPD: can be used with significant other CAPS: for significant other SAS: flexible, can be given to significant other, self-report available, good with psychosis |

Note. PERI = Psychiatric Epidemiology Research Interview (Dohrenwend et al. 1983). LIFE = Longitudinal Interval Follow-Up Evaluation (Keller et al. 1987). For other abbreviations, see Table 30–1.

choice because of limitations in range of functioning and applicability, as well as lack of a global measure. Groups 2 and 5 include many meritorious measures of symptoms and functioning. In fact, the Global Assessment Scale, the basis of the GAFS, is derived from the work of some of the same investigators who developed the instruments in Group 2.

In terms of user-friendliness, global ratings are given by instruments in Groups 2, 3, 6, and 7. All of these ratings, however, are based on fairly extensive interview schedules or structured self-reports. On the one hand, their structured formats make them reliable and recommend them for use in research; on the other hand, none of these measures could be regarded as simple enough for routine use in clinical practice.

Discussion

The approach to change for DSM-IV has been characterized as "conservative," requiring compelling arguments and extensive documentation to support alterations in the nosology (Frances et al. 1990). Although our review suggests a number of problems with the current GAFS, there are problems with all of the existing potential alternatives as well. Before considering a complete change in Axis V, there should be evidence of severe problems with GAFS and/or an outstanding new alternative. Considerable experience with GAFS (and its predecessor, the Global Assessment Scale) and its apparent simplicity made it a choice for DSM-III-R and argue for its retention, but with some significant modification.

As noted, the principal limitations of the GAFS are 1) the combination of symptoms and functioning on a single scale and 2) the rating of functioning based on mental impairment alone, rather than the combined effect of mental and physical impairments.

The GAFS could be modified to separate the rating of symptoms and psychological functioning from the rating of social and occupational functioning. We propose a field test of a modification of the current Axis V GAFS. (See Table 30–3 for examples of the modified scales.) The current GAFS has been divided into two separate scales, one to measure global symptomatology and psychological functioning, the other to measure social and occupational functioning. The modified GAFS in Table 30–3 retains the same scale points and many of the anchoring descriptors that are used in the current GAFS. It is hypothesized that this change will reduce confusion and improve the independence of the ratings of these domains. This hypothesis, as well as the reliability of the measures, should be assessed in a field trial of the modified GAFS. The results of the field trial may indicate a need for more elaborate anchoring descriptors, which could be developed at that time.

If the modified GAFS (GAFS-M, shown in Table 30–3) proves to be more reliable, to produce ratings on social and occupational functioning that are significantly more independent of Axis I than current GAFS ratings, and to be more acceptable to clinicians who use it in the field trial, then the GAFS-M should be used as a substitute for the existing GAFS.

The GAFS-M measure of social and occupational functioning (GAFS-M functioning rating) is similar conceptually to the original DSM-III Axis V measure of adaptive functioning. The GAFS-M measure of global symptomatology and psychological functioning (GAFS-M symptom rating) would be a new assessment. It might be included as a second rating on Axis V or rated on a separate axis. It is likely that ratings on this measure will be correlated highly with Axis I. To some extent it also may be redundant with proposed inclusion of severity ratings for each mental disorder (J. E. Mezzich, personal communication, February 1990).

The instruments in Group 7 should be examined further as potential substitutes in the future, especially if there are problems with the GAFS or the GAFS-M. If warranted by further examination, there should be a field trial of the best global measure(s) from Group 7 for use in general clinical practice without a standardized schedule.

A simple modification in the instructions for rating the GAFS could address the other problem with Axis V. As noted, when assessing certain patients, it is difficult (or impossible) to separate the effects of mental from physical impairments contributing to limitations in social and occupational functioning. Axis V in DSM-III did not instruct the rater to make any such distinction. In contrast, the instructions to the GAFS explicitly call for a rating of limitations of functioning due to mental impairments alone. We propose a field test of a modification of the instructions to the GAFS-M (functioning) to assess social and occupational functioning due to the combined effects of mental and nonmental medical impairments.

Recommendations

The options under consideration by the Work Group on Multiaxial Issues include some combination of changes in the basic structure of the GAFS as well as in the instructions. Our reviews of the relevant literature have suggested both of these potential modifications, following a conservative strategy for change. The final decision should be based on a field test of these recommendations. It is our hope that these modest changes will increase the utility and use of Axis V.

Table 30–3. Scale for measuring social and occupational functioning only and scale for measuring psychological symptoms only

Scale for Measuring Social and Occupational Functioning Only

Consider social and occupational functioning on a hypothetical continuum of mental health-illness. Do not include impairment in functioning due to physical (or environmental) limitations.[a]

HIGHEST LEVEL OF FUNCTIONING PAST YEAR: the highest level of functioning for at least a few months during the past year.

Code	
90 | 81	Good functioning in all areas, interested and involved in a wide range of activities, socially effective.
80 | 71	No more than a slight impairment in social or occupational functioning (e.g., misses a few deadlines or appointments) or school functioning (e.g., temporarily falling behind in school work).
70 | 61	Some difficulty in social or occupational functioning (e.g., frequent work absences, work is occasionally incomplete or judged "not up to standards") or school functioning (e.g., occasional truancy, or theft within the household), but generally functioning pretty well, has some meaningful interpersonal relationships.
60 | 51	Moderate difficulty in social, occupational, or school functioning (e.g., few friends, conflicts with co-workers, unable to complete work assignments, unsatisfactory work performance).
50 | 41	Serious impairment in social, occupational, or school functioning (e.g., no friends, unable to keep a job at expected or prior level of performance).
40 | 31	Major impairment in several areas, such as work or school, family relations, judgment (e.g., avoids friends, neglects family, and is unable to work; child frequently beats up younger children and is failing at school).
30 | 21	Inability to function in almost all areas (e.g., stays in bed all day; no job, home, or friends).
20 | 11	Occasionally fails to maintain minimal personal hygiene (e.g., smears feces); unable to function independently.
10 | 01	Persistent inability to maintain minimal personal hygiene; unable to function without harming self or others or without considerable external support (e.g., nursing care and supervision).

(continued)

Table 30–3. Scale for measuring social and occupational functioning only and scale for measuring psychological symptoms only *(continued)*

Scale for Measuring Psychological Symptoms Only

Consider psychological symptoms and impairments on a hypothetical continuum of mental health–illness.

SYMPTOMS—IMPAIRMENT PAST MONTH: If very recent onset, use past week.

Code

Code	
90 | 81	Absent or minimal symptoms (e.g., mild anxiety before an exam), generally satisfied with life, no more than everyday problems or concerns.
80 | 71	If symptoms are present, they are transient and expectable reactions to psychosocial stressors (e.g., difficulty concentrating after family argument).
70 | 61	Some mild symptoms (e.g., depressed mood and mild insomnia).
60 | 51	Moderate symptoms (e.g., flat affect and circumstantial speech, occasional panic attacks).
50 | 41	Serious symptoms (e.g., suicidal ideation, severe obsessional rituals, frequent shoplifting).
40 | 31	Some impairment in reality testing or communication (e.g., speech is at times illogical, obscure, or irrelevant).
30 | 21	Behavior is considerably influenced by delusions or hallucinations, serious impairment in communication or judgment (e.g., sometimes incoherent, acts grossly inappropriately, suicidal preoccupation).
20 | 11	Some danger of hurting self or others (e.g., suicide attempts without clear expectation of death, frequently violent, manic excitement) or gross impairment in communication (e.g., largely incoherent or mute).
10 | 01	Persistent danger of severely hurting self or others (e.g., recurrent violence) or serious suicidal act with clear expectation of death.

[a]Another option would be to include impairment in functioning due to physical limitations as well as mental impairments.

Following a less conservative strategy for change, several other avenues of research and scale development are indicated. First, there is a need to study the impact of various approaches to training on the reliability of measures of social and occupational functioning. Second, our review suggests the need for different measures for different areas of functioning. The conservative strategy and requirement for simplicity, applicable to multiaxial diagnosis and DSM, may be overly limiting for valid and useful measurements of functioning. A more multidimensional approach to measuring social and occupational functioning in individuals with mental disorders may be superior. The existing research literature suggests numerous more complex measures. Further investigation may produce simpler measures of each of the multiple dimensions of functioning that could be used in practice as well as research.

Leaders in general medicine have called for the use of simple measures of functioning in routine clinical practice to support the need for measures of clinical outcome (Ellwood 1988; Schroeder 1987; Tarlov et al. 1989). Feinstein et al. (1986) warned of the problems associated with these needed measures, that they be "sensible" as well as reliable and valid. The current Medical Outcomes Study (Tarlov et al. 1989) has been using a "short form" measure of several dimensions of functioning and health status (Stewart et al. 1988) and has adapted it for use in assessing outcomes in a variety of clinical conditions, including depression (Stewart et al. 1989; Wells et al. 1989). The field of psychiatry has growing experience with functional assessment and the measurement of medical outcomes. We have the opportunity to be in the forefront of this important area of health care research and practice.

References

American Psychiatric Association: Diagnostic and Statistical Manual of Mental Disorders, 3rd Edition. Washington, DC, American Psychiatric Association, 1980

American Psychiatric Association: Diagnostic and Statistical Manual of Mental Disorders, 3rd Edition, Revised. Washington, DC, American Psychiatric Association, 1987

Anthony WA, Cohen BF: Functional assessment in psychiatric rehabilitation, in Functional Assessment in Rehabilitation. Edited by Halpern A, Fuhrer M. Baltimore, MD, Brookes, 1984, pp 79–100

Baker R, Hall JM: Rehabilitation Evaluation of Hall and Baker (REHAB). Aberdeen, Scotland, Vine Publishing Ltd, 1983

Beiser M, Fleming JAE, Iacono WG, et al: Refining the diagnosis of schizophreniform disorder. Am J Psychiatry 145:695–700, 1988

Bronheim H, Strain JJ, Biller HF, et al: Psychiatric consultation on an otolaryngology service. Gen Hosp Psychiatry 11:95–102, 1989

Burnes AJ, Rosen SR: Social roles and adaptation to the community. Community Ment Health J 3:153–158, 1967

Ciarlo JA, Reihman J: The Denver Community Mental Health Questionnaire: Development of a Multi-Dimensional Program Evaluation Instrument. Denver, CO, Denver Mental Health Systems Evaluation Project, Northwest Denver Mental Health Center and the University of Denver, 1975

Ciarlo JA, Reihman J: The Denver Community Health Questionnaire: development of a multi-dimensional program evaluation instrument, in Program Evaluation for Mental Health: Methods, Strategies, and Participants. Edited by Coursey R, Spector G, Murrell S, et al. New York, Grune & Stratton, 1977, pp 131–167

Clare AW, Cairns VE: Design, development and use of a standardized interview to assess social maladjustment and dysfunction in community studies. Psychol Med 8:589–604, 1978

Clare AW, Cairns VE: A Manual for Use in Conjunction With the General Practice Research Unit's Standardized Social Interview Schedule. London, England, Institute of Psychiatry, 1979

Clayton P, Hirschfeld R: Personal Resources Inventory (PRI). St. Louis, MO, Washington University School of Medicine, 1977

Dohrenwend BS, Dohrenwend BP, Link B, et al: Social functioning of psychiatric patients in contrast with community cases in the general population. Arch Gen Psychiatry 40:1174–1182, 1983

Duncan-Jones P, Henderson S: Interview Schedule for Social Interaction (ISSI), 10th Edition. Canberra, Australia, Social Psychiatry Research Unit, Australian National University, 1978

Ellwood P: Shattuck lecture: outcomes management. N Engl J Med 318:1549–1556, 1988

Ellsworth RB, Foster L, Childers B, et al: Hospital and community adjustment as perceived by psychiatric patients, their families, and staff. J Consult Clin Psychology 32:1–41, 1968

Endicott J, Spitzer RL: Current and Past Psychopathology Scales (CAPPS): rationale, reliability, and validity. Arch Gen Psychiatry 27:678–687, 1972a

Endicott J, Spitzer RL: What! another rating scale? the Psychiatric Evaluation Form. J Nerv Ment Dis 154:88–104, 1972b

Evanson RC, Sletten I, Hedlund J: CAPS: an automated evaluation system. Am J Psychiatry 131:531–534, 1974

Fabrega H Jr, Pilkonis P, Mezzich J, et al: Explaining diagnostic complexity in an inpatient setting. Compr Psychiatry 31:5–14, 1990

Feinstein A, Josephy B, Wells C: Scientific and clinical problems in indexes of functional disability. Ann Intern Med 105:413–420, 1986

Fernando T, Mellsop G, Nelson K, et al: The reliability of Axis V of DSM-III. Am J Psychiatry 143:752–755, 1986

Frances A, Pincus HA, Widiger T, et al: DSM-IV: work in progress. Am J Psychiatry 147:1439–1448, 1990

Good-Ellis M, Fine S, Spencer J, et al: Developing a role activity performance scale. American Journal of Occupational Therapy 41:232–241, 1987

Gordon RE, Gordon KK: Relating Axes IV and V of DSM-III to clinical severity of psychiatric disorders. Can J Psychiatry 32:423–424, 1987

Gordon RE, Vijay J, Slote SG, et al: Aggravating stress and functional level as predictors of length of psychiatric hospitalization. Hosp Community Psychiatry 36:773–774, 1985a

Gordon RE, Jardiolin P, Gordon KK: Predicting length of hospital stay of psychiatric patients. Am J Psychiatry 142:235–237, 1985b

Gordon RE, Plutzky M, Gordon KK, et al: Using the Axis V scale to evaluate therapeutic outcome of psychiatric treatment. Can J Psychiatry 33:194–196, 1988

Gurland B, Yorkston N, Stone A, et al: The Structured and Scaled Interview to Assess Maladjustment (SSIAM), I: description, rationale, and development. Arch Gen Psychiatry 27:259–264, 1962a

Gurland B, Yorkston N, Goldberg K, et al: The Structured Scaled Interview to Assess Maladjustment (SSIAM), II: factor analysis, reliability, validity. Arch Gen Psychiatry 27:264–267, 1962b

Henderson S, Duncan-Jones P, Byrne D. Measuring social relationships: the Interview for Social Interaction. Psychol Med 10:1–12, 1980

Katz MM, Lyerly SB: Methods for measuring adjustment social behavior in the community, I: rationale, description, discriminative validity and scale development. Psychol Rep 13:502–535, 1963

Keller M, Lavori P, Friedman B, et al: The Longitudinal Interval Follow-Up Evaluation. Arch Gen Psychiatry 44:540–548, 1987

Kupfer D, Frank E: The KDS-15: a marital questionnaire. Pittsburgh, PA, Western Psychiatric Institute and Clinic, University of Pittsburgh, 1974

Liberman RP: Psychiatric Symptoms and the Functional Capacity to Work: Final Report (Social Security Administration Research Grant No 10-P-98193). Los Angeles, CA, Department of Psychiatry and Brentwood VA Medical Center, University of California at Los Angeles, 1990

Mellsop G, Peace K, Fernando T: Pre-admission adaptive functioning as a measure of prognosis in psychiatric inpatients. Aust N Z J Psychiatry 21:539–544, 1987

Mezzich AC, Mezzich JE, Coffman GA: Reliability of DSM-III vs DSM-II in child psychopathology. Journal of the American Academy of Child Psychiatry 23:273–280, 1985

Mezzich JE, Evancuk KJ, Mathias RJ, et al: Admission decisions and multiaxial diagnosis. Arch Gen Psychiatry 41:1001–1004, 1984

Mezzich JE, Fabrega H Jr, Coffman GA: Multiaxial characterization of depressive patients. J Nerv Ment Dis 175:339–345, 1987

Platt S, Weyman A, Hirsch S, et al: The Social Behavior Assessment Schedule (SBAS): rationale, content scoring and reliability of new interview schedule. Social Psychiatry 15:43–55, 1980

Remington M, Tyrer P: The Social Functioning Schedule: a brief semi-structured interview. Social Psychiatry 14:151–157, 1979

Rey JM, Plapp JM, Stewart G, et al: Reliability of the psychosocial axes of DSM-III in an adolescent population. Br J Psychiatry 150:228–234, 1987

Rey JM, Stewart GW, Plapp JM, et al: Validity of Axis V of DSM-III and other measures of adaptive functioning. Acta Psychiatr Scand 77:534–542, 1988

Russell AT, Cantwell DP, Mattison R, et al: A comparison of DSM-II and DSM-III in the diagnosis of childhood psychiatric disorders: multiaxial features. Arch Gen Psychiatry 36:1223–1226, 1979

Schooler N, Hogarty G, Weissman MM: Social Adjustment Scale II (SAS II), in Resource Materials for Community Health Program Evaluators (HEW Publ No ADM-79-328). Edited by Hargreaves WA, Attkisson CC, Sorenson JE. Washington, DC, U.S. Government Printing Office, 1979, pp 290–330

Schrader G, Gordon M, Harcourt R: The usefulness of DSM-III Axis IV and Axis V assessments. Am J Psychiatry 143:904–907, 1986

Schroeder S: Outcome assessment 70 years later: are we ready? N Engl J Med 316:160–162, 1987

Serban G. Social Stress and Functioning Inventory for Psychotic Disorders (SSFIPD): measurement and prediction of schizophrenics' community adjustment. Compr Psychiatry 19:337–347, 1978

Skodol AE, Link BG, Shrout PE, et al: Toward construct validity for DSM-III Axis V. Psychiatry Res 24:13–23, 1988a

Skodol AE, Link BG, Shrout PE, et al: The revision of Axis V in DSM-III-R: should symptoms have been included? Am J Psychiatry 145:825–829, 1988b

Spitzer RL, Forman JB: DSM-III field trials, II: initial experience with the multiaxial system. Am J Psychiatry 143:752–755, 1986

Spitzer RL, Endicott J, Fleiss J, et al: The Psychiatric Status Schedule: a technique for evaluating psychopathology and impairment in role functioning. Arch Gen Psychiatry 23:41–55, 1970

Spitzer RL, Gibbon M, Endicott J: Global Assessment Scale. New York, New York State Department of Mental Health, 1973

Stewart A, Hays R, Ware J: The MOS Short-Form General Health Survey. Med Care 26:724–735, 1988

Stewart A, Greenfield S, Hays R, et al: Functional status and well-being of patients with chronic conditions. JAMA 262:907–913, 1989

Strauss JS, Carpenter WT Jr: Prediction of outcome in schizophrenia, II: relationships between predictor and outcome variables: a report from the WHO International Pilot Study of Schizophrenia. Arch Gen Psychiatry 31:37–42, 1974

Strauss JS, Carpenter WT Jr: Prediction of outcome in schizophrenia, III: five-year outcome and its predictors. Arch Gen Psychiatry 34:159–163, 1977

Tarlov A, Ware J, Greenfield S, et al: The Medical Outcomes Study. JAMA 262:925–930, 1989

Trzepacz PT, Brenner R, Van Thiel DH: A psychiatric study of 247 liver transplantation candidates. Psychosomatics 30:147–153, 1989

Wallace CJ: Functional assessment in rehabilitation. Schizophr Bull 12:604–624, 1986

Weissman M, Bothwell S: Assessment of social adjustment by patient self-report. Arch Gen Psychiatry 33:1111–1115, 1976

Weissman MM, Sholomskas D, John K: The assessment of social adjustment, an update. Arch Gen Psychiatry 38:1250–1258, 1981

Wells K, Stewart A, Hays R, et al: The functioning and well-being of depressed patients. JAMA 262:914–919, 1989

Westermeyer J: DSM-III psychiatric disorders among refugees in the United States: a point prevalence study. Am J Psychiatry 143:197–202, 1986

Westermeyer J, Neider J: Social networks and psychopathology among substance abusers. Am J Psychiatry 145:1265–1269, 1988

Willer BS, Biggen P: Comparison of rehospitalized and nonrehospitalized psychiatric patients on community adjustment: self assessment guide. Psychiatry 39:239–244, 1976

Willer BS, Gustafero JR: Development of a computer-assisted record for psychiatry, in Goal Attainment Review, Vol 1. Edited by Garwick G. Minneapolis, MN, Program Evaluation Resource Center, 1974

Willer BS, Gustafero JR: Community Living Assessment Scale. Buffalo, NY, Transitional Services, 1985

Chapter 31

Patterns of Course of Illness

Juan E. Mezzich, M.D., Ph.D., and
Miguel R. Jorge, M.D., Ph.D.

Statement and Significance of the Issues

Standard psychopathological diagnosis has focused on symptomatological descriptions. More recently, interest has also been shown in considering the course of illness for a fuller diagnostic characterization. Some studies, such as that of F. Summers and Hersh (1983), have suggested that the diagnosis of chronicity is more crucial for the understanding of severe emotional disorders than the traditional symptom-based classification systems.

The two most important systems used to classify mental disorders—DSM-III-R (American Psychiatric Association 1987) and ICD-9 (World Health Organization 1978)—are based on symptom patterns. The DSM system includes some references to time-frame variables within the two axes on psychiatric disorders. However, no systematic assessment of course is provided across diagnoses.

One way to deal explicitly with the diagnostic delineation of course of illness corresponds to the multiaxial approach. This approach, as an alternative to the traditional single-label diagnostic model, summarizes the patient's condition in terms of several variables or axes that are thought to have high information value and are conceptualized and rated quasi-independently from each other (e.g., American Psychiatric Association 1980; Essen-Moller and Wohlfahrt 1947; Helmchen 1975; Leme Lopes 1954; Mogensen et al. 1986; Ottoson and Perris 1973; Rutter et al. 1975; Strauss 1975; Von Cranach 1977; L. Wing 1970).

A comparative synopsis of the time-frame variables covered in five multiaxial systems (Helmchen 1975; Mogensen et al. 1986; Ottoson and Perris 1973; Strauss 1975; Von Cranach 1977) is presented in Table 31–1. It can be seen that duration and episodicity are the only two variables included in all five multiaxial schemes. Progression and mode of onset come next, being listed in three of the five schemes.

Age at onset is mentioned only in Helmchen's system, which was proposed primarily for schizophrenic patients.

Also supporting the diagnostic importance of course of illness and the pertinence of the multiaxial approach for articulating it was an international consultation on multiaxial diagnosis sponsored by the World Psychiatric Association (Mezzich et al. 1985) that involved 175 expert diagnosticians from 52 countries. In this study, a list of 21 potential axes was presented to the participants who judged their value for four diagnostic purposes: describing the clinical condition, making treatment decisions, predicting illness outcome, and advancing theoretical development. The study showed that the five best-ranked axes for all purposes were psychopathological syndromes, personality disorders, physical disorders, episodicity/progression, and duration of illness. For specifically predicting illness outcome, episodicity/progression and duration of illness, along with psychiatric syndromes, had the highest score.

These indications of the importance of course of illness for a comprehensive diagnosis created interest in the possible inclusion of a systematic rating of course in DSM-IV. In this chapter, we review the psychiatric literature and DSM-III-R to elucidate patterns of course of illness and suggest options for incorporation in DSM-IV.

Method

For both the literature review and the analysis of DSM-III-R, the first step was to identify and define the key time-frame variables underlying the concept of course of illness. Five terms were chosen to represent this domain:

Table 31–1. Time-frame variables considered in published multiaxial systems

Multiaxial systems	Age at onset	Mode of onset	Duration	Episodicity	Progression
Otosson and Perris 1973			X	X	X
Helmchen 1975	X	X	X	X	X
Strauss 1975			X	X	
Von Cranach 1977		X	X	X	
Mogensen et al. 1986		X	X	X	X

1. *Age at onset* of the first manifestation of psychiatric disorder.
2. *Mode of onset* (e.g., abrupt or insidious) of the psychiatric disorder.
3. *Duration* or *chronicity,* referring to the period from the emergence of manifestations of the psychiatric disorder to the present.
4. *Episodicity,* referring to the presence of distinct periods of illness separated by intervals either free of symptoms or with clearly contrasting psychopathology (e.g., manic and depressive).
5. *Progression,* describing the general trend of the disorder over time (e.g., stationary, worsening, improving).

We conducted a Medline search in seven languages (English, French, German, Italian, Portuguese, Russian, and Spanish) for the period from 1970 to August 1989. For each of the time-frame variables listed, we searched for the intersection of the following key-word sets:

- *mental* or *psychiatric* or *psychopathological* and
- *illness* or *disorder* or *disease* or *syndrome* and
- *diagnosis* or *epidemiology.*

The manual search of the international literature comprised the following 11 journals from 1984 to 1989: *Acta Psiquiátrica y Psicológica de América Latina, Acta Psychiatrica Scandinavica, Annales Médico-Psychologiques, American Journal of Psychiatry, Archives of General Psychiatry, British Journal of Psychiatry, Canadian Journal of Psychiatry, Comprehensive Psychiatry, Journal of Nervous and Mental Disease, Psychological Medicine,* and *Psychopathology.*

The search identified 562 papers that were then processed through the following three consecutive selection steps: reading of the title, the abstract, and the whole paper. Through this process, 75 papers were finally selected that were clearly pertinent to course of illness. They were divided into two categories: overview and empirical papers. Each overview was cataloged by the diagnoses of its target population and the time-frame variables covered. The empirical studies were cataloged by country, target population (number and age of subjects), diagnostic system and evaluation instrument used, and diagnoses and time-frame variables covered.

Diagnostic systems were carefully inspected to identify references to key time-frame variables. The examination focused on the diagnostic criteria of the various DSM-III-R disorders, first in general and then with specific attention to subtyping rules.

Results

General Analysis of Course of Illness

Overview and empirical papers. The 75 papers we selected came from several countries and continents and were published in 23 different journals. Half of the papers appeared in the following four periodicals: *Acta Psychiatrica Scandinavica, American Journal of Psychiatry, Archives of General Psychiatry,* and the *British Journal of Psychiatry.*

Table 31–2 lists the 16 overview papers pertinent to course of illness; Table 31–3 lists the 59 empirical investigations of the topic. Most of the papers selected (67 of 75) were published after 1983, and 60% of the overview articles appeared during the period 1986–1989. The majority of the papers referred to schizophrenia and affective diagnoses. Most of the articles dealt with more than one time-frame

Table 31–2. Overview papers on course of illness

Study	Population diagnoses	Time-frame variables[a]
Mezzich 1979	Mental disorders	A,M,D,E
Zubin et al. 1983	Schizophrenia	E,P
Ciompi 1984	Schizophrenia-like psychotic phenomena	A,M,E
Petho 1984	Endogenous psychoses	E
Lipkowitz and Idupuganti 1985	Schizophrenia	A,M,D
Reich 1986	Anxiety disorders	A,D
Egeland et al. 1987	Major affective disorder	A
Kocsis and Frances 1987	Chronic depression	A,M,D
Alexopoulos et al. 1988	Depression	A,E
Angermeyer and Kuhn 1988	Schizophrenia, other functional psychosis	A,M
Galasko et al. 1988	Psychosis, depression	A
Lin and Kleinman 1988	Schizophrenia	M,D,P
Post et al. 1988	Affective disorder	A,D,E,P
Scott 1988	Chronic depression	D
Yassa et al. 1988	Bipolar disorder	A
Kendler et al. 1989	Psychotic disorders	A,D

[a] A = Age at onset. M = Mode of onset. D = Duration. E = Episodicity. P = Progression.

variable: 53 with age at onset, 20 with mode of onset, 43 with duration, 27 with episodicity, and 12 with progression.

The empirical studies (Table 31–3) were mostly conducted in industrialized countries, half of them in the United States. Although not all papers identified precisely the age of the study population, those that did covered children, adolescents, adults, and geriatric patients as groups. The diagnostic systems most frequently used were the DSM in 29 of 59 empirical studies, the Research Diagnostic Criteria (Spitzer et al. 1978) in 13 studies, the ICD in 11 studies, and the Feighner criteria (Feighner et al. 1972) in 6 studies. Interestingly, almost half of the studies using the DSM diagnostic system were done outside the United States. The two diagnostic assessment instruments used most were the Schedule for Affective Disorders and Schizophrenia (Endicott and Spitzer 1978) in 10 studies and the Present State Examination (J. K. Wing et al. 1974) in 6 studies.

DSM-III-R. From all 17 broad categories in DSM-III-R, only 2 (factitious disorders and psychological factors affecting physical condition) do not use any of the selected time-frame variables. None of the broad categories used all five variables but 2 (organic mental syndromes and child-onset disorders) used four variables and another 10 broad categories used more than one variable. Considering specific disorders (first 4-digit code), 204 (87%) of them used at least one time-frame variable in the diagnostic criteria, and 17 used it for subtyping.

Analysis of the Literature and the DSM-III-R by Individual Variables

Age at onset. Table 31–4 shows results of the analyses of the literature on age at onset. Of the papers reviewed, 70% dealt with age at onset. These papers tended to assess this variable as early versus late onset, and there was great variability in the cutoff point used across diagnostic categories. Table 31–5 shows the consideration of age at onset in DSM-III-R. The DSM-III-R diagnostic criteria for 68 disorders in five broad categories mention age at onset. More specifically, age at onset was used for subtyping purposes for the following disorders: autistic disorder, primary degenerative dementia of the Alzheimer type, schizophrenia, and dysthymia.

Mode of onset. Table 31–6 shows that mode of onset was mentioned in only 20 of the 75 papers reviewed. In most cases, the terms used were *acute* versus *insidious* onset. The small number of papers that defined cutoff points for individual diagnoses would not allow determination of consistent patterns even for the two categories most frequently considered: schizophrenia and affective disorders.

The review of the DSM-III-R presented in Table 31–7 indicates that mode of

Table 31–3. Empirical studies dealing with course of illness

Study	Country	N	Age	Diagnosis	Diagnostic system (Sys) and instrument (Ins)	Time-frame variables[a]
Murphy and Raman 1971	Mauritius	90	> 14	Schizophrenia		E
Kurashov 1972	USSR	56		Schizophrenia and affective disorders		A,M,D,E
Nuller et al. 1972	USSR	75		Manic-depressive psychoses		A,D,E
Angst et al. 1973	Canada, Denmark, Germany, Switzerland, Czechoslovakia	1,027		Monopolar depression and bipolar psychoses	Sys: ICD	A,D,E
Diebold and Haveisen 1978	Germany	152		Schizophrenia, endogenous depression, and psychopathia		A,D
Kulhara and Wig 1978	India	100	15–60	Schizophrenia	Sys: Schneider	E,P
Bovet 1980	Canada	1,116	> 15	Mental disorders		D
Akiskal et al. 1983	United States	82		Depressive illness	Sys: Feighner	A,D,E

Study	Country	N	Age	Diagnosis	System/Instrument	Codes
Armbruster et al. 1983	Germany	113		Schizoaffective, schizophreniform, and cycloid psychoses	Sys: Schneider, Kasanin, RDC, Retterstol, Angst, Leonard/Perris	M
Retterstol 1983	Norway	301		Paranoid psychoses		A,M,D,P
W. K. Summers 1983	United States	2	> 69	Mania	Sys: Feighner	A
F. Summers and Hersh 1983	United States	295	Mean, 33–37	Schizophrenia	Sys: DSM-III	D
Coryell et al. 1984	United States	354	Mean, 32–41	Depression	Sys: RDC Ins: SADS	P
Dube et al. 1984	India	140	15–44	Schizophrenia, manic-depressive psychosis, and psychoneurosis	Sys: ICD-8 Ins: PSE	E
Jonsson and Nyman 1984	Sweden	110		Schizophrenia		A,M,D,E
Joyce 1984	New Zealand	200		Bipolar affective disorder	Sys: DSM-III	A
Kovacs et al. 1984	United States	114	8–13	Depressive disorders	Sys: DSM-III Ins: ISC	A,D
Loranger 1984	United States	200		Schizophrenia	Sys: DSM-III	A
Atkinson et al. 1985	United States	36	53–76	Alcoholism	Ins: MacAndrew Scale	A
Ciompi 1985	Switzerland	289	> 65	Schizophrenia	Sys: Feighner, DSM-III	A,M,E

(continued)

Table 31–3. Empirical studies dealing with course of illness *(continued)*

Study	Country	N	Age	Diagnosis	Diagnostic system (Sys) and instrument (Ins)	Time-frame variables[a]
Eagles and Whalley 1985	Scotland		All	Affective disorder	Sys: ICD-8	A
Lee and Diclimente 1985	United States	70	Mean, 23–42	Problem drinking	Sys: DSM-III	A,D
Maj 1985	Sweden	94	23–51	Schizoaffective disorders and major affective disorders	Sys: RDC	A,D,E
Roy-Byrne et al. 1985	United States	95	19–69	Affective illness	Sys: RDC, DSM-III	A,D,E
Thyer et al. 1985	United States	423	Adults	Anxiety disorders	Sys: DSM-III	A
Young and Grabler 1985	United States	11	20–69	Depression	Sys: RDC Ins: SADS	A,M
Ambelas and George 1986	England	20		Mania	Sys: Feighner	A,E
Breier et al. 1986	United States	60	18–65	Agoraphobia and panic disorder	Sys: RDC, DSM-III Ins: SADS-L	A,M,D,E
Coryell and Tsuang 1986	United States	328	Mean, 54–62	Schizophreniform disorder and schizophrenia	Sys: Feighner, DSM-III	D

Patterns of Course of Illness

Hirschfeld et al. 1986	United States	38		Major depressive disorder	Sys: RDC Ins: SADS, LIFE	A,M,D,E
Keller et al. 1986	United States	101	Mean, 39–42	Nonbipolar major depressive disorder	Sys: RDC Ins: SADS, LIFE	D,E
Jonsson and Nyman 1986	Sweden	54	Mean, 38	Schizophrenia		A,M,D,P
Leon 1986	Colombia	76	15–44	Schizophrenia	Sys: ICD-8, ICD-9 Ins: PSE	A,M,D,E,P
McGlashan 1986	United States	163	16–55	Schizophrenia	Sys: New Haven, Feighner, DSM-III	A,M,D
Rabiner et al. 1986	United States	64	Mean, 23–28	Functional psychosis	Sys: RDC Ins: SADS, SCL–90, SADS-C, SADS-L	D
Fahndrich and Wirtz 1987	Germany	34		Affective psychoses	Sys: ICD-8	A,D
Huff et al. 1987	United States	165	Mean, 68	Alzheimer's disease		A,D,P
Makanjuola and Adepapo 1987	Nigeria	116	Mean, 27–33	Schizophrenia and schizophreniform disorders	Sys: DSM-III Ins: PSE, BPRS	A,D
Smeraldi et al. 1987	Italy, Sweden	525		Affective disorder	Sys: DSM-III, ICD-8	A

(continued)

Table 31–3. Empirical studies dealing with course of illness *(continued)*

Study	Country	N	Age	Diagnosis	Diagnostic system (Sys) and instrument (Ins)	Time-frame variables[a]
Asarnow and Ben-Meir 1988	United States	66	7–13	Schizophrenia spectrum and depressive disorders	Sys: DSM-III Ins: SADS-Children Camberwell	M
Bland et al. 1988	Canada	3,258	> 17	Mental disorders	Sys: DSM-III Ins: DIS	A
Christie et al. 1988	United States	18,572	> 17	Anxiety disorder, major depression, and substance use disorder	Sys: DSM-III Ins: DIS	A
Craig and Bregman 1988	United States	32	> 64	Schizophrenia-like illness	Sys: DSM-III	A,D
Hwu et al. 1988	China	127		Schizophrenia	Sys: ICD-9, DSM-III Ins: PSE	A,M,D,E
Maj 1988	Italy	120	22–54	Cycloid psychotic, affective and schizoaffective disorders	Sys: Perris/Brockington, RDC, DSM-III, ICD-9 Ins: CPRS	A,E
Marneros et al. 1988	Germany	72		Schizoaffective disorders	Sys: DSM-III-R Ins: PSE	A,D,E
McFarlane 1988	Australia	315	Mean, 35	Posttraumatic morbidity	Sys: GHQ-case Ins: GHQ	M,D

Study	Country	N	Age	Disorder	Instruments	Codes
McGlashan 1988	United States	66		Mania	Sys: DSM-III	A,D
Miklowitz et al. 1988	United States	23	18–30	Bipolar affective disorder	Sys: RDC, DSM-III	A,D,E
Opjordsmoen 1988	Norway	126		Delusional disorders	Sys: RDC, DSM-III, ICD-9, Kendler Ins: SADS-L	D
Sorensen et al. 1988	United States	497	18–69	Paranoid behavior	Ins: PIP	D
Watkins et al. 1988	United States	18	Children	Schizophrenia	Sys: DSM-III Ins: DSM-III, SRS, ACBC	A
Buydens-Branchey et al. 1989	United States	218	25–60	Alcoholism	Sys: DSM-III Ins: SCID, SADS	A,D
Hasin et al. 1989	United States	127		Major affective syndromes and alcoholism	Sys: RDC Ins: SADS	D
Lehmkuhl et al. 1989	Germany	93	5–19	Conversion disorder	Sys: DSM-III	A,D,P
Munk-Jorgensen and Mortensen 1989	Denmark	53	> 14	Schizophrenia	Sys: ICD-8, DSM-III, Bleuler, Schneider Ins: PSE	A,D
Robert et al. 1989	France	383		Psychoses	Sys: DSM-III	P

(continued)

Table 31–3. Empirical studies dealing with course of illness *(continued)*

Study	Country	N	Age	Diagnosis	Diagnostic system (Sys) and instrument (Ins)	Time-frame variables[a]
Robinson 1989	England	153	49–93	Organic brain syndrome, depressive illness, personality disorder, and schizophrenia		P

Note. RDC = Research Diagnostic Criteria. SADS = Schedule for Affective Disorders and Schizophrenia. PSE = Present State Examination. SADS-L = Schedule for Affective Disorders and Schizophrenia—Lifetime. LIFE = Longitudinal Interval Follow-Up Examination. SCL–90 = Symptom Checklist–90. BPRS = Brief Psychiatric Rating Scale. DIS = Diagnostic Interview Schedule. CPRS = Comprehensive Psychopathological Rating Scale. GHQ = General Health Questionnaire. PIP = Psychotic Inpatient Profile. SRS = Symptom Rating Scale. ACBC = Achenbach Child Behavior Checklist. SCID = Structured Clinical Interview for DSM-III.
[a]E = episodicity. A = age at onset. M = mode of onset. D = duration. P = progression.

onset was mentioned only in four broad categories (63 of 234 specific disorders), and for subtyping it was used only for posttraumatic stress disorder.

Duration. Table 31–8 shows that duration appeared in 43 (57%) of the papers reviewed. The DSM-III-R review in Table 31–9 shows duration mentioned in 101 specific disorders corresponding to 13 of the 17 DSM-III-R broad diagnostic categories. For subtyping purposes, it was used only for schizophrenia and major depression. Both tables show that, for most diagnoses, duration was dichotomized as short versus chronic. Across diagnostic categories, the most frequent cutoff points were 6 months and 2 years.

Episodicity. The literature review (Table 31–10) indicated that episodicity appeared in 27 papers. In 55% of them, a specific scale or categorization was given for

Table 31–4. Literature review on age at onset

Disorder	Early or late onset specified (N)	Cut-off age (years)	n	%
Schizophrenia	8	Not specified	4	50.0
		24	1	12.5
		25	1	12.5
		45	2	25.0
Affective disorders	17	Not specified	9	53.0
		20	2	11.7
		21	1	5.9
		25	1	5.9
		30	1	5.9
		45	2	11.7
		50	1	5.9
Other psychotic disorders	2	Not specified	0	
		30	1	50
		45	1	50
Neurotic disorders	3	Not specified	2	66.7
		20	1	33.3
Substance use disorders	5	Not specified	0	
		20	4	80
		40	1	20
Other disorders	2			
In general				
Scale unspecified: 23 papers (43.4%)				
Early- or late-onset specification: 30 papers (56.6%)				

Table 31–5. Consideration of age at onset in DSM-III-R

Disorder	Term (age in years)	Specific categories
A. Used in the diagnostic criteria of core disorders		
Disorders usually first evident in infancy, childhood, or adolescence		46
Mental retardation	Before age 18	4
Autistic disorder	Infancy or childhood	1
Attention-deficit/hyperactivity disorder	Before age 7	1
Separation anxiety disorder	Before age 18	1
Avoidant disorder of childhood or adolescence	At least age 2.5	1
Gender identity disorders	Reached puberty or not	3
Tic disorders	Before age 21	3
Elimination disorders	At least age 4 or 5	2
Reactive attachment disorder of infancy or early childhood	Before age 5	1
Without particular specification		29
Organic mental syndromes and disorders		8
Primary degenerative dementia of the Alzheimer type	Before or after age 65	6
Senile dementia not otherwise specified	After age 65	1
Presenile dementia not otherwise specified	Before age 65	1
Somatoform disorders		1
Somatization disorder	Before age 30	1
Sexual disorders		1
Pedophilia	At least age 16	1
Personality disorders	Early adulthood/ before age 15	12
Total		68
B. Used for subtyping		
Disorders usually first evident in infancy, childhood, or adolescence		
Autistic disorder: specify if childhood onset (after 36 months)		
Organic mental disorders		
Primary degenerative dementia of the Alzheimer type:		
senile onset (after 65)		
presenile onset (age 65 and below)		
Schizophrenia		
Schizophrenia: specify if late onset (after age 45)		
Mood disorders		
Dysthymia: specify early onset (before age 21) or late onset (age 21 or later)		

Table 31–6. Literature review on mode of onset

Disorder	Acute or insidious specified (N)	Cut-off point (age)	n	%
Schizophrenia	12	Not specified	9	75
		1 month	1	8.3
		1 year	1	8.3
		1–5 years	1	8.3
Affective disorders	5	Not specified	3	60
		2–4 weeks	1	20
		1–5 years	1	20
Other disorders	4			

In general
  Scale unspecified: 1 paper (5%)
  Acute or insidious onset specification: 17 papers (85%)
  Other specification : 2 papers (10%)

this variable; in most of these cases, it was formulated as episodic versus continuous.

DSM-III-R (Table 31–11) contains 39 specific disorders corresponding to 7 broad categories for which episodicity was mentioned in the diagnostic criteria. For subtyping, episodicity was used only for transient tic disorder, major depression, and conversion disorder. Throughout DSM-III-R, the episodicity terms most frequently used were *recurrent* and *persistent*.

Progression. The general literature (Table 31–12) shows that 12 of the 75 papers dealt with the concept of progression. By far the most frequent specification of this concept was in terms of the trichotomy worsening/stable/improving. Progression was mentioned with regard to several psychiatric disorders, particularly schizophrenia, affective disorder, and other psychotic and organic disorders.

Table 31–13 indicates that schizophrenia was the only DSM-III-R broad category specifically dealing with progression. Progression was used for subtyping in two ways: to refer to the acute exacerbation of a chronic or subchronic form, and to refer to a stable specification of paranoid schizophrenia.

Discussion

The review of the international psychiatric literature and of DSM-III-R provided considerable evidence for the interest in course of illness. Five specific variables underlying course were identified and used throughout the review (i.e., age at onset, mode of onset, duration, episodicity, and progression).

Table 31–7. Consideration of mode of onset in DSM-III-R

Disorder	Term	Specific categories
A. Used in the diagnostic criteria for core disorders		
Organic mental syndromes and disorders		51
Primary degenerative dementia of the Alzheimer type	Insidious onset	6
Psychoactive substance-induced organic mental disorder	Shortly following	45
Psychotic disorders not elsewhere classified		1
Brief reactive psychosis	Shortly after events	1
Dissociative disorders		2
Psychogenic fugue	Sudden	1
Psychogenic amnesia	Sudden	1
Adjustment disorder		9
Adjustment disorder	Within 3 months of onset of stressor	9
Total		63

B. Used for subtyping
Anxiety disorders
  Posttraumatic stress disorder: specifically if delayed onset (at least 6 months after the trauma)

Age at onset was frequently considered in the course of illness literature and in DSM-III-R, but its specification varied greatly across syndromes.

Mode of onset was considered in a small number of literature papers and in some DSM-III-R categories. It was often formulated as acute versus insidious, but specific definitions or cutoff points were rarely presented.

Duration was the course variable most frequently considered in both the literature and DSM-III-R. The most frequent cutoff points used were 6 months and 2 years. Consequently, it appears that three duration classes defined by these cutoff points could be used to scale this variable across diagnostic categories.

Episodicity was mentioned in a relatively sizable number of literature papers and DSM-III-R categories. Most frequently this variable was dichotomized as single episode or continuous versus recurrent or episodic.

Progression was the course variable least frequently considered in both the general literature and DSM-III-R. Its most encompassing formulation involved the trichotomy worsening/stable/improving. This trichotomy may also incorporate

Table 31–8. Literature review on duration

Disorder	Short or chronic specified (N)	Specification in time	n	%
Schizophrenia	10	Not specified	4	40
		6–12 months	1	10
		1 year	1	10
		2 years	1	10
		3 years	1	10
		Various	2	20
Affective disorders	9	Not specified	3	33.3
		2–6 months	1	11.1
		6 months	1	11.1
		2 years	4	44.5
Other psychotic disorders	3	Not specified	2	66.7
		6 months	1	33.3
Substance use disorders	2	Not specified	0	
		6 months	1	50
		10 years	1	50
Neurotic disorders	2	Not specified	2	100
Other disorders	3			

In general
  Scale unspecified: 17 papers (39.5%)
  Short or chronic specification: 22 papers (51.2%)
  Other specification: 4 papers (9.3%)

two other progression concepts: acute exacerbation may be included under worsening, and recovery may be housed under improving. In this way, the two concepts lose the sharp edges associated with episodicity and incorporate a connotation of gradualness that is in line with progression.

It appears that there could be two ways to include course variables in DSM-IV: through an additional diagnostic character across diagnostic categories, and considering course patterns disorder by disorder, either by defining formal course subtypes or through comments in the text.

Additional Diagnostic Character Across Diagnostic Categories

Given the frequency of interest in duration and the reasonably clear three-class scale that could be used uniformly across diagnostic categories, it appears that duration would be the most appropriate course variable to be considered in an additional diagnostic character. The three classes would be: less than 6 months, between 6 months and 2 years, and more than 2 years.

Table 31–9. Consideration of duration in DSM-III-R

Disorder	Term	Specific categories
A. Used in the diagnostic criteria of core disorders		
Disorders usually first evident in infancy, childhood, or adolescence		18
Disruptive behavior disorders	At least 6 months	5
Anxiety disorders of childhood or adolescence	At least 2 weeks/ 6 months or longer	3
Bulimia nervosa	At least 3 months	1
Pica	At least 1 month	1
Rumination disorder of infancy	At least 1 month	1
Transsexualism	At least 2 years	1
Gender identity disorder of adolescence or adulthood, nontranssexual type	At least 2 years	1
Tic disorder	More than 1 year / At least 2 weeks / No longer than 12 months	3
Functional encopresis	At least 6 months	1
Identity disorder	At least 3 months	1
Organic mental syndromes and disorders		5
Dementia associated with alcoholism	At least 3 weeks	1
Amphetamine or similar withdrawal	More than 24 hours	1
Cocaine withdrawal	More than 24 hours	1
Hallucinogen mood disorder	More than 24 hours	1
Phencyclidine or similar mood disorder	More than 24 hours	1
Psychoactive substance use disorder	At least 1-month long period of time	22
Schizophrenia	At least 6 months	5
Delusional disorder	At least 1 month	1
Psychotic disorder not elsewhere classified		3
Brief reactive psychosis	From few hours to 1 month	1
Schizophreniform disorder	Lasts less than 6 months	1
Schizoaffective disorder	At least 2 weeks	1
Mood disorders		6
Bipolar disorder, depressed	2-week period	1
Bipolar disorder not otherwise specified	2-week period	1
Major depression, single episode	2-week period	1
Major depression, recurrent	2-week period	1
Cyclothymia	At least 2 years/1 year	1
Dysthymia (or depressive neurosis)	At least 2 years/1 year	1

(continued)

Table 31–9. Consideration of duration in DSM-III-R *(continued)*

Disorder	Term	Specific categories
Anxiety disorders		3
Panic disorder	4-week period	2
	At least 1 month	
Posttraumatic stress disorder	At least 1 month	1
Somatoform disorders		1
Multiple personality disorder	Enduring pattern	1
Sexual disorders		9
Paraphilias	At least 6 months	9
Sleep disorders		7
Insomnia disorders	At least 1 month	3
Hypersomnia disorders	At least 1 month	4
Adjustment disorders	No longer than 6 months	9
Personality disorders	Long-term functioning	12
Total		101

B. Used for subtyping

Schizophrenia
  Subchronic (less than 2 years, but at least 6 months)
  Chronic (more than 2 years)

Mood disorders
  Major depression: specifically if chronic (has lasted 2 consecutive years)

Table 31–10. Literature review on episodicity

Disorder	Episodic or continuous specified (N)	Papers where number of episodes are specified	
		n	%
Schizophrenia	9	2	22.2
Affective disorders	6	1	16.7
Other disorders	3		

In general
  Scale unspecified: 12 papers (44.4%)
  Episodic or continuous specification: 15 papers (55.6%)

Table 31–11. Consideration of episodicity in DSM-III-R

Disorder	Term	Specific categories
A. Used in the diagnostic criteria of core disorders		
Disorders usually first evident in infancy, childhood, or adolescence		5
Bulimia nervosa	Recurrent/persistent	1
Gender identity disorder	Persistent/recurrent	3
Elective mutism	Persistent	1
Organic mental syndromes and disorders		11
Organic hallucinosis	Persistent or recurrent	3
Organic mood disorder	Persistent	4
Organic anxiety disorder	Recurrent	2
Organic personality syndrome	Persistent	2
Mood disorders		3
Cyclothymia	Numerous episodes and periods	1
Bipolar disorder not otherwise specified	At least one hypomanic episode and one major depressive episode	1
Major depression, recurrent	Two or more major depressive episodes	1
Dissociative disorders		1
Depersonalization disorder (or depersonalization neurosis)	Persistent or recurrent	1
Sexual disorders		10
Sexual dysfunctions	Persistent or recurrent	10
Sleep disorders		6
Hypersomnia disorders	Episodically	4
Sleep terror disorder	Recurrent episodes	1
Sleepwalking disorder	Repeated episodes	1
Impulse control disorders not elsewhere classified		3
Intermittent explosive disorder	Several discrete episodes	1
Kleptomania	Recurrent failure	1
Trichotillomania	Recurrent failure	1
Total		39
B. Used for subtyping		
Disorders usually first evident in infancy, childhood, or adolescence		
Transient tic disorder: specify single episode or recurrent		

(continued)

Table 31–11. Consideration of episodicity in DSM-III-R *(continued)*

Disorder	Term	Specific categories
Mood disorders		
Major depression		
single episode		
recurrent		
Somatoform disorders		
Conversion disorder: specify single episode or recurrent		

Table 31–12. Literature review on progression

Disorder	Progression specified (*n*)
Organic brain syndromes	2
Schizophrenia	10
Affective disorders	4
Other psychotic disorders	3
Other disorders	3
In general	
Worsening or stable or improving specification: 7 papers (58.3%)	
Recovered or nonrecovering specification: 3 papers (25%)	
Other specification: 2 papers (16.7%)	

Another course variable that could be appropriately considered for an additional diagnostic character is episodicity, given the noticeable level of interest in it and the widely endorsed scaling (single episode versus recurrent) that could be used across diagnostic categories.

Progression could also be accommodated within an additional diagnostic character by applying its trichotomy (worsening/stable/improving) to the intermediate and long-term specifications of duration of illness.

Mode of onset could have been a candidate for inclusion within an additional diagnostic character because its acute versus insidious classification was consistently recognized. However, the variation in the specific definitions and cutoffs for this classification across diagnostic categories decreases its suitability for a uniform formulation.

Table 31–13. Consideration of progression in DSM-III-R

Disorder	Term	Specific categories
A. Used in the diagnostic criteria of core disorders		
Schizophrenia	(Subchronic or chronic) with acute exacerbation	5
Total		5
B. Used for subtyping		
Schizophrenia		
Schizophrenia: fifth digit		
subchronic with acute exacerbation		
chronic with acute exacerbation		
Schizophrenia paranoid: specify if stable type (criteria have been met during all past and present active phases)		

In practical terms, the coding of duration, episodicity, and progression within an additional diagnostic character across diagnostic categories could be accomplished by combining their classes into the following 15 codes:

1. Single episode, less than 6 months.
2. Single episode, between 6 months and 2 years, worsening.
3. Single episode, between 6 months and 2 years, stable.
4. Single episode, between 6 months and 2 years, improving.
5. Single episode, more than 2 years, worsening.
6. Single episode, more than 2 years, stable.
7. Single episode, more than 2 years, improving.
8. Recurrent, less than 6 months.
9. Recurrent, between 6 months and 2 years, worsening.
10. Recurrent, between 6 months and 2 years, stable.
11. Recurrent, between 6 months and 2 years, improving.
12. Recurrent, more than 2 years, worsening.
13. Recurrent, more than 2 years, stable.
14. Recurrent, more than 2 years, improving.
15. Unspecified.

The value of the additional diagnostic character approach is principally that it would facilitate systematic attention to, and evaluation of, key course variables. Furthermore, it would promote gaining experience with these variables that would lead to insight into the unfolding of mental illness and interactions with the clinical care process. On the other hand, this approach has the disadvantage of adding another rating to be done. It may also be more suitable to define course subtypes specifically for certain individual syndromic categories. This leads to the next option for considering course in DSM-IV.

Consideration of Course, Disorder by Disorder

This approach allows the greatest flexibility for including considerations related to course of illness in DSM-IV. However, it would require laborious preparation of qualifiers for a number of diagnostic categories, for many of which conceptual and empirical bases for individual specifications may not be currently available. Even more importantly, this approach misses the opportunity of systematically assessing the course of all mental disorders that could be a significant innovation in DSM-IV.

This approach would be particularly appropriate for age at onset, the specification of which is quite dependent on the particular disorder, and for mode of onset, given the variation in the specification of its dichotomy across diagnostic categories.

Definition of formal course subtypes. The definition of course subtypes pertinent to each disorder could be prepared along the lines of those already available for some DSM-III-R categories (e.g., primary degenerative dementia of the Alzheimer type, senile onset; schizophrenia, chronic with acute exacerbation; major depression, single episode). It may be possible to prepare a list of course types for each disorder similar to the 15 listed earlier, or a subset of those most pertinent for each disorder. For instance, instead of recurrent major depression, we could consider specifying major depression, recurrent, with more than 2 years total duration and a worsening trend. Another example would be schizophrenia, chronic (more than 2 years duration) with a worsening trend.

Comments in the text. This would be a low-key and less systematic way of considering course variables to qualify mental disorders. Instead of a formal code for each course type, there would be some general guidelines for course variations pertinent to each disorder. For example, for schizophrenia, it could be indicated that course may be continuous or episodic, stable or progressive (with exacerbations), and of variable duration.

Recommendations

The DSM-III-R classification primarily focuses on symptomatological descriptions of disorders. Course features are characterized in two ways: 1) by the use of the severity modifiers "in full remission" or "in partial remission," and 2) by the use of disorder-specific course modifiers (e.g., "recurrent" in major depressive disorder, and "chronic with acute exacerbation" in schizophrenia). The literature review identified five course variables as being most important: 1) age at onset, 2) mode of onset (e.g., abrupt or insidious), 3) duration or chronicity, 4) episodicity, and 5) progression of illness. To emphasize the importance of the course of illness, the text section on course for each disorder should systematically consider each of these course variables. The possible use of more specific course modifiers for mood disorder is being tested in a field trail.

References

Akiskal HS, Walker P, Puzantian VR, et al: Bipolar outcome in the course of depressive illness: phenomenologic, familial and pharmacologic predictors. J Affect Disord 5:115–128, 1983

Alexopoulos GS, Young RC, Meyers BS, et al: Late-onset depression. Psychiatr Clin North Am 11:101–115, 1988

Ambelas A, George M: Predictability of course of illness in manic patients positive for life events. J Nerv Ment Dis 174:693–695, 1986

American Psychiatric Association: Diagnostic and Statistical Manual of Mental Disorders, 3rd Edition. Washington, DC, American Psychiatric Association, 1980

American Psychiatric Association: Diagnostic and Statistical Manual of Mental Disorders, 3rd Edition, Revised. Washington, DC, American Psychiatric Association, 1987

Angermeyer MC, Kuhn L: Gender differences in age at onset of schizophrenia: an overview. Eur Arch Psychiatry Neurol Sci 237:351–364, 1988

Angst J, Baastrup P, Grof P, et al: The course of monopolar depression and bipolar psychoses. Psychiatria, Neurologia, Neurochirurgia 76:489–500, 1973

Armbruster B, Gross G, Huber G: Long-term prognosis and course of schizoaffective, schizophreniform, and cycloid psychoses. Psychiatria Clinica 16:156–168, 1983

Asarnow JR, Ben-Meir S: Children with schizophrenia spectrum and depressive disorders: a comparative study of premorbid adjustment, onset pattern and severity of impairment. J Child Psychol Psychiatry 29:477–488, 1988

Atkinson RM, Turner JA, Kofoed LL, et al: Early versus late onset alcoholism in older persons: preliminary findings. Alcohol Clin Exp Res 9:513–515, 1985

Bland RC, Newman SC, Orn H: Age of onset of psychiatric disorders. Acta Psychiatr Scand 77 (suppl 338):43–49, 1988

Bovet P: La charge de la chronicité dans le secteur. Archives Suisses de Neurologie, Neurochirurgie et de Psychiatrie 126:275–282, 1980

Breier A, Charney DS, Heninger GR: Agoraphobia with panic attacks: development, diagnostic stability, and course of illness. Arch Gen Psychiatry 43:1029–1036, 1986

Buydens-Branchey L, Branchey MH, Noumair D: Age of alcoholism onset, I: relationship to psychopathology. Arch Gen Psychiatry 46:225–230, 1989

Christie KA, Burke JD Jr, Regier DA, et al: Epidemiologic evidence for early onset of mental disorders and higher risk of drug abuse in young adults. Am J Psychiatry 145:971–975, 1988

Ciompi L: Is there really a schizophrenia? the long-term course of psychotic phenomena. Br J Psychiatry 145:636–640, 1984

Ciompi L: Aging and schizophrenic psychosis. Acta Psychiatr Scand 71 (suppl 319):93–105, 1985

Coryell W, Tsuang MT: Outcome after 40 years in DSM-III schizophreniform disorder. Arch Gen Psychiatry 43:324–328, 1986

Coryell W, Lavori P, Endicott J, et al: Outcome in schizoaffective, psychotic, and nonpsychotic depression: course during a 6- to 24-month follow-up. Arch Gen Psychiatry 41:787–791, 1984

Craig TJ, Bregman Z: Late onset schizophrenia-like illness. J Am Geriatr Soc 36:104–107, 1988

Diebold K, Haveisen S: Objektivierende Untersuchungen zur Diagnosenänderung im Krankheitsverlauf von Fallen mit der Anfangs-Bzw: Enddiagnose "Schizophrenie," "Endogene Depression" Oder "Psychopathie." Psychiatria Clinica 11:34–46, 1978

Dube KC, Kumar N, Dube S: Long term course and outcome of the agra cases in the international pilot study of schizophrenia. Acta Psychiatr Scand 70:170–179, 1984

Eagles JM, Whalley LJ: Aging and affective disorders: the age at first onset of affective disorders in Scotland, 1960–1978. Br J Psychiatry 147:180–187, 1985

Egeland JA, Blumenthal RL, Nee J, et al: Reliability and relationship of various ages of onset criteria for major affective disorder. J Affect Disord 12:159–165, 1987

Endicott J, Spitzer RL: A diagnostic interview: the Schedule for Affective Disorders and Schizophrenia. Arch Gen Psychiatry 35:837–844, 1978

Essen-Moller E, Wohlfahrt S: Suggestions for the amendment of the official Swedish Classification of Mental Disorders. Acta Psychiatr Scand 27 (suppl 47):551–555, 1947

Fahndrich E, Wirtz W: Verlaufsprädikatoren Affektiver Psychosen: Eine Katamnestische Untersuchung. Schweizer Archiv für Neurologie und Psychiatrie 138:17–30, 1987

Feighner JP, Robins E, Guze SB, et al: Diagnostic criteria for use in psychiatric research. Arch Gen Psychiatry 26:57–63, 1972

Galasko D, Kwo-On-Yuen PF, Thal L: Intracranial mass lesions associated with late-onset psychosis and depression. Psychiatr Clin North Am 11:151–166, 1988

Hasin DS, Endicott J, Keller MB: RDC alcoholism in patients with major affective syndromes: two-year course. Am J Psychiatry 146:318–323, 1989

Helmchen H: Schizophrenia: diagnostic concepts in the ICD-8. Br J Psychiatry Special Publ No 10:10–18, 1975

Hirschfeld RMA, Klerman GL, Andreasen NC, et al: Psycho-social predictors of chronicity in depressed patients. Br J Psychiatry 148:648–654, 1986

Huff FJ, Growdon JH, Corkin S, et al: Age at onset and rate of progression of Alzheimer's disease. J Am Geriatr Soc 35:27–30, 1987

Hwu HG, Chen CC, Strauss JS, et al: a comparative study on schizophrenia diagnosed by ICD-9 and DSM-III: course, family history and stability of diagnosis. Acta Psychiatr Scand 77:87–97, 1988

Jonsson H, Nyman AK: Prediction of outcome in schizophrenia. Acta Psychiatr Scand 69:274–291, 1984

Jonsson H, Nyman AK: Non-regressive schizophrenia: prediction of regressive course. Acta Psychiatr Scand 74:440–445, 1986

Joyce PR: Age of onset in bipolar affective disorder and misdiagnosis as schizophrenia. Psychol Med 14:145–149, 1984

Keller MB, Lavori PW, Rice J, et al: The persistent risk of chronicity in recurrent episodes of nonbipolar major depressive disorder: a prospective follow-up. Am J Psychiatry 143:24–28, 1986

Kendler KS, Spitzer RL, Williams JBW: Psychotic disorders in DSM-III-R. Am J Psychiatry 146:953–962, 1989

Kocsis JH, Frances AJ: A critical discussion of DSM-III dysthymic disorder. Am J Psychiatry 144:1534–1542, 1987

Kovacs M, Feinberg TL, Crouse-Novak MA, et al: Depressive disorders in childhood, I: a longitudinal prospective study of characteristics and recovery. Arch Gen Psychiatry 41:229–237, 1984

Kulhara P, Wig NN: The chronicity of schizophrenia in North West India: results of a follow-up study. Br J Psychiatry 132:186–190, 1978

Kurashov AS: Characteristics of the affective states in the early stages of attack-like progressive schizophrenia with onset in adolescence. Zhurnal Nevropatologii I Psikhiatrii 72:1224–1229, 1972

Lee GP, Diclimente CC: Age of onset versus duration of problem drinking on the Alcohol Use Inventory. J Stud Alcohol 46:398–402, 1985

Lehmkuhl G, Blanz B, Lehmkuhl U, et al: Conversion Disorder (DSM-III 300.11): symptomatology and course in childhood and adolescence. Eur Arch Psychiatry Neurol Sci 238:155–160, 1989

Leme Lopes J: As Dimensoes Do Diagnóstico Psiquiatrico. Rio de Janeiro, Brazil, Agir, 1954

Leon CA: Curso Clínico y Evolución de la Esquizofrenia en Cali: un Estudio de Seguimiento de Diez Anōs. Acta Psiquiátrica y Psicológica de América Latina 32:95–136, 1986

Lin K, Kleinman AM: Psychopathology and clinical course of schizophrenia: a cross-cultural perspective. Schizophr Bull 14:555–567, 1988

Lipkowitz MH, Idupuganti S: Diagnosing schizophrenia in 1982: the effect of DSM-III. Am J Psychiatry 142:634–637, 1985

Loranger AW: Sex difference in age at onset of schizophrenia. Arch Gen Psychiatry 41:157–161, 1984

Maj M: Clinical course and outcome of schizoaffective disorders: a three-year follow-up study. Acta Psychiatr Scand 72:542–550, 1985

Maj M: Clinical course and outcome of cycloid psychotic disorder: a three-year prospective study. Acta Psychiatr Scand 78:182–187, 1988

Makanjuola ROA, Adepapo SA: The DSM-III concepts of schizophrenic disorder and schizophreniform disorder: a clinical and prognostic evaluation. Br J Psychiatry 151:611–618, 1987

Marneros A, Deister A, Rohde A: Syndrome shift in the long-term course of schizoaffective disorders. Eur Arch Psychiatry Neurol Sci 238:97–104, 1988

McFarlane AC: The longitudinal course of posttraumatic morbidity: the range of outcomes and their predictors. J Nerv Ment Dis 176:30–39, 1988

McGlashan TH: Predictors of shorter-, medium-, and longer-term outcome in schizophrenia. Am J Psychiatry 143:50–55, 1986

McGlashan TH: Adolescent versus adult onset of mania. Am J Psychiatry 145:221–223, 1988

Mezzich JE: Patterns and issues in multiaxial psychiatric diagnosis. Psychol Med 9:125–137, 1979

Mezzich JE, Fabrega H, Mezzich AC: An international consultation on multiaxial diagnosis, in Psychiatry—the State of the Art. Edited by Pichot P, Berner P, Wolfe R, et al. London, England, Plenum, 1985, pp 51–56

Miklowitz DJ, Goldstein MJ, Nuechterlein KH, et al: Family factors and the course of bipolar affective disorder. Arch Gen Psychiatry 45:225–231, 1988
Mogensen JT, Simonsen E, Mellergaard M: Multiaxial diagnosis in a department of adult psychiatry. Ugeskrift fur Laeger 148:2869–2872, 1986
Munk-Jorgensen P, Mortensen PB: Schizophrenia: a 13-year follow-up: diagnostic and psychopathological aspects. Acta Psychiatr Scand 79:391–399, 1989
Murphy HBM, Raman AC: The chronicity of schizophrenia in indigenous tropical peoples: results of a twelve-year follow-up survey in Mauritius. Br J Psychiatry 118:489–497, 1971
Nuller L, Kalinin OM, Rubtsova S: Use of factor analysis in studying the course of manic-depressive psychosis. Zhurnal Nevropatologii I Psikhiatrii 72:548–554, 1972
Opjordsmoen S: Long-term course and outcome in delusional disorder. Acta Psychiatr Scand 78:576–586, 1988
Ottosson JO, Perris C: Multidimensional classification of mental disorders. Psychol Med 3:238–243, 1973
Petho B: Dimensional assessment of the course of psychiatric illness. Psychopathology 17:110–116, 1984
Post RM, Roy-Byrne PP, Uhde TW: Graphic representation of the life course of illness in patients with affective disorder. Am J Psychiatry 145:844–848, 1988
Rabiner CJ, Wegner JT, Kane JM: Outcome study of first-episode psychosis, I: relapse rates after 1 year. Am J Psychiatry 143:1155–1158, 1986
Reich J: The epidemiology of anxiety. J Nerv Ment Dis 174:129–136, 1986
Retterstol N: Course of paranoid psychoses in relation to diagnostic grouping. Psychiatria Clinica 16:198–206, 1983
Robert P, Benoist P, Gueniffey S, et al: Évolution des psychoses: résultats d'une enquête clinique portant sur 383 cas suivis pendant 10 ans (1975–1985). Annales Medico-Psychologique 147:15–32, 1989
Robinson JR: The natural history of mental disorder in old age: a long-term study. Br J Psychiatry 154:783–789, 1989
Roy-Byrne P, Post RM, Uhde TW, et al: The longitudinal course of recurrent affective illness: life chart data from research patients at the NIMH. Acta Psychiatr Scand 71 (suppl 317):1–34, 1985
Rutter M, Shaffer D, Shepherd M: A Multiaxial Classification Of Child Psychiatry Disorders. Geneva, Switzerland, World Health Organization, 1975
Scott J: Chronic depression. Br J Psychiatry 153:287–297, 1988
Smeraldi E, Macciardi F, Holmgren S, et al: Age at onset of affective disorders in Italian and Swedish patients. Acta Psychiatr Scand 75:352–357, 1987
Sorensen DJ, Paul GL, Mariotto MJ: Inconsistencies in paranoid functioning, premorbid adjustment, and chronicity: question of diagnostic criteria. Schizophr Bull 14:323–336, 1988
Spitzer RL, Endicott J, Robins E: Research Diagnostic Criteria. Arch Gen Psychiatry 35:773–782, 1978
Strauss JS: A comprehensive approach to psychiatric diagnosis. Am J Psychiatry 132:1193–1197, 1975
Summers F, Hersh S: Psychiatric chronicity and diagnosis. Schizophr Bull 9:122–133, 1983
Summers WK: Mania with onset in the eighth decade: two cases and a review. J Clin Psychiatry 44:141–143, 1983

Thyer BA, Parrish RT, Curtis GC, et al: Ages of onset of DSM-III anxiety disorders. Compr Psychiatry 26:113–122, 1985

Von Cranach M: Categorical versus multiaxial classification. Paper presented at the 6th Symposium on Multiaxial Diagnosis, 6th World Congress of Psychiatry, Honolulu, HI, 1977

Watkins JM, Asarnow RF, Tanguay PE: Symptom development in childhood onset schizophrenia. J Child Psychol Psychiatry 29:865–878, 1988

Wing JK, Cooper JE, Sartorius N: The Measurement and Classification of Psychiatric Symptoms. London, England, Cambridge University Press, 1974

Wing L: Observations on the psychiatric section of the International Classification of Diseases and the British Glossary of Mental Disorders. Psychol Med 1:79–85, 1970

World Health Organization: International Classification of Diseases, 9th Edition. Geneva, Switzerland, World Health Organization, 1978

Yassa R, Nair NPV, Iskandar H: Late-onset bipolar disorder. Psychiatr Clin North Am 11:117–131, 1988

Young MA, Grabler P: Rapidity of symptom onset in depression. Psychiatry Res 16:309–315, 1985

Zubin J, Magaziner J, Steinhauer SR: The metamorphosis of schizophrenia: from chronicity to vulnerability. Psychol Med 13:551–571, 1983

Chapter 32

On Measuring Syndromic Severity

Juan E. Mezzich, M.D., Ph.D., and
Patrick F. Sullivan, M.D.

Statement and Significance of the Issues

Severity of illness is currently the focus of considerable attention in medicine in general and in psychiatry in particular. For the development of DSM-IV, a key issue was whether more specific criteria for measuring the severity of psychiatric syndromes was feasible and appropriate.

The interest in severity stems from several sources. In general medicine and surgery, the pursuit of cost containment and research interests have been the principal driving forces. The ubiquitous diagnosis-related group (DRG) system has been criticized for not adequately adjusting a given DRG for the degree of complexity of the illness (Eisenberg 1984). Several severity measures have been developed to make DRG reimbursement more equitable. For health care "consumers" (e.g., private patients, employees, or insurance companies), quality of care between various institutions can be compared if illness severity is taken into account, and the consumer can then patronize the institutions with the best "value." With regard to research, severity measures could be used to follow patients longitudinally to evaluate treatment efficacy. This "revolutionary" development may receive one billion dollars from the United States Congress for research support (Meyer 1989).

In psychiatry, severity and its measurement have received comparatively less attention. Severity, however, may be clinically important for better describing patients, for communication between practitioners, and for planning treatment. Moreover, the economic policies prevalent in other areas of medicine are increasingly impinging on psychiatry. In Pennsylvania, for example, a system for quantifying severity in psychiatric inpatients is under development. The intent of this system is to monitor quality of care, and it could easily be employed for utilization review with profound effects on the practice of inpatient psychiatry.

Method

For this review, we conducted manual and computer searches of the literature. Because of the potential for crossover and cross-fertilization in the development of severity measures, we covered both the psychiatric or mental health field and general medicine and surgery.

The manual search involved the review of key international journals such as *Acta Psychiatric Scandinavica, American Journal of Psychiatry, Archives of General Psychiatry,* and the *British Journal of Psychiatry.* The titles, abstracts, and, when pertinent, full papers in the selected journals were examined for 1981 to 1990.

The computer search was conducted through Medline, the computerized files of *Index Medicus.*

We considered additional papers brought to our attention as members of the psychiatric advisory panel for the Commonwealth of Pennsylvania Health Care Cost Containment Council for 1989 to 1991 and as members of the Work Groups for the development of the multiaxial systems in DSM-III (American Psychiatric Association 1980), DSM-IV, and ICD-10 (World Health Organization 1989).

Results

Severity: General Concepts

We begin by reviewing general ways in which severity can be conceptualized and then define the four aspects of severity on which we focus in the next two sections of this chapter.

Stein et al. (1987) viewed severity at three distinct levels. Physiological severity, although elusive, uses laboratory or physical data to indicate the biological impact of a disease. Functional severity measures the impact of a disease on an individual's capacity to perform age-appropriate roles or activities. Burden of illness estimates the influence of a disease on an individual's social unit or on society at large and corresponds to the extrapersonal implications of illness.

McMahon and Billi (1988) offered a somewhat different conceptual framework. A physiological perspective of severity estimates the likelihood of morbidity and mortality, a consideration mainly relevant to physical medicine. A psychological perspective examines the response of the patient and family to illness, principally physical illness. Finally, an economic perspective notes resource use.

Using a psychiatric multiaxial approach, we can articulate four measures of severity related to the functional severity of Stein et al. (1987) and the psychological perspective of McMahon and Billi (1988).

1. Syndromic severity estimates the symptomatological intensity of each psychi-

atric or physical condition identified in a multiaxial formulation.
2. Comorbid severity reflects the total pathological magnitude of a set of disorders experienced by an individual, taking into account the formulation of multiple disorders and the concept of illness complexity.
3. Functional impairment or disability measures deviation from some expected norm in interpersonal and occupational performance due to the cumulative effects of a person's various illnesses.
4. Overall severity is an all-encompassing concept, covering both symptomatological intensity and functional impairment.

Syndromic severity allows for delineation of the intensity of individual disorders. It may be useful to facilitate communication among clinicians about the seriousness of specific disorders. Syndromic severity may also be important in planning treatment. Results of the NIMH Treatment of Depression Collaborative Research Program (Elkin et al. 1989) are illustrative in this regard. For less severely depressed subjects, there were no significant differences in treatment response across the four modalities studied, whereas significant differences did exist for the more severely depressed subjects. An editorial by Kupfer and Rush (1983) on behalf of the depression research community described syndromic severity as an item of "highest priority" for describing a given sample in clinical research.

Comorbid severity attempts to capture the magnitude of all psychopathological and physical problems suffered by an individual by taking into account the plurality of disorders present. Possible approaches to this form of severity include totaling the number of psychiatric and general medical disorders present and combining the syndromic severity scores from individual disorders.

Functional impairment was incorporated as Axis V in DSM-III. Several issues concerning functional impairment have been identified. One is the time frame (i.e., the highest level in the past year, which has prognostic implications, versus current functioning, which is particularly pertinent to clinical management); another refers to scope (i.e., global adaptive functioning versus separate assessments by areas of functioning).

Overall severity would combine functional impairment with symptom status. In the context of a multiaxial system, it may prove difficult to develop a definition of this concept that is sufficiently independent of the other diagnostic axes. Still, an index of overall severity could be developed from information contained in various special-purpose axes and serve as a predictor of resource utilization.

Severity in Psychiatric Multiaxial Systems

Syndromic severity, comorbid severity, functional impairment, and overall severity appear in several multiaxial psychiatric classification systems (Table 32–1).

Ottosson and Perris (1973) viewed overall severity as referring to the following range: healthy, nonpsychotic mentally ill, occasionally psychotic, psychotic. These considerations cover information contained in their axis on symptoms.

Helmchen (1975) proposed a five-axis system to classify subjects with schizophrenia. His fourth axis is in a sense a measure of syndromic severity for schizophrenia.

Axes IV and V of Strauss (1975) addressed functional impairment with reference to personal relationships and work function, respectively. His was the first multiaxial system that clearly incorporated functional impairment and a rating scale (5 point).

DSM-III, as well as ICD-9 (World Health Organization 1978), explicitly considered syndromic severity only for mental retardation, where subtypes are defined by IQ level (e.g., mild mental retardation for an IQ of 50–70, moderate mental retardation for 35–49). Syndromic severity exists implicitly in the contrast between minor and major variants of certain disorders that are distinguished by symptom intensity. Examples include cyclothymic disorder and bipolar affective disorder; adjustment disorder with depressed mood, which Fabrega et al. (1987) call a "transitional" illness, and dysthymia versus major depression; or, on Axis II, personality "traits" when criteria for a particular personality disorder are not met. Syndromic severity is also found implicitly in the fifth digit codes for certain disorders. Primary degenerative or multi-infarct dementia each may be uncomplicated or with depression, delirium, or delusions. A major depressive episode may carry psychotic features or melancholia. A manic episode may also have psychotic features. DSM-III Axis V measures functional capacity with a 7-point composite of social relationships ("given greater weight"), occupational function, and use of leisure time. Reliability was moderate (Spitzer et al. 1979). Skodol et al. (1988) found that 19% of the variance in Axis I diagnosis was accounted for by Axis V ratings, suggesting the relative independence of these axes, a desirable feature for a multiaxial classification system (Mezzich 1979). Relatively few studies have addressed the predictive validity of Axis V (Williams 1985). Mezzich et al. (1984) found that Axis V rating was the strongest independent predictor of admission to psychiatric inpatient units from a psychiatric emergency room—the worse the adaptive function, the more likely the admission. Gordon et al. (1985a, 1985b) claimed to show a relationship between the ratio of DSM-III Axis IV/Axis V scores and length of inpatient admissions, but these two studies contained methodological limitations.

Comorbid severity is addressed principally by allowing multiple diagnoses for psychopathological disorders, personality conditions, and physical disorders. In this manner, dual diagnoses or comorbidity may be noted.

Mezzich and Sharfstein (1985), in a position paper prepared during the

Table 32–1. Comparison of psychiatric multiaxial systems that include severity

Study	Multiaxial proposition	Proposition addresses	How coded	Time frame for severity	Reliability	Validity
Ottosson and Perris 1973	4 axes	OS-severity axis	Healthy, nonpsychotic, occasionally psychotic, psychotic	Current	77%	Accepted by clinicians
Helmchen 1975	5 axes (for schizophrenia)	SS-axis on intensity of symptoms, course, and etiology	Not specified	Not specified	No data	No data
Strauss 1975	5 axes	FI-axis on quality of personal relationships FI-axis on level of work function	5-point scale 5-point scale	Not specified Not specified	No data No data	No data No data
American Psychiatric Association 1980	5 axes	FI-axis on highest level of adaptive functioning	1 = superior to 7 = grossly impaired	For a few months in past year	kappa = .8	See text
Mezzich and Sharfstein 1985	5 axes (DSM-III)	SS-each Axis I–III diagnosis	1 = no symptom to 4 = severe	Past month	No data	No data
American Psychiatric Association 1987	5 axes	SS-axis I–III (optional) FI-axis on global assessment of functioning, including symptoms	Mild to full remission 90 = min symptom to 1 = dangerous	Current Current and past year	No data ?	No data See text

(continued)

Table 32–1. Comparison of psychiatric multiaxial systems that include severity *(continued)*

Study	Multiaxial proposition	Proposition addresses	How coded	Time frame for severity	Reliability	Validity
Bech et al. 1987	5 axes (DSM-III/ICD-8 hybrid)	SS-axis I–III, how ill at this time? FI-DSM-III Axis V	1 = normal to 7 = most ill DSM-III above	At admission and discharge DSM-III above	kappa = .7–.8 DSM-III above	See text See text
Jenkins et al. 1988	4 axes	OS, CS-for each axis (psychological, supports, personality, physical)	0 = absent to 4 = severe	Not specified	No data	No data

Note. OS = overall severity. SS = syndromic severity. FI = functional capacity. CS = comorbid severity.

development of DSM-III-R (American Psychiatric Association 1987), proposed a modification to DSM-III in the form of a 4-point measurement of syndromic severity for each Axis I–III diagnosis. For example, 300.02-2 signifies generalized anxiety disorder with mild symptoms.

DSM-III-R considered syndromic severity in a limited manner. Any diagnosis can, at the clinician's judgment, be qualified as mild, moderate, severe, in partial remission/residual state, or in full remission according to the general criteria provided. No coding system was proposed, although a system like that of Mezzich and Sharfstein (1985) could readily be adapted. These five qualifiers are incomplete in that no "permanent remission" or "cure" is included. Some find this deficiency objectionable because it makes permanent labeling possible. To our knowledge, no data exist with regard to the reliability and validity of this schema, and it seems that many clinicians are unaware of this option.

DSM-III-R Axis V, Global Assessment of Functioning, is based on the Global Assessment Score (Endicott et al. 1976), modified for use with children as well as adults and deleting the highest range of function (scores 91–100). However, as Skodol et al. (1988) cautioned, inclusion of symptomatology in Axis V (e.g., 51–60: moderate symptoms—"flat affect and circumstantial speech" [American Psychiatric Association 1980, p. 12]) risked redundancy between Axes I and V, contrary to the purpose of a multiaxial system. Robert et al. (1989) seem to validate this warning: DSM-III-R Axis V explained 64% of the variance in Axis I diagnoses, a large degree of overlap. A possible solution may be to split Axis V into Axis Va (global function) and Axis Vb (global severity), analogous to the distinction we make between functional capacity and overall severity. There appears to be a need to delineate these constructs explicitly.

Bech et al. (1987) proposed a hybrid of DSM-III and ICD-8 (World Health Organization 1967), the international standard employed in the Scandinavian countries at that time. Axis I codes the 16 ICD-8 major psychiatric groupings, although only a single diagnosis seems to be allowed. Axis II has four categories for personality disorders, and Axis III codes physical disorders based on ICD-8. A 7-point measure of syndromic severity qualified each Axis I–III diagnosis in the clinician's total experience. Axis V, coded along the lines of DSM-III, estimated functional capacity at several points in time. Interrater reliability was moderate, and no validity data were presented, nor were the novel aspects of this proposal (i.e., the syndromic severity measure and its reliance on the degree of clinical experience) systematically evaluated.

Jenkins et al. (1988) proposed a classification system for mental disorders in patients presenting to primary care practitioners. The four axes were psychological conditions, social problems/supports, personality, and physical disorders. The severity of each axis is noted on a 5-point scale, thus estimating overall severity.

Comorbid severity is also assessed by listing and making a gross rating of the multiple psychological and physical conditions. No validity or reliability data for the severity aspects of this schema have been published.

Finally, an interesting approach to overall severity, although from an economic perspective and not in a clinical multiaxial system, is the Psychiatric Severity of Illness Index (Horn et al. 1989). Psychiatric inpatients are rated on a 4-point scale over seven dimensions: stage of principal diagnosis, complications, interactions, level of care, social support, rate of response to therapy, and resolution of acute symptoms. The modal score, or the average if no mode exists, determines the overall 4-point Psychiatric Severity of Illness Index. This index has been shown to be reliable and valid in that it may explain 34%–50% of the variation in inpatient length of stay, far more than the parallel DRG.

Severity Indices in General Medicine and Surgery

A sample of the most prominent severity indices from general medicine and surgery are summarized in Table 32–2. Several indices have been used in attempts to modify DRG reimbursement. Most are related to economics rather than facilitating patient care.

Acute Physiology and Chronic Health Evaluation (APACHE II) (Knaus et al. 1985), an index of overall severity based largely on physiological data, was designed to predict mortality of intensive-care unit patients and has been well validated clinically. Therapeutic Intervention Scoring System (TISS) (Keene and Cullen 1983), a rough measure of overall severity, is used to monitor and assign intensive-care unit resources, but data on its reliability and validity are sparse. Disease staging (Gonella et al. 1984) was designed to measure the physiological syndromic severity of particular diseases, but has been validated only with regard to economics. No method was presented for estimating overall severity for those with multiple diagnoses. MedisGroups (Brewster et al. 1985), an index of overall severity mandated in Pennsylvania, was designed to measure physiological severity and economic resource use, but has been validated only for the latter. Severity of Illness Index (SII) (Horn et al. 1986) was intended to measure overall severity and has been validated economically but not clinically.

Discussion

Proposals for Syndromic Severity

We now narrow the preceding discussion to focus on the possible incorporation of a syndromic severity measure in DSM-IV. First, we review the main points for

Table 32–2. Severity indices in internal medicine and surgery

Index	Reference	Definition of severity	Focus	Setting	Method	Validity
APACHE II (Acute Physiology and Chronic Health Evaluation)	Knaus et al. 1985	Risk of death while in hospital	Clinical (OS)	Intensive care unit	Sum of points for specific clinical and lab data, age, history of organ failure	Predicts mortality
TISS (Therapeutic Intervention Scoring System)	Keene and Cullen 1983	Therapeutic effort intensity	Clinical (OS)	Intensive care unit	Sum of all therapies provided, ranked for acuity	No data
Disease staging	Gonella et al. 1984	Likelihood of death or residual impairment	Clinical (SS)	Hospital inpatient	Expert panel created four "stages" for 420 diagnoses, from minimal to death	Economic, NOT clinical
MedisGroups	Brewster et al. 1985	Potential for organ failure	Clinical economic (OS)	Hospital inpatient	Proprietary algorithm summing "key clinical findings" yields final score	Economic ONLY
SII (Severity of Illness Index)	Horn et al. 1986	Subgroups homogeneous in severity of illness	Clinical economic (OS)	Hospital inpatient	Seven subscales combined for overall severity ranking	Economic ONLY

Note. OS = overall severity. SS = syndromic severity.

inclusion. The improved definition of disorders is a hallmark of DSM-III and DSM-III-R, and a measure of syndromic severity would contribute a vital missing element. Such measures would be relevant to treatment decisions and could help focus therapy or serve in its evaluation. Syndromic severity measures could also provide epidemiological natural history data concerning the longitudinal course of the illness. The argument for including a more extensive syndromic severity measure in DSM-IV is thus quite strong.

The argument against incorporating syndromic severity measures in DSM-IV is based on conceptual and practical concerns. It may prove difficult for clinicians to delineate accurately and conveniently the sources of severity. It may not be possible to develop a reliable, valid, and easy-to-use severity index by the projected release date of DSM-IV. Moreover, clinicians might perceive such a measure as an unreasonable burden.

If these obstacles are judged surmountable, several fundamental decisions regarding syndromic severity are required. First, the specific definition of "syndromic severity" needs to be closely considered to ensure its adequacy, including the time frame (i.e., current, last month, this episode, and so on). Second, the grounds for measuring this construct must be determined (i.e., based on symptom intensity alone or with functional impairment). Third, the form must be determined (see later). Fourth, reliability, content validity, and construct validity must be established empirically. Ideally, such measures would require minimal learning time and be easy to use.

There are several possible forms for a syndromic severity index. First, a sixth digit, either a number or an alphabetic character, could be added to the diagnostic code in the manner that is illustrated by Mezzich and Sharfstein (1985) or Bech et al. (1987), as discussed earlier in this chapter. Second, as discussed under DSM-III-R earlier, phrases that qualify the severity for each psychiatric disorder could be used.

The criteria for a syndromic severity measure pose an interesting problem. Generic guidelines similar to those in DSM-III-R may be too vague and lack rigor and reliability. At the other extreme, distinct guidelines for each disorder, found in DSM-III-R for several disorders, would lengthen DSM-IV considerably and might prove tedious to clinicians. Clearly, some balance needs to be found that satisfies these conflicting requirements.

Operationally, syndromic severity may also be approached from the perspective of diagnostic criteria or symptoms. Criterion-based syndromic severity would reflect the extent to which the diagnostic criteria for a given syndrome are met. Symptom-based syndromic severity refers to the intensity and persistence of current symptoms of a given syndrome. These approaches and a combination of both are now described in more detail.

Criterion-Based Severity

The intent of this approach to syndromic severity is to grade severity explicitly in relation to DSM-IV diagnostic criteria. The criteria for most diagnoses are composed of inclusion and exclusion criteria. Inclusion criteria are signs of symptoms that must be present for a diagnosis to be made, whereas exclusion criteria describe features that must be "ruled out" or absent for a diagnosis to be made. For example, of the diagnostic criteria for schizophrenia in DSM-III-R, A (psychotic symptoms), B (functional decline), and D (duration) are inclusion criteria whereas C, E, and F are exclusion criteria.

This approach assumes that the more severe the disorder, the more inclusion criteria are met. Usually, all specified criteria must be satisfied for a diagnosis to be made.

There are four grades of severity proposed here, plus an unspecified rating. *Asymptomatic* refers to patients for whom descriptive criteria were fully met at some point in the past but for whom criteria are not currently met at all (i.e., the disorder is in remission). *Marginal* describes a disorder in partial remission: full descriptive criteria were previously met but at present some criteria are not fully met. *Moderate* describes a disorder now present for which criteria are just sufficiently met but not abundantly so. With *severe,* the inclusion criteria for a disorder are not only met but are substantially exceeded. Finally, *unspecified* describes the situation when adequate data are unavailable. The criteria are summarized as follows:

- Asymptomatic. Disorder present in past, now in remission; diagnostic criteria are not met.
- Marginal. Disorder present in past, at present some diagnostic criteria are fully met while others are questionably met.
- Moderate. Disorder now present, all criteria are fully met, but just adequately so.
- Severe. Disorder now present, inclusion criteria abundantly met.
- Unspecified. Information inadequate.

For example, DSM-III-R major depressive episode has four criteria. Criteria B, C, and D describe exclusionary conditions. The inclusion criterion A requires that five of nine symptoms be present. If a major depressive episode had been present in the past but no criteria are now met, rate as asymptomatic. If three or four symptoms are currently present, rate as marginal. If five or six symptoms are currently present, rate as moderate. If seven to nine symptoms are present, rate as severe.

Symptom-Based Severity

This approach requires the clinician to grade the intensity and persistence of symptoms for a given disorder using a four-level scale. Each level assumes that at some point full diagnostic criteria were met, either in the past or currently. *Asymptomatic*, for a disorder previously diagnosed, characterizes a current state in which the symptoms are absent or rare. *Mild* refers to either slight but persistent or moderate but occasional symptoms. *Moderate* characterizes either persistently moderate or occasionally severe symptoms. *Severe* signifies severe and persistent symptoms. Finally, *unspecified* describes the situation where adequate data are unavailable. The criteria are as follows:

- Asymptomatic. Absent or rare symptoms; disorder present in past, but now in remission.
- Mild. Slight symptoms most of the time or moderate symptoms occasionally.
- Moderate. Moderate symptoms most of the time or severe symptoms occasionally.
- Severe. Severe symptoms most of the time.
- Unspecified. Information inadequate.

Hybrid Criterion/Symptom Severity

This severity coding schema combines the two previous methods. There are five levels, each with elements of the above two schemata. *Asymptomatic* refers to a disorder fully diagnosed at some point in the past but that presently fails to meet descriptive criteria or shows only rare symptoms: a disorder in remission. *Subthreshold* also refers to a disorder diagnosed in the past but for which some but not all diagnostic criteria are present and which has slight symptoms most of the time or moderate symptoms occasionally. *Moderate* conditions just meet diagnostic criteria and carry moderate symptoms most of the time or severe symptoms occasionally. *Severe* conditions abundantly meet diagnostic criteria and carry severe symptoms most of the time. Finally, *unspecified* describes the situation where adequate data are unavailable. The criteria are as follows:

- Asymptomatic. Disorder diagnosed in the past, now in remission; currently, diagnostic criteria are not met at all, and symptoms are virtually absent.
- Subthreshold. Disorder diagnosed in the past; currently, some but not all required diagnostic criteria are present, and symptoms are persistently slight or occasionally moderate.
- Moderate. Disorder now present, descriptive criteria just met, and symptoms are persistently moderate or occasionally severe.

- Severe. Disorder now present, descriptive criteria abundantly met, and symptoms are persistently severe.
- Unspecified. Information inadequate.

Comparative Comments

The major advantage of each of these three schemata is that they are generic and perhaps not difficult to learn. Clinicians could apply them from memory without having to resort to reference material.

The criterion-based approach is possibly the most clear of the three. It explicitly references diagnostic criteria and thus provides a more objective framework for a severity rating. For those with multiple diagnoses, it should also prove workable without requiring clinicians to parcel out severity in an arbitrary manner. However, its conception of severity may not correspond to that which clinicians typically employ. The severity of mania, for example, may relate clinically to the degree of elation or hyperactivity rather than to the number of diagnostic criteria displayed.

The symptom-based approach probably grades an aspect of severity distinct from that subsumed under the diagnosis itself and thus is less redundant. Moreover, it is probably closer to the typical clinician's conception of "severity" and thus possesses considerable face validity. However, for individuals with multiple diagnoses, it may require the clinician to perform a sort of mental gymnastics to match symptoms and diagnoses. For a hypothetical individual with overlapping symptomatology (e.g., a person with major depression, borderline personality disorder, and alcohol dependence), the rating of symptom-based syndromic severities may be problematic.

The hybrid approach shares the best and worst elements of its parents and may be more difficult to use without a handy reference manual. Some clinical presentations may fall between its cracks when symptom and criterion patterns do not correspond to the same level.

Generic Versus Specific Measurement of Syndromic Severity

The value of considering syndromic severity in DSM-IV was demonstrated earlier in this chapter, and it is assumed that it is possible to establish a basic scale, one having an agreed number of levels with conceptually consistent labels. The dilemma of generic (across diagnostic categories) versus specific (pertinent to individual diagnostic categories) definitions must be approached flexibly at this point. Diagnosis-specific definitions for the severity levels could be included whenever such definitions are feasible (e.g., for DSM-III-R mood disorders). Otherwise (for the majority of disorders), generic definitions, such as those offered in this chapter, could be considered.

Recommendations

In DSM-III-R, guidelines are provided for noting the severity of the mental disorders as "mild," "moderate," or "severe." In addition, if criteria for the disorder are not currently met, the modifiers "in partial remission" or "in full remission" can be used. After an unspecified duration of being in full remission, the clinician can consider the individual "recovered" (no current mental disorder). An alternative approach would be to have severity noted in a purely cross-sectional manner to separate ratings of severity from ratings of course. Under this proposal, the disorder would be rated as "asymptomatic," "subthreshold," "mild," "moderate," or "severe." The major problem with this proposal is its lack of familiarity and potential confusion about use of the term *subthreshold*. A less radical alternative that refines DSM-III-R usage would allow the clinician to differentiate three types of subthreshold case: 1) individuals *in partial remission* (a term already included in DSM-III-R); 2) individuals *in partial relapse* (a suggested new term for DSM-IV) who have met full criteria for a disorder in the past but who, after a period of full remission, develop symptoms at a subthreshold level; and 3) for individuals who have never met diagnostic criteria for the condition, the term *subthreshold* could be used as a modifier in the not otherwise specified category (e.g., depressive disorder not otherwise specified [subthreshold major depressive disorder]).

References

American Psychiatric Association: Diagnostic and Statistical Manual of Mental Disorders, 3rd Edition. Washington, DC, American Psychiatric Association, 1980

American Psychiatric Association: Diagnostic and Statistical Manual of Mental Disorders, 3rd Edition, Revised. Washington, DC, American Psychiatric Association, 1987

Bech P, Hjorts S, Lund K, et al: An integration of DSM-III and ICD-8 by global severity assessments for measuring multidimensional outcomes in general hospital psychiatry. Acta Psychiatr Scand 75:297–306, 1987

Brewster AC, Karlin BG, Hyde LA, et al: MEDISGRPS: a clinically based approach to classifying hospital patients at admission. Inquiry 22:377–387, 1985

Eisenberg BS: Diagnosis-related groups, severity of illness, and equitable reimbursement under Medicare. JAMA 251:645–646, 1984

Elkin I, Shea T, Watkins JT, et al: NIMH Treatment of Depression Collaborative Research Program: general effectiveness of treatments. Arch Gen Psychiatry 46:971–982, 1989

Endicott J, Spitzer RL, Fleiss J, et al: The Global Assessment Scale: a procedure for measuring overall severity of psychiatric disturbance. Arch Gen Psychiatry 33:766–771, 1976

Fabrega H, Mezzich JE, Mezzich AC: Adjustment disorder as a marginal or transitional illness category in DSM-III. Arch Gen Psychiatry 44:567–572, 1987

Gonella JS, Hornbrook MC, Louis DZ: Staging of disease: a case-mix measurement. JAMA 251:637–644, 1984

Gordon RE, Vijay J, Sloate SG, et al: Aggravating stress and functional level as predictors of length of psychiatric hospitalization. Hosp Community Psychiatry 36:773–774, 1985a

Gordon RE, Jardiolin P, Gordon KK: Predicting length of hospital stay of psychiatric inpatients. Am J Psychiatry 142:235–237, 1985b

Helmchen H: Schizophrenia: diagnostic concepts in the ICD-8. Br J Psychiatry Special Publ No 10:10–18, 1975

Horn SD, Horn RA, Sharkey PD, et al: Severity of illness within DRGs. Med Care 24:225–235, 1986

Horn SD, Chambrers AF, Sharkey PD, et al: Psychiatric severity of illness: a case mix study. Med Care 27:69–84, 1989

Jenkins R, Smeeton N, Shepard M: Classification of mental disorder in primary care. Psychol Med Monogr Suppl 12, 1988

Keene AR, Cullen DJ: Therapeutic intervention scoring system: update 1983. Critical Care Medicine 11:1–3, 1983

Knaus WA, Draper EA, Wagner DP, et al: APACHE II: a severity of disease classification system. Critical Care Medicine 13:818–829, 1985

Kupfer DJ, Rush AJ: Recommendations for scientific reports on depression. Am J Psychiatry 140:1326–1327, 1983

McMahon LF, Billi JE: Measurement of severity of illness and the Medicare prospective payment system. J Gen Intern Med 3:482–490, 1988

Meyer H: Outcomes management going nationwide. Am Med News, August 11, 1989, pp 1, 47

Mezzich JE: Patterns and issues in multiaxial psychiatric diagnosis. Psychol Med 9:125–137, 1979

Mezzich JE, Sharfstein SS: Severity of illness and diagnostic formulation: classifying patients for prospective payment systems. Hosp Community Psychiatry 36:770–772, 1985

Mezzich JE, Evanczuk KJ, Mathias RJ, et al: Admission decisions and multiaxial diagnosis. Arch Gen Psychiatry 41:1001–1004, 1984

Ottosson JO, Perris C: Multidimensional classification of mental disorders. Psychol Med 3:238–243, 1973

Robert P, Aubin V, Dumarcet M, et al: Effect of symptoms on assessment of social functioning. Psychiatrie et Psychologie 12:183–187, 1989

Skodol AE, Link BG, Shrout PE, et al: The revision of Axis V in DSM-III-R: should symptoms have been included? Am J Psychiatry 145:825–829, 1988

Spitzer RL, Forman JBW, Nee J: DSM-III field trials, I: initial interrater diagnostic reliability. Am J Psychiatry 136:815–817, 1979

Stein RE, Gortmaker SL, Perrin EC, et al: Severity of illness: concepts and measurements. Lancet 2:1506–1509, 1987

Strauss JS: A comprehensive approach to psychiatric diagnosis. Am J Psychiatry 132:1193–1197, 1975

Williams JBW: The multiaxial system of DSM-III: where did it come from and where should it go? II: empirical studies, innovations, and recommendations. Arch Gen Psychiatry 42:181–186, 1985

World Health Organization: Manual of the Eighth Revision of the International Classification of Diseases, Injuries, and Causes of Death (ICD-8). Geneva, Switzerland, World Health Organization, 1967

World Health Organization: Mental Disorders: Glossary and Guide to Their Classification in Accordance With the Ninth Revision of the International Classification of Diseases. Geneva, Switzerland, World Health Organization, 1978

World Health Organization: International Classification of Diseases, 10th Edition Draft. Geneva, Switzerland, World Health Organization, 1989

Chapter 33

Defense Mechanisms

Andrew E. Skodol, M.D., and
J. Christopher Perry, M.P.H., M.D.

Statement of the Issues

The purpose of this review is to determine whether there is sufficient empirical evidence to support inclusion of an axis for defense mechanisms in DSM-IV. A decision regarding a defense mechanism axis should be based on consideration of the following issues.

1. The DSM is designed for use by all mental health professionals. Concepts of defensive functioning have their origins in psychodynamic conflict theory and have largely been the domain of psychodynamically oriented practitioners. Will defense mechanisms be useful to clinicians of other theoretical and therapeutic persuasions?
2. An axis in DSM-IV must reflect a consensus on the domain being assessed. Is there a consensus on the relevant defense mechanisms and their definitions?
3. An axis represents a simplified, shorthand assessment of an area. Is there evidence supporting such a streamlined, global assessment of defensive func-

---

A version of this chapter titled "Should an Axis for Defense Mechanisms Be Included in DSM-IV?" by A. E. Skodol and J. C. Perry has previously been published in *Comprehensive Psychiatry* 34:108–119, 1993.

The authors thank the other members of the DSM-IV Multiaxial Issues Work Group (Co-Chair, Howard H. Goldman, M.D., Ph.D.; Alan M. Gruenberg, M.D.; Juan E Mezzich, M.D., Ph.D.; and Chair, Janet B. W. Williams, D.S.W.), the Advisers to the Work Group (Stephen F. Bauer, M.D.; Arnold M. Cooper, M.D.; Paul Crits-Christoph, Ph.D.; Paul Jay Fink, M.D., Lester Luborsky, Ph.D.; Roger A. MacKinnon, M.D.; Lawrence H. Rockland, M.D., and M. Katherine Shear, M.D.), and the ad hoc Committee on Defense Mechanisms (Michael Bond, M.D.; Steven Cooper, Ph.D.; Bram Fridhandler, Ph.D.; Co-Chair, Mardi Horowitz, M.D.; and George E. Vaillant, M.D.) for reviewing and commenting on this work.

tioning, and can it be shown to be reasonably representative of a more detailed, comprehensive assessment of defenses?
4. Axial ratings must be feasible on the basis of general clinical initial or intake interview procedures. Even if it requires several patient contacts, can an adequate assessment of defenses be made without highly specialized training or procedures?
5. A preliminary criterion for the acceptability of an axis is its reliability. Can defenses be rated reliably with the information available in an initial evaluation by clinicians of average training and experience?
6. An axis increases the complexity of the evaluation process, and its utility should warrant the extra effort. Is there evidence to support the validity (i.e., clinical utility) of defense mechanisms?
7. Because DSM-III-R (American Psychiatric Association 1987) already contains five axes, additional axes should add useful information not conveyed by the other five. Is there evidence that defense mechanisms contribute unique information over and above that provided by Axes I through V?

Significance of the Issues

The DSM-III (American Psychiatric Association 1980) approach to diagnosis was criticized by psychodynamically oriented clinicians from its inception for reliance on descriptive psychopathology to the exclusion of assessment of mental functioning. The earliest critique by Karasu and Skodol (1980) pointed out that the absence of a psychodynamic evaluation of personality structure and functioning severely restricted the usefulness of the classification system for planning treatment with psychotherapy. They argued that the validity of the DSM-III multiaxial evaluation system would be enhanced by the addition of a parallel sixth axis requiring a rating of each patient's conflicts, object relations, defenses, or coping mechanisms. Others (Giovacchini 1981; Strayhorn 1983; Vaillant 1984) have echoed this sentiment. DSM-III-R included an extensive list of defense mechanisms in its glossary of technical terms and suggested that habitual use of particular defenses might be indicated on Axis II. Nevertheless, disappointment was expressed by Cooper and Michels (1988) that DSM-III-R continues to lack "a richer or more textured understanding either of the patient or of the patient's illness" (p. 1300).

A multiaxial system of diagnosis was introduced in DSM-III because of recognition that a comprehensive assessment of mental disorder, useful in planning treatment and estimating prognosis, could not be adequately represented by simple, standard diagnostic categories (Mezzich 1979; Strauss 1975; Williams 1985). The additional axes were believed to capture important aspects of clinical heterogeneity not conveyed by Axis I or Axis II. How effective Axes III ("Physical Disorders and Conditions"), IV ("Severity of Psychosocial Stressors"), and V ("Highest Level of Adaptive Functioning") have been in accomplishing their stated purposes are open questions, but the idea of a sixth psychodynamic axis, now proposed solely for defense mechanisms, remains on the table for consideration for DSM-IV.

Method

Initially, we considered all articles reporting research on defense mechanisms measured by clinical interview, self-report questionnaire, or projective test. One of us had conducted a review previously (Perry and Cooper 1987); this update includes articles published through December 1990, identified with the assistance of the PsychLit computer search.

Results

The results of the literature review are presented in the following nine sections: assessment methods, general applicability, consensus on defenses, support for an axial rating, degree of complexity, reliability, clinical utility, relationship to other axes, and recent developments.

Assessment Methods

There are three methods that have been used for the empirical assessment of defense mechanisms: clinical interview, self-report questionnaire, and projective test (Perry and Cooper 1987). By far the method most widely used with patients has been the clinical interview, which includes the methods and instruments developed by Haan (1963), Jacobson et al. (1986a, 1986b), Perry and Cooper (1989), Semrad et al. (1973), Vaillant (1976), and Weintraub and Aronson (1962). These methods all rate interview material (live/recorded, transcribed, or abstracted) of from 10 minutes to 12 hours in length and employ explicit definitions, often with accompanying rating scales. The definitions and rating scales vary, however. These methods have placed a premium on the objective rating of defenses for research purposes. As of this writing, no researcher has used a method comparable to usual clinical practice (i.e., conducting an interview and rating defenses on the basis of what the patient has said) without the benefit of review of transcriptions or summaries of the material.

Two self-report instruments to assess a number of defenses from a classical perspective have been developed: the Defense Mechanism Inventory of Gleser and Ihilevich (1969) and the Defense Style Questionnaire (DSQ), developed by Bond et al. (1983). Self-report questionnaires have the advantage of potentially enhanced reliability through the elimination of observer judgment, but the disadvantage of accessing only conscious derivatives of defenses. Moreover, the applicability of results derived from a questionnaire to a DSM system based on clinician judgment is not immediately obvious, unless attempts have been made to relate questionnaire results to clinical assessments. In the case of the Defense Mechanism Inventory, a review of 40 studies by Cramer (1988) indicated few attempts to compare this questionnaire with other standardized defense measures, and only one study made use of clinical ratings as the criterion measure. Furthermore, the concurrent and predictive validity results from Defense Mechanism Inventory scales were rather poor.

Two studies have compared the DSQ with clinically measured defense styles. In the Vaillant et al. (1986) study, 50% of the DSQ items correlated significantly with the style, measured clinically 6–8 years earlier, that they purportedly represented. All of the correlations, however, were less than .30 and were not necessarily highest with the identical defense style. Bond et al. (1989) also attempted validation of the DSQ using Perry and Cooper's (1989) Defense Mechanism Rating Scales (DMRS). They found that immature defenses (the lowest level) rated from clinical interviews correlated significantly with the lowest three of the four DSQ defense styles (maladaptive, image-distorting, and self-sacrificing), but otherwise the defense levels from the two methods were not comparable. Thus, there is some doubt regarding how informative results based on the DSQ would be to a clinical rating of defensive functioning. Results at a gross level (i.e., styles or levels) may be more pertinent than results on specific defenses.

Several other self-report measures have been developed from the traditions of personality trait and social psychology. The Repression-Sensitization Scale (Byrne et al. 1963) has been used extensively. Repressors have been found to respond to negative affect by avoiding negative implications of information, consequently performing less well under stress and showing less empathy than sensitizers (Weinberger 1990). Another well-known self-report measure is the Ways of Coping Scale (Folkman and Lazarus 1985; Lazarus and Folkman 1984). This scale measures conscious strategies in coping with stress, including confrontive coping, distancing, self-controlling, seeking social support, accepting responsibility, escape avoidance, planful problem solving, and positive reappraisal (Folkman et al. 1986). These and other measures are more fully reviewed elsewhere (Paulhus et al., in press).

The third method used in research on defense mechanisms is the Rorschach test. There have been few empirical studies of defense mechanisms using the Rorschach, nor is there evidence, thus far, that it provides more valid data than a clinical interview. Furthermore, given current diagnostic practice, data based on projective test methods seem mostly irrelevant to a defense mechanism axis for DSM-IV.

General Applicability

A defense has been defined as a "psychological mechanism that mediates between an individual's wishes, needs, affects, and impulses on the one hand, and both internalized prohibitions and external reality on the other" (Perry and Cooper 1989, p. 444). Although the language of such a formulation is derived from psychoanalytic theory, other theories of psychological functioning include structures or mechanisms for managing stress or general adaptation, such as coping or cognitive styles or mechanisms. Even within psychoanalysis, broadening the concept of defense mechanisms to include not only management of intrapsychic conflict but also adaptation of the person to the demands and constraints of the external world theoretically links coping and defense. The most adaptive defenses are sometimes referred to as coping mechanisms.

As yet, however, no systematic research has been conducted to assess the relationship between psychodynamic and other theoretical processes for adaptation or stress management. Some views concerning the etiology or pathogenesis of mental disorders, such as the behavioral or the biological, may explain defenses in other ways, or not address them at all.

Consensus on Defenses

Although achieving a consensus on the identification and definition of relevant defenses has been a stumbling block in the past, those investigators currently working on empirical studies have reached considerable consensus. The strongest consensus appears to be that defenses can be grouped and arranged in a hierarchy, with so-called mature, more adaptive defenses at the top, and immature, more maladaptive defenses at the bottom. Most schemata, whether theoretical or empirical, have three (Andrews et al. 1989; Vaillant 1976; Vaillant and Drake 1985), four (Battista 1982; Bond et al. 1983), or five (Perry and Cooper 1989) general levels. At the level of individual defenses rated by clinical methods, reviews by Perry and Cooper (1987) and Perry (1993) show that there is considerable overlap among the systems currently in use. All include immature, neurotic, and mature levels. They differ most on inclusion or exclusion of groups of specific borderline or image-distorting defenses (Perry and Cooper 1989) or explicitly psychotic defenses (Battista 1982). Among those who use the defense construct, a widely accepted list of defenses, with definitions on which there is general agreement, seems feasible.

Support for an Axial Rating

Much of the empirical research designed to validate defense mechanisms has actually tested the validity of hierarchies of levels of defensive functioning, apart from the validity of individual defenses themselves. The studies by Vaillant (1976) and Vaillant and Vaillant (1990), for example, have shown that individual defenses pooled into a hierarchy of mature, intermediate, and immature defenses correlated highly with independent, objective measures of mental health. In Vaillant's work, as well as others' (Bond et al. 1989; Perry and Cooper 1989), clusters of defense mechanisms were associated with better reliability than were individual defenses. Thus, although the reliability of rating groups of related defenses or defense styles has not been tested, it seems likely than a scale with a limited number of defense styles arranged in a hierarchy would prove more reliable that a schema in which identification of individual defenses was required. Details of existing reliability and validity studies are described later.

Degree of Complexity

The complexity of a defense mechanism axis would be a function of the amount and kind of information necessary to make the ratings, the inherent difficulty in judging clinically relevant material, and the level of general and specific training required by potential raters. As mentioned earlier, one early clinical method was based on transcriptions of up to 12 hours of interviews (Haan 1963). Because of the time involved and the form of the data to be rated, such a system would not be usable in a diagnostic manual. Of the more widely used clinical methods, Vaillant's (1992) glossary of 18 defense mechanisms has most often been applied to prepared life vignettes extracted from interviews with subjects. Typically, 20 vignettes describing how subjects dealt with important events in their lives have been selected per subject. It is doubtful that so rich a database could be obtained in one or two clinical interviews. Vaillant's method, as well as one developed by Jacobson et al. (1986a, 1986b) for use with adolescents and Perry and Cooper's (1986a, 1986b, 1989) DMRS, have all been applied most often to written or videotaped case material. The feasibility of use of the systems following live interviews or with routine clinical notes has not been tested.

Historically, defense mechanism determination required psychodynamic or psychoanalytic training. Here empirical methods have made great progress. All empirical methods use glossaries to define individual defenses, and most employ rating scales to quantify the degree to which a particular defense is used. These methods have greatly reduced the mystique surrounding inferential judgments concerning defensive functioning by offering clear guidelines and examples. Consequently, perceptive persons without extensive formal training in psychodynamics can learn to make clinical ratings. The most developed method is the DMRS (Perry and Cooper 1989), which includes a definition for each of 28 defenses, a description of its function, comments on how to discriminate it from other defenses, and an accompanying 3-point rating scale, with examples of probable and definite uses of the defense. Training is comparable to that employed for structured diagnostic interviews, such as the Schedule for Affective Disorders and Schizophrenia (Endicott and Spitzer 1978) or the Structured Clinical Interview for DSM-III-R (Spitzer et al. 1990). One unresolved issue regarding the DMRS is that, to date, studies have been based on group consensus ratings. Whether single clinicians can be trained to use the instrument as reliably or validly as the consensus groups remains to be seen.

Reliability

The following summarizes reliability for scales measuring defenses based on clinical methods. Weintraub and Aronson (1962) rated 12 characteristics of speech obtained from 10-minute samples that are believed to be related to defenses. Interjudge reliability was good, but it is unclear whether the method measures defensive functioning, cognitive functioning, or both. Haan's (1963) method enabled clinically experienced raters to rate 10 defense and 10 coping mechanisms acceptably (mean reliability coefficient = .66 for male and .50 for female subjects). Because ratings were made on written summaries of up to 12 hours of patient interview, the reliability of these scales cannot be generalized to standard clinical data. The Ego Function Assessment of Bellak et al. (1973) originally yielded an r of .81 for a 13-point scale of overall effectiveness of defensive functioning, but a replication by Dahl (1984b) failed to find acceptable reliability ($r = .13$). Individual defenses were not rated. Ablon et al. (1974) found interrater reliability coefficients of from .49 to .89 on nine defense patterns derived from the 45-item Ego Profile Scale developed by Semrad et al. (1973). These ratings were based on extensive inpatient observations and have not been attempted using outpatients.

Vaillant's (1976) method yielded a mean reliability for 18 defense mechanisms of .56 (range, −.01–.95) when rated from life vignettes by raters who were blind to their subjects' childhood and adult adjustment. Rater agreement was higher for combined ratings of two independent judges compared with Vaillant's own judgments (mean, $r = .73$; range, .53–.96). The method that Jacobson et al. (1986a, 1986b) applied to interview transcripts yielded good intraclass correlation coefficients ($\geq .60$) for 7 of 12 defenses, three correlations in the fair range (.40–.59), and three poor correlations. Perry and Cooper's (1989) DMRS ratings of 22 defenses on videotaped psychodynamic interviews by nonprofessionals yielded a mean intraclass correlation coefficient of .37 for individual defenses (range, .11–.59) and .51 for five summary defense scales (range, .39–.65). When raters were grouped and consensus ratings compared between groups, mean reliability for individual defenses improved to .57 and for summary scales to .71 (range, .57–.78). Subsequently, eight additional mature defenses were found to have comparable consensus reliabilities when applied to life vignette data. Perry (1993) also derived a weighted average score for defenses identified from audiotapes and written psychotherapy session transcripts, based on the level of each defense in a seven-point defense mechanism hierarchy. For this overall maturity of defenses score, interrater reliability was found to be .89.

In summary, newer empirical methods for rating defenses have shown that they can be rated reliably given certain kinds of clinical data and adequate training of raters. Consensus ratings are more reliable than ratings by individual raters, suggesting that identifying defenses still requires some level of inference. Defense clusters, groups, or summary scales are more reliably identified than are individual defense mechanisms. Because reliability studies have been based exclusively on specially prepared data in the form of life vignettes, interview transcripts, and videotapes, the reliability of procedures for identifying defenses in live clinical interviews has yet to be determined.

Clinical Utility

Defense mechanisms are hypothesized to be good measures of adaptive capacity. This hypothesis has been tested by examining the relationship of defenses with measures of global functioning, course of psychiatric illness, and various indicators of success in adult life.

Five studies have employed clinical methods to test a model that conceptualizes defenses in a hierarchy from least to most adaptive. Vaillant (1976) longitudinally studied a cohort of college-age men, and Vaillant et al. (1986) studied a second group of inner-city men to examine the relationship of defenses to adult mental health. Battista (1982) examined the association of Vaillant's defenses and global mental health in inpatients. Jacobson et al. (1986a, 1986b) studied defenses and measures of ego development in diabetic adolescents and control subjects. Perry and Cooper (1986a, 1986b, 1989) examined the relationship of defenses to global functioning in patients with personality disorders or bipolar II disorder. In general, individual defenses hypothesized to be low in a hierarchy of adaptiveness were found to be negatively correlated with measures of global functioning. Middle-level defenses were negatively correlated but less strongly. In the case of the ubiquitous neurotic defenses, hardly any correlation was found (median, .04). Mature defenses, those hypothesized to be most adaptive, had the only consistently positive relationship to global functioning (median $r = .33$). When studies were combined and defenses considered in conceptually related groups, each level of the hierarchy bore a regular relationship to global functioning (Perry 1993), tending to validate the proposition that defenses can by hierarchically arranged according to their adaptiveness.

Using self-report data generated from the DSQ, Bond et al. (1983) found a strong negative correlation between his lowest defense style and independent measures of ego strength and ego development, somewhat negative correlations for his intermediate styles, and a positive correlation for his most mature level. These findings were partially replicated in a second sample (Bond et al. 1989) with the Health Sickness Rating Scale as the measure of functioning.

Ablon et al. (1974) have shown a relationship between maturity of defense used and improvement in hospitalized patients with affective disorders. Perry (1988, 1990) also found a relationship between low-level defenses and more severely symptomatic course and between obsessional defenses and a less severe course for patients with personality and affective disorders. Ellsworth et al. (1986) found that obese patients who were able to sustain weight loss following treatment had more mature defenses as measured by Vaillant's method.

Other measures found to be associated with mature levels of defenses are IQ (Haan 1963), upward social mobility (Snarey and Vaillant, 1985), and psychosocial maturity and social competence (Vaillant et al. 1986). In the latter study, the role of mature defenses seemed greatest among people who had the most difficult childhoods. Vaillant and Vaillant (1990) also found a relationship between maturity of defenses measured prospectively and physical health, adjustment, and satisfaction in late life among college-educated men in their mid-60s.

The studies reviewed suggest that defense levels are differentially related to psychosocial adjustment and functioning. It is not known whether a hierarchy of defenses would predict functioning better than other measures, although Vaillant and Vaillant (1990) continued to find an association with adjustment even after other predictor variables, including childhood strengths, were controlled. It is interesting that few studies have reported specifically on the ability of empirically determined defense styles or levels to select persons for psychodynamically oriented psychotherapy or to predict its outcome. One study by Piper et al. (1985) did find that defense style measured by the DSQ predicted some aspects of psychotherapy process and outcome.

Relationship to Other Axes

A good measure or predictor of functioning may not be necessary in a multiaxial evaluation system that already includes indicators for syndromic diagnoses, personality disorders, physical problems, stressors, and global functioning. Useful as defense mechanisms may prove to be, they might not be appropriate for an axis if they were redundant with existing designations that are more broadly accepted or easier to make. The evidence cited suggests that defenses are not redundant with existing Axes I–V.

With respect to Axis I and II diagnoses, an additional axial rating may show some regular relationship to diagnoses, but to be most useful should capture variability within diagnostic categories. Therefore, one would not expect a one-to-one relationship between diagnosis and defensive style.

Most of the studies of defense mechanisms and diagnosis have focused on the personality disorders. Vaillant and Drake (1985) found that 66% of inner-city men with any Axis II diagnosis used mostly immature level defenses as opposed to only 10% of those without an Axis II disorder. Maturity of defenses was negatively associated with personality disorder. Certain individual Axis II disorders were strongly associated with predictable individual defenses, such as paranoid with projection, schizoid with fantasy, and antisocial with acting out. Perry and Cooper (1986a) found predictable relationships between borderline personality disorder and defenses, such as the image-distorting defenses of splitting and projective identification ($r = .36$) and the action defenses of acting out, passive aggression, and hypochondriasis or help-rejecting complaining ($r = .26$). These findings were replicated by Bond (1990) using Perry's method. Antisocial personality disorder and bipolar II were also associated with particular defenses, but defenses alone were not able to separate the diagnostic groups in multivariate analyses. Dahl (1984a) found that patients with borderline personality disorder had higher defensive functioning than those with schizophrenia, comparable to patients with affective disorders, but lower than those with other personality disorders and neurotic disorders. Goldsmith et al. (1984) also found that defensive functioning differentiated borderline from neurotic patients.

Using the DSQ, Bond and Vaillant (1986) found that Bond's lowest three defense style levels distinguished psychiatric patients from control subjects, but the authors found no clear relationship between style and particular diagnosis. In a subsequent study, Bond (1990) could not discriminate between borderline personality disorder, other personality disorders, and control subjects without personality disorder on DSQ defensive style. Andrews et al. (1989) found a relationship between Bond's maladaptive style and Eysenck's Neuroticism Scale (Eysenck and Eysenck 1975) and an overall score on the SCL-90 (Derogatis 1977). Pollock and Andrews (1989) found a differential association between type of anxiety disorder (e.g., panic disorder, social phobia, obsessive-compulsive disorder) and DSQ defenses. Steiger et al. (1989) and Steiner (1990) found that patients with different eating disorders could be distinguished to a degree from each other and from control subjects based on their predominant defense style.

Apparently, no studies have examined the relationship between defense mechanisms and physical illness among psychiatric patients, although the longitudinal study of college men by Vaillant and Vaillant (1990) discussed earlier found a relationship between maturity of defenses and physical health in later life ($r = .19$). Bond and Vaillant (1986) found no relationship between the use of a particular defense style and a given level of psychosocial stressors rated on Axis IV.

The greatest possibility for redundancy with an existing DSM-III-R Axis would appear to be with Axis V, the Global Assessment of Functioning Scale. As reviewed earlier, hierarchies of defenses have been found to be regularly associated with measures of global functioning. In the study by Perry and Cooper (1989), the global measure was the Global Assessment Scale (Endicott et al. 1976), the forerunner and close counterpart of the Global Assessment of Functioning Scale. Close examination of the magnitude of the correlations (range, −.42–.22), however, would support the contention that these two measures tap related but not identical constructs. Studies are needed that use multivariate designs to compare ratings on the Global Assessment Scale or the Global Assessment of Functioning Scale with defense mechanism ratings in predicting outcomes.

Recent Developments

Since 1988, an ad hoc Committee on Defense Mechanisms[1] has been developing a proposal for a Defense Mechanisms Axis for consideration by the DSM-IV Multiaxial Issues Work Group. This committee has independently reviewed the literature, debated the individual definitions to be included, and mustered the empirical basis for a hierarchy. The committee considered whether the axis should identify individual defenses, defense styles representing common groupings (e.g., obsessional or hysterical), or an overall rating of defensive adaptation. The goals were to remain close to the clinical phenomena, preserve what is most useful to the clinician, and create a proposal that would not be largely redundant with global functioning.

The axis proposed for the *DSM-IV Options Book* (American Psychiatric Association 1991) reflects a decision not to propose rating overall level of defensive functioning based on the hierarchy of defenses, because such a rating would remove the detail most meaningful to the clinician and possibly be excessively redundant with the Global Assessment of Functioning Scale. Instead, clinicians would identify specific individual defenses (up to seven) characterizing, first, the patient's current functioning and, second, usual functioning (past year or longer prior to and excluding episodes of mental disorder) if different from current. In addition, the clinician would identify the current and usual styles or groups (up to three) that have been demonstrated empirically (e.g., high adaptive, obsessional, action). In each case, the most prominent defense would be listed first.

A defense mechanism axis is currently undergoing field testing at the Cambridge Hospital in Massachusetts, the Payne Whitney Clinic at Cornell University–

---

[1]Membership: Michael Bond, M.D., Steven Cooper, Ph.D., Bram Fridhandler, Ph.D., Mardi Horowitz, M.D. (Co-Chair), J. Christopher Perry, M.P.H., M.D. (Co-Chair), George E. Vaillant, M.D. Supported in part by the Program on Conscious and Unconscious Mental Processes of the University of California at San Francisco and the John D. and Catherine T. MacArthur Foundation.

New York Hospital, and the clinics of the University of Oslo. The field trial will focus on reliability under conditions of usual clinical practice and on clinical usefulness.

Discussion

Considerable progress has been made in defense mechanism research since the deliberations of the late 1970s that resulted in DSM-III. Empirical methods for rating defense mechanisms more reliably have been developed, and data on the clinical utility of such ratings have begun to accumulate. A consensus on definitions appears to be emerging in the research literature, and evidence exists supporting a hierarchy of defenses based on their adaptiveness.

Two advisers to the Multiaxial Work Group pointed out that belief in specific defenses arranged in a hierarchy is not universal among psychoanalysts. Some theorists propose that any ego activity can be used for the purpose of defense, and others believe that patients at all levels of psychopathology use defenses from all levels (i.e., that the differences in defenses between patients are quantitative rather than qualitative). These two advisers did concede, however, that the idea that maladaptive or "primitive" defenses dominate in syndromes of greater clinical severity, although as yet unproven, is the prevailing view of most psychodynamically oriented clinicians. One adviser believed that an overall assessment of ego functioning would be more useful than a focus solely on defense mechanisms.

Furthermore, although the Defensive Styles Rating Scale proposed in the *DSM-IV Options Book* represents the consensus of one group of researchers, other advisers took issue with particular conceptualizations of several of the listed levels of defenses. Some defenses at the high adaptive level were criticized for being ego functions (e.g., self-observation) and not necessarily defensive in nature. At the action level, several defenses were viewed as behaviors common to the failure of other defense styles. Questions were also raised about the terminology used to refer to several specific defenses (e.g., hypochondriasis as opposed to somatization). Thus, although general consensus is growing concerning defense mechanisms, a specific concrete proposal is likely to provoke some debate. A potential obstacle for a DSM defense mechanism axis is the assumed strong theoretical link of the concept of defense to psychodynamic theory. Among advisers, this point raised some controversy. Several suggested that clinicians without a primary psychodynamic orientation have already adopted or adapted psychodynamic ideas about how their patients habitually deal with stress and that defense mechanisms had reached the position of "common language" basic to all of psychiatry and psychology. Others were more skeptical. It remains a question whether clinicians without some training in the psychodynamic perspective would use the proposed axis. It is clear that one need not be a psychoanalyst to reliably rate defenses using the newer methodologies. But will the practitioner want to?

Another problem is that the new methodologies have not been tested under usual clinical conditions, with limited, "live" clinical data. Also, there appears to be a need for discussion with persons who know the patient well to make reliable ratings, although this may be a problem shared with other axes as well (e.g., personality disorders). Do existing results translate into comparable results for the individual clinician conducting a standard patient assessment? Answers to these questions should emerge from the field trials described in this chapter.

Recommendations

A viable option for DSM-IV might be the inclusion of a defense mechanism axis in an appendix of optional axes for use in special clinical and research settings. This choice would be especially appealing if similar recommendations are made for other new axes, such as an axis for Global Assessment of Relational Functioning, or if current or proposed Axes IV or V also become more "officially" optional.

Inclusion of a defense axis, at least as an option, appears to be warranted. In addition to providing dynamically meaningful diagnostic data, it would also facilitate expansion of the empirical database on a standardized measure of defenses that does not require cumbersome, research-oriented raw data or multiple raters. Studies of the utility of defense mechanism ratings for planning specific treatment interventions and for predicting outcomes should be a high priority. Pending the outcome of field trials, a sixth axis for defense mechanisms may prove to be justified.

References

Ablon SL, Carlson GA, Goodwin FK: Ego defense patterns in manic-depressive illness. Am J Psychiatry 131:803–807, 1974

American Psychiatric Association: Diagnostic and Statistical Manual of Mental Disorders, 3rd Edition. Washington, DC, American Psychiatric Association, 1980

American Psychiatric Association: Diagnostic and Statistical Manual of Mental Disorders, 3rd Edition, Revised. Washington, DC, American Psychiatric Association, 1987

American Psychiatric Association: DSM-IV Options Book: Work in Progress. Washington, DC, American Psychiatric Association, 1991

Andrews G, Pollock C, Stewart G: The determination of defense style by questionnaire. Arch Gen Psychiatry 46:455–460, 1989.

Battista JR: Empirical test of Vaillant's hierarchy of ego functions. Am J Psychiatry 139:356–357, 1982

Bellak L, Hurvich M, Gediman H: Ego Functions in Schizophrenics, Neurotics and Normals. New York, John Wiley, 1973

Bond M: Are "borderline defenses" specific for borderline personality disorders? Journal of Personality Disorders 4:251–256, 1990

Bond MP, Vaillant JS: An empirical study of the relationship between diagnosis and defense style. Arch Gen Psychiatry 43:285–288, 1986

Bond M, Gardner ST, Christian J, et al: Empirical study of self-rated defense styles. Arch Gen Psychiatry 40:333–338, 1983.

Bond M, Perry JC, Gautier M, et al: Validating the self-report of defense styles. Journal of Personality Disorders 3:101–112, 1989

Byrne D, Bary J, Nelson D: Relation of the revised Repression-Sensitization Scale to measures of self-description. Psychol Rep 13:323–334, 1963

Cooper AM, Michels R: Diagnostic and Statistical Manual of Mental Disorders, 3rd Edition, Revised (DSM-III-R) (book review). Am J Psychiatry 145:1300–1301, 1988

Cramer P: The Defense Mechanism Inventory: a review of research and discussion of the scales. J Pers Assess 52:142–164, 1988

Dahl AA: Ego function assessment of hospitalized adult psychiatric patients with special reference to borderline patients, in The Broad Scope of Ego Function Assessment. Edited by Bellak L, Goldsmith LA. New York, Wiley, 1984a, pp 167–176

Dahl AA: A study of agreement among raters of Bellak's Ego Function Assessment Test, in The Broad Scope of Ego Function Assessment. Edited by Bellak L, Goldsmith LA. New York, John Wiley, 1984b, pp 160–166

Derogatis LR: SCL-90 Revised Version Manual—1. Baltimore, MD, Johns Hopkins School of Medicine, 1977

Ellsworth GA, Strain GW, Strain JJ, et al: Defense maturity ratings and sustained weight loss in obesity. Psychosomatics 27:772–781, 1986

Endicott J, Spitzer RL: A diagnostic interview: the Schedule for Affective Disorders and Schizophrenia. Arch Gen Psychiatry 35:837–844, 1978

Endicott J, Spitzer RL, Fleiss J, et al: The Global Assessment Scale: a procedure for measuring overall severity of psychiatric disturbance. Arch Gen Psychiatry 33:766–771, 1976

Eysenck HJ, Eysenck SBG: Manual of the Eysenck Personality Questionnaire (Junior and Adult). Kent, England, Hodder & Stoughton, 1975

Folkman S, Lazarus RS: If it changes it must be a process: study of emotion and coping during three stages of a college examination. J Pers Soc Psychol 48:150–170, 1985

Folkman S, Lazarus RS, Dunkel-Shetter C, et al: Dynamics of a stressful encounter: cognitive appraisal, coping and encounter outcomes. J Pers Soc Psychol 50:992–1003, 1986

Giovacchini PL: The axes of DSM-III. Am J Psychiatry 138:119–120, 1981

Gleser GC, Ihilevich D: An objective instrument for measuring defense mechanisms. J Consult Clin Psychol 33:51–60, 1969

Goldsmith LA, Charles E, Feiner K: The use of EFA in the assessment of borderline pathology, in The Broad Scope of Ego Function Assessment. Edited by Bellak L, Goldsmith LA. New York, John Wiley, 1984, pp 340–361

Haan N: Proposed model of ego functioning: coping and defense mechanisms in relationship to IQ change. Psychological Monographs 77:1–23, 1963

Jacobson AM, Beardslee W, Hauser ST, et al: An approach to evaluating ego defense mechanisms using clinical interviews, in Empirical Studies of the Ego Mechanisms of Defense. Edited by Vaillant GE. Washington, DC, American Psychiatric Press, 1986a, pp 47–59

Jacobson AM, Beardslee W, Hauser ST, et al: Evaluating ego defense mechanisms using clinical interviews: an empirical study of adolescent diabetic and psychiatric patients. Journal of Adolescence 9:303–319, 1986b

Karasu BT, Skodol AE: VIth axis for DSM-III: psychodynamic evaluation. Am J Psychiatry 137:607–610, 1980

Lazarus RS, Folkman S: Stress, Appraisal and Coping. New York, Springer, 1984

Mezzich JE: Patterns and issues in multiaxial psychiatric diagnosis. Psychol Med 9:125–137, 1979

Paulhus DL, Fridhandler B, Hayes S: Psychological defense: contemporary theory and research, in Handbook of Personality Psychology. Edited by Hogan R, Johnson J, Briggs SR. San Diego, CA, Academic Press (in press)

Perry JC: A prospective study of life stress, defenses, psychotic symptoms and depression in borderline and antisocial personality disorders and bipolar type II affective disorder. Journal of Personality Disorders 2:49–59, 1988

Perry JC: Psychological defense mechanisms in the study of affective and anxiety disorders, in Comorbidity of Mood and Anxiety Disorders. Edited by Maser JD, Cloninger CR. Washington, DC, American Psychiatric Press, 1990, pp 545–562

Perry JC: Defenses and their effects, in Psychodynamic Treatment Research. Edited by Miller N, Luborsky L, Docherty J. New York, Basic Books, 1993, pp 274–307

Perry JC, Cooper SH: A preliminary report on defenses and conflicts associated with borderline personality disorder. J Am Psychoanal Assoc 34:863–893, 1986a

Perry JC, Cooper SH: What do cross-sectional measures of defenses predict?, in Empirical Studies of the Ego Mechanisms of Defense. Edited by Vaillant GE. Washington, DC, American Psychiatric Press, 1986b, pp 31–46

Perry JC, Cooper SH: Empirical studies of psychological defenses, in Psychiatry, Vol 1. Edited by Michels R, Cavenar JO Jr. Philadelphia, JB Lippincott, 1987, pp 1–19

Perry JC, Cooper SH: An empirical study of defense mechanisms, I: clinical interview and life vignette ratings. Arch Gen Psychiatry 46:444–452, 1989

Piper WE, de Carvfel FL, Szkrumelak N: Patient predictors of process and outcome in short-term individual psychotherapy. J Nerv Ment Dis 173:726–733, 1985

Pollock C. Andrews G: Defense styles associated with specific anxiety disorders. Am J Psychiatry 146:1500–1502, 1989

Semrad E. Grinspoon L, Fienberg SE: Development of an Ego Profile Scale. Arch Gen Psychiatry 28:70–77, 1973

Snarey JR, Vaillant GE: How lower and working-class youth become middle-class adults: the association between ego defense mechanisms and upward social mobility. Child Dev 56:899–910, 1985

Spitzer RL, Williams JBW, Gibbon M, et al: User's Guide for the Structured Clinical Interview for DSM-III-R (SCID). Washington, DC, American Psychiatric Press, 1990

Steiger H, van der Freen J, Goldstein C, et al: Defense styles and parental bonding in eating-disordered women. International Journal of Eating Disorders 8:131–140, 1989

Steiner H: Defense styles in eating disorders. International Journal of Eating Disorders 9:141–151, 1990

Strauss JS: A comprehensive approach to psychiatric diagnosis. Am J Psychiatry 132:1193–1197, 1975

Strayhorn JM Jr: A diagnostic axis relevant to psychotherapy and preventative mental health. Am J Orthopsychiatry 53:677–696, 1983

Vaillant GE: Natural history of male psychological health: the relation of choice of ego mechanisms of defense to adult adjustment. Arch Gen Psychiatry 33:535–545, 1976

Vaillant GE: The disadvantages of DSM-III outweigh its advantages. Am J Psychiatry 141:542–545, 1984

Vaillant GE: Vaillant's glossary of defenses, in Ego Mechanisms of Defense: A Guide for Clinicians and Researchers. Edited by Vaillant GE. Washington, DC, American Psychiatric Press, 1992, pp 243–251

Vaillant GE, Drake RE: Maturity of ego defenses in relation DSM-III Axis II personality disorder. Arch Gen Psychiatry 42:597–601, 1985

Vaillant GE, Vaillant CO: Natural history of male psychological health, XII: a 45 year study of predictors of successful aging at age 65. Am J Psychiatry 147:31–37, 1990

Vaillant GE, Bond M, Vaillant CO: An empirically validated hierarchy of defense mechanisms. Arch Gen Psychiatry 43:786–794, 1986

Weinberger DA: The construct validity of the repressive coping style, in Repression and Dissociation: Implications for Personality Theory, Psychopathology, and Health. Edited by Singer JL. Chicago, IL, University of Chicago Press, 1990, pp 337–386

Weintraub W, Aronson H: The application of verbal behavior analysis to the study of psychological defense mechanisms: methodology and preliminary report. J Nerv Ment Dis 134:169–181, 1962

Williams JBW: The multiaxial system of DSM-III: where did it come from and where should it go? I: its origins and critiques. Arch Gen Psychiatry 42:175–180, 1985

Section V

Family/Relational Problems

Introduction to Section V

Family/Relational Problems

Allen J. Frances, M.D., John F. Clarkin, Ph.D., and
Ruth Ross, M.A.

One of the major criticisms of DSM-III (American Psychiatric Association 1980) and DSM-III-R (American Psychiatric Association 1987) was that their exclusive focus on mental disorders as they occur in individuals has restricted the usefulness of the system in the diagnosis and treatment of problems that occur in the family and other relational units. For this reason, literature reviews on the utility and definitional features of a number of important relational and family problems were solicited from experts in the field. They were asked to examine the literature on these problems and to make recommendations as to whether such diagnoses should be included in DSM-IV.

The authors of these reviews were asked to follow the same format as was used for all the other DSM-IV literature reviews. However, these authors were given a somewhat different mandate: rather than trying to be simply objective, they were also asked to critique DSM-III-R with respect to its consideration of family and relational issues. They were therefore given more latitude to present their own perspective rather than a consensus position. For this reason, their recommendations are not always consistent with those that actually appeared in the *DSM-IV Options Book* (American Psychiatric Association 1991).

Relational Problem Related to a Mental Disorder or General Medical Condition

Goldstein et al. (Chapter 34) reviewed the literature on relational problems associated with high expressed emotion, defined as an index of the intensity of attitudes that one person, prototypically a relative, feels about another person, prototypically a patient. They considered the research data on high expressed emotion as a predictor of schizophrenic relapse and on the generalizability of high expressed emotion. They also examined the characteristics and determinants of high expressed emotion and the measures currently available for evaluating high expressed emotion. The authors note that the concept of high expressed emotion has been misinterpreted as "blaming" relatives. In reality, it describes a far more complex process that, understandably, is likely to emerge while caring for difficult, perplexing persons; nor is high expressed emotion a phenomenon that is at all specific to families of schizophrenic patients. Goldstein et al. concluded that high expressed emotion is best construed as a significant prognostic factor that is relevant to the course and contains treatment indications for a wide range of mental disorders and probably some physical disorders as well. For diagnostic purposes, they recommended that it be viewed as an indicator or marker of seriously dysfunctional interpersonal relationships that are not otherwise explicitly described, usually associated with bidirectional or multidirectional difficulties in the relationship. They concluded, based on empirical evidence, that high expressed emotion should be considered a transactional process that is not located exclusively in any individual and is typically associated with observable disturbed family interactions. The authors concluded that, despite uncertainties and gaps in the currently available research data, the evidence was sufficiently persuasive to justify including parent-child relational problem with high expressed emotion in DSM-IV. The authors were less sure of the most appropriate label for the category and considered alternative terms such as *emotionally intense interpersonal relationship* or *emotionally stressful interpersonal relationship*. They were also unsure of the most suitable location for it, but thought that the results of their review most strongly supported the inclusion of parent-child relational problem with high expressed emotion as a V code (ICD-10 [World Health Organization 1990] Z code) problem in the section on relational problems under "Other Conditions That May Be a Focus of Clinical Attention." The authors also recommended the inclusion of a parallel relational category of partner relational problem with high expressed emotion.

It was clear from the literature review by Goldstein et al. (Chapter 34) that relational problems can be associated with a wide range of disorders and may involve both parent-child and partner relationships. For this reason, the Task Force on DSM-IV is considering broadening the proposed category to be more clinically useful by dropping the term *expressed emotion* and including relational problems associated with general medical conditions as well as mental disorders. It is therefore proposed that the category "relational problem related to a mental disorder or a general medical condition" be included in the section for "Other Conditions That May Be a Focus of Clinical Attention."

Parent Inadequate Discipline

Chamberlain et al. (Chapter 35) examined the literature on the validity and clinical utility of parent inadequate discipline (PID) and its association with childhood and adult disorders. The authors also reviewed studies concerning social and contextual correlates and family relational patterns associated with PID and studies on the social acceptability of various discipline methods. Finally, they considered methodological issues that may affect the assessment of PID.

The authors found that both parents and children make unique contributions to discipline interchanges and exert influences on each other that affect the child's current adjustment and subsequent course of development. The authors identified five types of problem discipline interactions: 1) inconsistent discipline, including intraparent and interparent inconsistency; 2) irritable and explosive discipline; 3) low parent involvement and supervision; 4) inflexible and rigid discipline strategies; and 5) lack of planful discipline or discipline that is determined more by the parent's mood state or by the child's problem behavior, rather than by an overall plan to teach or socialize the child. The authors proposed including only the first four in the final criteria for PID in DSM-IV, because the fifth category is subsumed by the other four.

The authors found that, in several studies, problem discipline in childhood has been found to be related to adult criminal and psychiatric problems, with the former more relevant for males and the latter for females. Early PID has also been found to be related to later problems with parenting practices in women and with unstable employment and marital difficulties in men. The correlation is strong between PID and childhood disruptive behavior disorders, especially conduct disorder and oppositional defiant disorder. There is also evidence relating PID to childhood depression, academic problems, poor peer relations, and difficult child temperament.

The authors concluded that there is strong evidence for the predictive validity of PID, with early, severe disruptions in discipline appearing to bode poorly for the child's subsequent adjustment in adolescence and adulthood. Contextual factors such as the mental health and quality of the marital relationship of the parents have been shown to have both direct and indirect influences on discipline interactions. Several well-controlled treatment outcome studies have shown that helping parents improve their discipline practices results in at least short-term improvements in child and family adjustment.

The authors identified a number of methodological problems in evaluating PID. For example, several studies have found that parent reports are susceptible to systematic bias, with parents' stress level or depression likely to influence their reports of problem child behavior. The authors recommended that clinicians use a variety of sources and types of evaluation to diagnose PID.

The authors concluded that research on the etiology and treatment of childhood disorders would be enhanced by the inclusion of PID as a diagnostic category in DSM-IV.

Marital and Family Communication Difficulties

Clarkin and Miklowitz (Chapter 36) reviewed the literature on marital and family communication difficulties to see if there are data supporting the validity of these disturbances and reliable measures for evaluating them. They also considered data on the relationship between communication difficulties and Axis I and II mental disorders. They reviewed studies concerning spouse/spouse difficulties involving communication of information, affective expression, deficient problem solving, conflict and conflict resolution, and family structure. The authors then examined parent-child difficulties involving communication deviance, affective expression, family interactions, overinvolvement, coercive family processes, and deficits in family problem solving.

The authors concluded that the empirical data substantiate the existence of communication difficulties that can be reliably assessed and can cause malfunction in the family unit, may threaten the viability of the family, and may cause or exacerbate symptoms in vulnerable family members. They found that, with the exception of depression and schizophrenia, the data are sparse concerning the relationship between specific mental disorders and coexisting family communication difficulties.

The authors proposed four options for handling family communication difficulties in DSM-IV: 1) inclusion as a disorder in the DSM-IV diagnostic classification; 2) inclusion as a V code (Z code in ICD-10) under "Other Conditions That May Be a Focus of Clinical Attention"; 3) the creation of a separate axis for general family disruption, which would include communication and other family problems, to give special status to the family unit as an important factor in most individual pathology; and 4) ignoring family communication difficulties in the diagnostic system. The authors reviewed the pros and cons of including communication difficulties as a separate disorder. They noted that the option most likely to be accepted by the DSM-IV Task Force would be inclusion of family communication problems as a V code under "Other Conditions That May Be a Focus of Clinical Attention."

Partner Relational Problems With Physical Abuse

O'Leary and Jacobson (Chapter 37) reviewed the literature on partner relational problems with physical abuse to see if there are data supporting the validity and clinical utility of this category. They examined the following issues: the clinical and public health significance of partner relational problems with physical abuse, the adequacy of current diagnoses (e.g., intermittent explosive disorder, sadistic personality disorder, self-defeating personality disorder, posttraumatic stress disorder, battered woman syndrome) to describe these problems, the prevalence of physical aggression against an intimate partner, the sex ratio and impact of physical abuse, the age at onset of physical abuse, the responsibility for acts of physical aggression, the course of physical abuse, complications associated with physical abuse, familial patterns of abuse, and differential diagnostic issues. Based on this review, the authors proposed the following definition for partner relational problem with physical abuse: "Acts of physical aggression toward a partner such as slapping, kicking, beating, and choking. These acts do not necessarily result in physical injury requiring medical attention although in many cases they do. Often the acts are designed to force the individual to behave in a certain way."

The authors considered the adequacy of current assessment procedures to measure physical abuse and found that physical aggression against a partner can be reliably assessed with self and partner reports. The chapter ends with a list of pros and cons of including a diagnosis of partner relational problems with physical abuse in DSM-IV. The authors concluded that there is an urgent need for a diagnosis that covers the problems of physical abuse of partners and recommend its inclusion in DSM-IV.

Sibling Relational Problems

Kahn and Monks (Chapter 38) reviewed the literature on the validity and clinical utility of the category sibling relational problems. They noted that, although sibling rivalry is common, it can reach excessive proportions of violence, domination, and exploitation and can lead to severe psychological problems. Sibling relational problems appear to be the result of disruptions in parental functioning and may occur in the context of family conflict, crisis, or change. Abusive sibling relationships are frequently hidden from parental view.

The authors examined four main categories of sibling relational problems: 1) aggression, 2) incest, 3) illness, and 4) death. They considered their impact, course, sex ratio, age at onset, and familial pattern.

They found that sibling aggression is the most prevalent form of family violence. However, because its milder form is so common, it is often not viewed as a clinical problem. Of all homicides, 3% were sibling homicides. Sibling aggression increases as the family size increases, or as the availability of the parent decreases. The authors found that the data suggested that siblings who perpetuate violence against siblings are more likely to become violent adults and to engage in abusive relationships.

Concerning sibling incest, the data showed that sexually abused sisters are the usual informants of incest and experience more long-term effects than reported by their perpetrating brothers. The experience is more destructive the younger the child, the longer the duration of the incest, and the greater the degree of force used by the perpetrator. Symptoms experienced in the victim can include low self-esteem, guilt, depression, sexual dysfunction, fear of intimacy, difficulties in marriage, poor choice in marital partners, poor self-concept, lack of trust, and posttraumatic stress disorder.

The authors examined studies concerning the effects of a sibling's death on the family and the other children. They found that parents may not cope well with sibling grief and mourning because of their own grief, may become overprotective, or may seek to have the sibling replace the lost child. These responses can result in a variety of psychological problems, including guilt, confusion, depression, loneliness, anger, problems with schoolwork, a decrease in social competence, sleep disturbances, hallucinations of the deceased sibling, fear of death, and suicidal ideation. Intervention is needed to prevent long-term effects.

The authors also examined studies on the effects of a sibling's illness on the family and other children and found that the well sibling can experience feelings of social inadequacy, fear of contracting the illness or disability, anger, depression, a feeling of resentment or being unappreciated, and guilt.

The authors concluded that sibling relational problems (aggression, incest, illness, or death) can cause behavioral and emotional problems and can have a negative impact on the social and psychological development of the child and should be considered in treatment. They therefore recommend including sibling relational problems as a diagnostic category in DSM-IV.

Physical Abuse and Neglect of Children

Knutson and Schartz (Chapter 39) reviewed the literature on physical abuse and neglect of children to determine the potential utility of this category as a parent-child relational diagnosis for DSM-IV. The authors reviewed public policy concerning child abuse and neglect and its implications for possible diagnostic definitions. They then considered strategies for operationally defining abuse and neglect and examined the methodological limitations in the existing studies. They examined data on the epidemiology of physical abuse and neglect, characteristics of abused and neglected children (e.g., risk factors, behavioral characteristics, association with child and adolescent psychopathology), parent characteristics, the course and long-term consequences of physical abuse and neglect, and the possible association between childhood maltreatment and adult dysfunction.

The authors concluded that physical abuse and neglect of children by their parent(s) are important public health problems and that, even when stringent criteria are used to define abuse, the base rate of the problem is clearly sufficient to warrant attention. Because physical abuse and neglect appear to be chronic, they require intervention, and because they are strongly associated with child psychopathology or later behavioral deviance in adulthood, they are appropriate areas of interest for psychiatry. Because efforts to understand abuse by focusing on either the child or the parent have been relatively unsuccessful, the authors concluded, based on the available evidence, that it may be fruitful to conceptualize physical abuse and neglect as relational problems. They considered the clinical and research implications of including physical abuse and neglect as diagnostic categories in DSM-IV and the difficulties involved in establishing diagnostic guidelines. They concluded that physical abuse and neglect should be included as a relational diagnosis in DSM-IV because 1) a large amount of data strongly suggest that abuse and neglect are interactional problems involving a specific relationship, 2) it should improve the quality of research in the area relating abuse and neglect to other child and adult psychopathologies, and 3) most importantly, it should result in an improvement in services to children who are at great risk for many health and behavioral problems. The authors also discussed diagnostic standards for physical abuse and neglect.

Incest

Kaplan and Pelcovitz (Chapter 40) reviewed the literature on incest (the sexual abuse of a child under 18 by a family member) to determine if there was sufficient evidence to support its inclusion as a parent-child relational diagnosis in DSM-IV.

The authors reviewed 1) family studies that directly assessed functioning in incestuous families to see if there is empirical support for a specific family structure associated with incest; 2) studies concerning child and adolescent victims of incest, including emotional and behavioral difficulties in children and adolescents and the functioning of adult incest survivors; 3) studies of the nonoffending parent to see if there is empirical support for clinical descriptions of the nonabusive family member as a "cornerstone" of the pathological family process; 4) studies of the offending parent that evaluate the psychological, sexual, and interpersonal functioning of the incest perpetrator to determine if the incest reflects a pattern that is reactive to family pathology or exists outside of the family system as well; and 5) methodological criticisms of studies of incestuous families and their implications for including incest as a parent-child relational diagnosis in DSM-IV.

The authors found that clinical descriptions of incestuous families mentioned systems characterized by a high level of enmeshment, rigidity, traditional and sexually stereotyped family values, a tendency to parentify at least one child, and social isolation. The family dynamic most frequently described is that of a poor marital relationship with an absent and/or emotionally unavailable mother and a rigid controlling father. The authors did not find any large observational studies that systematically assessed characteristics of incestuous families compared with appropriate control groups. Although recent studies provided limited support for the presence of rigidity, poor parent-child relationships, and dysfunctional families, there was no evidence that these characterized the majority of incestuous families or were unique to incestuous families.

The authors found that a wide range of behavioral and emotional difficulties were reported in studies of incest victims younger than 12 years old including, in descending order of frequency, depressive symptoms and/or disorders, aggressive behavior, anxiety, sexualized behavior problems, cognitive and/or social functional impairment, low self-esteem, somatization, posttraumatic stress disorder symptoms, and dissociation. Symptoms and disorders reported in studies of sexually abused adolescents included, in descending order of frequency, sexualized behavior and/or gender identity disturbance, aggressive behavior, substance abuse, suicidal behavior, depression, low self-esteem, and impairment in social functioning. Symptoms and disorders reported in studies of adults who reported sexual abuse as children younger than 18 years old included, in descending order of frequency, sexual behavior problems including sexual dysfunction and gender identity disturbance, depressive symptoms or disorders, substance abuse, somatic concerns, suicidal or other self-destructive behavior, posttraumatic stress disorder symptoms, dissociation, social impairment, anxious behavior, aggressive behavior, low self-esteem, borderline personality disorder, and eating disorders.

The authors found that the empirical evidence did not support the many unsubstantiated claims in the literature that mothers generally know when their daughters are being abused; in fact, the evidence indicated that mothers generally take active steps to stop the abuse when they learn of its occurrence. The authors suggested that the early literature's emphasis on maternal psychopathology may have been in the tradition of blaming the victim seen in clinical descriptions of other victim groups.

The authors found that many of the assumptions concerning incest perpetrators in the clinical literature have not been supported by more recent empirical studies. For example, systematic studies have not found that fathers who commit incest were usually themselves victims of child sexual abuse, although higher than average rates of a history of physical abuse have been found. Most studies of psychopathology in incest perpetrators have failed to reveal a consistent pattern of psychological disturbance, although incest perpetrators do appear to be significantly more dependent than control or normative samples.

The authors identified a number of methodological problems in studies of incestuous families. They cautioned that although further studies are needed, it appears that any consideration of a relational disorder diagnosis for incestuous families should take into account the fact that, in a significant percentage of incestuous families, the deviant sexual behavior on the part of the father exists outside the context of the family and may have predated the formation of the family.

The authors concluded that it would be premature to include specific criteria for incest as a relational disorder both because the literature to date does not support a clear-cut family dynamic and because of the need for a high degree of accuracy in the area of child sexual abuse due to the potential for misuse in forensic settings. However, they recommended including incest as a V code problem, "parent-child relational problem with sexual abuse of child" in the section on "Other Conditions That May Be a Focus of Clinical Attention." They also recommended that incest be discussed in the diagnostic categories that involve the psychiatric sequelae of stress for the individual.

DSM-IV Options Book Proposals

All the authors of the literature reviews on family/relational problems recommended that these problems be included in some way in DSM-IV. Some favored inclusion as separate diagnostic categories; others as V code problems listed under "Other Conditions That May Be a Focus of Clinical Attention." The Task Force on DSM-IV will need to decide where it would be most appropriate to list family and relational problems. The proposal in the *DSM-IV Options Book* is that the following categories be assigned V codes (ICD-10 Z codes) and be listed under Relational (Family) Problems in the section for "Other Conditions That May Be a Focus of Clinical Attention:"

- Parent-Child Relational Problem
    With Physical Abuse of Child
    With Sexual Abuse of Child
    With Child Neglect

　　　　With Inadequate Parental Discipline
　　　　With Parental Overprotection
　　　　With Communication Problems
　　　　With High Expressed Emotion[1]
　　　　Unspecified

- Partner Relational Problem
　　　　With Physical Abuse
　　　　With Sexual Abuse
　　　　With Communication Problems
　　　　Other Partner Relational Problems

- Sibling Relational Problem

- Other Relational Problem

References

American Psychiatric Association: Diagnostic and Statistical Manual of Mental Disorders, 3rd Edition. Washington, DC, American Psychiatric Association, 1980

American Psychiatric Association: Diagnostic and Statistical Manual of Mental Disorders, 3rd Edition, Revised. Washington, DC, American Psychiatric Association, 1987

American Psychiatric Association: DSM-IV Options Book: Work in Progress. Washington, DC, American Psychiatric Association, 1991

World Health Organization: ICD-10 Chapter V: Mental and Behavioral Disorders Diagnostic Criteria for Research. Geneva, Switzerland, World Health Organization, 1990

---

[1]This proposed category may later be broadened to include both parent-child and partner relational problems and problems associated with general medical conditions as well as mental disorders.

Chapter 34

Relational Problem Related to a Mental Disorder or General Medical Condition

Michael J. Goldstein, Ph.D., Angus M. Strachan, Ph.D., and Lyman C. Wynne, M.D., Ph.D.

Introduction

As part of the effort to increase the usefulness of DSM-IV in the diagnosis and treatment of problems that occur in the family and other relational units, the extent to which family-related problems might affect the course or outcome of a mental disorder or general medical condition was considered. In this review, we focus on relational problems associated with high expressed emotion (EE). This was the original diagnostic category named by the DSM-IV Task Force in the *DSM-IV Options Book* (American Psychiatric Association 1991) and referred to a relational problem associated with a psychiatric disorder. This was the topic assigned to the authors of this review. After the review was submitted, the DSM-IV Task Force decided to make two changes in the category: 1) to drop the term *expressed emotion*, and 2) to include reference to general medical as well as psychiatric disorders.

Statement of the Issues

EE has been defined as an index of the intensity of attitudes that one person, protypically a relative, feels about another person, protypically a patient (Leff and Vaughn 1985). In this chapter, we address the question of whether relational problems with high EE should be considered for inclusion in DSM-IV. In our Results section, we focus on four major avenues of inquiry.

1. **Core research data on high EE as a predictor of schizophrenic relapse:** What is the strength of the core research evidence (predicting the course of schizophrenia) that validates the EE concept? That is, what is the sensitivity, specificity, and positive and negative predictive power of EE in predicting schizophrenic relapse?
2. **Research data on the generalizability of EE:** To what extent is the EE concept generalizable to nonschizophrenic disorders and to problems other than schizophrenic relapse? To what extent is EE relevant not only to parent-child relationships but also to marital relationships and to other familial and nonfamilial interpersonal relationships?
3. **Characteristics and determinants of EE:** To what extent is EE a function of the behavior and attitudes of the patient or "target" person? That is, what is the evidence that EE is a *transactional* or relational problem (between persons) and not primarily an individual characteristic (located within a relative or other person)? To what extent is EE determined by *contextual* variables such as the family constellation or the culture or ethnicity of the family? To what extent is EE a *stable* characteristic of individuals?
4. **Measurement and clinical criteria for high EE or an alternatively named category:** What is the reliability of the research measures of EE? What about alternative measures of EE?

Finally, in our Discussion and Recommendations section, we consider the implications of including such a relational disorder in DSM-IV and make recommendations regarding a relational disorder with high EE for DSM-IV and regarding clinical criteria.

Significance of the Issues

It has been more than 30 years since Brown (1959) suggested that aspects of the social environment, particularly the family affective climate, were related to the short-term course of a schizophrenic patient's disorder. This study and other early studies (Brown et al. 1958, 1962) identified the key construct, originally named *emotional overinvolvement* and subsequently renamed *expressed emotion,* and provided striking data on the impact of the family environment on relapse in schizophrenic psychosis. The EE construct was refined to reflect three kinds of negative attitudes—criticism, hostility, and emotional overinvolvement—and two kinds of positive attitudes—warmth and positive remarks. In addition, a method of measurement was developed: the Camberwell Family Interview (CFI) (Brown and Rutter 1966; Rutter and Brown 1966), a semistructured interview with a relative about the patient, which has subsequently been shortened to an hour-long interview.

We review the results of attempts to replicate the original findings during the ensuing three decades. These findings on relapse and remission are highly relevant to the DSM descriptions of "course" in the text for specific mental disorders. For many disorders, including schizophrenia, schizoaffective disorder, and schizophreniform disorder, the course of the illness is a crucial feature that helps to define diagnostic boundaries. However, even the most significant and valid prognostic indicators are not in themselves ordinarily considered to be "disorders" or diagnostic categories.

Therefore, to assess whether "relational problems associated with high expressed emotion" warrant inclusion in DSM-IV as a diagnostic category, it is necessary to go beyond the prognostic data and consider whether the potentially broad class of "Relational Disorders" or "Relational Problems" should be given diagnostic status. Insofar as high EE is a significant defining feature of such problems, this category could be regarded as an appropriate entry point for introducing the broader class of relational problems or disorders into DSM-IV. We evaluate the merits and weaknesses of this approach including, but going beyond, the predictive, prognostic data.

Method

A comprehensive, systematic search of the literature on EE and closely related concepts, such as affective style, was carried out using Medline and PsychLit and located 172 publications on this subject. We also located 71 additional writings in our personal reprint files: 42 articles in professional journals, 19 book chapters, and 10 unpublished manuscripts and abstracts.

Our review of the "core" research literature is based on those follow-up studies of EE and schizophrenic relapse that were peer reviewed and published through 1990. These studies have been conducted in Australia (Parker et al. 1988), Great Britain (Brown et al. 1972; MacMillan et al. 1986a, 1986b; Tarrier et al. 1988; Vaughn and Leff 1976), India (Leff et al. 1987), Switzerland (Barrelet et al. 1990), the United States (Hogarty et al. 1988; Karno et al. 1987; Moline et al. 1985; Nuechterlein et al. 1986; Vaughn et al. 1984), and West Germany (Dulz and Hand 1986; Kottgen et al. 1984 [both of which are based on the same study that we refer to as the Kottgen-Hand study]). We excluded one published naturalistic study of EE by McCreadie and Phillips (1988) because it was a retrospective study and did not start with an index episode. Further, we have not included data from samples who received systematically applied psychosocial interventions designed to modify the family environment. Although these studies provide important data on the construct validity of EE by showing that its modifiability affects the course of the disorder, they do not provide data on its predictive validity. However, we have included data from the naturalistic comparison groups in the psychosocial intervention studies. For those studies included in our review of core findings, we have sought additional unpublished data from many of the authors on variables that were not specifically reported in each publication. We are grateful to the investigators who were generous enough to share these data.

Results

A number of previous reviews of the literature on EE and schizophrenic relapse have appeared (Hatfield et al. 1987; Hooley 1985; Kanter et al. 1987; Koenigsberg and Handley 1986; Kuipers and Bebbington 1988; Leff and Vaughn 1985; Mintz et al. 1987; Strachan 1991), which have summarized the existing findings and discussed their implications for theory and treatment. However, they have not addressed the details of the samples and methods of data collection and data analysis that might account for discrepancies in results. As our first goal, this review attempts to do just that.

Issue 1: Core Research Data on High EE as a Predictor of Schizophrenic Relapse

Overview comments. Although the great majority of studies have replicated the original findings showing that high EE is a predictor of schizophrenic relapse, a few studies have failed to replicate. Further, some authors have suggested that the predictive value of a relative's EE attitudes is largely explainable by correlations with third variables reflecting some attribute of the patient's past or current clinical state (Hatfield and Lefley 1987; Hogarty et al. 1988; MacMillan et al. 1986a; Parker et al. 1988). Therefore, we think it is timely to examine the existing literature in detail to determine the effect of conditions on the predictive value of EE as an empirical starting point for deciding whether the construct is viable for inclusion in DSM-IV as a relational problem.

It is important to recognize immediately at least three points about EE. First, although EE is a broad construct referring to intense emotional attitudes, it has unfortunately been overly identified with data obtained with the original measurement technique, the semistructured CFI. The construct would have greater clinical meaning if it could be measured in a variety of ways, thus increasing its construct validity. We present some evidence that alternative forms of measurement are emerging that increase its utility as a clinical measure.

Second, it is important to recognize that, although EE is a measure assessed from a relative's speech, it is not only a measure of what goes on "inside" the relative. More accurately, it is a measure of a relative's relationship with the patient at a particular time in a particular setting. Therefore, EE may be better thought of as tapping a type of relationship based on characteristics of the relative, of the patient, and of the context. We make no assumptions about the causes of EE or the direction of effects. Measurable EE can best be thought of as a punctuation point in a series of interpersonal transactions or relational processes in which the "origin" or "cause" can be only arbitrarily identified. Recent research data confirm that EE indeed taps a transactional process. Strachan et al. (1989) presented data suggesting that EE correlates with *both* the relatives' and the patients' behavior in the interaction.

Third, although the original research assessed the EE of relatives toward a specific patient with whom they have been in close face-to-face contact, it is obvious, both conceptually and empirically, that clinically meaningful EE may exist in the attitudes of patients toward relatives and others who are not relatives but who are psychologically close.

Inclusion criteria: naturalistic and special population studies. We start by outlining the database of the core studies in which EE is used to predict relapse of schizophrenia. Table 34–1 lists all the peer-reviewed follow-up studies of EE and schizophrenia that had been published up to 1990.

Despite the similar research paradigms used in all these studies, there are some variations in both design and criteria for EE. We have taken these variations into account as carefully as possible to provide a clear comparison between studies. The inclusion criteria used in the studies reviewed in this chapter were

1. The study started with an index episode of schizophrenia in the patient.
2. The subjects were followed up for at least 9 months.
3. No special psychosocial intervention was given to either the patient or family members.
4. The patients were started on maintenance antipsychotic medication after hospital discharge.
5. The patients were reported to be living with a family member or in significant contact with them before and after discharge.

Further, we made a distinction between naturalistic studies and those involving special populations of patients who had to fit special criteria before they could enter

Table 34–1. Main results of studies of expressed emotion (EE) and relapse in schizophrenia: naturalistic studies and special populations

Study	Location	Partici-pants	Follow-up	Overall relapse rate (%)	High EE relapse rate (%)	Low EE relapse rate (%)	Significance of high-low EE difference (chi-squared)
Naturalistic studies							
Brown et al. 1972[a]	S. London, England	101	9 months	35	58 (26/45)	16 (9/56)	.001
Vaughn and Leff 1976	S. London, England	37	9 months	30	48 (10/21)	6 (1/16)	.006
Vaughn et al. 1984	Los Angeles, California	54	9 months	35	56 (20/36)	17 (3/18)	.006
Dulz and Hand 1986; Kottgen et al. 1984[b]	Hamburg, Germany	34	9 months	53	50 (7/14)	55 (11/20)	NS
Moline et al. 1985 (personal communi-cation 1989)	Chicago, Illinois	24	2 years	58	71 (12/17)	29 (2/7)	.06
Karno et al. 1987	Los Angeles, California	44	9 months	39	59 (10/17)	26 (7/27)	.03
Leff et al. 1987	Chandigarh, India	70	1 year	14	31 (5/16)	9 (5/54)	.03

Study	Location		Follow-up			p
Tarrier et al. 1988[b,c]	Manchester, England	48	9 months	38	48 (14/29)	21 (4/19)	.06
Parker et al. 1988	Sydney, Australia	57	9 months	51	48 (20/42)	60 (9/15)	NS
Barrelet et al. 1990	Geneva, Switzerland	36	9 months	22	33 (8/24)	0 (0/12)	.03
Special populations							
Nuechterlein et al. 1986	Los Angeles, California	26	1 year	30	37 (7/19)	0 (0/7)	.06
MacMillan et al. 1986b, 1987[d]	N. London, England	44	2 years	45	60 (12/20)	33 (8/24)	.08
Hogarty et al. 1988[e]	Pittsburgh, Pennsylvania	64	1 year	17	19 (7/36)	14 (4/28)	NS

Note. NS = not significant.
[a] EE criteria based on seven or more criticisms or behavior in joint interview.
[b] Excludes patients in treatment groups.
[c] Includes patients whose families received brief education.
[d] Excludes patients on placebo.
[e] Includes patients on standard or minimal dosages.

the EE phase of the study. We defined a *naturalistic study* as one in which the sample fit our inclusion criteria and in which the patient was discharged to an aftercare system for follow-up care that usually involved, at a minimum, maintenance pharmacotherapy. No other selection criteria were imposed on the samples, and sample attrition was therefore due to either a failure to locate patients or patients' refusal to participate in follow-up evaluation.

In a number of these studies, an effort was made to evaluate the role of medication compliance during the follow-up period as a modifier of the risk for relapse in high- and low-EE families. Unfortunately, because medication compliance was not controlled, interpretation of outcome data in relation to EE could be confounded by patient attributes or attributes of the family that predict medication compliance.

By contrast, in what we term the *special population studies,* stringent selection criteria were used to include only those patients who fit rigorous criteria for the stabilization of their symptoms and/or compliance with medication (Hogarty et al. 1988; MacMillan et al. 1986a, 1986b; Nuechterlein et al. 1986). In these studies, clinical stabilization was required before entry to the EE phase of the research. When random assignment to medication and compliance with medication both were required (Hogarty et al. 1988; Nuechterlein et al. 1986), the proportion of patients dropped from the study was much larger than in the naturalistic studies, because some patients' symptoms did not stabilize after discharge, some refused assignment to a particular medication condition, some had unmanageable side effects and had to be dropped from the study, and some did not comply with their medication. Thus, the patients in these three samples were a subset of those likely to enter the naturalistic studies, and we considered these patient groups as "special populations."

This raises the question of whether the results of these two types of studies are comparable with one another. In the special populations, the prognostic value of EE was evaluated on samples who made good clinical recoveries and who were compliant with their pharmacotherapy. In the naturalistic studies, by contrast, greater variability in patient clinical state and medication compliance was permissible and could covary freely with the EE status of the relatives. It may be that these special population studies, which appear to be ideal designs for assessing whether EE has an impact on relapse independent of drug compliance, possess serious limitations for testing the predictive validity of the EE construct because they restrict the samples to unusual cases. Hogarty et al. (1988), in their paper on the predictive validity of EE, stated: "Thus, this investigation is *not* another attempt to replicate the effects of EE on relapse, since a large number of patients who were unable to stabilize and, hence, at greater risk of relapse, were removed from the study by design" (p. 198).

For this review, the criterion for rating a relative as high EE on criticism was kept at a cutting score of six or more criticisms expressed during the CFI. To accomplish this for studies that reported cutting scores other than six, we either sought additional data from the authors or recalculated relapse rates for this cutting score from published data. Thus, all (except Brown et al. 1972) figures for high- versus low-EE families that are summarized in this review are based on a cutting score of six or more criticisms on the CFI.

The criterion for emotional overinvolvement also varied from study to study; some define high emotional overinvolvement as a score of three or more and some as four or more on the CFI (see Kuipers and Bebbington 1988). Because relatively few relatives are defined as high EE on the basis of emotional overinvolvement alone, and because most of these relatives in fact have a score of four or more, we have followed the cutting score used in each study for this review.

EE and relapse: main trends. Table 34–1 summarizes relapse rates for patients returning to high- or low-EE environments, the number of participants, the location of the study, and the length of follow-up. Most of the studies had follow-up at 9 months. Data from longer-term follow-ups were not included unless they were the only data available. We discuss longer-term follow-up data at the end of this section.

A variety of statistics were used to analyze the difference in relapse rates (Fisher's exact test, chi-squared, Yates corrected chi-squared, maximum likelihood chi-squared). We decided to reanalyze all of the data using the uncorrected chi-squared test. We chose this test because Monte Carlo simulation studies have found that the uncorrected chi-squared test best predicts the true probabilities in the larger population. For example, Grizzle (1967) studied a large number of randomly generated samples. The corrected and uncorrected chi-squared statistics were compared with the percentage points of the chi-squared distribution. It was found that when the sample size was small, the uncorrected chi-squared statistic was slightly conservative but the corrected chi-squared statistic was "so conservative as to be almost unclear" (p. 31).

Camilli and Hopkins (1978) examined randomly generated 2 × 2 tables with as few as eight observations. They found that Pearson's chi-squared test was very robust with such small expected cell frequencies and contradicted the standard textbook advice that the Yates continuity correction or the F-test be used.

Therefore, we used the uncorrected chi-squared test. It could be argued that we could have use one-tailed tests; but, because all the studies after the original one were replications, we decided to present the conservative two-tailed data.

Finally, note that because we reanalyzed the data from each study using the uniform criteria of six or more criticisms or used data only from certain subgroups as described earlier, the statistics reported here do not necessarily match those in the original publications.

These studies support three main conclusions. First, examination of Table 34–1 shows that, in most of the naturalistic studies (8 of 10), the relapse rates for patients returning to high-EE environments are greater than for those returning to low-EE environments. When we applied the chi-square test to these data, we found that six were significant at the .05 level and two were marginally significant at the .06 level. Only two studies are true nonreplications (the Kottgen-Hand study [Dulz and Hand 1986; Kottgen et al. 1984]; Parker et al. 1988). Relapse rates in these two special population studies are lower overall; this is expected because these populations were purified to remove those subjects who refused medication or were unstable or noncompliant. Nevertheless, in all the special population studies, the relapse rates are higher in the high-EE groups. However, when we reanalyzed these data, in only two studies did the differences between high- and low-EE cohorts approach statistical significance ($P < .08$ in MacMillan et al. 1986b; $P < .06$ in Nuechterlein et al. 1986).

Second, it can be seen in Table 34–1 that the relapse rates across the studies for the patients who returned to high-EE family units are very stable in comparison with greater variation in low-EE samples. If the two studies with very *low* overall relapse rates are excluded (Hogarty et al. 1988; Leff et al. 1987), both of which used very select populations, the relapse rates among high-EE samples vary from 71% to 40%, with most falling between 40% and 50%, whereas among low-EE samples the relapse rate varies from 50% to 0%. Thus, even in the nonreplication studies, the relapse rates for family units classified as high EE are very consistent. It is the extraordinarily *high* rate of relapse in some of the low-EE samples that sets the nonreplication studies apart.

Although most of the naturalistic studies give similar results, the data were not examined with four measures typically used in psychological or biological tests: sensitivity, specificity, positive predictive power, and negative predictive power. These measures are presented separately in Table 34–2 for the naturalistic and special population studies. In addition, we report the base rate for the incidence of family EE.

Sensitivity refers to the percentage of all relapsers who were classified correctly by a high-EE rating. More precisely, it is calculated as the ratio of high-EE relapsers to total relapsers. The percentage of all relapsers who were from the high-EE group varied from 39% to 100%, suggesting that most relapses occur in the high-EE rather than low-EE groups.

Specificity, the percentage of nonrelapsers in the low-EE group, varies from 21% to 82%; if we exclude the studies by Brown et al. (1972) and Karno et al. (1987), however, the number of patients who return to high-EE families who do *not* relapse is considerable. Thus, there are many false positives among the cohort from high-EE families who are predicted to relapse but do not.

The indices of positive predictive power (the relapse rate for high-EE cases) and negative predictive power (the rate of *non*relapse in patients returning to low-EE families) support this conclusion. Although positive predictive power averages only 50.2%, negative predictive power averages 76.2%.

One conclusion from these data is that knowing that a patient is returning to a low-EE environment is more informative than knowing that a patient is returning to a high-EE environment. Most previous studies have focused on the potentially aversive quality of a high-EE environment, ignoring the fact that this hypothesized aversiveness is *not* associated with relapse for the majority of cases. What has been lost in these discussions is the fact that the data point to the *protective* effects of a low-EE environment, effects that are remarkably stable across all studies except those of Kottgen and Dulz (Dulz and Hand 1986; Kottgen et al. 1984) and Parker et al. (1988). As yet, few studies have investigated the characteristics of low-EE family environments. Although it would seem that protective effects should be related to such characteristics as family warmth, relapse has rarely been found to correlate significantly with warmth rated on the CFI. This does not mean that factors such as warmth are insignificant in real life but that predictive variation in family functioning as assessed by this method is related to variation in the relative's description of emotionally charged interaction with the patient at a time of great stress in the family during or shortly after a hospitalization. This interview format probably "pulls" more variation in negative affect than in positive affect. More research is needed on the protective aspects of supportive family environments; low EE is a residual category that presumably includes both supportive environments and those that are emotionally disengaged or distant.

Third, it is noteworthy that if the relapse rate in a sample is over 50%, there is rarely a difference in relapse rates between low- and high-EE samples. The one exception to this is in the study by Moline et al. (1985), where an EE effect of borderline significance was found despite a 58% relapse rate. In fact, both of the nonreplication studies had samples in which the relapse figures were notably higher than those usually found for 9-month relapse rates in recently discharged schizophrenic patients. It appears that the EE effect is most likely to be robust when the overall sample relapse rate is between 30% and 50%. In settings where the overall relapse rate is higher, other factors contributing to high relapse presumably are more potent; if so, this would tend to obscure high-EE versus low-EE differences.

Relationship between patient characteristics and EE across the studies. Table 34–3 shows the wide range of sample characteristics in the various studies: some

Table 34–2. Measures of the predictive power of expressed emotion (EE) and relapse from schizophrenia: naturalistic studies and special populations

Study	High-EE families (%): base rate	Sensitivity (%)[a]	Specificity (%)[b]	Positive predictive power (%)[c]	Negative predictive power (%)[d]
Naturalistic studies					
Brown et al. 1972[e]	45	74	71	58	84
Vaughn and Leff 1976	57	91	58	48	94
Vaughn et al. 1984	67	87	48	56	83
Dulz and Hand 1986;[f] Kottgen et al. 1984	71	39	56	50	45
Moline et al. 1985 (personal communication 1989)	41	86	50	71	71
Karno et al. 1987	39	59	74	59	74
Leff et al. 1987	23	50	82	31	91
Tarrier et al. 1988[f,g]	60	78	50	48	79
Parker et al. 1988	74	69	21	48	40
Barrelet et al. 1990	67	100	43	33	100

Special populations

Nuechterlein et al. 1986	73	100	37	37	100
MacMillan et al. 1986a, 1986b, 1987[h]	45	60	67	60	67
Hogarty et al. 1988[i]	56	64	45	19	86

[a] Total relapses in high-EE groups.
[b] Nonrelapses in low-EE groups.
[c] High-EE group who do relapse.
[d] Low-EE who do not relapse.
[e] EE criteria based on seven or more criticisms or behavior in joint interview.
[f] Excludes patients in treatment groups.
[g] Includes patients whose families received brief education.
[h] Excludes patients on placebo.
[i] Includes patients on standard or minimal dosages.

are composed primarily of young patients, some of older patients; some contain mostly male patients, some mostly female; some contain predominantly chronic patients, some recent onset; some are mostly single, some are mostly married. Although some authors (e.g., Hogarty et al. 1988) suggest that the EE effect may be restricted to younger males who live with their parents, the data from the studies overall suggest that, in general, none of these variables is associated either with rates of high- or low-EE relatives or with the prognostic validity of the EE variable. The EE effect seems to be a robust phenomenon emerging from a heterogeneous aggregation of samples. We discuss this further later and argue that although there may be no simple connection between levels of EE and patient symptomatology, there is evidence that there are more subtle connections between patients' and their relatives' behavior.

Reliability of the EE categorization across the studies. It is a well-known fact in psychometrics that the validity of a test cannot exceed its reliability. If a measure such as EE is marginally reliable, then assessments of the EE status of a relative will produce numerous false positives and false negatives. This is particularly likely when a binary classification system (high versus low EE) is used. For respondents at the margin of the cutting score, with five or six criticisms for example, a low reliability in rating EE status could produce major reclassification errors so that the EE findings would be a "now you see it, now you don't" phenomenon.

The few data that are available suggest that, for the high- versus low-EE distinction, raters can agree quite well with reliabilities above 80% (Karno et al. 1987; Kottgen-Hand study [Dulz and Hand 1986; Kottgen et al. 1984]; Tarrier et al. 1988). The reliabilities of the specific components that make up these ratings are also quite reliable in the few studies where they are reported. It appears from the sparse reliability data available that variations across studies in the predictive value of the EE ratings cannot be explained by the degree of unreliability in the rating process. However, one should recognize the complex nature of the rating system and the facts that raters need not attain perfect reliability to be certified as trained, that rater drift is not routinely monitored, and that a single criticism can occasionally make the difference between a relative or family being classified as high or low EE. Therefore, it is not surprising that the number of false positives and false negatives can be considerable in any particular study, thereby reducing the prognostic validity of the EE variable. This is particularly salient in the studies by Dulz and Hand (1986), Kottgen et al. (1984), and Parker et al. (1988), where the nonreplications were primarily due to the very high relapse rates observed in the low-EE cohorts. The data for their high-EE samples were almost identical to all other studies. If these low-EE relatives were erroneously classified because of some unreliability in the method of assessment that tended to underscore criticisms, a

Table 34–3. Salient features of studies of expressed emotion (EE) and relapse from schizophrenia: naturalistic studies and special populations

Study	Assignment to sample	Mean age (years)	Gender (% male)	Married (%)	Living at home Before (months)[a]	Living at home After (yes/no)	First admission (%)	Persisting symptom patients excluded?
Naturalistic studies								
Brown et al. 1972[b]	All	75% over 45	48	46	3	Yes	57[c]	Yes
Vaughn and Leff 1976	All	33	41	35	3	Yes	59[c]	No
Vaughn et al. 1984	All	26	77	6	1	87%	17	Yes
Dulz and Hand 1986; Kottgen et al. 1984[d]	Half high-EE families excluded	23	65	7	?	?	69	No
Moline et al. 1985 (personal communication 1989)	All	24	67	8	3	Yes	67	Yes
Karno et al. 1987	All	26	57	14	1	Yes	30	Yes
Leff et al. 1987	All	?	?	28	3	Yes	100	Yes
Tarrier et al. 1988[d,e]	Half high-EE families excluded	35	35	35	3	Yes	30	No

(continued)

Table 34–3. Salient features of studies of expressed emotion (EE) and relapse from schizophrenia: naturalistic studies and special populations *(continued)*

Study	Assignment to sample	Mean age (years)	Gender (% male)	Married (%)	Living at home Before (months)[a]	Living at home After (yes/no)	First admission (%)	Persisting symptom patients excluded?
Parker et al. 1988	All	26	58	0	"In contact"	Yes	25	No
Barrelet et al. 1990	All	25	48	?	Frequent contact	Yes	100	No
Special populations								
Nuechterlein et al. 1986	Recent onset; medication-compliant for 1 year	23	77	?	1	?	73	Yes
MacMillan et al. 1986,[a] 1986,[b] 1987[f]	First admissions; placebo versus medication study plus some customary care	23	58	20	3	?	100	Yes

| Hogarty et al. 1988[g] | Stabilized for 6 months; medication compliant for 2 years; low- or high-dosage study | 28 | 57 | 29 | 1 | ? | 31 | Yes |

Note. ? = no information provided by authors.
[a]Minimum number of months in last 3 months.
[b]EE criteria based on seven or more criticisms or behavior in joint interview.
[c]Leff and Brown 1977.
[d]Excludes patients in treatment groups.
[e]Includes patients whose families received brief education.
[f]Excludes patients on placebo.
[g]Includes patients on standard or minimal dosages.

false picture of nonreplication results. In addition, it appears that fewer relatives were interviewed in these two studies than in others, so that they may have missed a high-EE relative. Most EE studies went to some length to interview as many relatives as possible. Thus, some cases identified by Kottgen-Hand and Parker as low EE may in fact have been high-EE families.

Influence of variation in relapse criteria across studies. The major outcome criterion in these studies was an indication of the return of psychotic symptoms of a schizophrenic disorder during a specified follow-up period. The term *relapse* is used to define this outcome criterion. The original EE studies (Brown et al. 1972; Vaughn and Leff 1976) specifically define relapse as the return of symptoms that were used to define the index episode of schizophrenic disorder as assessed by the Present State Examination (Wing et al. 1974) administered at either the time of a relapse or at the time of a fixed follow-up period, originally 9 months postdischarge.

The duration of the follow-up period has varied in more recent studies from 1 to 2 years after some specified start date (Hogarty et al. 1988; MacMillan et al. 1986b; Nuechterlein et al. 1986). In the two studies by Hogarty et al. and Nuechterlein et al., the follow-up period began not on the date of discharge but rather when (and if) clinical stabilization had occurred. Thus, the follow-up period in these studies was quite variable, depending on when this stabilization could be achieved, and the findings cannot be directly compared with the naturalistic studies in which the 9-month follow-up period began at the point of discharge for all patients.

Both the early and the more recent studies have rejected readmission to hospital as a criterion for relapse, recognizing that readmission may be for factors other than the return of schizophrenia and may not be independent of a relative's EE attitudes (e.g., high-EE relatives may be less tolerant of a patient's behavior and more likely to request rehospitalization than low-EE relatives).

In the original British studies, two types of relapses were recognized: Type I, in which a remission of schizophrenic symptoms at discharge is followed at some point by a return of these symptoms; and Type II, where there are notable symptoms persisting at discharge that worsen over the course of the follow-up period. In the Vaughn and Leff (1976) study, only 1 of 11 relapses was of Type II, and no patients were eliminated from the study because they showed high persisting symptoms throughout the 9-month follow-up period.

Since the original Vaughn and Leff (1976) study, many changes in the mental health system, particularly in the United States, interfered with attempts to replicate the British work. Most notable was a reduction in the length of hospitalization for an index episode of schizophrenia. Whether or not this is a major factor, subsequent studies have had to eliminate a larger number of patients from their follow-up analyses than was the case in the British studies, because the patients either were not capable of being discharged at all from the hospital or manifested high rates of persisting symptoms of schizophrenia throughout the 9-month follow-up period (e.g., Karno et al. 1987; Vaughn et al. 1984). Thus, the composition of the final samples in these later studies reflected a higher rate of sample attrition than was observed in either Brown et al. (1972) or Vaughn and Leff (1976). As indicated, this factor was even more pronounced in those special population studies in which an EE replication analysis was superimposed on another clinical trial. For example, in the Hogarty et al. (1988) study, about 30% of the sample who could potentially enter the EE study were eliminated because they could not achieve a level of stabilization on maintenance medication after hospital discharge. Another 30% were not subsequently compliant with their assigned medication. Thus, the samples of these studies are not comparable with those of the original naturalistic studies. For example, Hogarty et al. report a relapse rate that is notably lower than those found in the majority of naturalistic studies, presumably due to the fact that their ultimate sample was composed solely of clinically stable, medication-compliant patients.

There have also been some major changes in how the clinical status of patients has been evaluated during the follow-up period that could alter the estimates of relapse rates. In the two early British replication studies (Brown et al. 1972; Vaughn and Leff 1976), patients were reevaluated using the Present State Examination either at the time of the 9-month follow-up contact or at the time of a relapse. The status of patients in between these contacts was evaluated from the records of the aftercare clinics that patients attended after discharge or from hospital records. If a readmission occurred, the research team was alerted and a Present State Examination was administered. In a number of the subsequent replication studies in the United States (Karno et al. 1987; Nuechterlein et al. 1986; Vaughn et al. 1984), the clinical status of patients was monitored prospectively on a monthly basis using instruments such as the Brief Psychiatric Rating Scale (Overall and Gorham 1962) or the Psychiatric Assessment Schedule (Krawiecka et al. 1977). These ratings played a major role in defining whether or not a patient relapsed, because the changes in scale scores provided systematic criteria for a relapse. This operationalization of relapse criteria using standardized assessment instruments has increased the probability that, across various studies, the same phenomena are likely to be classified as a major change in the clinical state of a patient. Two nonreplications (Dulz and Hand 1986; Kottgen et al. 1984; Parker et al. 1988) did not monitor symptoms prospectively, and both report relapse rates for their samples that are notably higher than those reported where prospective monitoring was the case. As indicated previously, the EE effect was less likely to appear when the sample relapse rate exceeded 40%. Hence, these two replication failures may be a function of the particular relapse assessment procedures used.

Issue 2: Research Data on the Generalizability of EE

The original Vaughn and Leff (1976) paper showed that CFI ratings were highly predictive of relapse in depressed patients, although the cutoff score for distinguishing high- from low-EE relatives (almost all spouses) was lower than for schizophrenia. These findings were subsequently replicated by Hooley et al. (1986) with a comparable sample of previously depressed patients, where the same cutoff score of two criticisms (in contrast to six or more for relatives of schizophrenic patients) was the optimal one for predicting relapse. In a subsequent study, Hooley and Teasdale (1989) reported the interesting finding that the depressed person's rating of the perceived critical attitude of the spouse on a simple 5-point scale predicted relapse better than the more complex ratings derived from the CFI.

Miklowitz et al. (1988) found ratings on the CFI to be as predictive of relapse for young, bipolar manic patients of recent onset as for schizophrenic patients. In this study, the same cutting scores for criticism and emotional overinvolvement that were used with relatives of schizophrenic patients were the optimal ones for predicting bipolar recurrences.

Recently, there have been a number of attempts to use the EE concept to predict the incidence or course of childhood psychiatric disorders. Stubbe et al. (1993), in a community epidemiological survey, found that a brief method for rating EE, described later as the Five-Minute Speech Sample (FMSS) EE method, predicted the likelihood of a childhood disorder in that community sample. Asarnow et al. (1993) found that the FMSS EE method was highly predictive of the course of childhood-onset depression. Schwartz et al. (1990) applied EE ratings to an interview similar to the CFI and found that EE status was highly correlated with the incidence of psychiatric disorder in the offspring of depressed mothers. High-EE status independently contributed to the concurrent prediction of the child's psychiatric status beyond any association with parental diagnosis of affective disorder.

Overall, it appears that the EE construct measures an attribute of relatives' attitudes that is relevant to a wide range of psychiatric disorders and is not specifically connected to any one form of psychopathology. Therefore, it seems appropriate to consider EE as a risk factor for most psychiatric disorders, whether of adult or childhood onset.

A key issue is whether EE status predicts relapse because the construct is isomorphic with the presence of a diagnosable psychiatric disorder in a respondent. Goldstein et al. (1992) examined the psychiatric status of the relatives of recent-onset schizophrenic patients who had been independently assessed for EE using both the CFI and the FMSS methods, the latter administered 4–5 weeks after the patient's discharge from the hospital and the former during hospitalization. Only a slight relationship was found between the CFI status of a relative and lifetime estimates of moderate or severe psychiatric disorders in those same persons. There was a more significant association with the subsequent FMSS EE rating (62% of FMSS high-EE relatives received a diagnosis, whereas only 23% of the FMSS low-EE relatives did so). Considering the pattern of EE across assessments yields three groups: low CFI–low FMSS, high CFI–low FMSS, and high CFI–high FMSS. The rates of psychiatric disorder in these groups were 19%, 36%, and 71%, respectively, with almost all of the severe diagnoses (e.g., schizophrenia, bipolar, schizotypal, paranoid) found in the consistently high-EE group. It is unclear from these data whether the time of administration or the method (CFI or FMSS) is the significant factor in this high rate of psychopathology in the high-high group. If time is the factor, then it appears that those relatives whose high-EE attitudes carry over from the acute to the remitted state of a schizophrenic patient's disorder are most likely to be persons who appear vulnerable by virtue of a prior psychiatric disorder of their own. This was also suggested in a study by Hibbs et al. (1991) of parents of control children, obsessive-compulsive children, and disruptive children. The number of relatives rated high FMSS EE was significantly greater in the parents of the disturbed as contrasted with the control children. Similarly, the rates of psychiatric disorders were notably higher in the parents in these two pathological samples and frequently overlapped with FMSS high-EE status. However, the psychiatric disorders detected were not *currently* observable and represented past episodes, indicating that high-EE status is not a measure of concurrent psychopathology but could at times be a derivative of a past disorder. This is similar to data from the Goldstein et al. (1992) study cited earlier, where most disorders in FMSS high-EE relatives had been evident long before their offspring's initial episode of schizophrenia and the EE assessment.

Issue 3: Characteristics and Determinants of EE

Does EE index a transactional process between persons (such as patient and key relatives)? As discussed earlier, although EE is a measure assessed from a relative's speech, it is important to recognize that it is not only a measure of what goes on "inside" the relative. It may be better thought of as tapping a type of relationship based on characteristics of the relative, the patient, and the context.

In terms of characteristics of the patient that may help determine parental EE, most research has found little relationship between EE and the symptomatology of the patient. For example, Miklowitz et al. (1986) have shown no statistical relationship across a number of studies between EE and positive or negative schizophrenic symptoms (as measured by the Present State Examination or Brief Psychiatric Rating Scale). There have been some spotty findings suggesting that high levels of EE are associated with the patient's behavioral difficulties (Brown et al. 1972), depression (Strachan et al. 1986), and the anxiety/depression scale of the Brief Psychiatric Rating Scale (Glynn et al. 1990). However, the patient's contribution to EE may be more subtle than the presence of schizophrenic symptoms. Some relatives may have EE behaviors drawn out of them by more subtly troubling or irritating behavioral styles such as being oppositional, passive, or forgetful in response to simple concrete requests (Rosenfarb et al. 1995).

An important new direction in the study of the transactional nature of EE is the work on the patient's interactional behavior. Strachan et al. (1989) and Goldstein et al. (1989) presented data on how patients interact with relatives during a stressful discussion task. The patient's behavior was categorized according to his or her "coping style." There were significant relationships between the patient's coping style and parents' EE. Specifically, patients who had parents who were high EE showed more criticism themselves directed at their parents and fewer statements of autonomy than patients whose parents were low EE. These data suggest that EE may tap a transactional process. They do not, however, show whether the relatives' or patients' behavior is causative. We believe that neither is and that the process emerges from a combination of parental and patient influences.

EE may also be related to a variety of family factors: the level of relatives' understanding of schizophrenia and consequently their view of the causes of various behaviors they see, enduring personality characteristics of relatives and their distinctive roles in the family system, their characteristic responses to stress, other stressors in their lives, or aspects of temperament.

Thus, although the EE construct is operationalized in terms of the relative's expressed attitudes, it is more adequately conceptualized as a summary measure indexing complex transactional processes within emotionally meaningful, relatively enduring relationships.

In an effort to assess the transactional aspects of EE by direct observation and rating of interpersonal interaction, a number of studies (Hooley 1986; Hooley and Hahlweg 1986; Kuipers et al. 1983; Miklowitz et al. 1984; Strachan et al. 1986) have found that high-EE ratings on the CFI predict the interactional behavior of relatives during a family discussion task. Criticisms of the patient and guilt-inducing and intrusive remarks were far more frequent in CFI high as compared with CFI low relatives. In a study of young schizophrenic patients of recent onset, Miklowitz et al. (1989) found that the relationship between CFI EE measured during hospitalization and interactional behavior 4–5 weeks postdischarge was not so strong. However, FMSS EE measures obtained at the time of the interactional assessment were highly predictive of the levels of criticism and intrusiveness expressed by the relative toward the patient. The most averse interactions were noted in families where there was consistency in EE status across both the inpatient and outpatient periods.

These findings raise the question of the optimum time for assessing EE or its interactional analogue. Assessments during the inpatient period, when the patient is acutely ill and the relatives are under great stress, may not permit the separation of transient high-EE states from those that are more stably rated as high EE.

Although there have been fewer studies relating interactional data to the subsequent course of a disorder, the few studies completed to date are encouraging. Miklowitz et al. (1988) and Doane et al. (1986) both found that data based on observations of family interaction predicted relapse as well as CFI EE attitudes. It thus appears reasonable to pursue this line of study in clinical research, because clinicians usually have more ready access to samples of family behavior than to research measures of attitudes.

A major issue in shifting to behavioral assessments of EE is to define the construct in a fashion that is applicable to clinical interviews with families or other relational units. The studies cited all relied on structured interaction tasks in which a clinician was not present in the room.

Contexts of EE: culture, ethnicity, and family constellation. Given the interactional nature of the studies of EE, it is possible to examine the influence of culture, ethnicity, and family composition on the predictive nature of EE.

There is a remarkable stability in the predictive power of EE across a number of cultures: German, Swiss, Indian, British, and American. This stability supports using the same cutoff points for criticism and emotional overinvolvement. However, the predictive effect slightly strengthens using a lower cutoff of criticism for the Indian study. It is suggested that this may be due to a culture where criticism is less frequent so that even a small amount of criticism may be perceived as stressful. It is hard to know whether cultural norms regarding criticism can account for the unique findings in the Indian study, because Leff et al. (1987) used large rural families where the patient frequently lived with a dozen or so relatives. Because only one or two relatives were interviewed in these families, it may be that high-EE families were missed in this particular sample. We know of unpublished data and ongoing studies in several other cultures (e.g., Spain, Poland, Japan, France, and Italy).

There also seems to be remarkable stability of the predictive power of EE across ethnicity. Similar effects were found in studies in the United States with black (Moline et al. 1985), Mexican American (Karno et al. 1987), and Caucasian (Nuechterlein et al. 1986) subjects. Karno et al.'s study showed that, although the base rate for high EE was quite a bit lower among Mexican Americans, patient relapse was significantly associated with high-EE attitudes.

Finally, the family constellation may have a modulating influence on the relationship between EE and relapse. However, our review does not suggest that this is true in general: the effects seem to be independent of family type.

To what extent is EE a stable characteristic of individuals? EE has typically been assessed in prospective studies when the patient-relative was in an active phase of schizophrenia, usually during a period of inpatient stay. It is assumed that the attitudes tapped by the CFI interview carry over into the postdischarge period and thereby provide an indication of the probable family environment after discharge. It is not clear whether this assessment assumes that high- or low-EE status represents enduring trait-like characteristics of a person or a dispositional tendency to react in a particular way when faced with the stress of schizophrenia in a relative. Vaughn (1986) indicated that much of the early research was guided by the dispositional notion. Brown et al. (1972) carried out follow-up interviews within a year of the patient's discharge from the hospital. The number of criticisms decreased considerably, with the greatest reduction for patients who had shown the greatest improvement over that period. It appeared that reductions in criticism are more common than in cases where emotional overinvolvement was the basis for the high-EE rating.

Dulz and Hand (1986) reported on the stability of the CFI ratings in an untreated control group over a 9-month follow-up period. Unfortunately, there was considerable attrition in this sample, particularly in the low-EE group in which 12 of 29 respondents refused the 9-month CFI, whereas only 3 of 21 of the high-EE relatives did so. There was considerable stability in those low-EE relatives who did participate, but 50% of the relatives in the high-EE group changed status to a low-EE rating. This is a common finding in other studies where low-EE relatives appear consistent over time whereas high-EE relatives vary, often as a function of change in the patient's clinical state. Thus, it appears that EE as assessed by the CFI to some extent reflects the presence of active symptoms in a patient-relative and functions like a dispositional characteristic and not a stable trait.

A report by Leeb et al. (1991) examined the stability of the FMSS procedure (Magana et al. 1986) over a 5- to 6-week period in a German sample of the close relatives of schizophrenic patients. The initial assessment was made when the patient was hospitalized and the repeat measurement when the patient was in the community living with relatives. The magnitude of the association between the two assessments was .64 (phi coefficient). In this sample, 8 of 9 high-EE relatives were still high and 15 of 19 low-EE relatives were still low as well. In the short run, the FMSS method appears quite a stable indicator of affective attitudes held toward a patient-relative.

A problem in estimating the stability of the CFI over shorter time periods is that the focus of the interview is on the previous 3 months, and an attempt to repeat the procedure for less than a 6-month interval makes little sense.

These data indicate a curious paradox. EE as assessed during an acute episode of schizophrenia requiring hospitalization of a patient does not appear to reflect the concurrent severity or form of the patient's symptomatology. However, over longer periods of time, it appears that relatives' affective attitudes tend to fluctuate as a function of the variations in the patient's clinical state. Research by Goldstein et al. (1992) found that those relatives whose EE status remains constant from the inpatient to outpatient period have a prior history of some type of psychiatric disorder, suggesting a particular vulnerability to the stress of schizophrenia in a close family member that limits the range of affective response.

Issue 4: Measurement and Clinical Criteria for High EE or an Alternatively Named Category

Measurement issue: reliability. EE has most customarily been rated using the CFI. The CFI is a semistructured interview that covers major areas of a patient's behavior during the period beginning 3 months prior to an index admission to a hospital for a major mental disorder. The main areas covered are psychiatric history leading up to the hospitalization, a weekly time budget of face-to-face contact between patient and relatives, irritability of the patient, and psychiatric symptoms. The interviews are audiotaped and rated subsequently as follows: a count of the number of criticisms, the number of positive remarks, and ratings on a 6-point scale of emotional overinvolvement, a 6-point scale of warmth, and a 4-point scale of hostility.

Raters who conduct and score the CFI are qualified by a trainer, who runs a course and provides a set of 10 master training tapes. Raters must achieve a minimum correlation of .80 (Pearson's r) on all scales with the criterion rater to be certified as reliable. All of the studies reviewed here reported that coders were trained to reach this level of reliability. This would be important to consider if any clinical trials or brief measures are carried out. However, the degree to which this level of rater reliability has been sustained during a study has rarely been reported, nor have checks for rater drift over the course of a study and methods for controlling for such drift been reported.

Alternative measures of EE. It appears that an assessment of a relative's or family's EE level provides an important source of information for prognosis and planning psychosocial intervention strategies. However, the major method used for making this assessment, the CFI, poses major difficulties when introduced into clinical practice. The interview itself is very lengthy (1.5–2 hours to administer), and it is time consuming to learn and actually score the CFI. Thus, there is a strong need to develop alternative, economical methods of assessment that are more readily compatible with regular clinical work. Previously, we alluded to the FMSS EE approach, which adapts the 5-minute monologue method of Gottschalk and

Gleser (1969) using an instructional set suggested by Gift et al. (1985). Magana et al. (1986) developed a coding system for rating EE from these speech samples that produced a reasonable correlation with CFI EE. Subsequent studies with a Spanish-speaking sample in the United States (Magana et al. 1986), a German-speaking sample (Leeb et al. 1991), and English-speaking samples (Miklowitz et al. 1989) have produced essentially the same relationships between FMSS EE ratings and CFI ratings. The sensitivity and specificity of the FMSS to the CFI were evaluated by Leeb et al. in samples from the United States and Germany. Specificity was generally high (80%) in the sense that FMSS high-EE relatives are always CFI high EE; but the sensitivity (71%) was less than desired in both samples because a third of respondents who rated CFI high EE were rated low by the FMSS EE method.

As of this writing, there is only one study comparing the relative predictive validity of FMSS and CFI EE ratings, and full data are not available for this study. Also, the CFI and FMSS data were not collected at the same time, limiting the interpretation that can be drawn from the data in this study. Preliminary data indicate that the CFI predicts relapse somewhat better than the FMSS method, but the differences in prediction rates are not statistically significant.

The only other study with data on the predictive validity of the FMSS is that of Asarnow et al. (1993), which reported highly significant variations in the course of childhood-onset depressive disorder as a function of FMSS EE status of a parent.

The lack of data regarding the predictive validity of the FMSS limits our ability to recommend that it become a standard method for estimating EE in clinical practice, despite its simplicity and compatibility with normal interviewing procedure. However, it does appear to be a promising method for a field trial to ascertain applicability and validity. The fact that one needs training in scoring audiotapes of the FMSS samples should not be ignored, although numerous training courses have revealed that reliability of scoring can be achieved in a relatively short time.

A self-report method for EE would be the preferred solution. Friedmann and Goldstein (1993) developed a self-report adjective-rating system for relatives designed to measure their EE attitudes. Relatives rated 20 adjectives, 10 positive and 10 negative, on an 8-point scale (1 = never, 8 = always) on two forms, on one of which they rated their typical behavior toward the patient over the previous 3 months and on the other the relative's behavior toward them over the same time period. Patient-relatives were recent-onset schizophrenic or bipolar-manic patients. Relatives also received the CFI when the patient was in the hospital and the FMSS 4–5 weeks after discharge. Friedmann and Goldstein found highly significant associations between the adjective ratings and both CFI EE and FMSS EE ratings of relatives. The strongest relationship was with the FMSS data that were collected at the same family assessment session. When subtypes of EE were considered, very strong associations to EE status were found for relatives rated as high on criticism, but not for those rated as high EE by the overinvolvement criterion. Also, adjective ratings describing how the relative typically behaves toward the patient were just as related to the relative's EE status as ratings of the patient's typical behavior toward relatives. When Friedmann and Goldstein applied logistic regression methods to the adjective rating data, they found that ratings on the 10 negative adjectives correctly distinguished 70.9% of the FMSS low-EE from high-EE critical relatives. Discrimination of FMSS high overinvolvement relatives from either high critical or low-EE relatives proved more difficult. Interestingly, whatever discrimination was achieved for FMSS high-EE overinvolvement relatives was based on the 10 *positive* adjectives in which the overinvolvement relatives rated the patient more positively than the other two groups.

Hooley and Richters (1991) indicated that it was possible to use a 28-item Q-sort procedure to rate a full CFI, thereby avoiding the usual detailed rating system for that instrument. Undergraduates, largely naive about EE or schizophrenic research, agreed well with each other and with a trained criterion rater. However, the predictive validity of this global rating was not as good as that derived from a careful, expert scoring of the same CFI material. It remains to be seen how readily experienced clinicians can infer high-EE attitudes from interview material, whether structured or unstructured.

Discussion and Recommendations

Implications of Including Such a Relational Disorder in DSM-IV

Despite uncertainties and gaps in the currently available research data, our conclusion is that the overall weight of the evidence is sufficiently persuasive and clinically significant to justify inclusion in DSM-IV. However, we are less clear about the most appropriate label and most suitable location for such a category. As we have noted, the early papers focused explicitly on EE as measured by the CFI, especially the components of critical comments and emotional overinvolvement that were obtained under closely controlled conditions. EE was found to be predictive of relapse of florid psychotic schizophrenic symptoms within 9–12 months after hospital discharge. Despite the fact that, in one of the first reports (Vaughn and Leff 1976), EE was found to be a sensitive predictor of relapse of depression, high EE came to be viewed as primarily a characteristic of the relatives, especially the parents, of schizophrenic patients. The premature but still often misunderstood assumption was that parents were unilaterally "causing" the relapse. Despite efforts to refute the notion, EE has unfortunately been perceived as blaming these relatives for the relapse, rather than as a far more complex process that understandably is likely to emerge while caring for difficult, perplexing patients, a phenomenon not at all specific to the families of schizophrenic patients.

We have considered alternative terms such as *emotionally intense interpersonal relationship* or *emotionally stressful interpersonal relationship*. These terms have the disadvantage of not emphasizing the component of criticism that has been important in the EE literature. On the other hand, they would invite more detailed study of the components, which the recent research literature clearly indicates is desirable. The diagnostic criteria for these terms would need to be carefully specified so that only clear-cut cases are diagnostically recorded; otherwise there would be a hazard that the category could be trivialized by overusage.

A further problem is that there is no place in DSM-III-R (American Psychiatric Association 1987) where attention is focused explicitly on EE or its clinical counterpart. "Emotionally intense interpersonal relationships" could presumably be considered as a component of one or more of the existing V codes, especially "parent-child problem" or "marital problem." However, this concept is not mentioned as a possible example of these problems, and no operational diagnostic criteria of any kind are included for any of the V codes in DSM-III-R. This lack of specificity in the V codes has surely inhibited research on and clinical attention to EE, given the fact that the DSM-III-R has become the dominant framework for research and practice concerning psychopathology. Also, the DSM-III-R statement that the conditions in the V codes are "not attributable to a mental disorder" implies that a clear causal relationship between comorbid conditions can be established—something that is not expected when, for example, criteria are met for both an Axis I and an Axis II diagnosis.

The question needs to be considered as to where these relational problems can appropriately be located within the scope of the DSM-IV psychiatric classification: 1) as an *individual disorder* (located in the relatives who express intense feelings about a patient), or 2) as a *relational disorder* (in effect, an "illness" characterizing the relationship between persons), or 3) as a *relational problem* between persons.

Although DSM-III-R conceptualizes mental disorders as syndromes or patterns that occur "in a person," certain problems and conditions that have always been of clinical concern to mental health professionals cannot be adequately described in terms of individual functioning—emotionally intense interpersonal relationships are an example. Such problems are inherently relational; that is, they are better regarded as *between* people rather than as primarily *in* a person. Comprehensive biopsychosocial assessments include but go beyond individually located symptoms (Group for Advancement of Psychiatry Committee on the Family 1989).

The question of whether a category relevant to high EE should be viewed as a relational *disorder* or a relational *problem* hinges on the conceptualization of disorders and illness. Historically and cross-culturally, relational difficulties have not been regarded as being disorders or illnesses, even when such difficulties have been perceived as either causing or resulting from individual illness (Wynne and Shields, in press). The thrust of this review suggests that such a category would optimally be included in DSM-IV in the section on relational problems included in the "Other Conditions That May Be a Focus of Clinical Attention." Clinically, then, "emotionally intense interpersonal relationships" (or a similar term) would imply nothing about the source of the problem in one person versus another; the clinician would be sensitized to attend to feelings of burden or stress that are troublesome experiences in certain relationships. The clinician should be stimulated to explore the context of these feelings or attitudes, for example, recognizing that frustrated and critical attitudes often appear to be associated with the perception of a family member that a patient family member seems to be willfully failing to cooperate with home routines. With emotional support for the relative and educational input about how the patient's behavior is an expectable symptom of a clear-cut mental disorder, the relative may be relieved from subjective burden and become less intensely involved. Thus, the diagnostic assessment of these attitudes can have valuable clinical relevance, a result that would be more likely if this relational problem were specifically recognized in DSM-IV.

Recommendations Regarding a Relational Disorder With High EE

This review leads us to certain conclusions and recommendations for including the EE factor in DSM-IV. First, it does not seem reasonable to regard high-EE status in itself, out of context, as a diagnosable disorder, even in relational terms. High EE is best construed as a significant prognostic factor that is relevant to the course and contains treatment indications for a wide range of psychiatric disorders and probably some physical disorders as well. However, for diagnostic purposes, it can also be viewed as an indicator or marker of seriously dysfunctional interpersonal relationships that are not otherwise explicitly described. By formulating the diagnosis in this manner, one assumes that the presence of high EE, assessed as one person's attitudes toward another, is always, or at least usually, associated with bidirectional or multidirectional difficulties in the relationship. Here the evidence we reviewed earlier is crucial: individually measured high EE resonates as a transactional process that is not located exclusively in any individual and is typically associated with observable disturbed family interactions, which have been described under the heading of "affective style" (Doane et al. 1981) and "coping style" (Strachan et al. 1989).

Second, as we have noted, there is an arguable question as to whether this category should be labeled as a relational *disorder* or as a relational *problem*. If the

DSM-III-R definition of mental disorders as syndromes or patterns that occur "in a person" is rigidly retained in DSM-IV, then no category of relational disorder will be clinically useful. To make the diagnostic manual more clinically useful and more relevant to how assessment and treatment needs are actually met, in accord with a biopsychosocial medical model (Engel 1977, 1980), it has been recommended that a place for relational disorders be provided in DSM-IV (Group for Advancement of Psychiatry Committee on the Family 1989). This viewpoint would be consistent with a concept of "disorder" as patterned dysfunction. However, if the somewhat ambiguous term *disorder* is equated with *disease*, which implies an underlying pathophysiologic process, then the term *relational disorder* becomes more difficult to defend. If the concept of relational disorder is rejected for inclusion on Axis I, we recommend that this and perhaps other categories be included, in accord with ICD-10 (World Health Organization 1990) guidelines and codes, as "relational problems." If so included, they should be given Z codes with operational criteria, as for other diagnoses. The relegation of family and other relational problems to the V codes, as in DSM-III-R, where they carry no criteria and are almost completely ignored for clinical and research purposes, greatly impedes investigation and attention of these highly disruptive yet common human dysfunctions. An alternative approach is to have "relational problems" as a new axis, because research suggests that factors such as EE can have a significant impact on the course of many Axis I disorders.

Third, current research on methods for assessing high-EE status in more simplified, clinically usable ways needs to be continued. Although there are some promising methods under development (e.g., FMSS, questionnaires, adjective-rating forms), they are not yet at the stage where they are fully established for general clinical use. It seems likely that clinical assessment using a combination of an uninterrupted speech sample followed by certain key sections drawn from the CFI will be able to make a useful clinical distinction between high- versus low-EE attitudes.

Another quite different approach to assessment would be to bypass or supplement the evaluation of affective *attitudes of individuals* and base EE assessments on observation of *interpersonal interaction*. It would be necessary to define some situations in which clinicians could observe intrafamilial communication and rate the presence or absence of critical and intrusive behaviors. In fact, it has been our experience that it is easier to train personnel to evaluate behavior than the kinds of subtleties required to evaluate CFI EE, such as notable changes in voice tone and involvement in the patient's life. We believe it would be feasible to develop some rather simple rating scales, analogous to the Brief Psychiatric Rating Scale method for rating symptoms, that could be used to evaluate behavioral concomitants of high- and low-EE attitudes.

We recommend that a category termed *parent-child relational problem with high EE* be included in DSM-IV as suggested on Z62.8 of the *DSM-IV Options Book* (American Psychiatric Association 1991, p. U:3). However, we suggest two further modifications of this relational category.

1. Include a parallel relational problem category for partners as Z63.8, partner relational problem with high EE. The previous literature amply documents that this type of relational problem is frequently noted in partner relationships and has been found to have comparable prognostic value when a partner has a major mental disorder.
2. We also recommend that the relational disorder have three subtypes, one characterized by criticism, the second by emotional overinvolvement, and the third by a combination of the two. Thus, we suggest that the Z62.8, parent-child and partner relationship problems, has these subtypes as Z62.8.1 critical type, Z62.8.2 overinvolved type, and Z62.8.3 critical *and* overinvolved type. The literature review supports such a distinction because these different subtypes have different interactional correlates and responsivity to treatment.

If such a recommendation is accepted, it would be necessary and advisable to drop Z62.1, relational disorder with parental overprotection, from DSM-IV because it would be redundant with Z62.8.2.

Recommendations for Clinical Criteria for Relational Disorders Characterized by High EE

The specification of a person or relational group as high in EE reflects an ongoing, unsatisfying relationship in which one or more members of a family are unhappy with one another, usually because the performance of one family member is less than expected or desired. This disappointment may relate to the symptomatic status of a patient with a psychiatric disorder, his or her social role functioning, or a prior history of impaired functioning. Interactions in such families are characterized either by reciprocal criticism and escalation of hostile interchanges or by one-way criticism directed toward a relative with a psychiatric disorder that is not reciprocated. At times, such families show a different way of coping with the stress of the patient's disorder by becoming overinvolved in the patient's life and neglecting their own needs or relationships with other family members.

Specifically, the criteria that can be used to identify high EE as a marker of seriously disturbed relational functioning can be manifest in one of three subtypes, which are equally applicable to parent-child or partner relationships.

Z62.8.1 and Z63.8.1: high EE—criticism subtype. The relationship between two or more members of a family is characterized by *repeated and harsh criticisms of the patient that express affective attitudes marked by sustained hostility.* The criticism may be transactional in nature in the sense that the "target" of the criticism may be matched by criticism from the other. The behaviors and personal characteristics that are criticized may very well be dysfunctional, irritating to the average person, and hard to live with. Harsh criticism refers to statements in which the character, motives, or personality are impugned ("you are lazy," "you don't want to get well," "you just want to punish our family") or seem intended to make the other feel guilty ("you are killing your mother with your behavior," "you ruin every family outing"). The frequency and intensity of these criticisms is such that they are rarely absent from family transactions and they preclude most positive aspects of family life.

Z62.8.2 and Z63.8.2: high EE—emotional overinvolved subtype. The relationship manifests at least two of the following attitudes and/or behaviors.

1. One person's life is constricted so that it is focused exclusively on the other's needs.
2. An attitude of self-sacrifice or martyrdom as the reason for the marked involvement in the life of the other.
3. A marked tendency to intrude in conversations with the other by interrupting or telling the individual what his or her motives or feelings are without clues justifying such inferences.
4. A notable tendency to do all daily chores or self-care tasks for the other.
5. Repeated breakthrough of emotion such as tears or overt crying whenever the other is discussed.

To rate a family or other relational unit as emotionally overinvolved, it is necessary to consider the clinical state of the "targeted" person. Severely regressed patients with minimal self-care skills may demand a high degree of involvement from relatives as required by their condition, which would not be rated as overinvolvement. Similarly, in the relationship of parents with young children, the line between appropriate involvement and overinvolvement is a subtle one, although research with the FMSS method (Stubbe et al. 1993) has indicated that such a distinction can be made and that it relates to the form of a child's disorder.

Z62.8.3 and Z63.8.3: high EE with both critical and emotionally overinvolved subtypes. This involves families in which both attributes are present. These are of two types: 1) in which a single relative manifests both attitudes and vacillates between critical and emotionally overinvolved behavior at various times, and 2) in which two key relatives present with different attitudes and behaviors so that one satisfies the criteria for high EE critical and the other for high EE emotionally overinvolved. This second pattern is most frequently noted in parental families where an offspring is the focus of the relational problem and is often correlated with a history of preexisting chronic marital conflict.

Summary

The weight of evidence suggests that the construct of EE is a prognostic indicator of the course of psychopathology in a variety of cultures. We recommend that DSM-IV include a category called relational problems with high EE as a V code (ICD-10 Z code). We further recommend that the relational problem have three subtypes, one characterized by criticism, the second by emotional overinvolvement, and the third by a combination of the two. Finally, we recommend including parallel categories for relational problems with high EE for both parent-child and partner relationships.

Addendum

As we have found in this literature review, relational problems can be associated with a wide range of disorders and may involve both parent-child and partner relationships. The DSM-IV Task Force therefore decided that the category of "relational problem with high expressed emotion" was too specific and narrow and that a broader and more general category was needed to be clinically useful. For this reason, the final proposal for DSM-IV is to include a category for "Relational Problems Related to a Mental Disorder or a General Medical Condition" in the section for "Other Conditions That May Be a Focus of Clinical Attention" with the following description: "This category should be used when the focus of clinical attention is a pattern of impaired interaction that is associated with a mental disorder or a general medical condition in a family member."

References

American Psychiatric Association: Diagnostic and Statistical Manual of Mental Disorders, 3rd Edition, Revised. Washington, DC, American Psychiatric Association, 1987

American Psychiatric Association: DSM-IV Options Book: Work in Progress. Washington, DC, American Psychiatric Association, 1991

Asarnow JR, Goldstein MJ, Tompson M, et al: One year outcomes of depressive disorders in child psychiatric inpatients: evaluation of the prognostic power of a brief measure of expressed emotion. J Child Psychol Psychiatry 34:129–137, 1993

Barrelet L, Ferrero F, Szigethy L, et al: Expressed emotion and first admission schizophrenia nine-month follow-up in a French environment. Br J Psychiatry 156:357–362, 1990

Brown GW: Experiences of discharged chronic schizophrenic mental hospital patients in various types of living group. Millbank Memorial Fund Quarterly 37:105–131, 1959

Brown GW, Rutter M: The measurement of family activities and relationships: a methodological study. Human Relations 19:241–263, 1966

Brown GW, Carstairs GM, Topping GG: The post-hospital adjustment of chronic mental patients. Lancet 2:685–689, 1958

Brown GW, Monck EM, Carstairs GM, et al: Influence of family life on the course of schizophrenic illness. British Journal of Preventive and Social Medicine 16:55–68, 1962

Brown GW, Birley JLT, Wing JK: Influence of family life on the course of schizophrenic disorders: a replication. Br J Psychiatry 121:241–258, 1972

Camilli G, Hopkins K: Applicability of chi-square to 2×2 contingency tables with small expected cell frequencies. Psychol Bull 85:163–167, 1978

Doane JA, West KL, Goldstein MJ, et al: Parental communication deviance and affective style. Arch Gen Psychiatry 38:679–685, 1981

Doane JA, Goldstein MJ, Miklowitz DJ, et al: The impact of individual and family treatment on the affective climate of families of schizophrenics. Br J Psychiatry 148:279–287, 1986

Dulz B, Hand I: Short-term relapse in young schizophrenics: can it be predicted and affected by family (CFI), patient and treatment variables? an experimental study, in Treatment of Schizophrenia: Family Assessment and Intervention. Edited by Goldstein MJ, Hand I, Hahlweg K. Berlin, Heidelberg, Germany. Springer-Verlag, 1986, pp 59–75

Engel GL: The need for a new medical model: a challenge for biomedicine. Science 196(8):129–136, 1977

Engel GL: The clinical application of the biopsychosocial model. Am J Psychiatry 137:535–544, 1980

Friedmann MS, Goldstein MJ: Relatives' awareness of their own expressed emotion as measured by a self-report adjective checklist. Fam Process 32:459–472, 1993

Gift T, Cole R, Wynne LW: A hostility measure for use in family contexts. Psychiatry Res 15:205–210, 1985

Glynn SM, Randolph ET, Spencer F, et al: Patient psychopathology and expressed emotion in schizophrenia. Br J Psychiatry 157:877–880, 1990

Goldstein MG, Miklowitz DJ, Strachan AM, et al: Patterns of expressed emotion and patient coping styles that characterize the families of recent onset schizophrenics. Br J Psychiatry 155:107–111, 1989

Goldstein MJ, Talovic SA, Nuechterlein KH, et al: Family interaction versus individual psychopathology: do they indicate the same processes in families of schizophrenics? Br J Psychiatry 161:97–102, 1992

Gottschalk LA, Gleser GC: The Measurements of Psychological States Through Analysis of Verbal Behavior. Berkeley, CA, University of California Press, 1969

Grizzle JE: Continuity correction in the chi-square test for 2×2 tables. American Statistician 21:28–32, 1967

Group for the Advancement of Psychiatry Committee on the Family: The challenge of relational diagnoses: applying the biopsychosocial model in DSM-IV. Am J Psychiatry 146:1492–1494, 1989

Hatfield AB, Lefley HP: Families of the Mentally Ill: Coping and Adaptation. New York, Guilford, 1987

Hatfield AB, Spaniol L, Zipple AM: Expressed emotion: a family perspective. Schizophr Bull 13:221–226, 1987

Hibbs ED, Hamburger SD, Lenane M, et al: Determinants of expressed emotion in families of disturbed and normal children. Journal of Child Psychiatry 32:757– 770, 1991

Hogarty GE, McEvoy JP, Munetz M, et al: Dose of fluphenazine, familial expressed emotion, and outcome in schizophrenia: results of 2-year controlled study. Arch Gen Psychiatry 45:797–805, 1988

Hooley JM: Expressed emotion: a review of the critical literature. Clinical Psychology Review 5:119–139, 1985

Hooley JM: Expressed emotion and depression: interactions between patients and high- versus low-expressed-emotion spouses. J Abnorm Psychol 95:237–246, 1986

Hooley JM, Hahlweg K: The marriages and interaction patterns of depressed patients and their spouses: comparison of high and low EE dyads, in Treatment of Schizophrenia: Family Assessment and Intervention. Edited by Goldstein MJ, Hand I, Hahlweg K. Berlin, Germany, Springer, 1986, pp 85–96

Hooley JM, Richters JE: A tentative measure of EE: a methodology and competency note. J Abnorm Psychol 100:94–97, 1991

Hooley JM, Teasdale JD: Predictors of relapse in unipolar depressives: expressed emotion, marital distress, and perceived criticism. J Abnorm Psychol 98:229–235, 1989

Hooley JM, Orley J, Teasdale JD: Levels of expressed emotion and relapse in depressed patients. Br J Psychiatry 148:642–647, 1986

Kanter J, Lamb R, Loeper C: Expressed emotion in families: a critical review. Hosp Community Psychiatry 38(4):374–380, 1987

Karno M, Jenkins JH, de la Selva A, et al: Expressed emotion and schizophrenic outcome among Mexican-American families. J Nerv Ment Dis 175:143–151, 1987

Koenigsberg HW, Handley R: Expressed emotion: from predictive index to clinical construct. Am J Psychiatry 143:1361–1373, 1986

Kottgen C, Sonnichsen I, Mollenhauer K, et al: The family relations of young schizophrenic patients: results of the Hamburg Camberwell Family Interview Study 1. International Journal of Family Psychiatry 5:61–94, 1984

Krawiecka M, Goldberg D, Vaughn M: Standardized psychiatric assessment scale for rating chronic patients. Acta Psychiatr Scand 55:299–308, 1977

Kuipers L, Bebbington PE: Expressed emotion research in schizophrenia: theoretical and clinical applications. Psychol Med 18:893–908, 1988

Kuipers L, Sturgeon D, Berkowitz R, et al: Characteristics of expressed emotion: its relationship to speech and looking in schizophrenic patients and their relatives. Br J Clin Psychol 22:257–264, 1983

Leeb B, Hahlweg K, Goldstein MJ, et al: The cross-national reliability, concurrent validity, and stability of a brief method for assessing expressed emotion. Psychiatr Res 39:25–31, 1991

Leff JP, Brown GW: Family and social factors in the course of schizophrenia. Br J Psychiatry 130:417–418, 1977

Leff J, Vaughn C: Expressed Emotion in Families: Its Significance for Mental Illness. New York, Guilford, 1985

Leff J, Wig N, Ghosh A, et al: Influence of relatives' expressed emotion on the course of schizophrenia in Chandigarh. Br J Psychiatry 151:166–173, 1987

MacMillan JF, Crow TJ, Johnson AL, et al: The Northwick Park study of first episodes of schizophrenia, III: short-term outcome in trial entrants and trial eligible patients. Br J Psychiatry 148:128–133, 1986a

MacMillan JF, Gold A, Crow JT, et al: The Northwick Park study of first episodes of schizophrenia, IV: expressed emotion and relapse. Br J Psychiatry 148:133–143, 1986b

MacMillan JF, Crow TJ, Johnson AL, et al: Expressed emotion and relapse in first episodes of schizophrenia. Br J Psychiatry 151:320–323, 1987

Magana AB, Goldstein MJ, Karno M, et al: A brief measure for assessing expressed emotion in relatives of psychiatric patients. Psychiatry Res 17:203–212, 1986

McCreadie RG, Phillips K: The Nithdale Schizophrenic Survey, VII: does relatives' high EE predict relapse? Br J Psychiatry 95:60–66, 1988

Miklowitz DJ, Goldstein MJ, Falloon IRH, et al: Interactional correlates of expressed emotion in the families of schizophrenics. Br J Psychiatry 144:482–487, 1984

Miklowitz DJ, Strachan AM, Goldstein MJ, et al: Expressed emotion and communication deviance: the families of schizophrenics. J Abnorm Psychol 95:60–66, 1986

Miklowitz DJ, Goldstein MJ, Nuechterlein KH, et al: Family factors and the course of bipolar affective disorder. Arch Gen Psychiatry 45:225–231, 1988

Miklowitz DJ, Goldstein MJ, Doane JA, et al: Is expressed emotion an index of a transactional process? I: relative's affective style. Fam Process 28:153–167, 1989

Mintz LI, Liberman RP, Miklowitz DJ, et al: Expressed emotion: a call for participation among relatives, patients and professionals. Schizophr Bull 13:227–235, 1987

Moline RA, Singh S, Morris A, et al: Family expressed emotion and relapse in schizophrenia in 24 urban American patients. Am J Psychiatry 142:1078–1081, 1985

Nuechterlein KH, Snyder KS, Dawson ME, et al: Expressed emotion, fixed dose fluphenazine decanoate maintenance, and relapse in recent-onset schizophrenia. Psychopharmacol Bull 22:633–639, 1986

Overall JE, Gorham DR: The Brief Psychiatric Rating Scale. Psychol Rep 10:799–812, 1962

Parker G, Johnston P, Hayward L: Parental "expressed emotion" as a predictor of schizophrenic relapse. Arch Gen Psychiatry 45:806–813, 1988

Rosenfarb IS, Goldstein MJ, Mintz J, et al: Expressed emotion and subclinical psychopathology observable within the transactions between schizophrenic patients and their family members J Abnorm Psychol 104:259–267, 1995

Rutter ML, Brown GW: The reliability and validity of measures of family life and relationships in families containing a psychiatric patient. Social Psychiatry 1:38–53, 1966

Schwartz CE, Dorer DJ, Beardslee WR, et al: Maternal expressed emotion and parental affective disorder: risk for childhood depressive disorder, substance abuse, or conduct disorder. J Psychiatr Res 24:231–250, 1990

Strachan AM: Family management, in Handbook of Psychiatric Rehabilitation. Edited by Liberman RP. New York, Pergamon, 1991, pp 183–212

Strachan AM, Leff JP, Goldstein MJ, et al: Emotional attitudes and direct communication in the families of schizophrenics: a cross-national replication. Br J Psychiatry 149:279–287, 1986

Strachan AM, Feingold D, Goldstein MJ, et al: Is expressed emotion an index of a transactional process? II: patient's coping style. Fam Process 28:169–181, 1989

Stubbe DE, Zahner GE, Goldstein MJ: The diagnostic specificity of a brief measure of expressed emotion in a community sample of children and families. J Child Psychol Psychiatry 43:139–154, 1993

Tarrier N, Barrowclough C, Porceddu K, et al: The community management of schizophrenia: a controlled trial of a behavioural intervention with families to reduce relapse. Br J Psychiatry 153:532–542, 1988

Vaughn CE: Patterns of emotional response in families of schizophrenic patients, in Treatment of Schizophrenia: Family Assessment and Intervention. Edited by Goldstein MJ, Hand I, Hahlweg K. New York, Springer-Verlag, 1986, pp 97–108

Vaughn CE, Leff JP: The influence of family and social factors on the course of psychiatric illness: a comparison of schizophrenic and neurotic patients. Br J Psychiatry 129:125–137, 1976

Vaughn CE, Snyder KS, Jones S, et al: Family factors in schizophrenic relapse: replication in California of the British research on expressed emotion. Br J Psychiatry 41:1169–1177, 1984

Wing JK, Cooper JE, Sartorius N: The Description and Classification of Psychiatric Symptoms: An Instructional Manual for the Use of the PSE and Catego System. Cambridge, MA, Cambridge University Press, 1974

World Health Organization: ICD-10 Chapter V: Mental and Behavioral Disorders Diagnostic Criteria for Research. Geneva, Switzerland, World Health Organization, 1990

Wynne LC, Shields CG: Illness, family theory, and family therapy, II: the physical illness/mental illness distinction. Family Process (in press)

Chapter 35

Parent Inadequate Discipline

P. Chamberlain, Ph.D., J. B. Reid, Ph.D., J. Ray, B.A.,
D. Capaldi, Ph.D., and P. Fisher, Ph.D.

Statement of the Issues

The purpose of this chapter is to determine if there is sufficient scientific evidence for the validity and clinical utility of the category "parent inadequate discipline" (PID) to recommend that it be included as a subcategory of "parent-child relationship problems" in DSM-IV. We examine the case for the importance of PID as a determinant of serious personal dysfunction in children and adolescents and their parents. We review studies relevant to the predictive validity of PID, its associations with childhood and adult disorders, and its correlates and studies of family interactional patterns and social and familial factors characterizing families with PID. Finally, we discuss the social validity of various discipline methods and review methodological considerations and limitations of the studies.

Significance of the Issues

The classification of parental discipline problems along with individual child and parent diagnoses would facilitate systematic research on childhood disorders and risk factors. Such a classification would also help determine appropriate treatments for children and their families. Clinical trials have shown that treatments aimed at strengthening parents' capacity to be nonviolent or more effective in their use of

---

Research assistance was provided by Kathleen Reid and Allen Winebarger, and editorial and typing assistance by Judith Boler. Support was provided by Grant number MH 46690, Prevention Research Branch, National Institute of Mental Health, U.S. Public Health Service.

discipline have had positive results (Patterson et al. 1982) and are widely used by practitioners.

Studies have shown that the processes of parental restriction and control of their children, how and when parents attempt to use discipline, and the effectiveness of such attempts vary widely among families and predict child adjustment and outcomes. Parents and their children have been shown to exert mutual influences on each other during discipline transactions, and identifiable patterns of parent-child social interaction have been found to predict child psychiatric status and long-term outcomes. Although there has been substantial controversy and some good empirical studies on the relative importance of the contributions of parents and children in discipline transactions, there is consensus that both parents and children make unique contributions to such transactions and that these interchanges influence the current adjustment and later course of the child's development (Anderson et al. 1986; Grusec and Kuczynski 1980; Patterson et al. 1990).

Parent-child interactions occur in the context of the psychiatric and medical characteristics of the individual parent and child and in the context of influential social factors such as socioeconomic status, marital status/relationship, social networks, and educational level of the parent. All of these factors have been shown to affect parent-child interaction and child outcomes.

In past research, investigators have conceptualized discipline in a variety of ways. Early work by the Fels Research Program emphasized restrictiveness (control) versus permissiveness (Baldwin 1949). In the 1960s and 1970s, seminal studies were conducted that examined parental discipline styles, including power assertion, induction, and love withdrawal (Hoffman 1960), as well as authoritative, authoritarian, and permissive parenting (Baumrind 1968). Such "categories" of discipline styles were extremely global and typically included more than one specific type of discipline strategy used by parents who were classified into a given category. For example, a definition of power assertion is the use of techniques of force applied by a parent in a contest of wills with the child and includes both physical punishments and deprivation of material objects or privileges. The specific definitions used for the different categories of global style often vary from study to study. For example, restrictiveness has been defined in terms of directness, critical interference, and forceful intervention (Loeb et al. 1980; Londerville and Main 1981) and as consistent control and setting clearly defined limits (Coopersmith 1967; Lytton 1980; Pulkkinen 1982). As Grusec and Lytton (1988) pointed out, it is difficult to integrate research findings based on ratings of various parental discipline styles, because a variety of definitions have been used for the traits or styles being investigated.

To examine the specific characteristics and effects of types of problematic parental discipline, and to set the stage for more reliable identification of pathognomic patterns, we attempt to use specific descriptions of discipline strategies in this chapter. Parental discipline can be operationally defined as occurring during instances in which the parent attempts to give directions or commands to the child or to impose rules, restrictions, and controls. Within this context, five types of problem discipline have been identified in the literature: 1) inconsistent discipline, 2) irritable and explosive discipline, 3) low supervision and involvement, 4) inflexible and rigid discipline, and 5) mood-dependent (versus planful) discipline. In this chapter, we focus on problem discipline and discuss only incidentally the parental and child characteristics and correlates associated with effective discipline.

This chapter is intended to provide an overview of the literature on the predictive, concurrent, and social validities of PID. Studies of predictive validity examine the effects of poor early discipline on adolescent and adult adjustment. Concurrent validity studies examine the co-occurrence of PID with child and adult disorders and associated risk factors. Social validity studies examine the acceptability to parent, child, and treatment professionals of various forms of discipline. Although a number of controlled clinical trials targeting parent disciplinary practices have had relatively positive results (Forgatch and Toobert 1979; Patterson et al. 1982; Wahler and Fox 1980; Webster-Stratton and Hammond 1990), a review of the outcomes of these studies is beyond the scope of this chapter.

Method

Inclusion/Exclusion Criteria

In selecting studies to review, we were inclusive rather than exclusive in our criteria. However, studies that failed to contain either experimental designs or comparison/control groups were not included, with the exception of theoretical papers that were empirically based. In all, more than 300 studies were reviewed; 278 are included in this chapter. A summary of methodological considerations and problems with reliability is presented later.

Sources

Initially, studies were obtained through informal channels and a limited search of selected journals from 1988 to 1991 (e.g., the *Journal of the American Academy of Child and Adolescent Psychiatry, Journal of Consulting and Clinical Psychology, Journal of Family Violence,* and *Journal of Interpersonal Psychiatry and Child Development*). Next, we conducted a computer search using PsychLit and Medline. The PsychLit search included studies from 1974 to 1990, and the Medline search included studies from 1986 to 1991. As studies were reviewed, their reference lists were examined to locate other relevant articles that had been missed by the other methods. Additionally, we solicited papers from active researchers (e.g., Dornbusch, Elder, Conger, Larzelere, Gelles, Kendall, and Patterson).

Aggregation of Findings

In the Results section of this chapter, findings on the validity of PID are summarized in the following sections.

1. Definitions of types of PID that are identified in the literature.
2. The long-term predictive validity of PID in adolescent and adult clinical, "at-risk," and nonclinical populations.
3. The predictive validity of the relationship of PID to childhood disorders and other child characteristics.
4. Parental disorders and other parental characteristics associated with PID.
5. Social and contextual correlates of PID.
6. Parent-child interactional patterns associated with PID.
7. The social validity of various types of discipline.

We also review methodological considerations and the design characteristics of representative studies, including definition of the samples (diagnostic or selection criteria used), methods of data collection, source(s) of information, setting, and methods of subject selection.

Results: Validity

Definitions of PID

Types of PID that have been identified in the literature are reviewed in this section, along with available data relevant to their incidence in clinical and nonclinical populations.

Inconsistent discipline. Two primary types of parental inconsistent/incontingent discipline have been identified: intraparent inconsistency and interparent inconsistency. Within each of these types there are several variations.
Intraparent inconsistency includes the following types of behavioral patterns.

1. A parent's indiscriminate reactions to the child's positive and negative behaviors (e.g., punishing appropriate actions and rewarding prohibited behaviors).
2. Low or inconsistent follow-through (e.g., parent gives a request or command,

child argues, parent withdraws or does not follow through on the demand).
3. Giving in (e.g., child makes a request or demand, parent says no, child argues, parent gives in).
4. Unpredictably changing expectations and consequences for rule violations (e.g., provision of mixed, inconsistent sanctions for child misbehaviors).

Interparent inconsistency involves two parents, or their equivalents, acting differently over time on any of the following dimensions.

1. Discipline policies (e.g., basic house, homework, or curfew rules).
2. Monitoring of rule infractions (e.g., differences in tracking of the child's levels of day-to-day compliance with established rules).
3. Providing consequences for rule-breaking (e.g., following through on provision of sanctions for rule breaking).

In a number of studies, inconsistent parental discipline has been linked with child conduct problems (W. McCord et al. 1959; Patterson 1976; Rutter et al. 1975; Zucker 1976) and depression (Gelfand and Teti 1990). W. McCord et al. (1959) also found that parental inconsistency was a good predictor of the continuation of child conduct problems. Wahler and Sansbury (1990) cited correlational studies of mother-child interaction to show that maternal inconsistency acts as a maintenance factor of child aggressive and oppositional behavior (Dumas et al. 1989; Gardner 1989; R. G. Wahler, A. J. Williams, A. Cerezo: The compliance and predictability hypotheses: some sequential and correlational analysis of coercive mother-child interactions, unpublished manuscript, Knoxville, TN, University of Tennessee, 1989). In their retrospective analysis of the relationship between discipline practices experienced in childhood and adult depression and alcoholism, Holmes and Robins (1988) noted that mothers of adult patients tended to be less harsh but more inconsistent than fathers: the mothers "made up in inconsistency what they lacked in brutality" (p. 34).

A number of investigators speculated about specific and negative processes that result from parental inconsistency. Wahler and Dumas (1986) asserted that parents inadvertently "prime" their children's aggressive and oppositional actions through their inconsistent reactions to what the child says and does. Patterson (1976, 1979, 1982) suggested that inconsistent parents get caught in a "reinforcement trap," where short-term gains, such as peace and quiet, are bought at the expense of strengthening the child's difficult behavior through direct reinforcement and by increasing the resistance to extinction of the child's subsequent problem behavior. This hypothesis has received consistent empirical support in a number of studies (Gardner 1989; Sawin and Parke 1979).

Irritable and explosive discipline. Specific types of irritable and explosive discipline transactions that have been identified in the literature include the following.

1. The parent's frequent use of high-amplitude, high-intensity discipline strategies such as hitting, yelling, and threatening.
2. The increased likelihood that the child will respond to the parent's negative behavior with a counterattack (e.g., with aggressive or defiant behavior).
3. Relatively long episodes of parent-child conflict.
4. Escalating intensities of negative and punitive behaviors.
5. The parent's frequent use of negative or humiliating statements to or about the child.
6. The parent's high rate of use of direct commands, especially those that are not accompanied by rationales or reasoning.

Two general sets of factors relate consistently to parents' irritable and explosive reactions toward their children. One set involves individual and family factors such as parent and child psychological functioning, family characteristics such as size and structure, and characteristics of family interaction patterns. The other set of factors involves extrafamily social and contextual forces such as daily stress, unemployment, poverty, and social isolation. The most extreme and obvious negative outcome of irritable and explosive parental discipline is physical child abuse. There is substantial evidence suggesting that short of abuse, there are pathognomic effects on children whose parents' discipline strategies are chronically irritable and harsh. Elevated levels of parental irritability and anger have been shown in numerous studies to relate to child problems such as aggression (Hetherington and Martin 1979; Patterson 1982; Sears et al. 1957), hyperactivity (Stevens-Long 1973), child temperament (Lee and Bates 1985), and antisocial and delinquent behavior (Farrington 1978; Gleuck and Gleuck 1968; J. McCord 1979). Examples of parent characteristics that have been found to correlate with hyperirritability include parental depression (Gelfand and Teti 1990; Kochanska 1991; Rutter and Quinton 1984), antisocial patterns (Patterson and Capaldi 1991), and social isolation and stress (Wahler 1980).

Family factors that appear consistently related to levels of parental irritability include family size (Elmer 1967; Gil 1970), marital adjustment (DeSalvo and Zurcher 1984; Downey and Coyne 1990; Hops et al. 1990), and family structure (two parents versus a single parent) (Hetherington et al. 1989).

It is well documented that negative social and contextual factors play a key role in putting parents at risk for irritable exchanges with their children (Gelles 1978a) and that these stressors may act to amplify parental irritability and explosiveness (Elder et al. 1983; Larzelere and Patterson 1990).

Low supervision and involvement. Parenting characterized by low supervision or involvement includes the following.

1. Parents are unaware of the child's activities that are outside their direct supervision.
2. Parents do not know with whom their child is associating and/or their child's whereabouts when they are not being directly supervised.
3. Parents are unaware of their child's adjustment and/or performance at school, including homework assignments.
4. Parents rarely engage in joint activities with their child such as play, recreation, and conversation.
5. Parents may be aware that their child is associating with peers who may be engaging in antisocial behavior in the community, but they are unable or unwilling to provide close supervision of their child's activities and whereabouts.

Several well-conducted longitudinal studies have reported strong relationships between low parental supervision and delinquency. These are reviewed below. Additionally, poor supervision has been associated with a variety of problems including poor school achievement (A. C. Crouter, S. M. MacDermid, S. M. McHale: Parental monitoring and perceptions of children's school performance and conduct in dual- and single-earner families, unpublished manuscript, 1989), negative peer pressure (Dishion 1990; Steinberg 1986), physical fighting (Loeber and Dishion 1984), lying (Stouthamer-Loeber and Loeber 1986), drug use (Baumrind 1991), and antisocial and conduct disorders (Kazdin 1985). One study showed that 12- to 17-year-olds who received low parental supervision in homes where the father was absent showed a greater likelihood of conduct problems (i.e., both self-reported delinquency and teacher-reported school discipline problems) than their well-supervised counterparts from either father-absent or father-present families (Goldstein 1984).

The demonstration of significant associations, of course, does not prove a causal relationship. Empirically, it could be equally possible that the quality of parental supervision is determined by child characteristics and behavior. Those children and teenagers with more serious problems might present parents with more resistance to supervision, or the association could be found in only a subset of families where the parents had given up on the youth as a result of previous failed attempts to monitor his or her activities. Certainly as the child matures, the task of parental supervision of his or her activities, peer associations, and whereabouts becomes a more complicated and demanding task given that an increasing number of the child's activities occur outside of the direct observation of the parent.

For younger children (e.g., infants to preadolescents), parent involvement and responsiveness appear to play an important role in the child's compliance, cooperativeness (Clarke-Stewart 1973; Parpal and Maccoby 1985), and moral development (Kochanska 1991). For example, Pettit and Bates (1989) found that a paucity of affectional and educational interactions between mother and child at ages 12–24 months were predictive of high rates of behavior problems at age 4 years. They also found that mothers who rated their children as being "difficult" were more likely to ignore their children's bids for attention, even though these children were observed actually to make more positive overtures to their mothers than those who had been rated by their mothers as "easy." Several studies have investigated the relationship between joint mother-child activities and child conduct problems. Gardner (1989) found that, compared with mothers of preschoolers with conduct problems, mothers of control subjects spent nearly three times as much time in joint play and twice as much time in joint conversation with their children. In a nonclinical sample, Dunn and Kendrick (1982) found an inverse relationship between joint play and child behavior problems.

Again, correlational findings do not imply causality. Clear evidence exists supporting the notion that there are important differences between children in their behavioral tendencies that may influence the way parents treat them (Bell and Harper 1977; Plomin and Daniels 1987). As suggested by Patterson (1982) and Rutter (1981), these individual differences likely interact with parenting styles to potentiate the development of child disorders.

Inflexible and rigid discipline. Specific types of inflexible and rigid discipline that have been reported in the literature include the following.

1. Reliance on a single discipline strategy (or a limited number) for all types of transgressions.
2. Failure to take contextual or "extenuating" factors into account when dealing with child transgressions.
3. Failure to give rationales, or to use other induction techniques, in the context of discipline confrontations.
4. Failure to adjust the intensity of the discipline reaction to the severity of the infraction.

Child developmentalists have stressed the importance of the parents' ability to fit their discipline strategy to situational demands as well as to the child's age and level of cognitive functioning (Crockenberg 1987; Kuczynski 1982, 1984; Maccoby 1991). Research on nonclinical populations has shown that parents use different discipline strategies depending on whether their goals are oriented toward short-

or long-term child compliance. Long-term compliance implies internalization of rules and demands. Parental uses of induction and reasoning have been associated with the level of maturity of children's moral reasoning, confession and acceptance of blame, and altruism.

Shaffer and Brody (1981) reviewed studies on parental influences on moral development. They found generally positive evidence for the association of maternal induction and moral development (especially compared with power assertive techniques) and noted that maternal affection was consistently associated with children's altruism and their willingness to accept blame for wrongdoing. Neither the fathers' discipline practices nor affection related to morality indexes. In that review, the authors found that differences in the use of both induction and power assertive techniques were associated with parental socioeconomic status. Data from two studies showed that lower-class parents used more power assertion and less induction than did middle-class parents (Hoffman and Saltzstein 1967; Zussman 1978). They also noted that inductive techniques are more likely to be associated with measures of moral maturity in older versus younger children.

Studies that have examined discipline episodes over time or that have experimentally varied situational or child variables have shown that nonreferred parents use a combination of a number of different discipline strategies in various circumstances. Research on parent responses to specific types of transgressions has shown correlations between types of parental responses and types of child misbehaviors. For example, Zahn-Waxler and Chapman (1982) found that physical punishment was high for destruction of property and lapses of self-control relative to its use for incidents involving harm to persons, where explanations and reasoning were more often used. Holden (1983) found that mothers of 2.5-year-olds were more likely to use power assertive responses following a motor behavior from their child (e.g., reaching for items) than following a child's request (65% versus 11%, respectively).

Grusec and Kuczynski (1980) presented mothers of 4- to 5-year-old and 7- to 8-year-old children with 12 different hypothetical transgressions and asked them what discipline technique they would use. They found that it was more likely for the individual situations to elicit the same discipline techniques from different mothers than it was for a given mother to show consistency across situations. Mothers often endorsed the use of multiple discipline strategies, including power assertion and reasoning.

Trickett and Kuczynski (1986) studied parental responses to four types of child transgressions (i.e., initial noncompliance, high arousal transgressions, conventional social transgressions, and moral transgressions) in 20 abusive and 20 control families with 4- to 10-year-old children. For three of the four types of transgressions, interactions between discipline and family type were found. Control parents were more discriminating in their predominant choice of strategy; they used no one predominant strategy following noncompliance, punishment for high arousal transgressions, reasoning after social transgressions, and punishment and reasoning after moral transgressions. Abusive parents used punishment as their predominant strategy for all four types of transgressions. Interestingly, following high arousal transgressions, control parents were more likely to punish than were abusive parents. These data suggest that well-functioning parents are equipped with a repertoire of discipline strategies that they can use singly or in combination, depending on the child and the situation. Parents who have restricted skills or who are inflexible in their employment of discipline strategies are less able to be effective in their discipline interactions with their child.

Mood-dependent (versus planful) discipline. Mood-dependent discipline may be defined as discipline that is more determined by the mood state of the parent than by the behavior of the child. In extreme cases, parents have no systematic strategy for dealing with discipline confrontations.

Studies relating maternal mood states to child cooperation and compliance consistently find that negative maternal moods are associated with less positive child responses to maternal directions and commands (Jouriles et al. 1989; Maccoby 1991). In discipline attempts where parents react more to their own negative mood than to the child's actual misbehavior, it could be expected that the information being conveyed to the child would be less effective in teaching or socializing him or her. Parents experiencing negative mood states would be expected to be less able to use proactive discipline strategies and more likely to be irritably reactive to their children.

Investigators from the National Institute of Mental Health Laboratory of Developmental Psychology have conducted several studies that support the notion that dysphoric mood disrupts the capacity of parents to engage in effortful child-rearing interactions (Kochanska et al. 1987, 1989; Kuczynski 1984). The developmental stage of the child apparently affects the impact of maternal depression on the specific types of control strategies the mother employs. In interactions with toddlers, maternal depression was related to decreased parental assertiveness: depressed mothers used fewer direct commands and reprimands and more explanations. The same mothers and children at age 5 showed a different pattern in which depressed mothers used more direct commands than well mothers. Kochanska et al. (1989) concluded that these findings provide support for the "avoidance of effort" hypothesis; at age 2, it takes the mother less effort if she avoids making direct demands on her child, whereas at age 5, when the child is better able to follow parental directions, it takes the mother less effort to control her child through the use of direct commands.

The use of parental proactive strategies as a method of controlling child behavior was illustrated in an observational study of mother-child interaction in the supermarket (Holden 1983). The supermarket setting was selected because it was seen as providing a "triple threat" to mothers: food shopping had to be accomplished, the child had to be managed in a setting with a diverse array of enticing objects, and both mother and child were in the public eye. Community mothers and their 2- to 3-year-old toddlers were observed during two shopping outings. The children provided opportunities for maternal intervention almost once per minute, primarily by interrupting their mother's shopping with requests or by reaching for objects. Maternal proactive controls, such as verbal initiations by the mother or giving the child food or an object, were found to relate both to subsequent child compliance and to a reduced frequency of power struggles. Rather than waiting to react to their child's misbehavior, mothers structured the social interaction with their child as a preventive tactic. It is common to see well-trained preschool teachers use strategies such as actively leading, distracting, or providing direction for the child in potentially tempting or difficult situations. Vygotsky (1978) discussed the concept of "zone of proximal development" that suggests that children learn to behave in appropriate ways by being systematically guided through experiences.

Proactive strategies probably require more effort and planning than reactive ones. They also require that the parent be able to take on the role of socializer/teacher with the child. Dysphoric mood may limit the parent's ability to engage in such strategies and thereby limit his or her positive influence on the child's social development.

Predictive Validity of PID: Studies of Long-Term Effects

In this section, studies that investigated the effects of problem parental discipline on the subsequent adult psychiatric status and criminality of subjects are reviewed. In addition, the effects of a history of physically harsh discipline in the family of origin on the parents' current discipline practices with their own children and attitudes toward discipline are reviewed.

Problem discipline and adult psychiatric or criminal status. In their study of 200 adults (46 depressed, 54 alcoholic, and 100 control subjects) in the St. Louis Epidemiologic Catchment Area, Holmes and Robins (1988) examined reports of harsh or unfair punishment during the childhood years (6–13 years old) of individuals with adult diagnoses of alcohol abuse and/or dependence or major depressive episodes. A strong and positive relationship was found between earlier harsh discipline and alcoholism for men and depression for women. The association of harsh prior discipline and both disorders was the strongest for children with psychiatrically ill parents. The authors found that even when both parents were well and the home was lower class, poor discipline increased the risk for both disorders in adulthood. An earlier study by Robins (1966) found that children of antisocial or alcoholic parents were less likely to become antisocial themselves if they experienced good discipline in their homes. These authors concluded that "the implications for prevention would seem to be that special efforts should be made to provide a reasonable disciplinary environment for children who are at risk because their parents are depressed or alcoholic" (p. 32).

Two major longitudinal studies have implicated the poor discipline practices of grandparents in the subsequent development of antisocial behavior in adults (Elder et al. 1983; Huesmann et al. 1984). In the Oakland and Berkeley Growth studies (Elder et al. 1983), males whose parents reported that they had difficulty managing their child's temper tantrums were found to be significantly more likely to experience later erratic work histories ($\beta = .35$); erratic work lives in turn were related to child and spouse reports of angry and inadequate parenting ($\beta = .36$). Even after controlling for social class and educational level, these authors found a substantial relationship between childhood temper tantrums, adult male parenting difficulties, and erratic work life. Females' early temper problems were found to be directly related to their children's reports 30 years later of maternal anger and loss of control ($r = .34$) and to spouse reports of inadequate parenting ($r = .34$). Huesmann et al. also found significant correlations between grandparent discipline practices and antisocial behavior in their grandchildren.

Yesavage and Widrow (1985) examined correlates of inpatient self-destructive behavior for 45 depressed male inpatients. The best predictors for self-destructive acts were patient reports of childhood discipline factors (as compared with early childhood losses and conflict between parents); specifically, 63% of the total variance in self-destructive acts was accounted for by interparent inconsistency, with extremely severe discipline by the father and mild discipline by the mother. The authors reported that these results are quite similar to those found when dangerous behaviors reported in a schizophrenic sample were examined (Yesavage et al. 1983).

Burbach and Borduin (1986) reviewed 14 studies that retrospectively examined the parent-child relations of depressed adults. The findings relevant to the reports of discipline, including overprotectiveness and overpermissiveness, are summarized below. In instances where depressed psychiatric outpatients were the subjects, samples consisted of patients who received a diagnosis of either unipolar or bipolar depression. For community populations, some measure of depression had to have been used for studies to be included.

Parker (1979a, 1979b, 1981, 1982) conducted four studies that support a positive link between retrospective reports of high maternal (but not paternal) overprotectiveness and adult depression. Raskin et al. (1971) found that parents of depressed adults were more likely to report that their parents used negative child-rearing styles than nondepressed adults. Lamont et al. (1976) and Lamont and Gottlieb (1975) found that mothers of depressed adults were rated as using high guilt induction and being overintrusive. Fathers of depressed adults in these samples were rated as being unloving and authoritarian. Depressed adults in the study conducted by Crook et al. (1981) reported that they had experienced more negative sanctions and more withdrawal from their parents than did adults in the control comparison group.

The results of studies examining retrospective recall of parenting behaviors that adults have received are called into question by a comprehensive study by Lewinsohn and Rosenbaum (1987). They examined whether depressive adults' recall of parental behavior was a stable characteristic that persisted even during asymptomatic periods. A sample of 998 randomly selected adults recruited from county voter registration lists participated in a longitudinal design where subjects were tested at two times separated by an average of 8.3 months. Based on Research Diagnostic Criteria (Spitzer et al. 1978) for major, minor, or intermittent depressive disorder (i.e., pure major depression, bipolar disorder, anxiety disorders, substance abuse, and schizophrenia were excluded), subjects were divided into four diagnostic groups: 1) control subjects who were not now, nor ever had been, depressed; 2) subjects who had a history of depression, but were not depressed during the assessment periods; 3) subjects who became depressed during the course of the study; and 4) subjects who were depressed at both assessments. During the study, the Center for Epidemiologic Studies–Depression Scale (Radloff 1977) was administered to subjects every 3 months. Those scoring 18 or above were brought in for a diagnostic interview. A modified Children's Reports of Parental Behavior Inventory (Raskin et al. 1971)—measuring positive involvement, negative control, and lax discipline—was administered to all subjects as a retrospective measure of the parenting behavior they had experienced.

The results showed that the control subjects did *not* differ from subjects in group 2 (history of depression, but not currently depressed at either assessment) in their reports of past parenting practices, regardless of whether the formerly depressed subjects had had only one or two or more past episodes of depression. The currently depressed cases (i.e., group 4, who were also divided into subgroups based on frequency of past episodes) reported more parental rejection than control subjects. Comparing the controls with the subjects who became depressed during the study (i.e., group 3), a significant subject × sex-of-group interaction was found. Females who had become depressed during the study (group 3) rated their parents as being more rejecting than control subjects, whereas males in group 3 did not. However, males (versus females) in group 3 reported that their parents had used more firm discipline than did control subjects.

Like other studies on recall of depressed adults reviewed in this section, this study found that currently depressed individuals, in comparison with nondepressed control subjects and those whose depression was in remission, recalled their parents in more negative terms. The authors concluded that negative memories of early discipline experiences are not a stable trait or characteristic of individuals who have had one or more episodes of depression. Although the currently depressed individuals (regardless of depression history) recalled their parents as having been more rejecting, those whose depression was in remission did not differ from the never-depressed control subjects. This study demonstrated the phenomenon of mood-dependent retrieval of early childhood memories of parent practices. Current depressive states, not past experiences with depression, influenced the degree to which negative aspects of past parenting were recalled.

Criminality. In a follow-up study of males who had participated in the Cambridge-Somerville longitudinal study, J. McCord (1988) divided the 130 subjects who had been assigned to the experimental (i.e., treatment) group into three subgroups: 1) those with parents rated by social workers as being aggressive (e.g., parents who typically yelled, threw things, or attempted to injure someone when frustrated) ($n = 40$), 2) those without aggression but where at least one parent regularly used corporal punishment ($n = 59$), and 3) those who neither were aggressive nor used regular corporal punishment ($n = 31$). All subjects had lived in deteriorated, low socioeconomic neighborhoods between 1939 and 1945. Comparison of criminal records showed that men who had been raised by either aggressive or punitive parents were more likely to be convicted for index crimes as adults (i.e., 48% of aggressive subjects and 27% of punitive subjects versus 13% of nonaggressive/nonpunitive subjects).

In an earlier analysis using the full Cambridge-Somerville sample (i.e., treated and control cases), J. McCord (1979) found that specific child-rearing practices were reliable antecedents of criminal behavior in middle-age males. Low parental supervision, high parental conflict, and low maternal affection were all related to adult criminality. Additional studies examining the relationship of poor parental discipline to adolescent delinquency are reviewed below.

Widom (1989) matched 908 cases who had court-documented histories of extremely harsh physical punishment (abuse), lack of parental care (neglect), and sexual abuse from 1967 to 1971 with 667 children of the same sex, race, date of birth, and hospital of birth ($n = 229$) or school ($n = 438$) and compared their subsequent adult criminal histories. Overall, significantly more of the abused/neglected females than control females had adult arrest records (16% versus 9%), as did abused/neglected males (42% abused/neglected versus 33% of control males). In addition, abused/neglected males differed significantly from control males in the frequency of arrests for violent offenses.

Effects of problem discipline in family of origin on current parenting. Zeanah and Zeanah (1989) described the maltreated-maltreating cycle as the most striking example of the psychodynamic notion that early relationship experiences are carried forward and reenacted in subsequent relationships. Many have examined the hypothesis that there is a significant transmission of the effects of harsh physical punishment and/or abuse from one generation to the next. As Cappell and Heiner (1990) pointed out, violence in the family of origin is neither a necessary nor a sufficient condition for generating aggression in one's own family. Nevertheless, consistent correlational evidence exists for the cross-generational transmission hypothesis. Many of the earlier studies of this issue were seriously flawed by methodological problems, such as total reliance on self-reports and retrospective data, and the use of nonrepresentative samples or samples of convenience, such as those brought to the attention of the authorities (Gelles 1982). More recent studies (mostly conducted in the last decade) have used representative and well-matched comparison groups to examine whether there is reliable evidence that harsh parenting is transmitted across generations. Most of these studies (Egeland et al. 1987; Herrenkohl et al. 1983; Straus 1983; Straus et al. 1980) found that there is an increased probability of problem child-rearing practices, characterized by a tendency to use harsh and inflexible discipline, among mothers who received harsh discipline from their own parents.

Simons et al. (1991), in their study of 451 two-parent Iowa families, found that mothers' harsh parenting of sons and daughters, as well as fathers' harsh parenting of sons, were related to parent reports of harsh parenting practices of their mothers. Engfer (1986) used retrospective reports of mothers' attachment to their own parents and their own parents' marital satisfaction and irritability to predict maternal parenting competence in free-play interactions. She found that grandmother irritability was positively associated with maternal irritability, which in turn was associated with the increased likelihood that the mother used punishment during free play. A mother's "sensitivity" to her child was enhanced by having had a close relationship with her own mother and impaired by growing up in a home with an unhappy marriage and having a close attachment with her father. In a study of a subsample of the National Survey of Physical Violence in American Families (Straus 1980) sample of cohabiting adults (i.e., those with children), Cappell and Heiner (1990) found a significant association between maternal reports of being hit during childhood and hitting their own children. No such association was observed in that study for fathers.

Taken together, these findings lend some support to the notion that mothers' current use of harsh punishment is related to their discipline history with their own mothers. However, the study by Lewinsohn and Rosenbaum (1987) clearly shows that recall of parent practices is affected by current mood state. Caution should be exercised in interpreting parent reports of their own histories of receiving inadequate discipline, especially if they are currently depressed.

Compared with the evidence for mothers concerning the relationship between current problems in parenting and histories of harsh treatment during childhood, little such data are available for fathers. This is not surprising because historically a more central role in day-to-day parenting was typically played by mothers than fathers. Current trends for parents to share parenting tasks more equally will allow future studies to examine the effects of paternal discipline practices.

Predictive Validity: Relationship of PID to Childhood Disorders

Parental discipline and delinquency. Studies of precursors of delinquency typically implicate PID as an antecedent of subsequent antisocial behavior. In reviewing general population samples for which the collection of family measures antedated boys' convictions, Rutter and Giller (1984) concluded that

> The results of such studies are in good agreement in showing that the most important variables associated with both juvenile delinquency and adult criminality include parent criminality, poor parental supervision, cruel passive and neglecting attitudes, erratic or harsh discipline, marital conflict and large family size (Bahr 1979; [J.] McCord 1979; [W.] McCord et al. 1959; Wadsworth 1979; West and Farrington 1973, 1977; Wilson 1980). (p. 180)

Rutter and Giller (1984) also pointed out that where early literature on the association of parenting practices and delinquency was concerned with discipline methods and severity of punishment, more recent research has focused on rather different aspects of discipline. Patterson and his colleagues have conducted several studies on the relation of inept parent discipline and poor supervision to children's antisocial behavior (Patterson 1986; Patterson and Forgatch, in press). Inept parent discipline is viewed as part of a family cycle of coercive process in which parents negatively reinforce their children's aggressive behavior by failing to follow through on commands when their child responds aggressively. The parents of aggressive children also tend to give in to their child's aggressive demands, thus rewarding aggressive behavior. Patterson (1984) also argued that, in families with ineffective discipline, siblings play a substantial role in reinforcing the child's aggressive behavior. Male siblings in the families of socially aggressive boys were found to be significantly more likely than their control counterparts to have coercive interactions with the identified problem child. The results of correlational analyses have supported the relation between ineffective discipline, poor supervision, and antisocial behavior in both clinical and "at-risk" samples studied by Patterson and colleagues (Capaldi and Patterson 1991; Patterson et al. 1992). Cross-sectional analyses across three samples are summarized in Forgatch (1991a).

All the studies on the relation of discipline to delinquent behavior found some association between PID and delinquency or conduct problems. Samples and measures varied greatly, with some studies involving only the adolescents' report of parenting practices and their own delinquency. Like most research on delinquency, many of the samples included only boys. Longitudinal studies with measures of parenting collected during childhood and measures of delinquency collected during adolescence include those by Farrington (1978), Kolvin et al. (1988), Laub and Sampson (1988), and Wilson (1987). A study by Cohen et al. (1990) used measures of externalizing rather than delinquency at adolescence. Wilson (1987) found that for a sample of boys from high crime areas, 80% of the families who had shown lax supervision at age 10–11, compared with 30% of the families who demonstrated strict supervision during that developmental period, had one or more delinquent sons. Of all the family variables she examined, lax supervision was the most strongly associated with delinquency. Farrington (1978) found harsh discipline and poor parental supervision at age 8 to be significant precursors of aggression and violence in adolescence. In their reanalysis of the Gleuck and Gleuck (1950) data, Laub and Sampson (1988) found that maternal lack of supervision, parental discipline characterized by inconsistent use of threats and physical punishment, and low parental attachment were the most important predictors of serious and persistent delinquency. The study by Kolvin et al. (1988) was unusual in having measures of parenting in infancy and measures of later delinquency. They found that poor quality mothering or neglect was predictive of delinquency in both males and females; ineffective parenting, defined by lack of coping with family matters, was predictive of male delinquency. Cohen et al. (1990) found differential effects of various parenting dimensions, with power assertive punishment but not lax rules being associated with externalizing at adolescence, whereas maternal inattention was related to substance use.

The studies based on adolescent self-report again vary widely in their measures of discipline and supervision, but generally support the findings of the longitudinal studies. Several studies found that delinquency was lower with higher levels of parental supervision and control (Campbell 1987; Cernkovich and Giordano 1987; Wells and Rankin 1988) and higher with harshly punitive discipline (Campbell 1987; Wells and Rankin 1988; Welsh 1976) or lax and erratic discipline (Lempers et al. 1989; Wells and Rankin 1988).

One may conclude from these studies that ineffective discipline along with neglect and poor supervision are parenting variables or practices that are all related to conduct problems and delinquency. The direction of this relationship is still not entirely clear because of the good possibility that children with difficult temperaments make parenting harder. The findings of these studies highlight the relationship of inadequate parental supervision to delinquency. The powerful predictive validity may arise partly from the fact that good supervision implies family organization, and probably implies reasonable discipline as well. For parents to supervise a child well, they must be committed to parenting and be involved in their child's day-to-day activities. There must be at least implicit rules about matters such as where the child may go in the afternoon and evening and what time the child is expected home. To maintain good supervision, the parent must have some degree of effectiveness in dealing with rule violations.

Another reason why studies have found more support for the importance of the supervision aspect of PID has been poor measurement of discipline practices in the majority of studies. It is difficult to obtain good measures of the process and efficiency of discipline from parent and child reports for a number of reasons. Parents who are skillful in discipline use a variety of methods and adjust them to the nature of the transgression, the context, and the situation. Children of parents with a history of successful discipline probably respond to subtle cues and prompts when their behavior starts to go over the line. Also, children of parents who use good and consistent discipline act up infrequently, thus limiting opportunities to observe or document "good" discipline. In short, poor supervision is easier to measure than poor discipline.

Studies involving measures based on observation of parental discipline have been rare. They include the work by Patterson and colleagues (Patterson et al. 1982; Reid 1978) and a study by Gardner (1989), which involved a group of preschoolers with conduct problems and a matched control group and used home observations of mother and child. Mothers in the problem group were found to be eight times as likely to capitulate by not following through on commands compared with the control group.

In summary, the studies reviewed are generally consistent in finding that poor supervision along with inconsistent, ineffective, and possibly harsh parental discipline practices in childhood and adolescence are related to delinquency. In addition, these poor parenting practices are found more frequently in families where adverse contextual factors are present.

Parental discipline and child depression. As Rutter and Garmezy (1983) pointed out, findings relating parenting practices to child depression are weaker and less consistent than those for conduct problems and delinquency. There has also been considerably less work in this area, mainly because child depression has emerged as an area of study only rather recently. Approximately one-third of children with a diagnosis of major affective disorder also qualify for a diagnosis of conduct or related disorder (Kovacs et al. 1988). Rutter (1989) suggested that conduct problems and depression may share some common causal factors such as poor parenting practices. A review by Burbach and Borduin (1986) found relatively few studies on the topic of parenting and child depression. A study by Poznanski and Zrull (1970) was typical in finding that parents of depressed children were often detached, angry, punitive, and belittling in their relations with their children. Puig-Antich et al. (1978) found that 11 of 13 families of depressed children showed poor parent-child relations. Several of the parents were reported to be cruel, abusive, or violent toward their children. Four of the children had been sexually molested. Unfortunately, neither of these studies included a control group. In a more recent study, Puig-Antich et al. (1985) found that depressed children and their mothers had poorer communications and less affectionate relations than did nondepressed psychiatric control children and their mothers.

One of the problems in interpreting the results of these studies is that they did not control for the overlap or comorbidity of conduct problems and depression. It is not clear that the relationships between childhood depression and harsh parental discipline and/or neglect would still be found if children with conduct problems were excluded from the sample. In a nonclinical sample, Capaldi (1991) compared boys with elevated measures of both conduct problems and depression, boys who demonstrated only depressive symptoms, and boys who demonstrated only conduct problems. Parents of the conduct-plus-depression and the conduct-problem-only groups showed inconsistent and ineffective discipline along with poor parental supervision, whereas the depressive-symptoms-only group showed poor parental supervision and low parental involvement but not inconsistent discipline. It seems possible from this finding that depressed and conduct-problem children may both share backgrounds of poor discipline, but the specific dimensions of that poor discipline may differ.

Other Child Correlates of PID

In this section, childhood correlates of poor parental discipline are examined, including aggressive/antisocial behavior, noncompliance, poor peer relations, academic failure, difficult temperament, and accidents.

Aggressive and antisocial behavior. It has been well documented that parents of antisocial children tend to be irritable and harsh in their disciplinary practices, to use punishment (especially corporal punishment) frequently, and to behave aggressively toward their children (Gleuck and Gleuck 1968; W. McCord et al. 1961; Nye 1958). Maccoby and Martin (1983) reviewed early work on the relation between discipline and aggressive behavior in children (Becker et al. 1962; Hoffman 1960; Radke 1986; Sears et al. 1953; Yarrow et al. 1968) and concluded that

The bulk of evidence points to a tendency for power-assertive, punitive parenting to be associated with above-average levels of aggression in children, although the strength of the relationship varies greatly according to the nature of the sample, the setting in which measurements were taken, and the methods of assessments used. (p. 42)

Child abuse and spouse abuse have been found to be more likely in families with antisocial youths compared with clinic referrals and control subjects (Behar and Stewart 1982; Lewis et al. 1979, 1983). Parental disagreement on how to discipline and erratic shifting from lax to punitive control have also been associated with child aggression (Elder et al. 1984; Hetherington and Martin 1979). A number of studies have found that degree of aggression in both clinic and nonclinic samples of children was correlated with the severity of punishment used in the home (Forgatch 1991a; Sears et al. 1957).

In an analysis of family interactional data gathered in the homes of nonreferred and socially aggressive boys, Patterson (1976) compared the differential effectiveness of the use of aversive consequences by mothers, fathers, and siblings in stopping the boys' ongoing negative behavior. The conditional likelihood of the child stopping his negative/aversive behavior, given each of the family members' negative versus positive or neutral reactions, was calculated. For boys in both groups, the unconditional probability of immediately repeating or continuing a negative behavior was .33. The probability was the same for both mild and serious negative behaviors. When parents of nonreferred boys reacted negatively to *mildly* aversive child behaviors, there was no significant change in the probability that the boys would persist. However, when these parents reacted negatively to a more serious subclass of child misbehavior (i.e., aggression, hitting and teasing), the effect was to suppress substantially and significantly the probability that the boy would persist (i.e., from .33 to .12). A very different effect was observed in the families of socially aggressive children. When their parents gave negative reactions to their mild or more serious misbehavior, the probability of the children's persistence significantly increased (i.e., from .33 to .52). Thus, when parents of socially aggressive boys tried to punish them, it actually made things substantially worse. The study also showed that these parents punished more often but less effectively than parents of nonreferred boys.

These findings were replicated by Snyder (1977), who also compared clinically referred aggressive boys with control subjects. The acceleration of child aversiveness following parental negative reaction reliably discriminated the aggressive from the control sample. The magnitude of the effect was slightly less dramatic than was observed in the Patterson study.

Other studies of family interaction patterns in families of aggressive and antisocial children and in families of control (nonreferred) children have found that although irritable, negative exchanges occur in all families, they are more frequent and longer in families of aggressive children. Reid et al. (1981) examined the success of discipline episodes (defined as the parent's ability to terminate child problem behaviors quickly) in self-referred abusive families, families of aggressive boys, and nondistressed control families. Abusive mothers were successful 46% of the time, mothers of aggressive children (not abused) were successful 65% of the time, and mothers of nonreferred children were successful in 86% of their attempts to stop ongoing child problem behaviors. Longer and more unsuccessful attempts at parent discipline have been found to increase the amount, severity, and intensity of the type of parent discipline used. Reid (1986) showed that the more misbehavior shown by the child, the more likely it is that the parents will use high rates of high-amplitude negative behavior toward the child; the correlation between child aversive behavior and the rates with which their parents hit them during home observation sessions was .53 for mothers and .74 for fathers. The severity of parental discipline attempts also increased with the length of the discipline episode. Reid examined the proportion of high-amplitude, parent-negative reactions (e.g., hit, threaten harm, yell, or humiliate) that occurred in short (i.e., 1–11 seconds), intermediate (i.e., 12–23 seconds), and long (i.e., more than 23 seconds) episodes of parent-child conflict. He found that regardless of the clinical status of the family (abusive, aggressive, or control), longer episodes contained more high-amplitude, negative parental reactions. Overall, the reactions of parents of aggressive children and abusive parents in the context of these extended episodes were more often intense than the reactions of parents of nonreferred children.

Parents' ineffective attempts to control their children's behavior are clearly associated with increases in children's level of aggression, although there is substantially more evidence for this relationship for boys than for girls. There is some consensus that although the actions and reactions of both the child and the parent contribute to this process, in younger children, at least, the parent has a more controlling influence and their behavior makes a more powerful impact on the discipline process (Lytton 1979). Parental irritable, inconsistent, or erratic reactions to child aggression are consistently related to increases in their frequency and intensity.

Compliance and noncompliance. In nonclinical populations, maternal responsiveness, sensitivity, and involvement have been implicated as key elements in the development of child compliance (Clarke-Stewart 1973; Maccoby and Martin 1983; Parpal and Maccoby 1985). The amount and type of reasoning that is given to the child to encourage compliance has also been found to be related to subsequent rates and duration of compliance and to the specific socialization goals the mother has for her child in a given situation, which appears to affect the amount and type of reasoning she chooses to use (Kuczynski 1982, 1984). Additionally, there is evidence that maternal mood affects child compliance rates (Jouriles et al. 1989) as do the specific characteristics, such as frequency and wording, of the commands that are given (Forehand et al. 1978; Snyder and Huntley 1990). Events that occur immediately before the parent issues the command influence the child's compliance rates, as does maternal tone of voice and (negatively) simultaneous use of physical force (Lytton 1979). Further, the timing of parental commands predicts child compliance as does the intensity with which the rationale for the command is given (Pfiffner and O'Leary 1989). Although child compliance-noncompliance rates are apparently affected by a host of variables, fairly uniform rates of compliance have been observed in samples of nonreferred preschoolers and school-age children. A brief overview of these findings is presented here because they may provide useful guidelines to the practitioner who is making determinations about the presence of clinically significant levels of parent ineffective discipline and child noncompliance.

Whiting and Edwards (1988), in their cross-cultural studies on the formation of social behavior, observed and reported on child compliance rates in 12 cultures. Compliance was measured as the percentage of occasions where the child obeyed immediately or after an initial short delay. For each sex and age group, the number of compliant acts was divided by the number of compliances plus noncompliances to form compliance ratios. Across cultures, older children showed more compliance than younger ones—ranging from 72% compliance at ages 2–3, to 79% at ages 4–5, to 82% at ages 6–8. In general, girls were observed to be more compliant than boys. Of 28 girl-boy comparisons made, girls scored as being more compliant in 20 (with 1 tie, and boys being more compliant in the other 7). Two studies (Forehand et al. 1978; Lobitz and Johnson 1975) using a structured laboratory task found that children in nonclinic samples complied with maternal commands 74% and 62% of the time, respectively.

Snyder and Huntley (1990) found that the likelihood of child compliance varied given different qualities of maternal requests and maternal reactions to previous child compliance or noncompliance. Five mother-child dyads were observed for 1 hour each day for 8 days. The probability of child compliance (regardless of child compliance or noncompliance in the previous episode) increased with the clarity of the mothers' directives (i.e., given clear maternal commands, compliance was 67%; ambiguous commands yielded a compliance rate of 50%; and maternal requests were complied with 31% of the time). Mothers were also more likely to achieve child compliance when they had positively reinforced, rather than ignored or inadvertently punished, child compliance in the previous episode (i.e., positive reinforcement 78%, ignoring 65%, punishing 10%). Similarly, child compliance was more likely when mothers had previously punished, rather than ignored or positively reinforced, previous noncompliance. A multivariate analysis of these data, including the type of maternal request, maternal reaction to child compliance or noncompliance, and their interaction, found that 39%–43% of the variance in child compliance rates could be accounted for. This study highlights the importance of maternal-contingent responding in the child's development of patterns of rates of compliance. Patterson (1982) stressed the key role played by child noncompliance in the development of child antisocial and delinquent outcomes.

As noted by Kuczynski (1991), a focus on the simple occurrence of child noncompliance versus compliance neglects to discriminate between types of child reactions to parental demands that may be more or less adaptive to long-term child outcomes. For example, child negotiation with a parent is seen as a higher order skill than simple refusal or direct defiance. Externally motivated compliance (i.e., use of power techniques or rewards by the parents) is thought to be less conducive to child internalization of social norms. Inductive techniques (e.g., reasoning, guilt) are thought to motivate the child to behave responsibly outside of the purview of adults (Cheyne and Walters 1969; Hoffman 1970; Lepper 1981; Parke 1969). According to Kuczynski's developmental model of child compliance, certain types of noncompliance at the various developmental stages of the child are thought to foster appropriate levels of child autonomy and assertiveness. A skilled parent is not one who obtains uniformly high rates of child compliance, but one who has the ability to make appropriate choices given varied situations and the child's current level of developmental functioning.

Maccoby and Martin (1983) discussed the concept of receptive compliance—that is, the child's readiness to be guided by the parent and to be cooperative. Receptive compliance is thought not to be attributed to parental control, but to parent-child interactions in other contexts. Mothers who facilitate cooperative child behavior have been found to be responsive and sensitive to the child (Lay et al. 1989; Stayton et al. 1971). Maternal affective state (i.e., positive versus negative mood) has been shown to be reliably related to levels of child compliance in laboratory studies (Dix 1991; Jouriles et al. 1989; Kochanska 1991; Lytton 1979).

Poor peer relationships. The characteristics that are most consistently found in children who are rejected by their peers are aggressiveness and disruptive behavior (Coie and Asher 1990; Coie and Dodge 1988; Dodge 1983). Other associated characteristics are social and academic skills deficits and social-cognitive biases or distortions. Recent research in the peer relations area has followed the recommendation of Hartup (1983) to focus on the interrelation between children's family experiences and their peer relations. Within such an integrated approach, the etiological processes and/or risk factors associated with family variables that relate to children's acceptance by peers (and at school [see next section]) can be more broadly examined.

Dishion (1990) reviewed the literature linking parenting practices and peer relations. Two studies (McDonald and Parke 1984; Putallaz 1987) found a positive relationship between parents' controlling, negative behavior and children's abrasiveness with familiar and unfamiliar peers, respectively. Using a structural equation modeling approach, Dishion examined the association between parent discipline practices and peer rejection (as measured by classroom sociometric ratings). He found that the impact of poor discipline on peer relations was mediated through child antisocial behavior and academic success. The sample consisted of two cohorts of 9- to 10-year-old boys from the Oregon Youth Study. The results showed that although poor parental discipline skill (both supervision and negativity in interactions) was significantly correlated with negative peer relations ($r = .29$ and $r = .34$, respectively), when the contributions of level of child antisocial behavior and academic achievement were included, the predictive strength of the model was increased. The effect of poor discipline had an indirect effect on peer relations through its effects on child antisocial behavior and academic achievement. Correlational data of this sort provide evidence that parental discipline practices contribute to the quality of peer relationships outside the home. The link between parent-child and child-peer relationships, particularly in adolescence, has received support in recent studies (Mounts et al. 1991).

In addition to negative interactions with parents, poor parental supervision is also implicated in the child's association with antisocial peers. Supervision is thought to be a key skill for parents of adolescents. Methods of supervision, however, become more complex for parents as the child matures. Normative data show an increase in the child's amount of unsupervised time as she or he gets older (Patterson and Stouthamer-Loeber 1984), making it more difficult for parents to keep track of the adolescent's whereabouts and associates.

In a study comparing after-school supervision of 865 10- to 16-year-olds, Steinberg (1986) found that children whose parents did not know their whereabouts after school were more susceptible to negative peer pressure compared with children whose whereabouts were known by their parents or to those who were directly supervised by an adult.

K. J. Weintraub (The correlation of family monitoring and juvenile delinquency, Department of Sociology, University of Michigan, unpublished manuscript, 1989) examined parental supervision of 1,395 11- to 18-year-olds who had participated in the National Survey of Youth study (Gold and Reimer 1975). Supervision questions concerned whether the youths' parents knew where they were and who they were with when away from home. A significant and negative correlation was found between self-reported delinquency and supervision. Boys were less supervised than girls, and older children were less closely supervised than younger children. An interaction was found between the reported level of supervision and affection from fathers: given a low supervision level, the father's affection was associated with reduced delinquency; this association was not significant when the supervision level was high.

Studies examining the connection between the quality of the parental relationship and peer relationships show a moderate relationship between parent-child attachment measures and peer relations for preschoolers (Sroufe 1986). Attachment to the parent may well be a key factor in enhancing positive peer relationships or it may operate as a protective factor against association with deviant peers. However, Elliott et al. (1985) found that regardless of the strength of the adolescent's conventional bonding with family, association with deviant peers predicted subsequent delinquency. The discrepancy in findings may have to do with the differences in age groups (i.e., preschoolers versus adolescents) that were studied.

Lax parental supervision combined with rejection by peers puts the child at risk for association with peers who have nonconventional or deviant orientations (Dishion et al. 1991; Farrington 1978; Patterson and Stouthamer-Loeber 1984). Association with deviant peers has been found to be a strong predictor of delinquency and drug use (Elliott et al. 1985). Baumrind (1991) and Mounts et al. (1991) examined the relationship between parent supervision and adolescent drug and alcohol use. Consistent positive relationships have been found between strict supervision and abstinence or low usage.

There is some evidence that poor supervision has a more negative effect on boys than on girls. For example, A. C. Crouter et al. (unpublished manuscript, 1989) found that maternal employment outside of the home interacted with poor parental supervision to predict boys' (but not girls') school competence, academic achievement, and ratings of problem behaviors. Other studies have also shown gender-related effects of maternal employment (Banducci 1967; Gold and Andres 1978; Reese and Palmer 1970).

Academic achievement, cognitive competence, and school adjustment. There is some evidence that children who are exposed to ineffective parental discipline at home are likely to develop lower levels of cognitive competence and more problems at school. In particular, child antisocial behavior patterns that accompany children into the school setting bode poorly for future academic and social adjustment (Kazdin 1985; Wahler and Dumas 1986). Often a child's antisocial behavior at school may provide the first indication that he or she is at risk for school failure.

In an analysis of a subsample of 80 middle school subjects (the 39 most antisocial subjects and 41 randomly selected control subjects) from Patterson's

Oregon Youth Study (Capaldi and Patterson 1989), Ramsey et al. (1989) examined the relation of parental discipline and supervision to four categories of school adjustment determined by the presence or absence of school disciplinary contacts and acceptance ratings by peers. They found that scores on parental discipline, as measured by home observation data, parent interview items, and observer impressions, reliably differentiated children who were classified as antisocial at school (i.e., those who had had one or more documented discipline contacts with the school principal and who were being rejected by peers) from those who were not. In this sample of 10- to 12-year-old boys, parental supervision scores were moderately related to the school adjustment classification.

Using the full Oregon Youth Study sample ($N = 206$), Dishion et al. (1991) found significant correlations between poor parental discipline and supervision (both measured using multiple indicators from multiple agents) and a construct score for child academic achievement (including the child's reading level as measured on a standardized achievement test, plus teacher ratings of achievement on the Child Behavior Checklist) ($r = .33$ and $r = .24$, respectively).

A. C. Crouter et al. (unpublished manuscript, 1989) compared the effect of parental supervision on school grades and teacher ratings of children's school performance for children in single- and dual-earner families. Well-supervised boys (but not girls) had higher grade point averages than those who were less well supervised. Learning problems were also reported to be greater for less well-supervised children.

Baumrind (1968, 1971) described a typology of parental discipline and then compared discipline types with levels of child competence in a longitudinal study that assessed youngsters and their parents when the children were in preschool, in elementary school, and in early adolescence. An overview of the results of the first two assessments that are relevant to the development of children's cognitive competence is presented here. The three primary parent discipline types that she described are 1) authoritarian—parents who used firm enforcement of rules, made high maturity demands, were not democratic, and did not encourage free give and take between parent and child; 2) authoritative—parents who also used firm control but coupled it with reasoning and were affectively responsive to their child; and 3) permissive—parents who were less controlling, granted more autonomy, made fewer maturity demands, consulted with their children about family policy, and allowed their children to regulate their own activities as much as possible. At the preschool assessment, children with authoritarian and permissive parents looked alike; their competence profiles were indistinguishable. But when compared with children with authoritative parents, boys from authoritarian households were relatively hostile and resistant, and girls were relatively submissive and dependent. In permissive homes, both sexes were less achievement oriented than their counterparts from authoritative homes, and girls were less socially assertive. Authoritative discipline was associated with achievement-oriented behavior for girls and friendly cooperative behavior for boys. At the elementary-age assessment, when the children were 9 years old, Baumrind added two additional categories to her parent typology: 1) rejecting-neglecting—where parents were neither responsive nor demanding, and 2) traditional—where parents enacted sex-stereotyped roles. She reported that 67% of the boys raised by rejecting-neglecting parents were incompetent, and more than 85% of the children raised by authoritative parents were optimally competent. Overall, more girls from nondemanding families (i.e., permissive plus rejecting-neglecting) were incompetent and more girls from demanding families (i.e., authoritative plus traditional plus authoritarian) were optimally competent. There was a similar nonsignificant trend in this direction observed for boys, but for boys to be optimally competent, it was necessary for parents to be responsive as well as demanding.

Dornbusch et al. (1987) examined the relationship among three parenting styles previously identified by Baumrind (1971) and children's social and cognitive competence. In examining the relationship between adolescents' reports of authoritarian, authoritative, and permissive parenting styles and high school grades for almost 8,000 students, they found that both authoritarian and permissive parenting styles were significantly related to poor academic performance as self-reported by the students. In contrast to either authoritarian or permissive parenting, authoritative discipline styles (i.e., characterized by use of both firm control and democratic give-and-take) were associated with positive grade reports, except in the case of Asian students, who tended to excel in school and to report that their parents were quite authoritarian. The lowest grades were found among students whose parents' style was mixed and inconsistent, especially when parents sometimes used authoritarian practices. The authors noted that a weakness of the study is that all data came from one source (self-report of participating adolescents); therefore, results implicating authoritarian styles may reflect a general level of dissatisfaction with their parents among those students who do less well in school.

The effect of maternal control strategies on children's later school performance was examined in a longitudinal study by Hess and McDevitt (1984), who measured levels of maternal dominance in a laboratory teaching task and in an interview using hypothetical discipline situations when the child was 4 years old. When the child was 5–6 years old, several tests of school-relevant skills were given, and at age 12, standardized achievement tests in math and vocabulary were administered. Results showed positive correlations with later low school achievement by children whose mothers demanded compliance without reasoning and used physical threats to force compliance from their 4-year-old children. High levels of maternal commands at age 4 were related to achievement at ages 5–6, but not at age 12. Maternal use of authority was related to socioeconomic status ($r = -.25$), and use of direct commands was related to the mother's intelligence ($r = -.25$). The authors concluded that, for preschool children, the optimal amount of control needed is that which is required to direct the child's attention to the task, and that parental attempts to have the child generate ideas and solutions are related to future academic success. They concur with Baumrind's findings that it is not firm control per se that has negative consequences for the child's cognitive development, but the extreme uses of direct and firm control.

Difficult temperament. Several studies have found an association between maternal ratings of infant difficult temperament and later child behavior problems (Bates 1982; Camerson 1978; Pettit and Bates 1989). Knutson (1978) reviewed the relevant literature and concluded that child difficult temperament, combined with hyperreactivity of parents to common child aversive events and a limited repertoire of discipline strategies, may produce extreme forms of discipline such as physical abuse. Green et al. (1974) noted that, regardless of the documented characteristics of the child, physically punitive mothers perceived their abused child to be more aggressive, demanding, and difficult to handle than his or her siblings. Low birth weight (Fanaroff et al. 1972) and hyperactivity (Morse et al. 1970) have also been associated with high levels of maternal punitiveness.

Using a longitudinal design, Lee and Bates (1985) investigated the link between child temperament ratings and later and concurrent child behavior problems in a sample of 111 mother-child dyads recruited from city birth announcements. Mothers provided temperament ratings when the child was 6, 13, and 24 months old. At age 24 months, 4–6 hours of home observation data were collected that targeted conflict sequences between mother and child. Although some stability of maternal ratings over the three assessments was found, of the children classified as "difficult" at 24 months, only 50% had been so classified at 6 months. For "average" children, the stability of temperament ratings from 6 to 24 months was .49, and for children classified as "easy," .69. Both the 6- and 13-month ratings were modestly correlated with maternal use of physical restraint at age 2. Early maternal ratings of difficult temperament were somewhat predictive of subsequent rates of mother-toddler conflict. Concurrent data were more compelling: temperament ratings of 2-year-olds were related to significant differences in rates of maternal prohibitions, repeated prohibitions, and restraint or removal of the child. Further, child behavior differentiated the difficult from the average and easy groups; children who were rated as difficult were more likely to resist maternal efforts at control, and their mothers were more likely to give in following the child's resistance. The authors concluded that the mother's ratings of child difficultness could stem either from child characteristics or from ineffective parenting and a negative parental bias toward the child. At any rate, those children whose mothers perceived them as being more difficult appeared to be at more risk for developing later behavior problems than children rated as average or easy. In a later study that used a subsample of the above study, Pettit and Bates (1989) found that the absence of early positive interactions between mother and child at age 2 was a stronger predictor of child behavior problems at age 4 than earlier negative interchanges.

Recognition that temperamental factors are mediated by parent-child interactional processes has led to the development of the "goodness-of-fit" concept (Thomas and Chess 1984). The goodness-of-fit theory suggests that the factors placing the child at risk for psychopathology involve an interaction between child temperament and the demands of the physical and social environment, rather than only the attributes of the child.

The appeal of the goodness-of-fit conceptualization has been widespread, perhaps because it incorporates both individual and interactional perspectives. It has been included in theories of child psychopathology, child behavior problems, and school adjustment (Doelling and Johnson 1990; Lerner 1983; Martin 1989).

Accidents. There is empirical support for an association between the occurrence of childhood accidents and problem discipline and certain child characteristics. Implicated child characteristics include impulsivity, activity level, antisocial behavior, and risk taking. Not surprisingly, parents report that children who have frequent accidents are difficult to discipline and are disciplined more frequently than comparison children with fewer accidents (Langley et al. 1983; Manheimer and Mellinger 1967).

Adult Disorders Associated With PID and Parental Correlates of PID

There is a substantial body of research on relationships of maternal depression, schizophrenia, and antisocial disorders to maternal discipline skills. Although methodological problems limit the generalizability of many of the studies in this area (e.g., small, unrepresentative, heterogeneous samples; unverified parental reports of child problems; and insensitivity to child developmental stage), there is convincing evidence that some forms of parental psychopathology relate to specific deficits and excesses in types and amounts of parental discipline used.

Maternal depression and schizophrenia. In this section, we draw on detailed reviews conducted by Downey and Coyne (1990), Gelfand and Teti (1990), and Rutter (1990). Both interview and observational studies have shown that parenting by women diagnosed as depressed (unipolar and bipolar) or schizophrenic is of poorer quality than that of women with no mental illness (Cohler et al. 1980, 1987;

Weissmann 1983). Goodman and Brumley (1990) noted that both of these disorders share the affective symptom dimension of emotional unavailability. In addition, more negative affect expressed toward the child and less positive parent-child interaction has been found to occur more in disturbed than in nondisturbed mothers.

Goodman and Brumley (1990) examined the effects of maternal diagnosis (i.e., major depression, recurrent or dysthymic disorder $n = 25$; schizophrenia $n = 53$; well $n = 23$) and parenting behaviors on child IQ and social behavior. They concluded that the risk to the child from parental mental disorder stemmed more directly from poor discipline and a poor quality social environment (as measured by the Home Observation for Measurement of the Environment Inventory [Bradley and Cantwell 1979]) than from parent pathology per se. These researchers found that, when other factors were controlled for, the overall severity of the mother's illness played a minor role in accounting for differences in child outcomes. Specifically, maternal avoidance of punishment and discipline and poor physical environment were found to predict children's psychomotor intellectual functioning. In addition, maternal responsiveness (which was found to be significantly lower in schizophrenic mothers) was a strong predictor of social behavior. The importance of these factors becomes clear when considered in conjunction with self-reported data collected from adolescent children of schizophrenic parents involved in the Stonybrook High-Risk Project (Weintraub et al. 1986). Weintraub et al. reported that these children found their home environments cold and restrictive. In addition, children of schizophrenic parents reported that their parents were punitive, cold, and rejecting.

Other studies have shown that the specific type of maternal disorder may matter less than its severity (Seifer and Sameroff 1981; Weintraub et al. 1986; Zuravin 1979). For example, both unipolar and bipolar forms of depression are associated with increased child problems (Downey and Coyne 1990; Radke-Yarrow 1988).

The relation between maternal depression and patterns of either irritable and hostile or insensitive and disengaged (i.e., low involvement) child discipline has been well documented. Gelfand and Teti (1990) found that depressed mothers were markedly poor at tracking their infants' activities and in providing physical protection from potential hazards. Inconsistent and erratic shifts between uninvolved/oblivious and irritable/harsh patterns of discipline have also been observed in depressed mothers. Depressed mothers tend to choose control strategies that require less cognitive effort than do well mothers, including unilateral enforcement of obedience and withdrawal when faced with resistance from the child. In addition to being inconsistent, depressed mothers are less likely to negotiate solutions with their child and are more likely to use physical punishment (Ghodsian et al. 1984).

Not surprisingly, children of depressed parents have shown significantly higher rates of disruptive behavior disorders, including conduct disorders (Beardslee et al. 1987; Hammen et al. 1987; Klein et al. 1988; Patterson 1980), hyperactivity (Orvaschel et al. 1988), and symptoms of depression and antisocial behavior at ages 2 and 6 (Zahn-Waxler et al. 1988).

Because of the correlational nature of the research, the direction of causality between child disorders, PID, and adult psychopathology cannot be determined. However, a strong set of associations is implied by the findings. Studies using longitudinal data sets; multimethod, multiagent assessment strategies; and comprehensive analytic strategies such as structural equation modeling and latent growth curve modeling allow for more precise tests of hypotheses regarding the sequencing of risk variables and prediction of later child adjustment. For example, Forgatch (1991b) tested the hypothesis that maternal depression would have a negative future impact on harsh discipline and poor supervision. She found that this relation generalized across samples of both single mothers (who were recently divorced) and those from intact families. The variance that maternal depression accounted for in predicting harsh discipline 4 years later on ranged from 10% to 53% in single and intact homes, respectively. For single mothers, maternal depression also predicted future poor supervision, but this relationship was not observed for intact families.

Antisocial parents. Patterson et al. (1992) examined the relationship of parents' own antisocial behavior to their current discipline practices with their own children. They defined a parent antisocial construct score using three indicators: state records of arrests, Minnesota Multiphasic Personality Inventory scales for psychopathic deviance and hypomania, and records of driving violations. Parent antisocial behavior covaried significantly ($r = -.26$) with the parents' current use of irritable discipline based on observations in their homes. Patterson and Dishion (1988) then examined the relationship for 70 mothers and 64 fathers between parents' antisocial scores and constructs measuring social disadvantage, drug use, and depression with observed parent-to-child irritable discipline in the home. The maternal irritable discipline score was then regressed on maternal depression, social disadvantage, and maternal antisocial behavior. The standard partial betas reflected significant effects of the mothers' antisocial behavior ($\beta = -.29$) and social disadvantage ($\beta = .17$) on irritable discipline. There was a nonsignificant effect for maternal depression. For paternal irritable discipline, a similar finding was obtained: fathers' antisocial behavior ($\beta = -.24$) and social disadvantage ($\beta = .40$) both accounted for significant variance in paternal irritable discipline. Again, father depression was nonsignificant in this analysis. Next, the question of whether mothers' and fathers' irritable discipline scores covaried with child antisocial behavior was addressed. A Structural Equation Modeling approach was used to show that for fathers the effect of their antisocial behavior on their boys' antisocial behavior was mediated through the fathers' use of irritable discipline. For mothers, both their own antisocial behavior and their use of irritable discipline had direct effects on their boys' antisocial behavior.

These findings accord with those from a longitudinal study (Huesmann et al. 1984) that found a correlation of .24 between an individual's antisocial behavior as a child and self-reported use of physical punishment with his or her own child 30 years later. Early aggression had a higher correlation with aggression of the offspring than it did with the subject's own aggression at follow-up. Elder et al. (1983) examined some possible mechanisms that would account for stability in antisocial behavior across generations. They showed that explosive, irritable discipline practices of the father, and to a lesser degree of the mother, were a significant predictor of child antisocial behavior. Parental discipline practices and antisocial personality traits were key mediating variables.

Social and Contextual Factors Associated With PID

The effect of the impact of social and contextual factors—including daily stress, marital conflict, socioeconomic status, race, and gender-role traditionality—on parental discipline are reviewed here.

Stress. Higher levels of parental stress have been associated with inadequate parent discipline styles. Patterson (1982) reviewed literature that suggests that both chronic adversity and the presence of daily hassles have a direct effect on a mother's irritability with her child. He concluded that mothers who are irritable and negative are less able to deal consistently and effectively with their child in face-to-face discipline confrontations and in supervision of their activities and whereabouts. Dumas (1986) investigated the impact of mothers' social interactions outside the home on their irritability with their children. Home observations were conducted on 10 days, and mothers were interviewed about the frequency and nature of their adult contacts outside the home on those days. Dumas found that on days when mothers engaged in unpleasant encounters with welfare agencies and neighbors, they were more likely to behave irritably toward their children. Pleasant encounters had an inhibiting effect on maternal irritability. These results implicate the effect of daily stress on maternal discipline practices.

It should be noted that the connection between discipline and stress has generally been investigated in a somewhat indirect manner. The focus of most research has been on either a wide range of parenting problems, of which discipline is only one, or on the prediction of child problem behavior, where both parenting variables and stressors are treated as independent variables. Recent studies have implicated parenting variables (especially discipline) as being the primary mediators through which the effects of stress are transmitted to the child through the parent-child interactions and relationship.

Marital conflict. Emery (1982) suggested four alternative paths between interparent conflict and child behavior problems: 1) altered parental discipline practices; 2) modeling of aggressive behavior; 3) disruption of attachment bonds; and 4) other factors such as stress, child effects, and triangulation of the conflict through the child. Patterson (1982) hypothesized that child externalizing behavior problems result from parental conflict because such conflict inhibits effective parenting, especially in the areas of consistency of discipline and supervision. Subsequent studies have examined whether it is more appropriate to describe a direct path between marital discord and child problems or whether, as Patterson suggested, discord leads to parenting difficulties, which in turn lead to child problems. Support for the mediating effect of parental discipline on child adjustment in families with marital discord has been found in several studies (Fauber et al. 1990; Jouriles et al. 1988; Patterson and Stouthamer-Lorber 1984). It appears that marital discord may be an important family risk factor for the genesis of PID.

Socioeconomic status. It is commonly believed that differences exist in parental discipline methods across various strata of society (Straus et al. 1980). Most often this is expressed as a proclivity toward more severe, punitive discipline in the lower classes. Although there is empirical support for this conceptualization (Bronfenbrenner 1958; Straus et al. 1980), it is important to examine the existing research for the explanations that have been offered for these tendencies.

McLoyd (1990) conducted a comprehensive review examining the role of economic hardship and loss of socioeconomic status in black families in terms of parenting, psychopathology, and child problem behavior. She cited a number of studies showing that parental irritability, explosiveness, and punishing behavior are high among those who have experienced economic loss (Elder 1979; Lempers et al. 1989). McLoyd argued that, in addition to economic loss, general economic hardship is likely to lead to problematic discipline, and in both cases the relationship between socioeconomic status and discipline is mediated through psychological distress. Put simply, economic difficulties cause parents to become upset, thus interfering with their ability to provide consistent, effective discipline.

McLoyd (1990) noted that alternative explanations for class differences in discipline have existed for some time. These include the notion that stable personality traits among the lower classes lead to negative discipline and that causal arrows may run from psychological distress to poverty rather than in the reverse direction.

A variety of studies, however, have yielded data that run counter to this explanation (Buss and Redburn 1983; Kasl and Cobb 1979; Kessler et al. 1987). An additional and possibly related explanation discussed by McLoyd is that the experience of economic hardship may produce power assertive parenting styles, in which parents may adopt these strategies to teach children who are living in relatively dangerous environments. It has also been suggested that one reason lower socioeconomic status parents might discipline more negatively is because of their lack of insulation from the surrounding environment. Crowded living conditions, more contact with the legal system, and pervasive class and racial stereotypes increase the likelihood that inadequate discipline will be noticed and reported to authorities.

Race. Differences in parenting styles have been noted among racial groups, although results are mixed. For example, some investigators have found that black families expect children to be more independent at earlier ages (Bartz and Levine 1978); others have found the opposite pattern (Allen 1985). McLoyd (1990) commented that although child abuse mortality rates are three times higher for black children, it is unclear if this effect is independent of socioeconomic factors. Some studies have shown that black families score higher than their nonminority counterparts on measures of inadequate discipline (Allen 1985; Durrett et al. 1975; Hale 1982); others have found that black parents tend toward firm but supportive discipline (Bartz and Levine 1978; Baumrind 1972). McLoyd concluded that the extent to which black parents are characterized by harsh, arbitrary discipline is a function of a combination of cultural, environmental, and psychological factors.

Gender-role traditionality. Rigidity of male and female parenting roles has been linked to problem discipline and physical abuse in several studies (Star 1980; Straus et al. 1980). It has been suggested that excessive rigidity in these roles makes problem solving between parents more difficult (Straus and Kantor 1987). It has also been noted that the traditional male role may in some cases encourage the use of violence to resolve conflict (Fisher 1990). However, most parents who subscribe to traditional male and female parenting roles do not exhibit inadequate discipline styles, suggesting that other factors (e.g., individual, cultural, economic) interact with traditionality to produce problem discipline. Interestingly, parents at the opposite end of the continuum who subscribe to "alternative lifestyle" values may also have discipline problems because of their unwillingness to provide clear limits or structure for their child.

Parent-Child Interactional Patterns Associated With PID

With a few exceptions, most studies of parent-child social interaction have focused on dyadic interchanges. Although there is considerable clinical interest in, and practice of, interventions that target multiple members of the family, methodological and mathematical constraints have limited research on interactions involving three or more people. Our understanding of family interaction, at this point, is limited to "snapshots" of family dyads. Inferences about multiperson interactions within the family can be drawn only by making a collage of these dyadic shots. Considerable research has been conducted, however, on dyadic interchanges between parent and child in discipline episodes. Most studies have been conducted with mothers and preschoolers or elementary school-age children. Conditional probability studies have shown that the parent and the child exert mutual influences on each other and that these influences have an effect on their subsequent behavior. Examples of these are reviewed below.

There is substantial controversy about whether it is the parent or the child who primarily determines the discipline interaction. Hoffman (1963) noted that parents obviously have more power and the ability to initiate and direct the type of discipline they use. However, numerous studies have shown that child characteristics such as levels of aggression, resistance to discipline, and activity level are strong influences on the use of parental discipline.

Who determines discipline, the parent or the child? Eron et al. (1991) reported on a 3-year study in five countries (the United States, Australia, Finland, Poland, and Israel) on the relation of television habits and parenting practices to child aggression. Subjects were 6–8 years old. They found that in the United States, Finland, and Australia, the child's early aggression was a significant predictor of later parental punishment, even after the effects of early punishment had been partialed out. However, early punishment was not a significant predictor of later aggression once early aggression had been partialed out. They concluded that by the time a child is 6 years old, parental punishment seemed to be more of a response to aggression than a cause of it.

Laboratory studies have also demonstrated the effects of child characteristics on parental discipline. Mulhern and Passman (1981) found that children's simulated success or failure on a learning task was found to exert functional control over the intensities of punishment that their parents used. Stevens-Long (1973) showed that both overactive and underactive children evoked more severe punishment than children with average activity levels. Children labeled as emotionally disturbed evoked less punishment.

Child conduct problems have been shown to be predictive of parental discipline. Anderson et al. (1986) found that mothers of both nonproblem and conduct problem children directed more negatives and requests to conduct problem children than to nonproblem children. Conduct problem children were less compliant than nonproblem children regardless of the type of mother they were interacting with. The authors concluded that the child's (not the mother's) behavioral tendency was the major influence on conduct problems. Patterson et al. (1990) examined the contribution of preadolescent boys' antisocial behavior to later parental discipline practices. They used a Structural Equation Modeling analysis that controlled for the stability of both child antisocial behavior and parenting practices over time. They found that the more extreme the child's time 1 antisocial score was, the more problems his parents had with discipline and supervision at time 2. They concluded that the child's antisocial behavior forms a feedback loop that worsens the abilities of the parents to provide adequate discipline and supervision in the future. It is clear from these studies that child factors have at least some effect on parental discipline strategies. The strength of child effects probably increases with the child's age.

Conditional probability studies. Investigators have examined the presence of predictable patterns of parent-child social interaction by calculating a set of probabilistic connections between sequential interactional events. A pattern can be said to be identified when the probability of a reaction of one person to the action of another is greater than the unconditional probability or base-rate probability of the person's reaction. Of primary interest are questions of how these patterns develop, and once developed, how they change over time. For example, Snyder and Patterson (1986) conducted extended observations of the interactions of two mother-child dyads. First, they identified reliable mother action and child reaction patterns. Next, the effects of maternal consequences for child reactions on the probability of subsequent child reactions were studied. Positive maternal consequences for child compliance were associated with an increased probability of child compliance the next time the mother issued a command or request. Negative maternal consequences for child compliance were associated with a decreased probability of compliance given the next maternal command or request. If the child reacted in a coercive or defiant way to a maternal command or request and the mother gave in or reacted positively, the probability of child coercion or defiance in response to the next maternal command increased. Negative maternal reactions to child coercion or defiance decreased the likelihood of child coercion reoccurring in the next episode. Neutral maternal consequences had no amplifying or suppressing effect on child reactions in this study. The authors concluded that maternal consequences systematically and predictably influenced shifts over time in the probability of a child's compliance or noncompliance. These data imply that parental discipline reactions determine an orderly process that unfolds over time and affects the subsequent disposition of children to react in cooperative versus noncooperative ways to their parents.

Social Validity of Various Types of Discipline

The acceptability of various discipline techniques from the perspectives of adults and children has been examined in several studies reviewed below.

Children's perceptions of acceptable discipline practices appear to be influenced by several factors, such as the age and gender of the child, the gender of the parent, the gender of the transgressor, the nature of the transgression, and family marital discord. In general, young children give more approval to power assertion and directive techniques; with increasing age, induction is rated more highly. There is also evidence indicating that physical punishment is more accepted both by and for males than by and for females, and that overall children both expect and endorse the use of more coercive and/or power assertion techniques by their fathers than by their mothers.

Leahy (1979) interviewed children 6 and 11 years of age and asked how much they thought a peer who hit them should be punished by spanking. Regardless of age and mitigating circumstances (ranging from none to provocation to emotional maladjustment), both younger and older children thought that male transgressors should be punished more severely than female transgressors. Leahy suggested that this finding indicates that even at an early age, both males and females share stereotypes of advocating more severe punishment for males. Older children used more information about situational and personal factors in making their judgments, whereas younger children appeared to use an elementary rule of reciprocity of aggression and punishment to determine appropriate levels of physical discipline.

Eimer (1983) investigated the relationship between a child's age and his evaluation of the type of parental intervention used when the child physically abused a peer. Boys in three age groups (mean ages 5.8, 8.8, and 11.8 years) rated the acceptability of reasoning versus grounding by the father in this situation. He found age differences in the boys' evaluations of the fathers, but these differences were not a function of type of intervention. Older boys gave more positive evaluations of their fathers than did younger boys. Younger boys viewed both interventions to be equally noxious, whereas older boys tended to use more sophisticated judgments of intentionality and possible consequences in their rankings of the acceptability of these interventions.

Siegal and Barclay (1985) also explored children's evaluation of their fathers' discipline techniques by comparing the rankings of boys and girls (age range 5–18) of induction, physical punishment, love withdrawal, and permissiveness over a range of situations where a culprit was described as having transgressed. Overall, evaluations were determined more by the nature of the child making the evaluation than by the situation. Younger children (mean age 6.3) had no particular preference for one technique over another, whereas three older groups (mean ages 8.9, 12.1, and 17.0) rated both induction and physical punishment more favorably than the other two techniques. In none of these age groups was induction evaluated more favorably than physical punishment. Boys tended to evaluate fathers more highly than did girls, especially in the use of physical punishment in situations of simple disobedience. A previous study (Siegal and Cowen 1984) found that regardless of age, both boys and girls tended to endorse active parenting by their mothers, expressing strong approval of inductive techniques and only mild approval of physical punishment. These data suggest that although children approve of their mothers' use of physical punishment as a secondary discipline option, for the father it is seen as a primary tool, and that children's views of legitimate discipline vary with the gender of the parent.

Somewhat contradictory evidence of children's views of physical punishment is provided by Carlson (1986). This study asked 4th, 5th, and 6th graders, half male and half female, to choose from eight possible parental responses (ranging from doing nothing to hitting with a belt) to four types of misbehavior (i.e., disobeying a parent and losing a possession, stealing money, hitting a younger same-sex sibling, and physically fighting with a peer). Across all these situations, physical punishment was the least chosen option; of those who chose physical punishment, spanking using a hand was overwhelmingly (87%) endorsed. The discipline practices most favored were reasoning with children and talking to them about what they had done wrong. Across all situations, 87%–100% of boys and girls preferred some form of nonphysical punishment. Interestingly, in this sample, about the same percentages of boys and girls recommended physical punishment for the two most serious misbehaviors (13% of both sexes for hitting a sibling, 4% of the boys and 9% of the girls for physically fighting with a peer).

Further evidence that children prefer interventions of some type over permissiveness is provided by Dadds et al. (1987). Behavior-problem children and nonclinically referred control children were asked to rate the acceptability of five maternal discipline techniques (ranging from permissiveness to time out to physical punishment) across four different situations (three types of noncompliance and one instance of aggression toward others). There was no difference between these two groups of children; both rated permissiveness as less acceptable than any other response across most situations, and both rated it as unacceptable in absolute terms. Time out was rated equally with physical punishment, directed discussion, and quiet time. These authors pointed out that the apparent contradiction with earlier research by Kazdin (1987), in which children rated time out as the least acceptable practice, may be due to the younger age of this sample and the evidence that younger children typically prefer more directive parents (Siegal and Cowen 1984).

Although none of the previous studies identified contextual factors such as family composition, income, and education as being important in children's ratings of acceptable discipline, Dadds et al. (1990) found that the amount of marital discord in a child's family does appear to have a direct influence on the types of discipline techniques children prefer, and expect, both mothers and fathers to use. Compared with children from families characterized by low marital discord, children (and particularly boys) from families with high marital discord indicated that coercive behavior would and should be used more often by both parents. In addition, all children also approved of and expected more coercive behavior from fathers than from mothers. It is important to note here that, overall, these children indicated a preference for discussions and time out as discipline techniques, but several ratings by children in the high marital discord families indicated a preference for physical punishment. In accord with earlier findings, boys tended to endorse higher levels of coercive practices than did girls.

Adolescents' views of the acceptability of various parental control styles were addressed by Kelly and Goodwin (1983), using a questionnaire designed to measure the acceptability of autocratic, democratic, and permissive styles of parenting. They asked 100 adolescents first to describe their parents' styles and then to rate whether they would adopt those styles for raising their own children (a measure of acceptability). The study showed that 83% reported their parents were democratic (i.e., included the child in discussions of issues relevant to them), 11% reported having autocratic parents (i.e., did not allow children to express their views or regulate their own behavior), and 6% reported permissive parents (children have more influence in decisions than parents do). Patterns of rankings of acceptability reflect a clear preference for a democratic control style; only 16% and 27% of adolescents of autocratic and permissive parents, respectively, would choose their parents' styles for their own children, whereas 64% of the adolescents of democratic parents would raise their own child in the same manner. This study confirms earlier findings that with increasing age, children tend to prefer more inductive, less power-assertive parenting techniques.

The views of adults on the social validity of various discipline procedures are more congruent than those of children. Without exception, the adults assessed in the following studies reported that discipline techniques involving reinforcement of prosocial behaviors and some form of time out are more acceptable than those that involve more severe forms of power assertion (i.e., spanking, yelling). Several surveys of the general population (Bryan and Freed 1982; Gelles 1978b; Milner et al. 1990) indicated that 70%–95% of parents say that they subscribe to the use of mild physical punishment (spanking or slapping). However, when asked specific questions (e.g., what form of discipline is appropriate for a given problem; is it fair, reasonable, or intrusive, and consistent with conventional notions of what a treatment should be), parents are in agreement that physical punishment ranks last.

In two studies using undergraduate students as raters, Kazdin (1980a, 1980b) evaluated the acceptability of alternative treatment procedures used to suppress deviant child behavior. In the first study, treatments were clearly differentially distinguished, with reinforcement of appropriate or desirable behavior being most acceptable, followed, in order, by time out, drug therapy, and electric shock. Case severity interacted with judgments of acceptability of procedures, with all treatments being rated more acceptable for more severe cases. The second study evaluated the differential acceptability of time-out and reinforcement procedures and, in addition, explored whether the manner in which isolation techniques were implemented could increase the acceptability of isolation over reinforcement of appropriate behavior. Results indicated that reinforcement and nonexclusionary forms of time out were rated as more acceptable than isolation, although isolation was more acceptable when presented as part of a contingency contract and used to back up another form of time out than when used by itself. Kazdin (1980a) pointed out that these students' views of acceptable discipline practices may differ from those of people having more direct responsibility for the care of children.

Following up this work, Kazdin (1987) subsequently solicited evaluations from inpatient children, parents, and staff on the acceptability of four alternative treatments for children with severe behavior problems at home and at school. Judgments of the order of acceptability of the methods were exactly the same across all three groups, with reinforcement of appropriate behavior ranked highest, followed by practicing a positive behavior, medication, and time out. Furthermore, although practicing a positive behavior and medication were not rated differently on acceptability, each was significantly more acceptable than time out. Kazdin, however, is careful to point out that time out was not rated as unacceptable in terms of its absolute standing in the ratings and also that participants were not given the opportunity to judge these procedures against more intrusive corporal punishment procedures.

Norton et al. (1983) expanded the work of Kazdin (1980b) on the acceptability of time-out procedures by having teachers and parents evaluate the acceptability of five procedures. Overall, teachers rated all procedures as slightly more acceptable than did parents, but the two groups agreed on the order of acceptability. Reinforcement of appropriate behavior was rated as the most acceptable procedure, followed, in order, by isolation and contractual agreement, withdrawal, time out in the classroom, and lastly, isolation alone.

Additional evidence for the acceptability of reinforcement and time-out procedures is provided by Frentz and Kelley (1986). A nonclinical group of mothers of nonreferred children ages 2–12 rated the acceptability of five discipline practices in response to two situations differing in levels of severity (noncompliance and aggression). All techniques were rated as significantly more acceptable if applied to more severe misbehavior, but the severity level did not affect the ranking of order of acceptability. These mothers rated response cost as more acceptable than any of the other techniques, followed by time out, which was rated higher than any of the remaining techniques. Differential attention, time out with spanking, and spanking alone were not rated differently.

The effect of maternal race and income on the acceptability of five child management techniques was explored in a study by Heffer and Kelley (1987). Parents rated discipline techniques to be applied to an 8-year-old boy described as disobedient, argumentative, and physically and verbally aggressive toward his younger sister. Response cost was perceived as highly acceptable by black and white parents of all income levels, but parents' perceptions of time out were highly influenced by income level. Lower-income mothers ranked time out as less acceptable than positive reinforcement and response cost procedures, and equal in acceptability to spanking and medication. Middle-upper-income mothers, in contrast, saw time out, response cost, and reinforcement as equally acceptable, and as significantly more acceptable than spanking and medication. Analyses of those parents who viewed time out as acceptable revealed that a majority of low-income blacks rated time out as less than moderately acceptable, whereas the reverse was true of their ratings of spanking. Medication was also rated as acceptable by more than half of low-income mothers of both races. These findings suggest that impoverished families may have different formulations for dealing with child behavior problems. Although direct causal statements of the influence of race and income cannot be made from this sample because significant differences were seen on marital status and education across the groups (more middle-upper-income mothers were married, more white mothers were married, lower-income mothers had fewer years of education), these authors suggested that time out may not be a method of choice for low-income mothers because of lack of practicality (no room available in which to isolate the child) and the fact that higher levels of stressors in these families lead to the tendency to use more immediate forms of discipline.

From the perspective of most parents, three discipline techniques appear to be the most acceptable: reinforcement of appropriate behavior, response cost, and some form of time out. Lower-income parents differ somewhat in that they endorse reinforcement and response cost, but view time out as equal in acceptability to spanking. It should be pointed out that in all these studies the majority of the adults surveyed were females; fathers' views of the social acceptability of discipline may vary. Indeed, the evidence from children that fathers are expected to be more coercive than mothers, and that this behavior is endorsed, especially by their sons, would suggest that because fathers may behave differently than mothers, their views of socially acceptable discipline merit further study.

Methodological Considerations

Reliability. In this section, issues relating to the reliability of PID are reviewed, including 1) the stability of PID over time, 2) interparent agreement on reports of discipline practices, 3) systematic bias associated with parent reports of discipline practices, and 4) the use of multiagent and multimode assessments (versus single source reporting).

Stability. It is well documented that, at least for externalizing types of child problems, there is substantial stability over time. Olweus (1979, 1980) reviewed more than a dozen longitudinal studies that showed that such problems are stable over childhood and adolescence (i.e., a mean correlation of .63 over intervals that averaged 5 years). A key question is: Is there a parallel stability in parent discipline practices? The test-retest reliability of parent discipline practices has been examined in several studies. For example, analyses from the Oakland and Berkeley longitudinal studies (Elder et al. 1983) showed that disruptions in parental discipline were stable when tested in 1930 and again in 1933–1935 (i.e., correlation of .63). Schaefer and Bayley (1960) found significant stability in maternal reports of irritable reactions to their children (.64) over a 6- to 11-year interval. Dunn et al. (1986) found that mothers were quite stable in how they reacted to their children at 12 and 24 months of age. Patterson and Bank (1989) reported that parent discipline practices were significantly related to variance in child antisocial behaviors at two points in time: when the child was in grade 4 and in grade 6, accounting for 27.4% and 26.9% of the variance, respectively. Further, these investigators found that shifts in the mean levels of parental supervision over the 2-year period were associated with heightened or reduced probabilities that the child would have a police contact. At both points in time, parents with poor discipline had children with high scores on their antisocial construct, and those with good discipline had low scores on their antisocial construct. Very few of the parents in that study showed substantial shifts in their discipline practices. Supervision was considered separately from discipline and was more likely to shift from time 1 to time 2. This finding is in accord with others that show that parental practices regarding supervision apparently change as the child reaches adolescence.

Interparent agreement. The picture is less clear with regard to the level of agreement between parents on their discipline practices. Relatively little work was found on this topic; the studies that do exist indicate that mothers and fathers may use different forms of discipline with their children and so would not be expected to agree in their reporting (Smith 1983). As previously noted, most studies have been conducted with only mothers and children; therefore, data on fathers' reports are somewhat lacking. As can be expected, the more specific the questions about discipline and supervision put to parents, the more likely they are to agree with each other. For example, Capaldi and Patterson (1989) found that parents were in substantial agreement about how often they felt that their preadolescent boy completed his homework and was directly supervised by an adult after school. However, there was not close agreement on how often mothers and fathers talked with their boy about plans for the next day. This could reflect a real difference in the amount and type of talking mothers and fathers engaged in with their boy or it could reflect a difference in parental perceptions.

Bias associated with parent reports. Several studies have shown that parent reports are susceptible to systematic bias (Clement and Milne 1967; Schelle 1974). Most approaches to parent reporting require that parents aggregate their perceptions of their child over periods of a year or longer. Given the historical nature of such data, the reports are susceptible to all of the well-known problems with retrospective reports (Radke-Yarrow et al. 1968, 1970). Studies also show that parents who are stressed are more likely to report difficulties disciplining their child and that the child is likely to have more substantial problems than are children of parents who are less stressed. In fact, the data suggest that discrepancies between parent-reported child behavior and actual child behavior may be the greatest for those parents who are least able to separate their own attitudes and feelings from the behavior of their child (Reid et al. 1987). For example, Patterson (1980) and Forehand et al. (1987) found that maternal ratings of child problems were correlated with their own levels of depression; the more depressed, the worse they rated their child's behavior. Webster-Stratton and Hammond (1990) also found this effect for fathers. Friedlander et al. (1986) found that as maternal depression increased, mothers reported more behavior problems in boys (but not girls) on the Child Behavior Checklist (Achenbach 1991). In one study (Conrad and Hammen 1989), the investigators found that depressed mothers were actually more accurate reporters of their child's internalizing and externalizing problems than were nondepressed mothers. In that study, depressed mothers were less tolerant of child dysfunction and engaged in more critical and negative interactions with their child. The investigators concluded that mothers' "depressive realism" and coercive interactions with their children were forces that influenced each other and created a downward spiral of reciprocal events.

Laboratory and observational studies have shown that abusive parents tend to attribute malevolent motives to their children (Bauer and Twentyman 1985; Steele and Pollack 1968) and to give exaggerated reports of their child's poor behavior (Burgess and Conger 1978; Mash et al. 1983; Reid et al. 1987). Abusive parents have also been found to react more negatively to videotaped scenes of stressful child behaviors (Frodi and Lamb 1980; Wolfe et al. 1983). Negative and biased parent reports may come about for any number of reasons, such as low tolerance on the part of the parents due to constitutional factors or environmental stress or attempts to avoid the perception by authorities or relatives that they have inadequate parenting skills.

Multiagent, multimode versus single-agent-mode reports. In an effort to obtain data on parent-child discipline interactions that can be used to determine the presence or absence of a clinically significant problem, the practitioner would be well advised to make use of multiagent and multimethod sources of information. Each single reporting agent brings with him or her a certain bias or "error" that detracts from the "true score" of the variable being measured (Chamberlain and Bank 1989). These biases do not represent measurement error (i.e., reduced reliability) but rather *reliable* distortions introduced by the agents being queried. Likewise, each method of assessment (e.g., interviews, observations) has a built-in bias for measuring a given construct. Aggregation of data across agents (e.g., mother, child, father) and modes of assessment will partially control for biases or distortions introduced by each single data source. The result is a more reliable and generalizable score that can be used with greater confidence to determine clinical diagnosis and to suggest treatment planning.

Discussion

In this section, we include a brief discussion of familial patterns associated with PID, comments about gender differences found in the literature, comments on the pros and cons of including Parent-Child Relational Disorders in the DSM-IV (including previous work conducted on this topic), and suggestions for various options for items relating to PID and thresholds.

Familial Patterns

Studies on differences between clinical and control populations have highlighted differences in discipline interactions that are associated with current and future poor child adjustment. Contextual factors have been found to exert indirect and direct influences on discipline interactions. For example, antecedent maternal interactions with significant others and maternal and child mood have been shown to exert powerful direct effects on discipline interactions. The father's employment stability, family size, and marital relationship are examples of forces that exert more indirect influences. Promising statistical techniques, such as structural equation modeling, have recently allowed the simultaneous examination of direct and indirect effects.

Sex Differences

Evidence for differential gender effects has emerged from the studies reviewed throughout this chapter. Studies support the notion that parents tend to use different discipline strategies for boys and girls, with more power assertive techniques being used with males. There are apparently different male and female patterns of long-term negative outcomes of PID, with early harsh punishment related to alcoholism, erratic work histories, and downward mobility in males, and related to depression and irritable, harsh discipline of their own children in females. Sex differences have also been documented in what male and female children perceive as being fair and appropriate discipline. These differences are complicated by child-reported differences in what discipline strategies children see as appropriate coming from mothers versus fathers.

Previous Work on Including PID as a Diagnostic Category

Several groups of investigators (most recently Shaffer et al. [1991] and van Goor-Lambo et al. [1990]) have laid a foundation for establishing a classification for PID as a psychosocial situations category.

Shaffer et al. (1991) developed and reported on the reliability and validity of 17 psychosocial situation codes thought to cause or contribute to the development of various childhood psychiatric disorders. Of the 17 codes, 8 relate to elements of the family environment, and 2 relate to disturbance in school or work and extrafamilial stress. The codes were tested by 52 child psychiatrists in a carefully conducted study involving two case history exercises and a field study of cases from their clinical practices. The case histories were abstracted from hospital case records. The coding of the psychosocial situations was done in conjunction with the psychiatric and medical disorder codes of ICD-9 (World Health Organization 1978). Results showed that, overall, the reliability of the codes was low, with kappa values ranging from .14 to .62. The kappa value for inadequate or inconsistent parental control (IIPC) was .31. Reliability was also assessed, when raters were given access to a glossary that provided more specific information on the categories. Use of the glossary (compared with ratings made without it) improved the reliability of the IIPC from .31 to .36. Raters with access to the glossary were also significantly less likely to use the IIPC category, thereby increasing its discriminative validity. The IIPC category and discordant intrafamilial relationships were most frequently applied to children with a conduct disorder diagnosis. Children with a conduct disorder, compared with children diagnosed as having neurotic or emotional disorders, were also less likely to be rated as having overinvolved family relationships. The authors concluded that the overall findings were generally confirmatory and provided some support for discriminate validity.

van Goor-Lambo et al. (1990) reported on a revision of the *Guide to a Multiaxial Scheme for Psychiatric Disorders in Childhood and Adolescence* (Rutter et al. 1975). The revision was conducted by a World Health Organization working group (World Health Organization 1988). The authors argued in favor of separate coding of psychosocial stressors in contrast to the method offered by DSM-III (American Psychiatric Association 1980) and DSM-III-R (American Psychiatric Association 1987), which pools heterogeneous stressors and gives a severity rating. This revision differs from previous coding versions in that it includes a more detailed specification of criteria, has more explicit severity requirements for coding, and conceptually regroups the code categories. The time limit chosen for coding the presence of the categories was 6 months immediately preceding the assessment. In this system, it was decided to have each and every category coded as being absent, dubiously present, or definitely present. Five main categories include 42 specific codes. "Inadequate parental supervision/control" is included as a subcategory of "abnormal qualities of upbringing."

Cantwell and Baker (1989), in the context of a study on the natural history and stability of DSM-III diagnoses, reported on the natural history of the DSM-III V code, "parent-child problem." Their study supports the predictive value of parent-child problems; its natural history was as poor as or poorer than many of the psychiatric disorders. Of 15 children with initial parent-child problem, only 3 were well at follow-up 4–5 years later. The authors concluded that their follow-up data suggest that the parent-child problem may be a precursor to later full-blown psychiatric disorders.

Pros and Cons of Including PID in the DSM-IV

In this review, strong evidence has been presented for the predictive validity of PID. Early, severe disruptions in discipline appear to bode poorly for the child's subsequent adjustment in adolescence and adulthood. From a clinical practice perspective, several well-controlled treatment outcome studies suggest that helping parents to improve their child management practices, especially discipline, results in improved child and family adjustment (Kazdin 1985; Patterson et al. 1982; Wahler 1980; Webster-Stratton and Hammond 1990). Anecdotally, in treating child problems, it is well known that practitioners from various theoretical perspectives use family therapy approaches. The specification of discipline as a target area for intervention would aid the practitioner in determining appropriate treatments. Research on the treatment of child disorders would be improved by giving clearer definition to the necessary and sufficient components for effective treatments.

A primary disadvantage of including PID in the diagnostic nomenclature is that it is unknown whether the diagnosis of PID could be reliably made by different clinicians from varying theoretical perspectives. Studies reviewed earlier in this section indicate that initial attempts at classification of discipline problems have only moderate interrater reliabilities. Another disadvantage is the possibility that inclusion of the parent-child relational disorders could produce high rates of false positive errors in diagnosis. The study by Cantwell and Baker (1989) implicating family problems in poor future child adjustment argues against this point, but a concern still remains.

Recommendations

The Task Force on DSM-IV (American Psychiatric Association 1991) included a new category of "Relational (Family) Problems" in the *DSM-IV Options Book*. Under this category, inadequate parental discipline is proposed as one of eight parent-child relational problems to be designated with V codes (Z codes after ICD-10 [World Health Organization 1990] is implemented in the United States). The criteria for PID discussed in this review refer to the Task Force's proposal to include PID in DSM-IV. The authors of this review concur with the Task Force that the inclusion of family relational problems, and more specifically PID, in DSM-IV will enhance both the diagnosis and treatment of pathognomic patterns of parent-child interaction. We concur with the Coalition on Family Diagnosis that ideally this category should be connected with Axis I disorders.

Suggested assessment of PID includes a determination of the presence of the following symptoms.

1. The parent is inconsistent/noncontingent in his or her reactions to the child's behavior.
2. The parent is irritable or explosive in attempts to discipline the child.
3. The parent finds it difficult or is unwilling to supervise the child.
4. The parent disciplines the child based more on the parent's own mood than on the child's misbehavior.
5. The parent is limited in the type of discipline methods he or she uses and tends to use one (e.g., yelling) rather than multiple methods.

In addition to interviewing parent and child using a standard set of questions about each of these five areas listed, the reliability and validity of the assessment would be improved by conducting a brief observation of the parent and child interacting. Depending on the child's age, the structure of the interaction could be similar to one of the following. For 2- to 12-year-olds, have the mother and child engage in a play session with age-appropriate toys for 10–15 minutes; then instruct the mother to have the child put the toys away. For 12- to 18-year-olds, the parent and the child are asked separately to identify an area about which they have conflict. A listing of typical conflict areas could be provided to them as a prompt. Next they would be asked to talk about each area in turn for 5–7 minutes, working toward a resolution of the conflict.

Direct clinical observation of parent-child interaction would be expected to add meaningful information to the self-reports of discipline problems provided by the parent and child, giving the practitioner a broader, less-biased base from which to make a diagnosis.

The presence of discipline problems for at least the past 6 months is the time frame that has most commonly been used in previous diagnostic studies. The presence of PID should be diagnosed only if the problem is significantly more frequent and severe than in families with children of the same mental age as the child being assessed.

References

Achenbach TM: Manual for the Child Behavior Checklist 4-18. Burlington, VT, University of Vermont Department of Psychiatry, 1991
Allen W: Race, income, and family dynamics: a study of adolescent male socialization processes and outcomes, in Beginnings: The Social and Affective Development of Black Children. Edited by Spencer M, Bookins G, Allen W. Hillsdale, NJ, Lawrence Erlbaum Associates, 1985, pp 273–292
American Psychiatric Association: Diagnostic and Statistical Manual of Mental Disorders, 3rd Edition. Washington, DC, American Psychiatric Association, 1980
American Psychiatric Association: Diagnostic and Statistical Manual of Mental Disorders, 3rd Edition, Revised. Washington, DC, American Psychiatric Association, 1987
American Psychiatric Association: DSM-IV Options Book: Work in Progress. Washington, DC, American Psychiatric Association, 1991
Anderson KE, Lytton H, Romney DM: Mothers' interactions with normal and conduct-disordered boys: who affects whom? Dev Psychol 22:604–609, 1986
Bahr S: Family determinants and effects of deviance, in Contemporary Theories About the Family. Edited by Burr W, Hill R, Nye FI, et al. New York, Free Press, 1979, pp 96–123
Baldwin AL: The effect of home environment on nursery school behavior. Child Dev 20:49–61, 1949
Banducci R: The effects of mother's employment on the achievement, aspirations, and expectations of the child. Personnel and Guidance Journal 46:263–267, 1967
Bartz K, Levine E: Child rearing by black parents: a description and comparison to Anglo and Chicano parents. Journal of Marriage and the Family 40:709–719, 1978
Bates J: Temperament as a part of social relationships: implications of perceived infant difficultness. Paper presented at the International Conference on Infant Studies, Austin, TX, March 1982
Bauer WD, Twentyman CT: Abusing, neglectful, and comparison mothers' responses to child-related and non-child-related stressors. J Consult Clin Psychol 53:335–343, 1985

Baumrind D: Authoritarian versus authoritative parental control, in Adolescence, Vol 3, No 2. Edited by Kazdin A. New York, Libra Publishers, 1968, pp 255–272

Baumrind D: Current patterns of parental authority. Dev Psychol Monographs 4 (No 1, Pt 2):132–142, 1971

Baumrind D: An exploratory study of socialization effects on black children: some black-white comparisons. Child Dev 43:261–267, 1972

Baumrind D: Effective parenting during the early adolescent transition, in Family Transitions. Edited by Cowan PA, Hetherington EM. Hillsdale, NJ, Lawrence Erlbaum Associates, 1991, pp 111–163

Beardslee W, Schultz L, Selman R: Level of social cognitive development, adaptive functioning, and DSM-III diagnosis in adolescent offspring of parents with affective disorders: implications of the development of the capacity for mutuality. Dev Psychol 23:807–815, 1987

Becker WC, Peterson DR, Luria Z, et al: Relations of factors derived from parent-interview ratings to behavior problems of five-year-olds. Child Dev 33:509–535, 1962

Behar D, Stewart MA: Aggressive conduct disorder of children. Acta Psychiatr Scand 65:210–220, 1982

Bell RQ, Harper LV: Child Effects on Adults. Hillsdale, NJ, Lawrence Erlbaum Associates, 1977

Bradley R, Cantwell B: Home Observation for Measurement of the Environment: a revision of the preschool scale. American Journal of Mental Deficiency 84:235–244, 1979

Bronfenbrenner U: Socialization and social class through time and space, in Readings in Social Psychology. Edited by Maccoby EE, Newcomb TM, Hartley EL. New York, Holt, 1958, pp 90–109

Bryan JW, Freed FW: Corporal punishment: normative data and sociological and psychological correlates in a community college population. Journal of Youth and Adolescence 11:77–87, 1982

Burbach DJ, Borduin CM: Parent-child relations and the etiology of depression: a review of methods and findings. Clinical Psychology Review 6:133–153, 1986

Burgess RL, Conger RD: Family interaction in abusive, neglectful and normal families. Child Dev 49:1163–1173, 1978

Buss T, Redburn FS: Mass Unemployment: Plant Closings and Community Mental Health. Beverly Hills, CA, Sage, 1983

Camerson JR: Parental treatment, children's temperament, and the risk of childhood behavioral problems, II: initial temperament, parental attitudes, and the incidence and form of behavioral problems. Am J Orthopsychiatry 48:140–147, 1978

Campbell A: Self-reported delinquency and home life: evidence from a sample of British girls. Journal of Youth and Adolescence 16:167–177, 1987

Cantwell DP, Baker L: Stability and natural history of DSM-III childhood diagnoses. J Am Acad Child Adolesc Psychiatry 28:691–700, 1989

Capaldi DM: The co-occurrence of conduct problems and depressive symptoms in early adolescent boys: a longitudinal study of general adjustment and familial factors. Development and Psychopathology 3:277–300, 1991

Capaldi DM, Patterson GR: Psychometric Properties of Fourteen Latent Constructs From the Oregon Youth Study. New York, Springer-Verlag, 1989

Capaldi DM, Patterson GR: Relation of parental transitions to boys' adjustment problems, I: a linear hypothesis, and II: mothers at risk for transitions and unskilled parenting. Developmental Psychology 27:489–504, 1991

Cappell C, Heiner RB: The intergenerational transmission of family aggression. Journal of Family Violence 5:135–152, 1990

Carlson BE: Children's beliefs about punishment. Am J Orthopsychiatry 56:308–312, 1986

Cernkovich SA, Giordano PC: Family relationships and delinquency. Criminology 25:295–321, 1987

Chamberlain P, Bank L: Toward an integration of macro and micro measurement systems for the researcher and the clinician. Journal of Family Psychology 3:199–205, 1989

Cheyne JA, Walters RH: Intensity of punishment, timing of punishment, and cognitive structure as determinants of response inhibition. J Exp Child Psychol 7:231–244, 1969

Clarke-Stewart K: Interactions between mothers and their young children: characteristics and consequences. Monographs of the Society for Research in Child Development 38 (6–7, Serial No 153):326–372, 1973

Clement PW, Milne PC: Group play therapy and tangible reinforcers used to modify the behavior of 8-year-old boys. Behav Res Ther 5:301–312, 1967

Cohen P, Brook JS, Cohen J, et al: Common and uncommon pathways to adolescent psychopathology and problem behavior, in Straight and Devious Pathways From Childhood. Edited by Robins L, Rutter M. Cambridge, MA, Cambridge University Press, 1990, pp 62–75

Cohler B, Gallant D, Grunebaum, H, et al: Child care attitudes and development of young children of mentally ill and well mothers. Psychol Rep 46:31–46, 1980

Cohler B, Stott F, Musick J: From infancy to middle childhood: the Thresholds Mothers' Project. Paper prepared for the Schizophrenia Consortium Conference on Risk in Infancy, Newport, RI, May 1987

Coie JD, Asher JD (eds): Peer Rejection in Childhood. Cambridge, MA, Cambridge University Press, 1990

Coie JD, Dodge K: Multiple sources of data on social behavior and social status in the school: a cross-age comparison. Child Dev 59:815–829, 1988

Conrad M, Hammen C: Role of maternal depression in perceptions of child maladjustment. J Consult Clin Psychol 57:663–667, 1989

Coopersmith S: The Antecedents of Self-Esteem. San Francisco, CA, WH Freeman, 1967

Crockenberg S: Predictors and correlates of anger toward and punitive control of toddlers by adolescent mothers. Child Dev 58:964–975, 1987

Crook T, Raskin A, Eliot J: Parent-child relationships and adult depression. Child Dev 52:950–957, 1981

Dadds MR, Adlington FM, Christensen AP: Children's perceptions of time out and other maternal disciplinary strategies: the effects of clinic status and exposure to behavioural treatment. Behaviour Change 4:3–13, 1987

Dadds MR, Sheffield JK, Holbeck JF: An examination of the differential relationship of marital discord to parents' discipline strategies for boys and girls. J Abnorm Child Psychol 18:121–129, 1990

DeSalvo FJ, Zurcher LA: Defensive and supportive parental communication in a discipline situation. J Psychol 17:7–17, 1984

Dishion TJ: The family ecology of boys' peer relations in middle childhood. Child Dev 61:874–892, 1990

Dishion TK, Patterson GR, Stoolmiller M, et al: Family, school, and behavioral antecedents to early adolescent involvement with antisocial peers. Developmental Psychology 27:172–180, 1991

Dix T: The affective organization of parenting: adaptive and maladaptive processes, in Emotion and Parenting: The Heart of the Matter. Chaired by Dix T. Symposium conducted at the meeting of the Society for Research in Child Development, Seattle, WA, April 1991

Dodge KA: Behavioral antecedents: a peer social status. Child Dev 54:1386–1399, 1983

Doelling JL, Johnson JH: Predicting success in foster placement: the contributions of parent-child temperament characteristics. Am J Orthopsychiatry 60:585–593, 1990

Dornbusch SM, Ritter PL, Leiderman PH, et al: The relation of parenting style to adolescent school performance. Child Dev 58:1244–1257, 1987

Downey G, Coyne JC: Children of depressed parents: an integrative review. Psychol Bull 108:50–76, 1990

Dumas JE: Indirect influence of maternal social contacts on mother-child interactions: a setting event analysis. J Abnorm Child Psychol 14:205–216, 1986

Dumas JE, Gibson JA, Albin JB: Behavioral correlates of maternal depressive symptomatology in conduct-disorder children. J Consult Clin Psychol 57:516–521, 1989

Dunn J, Kendrick C: Siblings: Love, Envy and Understanding. Cambridge, MA, Harvard University Press, 1982

Dunn JF, Plomin R, Daniels D: Consistency and change in mothers' behavior toward young siblings. Child Dev 57:348–356, 1986

Durrett M, O'Brien S, Pennebaker J: Child rearing reports of white, black, and Mexican American families. Developmental Psychology 11:871–912, 1975

Egeland B, Jacobvitz D, Papatola K: Intergenerational continuity of parental abuse, in Biosocial Aspects of Child Abuse. Edited by Lancaster J, Gelles R. San Francisco, CA, Jossey-Bass, 1987, pp 612–636

Eimer BN: Age differences in boys' evaluations of fathers intervening to stop misbehavior. J Psychol 115:159–163, 1983

Elder G: Historical change in life patterns and personality, in Life Span Development and Behavior, Vol 2. Edited by Baltes P, Brim O. New York, Academic Press, 1979, pp 117–159

Elder GH, Caspi A, Downey G: Problem behavior in family relationships: a multigenerational analysis, in Human Development: Interdisciplinary Perspective. Edited by Sorensen A, Weinert F, Sherrod L. Hillsdale, NJ, Lawrence Erlbaum Associates, 1983, pp 93–118

Elder GH, Liker JK, Cross CE: Parent-child behavior in the Great Depression: life course and intergenerational influences, in Life Span Development and Behavior, Vol 6. Edited by Baltes PB, Brim OG. New York, Academic Press, 1984, pp 109–158

Elliott DS, Huizinga D, Ageton SS: Explaining Delinquency and Drug Use. Newbury Park, CA, Sage, 1985

Elmer E: Children in Jeopardy: A Study of Abused Minors and Their Families. Pittsburgh, PA, University of Pittsburgh Press, 1967

Emery RE: Interparental conflict and the children of discord and divorce. Psychol Bull 92:310–330, 1982

Engfer A: Intergenerational influences on the mother-child relationship. Paper prepared for the 11th International Congress on New Approaches to Infant, Child, Adolescent and Family Mental Health, Paris, France, July 1986

Eron LD, Huesmann LR, Zelli A: The role of parental variables in the learning of aggression, in The Development and Treatment of Childhood Aggression. Edited by Peplar DJ, Rubin KH. Hillsdale, NJ, Lawrence Erlbaum Associates, 1991, pp 267–289

Fanaroff A, Kennell J, Klaus M: Follow-up of low birth weight infants: the predictive value of maternal visiting patterns. Pediatrics 49:287–290, 1972

Farrington DP: The family backgrounds of aggressive youths, in Aggression and Antisocial Behaviour in Childhood and Adolescence. Edited by Hersov LA, Berger M, Shaffer D. Oxford, England, Pergamon, 1978, pp 73–93

Fauber R, Forehand R, Thomas AM, et al: A mediational model of the impact of marital conflict on adolescent adjustment in intact and divorced families: the role of disrupted parenting. Child Dev 61:1112–1123, 1990

Fisher PA: Predicting negative discipline in traditional families: a multi-dimensional stress model. Master's thesis, Eugene, OR, University of Oregon, 1990

Forehand R, Gardner H, Roberts N: Maternal response to child compliance and noncompliance: some normative data. J Clin Child Psychol 63:121–124, 1978

Forehand R, McCombs A, Brody GH: The relationship between parental depressive mood states and child functioning. Advances in Behavioral Research and Therapy 9:1–20, 1987

Forgatch MS: The clinical science vortex: a developing theory of antisocial behavior, in The Development and Treatment of Childhood Aggression. Edited by Pepler DJ, Rubin KH. Hillsdale, NJ, Lawrence Erlbaum Associates, 1991a, pp 291–316

Forgatch MS: The effect of divorce-related stressors on younger and older sons, in Impact of Life Stressors on Adult Relationships and Adolescent Adjustment. Chaired by Conger RD, Elder GE Jr. Symposium conducted at the meeting of the Society for Research in Child Development, Washington, DC, April 1991b

Forgatch MS, Toobert DJ: A cost-effective parent training program for use with normal preschool children. J Pediatr Psychol 4:129–145, 1979

Frentz C, Kelley ML: Parents' acceptance of reductive treatment methods: the influence of problem severity and perception of child behavior. Behavior Therapy 17:75–81, 1986

Friedlander S, Weiss DS, Traylor J: Assessing the influence of maternal depression on the validity of the Child Behavior Checklist. J Abnorm Child Psychol 14:123–133, 1986

Frodi AM, Lamb M: Child abusers' responses to infant smiles and cries. Child Dev 51:238–241, 1980

Gardner FEM: Inconsistent parenting: is there evidence for a link with children's conduct problems? J Abnorm Child Psychol 17:223–233, 1989

Gelfand DM, Teti DM: The effects of maternal depression on children. Clinical Psychology Review 10:329–353, 1990

Gelles RJ: Etiology of violence: overcoming fallacious reasoning in understanding family violence and child abuse, in Conference Proceedings From Child Abuse: Where Do We Go From Here? Edited by Clark D. Atlanta, GA, Children's Hospital National Medical Center, 1978a, pp 61–66

Gelles RJ: Violence towards children. Am J Orthopsychiatry 48:580–592, 1978b

Gelles RJ: Applying research on family violence to clinical practice. Journal of Marriage and the Family 17:9–19, 1982

Ghodsian M, Zajicek E, Wolkind S: A longitudinal study of maternal depression and child behavior problems. J Child Psychol Psychiatry 25:91–109, 1984

Gil DG: Violence Against Children: Physical Abuse in the United States. Cambridge, MA, Harvard University Press, 1970

Gleuck S, Gleuck E: Unraveling Juvenile Delinquency. Cambridge, MA, Harvard University Press, 1950

Gleuck S, Gleuck E: Delinquents and Nondelinquents in Perspective. Cambridge, MA, Harvard University Press, 1968
Gold D, Andres D: Developmental comparisons between ten-year-old children with employed and nonemployed mothers. Child Dev 49:75–84, 1978
Gold M, Reimer DJ: Changing patterns of delinquent behavior among Americans 13 to 16 years old—1972. Crime and Delinquency Literature 7:483–517, 1975
Goldstein HS: Parental composition, supervision, and conduct problems in youths 12–17 years old. Journal of the American Academy of Child Psychiatry 23:679–684, 1984
Goodman SH, Brumley HE: Schizophrenic and depressed mothers: relational deficits in parenting. Developmental Psychology 26:31–39, 1990
Green AH, Gaines R, Sandgrund A: Child abuse: pathological syndrome of family interaction. Am J Psychiatry 131:882–886, 1974
Grusec JE, Kuczynski L: Direction of effects in socialization: a comparison of the parent's versus the child's behavior as determinants of disciplinary techniques. Developmental Psychology 16:1–9, 1980
Grusec JE, Lytton H: Social Development: History, Theory, and Research. New York, Springer-Verlag, 1988
Hale J: Black Children: Their Roots, Culture, and Learning Styles. Provo, UT, BYU Press, 1982
Hammen C, Gordon G, Burge D, et al: Maternal affective disorders, illness, and stress: risk for children's psychopathology. Am J Psychiatry 144:741–763, 1987
Hartup WW: Peer relations, in Handbook of Child Psychology, Vol 4: Socialization, Personality, and Social Development. Edited by Gordon A. New York, John Wiley, 1983, pp 460–483
Heffer RW, Kelley ML: Mothers' acceptance of behavioral interventions for children: the influence of parent race and income. Behavior Therapy 2:153–163, 1987
Herrenkohl E, Herrenkohl R, Toedter L: Perspectives on the intergenerational transmission of abuse, in The Dark Side of Families: Current Family Violence Research. Edited by Finkelhor D, Gelles R, Hotaling G, et al. Beverly Hills, CA, Sage, 1983, pp 305–316
Hess RD, McDevitt TM: Some cognitive consequences of maternal intervention techniques: a longitudinal study. Child Dev 55:2017–2030, 1984
Hetherington EM, Martin B: Family interaction, in Psychopathological Disorders of Childhood, 2nd Edition. Edited by Quay HC, Werry JS. New York, John Wiley, 1979, pp 247–302
Hetherington EM, Stanley-Hagen M, Anderson ER: Marital transitions: a child's perspective. Am Psychol 44:303–312, 1989
Hoffman ML: Power assertion by the parent and its impact on the child. Child Dev 31:129–143 1960
Hoffman ML: Personality, family structure, and social class as antecedents of parental power assertion. Child Dev 34:869–884, 1963
Hoffman ML: Moral development, in Carmichael's Manual of Child Psychology, Vol 2. Edited by Mussne PH. New York, John Wiley, 1970, pp 72–96
Hoffman ML, Saltzstein HD: Parent discipline and the child's moral development. J Pers Soc Psychol 5:45–57, 1967
Holden GW: Avoiding conflict: mothers as tacticians in the supermarket. Child Dev 54:233–240, 1983
Holmes SJ, Robins LN: The role of parental disciplinary practices in the development of depression and alcoholism. Psychiatry 51:24–36, 1988

Hops H, Sherman L, Biglan A: Maternal depression, marital discord, and children's behaviors: a developmental perspective, in Depression and Aggression in Family Interactions. Edited by Patterson GR. New York, Lawrence Erlbaum Associates, 1990, pp 185–208

Huesmann LR, Eron LD, Lefkowitz MM, et al: Stability of aggression over time and generations. Developmental Psychology 20:1120–1134, 1984

Jouriles EN, Pfiffner LJ, O'Leary SG: Marital conflict, parenting, and toddler conduct problems. J Abnorm Child Psychol 16:197–206, 1988

Jouriles EN, Murphy CM, O'Leary KD: Effects of maternal mood on mother-son interaction patterns. J Abnorm Child Psychol 17:513–525, 1989

Kasl SV, Cobb S: Some mental health consequences of plant closings and job loss, in Mental Health and the Economy. Edited by Ferman L, Gordus J. Kalazamoo, MI, WE Upjohn Institute for Employment Research, 1979, pp 255–300

Kazdin AE: Acceptability of alternative treatments for deviant child behavior. J Appl Behav Anal 13:259–273, 1980a

Kazdin AE: Acceptability of time out from reinforcement procedures for disruptive child behavior. Behavior Therapy 11:329–344, 1980b

Kazdin AE: Treatment of Antisocial Behavior in Children and Adolescents. Homewood, IL, Dorsey Press, 1985

Kazdin AE: Treatment of antisocial behavior in children. Psychol Bull 102:187–203, 1987

Kelly C, Goodwin GC: Adolescents' perception of three styles of parental control. Adolescence 18:567–571, 1983

Kessler R, House J, Turner J: Unemployment and health in a community sample. J Health Soc Behav 28:51–59, 1987

Klein D, Clark D, Dansky L, et al: Dysthymia in the offspring of parents with primary unipolar affective disorder. J Abnorm Psychol 94:115–127, 1988

Knutson JF: Child abuse as an area of aggression research. J Pediatr Psychol 3:20–27, 1978

Kochanska G: Affective factors in mothers' autonomy-granting to their five-year-olds: comparison of well and depressed mothers, in Emotion and Parenting: the Heart of the Matter. Chaired by Dix T. Symposium conducted at the meeting of the Society for Research in Child Development, Seattle, WA, April 1991

Kochanska G, Kuczynski L, Radke-Yarrow M, et al: Resolutions of control episodes between well and affectively ill mothers and their young children. J Abnorm Child Psychol 15:441–456, 1987

Kochanska G, Kuczynski L, Maguire M: Impact of diagnosed depression and self-reported mood on mothers' control strategies: a longitudinal study. J Abnorm Child Psychol 17:493–511, 1989

Kolvin I, Miller FJW, Fleeting M, et al: Social and parenting factors affecting criminal-offense rates: findings from the Newcastle Thousand Family Study (1947–1980). Br J Psychiatry 152:80–90, 1988

Kovacs M, Paulauskas S, Gatsonis C, et al: Depressive disorders in childhood, III: a longitudinal study of comorbidity with and risk for conduct disorders. J Affect Disord 15:205–217, 1988

Kuczynski L: Intensity and orientation of reasoning: motivational determinants of children's compliance to verbal rationales. J Exp Child Psychol 34:357–370, 1982

Kuczynski L: Socialization goals and mother-child interaction: strategies for long-term and short-term compliance. Developmental Psychology 20:1061–1073, 1984

Kuczynski L: Emerging conceptions of children's responses to parental control, in New Perspectives in Child Compliance, Noncompliance, and Parental Control. Chaired by Kochanska G, Kuczynski L. Symposium conducted at the meeting of the Society for Research in Child Development, Seattle, WA, April 1991

Lamont J, Gottlieb H: Convergent recall of parental behaviors in depressed students of different racial groups. J Clin Psychol 32:9–11, 1975

Lamont J, Fischoff S, Gottlieb H: Recall of parental behaviors in female neurotic depressives. J Clin Psychol 32:762–765, 1976

Langley J, McGee R, Silva P, et al: Child behavior and accidents. J Pediatr Psychol 8:181–189, 1983

Larzelere RE, Patterson GR: Parental management: mediator of the effect of socioeconomic status on early delinquency. Criminology 28:301–323, 1990

Laub JH, Sampson RJ: Unraveling families and delinquency: a reanalysis of the Gluecks' data. Criminology 26:355–379, 1988

Lay K, Waters E, Park KA: Maternal responsiveness and child compliance: the role of mood as a mediator. Child Dev 60:1405–1411, 1989

Leahy RL: The child's conception of Mens REA: information mitigating punishment judgments. J Gen Psychol 134:74–78, 1979

Lee CL, Bates JE: Mother-child interaction at age two years and perceived difficult temperament. Child Dev 56:1314–1325, 1985

Lempers JD, Clark-Lempers D, Simons RL: Economic hardship, parenting, and distress in adolescence. Child Dev 60:25–39, 1989

Lepper MR: Intrinsic and extrinsic motivation in children: detrimental effects of superfluous social controls, in Minnesota Symposia in Child Psychology, Vol 14. Edited by Block J. Minneapolis, MN, University of Minnesota Press, 1981, pp 63–84

Lerner JV: The role of temperament in psychosocial adaptation in early adolescents: a test of a "goodness of fit" model. J Gen Psychol 143:149–157, 1983

Lewinsohn PM, Rosenbaum M: Recall of parental behavior by acute depressives, remitted depressives, and nondepressives. J Pers Soc Psychol 52:611–619, 1987

Lewis DO, Shanok SS, Pincus JH, et al: Violent juvenile delinquents: psychiatric, neurological, psychological, and abuse factors. Journal of the American Academy of Child Psychiatry 18:307–319, 1979

Lewis DO, Shanok SS, Grant M, et al: Homicidally aggressive young children: neuropsychiatric and experiential correlates. Am J Psychiatry 140:148–153, 1983

Lobitz WC, Johnson SM: Parental manipulation of the behavior of normal and deviant children. Child Dev 46:719–726, 1975

Loeb RC, Horst L, Horton PJ: Family interaction patterns associated with self-esteem in preadolescent girls and boys. Merrill-Palmer Quarterly 26:205–217, 1980

Loeber R, Dishion TJ: Boys who fight at home and in school: family conditions influencing cross-setting consistency. J Consult Clin Psychol 52:759–768, 1984

Londerville S, Main M: Security of attachment, compliance and maternal training methods in the second year of life. Developmental Psychology 17:289–299, 1981

Lytton H: Disciplinary encounters between young boys and their mothers and fathers: is there a contingency system? Developmental Psychology 15:256–268, 1979

Lytton H: Parent-Child Interaction: The Socialization Process Observed in Twin and Singleton Families. New York, Plenum, 1980

Maccoby EE: New perspectives in child compliance, noncompliance, and parental control, in New Perspectives in Child Compliance. Chaired by Kochanska G, Kuczynksi L. Symposium conducted at the meeting of the Society for Research in Child Development, Seattle, WA, April 1991

Maccoby EE, Martin J: Socialization in the context of the family: parent-child interaction, in Handbook of Child Psychology, 4th Edition, Vol 4: Socialization, Personality, and Social Development. Edited by Mussen P, Hetherington EM. New York, John Wiley, 1983, pp 1–101

Manheimer DE, Mellinger GD: Personality characteristics of the child accident repeater. Child Dev 38:491–513, 1967

Martin RP: Activity level, distractibility, and persistence: critical characteristics in early schooling, in Temperament in Childhood. Edited by Kohnstamm GA, Bates JE, Rothbart MK. New York, John Wiley, 1989, pp 23–36

Mash EJ, Johnston C, Kovitz K: A comparison of the mother-child interactions of physically abused and nonabused children during play and task situations. J Clin Child Psychol 12:337–346, 1983

McCord J: Some child-rearing antecedents of criminal behavior in adult men. J Pers Soc Psychol 37:1477–1486, 1979

McCord J: Parental behavior in the cycle of aggression. Psychiatry 51:14–23, 1988

McCord W, McCord J, Zola IK: Origins of Crime. New York, Columbia University Press, 1959

McCord W, McCord J, Howard A: Familial correlates of aggression in nondelinquent male children. Journal of Abnormal and Social Psychology 62:79–93, 1961

McDonald K, Parke R: Bridging the gap: parent-child play interaction and parent interactive competence. Child Dev 55:1265–1277, 1984

McLoyd VC: The impact of economic hardship on black families and children: psychological distress, parenting, and socioemotional development. Child Dev 61:311–346, 1990

Milner JS, Robertson KR, Rogers DL: Childhood history of abuse and adult child abuse potential. Journal of Family Violence 5:15–33, 1990

Morse C, Sahler O, Friedman S: A three-year follow-up of abused and neglected children. Am J Dis Child 120:439–446, 1970

Mounts N, Brown BB, Lamborn SD, et al: Parenting style and crowd membership: contributions to adolescent adjustment, in From Family to Peer: Family Influences on Peer Relations From Early Childhood Through Adolescence. Chaired by Brown BB. Symposium conducted at the meeting of the Society for Research in Child Development, Seattle, WA, April 1991

Mulhern RK Jr, Passman RH: Parental discipline as affected by the sex of the parent, the sex of the child, and the child's apparent responsiveness to discipline. Developmental Psychology 17:604–613, 1981

Norton GR, Austen S, Allen GE, et al: Acceptability of time out from reinforcement procedures for disruptive child behavior: a further analysis. Child and Family Behavior Therapy 5:251–263,1983

Nye FI: Family Relationships and Delinquent Behavior. New York, John Wiley, 1958

Olweus D: Stability of aggressive reaction patterns in males: a review. Psychol Bull 86:852–875, 1979

Olweus D: Familial and temperamental determinants of aggressive behavior in adolescent boys: a causal analysis. Developmental Psychology 16:644–660, 1980

Orvaschel H, Walsh-Allis G, Ye W: Psychopathology in children of parents with recurrent depression. J Abnorm Child Psychol 16:17–28, 1988

Parke RD: Effectiveness of punishment as an interaction of intensity, timing, agent, nurturance, and cognitive structure. Child Dev 40:213–235, 1969

Parker G: Parental characteristics in relation to depressive disorders. Br J Psychiatry 134:138–147, 1979a

Parker G: Parental deprivation and depression in a non-clinical group. Aust N Z J Psychiatry 13:51–56, 1979b

Parker G: Parental reports of depressives: an investigation of several explanations. J Affect Disord 3:131–140, 1981

Parker G: Re-searching the schizophrenogenic mother. J Nerv Ment Dis 170:452–462, 1982

Parpal M, Maccoby EE: Maternal responsiveness and subsequent child compliance. Child Dev 56:1326–1334, 1985

Patterson GR: The aggressive child: victim and architect of a coercive system, in Behavior Modification and Families. Edited by Mash EJ, Hamerlynck LA, Handy LC. New York, Brunner/Mazel, 1976, pp 267–316

Patterson GR: A performance theory for coercive family interactions, in Social Interaction: Methods, Analysis, and Illustration. Edited by Cairns R. Hillsdale, NJ, Lawrence Erlbaum Associates, 1979, pp 119–162

Patterson GR: Mothers: The Unacknowledged Victims. Monogr Soc Res Child Dev Vol 45, No 5, 1980

Patterson GR: Coercive Family Process. Eugene, OR, Castalia Publishing Co, 1982

Patterson GR: Siblings: fellow travelers in coercive family process, in Advances in the Study of Aggression, Vol 1. Edited by Blanchard RJ, Blanchard DC. Orlando, FL, Academic Press, 1984, pp 173–215

Patterson GR: Performance models for antisocial boys. Am Psychol 41:432–444, 1986

Patterson GR, Bank L: Some amplifying mechanisms for pathologic processes in families, in Systems and Development: The Minnesota Symposia on Child Psychology, Vol 22. Edited by Gunnar MR, Thelen E. Hillsdale, NJ, Lawrence Erlbaum Associates, 1989, pp 167–209

Patterson GR, Capaldi DM: Antisocial parents: unskilled and vulnerable, in Family Transitions. Edited by Cowan PA, Hetherington EM. Hillsdale, NJ, Lawrence Erlbaum Associates, 1991, pp 195–218

Patterson GR, Dishion TJ: Multilevel family process models: traits, interactions, and relationships, in Relationships Within Families: Mutual Influences. Edited by Hinde R, Stevenson-Hinde J. Oxford, England, Clarendon Press, 1988, pp 283–310

Patterson GR, Forgatch MS: Further explorations of mechanisms that maintain single mother depression, in Stress, Coping, and Resiliency in Children and the Family. Edited by Hetherington EM, Cowen P. Hillsdale, NJ, Lawrence Erlbaum Associates (in press)

Patterson GR, Stouthamer-Loeber M: The correlation of family management practices and delinquency. Child Dev 55:1299–1317, 1984

Patterson GR, Chamberlain P, Reid JB: A comparative evaluation of parent training procedures. Behavior Therapy 13:638–650, 1982

Patterson GR, Bank L, Stoolmiller M: The preadolescent's contributions to disrupted family process, in From Childhood to Adolescence: A Transitional Period? Edited by Montemayor R, Adams GR, Gullotta TP. Newbury Park, CA, Sage, 1990, pp 107–133

Patterson GR, Reid JB, Dishion TJ: A Social Learning Approach, IV: Antisocial Boys. Eugene, OR, Castalia Publishing Co, 1992

Pettit GS, Bates JE: Family interaction patterns and children's behavior problems from infancy to four years. Developmental Psychology 25:413–420, 1989

Pfiffner LJ, O'Leary SG: Effects of maternal discipline and nurturance on toddler's behavior and affect. J Abnorm Child Psychol 17:527–540, 1989

Plomin R, Daniels D: Why are children in the same family so different from one another? The Behavioral and Brain Sciences 10:1–15, 1987

Poznanski EO, Zrull JP: Childhood depression: clinical characteristics of overtly depressed children. Arch Gen Psychiatry 23:8–15, 1970

Puig-Antich J, Blau S, Marx N, et al: Prepubertal major depressive disorder: a pilot study. Journal of the American Academy of Child Psychiatry 17:695–707, 1978

Puig-Antich J, Lukens E, Davies M, et al: Controlled studies of psychosocial functioning in prepubertal major depressive disorders, II: interpersonal relationships after sustained recovery from the affective episode. Arch Gen Psychiatry 42:511–517, 1985

Pulkkinen L: Self-control and continuity from childhood to adolescence, in Life-Span Development and Behavior, Vol 4. Edited by Baltes PB, Brim OG. New York, Academic Press, 1982, pp 63–105

Putallaz M: Maternal behavior and children's sociometric status. Child Dev 58:324–340, 1987

Radke M: The relation of parental authority to children's behavior and attitudes (Monograph No 22). Minneapolis, MN, University of Minnesota Institute of Child Welfare, 1986

Radke-Yarrow M: Parental psychopathology and child risk. Paper presented at Utah State University, Logan, UT, June 1988

Radke-Yarrow M, Campbell JD, Burton RV: Child Rearing: an Inquiry Into the Research and Methods. San Francisco, CA, Jossey-Bass, 1968

Radke-Yarrow M, Campbell JD, Burton RV: Reliability of maternal retrospection: a preliminary report, in Readings in Child Socialization. Edited by Danziger K. Oxford, England, Pergamon, 1970, pp 63–76

Radloff LS: The CES-D scale: a self-report depression scale for research in the general population. Applied Psychological Measurement 12:385–401, 1977

Ramsey E, Walker HM, Shinn MR, et al: Parent management practices and school adjustment. School Psychology Review 18:513–525, 1989

Raskin A, Boothe HH, Reatig NA, et al: Factor analyses of normal and depressed patients' memories of parental behavior. Psychol Rep 29:871–879, 1971

Reese AN, Palmer FH: Factors related to change in mental test performance. Developmental Psychology Monograph 3, 1970

Reid JB (ed): A Social Learning Approach to Family Intervention, II: Observations in Home Settings. Eugene, OR, Castalia Publishing, 1978

Reid JB: Social-interactional patterns in families of abused and nonabused children, in Altruism and Aggression: Biological and Social Origins. Edited by Zahn Waxler C, Cummings EM, Iannotti R. New York, Cambridge University Press, 1986, pp 238–255

Reid JB, Taplin PS, Lorber R: A social interactional approach to the treatment of abusive families, in Violent Behavior: Social Learning Approaches to Prediction, Management, and Treatment. Edited by Stuart RB. New York, Brunner/Mazel, 1981, pp 83–101

Reid JB, Kavanagh KA, Baldwin DV: Abusive parents' perceptions of child problem behaviors: an example of parental bias. J Abnorm Child Psychol 15:457–466, 1987

Robins LN: Deviant children grown up: a sociological and psychiatric study of sociopathic personality. Baltimore, MD, Williams & Wilkins, 1966

Rutter DR: Stress, coping, and development: some issues and some questions. J Child Psychol Psychiatry 22:323–356, 1981

Rutter M: The comorbidity of aggression and depression: diagnostic issues and social cognitive processes. Discussant at the meeting of the Society for Research on Child Development, Kansas City, MO, April 1989

Rutter M: Commentary: some focus and process considerations regarding the effects of parental depression on children. Developmental Psychology 26:60–67, 1990

Rutter M, Garmezy N: Developmental psychopathology, in Handbook of Child Psychology, Vol 4: Socialization, Personality and Social Development. Edited by Mussen PH. New York, John Wiley, 1983, pp 775–912

Rutter M, Giller H: Juvenile Delinquency: Trends and Perspectives. New York, Guilford, 1984

Rutter M, Quinton D: Parental psychiatric disorder: effects on children. Psychol Med 14:853–880, 1984

Rutter M, Shaffer D, Sturge C: A Guide to a Multi-Axial Classification Scheme for Psychiatric Disorders in Childhood and Adolescence. London, England, University of London, 1975

Sawin DG, Parke RD: Inconsistent discipline of aggression in young boys. J Exp Child Psychol 28:525–538, 1979

Schaefer ES, Bayley N: Consistency of maternal behavior from infancy to preadolescence. Journal of Abnormal and Social Psychology 61:1–7, 1960

Schelle J: A brief report on invalidity of parent evaluations of behavior change. J Appl Behav Anal 7:341–343, 1974

Sears RR, Whiting JWM, Nowlis V, et al: Some child-rearing antecedents of aggression and dependency in young children. Genetic Psychology Monograph 47:125–234, 1953

Sears RR, Maccoby EE, Levin H: Patterns of Childrearing. Evanston, IL, Row & Peterson, 1957

Seifer R, Sameroff AJ: Adaptive behavior in young children of emotionally disturbed women. Journal of Applied Developmental Psychology 1:251–276, 1981

Shaffer DR, Brody GH: Parental and peer influences on moral development, in Parent-Child Interaction: Theory, Research, and Prospects. Edited by Henderson RW. New York, Academic Press, 1981, pp 83–125

Shaffer D, Gould MS, Rutter M, et al: Reliability and validity of a psychosocial axis in patients with child psychiatric disorder. J Am Acad Child Adolesc Psychiatry 30:109–115, 1991

Siegal M, Barclay MS: Children's evaluations of fathers' socialization behavior. Developmental Psychology 21:1090–1096, 1985

Siegal M, Cowen J: Appraisals of intervention: the mother's versus the culprit's behavior as determinants of children's evaluations of discipline techniques. Child Dev 55:1760–1766, 1984

Simons RL, Whitbeck LB, Conger RD, et al: Intergenerational transmission of harsh parenting. Developmental Psychology 27:1–13, 1991

Smith TE: Adolescent reactions to attempted parental control and influence techniques. Journal of Marriage and the Family 10:533–542, August, 1983

Snyder JJ: Reinforcement analysis of interaction in problem and nonproblem families. J Abnorm Psychol 86:528–535, 1977

Snyder J, Huntley D: Troubled families and troubled youth: the development of antisocial behavior and depression in children, in Understanding Troubled and Troubling Youth. Edited by Leone PE. Newbury Park, CA, Sage, 1990, pp 194–225

Snyder J, Patterson GR: The effects of consequences on patterns of social interaction: a quasi-experimental approach to reinforcement in natural interaction. Child Dev 57:1257–1268, 1986

Spitzer RL, Endicott J, Robins E: Research Diagnostic Criteria: rationale and reliability. Arch Gen Psychiatry 35:773–782, 1978
Sroufe LA: Attachment and the construction of relationships, in Relationships and Development. Edited by Hartup W, Rubin Z. Hillsdale, NJ, Lawrence Erlbaum Associates, 1986, pp 57–72
Star B: Patterns of family violence. Social Casework 61:339–346, 1980
Stayton DJ, Hogan R, Ainsworth MDS: Infant obedience and maternal behavior: the origins of socialization reconsidered. Child Dev 42:1057–1069, 1971
Steele BF, Pollack CB: A psychiatric study of parents who abuse infants and small children, in The Battered Child. Edited by Heifer RE, Kempe CH. Chicago, IL, University of Chicago Press, 1968, pp 89–133
Steinberg L: Latchkey children and susceptibility to peer pressure: an ecological analysis. Dev Psychol 22:433–439, 1986
Stevens-Long J: The effect of behavioral context on some aspects of adult disciplinary practice and affect. Child Dev 44:476–484, 1973
Stouthamer-Loeber M, Loeber R: Boys who lie. J Abnorm Child Psychol 14:551–564, 1986
Straus M: A sociological perspective on the prevention of wife-beating, in The Social Causes of Husband-Wife Violence. Edited by Straus M, Hofaling G. Minneapolis, MN, University of Minnesota Press, 1980, pp 97–129
Straus M: Ordinary violence, child abuse, and wife-beating: what do they have in common? in The Dark Side of Families: Current Family Violence Research. Edited by Finkelhor D, Gelles R, Hotaling G, et al. Beverly Hills, CA, Sage, 1983, pp 213–234
Straus MA, Kantor GK: Stress and child abuse, in The Battered Child, 4th Edition. Edited by Helfer RE, Kempe RS. Chicago, IL, University of Chicago Press, 1987
Straus M, Gelles R, Steinmetz S: Behind Closed Doors. New York, Anchor Books, 1980
Thomas A, Chess S: Genesis and evolution of behavioral disorders: from infancy to early adult life. Am J Psychiatry 141:1–9, 1984
Trickett PK, Kuczynski L: Children's misbehaviors and parental discipline strategies in abusive and nonabusive families. Developmental Psychology 22:115–123, 1986
van Goor-Lambo G, Orley J, Poustka F, et al: Classification of abnormal psychosocial situations: preliminary report of a revision of a WHO scheme. J Child Psychol Psychiatry 31:229–241, 1990
Vygotsky LS: Mind in Society: The Development of Higher Psychological Processes. Cambridge, MA, Harvard University Press, 1978
Wadsworth MEJ: Roots of Delinquency. New York, Barnes & Noble, 1979
Wahler RG: The insular mother: her problems in parent-child treatment. J Appl Behav Anal 13:207–219, 1980
Wahler RG, Dumas JE: Maintenance factors in coercive mother-child interactions: the compliance and predictability hypotheses. J Appl Behav Anal 13:207–219, 1986
Wahler RG, Fox JJ: Solitary toy play and time out: a family treatment package for children with aggressive and oppositional behavior. J Appl Behav Anal 13:23–39, 1980
Wahler RG, Sansbury LE: The monitoring skills of troubled mothers: their problems in defining child deviance. J Abnorm Child Psychol 18:577–589, 1990
Webster-Stratton C, Hammond M: Predictors of treatment outcome in parent training for families and conduct problem children. Behavior Therapy 21:319–337, 1990
Weintraub S, Winters KC, Neale JM: Competence and vulnerability in children with an affectively disordered parent, in Depression in Young People. Edited by Rutter M, Izard CE, Read PB. New York, Guilford, 1986, pp 205–220

Weissman MM: The depressed mother and her rebellious adolescent, in Children of Depressed Parents: Risk, Identification, and Intervention. Edited by Morrison HL. New York, Grune & Stratton, 1983, pp 99–113
Wells E, Rankin JH: Direct parental controls and delinquency. Criminology 26:203–235, 1988
Welsh R: Severe parental punishment and delinquency. Journal of Clinical Child Psychology, Spring 1976, pp 17–21
West DJ, Farrington D: Who Becomes Delinquent? London, England, Heinemann Educational Books, 1973
West DJ, Farrington D: The Delinquent Way of Life. London, England, Heinemann, 1977
Whiting BB, Edwards CP: Children of Different Worlds: The Formation of Social Behavior. Cambridge, MA, Harvard University Press, 1988
Widom CS: Child abuse, neglect, and adult behavior: research design and findings on criminality, violence, and child abuse. Am J Orthopsychiatry 59:355–367, 1989
Wilson H: Parental supervision: a neglected aspect of delinquency. British Journal of Criminology 20:203–235, 1980
Wilson H: Parental supervision re-examined. British Journal of Criminology 27:215–301, 1987
Wolfe DA, Fairbank JA, Kelly JA, et al: Child abusive parents' physiological responses to stressful and nonstressful behavior in children. Behavioral Assessment 5:363–371, 1983
World Health Organization: Mental Disorders: Glossary and Guide to Their Classification in Accordance With the Ninth Revision of the International Classification of Diseases. Geneva, Switzerland, World Health Organization, 1978
World Health Organization: Draft Multi-Axial Classification of Child Psychiatric Disorders: Axis 5: Associated Abnormal Psychosocial Situations (MNH/PRO/86.1, Revision 1). Geneva, Switzerland, World Health Organization, 1988
World Health Organization: ICD-10 Chapter V: Mental and Behavioral Disorders: Diagnostic Criteria for Research. Geneva, Switzerland, World Health Organization, 1990
Yarrow MR, Campbell JD, Burton RV: Child Rearing: an Inquiry Into Research and Methods. San Francisco, CA, Jossey-Bass, 1968
Yesavage JA, Widrow L: Early parental discipline and adult self-destructive acts. J Nerv Ment Dis 173:74–77, 1985
Yesavage JA, Becker JMT, Werner PW, et al: Family conflict, psychopathology and dangerous behavior by schizophrenics in hospital. Psychiatry Res 8:271–280, 1983
Zahn-Waxler C, Chapman M: Immediate antecedents of caretakers' methods of discipline. Child Psychiatry Hum Dev 12:179–192, 1982
Zahn-Waxler C, Mayfield A, Radke-Yarrow M, et al: A follow-up investigation of offspring of parents with bipolar disorder. Am J Psychiatry 145:506–509, 1988
Zeanah CH, Zeanah PD: Intergenerational transmission of maltreatment: Insights from attachment theory and research. Psychiatry 52:177–196, 1989
Zucker RA: Parental influences on the drinking patterns of their children, in Alcoholism Problems in Women and Children. Edited by Greenblatt M, Schuckit MA. New York, Grune & Stratton, 1976, pp 211–238
Zuravin SJ: Severity of maternal depression and three types of mother-to-child aggression. Am J Orthopsychiatry 59:377–389, 1979
Zussman JB: Relationship of demographic factors to parental discipline techniques. Developmental Psychology 14:685–686, 1978

Chapter 36

Marital and Family Communication Difficulties

John F. Clarkin, Ph.D., and
David J. Miklowitz, Ph.D.

Statement and Significance of the Issues

This chapter is concerned specifically with marital and family communication difficulties and their possible relevance as disorders or a modifying axis in DSM-IV. Several central issues guided this chapter. First, is there empirical support for including marital and family communication difficulties as a disorder in DSM-IV? Such a designation would require research isolating and describing spouse/family communication disturbances that can be reliably rated and show various forms of validity. Second, can diagnostic criteria for communication disturbances be articulated that are precise and observable and thus allow for reliable assessment?

In DSM-III (American Psychiatric Association 1980), couple and family malfunction were conceived as stressors on an individual with a diagnosed mental disorder (Clarkin et al. 1983). This approach was consistent with the general orientation of DSM-III and DSM-III-R (American Psychiatric Association 1987) to perceive disorders as residing in the individual, to consider stressors on an individual, and to construct V codes as possible foci for intervention with interpersonal stressors. In the development of DSM-IV, it was considered timely to review the empirical evidence supporting the introduction of various forms of family malfunction as a disorder either independent of or coexisting with other Axis I and II disorders in family members.

To be a disorder in its own right, marital and family communication difficulties must demonstrate not only reliability of measurement, but also various forms of validity (i.e., construct, concurrent, and predictive). This validity would involve the association of marital and family communication disorders with 1) serious personal dissatisfaction; 2) disruptive behavior such as family arguments leading to violence, separation, and divorce, lack of effective parenting behavior, and behavioral dysfunction in the offspring, and so on; and/or 3) temporal association with diagnosed Axis I and II disorders in family members.

Whatever the relationship between family communication difficulties and individual disorders, we suspect it may be more interactive than linear. This might suggest that treatment of family communication problems is legitimate and necessary in and of itself.

Scope and Method

This chapter on marital and family communication difficulties is limited to the empirical literature, with particular emphasis on marital or family interaction studies, as this literature is more relevant to generating criteria that can be reliably assessed. Published empirical studies were located via PsychLit and Medline computer search programs. Although the anecdotal clinical literature was noted, it was not used as a primary source. We chose this focus and priority on empirical and interactive family research for several reasons. First, to be consistent with the focus of DSM-IV, the emphasis had to be on data-driven information. Second, the empirical work on family interaction data was emphasized more than that on self-report data, as interactional behavior is what the clinician will be observing in assessing families for communication disorders, and self-report data are often suspected of being inaccurate.

In locating and defining specific marital and family communication constructs to review for possible generation of diagnostic criteria, we were guided by the constructs measured in family research questionnaires and rating scales (Clarkin and Glick 1989; Clarkin et al. 1983; Jacob and Tennenbaum 1988) and those isolated in family interaction research (Markman and Notarius 1987). In the forthcoming section, we review a number of relevant marital communication constructs, and in a later section, family communication constructs. Our approach implies that, although each construct can in itself constitute a marital/family communication disorder, a family communication disorder can also be composed of several of these constructs.

Results and Discussion: Spouse/Spouse Communication Difficulties

In examining the categories and constructs of communication difficulty between spouses (or significant others), we emphasize those constructs that 1) have shown reliable assessment in research and 2) have been found to distinguish distressed from nondistressed couples, or distinguish couples where one or both mates manifest significant individual pathology. Some constructs with theoretical importance were found to lack one or both of these criteria and were therefore not utilized in the current recommended criterion set.

All interpersonal behavior is relevant for the study of the marital pair. Benjamin's (1974) "structural analysis of social behavior" model is based on a theory of interpersonal behavior that has been derived from several interpersonal circumplex models (Leary 1957). These models typically assume two perpendicular dimensions of interpersonal behavior, an interdependent axis (domination to emancipation) and an affiliation axis (friendly to hostile), which can capture most salient interpersonal behavior in the resulting quadrants. This seminal organizing view suggests that the constructs we focus on should represent the quadrants defined by the two major axes in relationship to family communication patterns.

Many of the constructs to follow have been validated in patient groups that are defined by symptoms in one member of a pair (e.g., depression) or in which the couple is defined as distressed. Different studies use similar but differing criteria for defining the patient groups. Depression is often defined either in terms of a diagnosis or in terms of a cutoff score on an instrument such as the Hamilton Rating Scale for Depression (Hamilton 1960). Couples defined as distressed are those who complain of marital conflict and/or dissatisfaction and apply for treatment, and/or those who are above a certain cutoff on a marital satisfaction inventory such as the Dyadic Adjustment Scale (Spanier 1976) or the Marital Satisfaction Inventory (D. K. Snyder 1979, 1981).

Communication of Information

Definition and measurement. We consider here the general construct of verbal communication between two or more individuals, with the various aspects of articulation of information and information exchange, its amount and clarity, and the reception of this information by another. In contrast to clear communication, conflicting and double-bind messages have been conceptualized as detrimental to marital and family adjustment (Bateson et al. 1956).

As will be seen later in the family communication section, the concept of communication here is broader than the more narrow and specific concept of communication deviance articulated in reference to schizophrenia and the family environment. Although communication deviance is composed principally of verbal reasoning and cognitive-perceptual disturbances, the broader concept of communication implies the willingness to convey information, the accuracy and clarity of that information, and the accurate decoding of the information by the other.

In addition to the overt verbal communication, we also consider the cognitive constructs thought to be intimately related to the nature and quality of communication. A review (Baucom et al. 1989) delineates five areas of cognitive phenomena that are hypothesized to play important roles in marital communication and maladjustment: 1) selective attention, 2) attributions, 3) expectancies, 4) assumptions, and 5) standards. Not all of these areas have been investigated equally.

Communication can be measured using several family and marital questionnaires: 1) a communication subscale of the Family Assessment Measure (Skinner et al. 1983), 2) the Dyadic Adjustment Scale (Spanier 1976) with a dyadic cohesion subscale, and 3) the Primary Communication Inventory (Navran 1967) with its verbal communication subscale.

Ratings of interpersonal behavior involving self-disclosure, positive solution, negative solution, justification, direct expression, criticism, critique, positive communication, and negative communication can be seen as relating to the general category of communication skills (Markman and Notarius 1987). As an example, Kategoriensystem für Partner-Schafliche Interactions (KPI) (Hahlweg et al. 1984a) codings such as self-disclosure ("I'm too angry to listen to you at the moment"), positive solutions ("I'll sweep the floor if you play with the kids"), problem description ("I think we've got a problem with the kids"), and disagreement ("No, that's not true") provide concrete examples of communication aspects and their verbalizations.

Validity. The substantive research findings concerning the cognitive communication difficulties of distressed couples are presented in Table 36–1. The amount and quality of verbal communication, as measured on the Primary Communication Inventory verbal communication score, has differentiated distressed and nondistressed couples; treatment leads to an improvement in Primary Communication Inventory scores (Ely et al. 1973). In the area of information exchange, there are more inaccuracies in the communication of distressed than nondistressed couples, because of encoding rather than decoding errors. Distressed husbands were distinguished by more encoding and decoding errors as compared with nondistressed husbands (Noller 1981, 1984). Although both distressed and nondistressed couples are relatively inaccurate observers of their own interactional behavior, it is the distressed couples that are comparatively less reliable (Elwood and Jacobson 1982, 1988).

There is a growing literature on the cognitive aspects (e.g., selective attention, attributions, expectancies, assumptions, and standards) that are hypothesized to influence communication importantly. For example, the attributions that distressed partners make about each other's behavior has been explored. Distressed spouses tend to attribute their partner's undesired communication behavior as global and stable (Camper et al. 1988; Fincham and O'Leary 1983). Positive events

Table 36–1. Representative studies of spouse communication difficulties

Study	Type of couple	Results
Communication of information		
Noller 1981	Distressed	Distressed spouses poor on decoding mate's communication
Fincham and O'Leary 1983	Distressed	Distressed spouses attribute global causes for negative behavior
Camper et al. 1988	Distressed	Distressed spouses view negative partner behavior as global and stable
Expression of affect		
Jacobson et al. 1980	Distressed	Distressed spouses more reactive to displeasing behavior than control subjects
Hautzinger et al. 1982	Depressed spouse	Negative and asymmetrical communication, expression of dysphoric and uncomfortable feelings
Hahlweg et al. 1984a	Distressed spouse	Nondistressed couples showed more self-disclosure, agreement, and acceptance than distressed couples
Hooley 1986	Depressed spouse and low/high expressed emotion mate	High expressed emotion exhibit negative critical remarks, disagreement with and nonacceptance of mate
Kowalik and Gotlib 1987	Depressed spouse	Negativity
Gotlib and Whiffen 1989	Depressed versus nondepressed control subjects	Depressed couples characterized by negative affect and negative appraisal of spouse's behavior
Problem solving		
Birchler et al. 1975	Distressed	Distressed couples manifest more negative communication and less positive communication
Vincent et al. 1975	Distressed	Distressed couples admitted more negative problem-solving behavior and less positive problem-solving behavior than control couples
Gottman et al. 1976b	Distressed	Negative reciprocity involves mutual fault finding and cross complaining
Margolin and Wampold 1981	Distressed	Nondistressed couples had higher rates of problem solving and verbal positive and neutral behavior

(continued)

Table 36–1. Representative studies of spouse communication difficulties *(continued)*

Study	Type of couple	Results
Revenstorf et al. 1984	Distressed	Positive reciprocity is less frequent in distressed couples
Biglan et al. 1985	Depressed	Depressed women showed less problem solving and spouses showed less self-disclosure than control couples
Conflict and conflict resolution		
Gottman et al. 1977	Distressed	Chains of reciprocal disagreement and negative behavior
Billings and Moos 1982	Couples	Couples high in interpersonal conflict report more depression
Billings et al. 1983	Depressed spouse	Less cohesion and interpersonal expressiveness and more conflict
Gottman and Krokoff 1989	Couples low and high in marital satisfaction	Defensiveness, stubbornness, and withdrawal predict marital dissatisfaction
Christensen and Shenk 1991	Distressed versus nondistressed	Distressed couples show more avoidance of communication and more demand/withdrawal communication
Structure		
Merikangas et al. 1979	Depressed ($N = 9$)	Regardless of change in depression, significant increase in patient's power in the marriage over time
Barnett and Gotlib 1988	Depressed spouse in remission	Enduring interpersonal dependency

are ignored, and the partner is blamed for negative behavior that is seen as intentional, global, stable, and originating from internal factors. On the other hand, nondistressed individuals give each other credit for positive behavior and overlook and/or exonerate their spouses for negative behavior (Holtzworth-Munroe and Jacobson 1985; Jacobson et al. 1985). One can only speculate as to the evolution or developmental history of these cognitive sets. Because Markman's (1981) data suggest that premarital communication patterns predict later marital conflict, and because a positive set toward the other would be presumed at first marriage, it may be that certain forms of premarital communication predict a growing negative cognitive set toward the other.

In the area of distorted assumptions that can affect marital behavior, Epstein and Eidelson (1981) found that distressed spouses assume that their partners cannot change the relationship and that overt disagreement is destructive. Likewise, there are some data to suggest that unrealistic assumptions and standards about relationships are predictive of general marital distress (Epstein and Eidelson 1981; Jordan and McCormick 1987). In the area of expectations, J. L. Pretzer, N. Epstein, and B. Fleming (The Marital Attitude Survey: a measure of dysfunctional attributions and expectancies, unpublished manuscript, 1985) found that spouses' low efficacy expectations regarding their ability to solve their marital problems were associated with marital distress and depression.

Criteria.

1. Couple does not clarify mutual requests, provide information, and accurately describe problems.
2. Spouse(s) verbalize underlying attributions, assumptions, and expectations that are negative (e.g., spouse is globally negatively intentioned) or exaggerated (e.g., couples should never fight).

Expression of Affect

At its conceptual extremes, communication involves the transmittal of cognitive matters (information) and affective messages. Although in reality all messages have cognitive and emotional content and overtones, it is conceivable that marital pairs could be relatively proficient in one area while deficient and disturbed in the other. When spousal communication is very negative or pejorative, the marriage is likely to be at high risk, and symptoms may develop in one or both mates. Because the direct and indirect expression of affects such as anger, hostility, and resentment seems quite central to both poor problem-solving behavior and low marital satisfaction, we isolate affect from cognition for conceptual clarity and emphasis.

Definition and measurement. Under the heading of expression of affect, we discuss both the direct expression of affect ("I am angry and depressed") and the expression of affectively toned messages that involve evaluation (positive and negative). Family and marital questionnaires address affect in terms of *expressiveness*, a subscale of the Family Environment Scale (Moos and Moos 1981); *affective communication*, a subscale of the Marital Satisfaction Inventory (D. K. Snyder 1979, 1981); *affectional expression*, a subscale of the Dyadic Adjustment Scale (Spanier 1976); and the *affective expression* and *affective involvement* subscales of the Family Adjustment Measure (Skinner et al. 1983). For interaction research, it has been recommended that affect be coded by observing the affective content of both verbalizations and nonverbal behavior (Markman and Notarius 1987).

Validity: expression of dysphoric affect. Depressed and distressed spouses are more likely to express dysphoric affect than nondepressed and nondistressed spouses (Hautzinger et al. 1982; Kowalik and Gotlib 1987). In addition, distressed spouses exchange more negative affect than nondistressed spouses (Schaap 1984). As the expressed emotion literature suggests, not all but certainly a subgroup of spouses of depressed individuals exhibit negative and critical remarks and nonacceptance of the mate (Hooley 1986).

Validity: reactivity to stimuli. In general, distressed couples, as compared with nondistressed couples, are more affectively reactive to ongoing stimuli, whether negative or positive (Jacobson et al. 1980, 1982). There is a greater likelihood that distressed spouses as compared with nondistressed spouses will react negatively to displeasing behavior by the other spouse (Jacobson et al. 1980), and this type of behavior may predict longitudinal marital satisfaction (Markman 1981).

Validity: consequences of reactivity. There is a circular pattern in which negative communication and a lack of positive support and responsiveness to the depressed spouse's behavior elicits hostility and withdrawal from the partner, which in turn elicits more depression and more calls for reassurance by the depressed individual (Baucom and Epstein 1990; Birchler 1986; Hinchcliffe et al. 1978a, 1978b; Klerman et al. 1984). When spouses of depressed mates are rated as high in expressed emotion, their interaction with the depressed spouse is characterized by negative and critical remarks, disagreement with the spouse, and nonacceptance of what the spouse said to them. In turn, depressed spouses showed a low frequency of self-disclosure and a high level of neutral nonverbal behavior (Hooley 1986). Depressed couples, as compared with control couples, are characterized by negative affect following interaction and negative appraisals of spouses' behavior (Gotlib and Whiffen 1989). Couples with a depressed partner exhibit negative and asymmetrical communication, with frequent expressions of dysphoric and uncomfortable feelings (Hautzinger et al. 1982). Depressed couples are most characterized by negativity (Kowalik and Gotlib 1987).

Low self-disclosure. Distressed couples are distinguished from nondistressed counterparts by the relative paucity of disclosure of emotions, wishes, and needs (Hahlweg et al. 1984b). According to the literature on spousal communication related to depression, self-disclosure has been found to be low in the presence of depressed spouses. In addition, negative communication and criticism are frequently present.

Criteria.

1. Affective communication characterized by negative affect (e.g., anger, hostility, jealousy), critical remarks, disagreement with spouse, and nonacceptance of what spouse has communicated.
2. Low frequency of self-disclosure of thoughts, feelings, and wishes.

Deficient Problem Solving

Definition and measurement. Problem solving is a general construct related to how two or more people consider alternative lines of action and proceed to the most optimal action as demanded by a problem situation. One self-report instrument, the Marital Satisfaction Inventory (D. K. Snyder 1979), has a problem-solving communication subscale. In addition, problem-solving behavior is often sampled directly, both as it spontaneously occurs in free-flowing discussion and in the context of solving assigned tasks such as card sorting (Oliveri and Reiss 1981) or the Revealed Differences Technique (Strodbeck 1951) and its modifications (Ferreira 1963).

Validity. Distressed couples manifest more negative communication and fewer positive communication behaviors when solving problems, as rated by observational coding systems (Birchler et al. 1975; Gottman 1979; Gottman et al. 1977; Revenstorf et al. 1984; Schaap 1984; Vincent et al. 1979). Problem-solving behavior is less frequent in depressed couples (Biglan et al. 1985) and more negative in distressed couples (Vincent et al. 1975). Problem escalation (problem solving by spouse 1, followed by negativity by spouse 2, followed by negativity by spouse 1) is also more characteristic of distressed couples (Revenstorf et al. 1984). Furthermore, negative reciprocity, involving mutual fault finding, cross-complaining (Gottman et al. 1976a), and the communication of global and negative attributions, is also greater among distressed than nondistressed couples (Billings 1979; Gottman et al. 1976a; Margolin and Wampold 1981; Raush et al. 1974; Revenstorf et al. 1984). Positive reciprocity is more characteristic of nondistressed couples (Revenstorf et al. 1984), but not in all samples (e.g., Margolin and Wampold 1981).

Criteria.

1. Couple demonstrates inadequate problem solving characterized by poor problem definition, lack of task focus, mutual criticism and complaint, and negative escalation.

Conflict and Conflict Resolution

Conflict resolution is a specific subset of behaviors under the general rubric of problem solving, (i.e., resolving differences of opinion between two or more people).

Definition and measurement. Conflict as a general construct is measured on the dyadic consensus subscale of the Dyadic Adjustment Scale (Spanier 1976) and on the conflict subscale of the Family Environment Scale (Moos and Moos 1981). It is measured by way of self-report, in terms of disagreement about finances, sexual dissatisfaction, and conflict over child-rearing on the Marital Satisfaction Inventory (D. K. Snyder 1979). The Conflict Tactic Scales (Straus 1979) obtain self-report on strategies used to resolve conflicts in families, including reasoning, verbal aggression, and violence.

Interactional ratings of conflict are similar in content. Interactional ratings of agreement, disagreement, and sequences of positive and negative communication, such as on the KPI (Hahlweg et al. 1984a), are all under the umbrella of conflict (Markman and Notarius 1987). Conflict has also been operationalized in interactional speech samples as speech interruptions, simultaneous speech, agreement/disagreement ratios (Jacob 1975), and failure to reach agreement (Farina 1960). More psychodynamic notions of intrapsychic and interpersonal conflict as manifested in marriages (e.g., Dicks 1967) have not been adequately operationalized.

Markman and Notarius (1987) noted that there is much theoretical and operational overlap between the constructs of affect (reviewed earlier) and conflict. High conflict is typically associated with affect that is inappropriately suppressed or negative, whereas the absence of conflict is typically associated with neutral or positive affect.

Validity. Families low in cohesion and expressiveness and high in interpersonal conflict report more depressive symptoms (Billings and Moos 1982). Unipolar depressed patients, compared with nondepressed control subjects, have less supportive marital relationships, and their family environments are characterized by less cohesion and interpersonal expressiveness and more conflict (Billings et al. 1983). Marital distress and low social integration appear to be factors in the etiology of depression (Barnett and Gotlib 1988). In depressed women, interpersonal friction, inhibited communication, and expression of hostility may continue over 8 months despite symptom improvement (Paykel and Weissman 1973).

Although all couples, distressed or not, display conflict, chains of disagreement especially characterize distressed couples (Gottman et al. 1977; Hahlweg et al.

1984b; Margolin and Wampold 1981). The reciprocity of negative behavior, not the reciprocity of positive behavior, is what distinguishes distressed from nondistressed couples (Revenstorf et al. 1984; Schaap 1984).

Christensen and Shenk (1991) used a self-report instrument to investigate the role of constructive communication, avoidance of communication, and "demand withdrawal communication," in which demands by one partner are consistently met with withdrawal by the other partner. Distressed couples (composed of clinic couples and divorcing couples) had less mutual constructive communication, more avoidance of communication, and more demand/withdrawal communication than did nondistressed couples. It is important to note that the wife demand-husband withdrawal pattern was more likely to occur across all groups than the husband demand-wife withdrawal pattern.

In a longitudinal study of the role of conflict resolution in marriage, Gottman and Krokoff (1989) suggested that predictions of short-term and long-term marital satisfaction may be different. Although exchanges involving disagreement and anger relate to dissatisfaction in the short run, they may not be harmful across time. In contrast, longitudinal marital deterioration was best predicted by defensiveness, whining, stubbornness, and withdrawal from interaction.

Criteria.

1. Couple displays sequences of negative communication characterized by criticism, disagreement, negative listening, and refusal to agree.
2. Couple avoids conflict by withdrawal, lack of discussion, and subsequent nonresolution.

Structure

Definition and measurement. For the family to function as a unit, it requires leadership and distribution of functions. One manifestation of the organization and leadership of the family appears in the relative dominance of the marital partners. Leadership, dominance, and power distribution can all have a profound effect on the quality of interaction satisfaction, and on adequate functioning of the spouses, both in ordinary and in stressful circumstances.

Structure as defined here is measured in self-report instruments as a control subscale on the Family Assessment Measure (Skinner et al. 1983) and the Family Environment Scale (Moos and Moos 1981) and as an organizational subscale on the Family Environment Scale (Moos and Moos 1981). In interaction research it has been recommended (Markman and Notarius 1987) that dominance be measured in terms of procedures that assess the consequence of behavior (e.g., influence of dominant one on decisions) rather than who speaks first and/or for the greatest proportion of the time.

Validity. Dominance as measured by verbal frequency has not distinguished functional and dysfunctional families (Jacob 1975). When one spouse is depressed, the power distribution has not always been found to be as theoretically hypothesized (i.e., depressed spouse submissive to dominance of other). Contrary to expectation, Hooper et al. (1977) found that depressed patients produced substantial control-oriented communication with their spouses during an acute depressed episode. In another hospitalized sample, Merikangas et al. (1979) found that, during early sessions, the patient was strongly influenced by the behavior of his or her spouse, but by the last session, there was a more equal balance of power. However, interpersonal functioning involving introversion and interpersonal dependency are enduring abnormalities in the functioning of individuals with remitted depression (Barnett and Gotlib 1988). Because the validity of this construct remains questionable, we are not recommending diagnostic criteria concerning the construct of structure at this time.

Results and Discussion: Parent/Child Communication Difficulties

The literature on parent-offspring communication dysfunction bears a strong resemblance to the spousal communication literature. Many of the same disordered processes (i.e., expression of hostility or excessive criticism, poor information exchange, lack of conflict resolution) are presumed to disrupt healthy family functioning. However, the family communication literature has traditionally focused on family processes that appear to affect, or at least covary with, the appearance of psychopathology in one or more family members. Unlike the marital literature, the independent variable in family studies is often the presence or absence of psychopathology in an offspring or parent, rather than high or low levels of marital distress. In this section, those aspects of family communication disturbance that covary with certain specific Axis I disorders are surveyed.

Communication Deviance

Definition and measurement. Wynne and Singer (1963a, 1963b) observed that the transactional processes of families of concurrently hospitalized schizophrenic patients were often unclear, amorphous, fragmented, or unintelligible. In their research, these high levels of "communication deviance" discriminated parents of schizophrenic patients from parents of borderline, neurotic, antisocial, autistic, and control children (Singer and Wynne 1963, 1965a, 1965b). These writers believed that communication deviance was present prior to, and was etiologically associated with, the appearance of schizophrenia in genetically prone offspring. Subsequent research (Table 36–2) has confirmed the discriminability of parents of schizophrenic persons from parents of nonschizophrenic persons on the basis of high levels of communication deviance, although not always with the degree of group differentiation found in the original studies (Miklowitz and Stackman 1992).

Communication deviance appears to consist of two primary components: disorders of linguistic-verbal reasoning (i.e., unfinished phrases, unintelligibility, odd word usage) and perceptual-cognitive disturbances (i.e., inability to integrate multiple pieces of information into a coherent message, inability to perceive and describe an object or concept accurately). The majority of studies on communication deviance have relied on verbatim transcripts of projective test (i.e., the Rorschach [Rorschach 1949] or Thematic Apperception Test [Murray 1943]) responses from parents as the primary data source for coding communication deviance. Thus, a parent receives a score for unintelligibility if he or she is unable to produce a coherent Thematic Apperception Test story, or if stimuli within the cards are misperceived and then translated incorrectly (e.g., male figures in the cards are seen as female). Because of the reliance on projective data, other investigators have evaluated whether similar speech dysfunction occurs in a family interaction context. At least one study (Velligan et al. 1990) found a correspondence between levels of parental communication deviance as measured in a projective and in an interactional context, although not all forms of communication deviance were measurable in both contexts.

Validity. Are levels of communication deviance related to the onset of major mental disorders? In a 15-year follow-up of a cohort of disturbed, nonpsychotic adolescents, Goldstein (1987) found that the initial level of communication deviance among parents, as measured by Thematic Apperception Test responses, was the best individual predictor of the onset of "broad" schizophrenia spectrum disorders (schizophrenia or personality disorders with associated psychotic processes) among these adolescents followed into adulthood. Results were not explained by the level or type of disturbance initially shown by these adolescents. In parallel, other studies (Asarnow et al. 1988; Doane et al. 1982) demonstrated that high levels of communication deviance predict certain childhood syndromes (i.e., low social competence, schizotypal attributes, chronic disturbance) that may predispose children to develop schizophrenia in adulthood, although follow-up of these samples is incomplete.

Is communication deviance a reaction among parents to thought disorder or

Table 36–2. Representative studies of family communication difficulties

Study	Diagnosis	Results
Communication deviance		
Wynne et al. 1977	Psychiatric patients and family members ($N = 114$)	Parents of schizophrenic patients have higher levels of communication deviance than parents of borderline, neurotic, and control individuals
Goldstein 1987	Disturbed adolescents ($N = 64$)	Levels of parental communication deviance were strongly predictive of offspring schizophrenia spectrum disorder at 5-year follow-up
Nuechterlein et al. 1989	Schizophrenic patients ($N = 40$)	Levels of communication deviance in mothers associated with offspring attentional disturbance
Affective communication		
Kreisman et al. 1979	Schizophrenic patients ($N = 133$)	Self-reported parental rejection of patient associated with relapse at 18 months
Nuechterlein et al. 1986	Schizophrenic patients (recent-onset) ($N = 27$)	High parental expressed emotion criticism associated with increased relapse risk at 1-year follow-up
Hooley and Teasdale 1989	Nonpsychotic depressive patients ($N = 39$)	High spousal criticism and high levels of criticism perceived by patients associated with relapse at 9 months
Emotional overinvolvement		
Miklowitz et al. 1983	Schizophrenic patients ($N = 42$)	Parental emotional overinvolvement associated with poor premorbid adjustment and more residual symptoms in patients
Vaughn et al. 1984	Schizophrenic patients ($N = 57$)	Emotional overinvolvement (based on expressed emotion criteria) associated with relapse at 9-month follow-up
Zweig-Frank and Paris 1991	Borderline ($n = 62$) and nonborderline ($n = 99$) patients	Borderline patients reported their parents to have been more protective and less caring

(continued)

Table 36–2. Representative studies of family communication difficulties *(continued)*

Study	Diagnosis	Results
Coercive family processes		
J. J. Snyder 1977	Problem families ($n = 10$) and non-problem families ($n = 10$)	In problem families, aversive consequences for displeasing behavior increased its occurrence
Patterson 1982	Socially aggressive ($n = 34$), stealing ($n = 37$), and control ($n = 36$) children	Family members from clinical samples had higher rates of total aversive behavior
Deficits in family problem solving		
Blechman and McEnroe 1985	Families of school-age children ($N = 566$)	Families who were good at solving definite-solution problems generated more satisfactory solutions to indefinite-solution tasks and had more competent children
Reiss et al. 1986	End-stage renal disease patients and their families ($N = 23$)	Patients from families that demonstrated openness to new information when solving pattern-recognition problems were at lower risk for future medical complications
Forehand et al. 1990	Families of adolescents from intact and divorced homes ($N = 214$)	Parenting skills, particularly problem solving, discriminated mothers from intact and divorced homes and predicted adolescent functioning

severe psychopathology in the offspring? Levels of communication deviance in parents are only modestly correlated with levels of thought disorder in affected offspring, and parental communication deviance continues to predict offspring disturbance even when the offspring's level of speech deviance or severity of clinical condition is covaried (Goldstein 1987; Johnston and Holzman 1979; Wynne et al. 1977). However, because the majority of research on communication deviance has used samples already diagnosed with schizophrenia, this question deserves further exploration.

Is communication deviance a marker of a genetic predisposition to psychopathology? Because certain types of communication deviance suggest information-processing disturbances, the latter of which are presumed to be largely genetically acquired in schizophrenia (Nuechterlein and Dawson 1984), the question arises as to whether communication deviance is simply a reflection of a genetic vulnerability to schizophrenia in parents of affected offspring. One study suggested that parents of schizophrenic patients who show high levels of the perceptual-cognitive forms of communication deviance are themselves more likely to show dysfunction on information-processing tasks (Wagener et al. 1986). However, levels of communication deviance are uncorrelated with the presence or absence of DSM-III-R diagnoses in parents (current or past) or with level of functional impairment as measured by the Global Assessment Scale (Endicott et al. 1976; Goldstein et al. 1990). Furthermore, levels of parental communication deviance continue to predict offspring schizophrenia even when these parents' own levels of psychiatric disturbance are covaried (Wynne et al. 1977). However, it may be that communication deviance reflects a subclinical marker of psychopathology that is not always manifested as a diagnosable disorder.

Summary and criteria. Studies of communication deviance suggest that high levels of communication deviance are a correlate of severe psychiatric conditions and may influence the development of these conditions, although it is premature to refer to communication deviance as an etiological agent in schizophrenia or other disorders. High levels of communication deviance may be modifiable via family communication skills training (Velligan et al. 1991) and, therefore, deserve consideration by the clinician. The construct is operationalized as any one of the following, with the presumption that these characteristics are central, readily observable features of the family's transactional processes, occur reasonably frequently, and are not only a feature of the communication of the ill offspring.

1. Lack of shared focus of attention: there is no apparent agreement on the topic of conversation. The listener is confused as to what is being discussed. Persons, places, or things are frequently referred to as "that," "there," or "him," without any apparent agreement as to who or what is being discussed.
2. Unintelligibility: parents or other family members frequently use phrases that cannot be understood by a listener within the context of conversation.
3. Odd word usage: words are used in unusual ways, are out of expected order, or are left out of phrases. Alternatively, too many, often unnecessary words are used to complete phrases (e.g., "It's gonna be up and downwards along the process all the while to go through something like this").
4. Idea abandonment: sentences are not completed or are left trailing. The listener is confused as to whether a new topic or idea has been broached.
5. Tangential, inappropriate responses: speakers bring up irrelevant topics in

Marital and Family Communication Difficulties

response to, or do not acknowledge, each other's statements. Speakers are often distracted by irrelevant stimuli in the room and often use these stimuli to change topics.

Communication: Affective Domain

As in couples, families may be able to communicate clearly but may deliver messages that are highly critical, pejorative, hostile, or vilifying. Although some degree of this type of communication is to be expected in every family, an excessive number or duration of negatively toned interactions may become associated with disturbance in one or more family members. Although it is not unusual for one family member to be the primary source of hostile emotional communication and another the primary target, it is also common for other family members to "aid and abet" these types of interchanges.

Definition and measurement. Negatively toned communication can consist of intensely personal, "character-assassinating" remarks (e.g., "You are an incompetent person") or, alternatively, an excessive number of specifically delineated criticisms of a person's behavior (e.g., "You never try hard in school"). It is also common to see "negatively escalating cycles" in which criticism by one family member is countered by criticism from the family member who was the target of the first criticism, which, in turn, is followed by counter-criticism from the first family member. These cycles become increasingly pejorative and personal as they continue. Often, these cycles are accompanied by negative, defensive, nonverbal behavior that also escalates (Hahlweg et al. 1989).

In the literature (see Table 36-2), negatively toned communication has been measured primarily via structured interviews of individual family members (i.e., the Camberwell Family Interview for rating expressed emotion [Vaughn and Leff 1976]) and through observation and coding of family interactions (e.g., the affective style coding system [Doane et al. 1981, 1985] or the KPI [Hahlweg et al. 1984a, 1989]). Studies using self-report instruments have also yielded interesting results (Haas et al. 1988; Hooley and Teasdale 1989; Kreisman et al. 1979).

Validity: expressed emotion studies. There is now evidence from at least 12 studies to suggest that excessive criticism from key relatives, as measured by the individually administered Camberwell Family Interview (Vaughn and Leff 1976), is prospectively associated with the course of mental disorders, including schizophrenia (Brown et al. 1962, 1972; Jenkins et al. 1986; Moline et al. 1985; Nuechterlein et al. 1986; Tarrier et al. 1988; Vaughn and Leff 1976; Vaughn et al. 1984), bipolar affective disorder (Miklowitz et al. 1988), nonpsychotic depression (Hooley et al. 1986; Vaughn and Leff 1976), and obesity (Fischmann-Havstad and Marston 1984). This literature is reviewed by Goldstein et al. (Chapter 34, this volume).

Family Interaction Studies

There is also evidence for the prognostic utility of negatively toned family interactions. In the 15-year prospective study of nonpsychotic, disturbed adolescents discussed earlier (Goldstein 1987), affective negativity in parent-to-adolescent interactions was independently predictive (along with the family's level of communication deviance) of the severity of outcomes observed in these adolescents at 15-year follow-up. Affective negativity was defined as 1) at least one intensely personal parent-to-offspring criticism or guilt-inducing statement, or 2) an excessive number of "mind-reading" or intrusive statements, during a 10-minute family problem-solving discussion. In parallel, Doane et al. (1985), using similar procedures and construct definitions, found that the level of affective negativity during interaction of parents of schizophrenic patients, measured after the patient's hospital discharge, was associated with the risk of patient relapse at 9-month follow-up. Miklowitz et al. (1988) found a similar prospective relation in a sample of recently discharged bipolar affective patients. Finally, Doane et al. (1986), in a controlled family treatment study, found that family treatment was most effective in delaying new episodes of schizophrenia if it was successful in reducing the number of critical comments and intrusive, "mind-reading" statements observed among parents during pretreatment family interaction.

Several studies of families of diagnosable or at-risk offspring have observed consistencies in parental critical behavior when comparing data from structured interviews with that from family interactions. For instance, high expressed emotion, critical relatives, based on the Camberwell Family Interview, are also highly critical in direct interaction (Miklowitz et al. 1984, 1989; Strachan et al. 1986; Valone et al. 1983). Furthermore, high expressed emotion, critical attitudes among parents of schizophrenic patients are associated with negative escalation cycles that are mutually generated by the critical parent and target schizophrenic patient (Hahlweg et al. 1989; Strachan et al. 1989).

Self-report studies. Several studies suggest that emotional negativity in the family milieu can be measured via self-report instruments. Kreisman et al. (1979) reported in a large sample of schizophrenic patients a significant correlation between degree of rejection of the patient reported by relatives on a Likert scale and the patient's likelihood of rehospitalization 18 months after discharge. Hooley and Teasdale (1989) reported that the amount of criticism depressed patients reported they experienced from their spouses ("perceived criticism") was an even stronger predictor of depressive relapse at 9-month follow-up than was the spouses' actual level of expressed emotion or number of expressed emotion criticisms (although the latter measures were also prognostically significant). Similar prospective findings using self-report data were reported by Parker et al. (1979) for depressed patients, Haas et al. (1988) for affective patients, and Warner and Atkinson (1988) for schizophrenic patients.

Criteria.

1. *Undirectional* negative affective communication characterized by 1) markedly personal, hostile criticism or guilt-inducing statements (e.g., "You enjoy being mean to others") or 2) an excessive number of specific criticisms of another family member's behavior (i.e., more than five nonreciprocated criticisms in a 10-minute interaction). Criticism may be directed from parent to offspring or offspring to parent, but is rarely reciprocated by the targeted family member. Criticisms are rarely "constructive" and are not usually accompanied by suggestions for improving relations.
2. *Negatively escalating cycles* between parent and offspring, marked by *mutually produced, mutually reciprocated* "chains" of pejorative, hostile comments that become more personal as they continue. These cycles may be accompanied by negative nonverbal behavior (e.g., frowns, arms folded across chest) and are also frequently associated with low levels of self-disclosure of feelings, needs, or wishes on the part of both family members.

Communication: Overinvolvement

Some parent-offspring relationships are marked by unclear boundaries and overdependence, often inhibiting the offspring's ability to separate, individuate, or recover from illness (Minuchin 1974). With respect to psychiatric disorders, it is not unusual to see a pairing of an overprotective, "overinvolved" parent with a highly disabled, passive, withdrawn offspring (Table 36–2). Because ill offspring in these families often elicit such responses, an overinvolved relationship is best thought of as a dyadic attribute rather than a problem generated by a parent. Overinvolvement is difficult to define or assess in parents of school-age children, although it may indeed characterize such parents as well as those of adolescents (Asarnow et al. 1987).

Definition and measurement. Parental overinvolvement has been defined in various ways in the psychiatric literature (Parker 1982), but the criteria used within the expressed emotion coding system (Leff and Vaughn 1985) are the best operationalized: a tendency to be overprotective, overly concerned about, or overly controlling of or domineering toward an offspring; to engage in numerous "self-sacrificing" behaviors in the name of good parenting (e.g., the parent denies him- or herself social relationships to satisfy the needs of the offspring); to engage in "intrusive," boundary-crossing interactions with the offspring; and to react to minor events affecting the child with exaggerated emotional responses and to overdramatize these incidents. In return, the offspring may react with overt struggles for independence or autonomy, or, in contrast, passivity, withdrawal, and overdependency.

Early research on overprotectiveness among parents of schizophrenic patients relied almost exclusively on retrospective case reports. The expressed emotion criteria cited have improved on this situation to some degree, as has the Doane et al. (1981) definition of excessive "intrusiveness" during parent-offspring family discussions: a tendency for the parent to frequently talk *for* the offspring and interpret his or her feelings, thoughts, or needs without the offspring expressing these internal states or even agreeing to their existence. Furthermore, Parker et al.'s (1979) well-validated Parental Bonding Instrument has provided a working definition of overprotection: parental overcontrol, intrusion, excessive contact, and preventing the child from acting independently (Parker 1983). Judging an overinvolved relationship, however, still requires a degree of abstraction on the part of the observer.

Validity. A number of studies in the 1950s and 1960s indicated that overprotectiveness characterized the parents of schizophrenic patients (Parker 1982). However, many of these studies were uncontrolled (Clardy 1951; Lidz et al. 1964; Reichard and Tillman 1950; Tietze 1949; Wahl 1954, 1956), and others contained control or comparison groups that were inadequately matched (Alanen 1958, 1966; Freeman and Grayson 1955; Garmezy et al. 1961; Gerard and Siegel 1950; Horowitz and Lovell 1960; Kohn and Clausen 1956; Lane and Singer 1957; Lu 1961; Mark 1953; McGhie 1961a, 1961b; McKeown 1950). Nonreplications were also reported (Gardner 1967; Waring and Ricks 1965; Zuckerman et al. 1958). The findings of these studies were often compromised by observer biases, sample selection biases, reliance on retrospective data, diagnostic ambiguities, unclear definitions of overprotectiveness, and inadequate handling of third variables.

More recent studies of expressed emotion suggest that overinvolvement is a risk factor for later episodes of psychosis among diagnosed schizophrenic patients, independent of the level of criticism demonstrated by the family (Brown et al. 1972; Leff and Vaughn 1985; Vaughn and Leff 1976; Vaughn et al. 1984). Subsequent expressed emotion studies and studies of family interaction have delineated other characteristics of overinvolved relationships in families of schizophrenic patients.

Schizophrenic patients in emotionally overinvolved families are more likely than those from normally involved families of schizophrenic patients to have had poor premorbid social adjustment and a high level of residual symptoms between episodes (Miklowitz et al. 1983).

Overinvolvement is infrequently observed among parents of recent onset schizophrenic patients (Nuechterlein et al. 1986). However, it is reasonably common among families of chronic patients (Miklowitz et al. 1986).

Emotionally overinvolved parents of schizophrenic patients are more likely than normally involved parents of schizophrenic patients to use an excessive number of intrusive, "mind-reading" statements in direct family interaction (Miklowitz et al. 1984). They are also characterized by high levels of communication deviance (Miklowitz et al. 1986).

Other investigators have evaluated whether a patient's recollections of an overprotective relationship with a parent are related to specific psychiatric conditions. Parker (1979, 1983) compared 50 adult patients with "neurotic depression" and 50 patients with manic depression with 50 matched control subjects on their recollections of the parenting behavior of their natural (rearing) parents, based on the self-report Parental Bonding Instrument. Patients with neurotic depression were more likely to rate their parents as overprotective and low in caring than were parents from either of the other two groups. Similarly, Zweig-Frank and Paris (1991), also using the Parent Bonding Instrument, reported that patients with borderline personality disorder rated both parents as more protective and less caring than did nonborderline patients. Of course, the effects of retrospective bias in reporting early parenting experiences cannot be ruled out in these studies.

Criteria.

1. Parental attitudes, whether directly stated or implied, that suggest overprotectiveness, overconcern, exaggerated emotional responses, overdependence, domination, self-sacrifice, or poorly defined boundaries in the relationship with the target offspring.
2. An excessive number (i.e., more than five in a 10-minute discussion) of intrusive statements in direct interaction with the offspring, that is, statements that imply the parent has knowledge of the offspring's inner feelings, thoughts, or aspirations beyond what the offspring has actually stated (e.g., "You know you really want to be an assertive person").
3. The offspring frequently complains about lack of autonomy or lack of privacy, but complies with the parents' attempts at domination. Alternatively, the offspring is passive, withdrawn, dependent, and socially avoidant and defers to the judgment of the parent on most matters.

Communication: Coercive Family Processes

Definition and measurement. When two individuals within a family (i.e., a parent and child) are controlling each others' behavior via aversive stimuli or responses, responses that are perceived by these individuals and/or by others in the family as unpleasant, a "coercive entrapment" has developed (Patterson 1982) (Table 36–2). The key ingredient to such entrapment is negative reinforcement. In this model, children first learn to perform mild, relatively innocuous aversive behaviors (e.g., whining, teasing, running back and forth, negativism) as a way of terminating aversive behaviors from a parent (e.g., scolding, issuing negative commands). The result is that the parent eventually responds in a neutral or positive way to terminate the child's aversive behavior. For the child, his or her aversive behavior has terminated the original aversive parental behavior (e.g., scolding). For the parent, his or her acquiescence has terminated the child's aversive behavior (e.g., whining). In this manner, the parent's attempts to discipline the child often have the effect of reinforcing the child's coercive behaviors (Patterson et al. 1991).

In families, coercive entrapment between a parent and child is believed to reinforce aggressive behavior in the child, aggression that may generalize to other settings (Patterson 1982). In addition, the aversive behaviors on the part of the child may escalate as this family interactional pattern continues, from minor coercive behaviors (e.g., whining) to more intense (if less frequent) coercive behaviors (e.g., hitting, temper tantrums, stealing). Indeed, coercive exchanges can be thought of as a series of "rounds" that escalate in severity and increase the probability that one or more family members (the child or the parent) will react aggressively (Robinson and Jacobson 1987).

Measurement. Measurement of coercive processes usually requires that the observer watch the family interact directly, because these processes often occur on a "behavior-exchange" rather than a "verbal-exchange" level. In this way, coercive processes are to be distinguished from affectively negative verbal exchanges.

Perhaps the best-known system for coding coercive processes is the Family Interaction Coding System (Patterson 1982; Patterson et al. 1969). This system is a home observation system in which positive, neutral, and negative behaviors on the part of all family members are coded sequentially by live observers, in contiguous 6-second time blocks. Interrater reliabilities for the system have been consistently high across studies (Robinson and Jacobson 1987).

Validity. The following research studies are a sample of those that provide validation for the association between highly coercive family relationships and antisocial or aggressive behavior in offspring.

Members of families (mothers, fathers, siblings) containing children who are socially aggressive ($n = 34$) or who are stealers ($n = 37$) engage in higher rates of aversive behavior than do members of families containing control children ($n = 36$) (Patterson 1982; Patterson et al. 1991). In other studies, mothers of children with conduct problems have been found to be more likely to initiate and continue unpleasant, aversive interchanges with the index child than mothers of control children (Lobitz and Johnson 1975; Patterson 1982; Patterson and Cobb 1970). In parallel, behavior-problem children are more likely to continue coercive interchanges with their mothers than are control children (Patterson 1982).

In a sample of 10 "problem" families (families containing a disturbed child or characterized by marital disturbance) and 10 nonproblem families completing a 45-minute interaction task (J. J. Snyder 1977), members of problem families (mothers, fathers, index children) were found to produce "displeasing" behaviors at a rate twice that of members of nonproblem families. Furthermore, among problem families, aversive consequences (punishment) for the "displeasing" behavior of one family member actually led to an increase in the recurrence of these behaviors in this family member over baseline. In nonproblem families, aversive consequences tended to decrease the recurrence of aversive behaviors.

Approximately 22% of the aversive behavior of aggressive children is negatively reinforced by parents (i.e., the aversive child behavior terminates a negative parental behavior), in comparison with approximately 13%–16% of the behavior of control children (Patterson 1982). However, this may be due in part to the higher base rate of aversive behavior among families of aggressive children (Robinson and Jacobson 1987).

The parents of problem children provide more positive consequences for aversive or deviant child behavior than do the parents of nonproblem children (Sallows 1972; Shaw 1971). In parallel, problem children are more likely to be punished for positive behavior than are nonproblem children (Shaw 1971; Taplin 1974).

In comparison with nonproblem children, aggressive children are more likely to respond to aversive maternal behavior with an increase in their own aversive behavior (a coercive cycle), acting as if the mother's aversive behavior were a reward. In contrast, aversive maternal behavior tends to suppress prosocial behavior on the part of the aggressive child (Kopfstein 1972; Patterson and Cobb 1970; Wahler and Dumas 1987). This pattern of aversive parental behavior following a prosocial child behavior is less frequently observed in families of nonproblem children (J. J. Snyder 1977).

"Bursts" of coercive responding in aggressive children, initially triggered by aversive parental behavior, usually lead to positive behavior on the part of mothers or at least to a discontinuation of maternal aversive behavior (Patterson 1976).

When mothers and their aggressive children show evidence of bidirectional "coercive entrapment," a lower number of positive interchanges is observed than in families with no entrapment (Burgess and Conger 1978). Perhaps as a consequence, coercive relationships are frequently associated with depression in one or more family members (Patterson 1980).

Criteria.

1. In identifying coercive processes within a family, the observer must look for strings of negative reinforcement contingencies. A clue to these processes is a high rate of escalating negative interchanges. The key events are cycles in which an aversive behavior is emitted by one family member (often a parent), followed by an equally aversive or more aversive behavior from another family member (often a child). The second family member's behavior serves to decrease the probability that the first member's behavior will occur again.
2. Aversive behaviors in children may include whining, verbal negativism, refusal to comply with a command, teasing, yelling, crying, ignoring, physical aggression, increased motor activity, and other behaviors. In adults, aversive behaviors may include threats, scolding, insults, humiliations, negative commands, yelling, and in extreme cases, various forms of corporal punishment (Patterson 1982; Robinson and Jacobson 1987).
3. Coercive processes may be accompanied by any of the following: 1) *crossover:* one family member initiates a negative interchange after another family member has performed a neutral or prosocial behavior; 2) *counterattack:* one family member issues an aversive response and a second family member issues an equally or more aversive consequent; 3) *punishment acceleration:* an aversive interaction is followed by the performance of a behavior by one family member that increases the probability that additional aversive responses by other family members will result; and 4) *persistence:* one or more family members continue or increase their rate of aversive responses even if other family members have attempted to end the negative interchange (Wahler and Dumas 1987).

Deficits in Family Problem Solving

Definition. It is common for families who seek treatment to be unable to solve major family problems; this is often the very reason they seek treatment. However, when families do not have the *skills* for solving problems in general, such as the ability to define a problem or generate possible solutions to it, they may become "stuck" in ways that prevent the growth or individuation of one or more members (Table 36–2).

To solve family problems adequately, several conditions and steps must take place: 1) all concerned family members must demonstrate a *willingness* at least to try to solve the problem, 2) the problem must be adequately *defined*, 3) possible *solutions* must be generated and realistically evaluated, 4) an *agreement* must take place in which multiple family members choose a solution or combination of solutions that is deemed best for all concerned, and 5) steps are taken to *implement* these solutions (Falloon et al. 1984; Liberman 1988).

When a family is deficient in solving problems, the tension level in the household is likely to increase, and conflict between members tends to escalate. In such a family climate, developing children do not learn to recognize the steps necessary to solve interpersonal problems and may develop psychiatric problems, or their social or academic competence may suffer (Blechman 1991).

Measurement. In the family literature, measurement of problem-solving skills has typically involved an unstructured task such as a directed family problem-solving exercise (Strodbeck 1954) or a semistructured family task such as attempting as a family to build a tower using building blocks (Goldberg and Maccoby 1965). Criterion variables generated by these tasks have included tabulations of problem-solving enhancement statements during direct interaction (Doane et al. 1986), the number of blocks the family puts together to build a tower (Blechman and McEnroe 1985), the number of questions necessary to resolve (as a family) a 20-questions task (Taylor and Faust 1952), or the family's self-rated satisfaction with an indefinite-solution task such as planning a vacation together (Blechman and McEnroe 1985).

In other studies, family members work independently in attempting to solve problems but can consult each other (Reiss et al. 1986). In these studies, problem solving may be measured by such attributes as the level of coordination shown by family members in solving a given problem (e.g., recognizing patterns in an array of symbols) or the family's openness to new information from each other or its ability to change solutions to accommodate new data ("delayed closure") (Reiss et al. 1986).

Validity. Using a pattern-recognition procedure, Reiss et al. (1986) found that, among 23 families in which one member had end-stage renal disease requiring long-term hemodialysis, "delayed closure" family problem-solving scores were associated with lack of medical complications over a 9-month prospective follow-up period. That is, those "environment-sensitive" families (Reiss 1971) who showed an openness to new information and an unwillingness to accept "quick fix" solutions were the most willing to recognize and seek help for early signs of medical complications in the affected family member.

In general, a strong relation has been found in the literature between the way parents solve socialization problems of their children and the cognitive abilities of these children (Al-Khayyal 1980; Baumrind 1975; Bee et al. 1982; Bradley and Caldwell 1980; Gottfried and Gottfried 1983; Hess and Shipman 1965). For example, in a study of 566 school-age children, Blechman and McEnroe (1985) found that those families who built the tallest towers in a cooperative task were those with the most academically and socially competent children. Perhaps more significant was their finding that a family's combined performance on the two definite solution tasks (tower building and 20 questions) was the best predictor of its performance on the indefinite solution, plan-something-together task, suggesting a degree of cross-situational stability in family problem-solving skills. Finally, similar to the Reiss et al. (1986) study, families who were effective at the two definite-solution tasks were slower to generate solutions to the indefinite solution task, whereas families ineffective at definite-solution tasks approached the indefinite solution task with quick solutions that were generally rated as unsatisfactory by the family.

Among 22 families of diabetic adolescents, 35 families of previously psychiatrically hospitalized adolescents, and 39 nonproblem adolescents, Powers et al. (1985) found that families of psychiatric patients were more passive and expressed less confidence in their coping and problem-solving strategies than the other samples.

Among 214 young adolescents from intact ($n = 121$) and recently divorced ($n = 93$) families, Forehand et al. (1990) found that, during direct interaction between mothers and these adolescents, mothers' problem-solving scores (i.e., ability to define a problem clearly and propose alternative solutions) and positive communication scores (i.e., acknowledgments, openness to others' opinions) were higher when these mothers were from intact than from divorced families. Conflict initiation occurred more frequently among divorced than married mothers. Perhaps most significantly, these parenting skills predicted adolescent functioning in the domains of cognitive and social competence.

Falloon et al. (1984) found that a communication and problem-solving-oriented family treatment (behavioral family management) was far more effective in delaying episodes of psychosis among 36 recently hospitalized schizophrenic patients than was an individual treatment for the patient of similar duration. In a reanalysis of the Falloon et al. data, Doane et al. (1986) found a marked increase, from baseline to 3-month follow-up, in the number of spontaneously occurring problem-solving statements among families in family treatment. Little or no change in the frequency of these statements occurred among families in which patients received individual treatment, even though a number of these patients had improved symptomatically during this same time period. Furthermore, increases in problem-solving ability were most notable when a decrease in emotional negativity among parents, as measured by number of critical and intrusive statements (negative affective style), was also observed. Thus, an improved ability by the family to address problems in a structured manner may reduce its need to "ventilate."

Criteria. Problem-solving deficits are suggested by *three or more* of the following.

1. A family raises issues as problems for discussion but then overtly expresses an unwillingness to solve them.
2. A family is unable to define a problem without resorting to changing the subject or bringing in vague generalities (e.g., "The thing is, she's just not a nice person"), or insists on defining problems so broadly as to exclude the possibility of concrete solutions (e.g., "The problem is one of motivation—he has none and never will have any"). The family resists attempts by the clinician to guide solution definition.
3. The family is unable to generate or evaluate the viability of potential solutions to problems. The family "draws a blank" when attempting to generate solutions or cannot distinguish between the value of one solution and another. As a result, solutions to problems are rarely accepted by the family as satisfactory.
4. The family is unable to implement solutions to problems. Solutions are often forgotten, or the steps necessary to implement solutions are never taken.

Two caveats should be applied to the above criteria: 1) the clinician should be able to observe these deficits when the family discusses a wide range of different problems, and 2) it is not necessary that the clinician adopt a "problem-solving skills" orientation to sessions to observe these deficits. Instead, the clinician should be able to glean evidence for these criteria from general discussions of family matters, aided by questions such as "How was that a problem for you?" "Did that problem ever get solved?" and "Did that solution work?"

Comparison of Spouse/Spouse and Parent/Child Communication Deficits

Now that the constructs for spouse/spouse and parent/child communication deficits have been isolated, it is instructive to compare the results (Table 36–3 and Table 36–4). The two areas of affective communication and conflict resolution are almost identical in conceptualization, behavioral criteria, and importance in the spouse/spouse and parent/child communication domains.

There are three rather sharply defined constructs in the parent/child literature that are not represented in the spouse/spouse work: communication deviance, overinvolvement, and coercive process. In the cognitive realm, the communication deviance construct has been investigated with children and parents, but comparable work has not been done with couples. The more general construct of communication has been explored with marital couples, with no theoretical link to thought disorder and schizophrenia. Likewise, the overinvolvement construct has been seen as most relevant with children and parents, and has little predictive utility in samples of adult couples (Hooley et al. 1986; Vaughn and Leff 1976). Coercive processes, the shaping of the behavior of parents by negative behavior on the part of the child, is similar to negative escalation in couples. Although not yet investi-

Table 36–3. Comparison of spouse/spouse and parent/child communication difficulty constructs

Spouse/Spouse	Parent/Child
Communication of information	Communication deviance (related to schizophrenia)
Negative affective communication	Negative affective communication
Deficient problem solving	Deficient problem solving
Deficient conflict resolution	
Structure	Overinvolvement
	Coercive process (similar to negative escalation in couples)

Table 36–4. Representative studies of spouse/spouse and parent/child communication difficulties

Study	Diagnosis	Results
Billings 1979	Distressed ($N = 24$)	Negative reciprocity is greater among distressed as compared with nondistressed couples
Wegener et al. 1979	Distressed ($N = 30$)	Although direct expression of feelings did not differentiate, facilitating listener behavior distinguished the nondistressed couples
Markman 1981	Nondistressed ($N = 9$)	Initial impact ratings of couples' communication predicted marital satisfaction 5.5 years later
Hahlweg et al. 1984b	Distressed ($N = 50$)	Marital treatment resulted in increase in direct expression and accepting/agreeing and decrease in critique and refusal

gated in couples, it is quite conceivable that one spouse could effectively utilize a coercive process with the other spouse.

The area of structure that was explored in the marital literature does not have a comparable literature in the family domain. It would seem that the concept of structure, with the issues of leadership, dominance/submission, and distribution of functions, is equally relevant to marriages and to the entire family. However, this area does not merit criteria at this time because of its unproven validity. This is an area that needs further exploration in reference to both couples and the entire family.

Discussion and Recommendations

The empirical data reviewed here substantiate the existence of communication difficulties that can be reliably assessed. With depression and schizophrenia as exceptions, the data are sparse with reference to each DSM disorder and the coexisting family communication difficulties.

Given the extent and limitations of our current empirical knowledge, one option would be to formulate a set of criteria for a family *disorder* using those general criteria defining communication difficulties that span across diverse individual diagnoses. This set of criteria articulates a "disorder" in the sense that 1) once they begin, these communication difficulties tend to be perpetuating and chronic; 2) the communication difficulties are frequently contemporaneous with or are followed by other serious problems, such as depression or divorce; and 3) the family communication difficulties, even when they apparently result from one member's attempts to cope with a disorder in another family member, have consequences and form a legitimate focus for intervention in and of themselves.

Arguments for considering family communication difficulties as a *disorder* would include the following:

1. At a certain level of severity, family communication difficulties are serious in terms of their consequences, whether or not a disorder in one individual has yet appeared. These family difficulties cause malfunction in the family unit, may threaten the viability of the social unit, and may create stress that causes symptoms to begin to appear in the most vulnerable members of the family. Although not residing in one individual (although it may be mostly dependent on one individual in the family), the family communication disorder is seen as serious in and of itself and potentially leads to or exacerbates symptoms in individuals and in many cases threatens the dissolution of the family unit. It may be diagnosed either in the presence or in the absence of an individual DSM

disorder. The strength and direction of causality between the individual and family disorder is in general empirically undetermined, but this empirical work will be fostered by making family disorders a focus of diagnosis.
2. If individual disorders alone are noted while family/marital disorders are ignored, family pathology can go undiagnosed and therefore will not receive intervention. Clinicians are less likely to apply a V code rather than a bona fide diagnosis and, as a result, may miss important features of the family that bear on the presenting Axis I disorder. Furthermore, family communication difficulties will likely be neglected by the research community, who can obtain federal funding for intervention studies only with DSM-defined disorders.
3. If family communication problems are not made a disorder but rather a V code, the V code implies that the relational disorders are secondary to the individual disorders. Current data suggest that this would be accurate as applied to an Axis I diagnosis of schizophrenia. On the other hand, if a couple presents with a marital conflict problem, a subsequent (in terms of time sequence) individual disorder such as Axis I depression might best be considered secondary to the marital conflict.

The arguments against including spouse/family communication difficulties as a disorder would include the following:

1. Only individual disorders should be included in the diagnostic manual, as it is traditional in medicine to diagnose disorders that reside in an individual. This argument rests on the notion that there is wisdom in tradition.
2. A spouse/family communication disorder would be conceptually different from all other individual disorders in DSM-IV and could set an unfortunate precedent of "diagnosing" multiple social units (e.g., extended family disorders, unmarried cohabitating partners disorder, bridge club interactional disorders, and school classroom disorders).
3. In the absence of data indicating that family disruption exceeds the (diagnosable) pathology in its individual members, the conservative and correct approach, akin to Ocham's razor, is to limit diagnosed disorders to individuals.
4. There is insufficient empirical investigation of the communication disorders as *precursors* of individual pathology. Most of the existing research selects disturbed family units in which one member has an existing disorder (e.g., schizophrenia, acting-out adolescent) and examines the communication difficulties that accompany the disorder. Thus, cause-and-effect relationships between individual disorders and communication difficulties have not been specified experimentally.

It can be argued, however, that parallel situations already exist in DSM-III-R. For example, the frequent comorbidity of depression and alcohol dependence is well documented, although the causal primacy of one disorder over the other is a topic of debate.

A second option would be to include family communication difficulties not as a disorder but as a V code, indicating that family communication difficulties are an important environmental variable that influences the individual who is the locus of diagnosable disorders. This option would be most congenial to those who espouse the arguments against a family communication *disorder* noted earlier, but who also take seriously the empirical examination of family variables in relationship to individual pathology noted in this review. This option seems most congenial to the framers of the *DSM-IV Options Book* (American Psychiatric Association 1991), who list family communication disorders as a V code (to be Z codes in ICD-10).

A third option, independent of treating family communication dysfunction as a disorder, would be the creation of an axis for general family disruption (communication and other family issues covered in other sections of DSM) in the interest of treatment planning when an Axis I or II disorder has been diagnosed in an individual residing in a nuclear family unit. Such an axis would recognize that, when present, family communication difficulties are relevant to all the disorders, either as a contributing cause, as a maintaining variable, or as a means of coping with the disorder. This axis would give special status to the family unit as an important factor in most individual pathology.

A final option would be to totally ignore family communication difficulties in the diagnostic system and leave it up to the individual clinician to consider these data.

Threshold

At what point of severity, frequency, and chronicity do family communication difficulties become a "disorder"? It is conceivable that as family communication difficulties vary in severity and frequency, in some situations family communication difficulties are accompanied by little dysfunction, whereas in other situations dysfunction is quite severe. First, some level of behavioral dysfunction in the presence of family communication difficulties should be used as part of the set of criteria. Second, there is the issue of generalization: do those who manifest communication problems with a spouse/family member manifest these same problems with others and in other contexts? If so, the communication difficulties would reduce to an individual disorder, possibly on Axis II. The literature on this issue is only preliminary, but the available data suggest that some individuals manifest clear communication difficulties with their spouses or other family members and do not manifest these problems with persons outside the family. These findings would argue for a specific marital/family communication disorder, at least in some cases.

Expressed Emotion

Although the DSM-IV Task Force has solicited reviews on multiple areas of family dysfunction for this *Sourcebook,* we think some collapsing across areas would be more helpful and parsimonious for the diagnostic criteria themselves. Most specifically, related to the present review, we recommend that the expressed emotion literature be a specific subset of investigations in the general category of family communication dysfunction. Not content with the Camberwell methodology (Vaughn and Leff 1976) of asking family members how they communicate, many researchers have investigated the actual communication behavior of subjects with various expressed emotion designations (Hooley 1986; Miklowitz et al. 1984; Valone et al. 1983). Most important for diagnostic criteria are the actual communication behaviors observed, which are included in the present review.

Criteria

Total set of criteria for spouse/spouse communication disorder. For a substantial period of time (at least 3 months), functional impairment (e.g., interference with job functioning, poor parenting, symptoms in one or both spouses), and several (*at least two*) of the following.

1. Couple does not clarify mutual requests, provide information, or accurately describe problems.
2. Spouse(s) verbalize underlying attributions, assumptions, and expectations that are negative (e.g., spouse is globally negatively intentioned) or exaggerated (e.g., couples should never fight).
3. Affective communication characterized by negative affect (e.g., anger, hostility, jealousy), critical remarks, disagreement with spouse, and nonacceptance of what the mate has communicated.
4. Low frequency of self-disclosure of thoughts, feelings, and wishes.
5. Couple demonstrates inadequate problem solving characterized by poor problem definition, lack of task focus, mutual criticism and complaint, and negative escalation.
6. Couple displays sequences of negative communication characterized by criticism, disagreement, negative listening, and refusal to agree.
7. Couple avoids conflict by withdrawal, lack of discussion, and subsequent nonresolution.

Associated Features. Associated features of marital communication difficulties/disorders include poor reported marital satisfaction, depression in one or more spouses, threatened and contemplated separation and divorce, or concentration and job performance difficulties.

Total set of criteria for family communication disorders. For at least a 3-month period: functional impairment of family member(s) (e.g., at least one child has psychiatric symptoms or is functioning at a low level of academic or social competence; interference with parents' job functioning; symptoms in parents) and *at least two* of the following.

1. Family is unable to communicate clearly, cannot communicate closure, or cannot share a focus of attention (communication deviance).
2. Family communication is characterized by unidirectional hostility or frequent criticism or by bidirectional, negatively escalating cycles of pejorative or critical comments.
3. Parent-offspring relationships are characterized by overprotectiveness, overconcern, unnecessarily self-sacrificing behaviors, intrusiveness, or overdependence (emotional overinvolvement).
4. Parent-offspring interchanges are marked by negatively reinforcing "coercive cycles" that tend to perpetuate antisocial or aggressive behavior in one or more family members.
5. A broad array of family problems cannot be solved because of the family's inability to agree to try to solve, define, generate, or evaluate solutions to, or implement solutions to, existing problems.

Associated Features. The associated features of parent/child communication difficulties/disorder include adolescent acting-out and disruptive behavior, major psychiatric disorders in one or more family members (e.g., schizophrenia, affective disorder), poor parental morale, and parenting dissatisfaction.

References

Alanen YO: The mothers of schizophrenic patients. Acta Psychiatr Scand Suppl 124:1–361, 1958
Alanen YO: The family in the pathogenesis of schizophrenic and neurotic disorders. Acta Psychiatr Scand Suppl 190:1–654, 1966
Al-Khayyal M: Healthy parental communication as a predictor of child competence in families with a schizophrenic and psychiatrically disturbed nonschizophrenic patient. Unpublished doctoral dissertation, University of Rochester, Rochester, NY, 1980
American Psychiatric Association: Diagnostic and Statistical Manual of Mental Disorders, 3rd Edition. Washington, DC, American Psychiatric Association, 1980
American Psychiatric Association: Diagnostic and Statistical Manual of Mental Disorders, 3rd Edition, Revised. Washington, DC, American Psychiatric Association, 1987
American Psychiatric Association: DSM-IV Options Book: Work in Progress. Washington, DC, American Psychiatric Association, 1991

Asarnow JR, Ben-Meir SL, Goldstein MJ: Family factors in childhood depressive and schizophrenia-spectrum disorders: a preliminary report, in Understanding Major Mental Disorder: the Contribution of Family Interaction Research. Edited by Hahlweg K, Goldstein MJ. New York, Family Process Press, 1987, pp 123–138

Asarnow JR, Goldstein MJ, Ben-Meir S: Parental communication deviance in childhood onset schizophrenia spectrum and depressive disorders. J Child Psychol Psychiatry 29:825–838, 1988

Barnett PA, Gotlib IH: Psychosocial functioning and depression: distinguishing among antecedents, concomitants, and consequences. Psychol Bull 104:97–126, 1988

Bateson D, Jackson DD, Haley J, et al: Towards a theory of schizophrenia. Behav Sci 1:251–264, 1956

Baucom DH, Epstein N: Cognitive-Behavioral Marital Therapy. New York, Brunner/Mazel, 1990

Baucom DH, Epstein N, Sayers S, et al: The role of cognitions in marital relationships: definitional, methodological, and conceptual issues. J Consult Clin Psychol 57:31–38, 1989

Baumrind D: The contributions of the family to the development of competence in children. Schizophr Bull 14:12–37, 1975

Bee HL, Barnard KE, Eyres SJ, et al: Predictions of IQ and language skill from perinatal status, child performance, family characteristics, and mother-infant interaction. Child Dev 53:1134–1156, 1982

Benjamin LS: Structural analysis of social behavior. Psychol Rev 81:392–425, 1974

Biglan A, Hops H, Sherman L, et al: Problem-solving interactions of depressed women and their husbands. Behavior Therapy 16:431–451, 1985

Billings A: Conflict resolution in distressed and nondistressed married couples. J Consult Clin Psychol 47:368–376, 1979

Billings A, Moos RH: Social support and functioning among community and clinical groups: a panel model. J Behav Med 5:295–311, 1982

Billings A, Cronkite RC, Moos RH: Social-environmental factors in unipolar depression: comparisons of depressed patients and nondepressed controls. J Abnorm Psychol 92:119–113, 1983

Birchler GR: Alleviating depression with "marital" intervention. Journal of Psychotherapy and the Family 2:101–116, 1986

Birchler G, Weiss R, Vincent J: Multimethod analysis of social reinforcement exchange between maritally distressed and nondistressed spouses and partners. J Pers Soc Psychol 31:349–360, 1975

Blechman EA: Effective communication: enabling multi-problem families to change, in Advances in Family Research, Vol 2. Edited by Cowan P, Hetherington ME. New York, Lawrence Erlbaum Associates, 1991, pp 219–244

Blechman EA, McEnroe MJ: Effective family problem solving. Child Dev 56:429–437, 1985

Bradley RH, Caldwell BM: The relation of home environment, cognitive competence, and IQ among males and females. Child Dev 51:1140–1148, 1980

Brown GW, Monck EM, Carstairs GM, et al: Influence of family life on the course of schizophrenic illness. Br J Prev Soc Med 16:55–68, 1962

Brown GW, Birley JLT, Wing JK: Influence of family life on the course of schizophrenic disorders: a replication. Br J Psychiatry 121:241–258, 1972

Burgess RL, Conger RD: Family interaction in abusive, neglectful, and normal families. Child Dev 49:1163–1173, 1978

Camper PM, Jacobson NS, Holtzworth-Munroe A, et al: Causal attributions for interactional behaviors in married couples. Cognitive Therapy and Research 12:195–209, 1988

Christensen A, Shenk JL: Communication, conflict, and psychological distance in nondistressed, clinical, and divorcing couples. J Consult Clin Psychol 59:458–463, 1991

Clardy ERA: A study of the development and course of schizophrenic children. Psychiatr Q 25:81–90, 1951

Clarkin JF, Glick ID: Instruments for the assessment of family malfunction, in Measuring Mental Illness: Psychometric Assessment for Clinicians. Edited by Wetzler S. Washington, DC, American Psychiatric Press, 1989, pp 213–227

Clarkin JF, Frances AJ, Perry S: Family classifications and DSM-III, in Group and Family Therapy 1983. Edited by Wolberg LR, Aronson ML. New York, Brunner/Mazel, 1983, pp 220–237

Dicks HV: Marital Tensions. London, England, Routledge & Kegan Paul, 1967

Doane JA, West KL, Goldstein MJ, et al: Parental communication deviance and affective style: predictors of subsequent schizophrenia-spectrum disorders in vulnerable adolescents. Arch Gen Psychiatry 38:679–685, 1981

Doane JA, Jones JE, Fisher L, et al: Parental communication deviance as a predictor of competence in children at risk for adult psychiatric disorder. Fam Process 21:211–223, 1982

Doane JA, Falloon IRH, Goldstein MJ, et al: Parental affective style and the treatment of schizophrenia: predicting course of illness and social functioning. Arch Gen Psychiatry 42:34–42, 1985

Doane JA, Goldstein MJ, Miklowitz DJ, et al: The impact of individual and family treatment on the affective climate of families of schizophrenics. Br J Psychiatry 148:279–287, 1986

Elwood RW, Jacobson NS: Spouse agreement in reporting their behavioral interactions: a clinical replication. J Consult Clin Psychol 50:783–784, 1982

Elwood RW, Jacobson NS: The effects of observational training on spouse agreement about events in their relationship. Behav Res Ther 26:159–167, 1988

Ely AL, Guerney BG, Stover L: Efficacy of the training phase of conjugal therapy. Psychotherapy: Theory, Research & Practice 10:201–207, 1973

Endicott J, Spitzer RL, Fleiss JL, et al: The Global Assessment Scale. Arch Gen Psychiatry 33:766–771, 1976

Epstein NB, Eidelson RJ: Unrealistic beliefs of clinical couples: their relationship to expectations, goals, and satisfaction. Am J Fam Ther 9:13–22, 1981

Falloon IRH, Boyd JL, McGill CW: Family Care of Schizophrenia. New York, Guilford, 1984

Farina A: Patterns of role dominance and conflict in parents of schizophrenic patients. J Abnorm Social Psychol 61:31–38, 1960

Ferreira AJ: Decision-making in normal and pathological families. Arch Gen Psychiatry 13:68–73, 1963

Fincham FD, O'Leary KD: Causal inferences for spouse behavior in maritally distressed and nondistressed couples. J Social Clin Psychol 1:42–57, 1983

Fischmann-Havstad L, Marston AR: Weight loss maintenance as an aspect of family emotion and process. Br J Clin Psychol 23:265–271, 1984

Forehand R, McCombs TA, Wierson M, et al: Role of maternal functioning and parenting skills in adolescent functioning following parental divorce. J Abnorm Psychol 99:278–283, 1990

Freeman RV, Grayson HM: Maternal attitudes in schizophrenia. J Abnorm Soc Psychol 50:45–52, 1955

Gardner GG: The role of maternal psycho-pathology in male and female schizophrenics. J Consult Psychol 31:411–413, 1967

Garmezy N, Clarke AR, Stockner C: Child rearing attitudes of mothers and fathers as reported by schizophrenics and normal patients. J Abnorm Soc Psychol 63:176–182, 1961

Gerard DL, Siegel J: The family background of schizophrenia. Psychiatr Q 24:47–73, 1950

Goldberg MH, Maccoby EE: Children's acquisition of skill in performing a group task under two conditions of group formation. J Pers Soc Psychol 2:898–902, 1965

Goldstein MJ: Family interaction patterns that antedate the onset of schizophrenia and related disorders: a further analysis of data from a longitudinal prospective study, in Understanding Major Mental Disorder: the Contribution of Family Interaction Research. Edited by Hahlweg K, Goldstein M. New York, Family Process Press, 1987, pp 11–32

Goldstein MJ, Talovic SA, Nuechterlein KH: Family interaction vs individual psychopathology: do they indicate the same processes in the families of schizophrenics? Paper presented at the Third International Schizophrenia Symposium, Transactional Processes in Onset and Course of Schizophrenic Disorders, Bern, Switzerland, 1990

Gotlib IH, Whiffen VE: Depression and marital functioning: an examination of specificity and gender differences. J Abnorm Psychol 98:23–30, 1989

Gottfried AW, Gottfried AE: Home environment and mental development in young children of middle-class families, in Home Environment and Early Mental Development: Longitudinal Research. Edited by Gottfried AW. New York, Academic Press, 1983

Gottman JM: Marital Interaction: Empirical Investigations. New York, Academic Press, 1979

Gottman J, Krokoff LJ: Marital interaction and satisfaction: a longitudinal view. J Consult Clin Psychol 57:47–52, 1989

Gottman J, Notarius C, Markman H, et al: Behavior exchange theory and marital decision making. J Pers Soc Psychol 34:14–23, 1976a

Gottman J, Notarius C, Gonso J, et al: A Couple's Guide to Communication. Champaign, IL, Research Press, 1976b

Gottman J, Markman H, Notarius C: The topography of marital conflict: a sequential analysis of verbal and nonverbal behavior. J Mar Fam 39:461–477, 1977

Haas GL, Glick ID, Clarkin JF, et al: Inpatient family intervention: a randomized clinical trial, II: results at hospital discharge. Arch Gen Psychiatry 45:217–224, 1988

Hahlweg K, Reisner L, Kohli G, et al: Development and validity of a new system to analyze interpersonal communication (KPI), in Marital Interaction: Analysis and Modification. Edited by Hahlweg K, Jacobson NS. New York, Guilford, 1984a, pp 182–198

Hahlweg K, Revenstorf D, Schindler L: Effects of behavioral marital therapy on couples' communication and problem-solving skills. J Consult Clin Psychol 52:553–566, 1984b

Hahlweg K, Goldstein MJ, Nuechterlein KH, et al: Expressed emotion and patient-relative interaction in families of recent-onset schizophrenics. J Consult Clin Psychol 57:11–18, 1989

Hamilton M: A rating scale for depression. J Neurol Neurosurg Psychiatry 23:56–61, 1960

Hautzinger M, Linden M, Hoffman N: Distressed couples with and without a depressed partner: an analysis of their verbal interaction. J Behav Ther Exp Psychiatry 13:307–314, 1982

Hess RD, Shipman, VC: Early experience and the socialization of cognitive modes in children. Child Dev 36:869–886, 1965

Hinchcliffe M, Vaughn PW, Hooper D, et al: The melancholy marriage: an inquiry into the interaction of depression, III: responsiveness. Br J Med Psychol 51:1–13, 1978a

Hinchcliffe M, Hooper D, Roberts FJ, et al: The melancholy marriage: an inquiry into the interaction of depression, IV: disruptions. Br J Med Psychol 51:15–24, 1978b

Holtzworth-Munroe A, Jacobson ND: Causal attributions of married couples: when do they search for causes? What do they conclude when they do? J Per Soc Psychol 48:1398–1412, 1985

Hooley JM: Expressed emotion and depression: interactions between patients and high versus low EE spouses. J Abnorm Psychol 95:237–246, 1986

Hooley JM, Teasdale JD: Predictors of relapse in unipolar depressives: expressed emotion, marital distress, and perceived criticism. J Abnorm Psychol 98:229–235, 1989

Hooley JM, Orley J, Teasdale JD: Levels of expressed emotion and relapse in depressed patients. Br J Psychiatry 148:642–647, 1986

Hooper D, Roberts FJ, Hinchliffe MK: The melancholy marriage: an inquiry into the interaction of depression. Br J Med Psychol 50:113–124, 1977

Horowitz FD, Lovell LL: Attitudes of mothers of female schizophrenics. Child Dev 31:299–305, 1960

Jacob T: Family interaction in disturbed and normal families: a methodological and substantive review. Psychol Bull 82:33–65, 1975

Jacob T, Tennenbaum DL: Family Assessment: Rationale, Methods, and Future Directions. New York, Plenum, 1988

Jacobson NS, Waldron H, Moore D: Toward a behavioral profile of marital distress. J Consult Clin Psychol 48:696–703, 1980

Jacobson NS, Follette WC, McDonald DW: Reactivity to positive and negative behavior in distressed and nondistressed married couples. J Consult Clin Psychol 50:706–714, 1982

Jacobson NS, McDonald DW, Follette WC, et al: Attributional processes in distressed and nondistressed married couples. Cognitive Therapy and Research 9:35–50, 1985

Jenkins JH, Karno M, Selva ADL, et al: Expressed emotion, maintenance pharmacotherapy, and schizophrenic relapse among Mexican-Americans. Psychopharmacol Bull 22:621–627, 1986

Johnston MH, Holzman PS: Assessing Schizophrenic Thinking. San Francisco, CA, Jossey-Bass, 1979

Jordan TJ, McCormick NB: The role of sex beliefs in intimate relationships. Paper presented at the annual meeting of the American Association of Sex Educators, Counselors, and Therapists, New York, April 1987

Klerman GL, Weissman MM, Rounsaville BJ, et al: Interpersonal Psychotherapy of Depression. New York, Basic Books, 1984

Kohn M, Clausen JA: Parental authority behavior and schizophrenia. Am J Orthopsychiatry 26:297–313, 1956

Kopfstein D: The effects of accelerating and decelerating consequences on the social behavior of trainable retarded children. Child Dev 43:800–809, 1972

Kowalik D, Gotlib H: Depression and marital interaction: concordance between intent and perception of communications. J Abnorm Psychol 96:127–134, 1987

Kreisman DE, Simmens SJ, Joy VD: Rejecting the patient: preliminary validation of a self-report scale. Schizophr Bull 5:220–222, 1979

Lane RC, Singer JL: Familial attitudes in paranoid schizophrenics and normals from two socioeconomic classes. J Abnorm Soc Psychol 59:328–329, 1957

Leary T: Interpersonal Diagnosis of Personality. New York, Ronald, 1957

Leff J, Vaughn C: Expressed Emotion in Families. New York, Guilford, 1985
Liberman RP: Behavioral family management, in Psychiatric Rehabilitation of Chronic Mental Patients. Edited by Liberman RP. Washington, DC, American Psychiatric Press, 1988, pp 199–244
Lidz T, Cornelison AR, Singer MT, et al: The mothers of schizophrenic patients, in Schizophrenia and the Family. Edited by Lidz T, Fleck S, Cornelison AR. New York, International Universities Press, 1964, pp 290–335
Lobitz WC, Johnson SM: Parental manipulation of the behavior of normal and deviant children. Child Dev 46:719–726, 1975
Lu Y-C: Mother-child role relations in schizophrenia. Psychiatry 24:133–142, 1961
Margolin G, Wampold BE: Sequential analysis of conflict and accord in distressed and nondistressed marital partners. J Consult Clin Psychol 49:554–567, 1981
Mark JC: The attitudes of the mothers of male schizophrenics towards child behavior. J Abnorm Soc Psychol 48:185–189, 1953
Markman HJ: The prediction of marital distress: a five year follow-up. J Consult Clin Psychol 49:760–762, 1981
Markman HJ, Notarius CI: Coding marital and family interaction: current status, in Family Interaction and Psychopathology. Edited by Jacob T. New York, Plenum, 1987, pp 329–390.
McGhie A: A comparative study of the mother-child relationship in schizophrenia. Br J Med Psychol 34:195–208, 1961a
McGhie A: A comparative study of the mother-child relationship in schizophrenia, II: psychological testing. Br J Med Psychol 34:209–221, 1961b
McKeown JE: The behavior of parents of schizophrenic, neurotic, and normal children. Am J Sociol 56:75–179, 1950
Merikangas KR, Ranelli CJ, Kupfer DJ: Marital interaction in hospitalized depressed patients. J Nerv Ment Dis 167:689–695, 1979
Miklowitz DJ, Stackman D: Communication deviance in families of schizophrenia and other psychiatric patients: current state of the construct. Prog Exp Pers and Psychopathol Res 15:1–46, 1992
Miklowitz DJ, Goldstein MJ, Falloon IRH: Premorbid and symptomatic characteristics of schizophrenics from families with high and low levels of expressed emotion. J Abnorm Psychol 92:359–367, 1983
Miklowitz DJ, Goldstein MJ, Falloon IRH, et al: Interactional correlates of expressed emotion in the families of schizophrenics. Br J Psychiatry 144:482–487, 1984
Miklowitz DJ, Strachan AM, Goldstein JA, et al: Expressed emotion and communication deviance in the families of schizophrenics. J Abnorm Psychol 95:60–66, 1986
Miklowitz DJ, Goldstein MJ, Nuechterlein KH, et al: Family factors and the course of bipolar affective disorder. Arch Gen Psychiatry 45:225–231, 1988
Miklowitz DJ, Goldstein MJ, Doane JA, et al: Is expressed emotion an index of a transactional process? I: parents' affective style. Fam Process 28:153–167, 1989
Minuchin S: Families and Family Therapy. Cambridge, MA, Harvard University Press, 1974
Moline RA, Singh S, Morris A, et al: Family expressed emotion and relapse in schizophrenia in 24 urban American patients. Am J Psychiatry 142:1078–1081, 1985
Moos R, Moos BS: Family Environment Scale: Manual. Palo Alto, CA, Consulting Psychologists Press, 1981
Murray HA: Thematic Apperception Test: Manual. Cambridge, MA, Harvard University Press, 1943

Navran L: Communication and adjustment in marriage. Fam Process 6:173–184, 1967
Noller P: Gender and marital adjustment level differences in decoding messages from spouses and strangers. J Per Soc Psychol 41:272–278, 1981
Noller P: Nonverbal Communication and Marital Interaction. New York, Pergamon Press, 1984
Nuechterlein KH, Dawson ME: Information processing and attentional functioning in the developmental course of schizophrenic disorders. Schizophr Bull 10:160–203, 1984
Nuechterlein KH, Snyder KS, Dawson ME, et al: Expressed emotion, fixed dose fluphenazine decanoate maintenance, and relapse in recent-onset schizophrenia. Psychopharmacol Bull 22:633–639, 1986
Nuechterlein KH, Goldstein MJ, Ventura J, et al: Patient-environment relationships in schizophrenia: information processing, communication deviance, autonomic arousal, and stressful life events. Br J Psychiatry 155:84–89, 1989
Oliveri ME, Reiss D: A theory-based empirical classification of family problem-solving behavior. Fam Process 20:409–418, 1981
Parker G: Parental characteristics in relation to depressive disorders. Br J Psychiatry 134:138–147, 1979
Parker G: Re-searching the schizophrenogenic mother. J Nerv Ment Dis 170:452–462, 1982
Parker G: Parental Overprotection: a Risk Factor in Psychosocial Development. New York, Grune & Stratton, 1983
Parker G, Tupling H, Brown LB: A parental bonding instrument. Br J Med Psychol 52:1–10, 1979
Patterson GR: The aggressive child: victim and architect of a coercive system, in Behavior Modification and Families, 1: Theory and Research. Edited by Nash EJ, Hamerlynck LA, Handy LC. New York, Brunner/Mazel, 1976, pp 267–316
Patterson GR: Mothers: the unacknowledged victims. Monographs of the Society for Research in Child Development 45:5, 1980
Patterson GR: A Social Learning Approach to Family Intervention, III: Coercive Family Process. Eugene, OR, Castalia, 1982
Patterson GR, Cobb JA: A dyadic analysis of "aggressive" behaviors, in Minnesota Symposia on Child Psychology, Vol 5. Edited by Hill JP. Minneapolis, MN, University of Minnesota Press, 1970, pp 72–129
Patterson GR, Ray RS, Shaw D: Manual for the coding of family interactions. (Available from ASIS National Auxiliary Publications Service under Document No 01234), 1969
Patterson GR, Capaldi D, Bank L: An early starter model for predicting delinquency, in The Development and Treatment of Childhood Aggression. Edited by Pepler DJ, Rubin KH. Hillsdale, NJ, Lawrence Erlbaum Associates, 1991, pp 139–168
Paykel ES, Weissman MM: Social adjustment and depression. Arch Gen Psychiatry 28:659–663, 1973
Powers SI, Dill D, Havser S, et al: Coping strategies of families of seriously ill adolescents. J Early Adol 5:101–113, 1985
Raush HL, Barry WA, Hertel RK, et al: Communication, Conflict and Marriage. San Francisco, CA, Jossey-Bass, 1974
Reichard S, Tillman C: Patterns of parent-child relationships in schizophrenia. Psychiatry 13:247–257, 1950
Reiss D: Varieties of consensual experience, II: dimensions of a family's experience of its environment. Fam Process 10:28–35, 1971

Reiss D, Gonzalez S, Kramer N: Family process, chronic illness, and death. Arch Gen Psychiatry 43:795–804, 1986

Revenstorf D, Hahlweg K, Schindler L, et al: Interactional analysis of marital conflict, in Marital Interaction: Analysis and Modification. Edited by Hahlweg K, Jacobson NS. New York, Guilford, 1984, pp 159–181

Robinson EA, Jacobson NS: Social learning theory and family psychopathology: a Kantian model in behaviorism? in Family Interaction and Psychopathology. Edited by Jacob T. New York, Plenum, 1987, pp 117–162

Rorschach H: Psychodiagnostics. New York, Grune & Stratton, 1949

Sallows G: Comparative responsiveness of normal and deviant children to naturally occurring consequences. Unpublished doctoral dissertation, University of Oregon, Eugene, OR, 1972

Schaap C: A comparison of the interaction of distressed and nondistressed married couples in a laboratory situation: literature survey, methodological issues, and an empirical investigation, in Marital Interaction: Analysis and Modification. Edited by Hahlweg K, Jacobson NS. New York, Guilford, 1984, pp 133–158

Shaw D: Family maintenance schedules for deviant behaviors. Unpublished doctoral dissertation, University of Oregon, Eugene, OR, 1971

Singer M, Wynne L: Differentiating characteristics of parents of childhood schizophrenics, childhood neurotics, and young adult schizophrenics. Am J Psychiatry 120:234–243, 1963

Singer M, Wynne L: Thought disorder and family relations of schizophrenics, III: methodology using projective techniques. Arch Gen Psychiatry 12:187–200, 1965a

Singer M, Wynne L: Thought disorder and family relations of schizophrenics, IV: results and implications. Arch Gen Psychiatry 12:201–212, 1965b

Skinner HA, Steinhauer PD, Santa-Barbara F: The Family Assessment Measure. Can J Comm Men Health 2:91–105, 1983

Snyder DK: Multidimensional assessment of marital satisfaction. J Mar Fam 41:813–823, 1979

Snyder DK: Marital Satisfaction Inventory (MSI) Manual. Los Angeles, CA, Western Psychological Services, 1981

Snyder JJ: Reinforcement analysis of interaction in problem and nonproblem families. J Abnorm Psychol 86:528–535, 1977

Spanier GB: Measuring dyadic adjustment: new scales for assessing the quality of marriage and similar dyads. J Mar Fam 38:15–30, 1976

Strachan AM, Leff JP, Goldstein MJ, et al: Emotional attitudes and direct communication in the families of schizophrenics: a cross-national replication. Br J Psychiatry 149:279–287, 1986

Strachan AM, Feingold D, Goldstein MJ, et al: Is expressed emotion an index of a transactional process? II: patient's coping style. Fam Process 28:169–181, 1989

Straus MA: Measuring intrafamily conflict and violence: the conflict tactics (CT) scales. J Mar Fam 41:75–88, 1979

Strodbeck FL: Husband-wife interaction over revealed differences. Am Sociological Rev 16:468–473, 1951

Strodbeck FL: The family as a three-person group. Am Sociological Rev 19:23–29, 1954

Taplin P: Changes in parental communication as a function of intervention. Unpublished doctoral dissertation, University of Oregon, Eugene, OR, 1974

Tarrier N, Barrowclough C, Vaughn C, et al: The community management of schizophrenia. Br J Psychiatry 153:532–542, 1988

Taylor DW, Faust WL: Twenty questions: efficiency in problem solving as a function of size of group. J Exp Psychol 44:360–368, 1952

Tietze T: A study of mothers of schizophrenic patients. Psychiatry 12:55–65, 1949

Valone K, Norton JP, Goldstein MJ, et al: Parental expressed emotion and affective style in an adolescent sample at risk for schizophrenia spectrum disorders. J Abnorm Psychol 92:399–407, 1983

Vaughn CE, Leff JP: The influence of family and social factors on the course of psychiatric illness. Br J Psychiatry 129:125–137, 1976

Vaughn CE, Snyder KS, Jones S, et al: Family factors in schizophrenic relapse: replication in California of British research on expressed emotion. Arch Gen Psychiatry 41:1169–1177, 1984

Velligan DI, Goldstein MJ, Nuechterlein KH, et al: Can communication deviance be measured in a family problem-solving interaction? Fam Process 29:213–226, 1990

Velligan DI, Goldstein MJ, Falloon IRH: The impact of individual and family treatment on communication deviance in the families of schizophrenic patients. Paper presented at the International Congress on Schizophrenia Research, Tucson, AZ, April 1991

Vincent JP, Weiss RL, Birchler GR: A behavioral analysis of problem solving in distressed and nondistressed married and stranger dyads. Behavior Therapy 6:475–487, 1975

Vincent JP, Friedman LC, Nugent J, et al: Demand characteristics in observations of marital interaction. J Consult Clin Psychol 47:557–566, 1979

Wagener DK, Hogarty GE, Goldstein MJ, et al: Information processing and communication deviance in schizophrenic patients and their mothers. Psychiatry Res 18:365–377, 1986

Wahl CW: Some antecedent factors in the family histories of 392 schizophrenics. Am J Psychiatry 110:668–676, 1954

Wahl CW: Some antecedent factors in the family histories of 568 male schizophrenics of the U. S. Navy. Am J Psychiatry 113:201–210, 1956

Wahler RG, Dumas JE: Family factors in childhood psychology: toward a coercion-neglect model, in Family Interaction and Psychopathology. Edited by Jacob T. New York, Plenum, 1987, pp 581–627

Waring M, Ricks D: Family patterns of children who become adult schizophrenics. J Nerv Ment Dis 140:351–364, 1965

Warner R, Atkinson M: The relationship between schizophrenic patients' perceptions of their parents and the course of their illness. Br J Psychiatry 153:344–353, 1988

Wegener C, Revenstorf D, Hahlweg K, et al: Empirical analysis of communication in distressed and nondistressed couples. Behav Anal Modif 3:178–188, 1979

Wynne LC, Singer MT: Thought disorder and family relations of schizophrenics, I: a research strategy. Arch Gen Psychiatry 9:191–198, 1963a

Wynne LC, Singer M: Thought disorder and family relations of schizophrenics, II: a classification of forms of thinking. Arch Gen Psychiatry 9:199–206, 1963b

Wynne L, Singer M, Bartko J, et al: Schizophrenics and their families: recent research on parental communication, in Developments in Psychiatric Research. Edited by Tanner JM. London, England, Hodder & Stoughton, 1977, pp 254–286

Zuckerman M, Oltean M, Monashkin I: The parental attitudes of mothers of schizophrenics. J Consult Psychol 22:307–310, 1958

Zweig-Frank H, Paris J: Parents' emotional neglect and overprotection according to recollections of patients with borderline personality disorder. Am J Psychiatry 148:648–651, 1991

Further Suggested Readings

Baucom DH, Adams A: Assessing communication in marital interaction, in Assessment of Marital Discord. Edited by O'Leary KD. Hillsdale NJ, Lawrence Erlbaum Associates, 1987, pp 139–181

Gray-Little B, Burks N: Power and satisfaction in marriage: a review and critique. Psychol Bull 93:513–538, 1983

Chapter 37

Partner Relational Problems With Physical Abuse

K. Daniel O'Leary, Ph.D., and
Neil S. Jacobson, Ph.D.

Statement of the Issues

In this chapter, we examine evidence for the validity and clinical utility of establishing *partner relationship problems with physical abuse* as a diagnostic category in DSM-IV. We address the following issues:

1. The significance of partner relational problems with physical abuse as important clinical and public health problems
2. The adequacy of current diagnoses to cover problems of physical abuse between partners
3. The prevalence of physical aggression against an intimate partner
4. The sex ratio and impact of physical abuse
5. The age at onset of physical abuse
6. The responsibility for acts of physical aggression
7. The course of physical abuse
8. Complications of physical abuse
9. Familial patterns of abuse
10. Differential diagnoses

We then provide a definition of partner relational problems with physical abuse and discuss the adequacy of current assessment procedures to measure physical abuse. We conclude with our recommendations, note arguments that might be raised for alternative diagnoses, and discuss why we believe that the diagnoses we propose are best able to address the problems of physical abuse in intimate relations.

We thank Dr. Susan O'Leary for substantive and editorial feedback on several versions of this manuscript.

Significance of the Issues

Severe and repeated physical abuse is a serious public health problem in the United States that is currently receiving long overdue attention. In 1985, Surgeon General C. Everett Koop called for national attention to this problem by sponsoring a conference on family violence. Koop noted that health problems are usually given priority based on the frequency with which they lead to death. Although homicide ranks 11th among the leading causes of death, when one considers "years of life lost prematurely" homicide ranks fourth, and violence within intimate relationships is a major contributor to that homicide statistic. In 1988, the *Journal of Consulting and Clinical Psychology* ran a special series, "Violence in the Home," with two articles devoted specifically to physical aggression in marriage (Maiuro et al. 1988; Margolin et al. 1988a). The American Medical Association (AMA) published a firsthand account of a female physician who was repeatedly beaten by her husband (Whitehall 1989). In 1992, the AMA published a compendium, *Violence,* from *JAMA, American Medical News,* and specialty journals of the AMA. In addition, the AMA began a national media campaign (e.g., *Time,* February 24, 1992) to heighten public awareness of physical abuse. Political organizations and women's groups have been working with Senator Joseph Biden of Delaware and others to sponsor national legislation that will provide more services to individuals who are physically abused. Indeed, at least a dozen bills that contain provisions for services for victims of physical abuse have been considered by Congress.

Physical abuse exacts a tremendous physical and mental health toll on its victims as well as their family members. Repeated and severe physical abuse is experienced by approximately 3%–4% of men and women in the United States (Straus and Gelles 1990). Physical abuse led to the murders of approximately 1,000 wives and 700 husbands per year over the last decade (M. Cascardi and K. D. O'Leary: Gender differences in intimate homicide across a decade, State University of New York, Stony Brook, NY, unpublished manuscript, 1991). Unfortunately, increases in the availability of legal and psychological services for women have not been associated with reductions in male-perpetrated homicide against a partner (Browne and Williams 1989). Children who witness physical aggression between their parents are also at risk for varied forms of psychopathology, and the victims of physical abuse suffer serious individual problems such as anxiety and depression (Stark and Flitcraft 1988). Moreover, physical aggression is one of the most frequent reasons for dissolution of marriages (O'Leary and Arias 1988), and "decline of the nuclear family" was seen as the single biggest threat to the mental health of Americans in a survey of the American Psychological Association (Hamilton 1991). Societal costs associated with this problem—police actions, court actions, shelters for victims, and services for medical and psychological treatment—are impossible to measure, but they clearly are escalating rapidly.

There is no diagnostic category in DSM-III-R (American Psychiatric Association 1987) that directly covers the problem of physical abuse (O'Leary and Murphy 1992). We briefly review the ways existing diagnostic categories are most commonly used in assessing the abuser and the victim. In accord with federal guidelines as well as those of states like Connecticut that have developed gender-neutral policies regarding treatment of victims of physical abuse (Lewin 1992), we propose a diagnosis that is gender neutral. However, there are large bodies of clinical and research literature that clearly pertain to gender-related problems associated with physical abuse. Consequently, under the overall diagnosis of partner relational problems with physical abuse, there will be subcategories of *aggressor, victim,* and *mutual.* These terms reflect the need to place responsibility on the individual who repeatedly victimizes another person. Such categorization will allow for use of these diagnoses in homosexual relationships in which males and females may be aggressors or victims, or in which both partners are mutually aggressive. Finally, these subcategories can be used in the small number of circumstances in which the male in a heterosexual relationship is unilaterally and repeatedly victimized in a way that results in physical injury.

Method

We compiled material for this chapter by first reviewing articles and book chapters in our own files. Then we performed a PsychLit search for the period 1983–1992 using the keywords *battering, physical abuse,* and *spouse abuse.* Finally, recent evidence (1992 and in press articles) with which the authors were familiar was added as deemed appropriate. Although each article found in the literature search is not cited here, we have included those articles that seemed to best present empirical evidence pertaining to the issues discussed.

Results: Adequacy of the Current Diagnoses

Perpetrator Diagnoses

First we consider the diagnoses used most frequently to describe the behavior pattern of the individuals who physically assault their partners. We attempt to use gender-neutral terms in describing patterns of physical abuse, but as we emphasize later, the perpetrator of serious physical assaults that result in injury is much more likely to be the male and the victim of such assaults is more commonly the female.

Therefore, the terms *perpetrator* and *victim* are not synonymous with the terms *male* and *female*, respectively, but they are certainly very highly correlated.

Intermittent explosive disorder. The diagnosis of intermittent explosive disorder has been used to describe the behavior pattern of the aggressor. DSM-III-R defines this disorder as

> Discrete episodes of loss of control of aggressive impulses resulting in serious assaultive acts or destruction of property. The degree of aggressiveness expressed during the episodes is grossly out of proportion to any precipitating psychological stressors. There are no signs of generalized impulsivity or aggressiveness between the episodes. (American Psychiatric Association 1987, p. 321)

However, this diagnosis does not fit the facts of spouse abuse. The latter criterion, that the aggressiveness be episodic and not occur between episodes, does not fit the behavior described in the clinical and empirical spouse abuse literature. Verbal aggressiveness and aggressiveness as a personality style have been found to be clear correlates and/or precursors of physical aggression against partners (Hamberger and Hastings 1986; Murphy et al. 1993; O'Leary et al. 1990). Moreover, as amply illustrated in many clinical depictions of male batterers, there is a unifying theme of coercive control that is seen throughout the diverse behaviors of these men. Common forms of coercion include verbal threats and postures, demeaning comments, sexual coercion and often rape, as well as pervasive attempts to monitor the partner's movements (Follingstad et al. 1990; Sonkin et al. 1985).

Sadistic personality disorder. Sadistic personality disorder was included in DSM-III-R in the appendix for "Proposed Diagnostic Categories Needing Further Study." However, according to Spitzer et al. (1991), there has been little systematic study of the disorder. Mental health professionals suggested sadistic personality disorder to describe individuals who had a long-standing pattern of cruel and aggressive behavior toward others but whose personality characteristics were not adequately described by the DSM-III personality disorders.

To evaluate the potential usefulness of sadistic personality disorder, Spitzer et al. (1991) sent questionnaires to 1,390 members of the American Academy of Psychiatry and the Law; of these, 279 questionnaires were returned in usable form. Approximately 50% of the psychiatrists had at some time evaluated an individual who met the criteria for this disorder, and 4% of the psychiatrists who had ever seen a case of sadistic personality disorder had done so in the last year. Almost all cases of sadistic personality disorder were men who had experienced parental loss and childhood abuse. Sadistic personality disorder was seen as a diagnostic category with significant potential for misuse in legal settings. In fact, the most frequent concern about misuse was in child or spouse abuse cases in which criminal responsibility might be mitigated.

The diagnostic criteria for sadistic personality disorder clearly have some overlap with the types of behaviors exhibited by individuals who abuse their partners. Specifically, an individual who physically abuses another often 1) uses violence for the purposes of establishing dominance in a relationship, 2) treats someone under his or her control unusually harshly (e.g., child or student), 3) gets other people to do what he or she wants by frightening them, and 4) restricts the autonomy of people with whom he or she has a close relationship. On the other hand, most individuals who abuse their partners 1) are not fascinated by violence, weapons, or torture; 2) are not amused by the physical suffering of others; 3) do not lie for the purpose of inflicting pain; and 4) do not humiliate people publicly. It has been proposed that sadistic personality disorder not be continued as a provisional diagnosis in DSM-IV. However, using the provisional DSM-III-R sadistic personality disorder diagnosis, Gay and Feister (1990) and Spitzer et al. (1991) found that individuals with sadistic personality disorder had themselves suffered physical abuse in approximately half the cases. It has been repeatedly documented that individuals who seriously physically abuse their partners were physically abused by their parents (Gayford 1975; Rosenbaum and O'Leary 1981).

Victim Diagnoses

Clinicians offering services to battered women have documented the consequences of severe and repeated victimization for over a decade (e.g., Walker 1979). To describe the behavior patterns of individuals (usually women) who are the victims of spouse abuse, two DSM-III-R diagnostic categories, self-defeating personality disorder and posttraumatic stress disorder, have sometimes been used, but they have very clear limitations.

Self-defeating personality disorder. Self-defeating personality disorder was included in the DSM-III-R appendix for "Proposed Diagnostic Categories Needing Further Study" in order "to facilitate further systematic clinical study and research" (American Psychiatric Association 1987, p. 367). The defining characteristics of self-defeating personality disorder are

> A pervasive pattern of self-defeating behavior, beginning by early adulthood and present in a variety of contexts. The person may often avoid or undermine pleasurable experiences, be drawn to situations or relationships in which he or she will suffer, and prevent others from helping him or her. (American Psychiatric Association 1987, p. 371)

A diagnosis of self-defeating personality disorder is based on the presence of at least five of the following criteria:

1. chooses people and situations that lead to disappointment, failure, or mistreatment even when better options are clearly available
2. rejects or renders ineffective the attempts of others to help him or her
3. following positive personal events . . . , responds with depression, guilt, or a behavior that produces pain . . .
4. incites angry or rejecting responses from others and then feels hurt, defeated, or humiliated . . .
5. rejects opportunities for pleasure, or is reluctant to acknowledge enjoying himself or herself . . .
6. fails to accomplish tasks crucial to his or her personal objectives despite demonstrated ability to do so . . .
7. is uninterested in or rejects people who consistently treat him or her well . . .
8. engages in excessive self-sacrifice that is unsolicited by the intended recipients of the sacrifice. (American Psychiatric Association 1987, pp. 373–374)

Many individuals in physically abusive relationships certainly are able to accomplish tasks crucial to their own personal objectives (e.g., pursue advanced education, advance on a job ladder). They do not incite others (e.g., coworkers, children, and relatives) to anger, and they often have good friends. Alternatively stated, they do not characteristically choose people and situations that lead to disappointment, failure, and mistreatment.

The diagnosis of self-defeating personality disorder is not to be made if all the characteristics noted in the criteria above are "in response to, or in anticipation of, being physically, sexually, or psychologically abused" (American Psychiatric Association 1987, p. 374). That is, if the physical abuse leads someone to fail to accomplish tasks crucial to his or her own personal development or to feel uninterested in people who treat her or him well, then a diagnosis of self-defeating personality disorder would not be applicable under DSM-III-R criteria. In essence, the diagnosis is to be made when the above criteria are seen as long-standing personality styles or traits. Although there may be a few individuals who display such behavior and later in life enter abusive relationships, many physically abused individuals, be they men or women, do not have the self-defeating personality styles described in the criteria for this disorder.

In an often-cited study published more than 30 years ago that predates studies of self-defeating personality disorder, Snell et al. (1964) evaluated 12 couples in which the husband had been charged with assault and battery by the wife. On average, the couples had been married 18 years, and physical abuse was reported throughout the marriage. The husbands were described as steadily employed alcohol abusers; the wives were described as fitting into a systemic role in the marriage in which physical abuse fulfilled their own masochistic needs and the abuse functioned to maintain complete equilibrium. The Snell et al. study has been criticized by many (cf., Brown 1987; Margolin et al. 1988b; Rosewater 1987) for placing blame on battered women for their plight and for failing to recognize that many of the behavioral styles or traits ascribed to battered women could be the sequelae of abuse, not the causes. Moreover, Brown (1987) argued for a diagnosis of "abuse or oppression artifact disorder" rather than self-defeating personality disorder for victims of physical abuse as well as for victims of other kinds of oppression (e.g., hostages).

Few studies addressed whether the diagnosis of self-defeating personality disorder characterizes most abused women. Snyder and Fruchtman (1981) assessed 119 women from a battered women's shelter and found that one subgroup of these women had patterns of interacting that were consistent with a self-defeating personality disorder. However, this group of women was only one of five groups who were identified, and, as is evident later in our discussion of male abusers, there does not appear to be a single type of individual that characterizes either gender in abusive relationships.

Widiger and Frances (1989), in their review of research on self-defeating personality disorder, discussed concerns with the use of this diagnosis as sex bias and the fact that the DSM-III-R diagnoses favor organic pathology and do not adequately address relationship factors. They emphasized, however, that the self-defeating personality disorder diagnosis is meant to be descriptive, not explanatory. Thus, this diagnosis might be readily understood as an underlying cognitive style, a subaffective disorder, or a result of sex-role indoctrination, rather than as masochism. Despite the concerns about misuse of self-defeating personality disorder with abused women, Widiger and Frances argued that this issue does not justify ignoring the possible association of personality traits and responses to victimization. Instead, they aptly argued that we should be sensitive and cautious when applying personality disorder diagnoses to abused women.

Posttraumatic stress disorder. Posttraumatic stress disorder is another DSM-III-R diagnosis that is relevant to individuals, especially women, in abusive relationships. Posttraumatic stress disorder, a subcategory of anxiety disorders, is diagnosed when 1) an individual has "experienced an event that is outside the range of usual human experience" (e.g., a serious threat to one's life), 2) "the traumatic event is persistently reexperienced," 3) "persistent avoidance of stimuli associated with the trauma or numbing of general responsiveness" is present, 4) "persistent symptoms of increased arousal" are present, and 5) "duration of the disturbance [is] at least one month" (American Psychiatric Association 1987, pp. 250–251).

There are very few empirical studies of the use of the posttraumatic stress disorder diagnosis with physically abused individuals, and we do not know whether this or another diagnostic category best differentiates and characterizes abused women. The most appropriate diagnosis for these women remains debatable. Houskamp and Foy (1991) evaluated 26 battered women attending domestic violence clinics for posttraumatic stress disorder. Using the structured clinic interview for the DSM-III-R, 45% of the women were rated as having posttraumatic stress disorder. Using a symptom checklist, 43% of the women were rated as having posttraumatic stress disorder. Moreover, exposure to violence was associated with posttraumatic stress disorder symptomatology. However, more research is necessary to indicate the percentage of battered women for whom the diagnosis is applicable.

Battered woman syndrome. A possible diagnosis that could be used for the problem of physical abuse in relationships is the battered woman syndrome. This diagnosis has been championed by Walker (1989), who described two essential features: 1) fear of unavoidable physical aggression and 2) fear of unpredictable physical aggression. The syndrome has been officially recognized and permitted in courts in all states for cases of murder of husbands by women (Pesce 1990). Until 1990, Ohio, Wyoming, Oregon, and Washington, DC, were the only United States jurisdictions that did not allow the battered woman syndrome as evidence in court. In March 1990, however, the Ohio State Supreme Court ruled that expert testimony on the battered woman syndrome could be presented as evidence and acknowledged that the state of mind of the defendant at the time of the crime could be considered. In December 1990, the battered woman syndrome received national attention in the media when Governor Richard Celeste commuted the life sentences of 25 women who had been convicted of and were imprisoned for killing their battering husbands. The assistant to Governor Celeste, attorney Linda Ammons, was particularly influenced by two books, *Terrifying Love* by Walker (1989) and *Justifiable Homicide: Battered Women, Self-Defense, and the Law* by Gillespie (1989). In about 50 additional cases, applications for clemency were rejected, and another 30 were sent back for additional review. In several cases in which release was granted, Governor Celeste required a minimum time in prison before the release, and in all cases he required 200 hours of community service in battered women's programs (Blum 1991). Because of its growing legal acceptance, we try to incorporate elements of this syndrome into our definition of physical abuse.

According to federal guidelines, national legislation has to be written in gender-neutral terms unless the legislation specifically applies to one gender. The guidelines for DSM-IV also call for diagnostic labels that are gender neutral. The battered woman syndrome is obviously not gender neutral, nor have its reliability and validity been empirically supported. Moreover, it may exclude individuals who are victims of physical aggression but who may be able to predict when the aggression of their partner may occur. Yet the work of Walker (1989) and others who have championed the cause of battered women certainly should not go unnoticed. A proposed diagnosis that is consistent with the battered woman syndrome will allow defense attorneys and expert witnesses to apply this new diagnostic label in murder cases without the opposition arguing that the syndrome is inconsistent with DSM-IV.

Some legal experts have seriously questioned the legitimacy of Walker's (1989) claims about the cycle of violence and criticized her failure to conduct controlled research (Faigman 1989). Nonetheless, Walker opened a field for systematic inquiry that had been ignored for decades, and her descriptive accounts of the battering cycle provide very fertile ground both for researchers and for legal experts.

Prevalence and Risk of Physical Aggression Against an Intimate Partner

Large representative community samples indicate that the prevalence of at least one act of physical aggression during a year against a woman or a man is approximately 11%–12% (Table 37–1). The lifetime prevalence rate of such aggression is approximately 28% (Gelles and Straus 1986; Straus et al. 1980). The prevalence of life-threatening aggression (i.e., kicking, biting and hitting, beating, threatening with a knife or gun, and using a knife or gun) is approximately 3%–5% per year (Straus and Gelles 1990).

Self-reported rates of physical aggression in community samples are often equal for men and women, and these figures can easily spark very heated debates. Straus and Gelles (1990) and O'Leary and Vivian (1990) pointed out that the similarity of rates of physical aggression should not lead one to conclude that they have equal impact on men and women. As is documented later, physical aggression by men toward women clearly has more adverse consequences.

Written self-reports asking whether very specific aggressive behaviors occurred yield much higher rates of physical abuse than do interviews in which individuals are asked whether physical abuse or violence is a problem in their relationship. In a marital clinic setting, data on 132 couples indicated that 53% of the women reported some physical aggression during the preceding year, and 21% of the women reported severe physical aggression (O'Leary et al. 1992). These figures were based on self-report questionnaires designed to assess specific aggressive behaviors in an intimate relationship (Straus 1979). The high rates of aggression were surprising because in the written reports of predominant problems only 6% of the women attending the marital clinic indicated that physical aggression or abuse was a major problem in their marriages. Even when anger was included as a major problem, the rate of reporting physical aggression and/or anger did not increase

Table 37–1. Marital violence indices: comparison of 1975 and 1985, in percent

Violence index	1975	1985
Husband to wife		
Overall violence	12.1	11.3
Severe violence	3.8	3.0
Wife to husband		
Overall violence	11.6	12.1
Severe violence	4.6	4.4

Note. These data are based on a sample of 2,143 individuals in 1975 and 4,032 individuals in 1985.
Source. Adapted from Straus and Gelles 1990, p. 118.

above 15%. The import of this study as well as related studies (cf., Holtzworth-Munroe et al. 1992) is that direct assessment of aggressive behavior is necessary if one wishes to ascertain whether violence is a problem in a marriage. Physical aggression is common among couples seeking treatment for problems other than violence.

Sex Ratio and Impact of Abuse

When one considers the lower levels of physical aggression in marriage, such as slapping, pushing, and shoving, the rates in representative community samples are approximately the same for men and women (Gelles and Straus 1986; Straus et al. 1980). However, in one of these nationally representative community samples, the rate of physical injury of women by their husbands was much greater than the rate of physical injury of men by their wives. Of the physically victimized women, 3% reported needing medical attention compared with only 0.4% of physically victimized men (Stets and Straus 1990). A study of 93 couples seeking marital therapy indicated that approximately 15% of wives who reported being victims of physical aggression in the preceding year experienced serious physical injuries; in contrast, only 2% of the men reported serious physical injuries when they were the targets of physical aggression (M. Cascardi and K. D. O'Leary, unpublished manuscript, 1991). In a sample of 284 couples assessed for a domestic violence containment program in the military, 23% of the wives reported injuries requiring medical attention compared with 5% of the husbands. Interestingly, the overall rates of severe physical aggression in men and women were also approximately the same, but serious physical injury clearly was different for men and women (Cantos et al. 1994). Further, as noted earlier, men murder their wives more frequently than vice versa (M. Cascardi and K. D. O'Leary, unpublished manuscript, 1991). In summary, the rates of physical aggression in men and women may not differ, but there is very common agreement that physical aggression exacts a much more serious toll on women than on men.

Onset of Physical Abuse

Physically aggressive behavior is most common in early marriage (Straus et al. 1980). Where it escalates to severe physical aggression, it appears to have started in the first 3 years of marriage in approximately 75% of cases (Rosenbaum and O'Leary 1981). Low levels of physical aggression often precede the use of more violent forms, and early intervention is very important from a preventive stance. Anger or negative emotional states characterize abusive men, as does heightened physiological arousal (Margolin et al. 1988a); both are reliable predictors of later physical aggression.

Responsibility for Acts of Physical Aggression

Physical aggression toward a partner is a behavior that is under volitional control, not one of which the perpetrator is unaware or unconscious, and individuals who engage in physically aggressive behaviors must be held accountable. The fact that behaviors labeled "spouse abuse" are placed under the diagnostic label "relational problems" does not mean that there should be any mitigation of responsibility unless the act can truly be seen as one of self-defense.

Course

The typical age at onset of physically aggressive behavior against a partner is 18–25 years. Psychological aggression generally precedes the onset of physical aggression. Depending on the precipitant, the course may be insidious, as with arguments over in-laws, or abrupt, as with arguments over an affair.

Low levels of physically aggressive behavior such as slapping, pushing, and shoving may occur in a single episode, but if such behavior occurs several times over a 2-year period, the likelihood of further physical aggression in young married men is approximately 60% (O'Leary et al. 1989). Moreover, long periods without physical aggression are uncommon for seriously abused women. Indeed, women who suffer serious physical abuse commonly report a dozen or more attacks by their husband a year (Cascardi and O'Leary 1992). Thus, serious physical aggression against a partner is generally recurrent.

Without therapeutic or legal intervention, serious physical aggression against a partner is unlikely to decrease in frequency. In fact, even when physically abusive men are placed in court-mandated programs, the likelihood is only 50%–70% that they will stop (O'Leary and Vivian 1990).

Complications

Correlates of both severe forms and recurrent low levels of physical aggression include episodic binge drinking and/or alcoholism, poor self-esteem, and depression (Goldstein and Rosenbaum 1985; Neidig et al. 1986). Severe marital discord occurs in 75%–95% of marriages in which there is severe physical abuse (cf., Cascardi and O'Leary 1992; Rosenbaum and O'Leary 1981). Marital separations are very common in such relationships, and physical aggression is one of the most common reasons for divorce (O'Leary and Vivian 1990). Murder of wives by husbands occurs as the end result of a series of physically aggressive behaviors. Murder of women by their husbands appears to be a way to punish a partner, whereas murder of men by their wives appears to be characteristically self-defensive (Cascardi and O'Leary 1992).

Familial Patterns

There is a clear statistical association between violence in one's family of origin and use of physical aggression against a wife (Kalmus 1984; Rosenbaum and O'Leary 1981; Straus et al. 1980). Both observing parents fighting and being the victim of physical abuse are associated with wife abuse. In general, the more severe the form of violence against a wife, the more likely the individual will have come from a violent home. For example, approximately 15% of young married men who slap and shove their partners experienced violence in their families of origin (O'Leary and Arias 1988). Approximately 66% of men whose wives attended a county violence center encountered violence in their family of origin (Rosenbaum and O'Leary 1981).

Differential Diagnosis

Individuals who physically abuse their partners often have varied psychiatric problems. Alcohol abuse, drug abuse, depression, and anxiety are present in rates much higher than in the general population. As a general rule, the more severe the abuse, the more likely the individual will have concurrent psychiatric problems. In one study, almost none of the young men who slapped, pushed, or shoved their wives reported clinical levels of depressive symptomatology (O'Leary et al. 1989). But husbands who were in treatment programs for batterers evidenced higher levels of depressive symptomatology than men in a comparison group (Maiuro et al. 1988). Moreover, husbands who seek treatment in marital therapy and who have been physically aggressive sometime in the past year have higher levels of depressive symptomatology than men whose marriages are discordant but who are not physically aggressive (Cascardi et al. 1991).

Alcohol use is statistically associated with physical aggression by young men against their partners, but the association is small. Further, in young men, the results are not consistent across measures of alcohol use or abuse (Leonard and Senchak 1990). For men in general, heavy episodic drinking rather than daily consumption of moderate amounts of alcohol are most associated with physical aggression. In male alcoholic samples, 50% of the men report having been physically violent to their partners during the preceding year (O'Farrell and Choquette 1990). This finding would appear to implicate alcohol use as a factor in the etiology of spouse abuse. But of the marital cases at a university clinic in which there were few alcoholic individuals, marital discord was associated with spousal violence 70% of the time. Thus, it appears that marital discord is the more crucial etiological factor.

Marital discord is the strongest correlate of physical abuse. When one assesses samples of women attending county agencies for the treatment of domestic violence, between 90% and 100% of the women report severe marital discord (O'Leary and Curley 1986; Rosenbaum and O'Leary 1981). Severe marital discord, however, is not a necessary condition for spouse abuse; for many couples, abuse starts during the engagement or honeymoon period (O'Leary et al. 1989; Walker 1989).

Personality disorders are definitely more common among men in abusive relationships than in the general population. However, there is no single personality profile of the spouse abuser. Hamberger and Hastings (1986) used the Millon Clinical Multiaxial Inventory (Millon 1987) to assess 99 men who attended a domestic violence abatement program and identified three profiles: 1) schizoid/borderline, 2) narcissistic/antisocial, and 3) possessive/dependent/compulsive. Men referred for voluntary treatment have lower sociopathy and depression scores than men mandated to treatment (Coates et al. 1987).

Murphy et al. (1993) compared men attending a program for batterers with a sample of men whose marriages were seriously discordant but nonviolent to determine the types of personality disorders that would differentiate these two groups. The Axis II disorders were assessed with the Millon Clinical Multiaxial Inventory-II (Millon 1987). The sum of standardized z scores on the scales for antisocial, narcissistic, and aggressive/sadistic personality provided a measure of autonomous personality disturbance. The sum of standardized scores on the histrionic, passive aggressive, and borderline scales provided a measure of expressive personality disturbance. The physically abusive men evidenced more autonomous and expressive personality disturbance than the discordant nonabusive men. Patterns of affective dysregulation and antisocial/narcissistic tendencies were consistently prominent in the physically abusive men.

Head injury or brain dysfunction has occasionally been implicated as a cause or contributor to wife abuse and family violence (cf., Elliott 1977). However, the only systematic controlled research is that of Rosenbaum and colleagues (Rosenbaum and Hoge 1989; Rosenbaum et al. 1994), who found that head injury is almost twice as common in physically abusive men as in discordant, nonabusive men. Rosenbaum and colleagues pointed out, however, that these data should not detract from the importance of psychosocial and cultural influences on aggressive behavior toward a partner; rather, they simply point to the need not to overlook the brain-behavior relationship. Head injury per se does not cause a man to batter his wife but may impair his ability to control his aggression.

Definition

We propose the following definition for "partner relational problem with physical abuse": Acts of physical aggression toward a partner such as slapping, kicking, beating, and choking. These acts do not necessarily result in physical injury requiring medical attention, although in many cases they do. Often the acts are designed to force the individual to behave in a certain way.

Defining characteristics.

1. The acts of physical aggression against a partner occur in anger; they are not made in self-defense.
2. The acts of physical aggression usually include behaviors such as slapping, pushing, shoving, kicking, throwing an object, beating, and threatening with a weapon. In addition, use of physical force to obtain sexual gratification may also be part of the physical abuse (see the proposed DSM-IV category, "partner relational problems with sexual abuse" [American Psychiatric Association 1991]).
3. Acts of physical aggression, such as slapping, pushing, and shoving, that occur more than once per year; or acts of physical aggression that result in physical injury requiring medical attention; and/or physically aggressive acts involving threats and intimidation so that the victim is almost always fearful of the perpetrator.
4. Generally, the acts of physical aggression are unpredictable and unavoidable by the victim of the aggression.

Adequacy of Assessments for Physical Abuse

Physical aggression against a partner can be reliably assessed with self-reports and partner reports such as the Conflict Tactics Scale (Straus 1979) and its many modifications. Although men seem to underreport physical aggression (Arias and Beach 1987; Jouriles and O'Leary 1985; Riggs et al. 1989), the specificity of behaviors on the Conflict Tactics Scale allows it to be used in a fashion that permits moderately good agreement levels (Kappas and Pearson) between husbands' and wives' reports of aggressive behavior (Cantos et al. 1994; Jouriles and O'Leary 1985). Therefore, physical aggression against a partner can be reliably assessed with the Conflict Tactics Scale, and modifications and extensions of this scale can be used to assess impact and injury associated with physical aggression. Nonetheless, it is advisable also to assess the presence and context of physical aggression with individual interviews, because some physical aggression is not reported on written self-report assessments. Moreover, interviews are helpful in assessing intimidation by the husband and the fear one individual has of the other. In sum, there is clearly a methodology that is readily available to practitioners for assessing physical aggression against a partner.

Recommendations

Arguments for including a diagnosis of partner relational problems with physical abuse in DSM-IV include the following:

1. Severe physical abuse in the form of behaviors such as hitting, kicking, and beating occur in at least 4%–5% of marriages per year.
2. Victims of physical abuse suffer serious mental and physical consequences: depression, alcoholism, and suicide attempts.
3. Organizations such as the American Psychological Association and the AMA have featured special issues on family violence, and these special issues will alert the public to the importance of physical abuse in relationships. Moreover, the AMA has taken space in national media (i.e., *Time*, February 24, 1992) to alert the public to the issues of spouse abuse and has published a firsthand account of a physician who was repeatedly beaten by her husband.
4. Federal legislation has been sponsored by Senator Biden to mandate funds for treatment services and protection of women who are the victims of spouse abuse.
5. There is no diagnostic category that adequately addresses the problems of individuals in physically abusive relationships.
6. There are self-report questionnaires that reliably assess physical abuse in relationships.
7. There is a body of research literature accumulated over the past decade on the subject of physical abuse of partners that gives validity to the concept of physical abuse. Its correlates, precursors, and sequelae are well described by clinicians and have reasonable documentation by researchers.

There have not been any published debates about the possible inclusion of a diagnostic category of partner relational problems with physical abuse. Nonetheless, arguments against such a diagnostic category (along with our rebuttals) might include the following:

1. Diagnostic categories should more readily capture the gender-specific problems of women in physically abusive relationships. For example, the category might be called *partner relational problems with physical abuse of women*. In fact, we initially used this phrase, but we were encouraged to develop gender-neutral diagnostic labels. We complied with that suggestion because of the format of DSM-IV and because of the desire of federal legislators for language that is gender neutral.
2. There are more specific diagnoses that could capture the problems of physical abuse of women (e.g., battered woman syndrome). This diagnosis was considered at length, and it was incorporated into the recommended diagnosis. However, because of arguments noted regarding gender-neutral language, because there is relatively little empirical research on the validity of this diagnosis, and because some individuals who are the victims of physical aggression will not meet the criteria for the battered woman's syndrome, we do not recommend it as a diagnostic category. Instead, we recommend inclusion of much of the substance of the battered woman's syndrome within the framework of the diagnosis we propose.
3. There may be a more overarching diagnosis that captures the problems of abuse. For example, *relational problem with high expressed emotion* might also describe individuals in abusive relationships. The review by Goldstein et al. (Chapter 34, this volume) indicates that relationships characterized by high expressed emotion are predictors of relapse across several different types of adult disorders, including schizophrenia and unipolar and bipolar affective disorders. Further, there is a large body of literature on spouse abuse that suggests that victims do indeed have partners who have high expressed emotion (i.e., highly critical attitudes toward a partner). Such a category, however, seems very unlikely to capture the specific problems of spouse abuse. It is a generic category that appears to cut across many disorders.
4. It may be argued that giving relational diagnoses to some aggressive individuals, especially males, may be seen as mitigating responsibility for the aggression. For example, some men may be repeatedly aggressive after drinking or after a head injury, and there may be no relational problem that is very relevant to the aggressive behavior. In such cases, it is important for the clinician to recognize that a primary diagnosis of alcoholism or a neurological disorder may be most appropriate. Even with subcategories of aggressor, victim, and mutual under

the main diagnosis of partner relational problem with physical aggression, some may argue that there is too little individual emphasis on the aggressor, because the diagnosis falls under the rubric of relational problems. This issue is debatable, and we could envision different headings such as physical abuse of women and physical abuse of men. However, these categories do not allow for easy use in homosexual relationships, and they do not address the problem of mutual aggression.

Considering the arguments for and against, we conclude that there is an urgent need for a diagnosis that covers the problems of physical abuse of partners, and we recommend the proposed diagnosis: partner relational problems with physical abuse, with three subcategories, victim, perpetrator, and mutual. We believe that these categories adequately cover the substantive issues of physical abuse in heterosexual and homosexual relationships.

References

American Psychiatric Association: Diagnostic and Statistical Manual of Mental Disorders, 3rd Edition, Revised. Washington, DC, American Psychiatric Association, 1987

American Psychiatric Association: DSM-IV Options Book: Work in Progress. Washington, DC, American Psychiatric Association, 1991

Arias I, Beach SRH: Validity of self-reports of marital violence. Journal of Family Violence 2:82–90, 1987

Blum J: Celeste's clemency for 25. Columbus Monthly, March 1991, pp 55–58

Brown L: Toward a new conceptual paradigm for the Axis II diagnosis. Paper presented at the DSM-III symposium conducted at the 95th Annual Convention of the American Psychological Association, New York, August 1987

Browne A, Williams K: Exploring the effect of resource availability and the likelihood of female perpetrated homicide. Law and Society Review 23:75–90, 1989

Cantos A, Neidig P, O'Leary KD: Gender differences in injury rates in domestic violence. Journal of Family Violence 9:113–124, 1994

Cascardi M, O'Leary KD: Depressive symptomatology, self-esteem, and self-blame in battered women. Journal of Family Violence 7:249–259, 1992

Cascardi M, Langhinrichsen JL, Vivian D: Marital aggression: impact, injury, and health correlates for husbands and wives. Arch Intern Med 152:1178–1184, 1991

Coates CL, Leong DJ, Lindsey M: Personality differences among batterers voluntarily seeking treatment and those ordered to treatment by the court. Paper presented at the 3rd National Family Violence Research Conference, Durham, NH, July 1987

Elliott FA: The neurology of explosive rage, in Battered Women: a Psychosocial Study of Domestic Violence. Edited by Roy M. New York, Van Nostrand Reinhold, 1977, pp 98–109

Faigman DL: The battered woman syndrome and self-defense: a legal and empirical dissent, in Representing Battered Women Who Kill. Edited by Johann SL, Osanka F. Springfield, IL, Charles C Thomas, 1989, pp 333–362

Follingstad DR, Rutledge LI, Berg BJ, et al: The role of emotional abuse in physically abusive relationships. Journal of Family Violence 5:107–120, 1990

Gay M, Feister S: Sadistic personality disorder, in Psychiatry, Vol 1. Edited by Cavenar JO, Michaels R, Cooper AM, et al. New York, Basic Books, 1990

Gayford J: Wife battering: a preliminary survey of 100 cases. BMJ 1:195–197, 1975

Gelles RJ, Straus MA: Societal changes and change in family violence from 1975 to 1985 as revealed by two national surveys. Journal of Marriage and the Family 48:465–479, 1986

Gillespie CK: Justifiable Homicide: Battered Women, Self-Defense, and the Law. Columbus, OH, Ohio State University Press, 1989

Goldstein D, Rosenbaum A: An evaluation of self-esteem of maritally violent men. Family Relations 34:425–428, 1985

Hamberger LK, Hastings J: Personality correlates of men who abuse their partners: a cross validation study. Journal of Family Violence 1:323–341, 1986

Hamilton D: Psychological risk assessment. Science 251:1566, 1991

Holtzworth-Munroe A, Waltz J, Jacobson NG, et al: Recruiting nonviolent men as control subjects for research on marital violence: how easily can it be done? Violence and Victims 7:79–88, 1992

Houskamp BM, Foy DW: The assessment of posttraumatic stress disorder in battered women. Journal of Interpersonal Violence 6:367–375, 1991

Jouriles EN, O'Leary KD: Interspousal reliability of reports of marital violence. J Consult Clin Psychol 53:419–421, 1985

Kalmus D: The intergenerational transmission of marital aggression. Journal of Marriage and the Family 46:11–19, 1984

Koop CE: The Surgeon General's Workshop on Violence and Public Health: Source Book. Leesburg, VA, U.S. Public Health Service/DHHS, October 1985

Leonard KE, Senchak M: Alcohol and spousal aggression in newlyweds. Paper presented at the 98th Annual Convention of the American Psychological Association, Boston, MA, 1990

Lewin T. Battered men sounding equal rights battle cry. The New York Times, April 20, 1992, p A12

Maiuro RD, Cahn TS, Vitaliano PP, et al: Anger, hostility, and depression in domestically violent versus generally assaultive men and non-violent control subjects. J Consult Clin Psychol 56:17–23, 1988

Margolin G, John RS, Gleberman L: Affective responses to conflictual discussions in violent and non-violent couples. J Consult Clin Psychol 56:24–33, 1988a

Margolin G, Sibner LG, Gleberman L: Wife battering, in Handbook of Family Violence. Edited by Van Hasselt VB, Morrison RL, Bellack AS, et al. New York, Guilford, 1988b, pp 89–117

Millon T: Millon Clinical Multiaxial Inventory-II: Manual for the MCMI-II, 2nd Edition. Minneapolis, MN, National Computer Systems, 1987

Murphy CM, Meyer S, O'Leary KD: Family of origin violence and MCMI-II psychopathology among partner assaultative men. Violence and Victims 18:165–176, 1993

Neidig PH, Friedman DH, Collins BS: Attitudinal characteristics of males who have engaged in some spouse abuse. Journal of Family Violence 1:223–233, 1986

O'Farrell TJ, Choquette KA: Marital violence in the year before and after spouse-involved alcoholism treatment. Paper presented at the 98th Annual Convention of the American Psychological Association, Boston, MA, August 1990

O'Leary KD, Arias I: Prevalence, correlates, and development of spouse abuse, in Marriage and Families: Behavioral Treatments and Processes. Edited by Peters R deV, McMahon RJ. New York, Brunner/Mazel, 1988, pp 104–127

O'Leary KD, Curley AD: Assertion and family violence: correlates of spouse abuse. Journal of Marital and Family Therapy 12:281–289, 1986

O'Leary KD, Murphy CM: Clinical issues in the assessment of spouse abuse, in Assessment of Family Violence: A Clinical and Legal Sourcebook. Edited by Ammerman RT, Hersen M. New York, John Wiley, 1992, pp 26–46

O'Leary KD, Vivian D: Physical aggression in marriage, in The Psychology of Marriage: Basic Issues and Applications. Edited by Fincham F, Bradbury TN. New York, Guilford, 1990, pp 323–348

O'Leary KD, Barling J, Arias I, et al: Prevalence and stability of physical aggression between spouses: a longitudinal analysis. J Consult Clin Psychol 57:263–268, 1989

O'Leary KD, Malone J, Tyree A: Physical aggression in early marriage: prerelationship and relationship effects. J Consult Clin Psychol 62:594–602, 1990

O'Leary KD, Vivian D, Malone J: Assessment of physical aggression in marriage. Behavioral Assessment 14:5–14, 1992

Pesce C: Inmates hope for freedom to start over. USA Today, October 4, 1990, p 1

Riggs DS, Murphy CM, O'Leary KD: Intentional falsification in reports of interpartner aggression. Journal of Interpersonal Violence 4:220–232, 1989

Rosenbaum A, Hoge SK: Head injury and marital aggression. Am J Psychiatry 146:1048–1051, 1989

Rosenbaum A, O'Leary KD: Marital violence: characteristics of abusive couples. J Consult Clin Psychol 49:63–71, 1981

Rosenbaum A, Hoge SK, Adelman SA, et al: Head injury in partner abusive men. J Consult Clin Psychol 62:1187–1193, 1994

Rosewater L: A critical analysis of the proposed self-defeating personality disorder. Journal of Personality Disorders 1:190–195, 1987

Snell J, Rosenwald R, Robey A: The wifebeater's wife: a study of family interaction. Arch Gen Psychiatry 11:107–112, 1964

Snyder D, Fruchtman L: Differential patterns of wife abuse: a data based typology. J Consult Clin Psychol 49:878–885, 1981

Sonkin DJ, Martin D, Walker LE: The Male Batterer. New York, Springer, 1985

Spitzer RL, Feister S, Gay M, et al: Results of a survey of forensic psychiatrists on the validity of the sadistic personality diagnosis. Am J Psychiatry 148:875–879, 1991

Stark E, Flitcraft A: Violence among intimates: an epidemiological review, in Handbook of Family Violence. Edited by Van Hasselt VB, Morrison R, Bellack A, et al. New York, Plenum, 1988, pp 293–317

Stets JE, Straus MA: Gender differences in reporting marital violence and its medical and psychological consequences, in Physical Violence in American Families: Risk Factors and Adaptations to Violence in 8,145 Families. Edited by Straus MA, Gelles RJ. New Brunswick, NJ, Transaction Press, 1990, pp 151–164

Straus MA: Measuring intrafamily conflict and violence: The Conflict Tactics Scale. Journal of Marriage and the Family 41:75–78, 1979

Straus MA, Gelles RJ, Steinmetz SK: Behind Closed Doors: Violence in the American Family. Garden City, NY, Anchor/Doubleday, 1980
Straus MA, Gelles RJ (eds): Physical Violence in American Families: Risk Factors and Adaptations to Violence in 8,145 Families. New Brunswick, NJ, Transaction Press, 1990
Walker L: The Battered Woman. New York, Harper & Row, 1979
Walker L: Terrifying Love: Why Battered Women Kill and How Society Responds. New York, Harper & Row, 1989
Whitehall JA: A piece of my mind (letter). JAMA 261:3460, 1989
Widiger TA, Frances AJ: Controversies concerning the self-defeating personality disorder, in Self-Defeating Behaviors: Experimental Research, Clinical Impressions, and Practical Implications. Edited by Curtis R. New York, Plenum, 1989, pp 289–309

Chapter 38

Sibling Relational Problems

Michael D. Kahn, Ph.D., and
Genevieve Monks, M.A.

Statement of the Issues

In DSM-III-R (American Psychiatric Association 1987), sibling relationship problems were identified with a V code as "other specified family circumstances." In this chapter, we examine the evidence concerning the validity and clinical utility of "sibling relationship problems" as a potential Axis I or Axis II disorder in DSM-IV.

Significance of the Issues

Until recently, sibling relationship problems have received little attention. Because of the large number of permutations (e.g., family size, birth order, age spacing, gender distribution, physical endowments), uniform assumptions are difficult to make. However, sibling relationships can be considered unique and contribute in important ways to the psychological development of the individual. Toman (1988) reported that studies indicate that sibling birth order accounts for 10%–20% of the differences in a person's social behavior, social interests, and preferences. Dysfunctional sibling relationships can result in severe psychological problems and are often found to exist when there are disruptions in caretaking by parents. For example, Jesse (1988) reported that alcoholic parents can negatively affect the sibling relationship by increasing sibling rivalry. Although sibling rivalry is commonplace, Jesse reported it may reach excessive proportions of violence, domination, and exploitation in an alcoholic family. Roberto (1988) reported that children in families with eating disorders have parents who are so threatened by the sibling relationship between their children that they discourage any sibling bonding and intimacy. Abusive sibling relationships are abundant and are frequently hidden from parental view (Dickstein 1988). The abusive sibling's family may also be experiencing a major conflict, crisis, or change (Rosenthal and Doherty 1984).

Method

Although in this chapter we focus on the available experimental designs, comparison/control groups, or observational studies, we also include some case studies and anecdotal literature, because empirical research in this area of family malfunction is sparse. Four main categories of sibling relational problems are discussed: 1) sibling aggression, 2) sibling incest, 3) sibling illness, and 4) sibling death. We consider the impact of the problem, course, sex ratio, age at onset, and familial pattern.

Results

Sibling Aggression

Sibling aggression is the most prevalent form of family violence (Straus et al. 1980). Milder forms are so common that they are often not viewed as a clinical problem but erroneously presumed to be normative. In fact, it is only in the last 25 years that sibling aggression has been systematically researched (Adelson 1972). Research also indicates that a firstborn child's reaction to the birth of a sibling is often one of considerable distress (Dunn and Kendrick 1980; Dunn et al. 1981). Symptoms include an increase in sleep disturbances, toilet training problems, excessive crying, changes in demanding behavior, negative behavior toward the mother, and withdrawal. Negative or demanding behavior was not associated with later sibling conflicts, whereas withdrawal was (Dunn et al. 1981). Aggression toward a younger sibling includes attempts to cause serious physical harm by poisoning or breaking bones or even attempts to murder the younger sibling (Gill 1982).

In a study of 2,143 families (Straus et al. 1980), of which 733 had at least two children between 3 and 17 years old living at home, those children engaged in the following behaviors in the period of 1 year: 1) 16% beat up a sibling, 2) 0.8% threatened the sibling with a knife or gun, and 3) 0.3% used a knife or gun on a sibling. Younger siblings, who are not as socialized, are more violent than older siblings, yet the younger siblings, by virtue of their smaller stature, are generally reported to be more abused. Whereas most violence decreases as the child matures, use of a knife or gun increased from 2.6% of preschoolers to 6.5% of high schoolers (Straus et al. 1980). Sibling murder is often committed without much remorse (Sargent 1962). In 1965, 3% of all New York homicides were sibling homicides (Bard 1971). In a study of aggressive children, results indicate that aggressive siblings engaged in longer coercive chains of belligerent behavior than nonsibling aggressive children (Loeber and Tengs 1986).

Prevalence and risk of sibling aggression. Steinmetz (1977) reported that in a 1-week period, parents in 49 families recorded a total of 131 sibling conflicts. The parents in these families worked outside the home, thus their reports likely underestimated the number of conflicts. Steinmetz also suggested that recording techniques may have caused an underestimation of conflicts. In a study of 360 5- to 6-year-old children with one sibling, the parents reported that 28.4% engaged in severe and frequent quarreling, 36% engaged in moderate quarreling, and 35.5% had very rare altercations (Koch 1960).

Sex ratio and impact of sibling aggression. Roscoe et al. (1987) investigated the precursors to sibling violence, types of violent behavior and antagonistic interactions, the type of conflict resolution most frequently used, and the relationship between sex of sibling pair and type of negative reaction. They found more similarities than differences according to gender. Boys were more likely to use more severe types of physical force to solve conflicts, whereas girls were more likely to use an ignoring strategy to deal with sibling conflict. Although the use of physical force was high, various forms of yelling and ignoring were used more often. Straus et al. (1980) found sex differences to be relatively small, but boys were slightly more aggressive than girls. However, in an observational study of same-sex siblings, Abramovitch et al. (1979) found that brothers were more physically aggressive than sisters. With dyads of mixed-sex siblings, Abramovitch et al. (1980) found no sex differences on any measure of aggression. A later study of dyads of mixed-sex and same-sex pairs showed few effects of sex composition of the dyads on antagonistic behavior (Abramovitch et al. 1986).

In the previously mentioned study of 360 5- to 6-year-old children with one sibling, Koch (1960) reported that firstborn children were less likely to report infrequent quarreling when their sibling was male. However, second-born boys reported more frequent quarreling with an older sister close in age than with an older brother close in age. Minnett et al. (1983) found that cheating, aggression, and dominance were more characteristic of children's behavior with a same-sex sibling than with an opposite-sex sibling.

Age and type of onset. Minnett et al. (1983) reported that 7- to 8-year-old children were more aggressive with a closely spaced sibling than with siblings whose age difference was greater. Furman and Buhrmeister (1985) found that siblings who were closer in age (which Bank and Kahn [1982] have labeled high access) reported more conflict than siblings who are spaced farther apart. Siblings perceived older children of the same sex to be more dominating than those of the opposite sex. Younger siblings were also more likely to report that their older siblings were more favored by the parent(s).

Other research indicates that older children initiated both agonistic and prosocial behavior more than younger siblings (Abramovitch et al. 1979, 1980, 1986). In contrast, other researchers have found that, as children grow older, use of openly witnessed violence to resolve conflicts decreases (Steinmetz 1977; Straus et al. 1980). Steinmetz suggested that this may occur because their conflicts are less likely to be observed and mediated by parents, but that the siblings will use violence in a clandestine manner.

Course. Whether sibling aggression is a stable pattern in children has important clinical relevance. To explore the continuity of this aspect of sibling relationships from a developmental perspective, Stillwell and Dunn (1985) examined children's initial interest in a newborn sibling, children's behavior (aggressive or positive) toward the same sibling 14 months later, and the behavior toward the sibling when the firstborn reached 6 years in age. The results of their study suggest that the quality of firstborn children's initial behavior toward younger siblings is positively correlated with their behavior 3–4 years later. Gully et al. (1981) explored how siblings themselves contribute to later violent behavior. Their results suggest that violence involving siblings, especially as perpetrators, may be more predictive of later adult violence than any other familial interaction. Bank and Kahn (1982) strongly indicated that lack of adequate parental caretaking dramatically increases the probability of sibling aggression. Aggressive children continue with their aggression once it starts, whereas when nonaggressive children are aggressive, they usually have only one aggressive behavioral episode at a time and then use developed mechanisms or rituals to cease the aggression (Loeber and Tengs 1986).

Familial patterns of sibling aggression. Sibling aggression increases with family size or as the availability of the parent decreases, requiring siblings to resolve their own conflicts (Bank and Kahn 1982).

A review of five case studies of highly abusive siblings revealed that the parents showed one or more of the following characteristics: 1) divorced or separated, 2) high interparental conflict, 3) psychopathology exhibited and/or abuse perpetuated against at least one spouse by the other, and 4) disinterest in the children. The mothers were often socially isolated and lacked an adequate support system (Green 1984). Green also reported that all five abusing siblings had been abused and were the first and only child when the victim sibling was born or the half-sibling joined the family. Their mothers were emotionally unavailable to them while they focused what resources they had on nurturing the younger children.

Crittendon (1984) found that children as young as 2 years old display the same patterns of interaction (maltreating or nonmaltreating) with their siblings as their mothers did.

Felson and Russo (1988) investigated whether parents may influence aggression between siblings through the use of punishment. They hypothesized that when siblings fight, boys who fight with their sisters are more likely to receive parental punishment, as is a much older child. The results supported these hypotheses and also showed that when a child 4 years older than his or her sibling is punished for aggression while the younger is not, the younger sibling is more likely to initiate aggression on subsequent occasions. Aggression was also found to be more frequent when male or older siblings were punished. In an exploratory study, Loeber and Tengs (1986) found that mothers of aggressive children were more inconsistent and tended not to complete their intervention when aggression continued. In a longitudinal study of 174 nondelinquent aggressive boys and their families, McCord et al. (1970) found the following familial conditions: 1) the boys' parents were rejecting, punitive, or used frequent threats; 2) control of the boys was ineffective, with the mother showing either overcontrol or undercontrol, or low demands for self-control; 3) there was lack of adequate supervision; 4) the parental model was socially deviant; and 5) the parental relationship involved a high degree of conflict, lacked mutual esteem, was unaffectionate, and was characterized by dissatisfaction with the parents' roles in life. Sears et al. (1957) found similar results. In a small study of 10 abusive siblings, Rosenthal and Doherty (1984) observed three situations: 1) parents chronically abused the child, 2) parents' unconscious behavior allowed the sibling abuse to continue, and 3) parents identified the abused child with some abusive person in the parent's life.

Sibling Incest

Sibling incest is differentiated from the comparison and exploration involved in early childhood sexual play. Finkelhor (1980) defined sex "play" as "activities of young children of the same age, engaged in mutually, that are limited to the showing and touching of genitals, and that go on for short periods of time" (p. 172). Sibling incest can be categorized in two major groups: 1) a less pathogenic variety with nurturance as motive and 2) a power-oriented variety that is violent, exploitative, and coercive with debilitating consequences (Bank and Kahn 1982). Researchers acknowledge that sibling incest can be nonabusive (Russell 1986), and, in fact, it has been viewed by some researchers as sometimes being a beneficial experience (Finkelhor 1980; Fox 1980). Finkelhor (1979) reported that approximately one-third of his sample described their sibling sexual experience as positive, one-third as negative, and one-third as neutral. However, more females reported the experience as unpleasant than did males (35% to 22%). While 30% of the subjects reported the experience as positive, only 12% reported that they had ever told anyone about the experience; not a single child who had sex with a much older sibling told anyone. Finkelhor and Hotaling (1984) defined incestuous abuse as any kind of sexual contact involving 1) a child younger than 13 years old and the perpetrator at least 5 years older than the victim; 2) a child 13–16 years old and the perpetrator at least 10 years older than the victim; or 3) any kind of force, threat, or deceit, no matter what the age of the perpetrator or victim. Johnson (1988) reported that almost half of the victims of 47 perpetrating boys were siblings, the most available targets for sexual abuse. Bank and Kahn (1982) and Russell (1986) suggested that one reason sibling incest has not been given the same attention as parent-child incest is the belief that the power differential is much less than in parent-child incest. Russell pointed out, however, that an age difference of even 7 years represents a considerable power differential for children or adolescents. Russell's study indicated that, in most cases, brother-sister incest is not mutually desired.

The experience is more destructive the younger the child, the longer the duration of the incest, and the greater the degree of force used by the perpetrator (Bank and Kahn 1982). Finkelhor (1980) found that 64% of the children who reported that force was used described the experience as negative and that the greater the age difference, the more likely the experience was negative. De Jong (1989) reported that 10% of 35 sibling incest cases involved documented injury. Short- and long-term effects experienced by the victim can include guilt, mistrust, low self-esteem (Courtois 1988; Laviola 1989; Lindberg and Distad 1985), depression, substance abuse, sexual dysfunction, poor self-concept, suicide attempts (Jehu 1989; Laviola 1989; Lindberg and Distad 1985), anxiety, sleep disturbances, hypervigilance, isolation (Lindberg and Distad 1985), fear of intimacy (Courtois 1988; Laviola 1989), difficulties in relationships or marriage, and poor choice in marital partners (Meiselman 1978; Russell 1986). Reports of case studies also confirm the existence of these symptoms (Canavan et al. 1992). Symptoms of posttraumatic stress disorder may also appear in the victim (Dickstein 1988; Lindberg and Distad 1985). Although not quite statistically significant, 47% of the sibling incest victims in Russell's (1986) study never married compared with 27% of all other incest victims combined. Some investigators suggest that sibling incest is harmful only when the brother is 5 or more years older than the sister (Finkelhor 1980; Russell 1986). Others propose that it is always harmful, whatever the age difference, because males are usually exercising a power differential (Cole 1982; Laviola 1989).

Women who are victims of brother-sister incest report significantly higher levels of revictimization than do women who have never been the victim of incest ($P < .01–.05$). The revictimization experiences included 1) having a husband be physically violent toward them, 2) having an unwanted sexual experience with an authority figure or with a girl or woman, 3) being upset on the street by men's sexual comments or advances, 4) being asked to pose for pornographic pictures, and 5) being upset by a "peeping Tom" or exhibitionist (Russell 1986).

Russell (1986) also found that victims of sibling incest had a significantly greater fear of sexual assault as adults than did women who had never been incestuously abused ($P < .001$). She also found that victims of brother-sister incest reported a significantly higher rate of defection from their original religion than women who had never been incestuously abused ($P < .01$).

Prevalence and risk of sibling incest. In a survey of 796 New England college undergraduates, 15% of females and 10% of males reported sibling sexual activity. Of these subjects, 74% reported heterosexual-type experiences; 16% of the incest cases were between brothers and 10% were between sisters (Finkelhor 1980). Gebhard et al. (1965) estimated sibling abuse to be five times as great as parent-child abuse. Russell (1986) reported that 2% (19 of 930) of women reported at least one incident of sexual abuse by a brother before the age of 18. One woman reported that she had been abused by three of her brothers and another reported that five of her brothers abused her. Thus there were 21 cases of brother-sister incest abuse. Russell speculated that this 2% prevalence rate underestimates the problem, because many girls have no older brother and are therefore not at risk for sibling incest abuse. She also suggests that prevalence rates should be based only on girls with at least one older brother, because most sibling abuse involves an older brother and younger sister. However, Meiselman's (1978) study of psychotherapy cases found that father-daughter incest occurred four times as often as brother-sister incest. Meiselman suggested this could indicate that women involved in brother-sister incest are less frequently disturbed as adults and therefore do not feel the need for therapy. Another study found that 75% of female psychiatric inpatients had a history of physical or sexual abuse (Bryer et al. 1987). Although that study does not directly implicate sibling incest, Meiselman reported studies that found an association between sibling incest and psychiatric illness. However, she noted that incest reports given by psychotic persons need to be weighed carefully, because psychosis implies the inability to perceive reality accurately and therefore to give accurate self-reports. Results of a study by Becker et al. (1986) suggest that perpetrators of adolescent incest with siblings committed more sexual crimes than they had been charged with. Of the 22 subjects studied, 31.8% denied all deviant sexual behavior; 41% of the subjects were identified as paraphiliacs (their victims were 5 years younger or more) and reported that they had engaged in other, nonincest sex with minors.

Sex ratio and impact of sibling incest. Females are more likely to be victims of exploitative sex than males (Bank and Kahn 1982; Finkelhor 1980; Smith and Israel 1987). In a study of 25 families, Smith and Israel reported that 20% of sibling perpetrators were female and 80% were male. In most studies, a small percentage of females are the perpetrators. Sexually abused sisters are the usual informants of sibling incest (Finkelhor 1979; Forward and Buck 1978; Meiselman 1978), and they experience more long-term effects than reported by their perpetrating brothers (Bank and Kahn 1982; Cole 1982; Finkelhor 1980). Finkelhor also reported that females were the victims in 82% of the cases where force or coercion was used. Russell (1986) found a significant difference ($P < .05$) in the use of force as a primary strategy for obtaining incest. In 44% of brother-sister incest cases, the brothers used force as the primary strategy compared with 25% of all other cases of incest combined. If only exhibition of genitals without touching was involved, the experience was more likely to be remembered as positive (Finkelhor 1980).

James and MacKinnon (1990) criticized the family systems theory of incest because of the failure to note power differentials due to gender. They believe a sister, regardless of age difference, will find it hard to refuse sexual contact with a brother even if they are close in age, because females are not accustomed to exercising power and assertion and, as Gilligan (1982) stated, are conditioned to nurture others at the expense of the self. The power advantages of males, socially sanctioned and owing to their physical advantages, encourage possibility for the occurrence of incest. Of the perpetrators of adolescent incest in the study by Becker et al. (1986), 17 were identified as pedophiles (their victims were 5 years younger or more), with 64.7% victimizing females and 35.3% victimizing males. In the study by Russell (1986), there was a significant difference in the level of severity of abuse between the sibling incest cases and other types of intrafamilial sexual abuse ($P < .01$). Only 12% of the sibling incest cases were mild cases compared with 40% of all other types of incest combined. She suggested that this dispels the myth that sibling incest is benign.

Age and type of onset. Case history reports include incidents of children as young as 5 or 6 years old having a sexual relationship or being raped by a brother 3–11 years older (Bank and Kahn 1982; Forward and Buck 1978). In the sample of 796 undergraduates described earlier, Finkelhor (1980) reported that 40% of respondents who reported sibling incest were under 8 years old at the time of abuse and that the median age of both victim and perpetrator was 10.2 years. Finkelhor also reported that younger children are more likely to engage in genital exhibition, whereas older children are more likely to engage in intercourse or attempted intercourse. He found that more experiences were reported between the ages of 8 and 11. De Jong (1989) reported the mean age of the victim in 35 cases of sibling incest as 7.4 years and the mean age of the perpetrator as 15.5 years. The mean of the victim/perpetrator age difference was 8.1 years. Smith and Israel (1987) reported the average age of the victim in 25 cases of sibling incest as 9.1 years and the average age of the sibling perpetrator as 13.2 years. Russell (1986) reported the mean age of female victims of sibling incest as 10.7 years and the mean age of their perpetrating brothers as 17.9 years.

Course. De Jong (1989) reported that 49% of sibling sexual abuse involved a single episode and 51% involved multiple episodes. Russell (1986) indicated that sibling abuse is significantly less likely to occur for more than a year compared with abuse by all other perpetrators (16% versus 30%; $P < .05$). However, Bank and Kahn (1982) reported cases with a duration of as long as 12 years.

Familial patterns. Meiselman (1978) reported that most families of children who engage in brother-sister incest have parents who provide poor supervision, especially regarding their sex play. Other researchers reported that incestuous siblings often have parents who 1) are distant, inaccessible, or neglectful; 2) encourage a sexually exploitative atmosphere in the home; and 3) are inadequate in general (Bank and Kahn 1982; Jehu 1989; Smith and Israel 1987). Meiselman (1978) reported other studies that corroborate these findings. The parent may also have been sexually abused as a child, or the sibling may be directed to keep family secrets about extramarital affairs (Smith and Israel 1987). Of the siblings in Smith and Israel's study, 48% witnessed their parents engaging in sexually provocative behavior. Case studies of sibling incest also support the finding that the parents are neglectful, rejecting, discouraging, or incapable of open communication (Ascherman and Safier 1990; Laviola 1989); have a history of physical or sexual abuse themselves (Friedrich 1990); and allow or engage in seductive behavior in the home (Daie et al. 1989; Friedrich 1990). Finkelhor (1979) found that female sibling incest victims were likely to come from large families, suggesting that poverty, inadequate parental supervision, and poor physical and psychological boundaries contribute to the incidence rate. Consistent with these findings, Russell (1986) found a significant difference ($P < .001$) in the number of people dependent on the family income at the time of the abuse. Of female victims of sibling incest, 77% came from families with 6 or more people dependent on the family income, compared with 32% of the victims of other types of incest. Russell also reported that only 5% of sibling victims were aware that their brothers were sexually abusing another relative compared with 35% of the victims of other types of incest ($P < .05$).

Sibling Death

The death of a child is usually overwhelming to the family and can strain family relationships. The surviving siblings become vulnerable to emotional unrest, and their social relationships can be disturbed (Adams and Deveau 1987). Children under 8 or 9 years old are generally incapable of understanding the finality of death (McCown and Pratt 1985; Williams 1981). However, in one study of 60 subjects, the majority of children expressed some belief in personal mortality by age 6 (Reilly et al. 1983). Psychological symptoms that often follow a sibling's death include guilt, confusion, depression, loneliness, anger, problems with schoolwork, an increase in behavior problems, an increase in aggression, social withdrawal, decrease in social competence, sleep disturbances, disruptions in eating habits, hallucinations of the deceased sibling, distortions in cognitive functioning, death phobias, accident proneness, increased dependence on parents, suicidal ideation, and disturbed attitudes toward doctors and hospitals (Atuel et al. 1988; Balk 1983; Binger et al. 1969; Cain et al. 1964; Davies 1988; Mandell et al. 1983, 1988; McCown and Pratt 1985; Williams 1981). Guilt reactions were experienced for the following reasons: 1) for being alive when the sibling was dead, 2) for having wished the sibling dead, and 3) for having been well when the sibling was ill (Rosen 1984–1985).

These symptoms can be exacerbated by such circumstances as 1) the unavailability of the mother while the terminally ill sibling is hospitalized, 2) the suddenness of the death, 3) witnessing or discovering the death, 4) the parents' reactions, 5) inadequate or confusing parental explanations of the death, 6) the degree to which the siblings were attached to each other (such as in an undifferentiated relationship), and 7) in some cases funeral attendance for preoedipal surviving siblings (Cain et al. 1964; Mandell et al. 1988; Williams 1981). Suddenness of death was associated with more separation themes in projective test stories in children from the Philippines (Atuel et al. 1988).

The death can affect the family structure in the following ways: 1) loss of a playmate or companion, 2) loss of an older brother who protected the younger sibling, 3) loss of a baby that an older child needed to mother, 4) loss of an ally against a mentally ill parent, or 5) loss of a younger sibling who could be dominated (Cain et al. 1964). The parent-child relationship can be changed or disrupted in the following ways: 1) the surviving sibling may blame the parents, 2) the sibling may ask difficult and painful questions that strain the relationship, 3) the sibling may become the reassuring one, or 4) the sibling may be used as a substitute for the deceased child (Best and VanDevere 1986; Mandell et al. 1983).

Sex ratio and impact of sibling death. There are few significant sex differences in behavior problems of the surviving sibling. If the deceased sibling was male, there was an increased probability of behavior problems in the surviving sibling (McCown and Pratt 1985). Sex of the child and the nature of the sibling's death (sudden or anticipated) was not significant (Atuel et al. 1988). In one study, confusion at the time of the interview was significantly greater in females ($P < .01$) (Balk 1983).

Age and type of onset. Rosen (1986) reported that a sense of loss was more likely to be felt in children who were older than 5 years at the time of death. Likewise, the death of an older child is more disruptive to surviving siblings than the death of a younger child or a perinatal death where the child was never seen by its siblings, thus making it harder to experience the death as real (Leon 1986). Atuel et al. (1988) found that the age of the deceased child significantly influenced the ease with which siblings moved through the various stages of grief. A higher proportion of children who experienced the death of a younger sibling were still in the earlier stages of grief reaction.

Course. For many children, adjustment to the death of a sibling may last for 6 months after the death (Williams 1981). With some children, there were still problematic behaviors after 1 year (Mandell et al. 1983). Atuel et al. (1988) reported that a higher proportion of children who experienced a recent death, and had a lower social status, were still in the earlier stages of grief and had not yet come to the stage of acceptance of the death. Although not statistically significant, more children whose siblings died suddenly versus those who anticipated their siblings' death were still in the earlier stages of grief (66% versus 50%). Rosen (1986) found a significant correlation between family communication at the time of death and the amount of contact between the family members (especially contact with mothers) as adults.

Familial patterns. The child's adjustment to a sibling's death is influenced by the parent's grief. Parents can often overlook sibling grief because of their own intense grief reactions (Bank and Kahn 1982). The surviving sibling's grief can be met with silence or irritation by the parent (Williams 1981), which the surviving child may interpret as blame that he or she caused the death. This imposed silence communicates to the sibling the need to deny feelings, thus preventing mourning and resolution of grief. Rosen (1986) found that 76% of adults who had lost a sibling in childhood had not spoken about their feelings to anyone prior to their participation in the study. Rosen identified three factors that contributed to the silence: 1) failure on the part of those intimately connected with the family to acknowledge and support the need to mourn; 2) the surviving siblings' own feeling that they must spare the grieving parents any more pain that would result from talking about their own grief; and 3) admonitions to the surviving siblings from extended family, neighbors, teachers, or adult friends to be "strong" and help their parents.

Factors significantly influencing the relative amount of helpful communication by parents with their children in one study were 1) the time spent at home by the dying child during the terminal stages of the illness, 2) the extent of communication, 3) discussions about the actual process of dying, and 4) religious faith (Graham-Pole et al. 1989). However, there was a lack of association between the perceived helpfulness of communication and the siblings' later mood, indicating that the siblings remained angry, sad, fearful, or in denial despite the discussions.

Graham-Pole et al. suggested that siblings may need discussion that focuses specifically on their subjective sense of loss. Parental overprotectiveness of the surviving siblings can also occur and can stifle the child's healthy struggle for separation (Bank and Kahn 1982). Later, in rebellion against this, the sibling can engage in risk-taking behavior to prove he or she is invulnerable to the deceased sibling's fate. In an effort to replace the lost child, parents may try to make the surviving sibling the embodied representative of the dead sibling or may conceive a child specifically for that reason. Parents who lose an infant may also want to retain infant behavior in the surviving sibling (Mandell et al. 1988). The child often then struggles in his or her efforts to live two identities, with resultant low self-esteem and a sense of burden or guilt. Davies (1988) reported that, following the death of a sibling, there was an initial increase in behavior problems in children, but that, 3 years after the death, there were fewer behavior problems if the family was cohesive, engaged in active recreation, and was religious. Likewise, if the family encouraged intellectual or cultural activity, the surviving children showed more adaptive behavior and social competence as a result of more social involvement. Family size was negatively correlated with behavior problems (McCown and Pratt 1985). Communication appeared easier in families whose religious beliefs were a source of support (Graham-Pole et al. 1989). In the extreme instances of suicide in adolescents, the siblings are usually deeply affected (McIntosh and Wrobleski 1988).

Sibling Illness

There are 35 million disabled people in the United States, of which half are adolescents or younger children. Approximately 10% of children under age 18 suffer from a physical handicap or chronic disease (Tolmas 1986). A sibling's illness can cause major disruptions in family functioning (Abramovitch et al. 1987; Burton 1975). Well siblings may resent the ill sibling because of added responsibilities, such as caring for younger siblings, more house chores to do, and being left to fend for themselves (Bank and Kahn 1975, 1982; Bendor 1990). Well or nonhandicapped siblings may experience feelings of social inadequacy (Israelite 1986), increased levels of anxiety, a desire to become ill, loneliness (Bendor 1990), feelings that parents value them less than the sick sibling, anger, guilt (Bendor 1990; Seligman 1983), fear of contracting the illness or disability (Seligman 1983), increased interpersonal aggression with peers and at school (Breslau et al. 1981), increased maladjusted school behavior (Tew and Laurence 1973), and symptoms of depression (Breslau and Prabucki 1987). Information obtained via maternal report indicates that well siblings of handicapped children experience increased depression, aggression, and somatic complaints (Lobato et al. 1987). Findings in a study by

Lavigne and Ryan (1979) indicate that siblings of ill or disabled children tend to be more socially withdrawn and irritable than children from healthy families and that this was especially true of siblings of children who had plastic surgery. Lavigne and Ryan also found that siblings between the ages of 3 and 6 years were more likely to show elevations in psychopathology, with siblings of plastic surgery patients showing the highest incidence of psychopathology. In the 7- to 13-year-old group, Lavigne and Ryan found that male siblings of hematology patients showed more likelihood of emotional problems than female siblings of hematology patients. Breslau and Prabucki (1987) reported that siblings of disabled children displayed more depressive symptomology than control subjects, but did not display a higher rate of major depression. Even though a well child's relationship with a disabled sibling can be positive, the well child's problems are often less observable and more troublesome (McHale and Gamble 1987). McHale and Gamble (1989) reported that children, especially girls, with mentally retarded siblings experienced increased psychological problems, although these were not clinically significant. Breslau et al. (1981) also reported that siblings of disabled children did not show higher proportions of severe psychological problems or greater overall symptomatology than control subjects.

There are many clinical reports of the pernicious effects of seriously emotionally disturbed children and adolescents on their siblings. For example, Bank and Kahn (1982) indicated that there is a fear of contagion, anxiety about being viewed as similar, antisocial or antiparental behavior, and repeated misjudgments by parents as to which child was culpable for rule breaking and misbehavior in the home. Roeder (1990) reported that the high access siblings of psychiatrically hospitalized adolescents suffered from lower self-esteem and poorer ego controls than control subjects of nonhospitalized high school students. Parents may polarize the perceived identities of their children into the "bad" child and the "good" child, which Schacter (1985), in a study of clinic patients, has referred to as "devils versus angels." In a study of schizophrenic and affectively disturbed young adults, Harris (1988) found that siblings were anxious about involving themselves in the hospital treatment and often displayed psychological symptoms of their own. Neuman (1966) found the younger brothers of schizophrenic patients to have many similar problems.

Vance et al. (1980) found no evidence of serious disturbance in siblings of children with nephrotic syndrome. However, their results indicated that these siblings did approach abnormality more than the control children. For example, siblings of nephrotic children demonstrated diminished school achievement (20.7% versus 9.4% for control subjects), increased embarrassment in the presence of the other (11.3% versus 3.8%), below average school performance (18.6% versus 1.6%), and decreased physical and emotional health as compared with control siblings. However, fighting was generally less common with nephrotic siblings (51.9% versus 75.9%). Other evidence suggests that ongoing interactions between mentally retarded children and their older siblings are neither more negative nor more positive than those between comparison siblings (Stoneman et al. 1987). McHale et al. (1986) also found children with autistic or mentally retarded siblings did not differ from children with nonhandicapped siblings on their self-reports, except that siblings of nonhandicapped children reported that their families were slightly more cohesive. Grakliker et al. (1962) found no negative effects on siblings of mentally retarded children. Trevino (1979) stressed that the siblings of handicapped children are often themselves at greater risk for psychological and physical problems.

Additional research suggests that sibling illness is not correlated with psychological maladjustment in well siblings if the data are not obtained via maternal report or when the family has an adequate support system (Lobato et al. 1987, 1988). However, Lobato et al. (1987) pointed out that the caretaking role given to female siblings may be a confounding factor, as male siblings who are not given a caretaking role but are given more privileges and more freedom during the period of illness show higher levels of depression. In addition, the psychological health of the female siblings may only be temporary, as sisters may become depressed and anxious as they become older children and adults. Simeonsson and Bailey (1986) reviewed 19 studies and concluded that siblings of handicapped children can experience both negative and positive effects.

Prevalence and risk of problems due to sibling illness. Information on this topic is not available.

Sex ratio and impact of sibling illness. McHale and Gamble (1989) reported that sisters of disabled siblings spend the most time in caregiving activities compared with brothers and sisters of nondisabled siblings and brothers of disabled siblings. They reported that brothers of disabled siblings do perform just as much caregiving as do sisters with nondisabled siblings, and brothers of nondisabled siblings spend the least amount of time in caregiving (McHale and Gamble 1989; Seligman 1983). A study of sisters of developmentally disabled persons found that the greater the dependency of the disabled sibling, the greater the sister's caretaking role and the less intimate the relationship (Begun 1989). Other evidence showed that sisters were more likely to show evidence of psychological problems if they were older than the ill or disabled child (Breslau et al. 1981; Gath 1974). However, Begun found that older sisters of disabled siblings may experience satisfaction with their relationship. Breslau et al. found that only younger, male siblings showed more impairment. They did not find that well siblings' level of adjustment was associated with the severity of illness or disability in the affected sibling.

Age and type of onset. Begun (1989) reported that siblings who were closer in age to developmentally disabled siblings expressed more conflicted relationships than those who were more removed in age from developmentally disabled siblings. His findings also indicate that older siblings who were widely spaced in age were more satisfied with the relationship with a developmentally disabled sibling than younger siblings who were widely spaced in age. Allan et al. (1974) reported that the child who was next youngest to a sibling disabled with cystic fibrosis was most vulnerable. Lavigne and Ryan (1979) found that preschool children tend to withdraw and be irritable, whereas older children act out socially.

Related to sibling illness is sibling drug use. Needle et al. (1986) found that older siblings are frequently a source of drugs and substance use for younger siblings, even though peers are the main source of substances and the most likely group with whom substances are used. They found that adolescents with older siblings who used drugs were statistically more likely to report having used substances than adolescents whose older siblings did not use drugs. Their findings suggest that older siblings are more important role models than parents and that younger siblings with older siblings who use substances are more likely to use substances earlier. Brook et al. (1983) also found that older brothers were influential in their younger siblings' drug use.

Course. The results of a study by Breslau and Prabucki (1987) indicate that the healthy siblings in families of disabled children respond to the ongoing stress with behavioral and emotional symptoms, such as social isolation, that can affect children's long-term adjustment.

Familial patterns. The stress is greater in lower socioeconomic-status families and smaller families where the fewer well siblings are given more household responsibilities (Gath 1974; Seligman 1983). Breslau and Prabucki (1987) found that mothers of disabled children showed more depressive symptomology than control subjects but did not show a higher rate of major depression. Daniels et al. (1987) described evidence for an increase in problems in siblings of children with chronic illness when there was an increase in parental and ill sibling dysfunction, when there were more family stressors, and when there was less family communication and unity. Israelite (1986) reported that siblings who expressed negative feelings toward their hearing-impaired siblings demonstrated negative affect throughout the interview.

Discussion and Recommendations

The sibling relationship is a distinct subsystem within the family system. Siblings have a very strong need to interact with each other, and their relationship is one of the means by which a person develops a sense of a cohesive self. High access siblings often try to "find affirmation of emerging self organization in each other" (Kahn 1988, p. 22). However, there are toxic agents that have the ability to disrupt the system. It is for this reason that sibling aggression, sibling illness, sibling death, or sibling incest, although not by themselves a mental illness any more than spousal death or illness is a marital problem, have the capacity to cause behavioral and emotional problems in the surviving or victim sibling. From a systemic point of view, these factors need to be considered in treating a child who is experiencing these problems, because these experiences can have a negative impact on the social and psychological development of the child. Research also indicates that these problems can extend into adulthood in exceptional cases and affect adult personality and functioning.

In summary, conflicts and losses within the sibling relationship can be a powerful determinant of emotional difficulties in children and adolescents. We recommend the inclusion of sibling relational problems as a diagnostic category in DSM-IV.

References

Abramovitch R, Corter C, Lando B: Sibling interaction in the home. Child Dev 50:997–1000, 1979

Abramovitch R, Corter C, Pepler DJ: Observations of mixed-sex sibling dyads. Child Dev 51:1268–1271, 1980

Abramovitch R, Corter C, Pepler DJ, et al: Sibling and peer interaction: a final follow-up and a comparison. Child Dev 57:217–219, 1986

Abramovitch R, Stanhope L, Pepler D, et al: The influence of Down's syndrome on sibling interaction. J Child Psychol Psychiatry 28:865–879, 1987

Adams DW, Deveau EJ: When a brother or sister is dying of cancer: the vulnerability of the adolescent sibling. Death Studies 11:279–295, 1987

Adelson L: The battering child. JAMA 222:156–161, 1972

Allan J, Townley R, Phelen P: Family response to cystic fibrosis. Australian Pediatric Journal 10:136–146, 1974

American Psychiatric Association: Diagnostic and Statistical Manual of Mental Disorders, 3rd Edition, Revised. Washington, DC, American Psychiatric Association, 1987

Ascherman LI, Safier EJ: Sibling incest: a consequence of individual and family dysfunction. Bull Menninger Clin 54:311–322, 1990

Atuel TM, Williams PD, Camar MT: Determinants of Filipino children's responses to the death of a sibling. Sigma Theta Tau International Research Conference, Maternal Child Nursing Journal 17:115–134, 1988

Balk D: Effects of sibling death on teenagers. Journal of School Health 53:14–18, 1983

Bank SP, Kahn MD: Sisterhood-brotherhood is powerful: sibling sub-systems and family therapy. Fam Process 14:311–337, 1975

Bank SP, Kahn MD: The Sibling Bond. New York, Basic Books, 1982

Bard M: The study and modification of intra-family violence, in The Control of Aggression and Violence. Edited by Singer JL. New York, Academic Press, 1971, pp 149–163

Becker JV, Kaplan MS, Cunningham-Rathner J, et al: Characteristics of adolescent incest sexual perpetrators: preliminary findings. Journal of Family Violence 1:85–97, 1986

Begun AL: Sibling relationships involving developmentally disabled people. American Journal on Mental Retardation 93:566–574, 1989

Bendor SJ: Anxiety and isolation in siblings of pediatric cancer patients: the need for prevention. Soc Work Health Care 14:17–35, 1990

Best EK, VanDevere C: The hidden family grief in the family following perinatal death. International Journal of Family Psychiatry 7:419–437, 1986

Binger CM, Ablin AR, Feuerstein RC, et al: Childhood leukemia, emotional impact on patient and family. N Engl J Med 280:414–418, 1969

Breslau N, Prabucki K: Siblings of disabled children: effects of chronic stress in the family. Arch Gen Psychiatry 44:1040–1046, 1987

Breslau N, Wietzman M, Messinger K: Psychologic functioning of siblings of disabled children. Pediatrics 67:344–353, 1981

Brook JS, Whiteman M, Gordon AS, et al: Older brother's influence on younger sibling's drug use. J Psychol 114:83–90, 1983

Bryer JB, Nelson BA, Miller JB, et al: Childhood sexual and physical abuse as a factor in adult psychiatric illness. Am J Psychiatry 144:1426–1430, 1987

Burton L: The Family Life Of Sick Children. London, England, Routledge & Kegan Paul, 1975

Cain AC, Fast I, Erickson ME: Children's disturbed reactions to the death of a sibling. Am J Orthopsychiatry 34:741–752, 1964

Canavan MM, Meyer WJ, Higgs DC: The female experience of sibling incest. Journal of Marital and Family Therapy 18:129–142, 1992

Cole E: Sibling incest: the myth of benign incest. Women and Therapy 1:79–89, 1982

Courtois CA: Healing the Incest Wound: Adult Survivors In Therapy. New York, WW Norton, 1988

Crittenden P: Sibling interaction: evidence of a generational effect in maltreating infants. Child Abuse Negl 8:433–438, 1984

Daie N, Wilztum E, Eleff M: Long term effects of sibling abuse. J Clin Psychiatry 50:428–431, 1989

Daniels D, Moos RH, Billings AG, et al: Psychosocial risk and resistance factors among children with chronic illness, healthy siblings, and healthy controls. J Abnorm Child Psychol 15:295–308, 1987

Davies B: The family environment in bereaved families and its relationship to surviving sibling behavior. Children's Health Care 17:22–31, 1988

De Jong AR: Sexual interactions among siblings and cousins: experimentation or exploitation? Child Abuse Negl 13:271–279, 1989

Dickstein LJ: Spouse abuse and other domestic violence. Psychiatr Clin North Am 11:611–628, 1988

Dunn J, Kendrick C: The arrival of a sibling: changes in patterns of interactions between mother and first-born child. J Child Psychol Psychiatry 21:119–132, 1980

Dunn J, Kendrick C, MacNamee R: The reaction of first-born children to the birth of a sibling: mothers' reports. J Child Psychol Psychiatry 22:1–18, 1981

Felson RB, Russo N: Parental punishment and sibling aggression. Social Psychology Quarterly 51:11–18, 1988

Finkelhor D: Sexually Victimized Children. New York, Free Press, 1979

Finkelhor D: Sex among siblings: a survey on prevalence, variety, and effects. Arch Sex Behav 9:171–194, 1980

Finkelhor D, Hotaling GT: Sexual abuse in the national incidence study of child abuse and neglect: an appraisal. Child Abuse Negl 8:23–33, 1984

Forward S, Buck C: Betrayal of Innocence: Incest and Its Devastation. New York, Dutton, 1978

Fox RJ: The Red Lamp of Incest. New York, Dutton, 1980

Friedrich WN: Psychotherapy Of Sexually Abused Children And Their Families. New York, WW Norton, 1990

Furman W, Buhrmeister D: Children's perceptions of the qualities of sibling relationships. Child Dev 56:448–461, 1985

Gath A: Sibling reactions to mental handicap: a comparison of the brothers and sisters of Mongol children. J Child Psychol Psychiatry 15:187–198, 1974

Gebhard PH, Gagnon JH, Pomeroy WB, et al: Sex Offenders: An Analysis of Types. New York, Harper & Row, 1965

Gill DG: Sibling induced injury? Ir Med J 75:12, 1982

Gilligan C: In A Different Voice. Cambridge, MA, Harvard University Press, 1982

Graham-Pole J, Wass H, Eyberg SM, et al: Communicating with dying children and their siblings: a retrospective analysis. Death Studies 13:465–483, 1989

Grakliker BV, Fisher K, Koch R: Teenage reaction to a mentally retarded sibling. American Journal of Mental Deficiency 66:838–843, 1962

Green AH: Child abuse by siblings. Child Abuse Negl 8:311–317, 1984

Gully KJ, Dengerink HA, Pepping M, et al: Research note: sibling contribution to violent behavior. Journal of Marriage and the Family 43:333–338, 1981

Harris EG: My brother's keeper: siblings of chronic patients as allies in family treatment, in Siblings in Therapy: Life Span and Clinical Issues. Edited by Kahn MD, Lewis KG. New York, WW Norton, 1988, pp 314–337

Israelite NK: Hearing-impaired children and the psychological functioning of their normal-hearing siblings. Volta-Review 88:47–54, 1986

James K, MacKinnon L: The incestuous family revisited: a critical analysis of family therapy myths. Journal of Marital and Family Therapy 16:71–88, 1990

Jehu D: Sexual dysfunctions among women: clients who were sexually abused in childhood. Behavioral Psychotherapy 17:53–70, 1989

Jesse RC: Children of alcoholics: their sibling world, in Siblings in Therapy: Life Span and Clinical Issues. Edited by Kahn MD, Lewis KG. New York, WW Norton, 1988, pp 228–252

Johnson TC: Child perpetrators: children who molest other children: preliminary findings. Child Abuse Negl 12:219–229, 1988

Kahn MD: Intense sibling relationships, in Siblings in Therapy: Life Span and Clinical Issues. Edited by Kahn MD, Lewis KG. New York, WW Norton, 1988, pp 3–24

Koch HL: The relation of certain formal attributes of siblings to attitudes held toward each other and toward their parents. Monogr Soc Res Child Dev 24(4):Serial No 78, 1960

Lavigne JV, Ryan M: Psychologic adjustment of siblings of children with chronic illness. Pediatrics 63:616–627, 1979

Laviola M: Effects of older brother-younger sister incest: a review of four cases. Journal of Family Violence 4:259–274, 1989

Leon IG: The invisible loss: the impact of perinatal death on siblings. Journal of Psychosomatic Obstetrics and Gynecology 5:1–14, 1986

Lindberg FH, Distad LJ: Post-traumatic stress disorders in women who experienced childhood incest. Child Abuse Negl 9:329–334, 1985

Lobato D, Barbour L, Hall LJ, et al: Psychosocial characteristics of preschool siblings of handicapped and nonhandicapped children. J Abnorm Child Psychol 15:329–338, 1987

Lobato D, Faust D, Spirito A: Examining the effects of chronic disease and disability on children's sibling relationships. J Pediatr Psychol 13:389–407, 1988

Loeber R, Tengs T: The analysis of coercive chains between children, mothers, and siblings. Journal of Family Violence 1:51–70, 1986

Mandell F, McAnulty EH, Carlson A: Unexpected death of an infant sibling. Pediatrics 72:652–657, 1983

Mandell F, McClain M, Reece R: The sudden infant death syndrome: siblings and their place in the family. Ann N Y Acad Sci 533:129–131, 1988

McCord W, McCord J, Howard A: Familial correlates of aggression in nondelinquent male children, in The Dynamics of Aggression. Edited by Megargee EI, Hokanson JE. New York, Harper & Row, 1970, pp 41–65

McCown DE, Pratt C: Impact of sibling death on children's behavior. Death Studies 9:323–335, 1985

McHale SM, Gamble WC: Sibling relationships and adjustment of children with disabled brothers and sisters. Journal of Children in Contemporary Society 19:131–158, 1987

McHale SM, Gamble WC: Sibling relationships of children with disabled and non disabled brothers and sisters. Developmental Psychology 25:421–429, 1989

McHale S, Sloan J, Simeonsson RJ: Sibling relationships of children with autistic, mentally retarded, and nonhandicapped brothers and sisters. J Autism Dev Disord 16:399–413, 1986

McIntosh JL, Wrobleski A: Grief reactions among suicide survivors: an exploratory comparison of relationships. Death Studies 12:21–39, 1988

Meiselman KC: Incest: A Psychological Study of Causes and Effects With Treatment Recommendations. San Francisco, CA, Jossey-Bass, 1978

Minnett AM, Vandell DL, Santrock JW: The effects of sibling status on sibling interaction: influence of birth order, age, spacing, sex of child, and sex of sibling. Child Dev 54:1064–1072, 1983

Needle R, McCubbin H, Wilson M, et al: Interpersonal influences in adolescent drug use: the role of older siblings, parents and peers. Int J Addict 21:739–766, 1986

Neuman G: Younger brothers of schizophrenics. Psychiatry 29:146–151, 1966

Reilly TP, Hasazi JE, Bond LA: Children's conceptions of death and personal mortality. J Pediatr Psychol 8:21–31, 1983

Roberto LG: The vortex: siblings in the eating disordered family, in Siblings in Therapy: Life Span and Clinical Issues. Edited by Kahn MD, Lewis KG. New York, WW Norton, 1988, pp 297–313

Roeder KA: A comparison of adolescent psychiatric patients and their siblings with regard to ego development and self-esteem. Unpublished doctoral dissertation, University of Hartford, West Hartford, CT, 1990

Roscoe B, Goodwin MP, Kennedy D: Sibling violence and agonistic interactions experienced by early adolescents. Journal of Family Violence 2:121–137, 1987

Rosen H: Prohibitions against mourning in childhood sibling loss. Omega Journal of Death and Dying 15:307–316, 1984–1985

Rosen H: When a sibling dies. International Journal of Family Psychiatry 7:389–396, 1986

Rosenthal PA, Doherty MB: Serious sibling abuse by preschool children. Journal of the American Academy of Child Psychiatry 23:186–190, 1984

Russell DEH: The Secret Trauma: Incest in the Lives of Girls and Women. New York, Basic Books, 1986

Sargent D: Children who kill. Social Work 7:35–42, 1962

Schacter FF: Sibling deidentification in the clinic: devil vs angel. Fam Process 24:415–427, 1985

Sears RR, Maccoby EE, Levin H: Patterns of Child-Rearing. New York, Harper & Row, 1957

Seligman M: Sources of psychological disturbance among siblings of handicapped children. Personnel and Guidance Journal 61:529–531, 1983

Simeonsson RJ, Bailey DB: Siblings of handicapped children, in Families of Handicapped Persons. Edited by Gallagher JJ, Vietze PM. Baltimore, MD, Brookes, 1986, pp 67–77

Smith H, Israel E: Sibling incest: a study of the dynamics of 25 cases. Child Abuse Negl 11:101–108, 1987

Steinmetz SK. The Cycle of Violence: Assertive, Aggressive and Abusive Family Interaction. New York, Praeger, 1977

Stillwell R, Dunn J: Continuities in sibling relationships: patterns of aggression and friendliness. J Child Psychol Psychiatry 26:627–637, 1985

Stoneman Z, Brody GH, Davis CH, et al: Mentally retarded children and their older same-sex siblings: naturalistic in-home observations. American Journal on Mental Retardation 92:290–298, 1987

Straus MA, Gelles RJ, Steinmetz SK: Behind Closed Doors: Violence in the American Family. New York, Anchor Books, 1980

Tew BJ, Laurence KM: Mothers, brothers and sisters of patients with spina bifida. Dev Med Child Neurol 15 (suppl 29):69–76, 1973

Tolmas HC: Adolescent disability and family dynamics. International Journal of Adolescent Medicine and Health 2:197–209, 1986

Toman W: Basics of family structure and sibling position, in Siblings in Therapy: Life Span and Clinical Issues. Edited by Kahn MD, Lewis KG. New York, WW Norton, 1988, pp 46–65

Trevino F: Siblings of handicapped children: identifying those at risk. Social Casework 60:488–493, 1979

Vance JC, Fazan LE, Satterwhite B, et al: Effects of nephrotic syndrome on the family: a controlled study. Pediatrics 165:948–955, 1980

Williams ML: Sibling reaction to cot death. Med J Aust 2:227–231, 1981

Chapter 39

Physical Abuse and Neglect of Children

John F. Knutson, Ph.D., and
Helen A. Schartz, Ph.D.

Statement and Significance of the Issues

The purpose of this chapter is to consider evidence for the utility of including physical abuse and neglect as parent-child relational diagnoses in DSM-IV. In considering the potential utility of these diagnostic categories, we first focus on public policies relevant to physical abuse and neglect and the implications of this public policy context for possible psychiatric diagnostic categories. Second, various strategies for operationally defining abuse and neglect are considered. Although defining abuse or neglect might seem to be the final component of such a review, it is the operational definitions adopted by investigators and service agencies that have determined the data that are available, including the prevalence or incidence estimates that can be made. Although the operational definitions of abuse and neglect that have been adopted in the research literature can limit the utility of the research, the definitions are not the only limiting factor affecting this review. Child abuse and neglect research is affected by a host of severe methodological limitations; these too are considered before we examine the actual data that are available. Following a summary of the existing data on the incidence of physical abuse and neglect, characteristics of abused and neglected children are reviewed. We include considerations of such child characteristics as risk factors, behavioral characteristics of abused and neglected children, and the association of abuse and neglect with child and adolescent psychopathology. A review of parent characteristics then follows as well as a review of evidence on the course of maltreatment, apparent long-term consequences of physical abuse and neglect, and the possible association between childhood maltreatment and adult dysfunction. Finally, we focus on issues related to abuse and neglect diagnoses, the clinical and research implications of including physical abuse and neglect as diagnostic categories in DSM-IV, the desirability of including physical abuse and neglect in DSM-IV, and recommended guidelines for establishing diagnostic criteria.

Method

The articles reviewed were identified by a variety of means: computerized searches (e.g., PsychLit and Medline), annotated bibliographies, journals that typically publish articles on child abuse and neglect, individual libraries of the authors, and personal communications with researchers. Searches of PsychLit from January 1973 through December 1990 and Medline from January 1988 through May 1991 yielded 1,936 citations. A considerable number of articles were identified and discarded ($n = 323$) because they did not actually deal with physical abuse or neglect of children, although the articles may have used those individual words in their titles, keywords, or abstracts. Some duplication ($n = 246$) among the computerized searches also resulted in a reduction in the number of sources to be examined. It was still necessary to establish guidelines to choose only those articles from among the remaining 1,367 citations that were most appropriate for a consideration of child abuse and neglect as a relational diagnosis.

Studies conducted to investigate types of maltreatment other than physical abuse or neglect (e.g., sexual abuse, elder abuse, domestic violence, fetal abuse, or institutional abuse) were disregarded unless they contained a comparison group of physically abused or neglected children and could address issues relevant to the inclusion of a relational diagnosis, as opposed to merely providing comparisons among types of maltreatment. Approximately 300 articles were excluded because they dealt primarily with abuse that could not be classified as physical abuse or neglect of children by parents.

Because mental disorders are assumed to transcend cultural differences and because of the relation between DSM-IV and ICD-10 (World Health Organization 1990), DSM-IV diagnoses should be formulated in a manner that is not culturally bound. Of course, the expression of the disorder often reflects the cultural context. With respect to abuse and neglect, there are significant cross-cultural differences in child care standards and the provision of services that can influence abuse detection (e.g., S. Cohen and Warren 1990); therefore, research samples drawn from different cultures can be difficult to compare. Moreover, the establishment of statutory-based mandatory reporting of suspected maltreatment has had a significant impact on both epidemiology and the defining of maltreatment. Thus, data from countries in which mandatory reporting was not in force would not be comparable to data from countries in which mandatory reporting of maltreatment was required (e.g., Doek 1984; Pieterse and Van-Urk 1989). As a result of these considerations, studies based on samples from outside North America were generally excluded unless they provided data that replicated North American studies or that amplified existing data. Thus, although work conducted in the United Kingdom and Europe is represented, 167 of the references identified from the computerized searches were eliminated because the samples were drawn from populations that would preclude generalization to the samples that characterized most of the reviewed research. In addition, virtually all research published in unedited journals, nonarchival journals, or newsletters that would not be generally available to a reader was excluded.

Computerized searches were supplemented with examinations of many annotated bibliographies available from the Clearinghouse of the National Center for Child Abuse and Neglect. These included bibliographies pertaining to risk factors, ethnicity, religious immunity, physical abuse, neglect, child fatalities, shaken baby syndrome, child characteristics, parental characteristics, effects of maltreatment, longitudinal studies, and studies of homeless and runaway children. Additionally, the tables of contents and indices of journals that often publish articles pertaining to child abuse and neglect (e.g., *American Journal of Psychiatry, American Journal of Orthopsychiatry, Child Abuse and Neglect, Developmental Psychology, Journal of Abnormal Psychology, Journal of Consulting and Clinical Psychology, Child Development,* and *Child Welfare*) were reviewed. Also, reference lists of articles were routinely examined for papers that might have been overlooked.

The process for identifying potentially useful citations was designed to result in a comprehensive list of articles pertaining to physical abuse or neglect of children. More than 800 articles that had not been excluded using the guidelines described above were then examined to determine whether they provided original data or innovative analyses of existing large data sets. Many were eliminated because they did not contain any empirical evidence. With few exceptions, studies that provided no *original* data were excluded. Because of problems generalizing from case studies, virtually all articles based on case studies were also eliminated. A few articles concerning important theoretical considerations, methodological critiques, reviews, or rare but possibly important case studies were retained in the review. However, more than 300 articles were eliminated because either they were descriptions of case studies or they contained no original data. Even with this systematic approach to reviewing the literature, it is likely some relevant articles were overlooked. However, it is improbable that any such omitted article would be so significant as to change the scope and thrust of this review. Therefore, we believe that the present review provides comprehensive coverage of the available empirical evidence directly related to the inclusion of the physical abuse or neglect of children by parents as relational psychiatric diagnoses in DSM-IV.

Results

Public Policy Issues

When considering the possibility of including physical abuse and neglect of children as a relational problem in DSM-IV, it is important to recognize that this diagnosis has legal and public policy implications. Such a DSM-IV diagnostic category could both reflect public policy and influence public policy to an extent that might exceed that of any other psychiatric diagnoses. Moreover, because the existing data on physical abuse and neglect are determined to some extent by existing public policy, a consideration of public policy issues in this review seemed critical.

Historically, it is possible to identify articles relevant to abuse and neglect in the late 19th and early 20th centuries. However, the maltreatment of children by parents was largely an ignored topic until the publication of "The battered-child syndrome" (Kempe et al. 1962). This article resulted in a dramatic growth of professional interest in child abuse and neglect, and, perhaps more importantly, the article attracted popular media attention to the problem, thereby setting the stage for a new child-related political agenda (e.g., B. J. Nelson 1984). In the United States, the new political agenda ultimately led to the passage in 1974 of the Child Abuse Prevention and Treatment Act (PL 93-247), a federal initiative that charged states with the responsibility to develop standards for defining abuse, to establish mandatory reporting of suspected abuse, and to identify the agency responsible for investigating abuse allegations. In addition, PL 93-247 provided for research and educational initiatives to reduce the incidence of child abuse. This initial federal legislation has been followed closely by legislation in each state that provides statutory definitions of child maltreatment as well as provisions to attempt to meet the needs of maltreated children and their families. Subsequent federal legislation (e.g., Title I of PL 95-266) and the Child Abuse Amendments of 1984 (PL 98-457) resulted in an expansion of the abuse domain to include sexual exploitation as well as the requirement to provide medical treatment for disabled infants with life-threatening conditions (i.e., Baby Doe regulations). Although the scope of abuse legislation has been expanded, those expansions have not always met with widespread approval, and challenges to public policy or abuse legislation do occur (see Newman 1989). In general, federal and state legislative actions have had such far-reaching effects on professional activities and research concerning child maltreatment that it can be reasonably argued that the entire field, at least within the United States, is essentially less than two decades old. Additionally, continuing legislative activity (e.g., PL 100-294, the Child Abuse Prevention, Adoption, and Family Services Act of 1988) has been setting research agenda, suggesting that the field of child abuse and neglect will continue to be in a state of transition and will be embedded in public issues for some time to come.

Several aspects of all this legislation have had a direct effect on the research reviewed in this chapter. One of the most important influences has been the establishment of mandatory reporting laws and their effects on both operational definitions of abuse and existing epidemiological assessments. Because abuse victims and their families come to the attention of researchers from the mandatory reporting system, it is clear that the current database is largely determined by the mandatory reporting statutes. Mandatory reporting statutes identify specific professions or occupational roles that are required to report *suspicions* of maltreatment of a child and the specific agency that is charged with the responsibility of investigating any abuse allegation. Because the laws were motivated by the desire to aid children who might be at risk for being harmed, the statutes specify relatively low standards of evidence necessary to evoke a suspicion, with higher standards being required for substantiation of an allegation by an investigating agency. In turn, this standard for substantiating maltreatment by a child protective service (CPS) agency is less stringent than the judicial standards in juvenile court proceedings for establishing the occurrence of abuse (i.e., "preponderance of evidence"). However, even judicial standards of evidence of abuse can reflect considerable variance. For example, if the child in question were a Native American, because of the Indian Child Welfare Act (PL 95-608), a more stringent evidential standard of "clear and convincing" must be met. Thus, because of statutes, the data on abuse among Native Americans may not be comparable to the data on abuse among other ethnic groups in the United States (Kessel and Robbins 1984; Wichlacz and Wechsler 1983).

Another public policy influence on existing data reflects inconsistencies between laws related to the needs of abused or neglected children and other clinical service statutes. For example, until the Federal Alcohol and Drug Abuse Confidentiality Act was amended in 1986 (PL 99-401), clinicians providing services to substance-abusing clients were prohibited by federal regulations from reporting the suspected abuse of a child by the substance-abusing client (Blume 1987; Bromley and Riolo 1988; Saltzman 1986). Thus, the epidemiological database might have underrepresented alcohol- and drug-abusing perpetrators between 1978 and 1986, because of conflicting public policy between a federal effort to protect the confidentiality of one class of clients and the mandatory reporting requirements of the states. Another example of public policy influences on abuse research and clinical practice is the passage of religious exemptions to child neglect laws in many states (Skolnick 1990). These laws stipulate that some parental actions may be exempt from maltreatment standards if the parental acts are consistent with "sincere" religious beliefs. However, even in states specifying religious exemptions to neglect statutes, child fatalities following unsuccessful but sincere faith-healing efforts can result in prosecution (e.g., Bussiere 1988).

One of the questions related to public policy that will have to be addressed in considering a psychiatric diagnosis of physical abuse or neglect is whether the diagnosis should be isomorphic with standards for suspicions in mandatory reporting statutes or whether a more stringent standard for diagnosis would have to be met. Related to this issue, the distinction among standards of abuse is often based on the difference between "harm" and "endangerment." Although either standard might be applicable for establishing a suspicion, substantiation of maltreatment may require the standard of harm, depending on the jurisdiction and the circumstances of the assessment. If a DSM-IV diagnosis for neglect and physical abuse were adopted, and if the diagnostic criteria establish a standard that exceeds that of the state mandatory reporting requirements, diagnosticians may be confronted with a demand to refer (submit a mandatory report of abuse suspicions) despite inadequate evidence to support a diagnosis. This is just one of many issues that must be considered in the public policy implications of a DSM-IV physical abuse and neglect diagnosis.

Because sexual abuse criteria are represented in the criminal codes of most states and because of the demand for prescribed prison terms for sex offenders, sexual abuse statutes tend to reflect a high degree of specificity. In contrast, the statutory definitions of physical abuse and neglect are necessarily vague, because they are designed to cover a remarkably broad range of endangering or harmful acts directed at children. Moreover, there is considerable variability among states (C. R. Flango 1988; Hartley 1981). Although the need to have a broad statutory base for defining abuse may be apparent, the possibility of adverse consequences has been the focus of considerable debate. Some have lamented the effects of these broad and vague definitions on research and called for more narrow definitions of abuse (e.g., Besharov 1981; Giovannoni and Becerra 1979; Mele-Sernovitz 1980); others have argued in favor of the broad definitions for both clinical and research purposes (e.g., Gelles 1982). In addition, the statutory definitions have been criticized for their clinical and legal implications. For instance, Guyer (1982) outlined the problems associated with a criterion of "reasonableness" in both clinical and judicial decision making in abuse cases. Similarly, Christophersen (1983) and Wasserman and Rosenfeld (1985) questioned the impact of the vague statutes on both clinical decision making and clinical practice. Wald (1975, 1976, 1982), considering legal and clinical implications of abuse statutes, argued for very stringent standards for defining abuse in terms of the harmful consequences of the abusive act. However, arguments such as those offered by Wald do not seem to have been persuasive in state legislatures. The political agenda has continued to embrace a broad and nonspecific approach to defining abuse and neglect in child protection statutes.

Changes in statutes, perhaps driven by various political agendas, can compromise the long-term epidemiological database. For example, the Amendment to the Child Abuse Act in 1984 added the "Baby Doe" requirements to neglect statutes, thereby adding failure to provide medical services to critically ill disabled infants to the forms of neglect (Bopp 1985; Bopp and Balch 1985). Although the rate of this form of neglect is probably too low to influence the existing statistics on physical abuse and neglect, it illustrates how the political agenda and public policies can affect research.

The statutory, judicial, and apparent public support for corporal punishment in the schools of most states is another public policy that may influence a possible physical abuse diagnosis (Reitman 1988). Although corporal punishment in the schools is prohibited by statute in several states, the codes of most states are either silent on corporal punishment or explicitly authorize it. When the laws of a state do not prohibit corporal punishment in the schools, the courts have treated statutory silence as support for the use of corporal punishment (Connors 1979). A Department of Education survey estimates that there were more than 1.4 million episodes of corporal punishment in schools in the United States in 1980. The use of corporal punishment was most common in southern and southeastern states and least common in the northeastern states (McCluney 1987; Van Dyke 1983). With widespread support for the use of corporal punishment in the schools, diagnostic standards for physical abuse by parents could be influenced by the standards of corporal punishment established for school personnel. The guidelines for corporal punishment, however, are also often vague or nonexistent (McCluney 1987), and the limits on corporal punishment in the schools have been based largely on judicial rulings.

Two Supreme Court decisions have been pivotal in establishing guidelines for the use of corporal punishment in the schools, and these may have implications for diagnostic standards of physical abuse. In a 5–4 decision, the 1977 *Ingraham v. Wright* (430 U.S. 651, 97 S. Ct. 1401, 51 L. Ed. 2d 711) ruling established that corporal punishment in the schools is not cruel and unusual punishment and, therefore, is not a violation of the Eighth Amendment. Moreover, the ruling established that the corporal punishment meted in that case did not violate due process standards and that a hearing prior to the imposition of corporal punishment was not required. In *Baker v. Owen* (395 F. Supp. 294 [M. D. N. C.] [1975], aff'd 423 U.S. 907 [1976]) the Supreme Court let stand an Appellate Court ruling that outlined minimal due process requirements for corporal punishment in the schools. Essentially, unless the transgressions are extreme, corporal punishment should not be applied on a first offense basis, students should be apprised of the corporal consequences of their offenses, punishment should be administered in the presence of another school official, and parents may request a written explanation of the reasons for the punishment and who was present during its administration. These guidelines do not directly address the issue of severity of punishment.

Based on a review of relevant statutes, state and local regulations, and judicial decisions, Hudgins and Vacca (1985) provided guidelines for corporal punishment in the schools that might have implications for diagnostic standards of physical abuse in homes. First, the goal of the punishment should be for "correction" and be the best means for achieving child obedience; it should not involve any malice. Second, the punishment should not be considered cruel and unusual. The dissenting opinion in *Ingraham v. Wright* noted that the injurious punishment experienced by the plaintiff in that case would clearly be unacceptable in criminal proceedings. Moreover, in a family court context, the discipline considered acceptable in *Ingraham v. Wright* would almost certainly be seen as abusive. According to Hudgins and Vacca, corporal punishment in the schools that would meet contemporary standards of "acceptability" would have the following characteristics: appropriate for the age and sex of the child, resulting in no lasting or permanent injury, and incorporating an appropriate instrument at an appropriate locus of impact. Similarly, Connors (1979) indicated that contemporary guidelines for *excessive* corporal punishment in the schools would entail more than three blows with a paddle, blows that left bruises or marks, blows applied anywhere other than the buttocks, and discipline that resulted in temporary or permanent physical injury. Public policy support for physical discipline in the schools, coupled with the widespread public support for physical discipline in the home (e.g., Erlanger 1974), caused Zigler (1979) to be pessimistic about the prospects of reducing physical abuse of children in the home. Whether there really are public policy limitations on efforts to reduce abuse, it is clear that any decisions regarding the inclusion of physical abuse and neglect as a diagnosis in DSM-IV will have to be made with an awareness of the broader public policy issues of maltreatment and corporal discipline. Moreover, if a diagnosis of abuse or neglect were included in DSM-IV, the complex relation of a psychiatric diagnosis to judicial decisions would also have to be recognized (see Goodman 1989; J. E. B. Myers and Carter 1988).

Defining Physical Abuse and Neglect

Physical abuse. The available evidence on the physical abuse and neglect of children is limited by the wide range of operational definitions adopted by researchers. Not surprisingly, some of those definitions are direct reflections of statutes, regulations, or local policies, but others reflect the methodological or theoretical positions of investigators (e.g., Besharov 1981; Finkelhor and Korbin 1988; Gelles 1982; Giovannoni and Becerra 1979; O'Toole et al. 1983; Parke 1977; Parke and Collmer 1975; Rosenthal 1988; U.S. Department of Health and Human Services 1988).

Physical abuse is typically defined as an act of commission by a parent or a child's caretaker that is associated with some specifiable consequence. Thus, the abuse definition may specify an act, an act and a consequence, or merely a consequence of parental action. When the act alone is the defining characteristic, abuse has been defined as striking a child with some object, specific types of blows (e.g., with closed fist), or blows directed at specified body loci (e.g., Berger et al. 1988; Straus 1980). When the definition of abuse is based on consequences of parental acts, tissue damage ranging from bruises and abrasions to fractures, disfigurement, need for medical services, or life-threatening injury has been used. Although the consequence approach to defining abuse seems straightforward, setting defining criteria for abuse in terms of degree of tissue damage only seems simple (Wald 1982). Because of the difficulty in setting a tissue damage standard or because of concerns that it is too stringent, "endangerment" as a consequence has also been adopted as an operational definition of abuse (Office of Human Development Services 1988; Sedlak 1990). Such a definition suggests that some acts pose a clear and present danger, albeit they might not have actually resulted in injury. Thus, the endangerment definition reflects a blending of defining abuse in terms of acts and outcome standards. In practice, the combination of acts and consequences is probably the most common strategy for operationally defining physical abuse.

One of the major issues in defining physical abuse has been the importance of the intentionality of the act. In a study of hospital personnel and their ratings of events as abusive, Snyder and Newberger (1986) demonstrated that the intentionality of the alleged perpetrator was important in determining whether physicians, social workers, psychologists, and nurses classified events as abuse. Intention is typically considered as the will to harm the victim, but it is often determined by expressions of socially desirable goals offered by perpetrators or indications that the injurious event was accidental. Of course, determining that an injury was accidental is difficult (e.g., C. F. Johnson 1990).

In court proceedings, the presumed intention of an abuse perpetrator is crucial. For example, youngsters could be brought to medical attention because of subdural hematoma or retinal hemorrhages that are the direct result of shaking (e.g., Alexander et al. 1990a, 1990b; Caffey 1972; Levin et al. 1989). If the act were determined to be in a disciplinary context, it would be viewed as physical abuse; however, if the act were determined to have occurred in a playful interaction, it would probably not be labeled physical abuse. The health consequence to the child would be indistinguishable, but whether CPS agencies would intervene might well be a function of a determination of the intention of the perpetrating parent. Finkelhor and Korbin (1988) argued that abuse should be defined as injurious acts that are proximal, proscribed, and preventable. Moreover, according to Finkelhor and Korbin, the intentionality of the act is critical for it to be termed abuse.

This concern with intention in operational definitions has a long history in aggression research (e.g., Buss 1961; Dollard et al. 1939; Feshbach 1971; Knutson 1973). There are those who argue that aggression must be defined in terms of intentionality (e.g., Berkowitz 1983; H. Kaufman 1970) and those who argue that intentions, because they cannot be assessed unequivocally, should not determine whether an act is aggressive (Buss 1961; Knutson 1973). Thus, by the latter approach, whether an act is defined as aggressive would not be a function of expressions of social desirability or subjective ratings of inadvertence. Knutson (1978, 1988) advanced the same argument while considering definitions of physical abuse. The social desirability of an act would be ignored; the accidental nature of the episode could be determined probabilistically or through an assessment of the setting in which the event occurred. If an injury occurred during rule-consistent activity (e.g., struck by a pitched ball), the probability of the injury being an accident would be enhanced. It has also been suggested that base rate information regarding accidents could be derived from consumer product safety data to distinguish between the probability of a particular injury occurring as an accident or as an abusive episode (Wissow and Wilson 1988).

Another approach to defining abuse operationally in terms of consequences is to incorporate the emotional or psychological sequelae of acts that have not resulted in significant tissue damage. Although this approach has been criticized for its vagueness (e.g., E. W. Browne and Penny 1974; B. J. Nelson 1984; Wald 1982), some investigators (e.g., Garbarino and Stocking 1980; Hart and Brassard 1987; Rohner and Rohner 1980) have argued that psychological consequences are at the heart of all maltreatment and could serve as the defining characteristics of physical abuse as well (e.g., Garbarino and Gillian 1980). Some authors have even argued that the presence of some psychiatric symptoms, such as multiple personality disorder in children, are prima facie evidence for abuse (e.g., Elliott 1982). Unfortunately, in the context of a psychiatric diagnosis of relational problems, determining the consequences of maltreatment, or the comorbidity of behavioral problems with maltreatment, such an approach would confuse outcomes with presenting problems. Moreover, as is noted later, research has yet to establish any behavioral or psychiatric markers of physical abuse or neglect with acceptable specificity and reliability.

Another strategy for defining physical abuse has been to adopt criteria based on contemporary social norms. For example, Sapp and Carter (1978) surveyed a representative sample of Texans and established their personal definitions of abuse by asking respondents to classify parent-child acts as abusive or nonabusive. If the criteria for physical abuse were based on a majority of respondents from the Sapp and Carter survey, striking children with some objects (e.g., belts, wooden paddles) would not be abuse, but striking children with other objects (e.g., coat hangers, belt buckles) would. According to a majority of Texans surveyed, any acts that resulted in injury to the child would also be considered abuse. In view of the regional differences in the acceptability of corporal punishment in the schools, it might be expected that there would be regional differences in rating different parenting behaviors as abusive that would thus confound a set of national criteria such as DSM-IV. It should be noted, however, that an assessment by Polansky et al. (1983) of community subcultural differences in rating parental acts as maltreatment did not identify any major group differences; in addition, a survey by Bower (1991) of university students in Iowa yielded ratings of parental acts that were generally comparable to those from Sapp and Carter.

Neglect. Where physical abuse has typically been operationalized as an act of commission, neglect has usually been defined in terms of acts of omission or in terms of more indirect pernicious influences than physical abuse. For example, in a widely cited paper, Polansky et al. (1975) defined neglect as a

> Condition in which a caretaker responsible for the child either deliberately or by extraordinary inattentiveness permits the child to experience available present suffering and/or fails to provide one or more of the ingredients generally deemed essential for developing a person's physical, intellectual and emotional capabilities. (p. 5)

In many respects the same issues and problems with the definition of physical abuse apply to operational definitions of neglect. With few exceptions, the literature on neglect tends to be vague in its definitions (e.g., Zuravin 1989). Like physical abuse, neglect has often been defined in terms of its consequences, especially harm or endangerment. Although some research incorporates clearly specified standards of both harm and endangerment (e.g., Office of Human Development Services 1988), it is often unclear in the research literature whether the neglected children experienced harm or endangerment. Clearly, diagnostic standards that incorporate consequences would have to specify either a harm or an endangerment standard.

Just as some definitions of physical abuse enumerate specific abusive acts, some definitions of neglect have been structured as taxonomies of deficient and neglectful parenting (e.g., Giovannoni 1985; Hegar and Yungman 1989; Office of Human Development Services 1988) under a general model of failure to meet parenting requirements according to prevailing cultural or professional norms. It is important to note, however, that "prevailing cultural norms" can vary according to time, gender, educational background, and occupation (e.g., Ringwalt and Caye 1989), as can "professional norms" (e.g., Snyder and Newberger 1986). Thus, the taxonomies can be quite complicated.

One influential approach to a taxonomy of neglect was provided by the second National Incidence Study (NIS-2) (Office of Human Development Services 1988). The NIS-2 distinguished among physical neglect, educational neglect, and emotional neglect, as well as whether harm or endangerment occurred. In addition, there was an unspecified category for classifying forms of neglect that could not be placed in the three specific categories. Included under the physical neglect classification were 1) health care refusal, 2) delay in seeking health care, 3) abandonment, 4) expulsion, 5) other custody issues, 6) inadequate supervision, and 7) other physical neglect. For each of these parental actions (or inactions), there had to be some occurrence of injury or clear risk of injury. Educational neglect entailed 1) permitting chronic truancy, 2) failure to enroll, and 3) inattention to a special education need. The emotional neglect category subsumed 1) inadequate nurturance or affection, 2) chronic or extreme violence in the child's environment, 3) permitting drug or alcohol abuse, 4) permitting maladaptive behavior, 5) refusal of psychological care, 6) delay in obtaining psychological care, and 7) other inattention to developmental needs.

Other defining strategies have followed somewhat different organizational structures and placement of specific neglectful actions (e.g., Hegar and Yungman 1989; Zuravin 1989). Regardless of the specific structure, it is clear that a broad range of parental acts or failures to act can be represented in neglectful parenting. As in research on physical abuse, decisions to include or exclude specific components can have a significant influence on data and possible diagnostic criteria.

The distinction between actual harm and endangerment has been important in public policy decisions, clinical service, and research. Some have argued for a high standard of harm to define neglect (e.g., Wald 1982), and others have argued for broader endangerment standards (e.g., Lally 1984; S. M. Smith 1984; Wolock and Horowitz 1984). If the former approach were uniformly adopted, home safety (e.g., Tertinger et al. 1984) or home cleanliness (e.g., Watson-Perczel et al. 1988) could not be used to define neglecting families.

Defining neglect in terms of acts of omission or the possibility that neglect reflects a lack of knowledge implies that the intention of the neglecting parent would be relevant to operational definitions. In fact, intention has been very important for some investigators in defining neglect. For example, Junewicz (1983) and Rohner and Rohner (1980) both noted the importance of hostility and rejection, and some states define neglect in terms of the volitional acts of parents. Of course, unequivocal determination of intention is no easier in diagnosing neglect than it is in physical abuse.

One clear intentional aspect of definitions of physical neglect relates to religious exemptions in the medical neglect statutes of many states (cf., Flowers 1984; Skolnick 1990). In most jurisdictions, depending on the degree of harm or endangerment, refusal of medical services in favor of faith healing may not be treated as neglect. Interestingly, sincerity of belief is also important in some jurisdictions, clearly implying another intentional caveat to the definition of neglect. Although state laws and courts often treat membership in a "recognized" church as a mark of sincerity, direct assessments of the sincerity of parents espousing faith healing have also been attempted.

Included among some classifications of neglect are children presenting with nonorganic failure to thrive (NO-FTT). Schmitt and Mauro (1989) noted, however, that NO-FTT is operationally defined in various ways, and not all NO-FTT can be considered to be a function of neglectful parenting. Ayoub and Milner (1985) also argued that there were distinguishing features that separated NO-FTT families from physically abusive and neglecting families. It is important to note that the widely publicized cases of NO-FTT involving deliberate parental acts that result in severe malnutrition probably account for fewer than 1% of the NO-FTT cases (Schmitt and Mauro 1989); those cases, however, seem to have had a significant public policy impact.

In this review, we focus on physical neglect rather than educational, emotional, or developmental neglect. However, the boundaries among various classes of neglect are not necessarily firm. For example, lack of supervision (e.g., "latchkey children" [Fosarelli 1984]) could be included in emotional neglect in some systems; if the child were to be at risk of injury, this lack of supervision would be placed in the category of physical neglect; if the lack of supervision were associated with truancy, then the neglect would be educational. Thus, specific "neglectful" acts of parenting may not be as defining as are the proximal consequences of those parenting acts. Perhaps because of the occurrence of overlapping classifications, there has been a tendency in both research and public policy to blend physical abuse and neglect into a single category of physical child maltreatment. Indeed, many studies with samples of physically abused, neglected, and sexually abused children place all groups in a category of maltreated children. Such an approach poses considerable difficulties for reviewers attempting to relate specific types of child maltreatment to psychological dysfunction, health consequences, or comorbidity with psychiatric diagnoses. Definitional inconsistencies have caused many research difficulties, but definitional problems are certainly not the only methodological limitations in contemporary child abuse research.

Methodological Problems in Abuse and Neglect Research

Research on clinical problems is often compromised by a variety of methodological constraints, and research on psychiatric problems is often associated with additional limitations. Research on the physical abuse and neglect of children, even among difficult areas of investigation, seems to be characterized by more than the usual number of difficulties. Indeed, review articles in the area routinely call attention to methodological problems and the manner with which conclusions are compromised by the quality of the research (e.g., Besharov 1981; Franks 1982; Gelles 1982; Hallett 1988; Knutson 1988; Leventhal 1981, 1982; Widom 1988). Although there seems to have been considerable improvement in the overall quality of research, we must consider the widespread limitations in the database before directly addressing the evidence that bears on abuse and neglect as a DSM-IV relational diagnosis.

One of the major problems is poorly defined samples. As suggested by the previous section, operationally defining abuse and neglect for research purposes can be a challenge. An additional problem is the aggregating of physical abuse, neglect, and sexual abuse into a single category of child maltreatment (e.g., Carlson et al. 1989). Although physical abuse, neglect, and sexual abuse might have common characteristics and outcomes (e.g., Cicchetti 1990; R. C. Herrenkohl and Herrenkohl 1981; Smetana et al. 1984), there are data to suggest that important epidemiological, causal, and outcome differences exist among these types of maltreatment (e.g., Goldston et al. 1988; Rohrbeck and Twentyman 1986; Widom 1989a, 1989b). Thus, aggregating samples at the present time may limit the progress in the field. Certainly, from the standpoint of establishing the need for diagnoses or establishing diagnostic standards, specification of samples with respect to the type of maltreatment is important. On occasion, samples are described so vaguely that it is impossible for the reader to know the maltreatment to which the child has been exposed, or even whether they have actually been exposed to abuse or neglect. That is, often samples are described as "high-risk" families, without indicating how the risk was established, or simply described as "abused" children. In the present review, descriptions of the samples were important factors in evaluating the potential utility of an article.

In much of the child abuse and neglect literature, the investigator leaves the operational definition of abuse or neglect to a referral source rather than making an independent assessment. Unfortunately, because a relatively large body of research suggests that standards for reporting suspicions of physical abuse and neglect differ among professionals and nonprofessionals and among geographical locations (e.g., Alter 1985; Deitrich-MacLean and Walden 1988; Dukes and Kean 1989; Giovannoni and Becerra 1979; Misener 1986; O'Toole et al. 1983; Snyder and Newberger 1986), the referral source may not be a reliable approach to defining abuse operationally. Similarly, differences between suspicions of abuse and substantiation of abuse can be considerable, and that distinction is not always made by the researcher when the referral source determines the abuse or neglect status of the subjects. Moreover, as detailed in the section on public policy, there can be important differences among jurisdictions in setting criteria for abuse occurrences. Just as aggregating types of maltreatment may limit the utility of research, aggregating referral sources (e.g., courts, CPS agencies, Parents Anonymous) can yield samples that may obscure the influence of important variables.

Dependency on a referral source to define a sample can also result in sampling bias. This is one of many causes of sampling bias discussed by Widom (1988) in a review article that focused on the implications of sampling biases and the resulting limitations of the knowledge base in the area of abuse. According to Widom (1988), there are two basic biasing influences: method selection and criterion selection. In the former, the common methodologies adopted by abuse investigators (e.g., using agency records, emergency rooms, families in treatment, self-report measures) yield data of unknown generality. When samples are selected on the basis of some criterion-related events (e.g., neurological impairment, biological family members), biased data on abuse-related events may result. Because of such problems in sampling bias, A. Browne and Finklehor (1986) have argued for using "natural collectivities." Such an approach has been used in some laboratories (e.g., Berger et al. 1988; Goldston et al. 1988), but it is not widely implemented. One important sampling bias that exists in the literature is the limited representation of fathers. As J. A. Martin (1984) and Bradley and Lindsay (1987) noted, although fathers are well represented as perpetrators of physical abuse, they are poorly represented in the research literature, especially the treatment literature; mothers have even participated as subjects in studies of maltreating parents when the perpetrator was the father.

Another methodological problem that characterizes the area of abuse and neglect is the limited original data. When Plotkin et al. (1981) reviewed the methodology of 270 representative articles related to causal variables in child abuse, they concluded that only 25% of the articles presented original data that had been collected by the authors. Occasionally, a data set is extensive, unique, or too costly to reproduce, so reanalysis might be actively encouraged (such as NIS-2). Similarly, by archiving unique data sets (e.g., National Data Archive on Child Abuse and Neglect, Cornell University, Ithaca, New York), creative new strategies of analysis might be permitted. Nevertheless, repeated reanalyses of the same data sets can yield limited understanding of important epidemiological factors while multiplying the influence of any sampling biases that exist. For that reason, Gelles (1982) discussed misattributions that were made regarding Light's (1973) reexamination of Gil's (1970) data set. Interestingly, there have been at least two other reanalyses of the Gil data (Daley and Piliavin 1982; Seaberg 1987).

The occasional need for repeated use of a single sample has been considered in the area of depression research (Garfield 1983; Kupfer and Rush 1983). Although repeated use of and multiple publications from a single sample can be acceptable, the requirement has been established that researchers should clearly identify any prior reports that were based on the sample described. This same standard should apply to child maltreatment research, but such a standard does not characterize the abuse field. We have often identified multiple articles from individual investigators that *seem* to have been based on a single sample (e.g., identical sample sizes, demographic characteristics, results and/or procedures). Because of the multidisciplinary nature of abuse research and the large number of journals in which abuse research is published, such papers were usually distributed among many different journals, so most editors and most single discipline readers would probably not notice the apparent overlap. In an extensive literature search, such as that undertaken for this chapter, such possible repeated use of a sample becomes quite apparent. When apparent duplicative use of data seemed to exist, we generally selected only articles based on original use (earliest citation) of the data. When reanalyses provide significant new information, later articles seemingly based on a single sample were, of course, included.

Although the present review is not focused on the utility of treatment for physically abusive or physically neglectful families, research on treatment is considered because it can provide information on comorbidity, outcome, and probable course. Control or comparison groups are often lacking in abuse research (e.g., Plotkin et al. 1981), but this lack is most apparent in treatment studies. J. H. Fantuzzo (1990) reported identifying more than 1,500 intervention articles in the abuse and neglect area through several standard database literature searches. Among these articles, J. H. Fantuzzo reported being able to identify only two treatment studies that met minimal standards of experimental design. Such a state of affairs clearly limits the empirical basis for intervening on behalf of maltreated children, but it does not necessarily compromise information regarding the possibility of including abuse or neglect as a relational problem. That is, despite the lack of adequate control groups to assess the effectiveness of the treatment, some treatment studies do provide outcome and recidivism data that are useful to the present review.

Beyond the treatment literature, there is a remarkable absence of experimental research involving group designs (Plotkin et al. 1981). Only about one-third of the studies in the abuse or neglect areas provide a control group. When control groups are included, they are often not matched on potentially relevant variables (e.g., Plotkin et al. 1981; Widom 1988). Similarly, although there have been repeated critiques of an excessive reliance on very small samples or individual case studies, such articles are ubiquitous in the contemporary abuse literature. As noted, unless there was a compelling reason associated with a unique diagnostic issue or a unique methodological issue, we did not include case studies. Coupled with the widespread use of case study material is the frequent use of measures of unknown reliability and validity, the use of subjective impressions as a source of data, or the use of nonquantitative descriptions of abuse-related events. Again, such articles were not included in the present review.

Although the child abuse reporting statutes have been in effect for close to two decades, and although large numbers of physically abused and neglected children have come to the attention of service agencies, there has been a remarkable paucity of long-term follow-up research with these populations. As a result, some of the more important questions regarding course and outcome are not easily answered. Moreover, few prospective studies (e.g., Egeland et al. 1980; E. C. Herrenkohl and Herrenkohl 1979; R. C. Herrenkohl and Herrenkohl 1981)) have been developed to eliminate the sampling biases noted by Widom (1988). Thus, methodological limitations continue to compromise the knowledge base in important theoretical and practical domains.

The development of central registries of abuse and neglect incidents was one of the consequences of early child abuse legislation. Among public officials, some investigators, and some clinicians, the registries are assumed to be major contributors to epidemiological and outcome data. Indeed, they are often thought to provide an opportunity to develop subject pools and cross-sectional studies. Unfortunately, as noted by several surveys reported since 1979 (e.g., American Humane Association 1979, 1983, 1988; V. E. Flango et al. 1988; National Center on Child Abuse and Neglect 1980), there is remarkable variability among state registries, and their research utility has been quite limited. For example, in most states, central registries are not likely to include events involving extrafamilial maltreatment, because such events typically proceed through law enforcement agencies, and law enforcement agencies do not routinely submit reports to central registries in most states (V. E. Flango et al. 1988). Although that omission in epidemiological evidence would not be critical for determining the feasibility of abuse and neglect as a parent-child relational problem, it certainly poses difficulties for other aspects of understanding abuse by child caretakers and nonfamilial perpetrators.

Despite the numerous methodological difficulties in the physical abuse and neglect research, evidence is available that is relevant to whether a parent-child relational diagnosis is supportable. In addition, studies that are inadequate in some respects may still provide useful information for the questions being addressed in the present review. For example, therapy outcome studies lacking appropriate control groups may not provide adequate data for supporting the use of a therapy, but data presented on recidivism of treated families can contribute to knowledge of the chronicity of abuse or neglect. Thus, although numerous articles were examined and discarded, there remains a very large body of research that is relevant to the desirability of including physical abuse and neglect in DSM-IV as a parent-child relational problem.

Epidemiology

As the discussion of definitions of abuse and neglect would suggest, the available epidemiological data on physical abuse and neglect are determined by the definitions adopted. As a result, depending on whether conservative or liberal criteria were adopted, prevalence estimates vary widely among studies (e.g., Fontana and Besharov 1979; Gil 1970; Light 1973; Straus and Gelles 1986; Straus et al. 1980). Epidemiological estimates of abuse and neglect are usually based on data obtained from national reporting statistics. As Finkelhor and Hotaling (1984) noted, there are five different levels of information that are potentially available regarding maltreatment statistics, and prevalence estimates are a function of the degree to which these different levels are assessed. The first level of information includes those cases that are known to the state CPS agency; such cases may be substantiated or unsubstantiated. The second level includes those cases that are known to other agencies providing services to children, but these agencies do not necessarily target these children for abuse-specific services. Very often these level-two maltreated children involve extrafamilial cases, law enforcement agencies, or the courts, and there may be some procedural conflicts or overlapping responsibilities among the agencies serving such cases. The third level of information involves children known to service agencies or professionals that are either unaware of their responsibility to submit reports or choose not to report the case to the appropriate CPS agency. Thus, level-three maltreated children would be known to some professionals, but they would not be represented in any official agency statistic as abused children. The fourth level of information involves abuse episodes known to someone not represented in the first three levels, such as a neighbor, a member of the community, or a family member. The fifth level involves abuse in which the incident is known only to the perpetrator and the victim, but the episode is not recognized as abuse by anyone, including the perpetrator and victim. Although it might seem improbable that victims could be involved in truly abusive interactions without recognizing it, only 25% of samples of adolescent and adult subjects meeting conservative criteria for physically abusive childhood experiences describe those experiences as abusive (e.g., Berger et al. 1988; Rausch and Knutson 1991). Moreover, even adolescents who were adjudicated abused are unlikely to label their experiences as physically abusive (Berger et al. 1988). Obviously, the prevalence or annual incidence estimates will be a joint function of the informational levels used and the manner with which they are assessed. It is also the case that local incidence rates may depart significantly from national estimates (e.g., Pless et al. 1987).

There have been several major national studies of the incidence of abuse and neglect, each of which adopted somewhat different definitions of abuse and obtained data from different levels of abuse information. Since 1975, the American

Humane Association has completed an annual report of child abuse and neglect data obtained from state CPS registries. Thus, these reports reflect only level-one data. Moreover, because there are definitional differences among states and because some states do not provide data for the reports, the American Humane Association reports are limited in their contribution to general prevalence estimates.

There have been two national incidence studies commissioned by the National Center on Child Abuse and Neglect. The first National Incidence Study (NIS-1) was completed in 1980, and the second (NIS-2) was completed in 1986 (Office of Human Development Services 1988). Each study was designed to obtain data from the first three levels of information noted. Although NIS-2 used expanded definitions of abuse and neglect relative to those of NIS-1, by using the original definitions as well as the new definitions, the structure of NIS-2 permitted an assessment of changes in the incidence of abuse over time. Straus et al. (1980) and Straus and Gelles (1986) obtained level-four information in 1975 and again in 1985. Their approach incorporated a telephone survey of a nationally representative sample of 2,000 two-parent families that had one or more children older than 3 years old. Although this research is directed at the fourth level of information, the restriction to households with telephones compromises the generalizablility of the data somewhat.

In addition, there are many studies that identify more limited samples and assess the prevalence of abuse in those samples through various self-report measures. Such studies typically obtain data related to level-four or level-five information, but they are typically not nationally representative. Thus, it is likely that the most accurate epidemiological estimates will require an integration of many different data sources.

The most important single epidemiological study available is the NIS-2. A total of 29 counties were selected to be nationally representative of geographic regions of the United States and the degree of county urbanization. Within each of the county areas, the CPS agency and a large sample of public and private child service agencies provided data on incidents of maltreatment known to them during a 3-month period. The submitted records were assessed to determine the "countability" of the incidents according to both NIS-1 definitional standards (harm) and new NIS-2 definitional standards (harm and endangerment) as well as to eliminate instances of record duplication. Then the data were weighted using algorithms to adjust for sampling errors and incomplete participation and to produce an annualized estimate from a 3-month sample. An annualized incidence rate was established for each of the specific forms of maltreatment operationalized for the study according to both harm and endangerment standards. With respect to the former standard, the NIS-2 (Sedlak 1990) estimated the annual incidence of physical abuse at 4.3 per 1,000 children and of physical neglect at 2.7 per 1,000 children. The combined incidence of seriously and moderately injured was 13 per 1,000 children. The incidence rates based on the endangerment standard was 4.9 per 1,000 children for physical abuse and 8.1 per 1,000 children for physical neglect. These estimates yield a combined total of 437,500 children harmed per year by physical abuse or physical neglect and an additional 819,200 endangered by physical abuse and physical neglect.

When contrasted with the 1980 NIS-1, the NIS-2 data indicated a large increase in the incidence of harmful maltreatment since 1980. Because the incidence of fatal maltreatment or severe injury had not changed since 1980, and because fatal or severely injurious maltreatment is unlikely to be undetected, the NIS-2 report concluded that the increase in the incidence of maltreatment of NIS-2 relative to NIS-1 probably reflected a greater professional awareness of the problem and greater recognition of individual cases. Indeed, the NIS-2 report concluded that agencies were reporting far more episodes of maltreatment in 1986 than in 1980. These data are not unlike the American Humane Association (1988) report that there was a 212% increase in reports of maltreatment between 1976 and 1986. Based on a review of 382 maltreatment cases seen at a county pediatric clinic over a 30-month period, Marshall et al. (1988) also concluded that there is greater public and professional awareness that has increased the referral rates of abused and neglected children. Although more cases are being recognized by service providers, the evidence provided by NIS-2 also suggested that fewer than half the recognized cases are actually reported to CPS agencies. Thus, although the NIS-2 indicates that there has been an increase in recognition of maltreatment, the agencies charged with the responsibility of investigating maltreatment allegations are aware of fewer than half the cases known to noninvestigatory child-service agencies. Moreover, epidemiological data that are based on CPS data, such as central registries, are likely to be significant underestimates of the "true incidence" of physical abuse and neglect, because they include only level-one information.

The apparent stability of child maltreatment between 1980 and 1986 reflected in the NIS-2 is not consistent with the two national surveys completed by Straus and Gelles (1986) in 1975 and 1985. In those surveys, the Conflict Tactics Scale (Straus 1979) was administered by telephone to households characterized by couples with a child younger than 3 years old. The data from white families suggested a significant decline in severe coercion directed at the child, but no change in moderate coercion. Although it was reported that there were some increases in coercion directed at children in black households, these increases were not statistically significant. Hampton et al. (1989) argued that this increase in child-directed violence, although not statistically significant, might be important; there are several factors, however, that argue for replication before asserting either the increase in black families or the decrease in white families. Although these studies can provide useful data on family violence, the Conflict Tactics Scale was not designed as an index of physical child abuse, and many parenting patterns are not represented on it. Moreover, the telephone survey approach and restricting the sample to two-parent households with telephones results in a very limited epidemiological base to estimate change.

In addition to establishing an overall estimate of the annual national incidence of maltreatment, the NIS-2 provided analyses of several demographic characteristics that could influence the epidemiology of maltreatment. Although sex of the victim plays an important role in the incidence of sexual abuse, no statistically significant differences were identified in physical abuse or neglect. For males and females, physical abuse was the most prevalent form of abuse. Although females were seen to be at greater risk for injury due to abuse, this difference was attributable to the much higher rate of sexual abuse of girls and the attendant risk for injury in many sexually abusive acts. In another large epidemiological study based on 30,901 confirmed reports in the Colorado Central Registry between July 1977 and June 1984, Rosenthal (1988) concluded that males were at greater risk for injury and serious injury. Although these differences were statistically reliable, they were modest in their absolute value.

With respect to age of victims, according to NIS-2, there was a higher incidence of physical abuse resulting in harm in the 3- to 5-year-old group than in the 0- to 2-year-old group. There was considerable variability in physical harm as a function of age among the older children, with no significant differences obtained among groups from 3 to 17 years of age. When the endangerment standard was applied, a significant increase in physically abusive endangerment was associated with the 12- to 14-year-old group relative to the other groups who were 3 years and older. Contrasts between the NIS-1 and NIS-2 data with respect to physical abuse and age indicated that there was a greater likelihood of reported abuse of older children in 1986 than in 1980. Thus, the assumption that only young children are at risk for physical abuse is seriously questioned by both the NIS-1 data (cf., Olsen and Holmes 1986) and the NIS-2 data. Not surprisingly, there is a marked decline in risk for fatal maltreatment (physical abuse or neglect) from 0.08 per 1,000 in the 0- to 2-year-old group to nearly 0 per 1,000 in the 6- to 8-year-old group. Similar age-related patterns of fatal abuse were reported by Jason and Andereck (1983). There was an increase in overall neglect associated with increasing age; however, this pattern was attributable to increases in educational and emotional neglect and not attributable to increases in physical neglect with age.

Although there were no family size influences on the various forms of maltreatment when a standard of harm was incorporated, data based on the endangerment standard indicated that large families were significantly more likely to evidence physical abuse. Although large families evidenced nearly double the rate of endangering physical neglect evidenced by small families, this difference only approached conventional levels of statistical significance. Overall, the NIS-2 report concluded that there were qualitative family differences beyond limited resources that increased the risk of physical abuse and physical neglect of children from large families. These data are similar to data collected in the United Kingdom between 1977 and 1982, in which large families were associated with greater risk for physical abuse and neglect (Creighton 1985). In a study of fatal child neglect and abuse in a single state between January 1980 and May 1988, Margolin (1990) reported that fatal neglect was associated with larger families than was fatal abuse. In that study, it is important to note that most of the fatal neglect reflected a single incident that could be characterized as a consequence of inadequate supervision rather than persistent physical neglect. Such data are relevant to considerations of including inadequate supervision as a form of endangering physical neglect in a DSM-IV diagnosis.

Among the demographic characteristics that have been widely investigated in studies of physical abuse and neglect is socioeconomic status (e.g., Garbarino and Crouter 1978; Garbarino and Sherman 1980; Gil 1970; Spearly and Lauderdale 1983). Interestingly, although there is a relatively large literature implicating poverty as a variable in child maltreatment, there is considerable controversy about the role of economic status in child maltreatment. The controversy relates in part to how socioeconomic status is measured (e.g., Brown 1984), in part to concerns about sampling biases in research, and in part to public policy issues (cf., Pelton 1978). Within the NIS-2, dividing the sample at a family income of $15,000 indicated that lower-income children were 4 times as likely to be physically abused and nearly 12 times as likely to be physically neglected. Such data are not unlike those described by Garbarino and Crouter (1978) and Zuravin (1989), who used census tract measures to assess poverty and found that neglect was strongly influenced by poverty. When indirect indices of economic disadvantage are used, such as the presence of a telephone or access to shopping and recreation (e.g., Dubowitz et al. 1987), or the presence of vacant homes in the census tract area (Zuravin 1989), poverty is strongly implicated in both physical abuse and physical neglect. In addition, Alperstein et al. (1988) indicated that homeless children evidenced higher rates of abuse and neglect than similar lower-socioeconomic status comparison children.

Although there is a substantial database that implicates economic disadvantage in the occurrence of physical abuse and physical neglect, it is important to recognize that large segments of economically disadvantaged children are not physically abused or neglected (e.g., Farber and Egeland 1987). Some data suggest that children from certain economically disadvantaged groups, such as migrant workers (Larson et al. 1987, 1990), may be at higher risk for abuse or neglect than other children from that socioeconomic stratum. But it is also the case that there is considerable evidence that physical abuse and neglect are represented in all economic strata (e.g., Lynch and Roberts 1982; Steele and Pollack 1974; Straus 1980; Van Stolk 1972). In the light of these data, it has been asserted that child maltreatment is classless and that impoverished groups are overrepresented because of sampling biases.

The overrepresentation of economically disadvantaged groups in central registry data is often attributed to the disadvantaged groups' reliance on public facilities and the use of service agencies that are more vigilant in reporting maltreatment. For example, Knudsen (1989) reported that 47% of the CPS reports in Indiana reflected reports on children already known to CPS. Although some data exist to suggest that hospitals do underreport abuse in higher-income groups (e.g., Hampton and Newberger 1985), there is also some evidence that supports Pelton's (1978) position that the sampling bias is overrated. For example, a study based on a 2-year sample from a metropolitan county in Arizona reported that a majority of the maltreating adolescent parents were receiving no public assistance (Bolton and Laner 1986). Similarly, Rivara (1985) examined the histories of 74 consecutive cases involving physical abuse of a child younger than 25 months old; for 77% of the cases, there was no involvement with the social service department prior to the abuse episode. Although it might be expected that detection and reporting biases might be evidenced in the effect of the metropolitan status of a county, the NIS-2 did not identify any metropolitan influence on the incidence of maltreatment.

Additional data that implicate socioeconomic factors beyond any sampling bias are those related to fatalities. Because underreporting of fatalities is less likely, distributions of fatal events provide a less biased estimate of class-related maltreatment. Nixon et al. (1981) noted that there was a greater rate of nonaccidental injurious child fatalities in lower classes but an equivalence of intentional child homicidal death across classes. Although the rate of fatal incidents in the lower economic group of NIS-2 was three times that of the upper income group, this difference was only marginally significant. Nevertheless, the fatality data certainly implicate socioeconomic variables in severe physical abuse and severe physical neglect.

Several studies have attempted to examine subcultural differences and economic status by using abuse data from military installations. The pattern of data from military settings suggests that the incidence of abuse and neglect is comparable to that in civilian settings (e.g., Acord 1977; Dubanoski and McIntosh 1984; K. K. James et al. 1984; S. S. Myers 1979). Lower enlisted grades were overrepresented in the abuse statistics, as were minority group members.

Ethnicity has been examined in several contexts of the epidemiology of maltreatment. In general, data have been reported as incidence rate differences among various subgroups. Often, these subgroups differ on variables other than ethnicity that seriously compromise any conclusions that can be made. The NIS-2 failed to identify any significant associations between incidence rates for various types of maltreatment and child victims classified as black, white, or other. Although there are studies that report that African Americans and groups with Spanish surnames may be overrepresented in abuse and neglect statistics (e.g., Bolton and Laner 1986; Spearly and Lauderdale 1983), it has been argued that this pattern of data probably reflects the influence of biased reporting. Buriel et al. (1979) noted that, within a random sample of confirmed cases of child abuse and neglect in southern California, Mexican Americans were more often referred to CPS by professional, as opposed to nonprofessional, community agencies than Anglo-American abusers. Hampton and Newberger (1985) also provided data strongly suggesting that a race bias in reporting could account for the existing data on ethnic differences in maltreatment rates. Moreover, when Hampton (1987) completed a subsequent analysis of the NIS-2 data using only "substantiated" cases, he concluded that the overrepresentation of minorities in maltreatment statistics can best be understood as a reflection of economic adversity and discrimination. Similarly, A. L. Wilson (1990) analyzed infant mortality in South Dakota and contrasted it with national statistics; the mortality of nonwhite infants in South Dakota was four times that of white infants, but the article noted that these differences reflected the role of socioeconomic factors in abuse and neglect rather than ethnic contributions per se.

In another study of the contribution of ethnicity to incidence estimates, Eckenrode et al. (1988) examined 5% of the abuse and neglect reports submitted to the New York Central Registry during a 5-month period and found that minority group membership was among the factors that significantly predicted substantiation of physical abuse reports. They interpreted this influence of ethnicity as a reflection of process variables rather than a static influence of ethnicity on abuse. The Eckenrode et al. data are certainly consistent with Hampton's (1987) call for studies of maltreating and nonmaltreating families within ethnic groups to determine empirically specific environmental and social factors that could be contributing to minority overrepresentation in *some* child maltreatment statistics. When studies of maltreatment have been conducted within minority groups, the data are often characterized by considerable variance. For example, within an American Indian culture, White and Cornely (1981) reported annual incidence rates of 10.34 per 1,000 for adjudicated or substantiated abuse or neglect among children younger than 9 years old living on Navajo reservations. However, within the reservations that were sampled, annual incidence rates ranged from 6.72 to 15.75 per 1,000. Such data indicate the amount of variance that can exist within an ethnic group and strongly suggest that variables other than ethnicity play a role in determining the occurrence of abuse or neglect.

Another area of concern about the current epidemiological estimates of physical abuse and neglect is the lack of representation of children who do not reside in established households. Census information suggests that large numbers of children are living on the streets with their homeless families. By many standards of harm or endangerment, many of these children probably qualify as neglected but have not been included in statistics on child abuse and neglect. In addition to homeless families, many runaway youths are not represented in official national samples. Descriptive reports based on interviews with youths living on the streets (Kufeldt and Nimmo 1987) and adolescents presenting at youth shelters (McCormack et al. 1988; Powers et al. 1990; Stiffman 1989) suggest that a significant proportion of these youth report experiencing physical abuse in the homes that they have left. Based on street interviews for five consecutive nights per month for 12 months in a major Canadian city, Kufeldt and Nimmo reported that 27.8% of the adolescents described being physically abused at home. Stiffman found that 43.9% of the 291 youths interviewed at shelters for adolescents reported being physically abused at home. The procedures of Stiffman, however, required that parental consent be gained by telephone from the guardians of all participating youths. This procedure suggests that many youngsters or families may have refused to participate, yielding a potentially unrepresentative sample. Unfortunately, information on the rate of refusal was not provided. The Powers et al. study reported that 60% of the sample of adolescents presenting at youth shelters in New York during 1986–1987 reported being physically abused; McCormack et al. indicated 43% of the sample from a Toronto shelter reported physical abuse.

In addition to socioeconomic status and ethnicity, epidemiological estimates are often influenced by the substantiation rates of suspected abuse by the state CPS agency. Several studies have examined substantiation rates to determine whether mandatory and permissive reports differ in their substantiation rates and whether substantiation was influenced by characteristics of the child. Although the overall substantiation rates are generally less than 50% (e.g., Eckenrode et al. 1988; Faller 1985; Kotch and Thomas 1986; Powers and Eckenrode 1988; Zuravin et al. 1987), the substantiation rates for anonymous reports (Zuravin et al. 1987) are only 15.5%. Similarly, professional reports are substantiated at a rate 23% higher than nonprofessional reports (Eckenrode et al. 1988). Not surprisingly, voluntary reports of neglect have the lowest substantiation rate. For physical abuse and neglect, substantiation rates decline with the age of the child, whereas sexual abuse substantiation rates increase with age. Although patently false accusations of maltreatment do occur (Schuman 1986), they account for only a small percentage of the unsubstantiated allegations.

In addition to the studies based on agency records, there have been a number of attempts to assess the epidemiology of physical abuse by gathering self-report data regarding personal experiences. In conducting such research, it is important that natural collectivities of subjects be used (A. Browne and Finkelhor 1986) to avoid the sampling biases noted. Based on questionnaire surveys completed by 600–1,600 undergraduates per year between 1979 and 1990, a conservative lifetime prevalence estimate of approximately 8% was established (Berger et al. 1988; Knutson and Mehm 1988; Knutson et al. 1991; Rausch and Knutson 1991; Zaidi et al. 1989). Moreover, there has been no obvious systematic change in the reports of physically punitive childhoods during the period during which these studies were conducted. Thus, the data are consistent with the hypothesis that the actual occurrence of abuse has not been changing significantly during the recent past. Consistent with these undergraduate data, based on a self-report survey of 3,998 adolescents attending middle school and high school in a midwestern city, Hibbard et al. (1990) reported that 9% indicated they had been physically abused, whereas an additional 5.2% described being physically and sexually abused. Other studies with college students (e.g., K. A. Miller and Miller 1983) have yielded data that are not unlike the Berger et al. (1988) data.

The existing epidemiological data do not permit an unequivocal conclusion regarding the "true prevalence" of physical abuse and physical neglect in the population, but the data do indicate that the problem is of sufficient magnitude to be a significant health risk for children. For the purposes of this chapter, the critical question is whether there is an important association between physical abuse and neglect and psychological dysfunction. Data from clinics suggest that abuse and neglect may be important factors in populations seeking services at child psychiatric facilities. For example, based on consecutive referrals to a tertiary-care psychiatric facility, 24% of the children seen had unequivocal evidence of physical abuse in their histories (Zaidi et al. 1989). Similarly, Leal (1976) reported that one-sixth of 3,600 admissions of children younger than age 5 to an inner-city child psychiatric facility had been physically abused or neglected. When contrasting adult and adolescent admissions to an emergency psychiatric facility, Hillard et al. (1988) concluded that recent physical abuse was the second most important determinant of adolescent admissions. In the pediatric clinic, 27% of the infants referred for psychological evaluations had been physically abused or severely neglected. Thus, admissions data from several psychiatric clinics suggest that physical abuse and neglect might be an important factor in child psychiatric services.

Characteristics of Abused or Neglected Children and Their Families

In this chapter, we focus on the issue of including physical child abuse and neglect as a relational diagnosis in DSM-IV. There is growing support in the abuse and neglect literature for models of maltreatment that reflect the interaction of parent characteristics, child attributes, and environmental factors in the occurrence of abuse or neglect (e.g., Belsky 1984; Cicchetti 1990; Kempe and Helfer 1972). Such an approach is consistent with other research related to parent-child interactions and the emergence of deviant behavior (e.g., Bell 1968; Lamb 1981; Patterson 1982). In addition to the conceptual appeal of the interactive models of abuse, the appeal of the broader approach has been facilitated by the general failure to identify significant psychopathology or other common deviant attributes among maltreating parents (Berger 1985; Parke and Collmer 1975). As a result, recent child abuse research has focused on a broad range of child attributes that could be contributing factors in the emergence of abuse or neglect, as well as parental attributes outside the domain of diagnosable psychopathology.

Child characteristics as contributing factors. There are many developmental difficulties that have been associated with physical abuse and neglect of children (Augoustinos 1987). Like other problems, they can be considered either antecedents or consequences of abuse and neglect, depending on their temporal relation to the maltreating episode. One of the more widely investigated developmental factors in abuse and neglect has been the neonatal risk factors of prematurity and low birth weight. Many early studies in the area (e.g., Faranoff et al. 1972; Frodi 1981; Goldberg 1979; E. C. Herrenkohl and Herrenkohl 1979; R. C. Herrenkohl and Herrenkohl 1981; Klein and Stern 1971; H. P. Martin 1976; S. M. Smith 1976) provided evidence that low-birth-weight or prematurity placed infants at great risk for physical abuse. Leventhal (1981), however, challenged this conclusion following a review of the methodological problems characterizing this literature. Moreover, based on a review of 11 longitudinal cohort studies, Leventhal (1988) concluded there was only limited utility in attempting to predict maltreatment from perinatal conditions. Yet Leventhal et al. (1989), examining the 4-year outcome of high-risk infants identified by clinicians, demonstrated that the high-risk infants were more likely to be abused or neglected than the matched comparison group. Other studies (e.g., Egeland and Brunnquell 1979; Egeland and Vaughn 1981; Gaines et al. 1978; Starr 1988) failed to establish the link between the premature birth of the infant and later abuse. Similarly, Benedict et al. (1985) compared a cohort of 532 abusive mothers with a case-matched control group based on birth records in Maryland and failed to identify any pregnancy history, labor, or delivery factors that were predictive of abuse.

Although direct evidence is inconclusive, there are some data to suggest that low birth weight or prematurity might have an indirect influence on the emergence of abuse or neglect through a disruption of the parent-child attachment process (e.g., Goldberg 1979). This disruption could be a function of mother-infant separation occasioned by intensive pediatric services, but evidence has been offered that prenatal stress and negative attitudes toward the pregnancy might also contribute (e.g., E. C. Herrenkohl and Herrenkohl 1979). Other data to support an interactive model of the association of physical abuse or neglect with prematurity or low birth weight come from the work of Frodi et al. (1978, 1981). This research demonstrated that premature infants emit vocalizations that are more irritating to listeners than those of full-term infants. Moreover, these irritating cries evoke different responses from abusive and nonabusive parents. It has been hypothesized that such irritating cries could impair the attachment process, resulting in the resistant-avoidant attachment characterizing some abused infants (e.g., Egeland and Sroufe 1981; Lyons-Ruth et al. 1987). It should be noted, however, that not all abused infants evidence irritating cries. Egeland et al. (1980) also noted that abused infants sometimes appear to be less responsive than nonabused infants.

Concerning specific attachment styles, Egeland and Sroufe (1981) were able to demonstrate an anxious-resistant type of impaired mother-child attachment in neglected children. Although Schneider-Rosen and Cicchetti (1984) and Crittenden (1988) documented impaired attachment in abused and neglected children, these studies were not able to make an unequivocal determination of a relation between type of maltreatment and the specific form of disrupted attachment. Schneider-Rosen and Cicchetti (1984) noted impaired visual self-recognition and impaired cognitive affective aspects of the attachment process for both neglected and abused children. In contrast to these studies, Crittenden (1988) noted that abused, and abused and neglected, children were more compulsively compliant, whereas the neglected children evidenced a more passive style of interaction with their mothers. According to Crittenden (1988), the abusive mothers were more controlling and the neglectful mothers were less responsive to their infant's signals.

Although a high rate of insecure attachment between abusive mothers and infants has been replicated in Britain (e.g., D. Browne and Saqi 1988), there has been considerable controversy regarding the relation between type of attachment and the occurrence of abuse. Moreover, studies have identified apparently securely attached infants who had experienced abuse, as well as insecurely attached infants who were not abused (e.g., D. Browne and Saqi 1988; Schneider-Rosen and Cicchetti 1984; Schneider-Rosen et al. 1985). Work by Carlson et al. (1989) suggests that the apparent inconsistencies regarding abuse and attachment could be due to the limitations of the commonly used three-category attachment classification system that is based on the work of Ainsworth et al. (1978). Carlson et al. added a disorganized-disoriented category to the original taxonomy and were able to identify that attachment pattern among many maltreated infants. Because these abused infants would not have been categorized as anxious-avoidant or anxious-ambivalent, they would have been erroneously classified as "securely attached" in the three-category system.

The possibility of early behavioral risk factors, such as low birth weight or prematurity, combining with maternal characteristics to yield an abusive pattern of parenting has been suggested by the prospective work of Egeland et al. (1980) and is consistent with research on child temperament (e.g., Plomin 1983) and child reactions to angry adult behavior (e.g., El-Sheikh et al. 1989). Thus, although it is impossible to assert that neonatal difficulties yield abuse or neglect, there are some data consistent with neonatal difficulties as risk factors that may combine with parental risk factors to yield abuse or neglect. In addition, abuse or neglect can exacerbate the health and developmental problems of high-risk infants.

In a prospective 4.5-year follow-up study of 129 infants with birth weights less than 1,251 grams, adverse neurological and cognitive outcomes were associated with intracranial hemorrhage. Neglectful or abusive parenting, however, was the most important risk factor in cognitive or neurological dysfunction of these children (Leonard et al. 1990). It should be noted that this study may be severely compromised by sample attrition. It began with 203 surviving infants of 326 admitted infants; from the 203, 74 were lost to various sources of attrition. Despite these sample limitations, the data suggest that abuse or neglect of low-birth-weight children poses a serious health risk beyond the risks associated with low birth weight per se.

Another risk factor about which there is considerable controversy is child illness. Early work (e.g., Lynch 1975) yielded speculation that childhood illness could be a stressor that contributes to the emergence of abuse. A prospective study by Sherrod et al. (1984) evaluated the contribution of many child characteristics to the emergence of physical abuse, neglect, or failure-to-thrive. During the first 3 years of life, the abused children were more likely to have experienced illness and accidental injuries, as well as maltreatment, than the control group. The greater incidence of accidental injury in the abused group relative to the neglected group is interesting in the context of the common assumption that it is neglect that increases risk for accidental injury. Based on a retrospective case-controlled study, Starr (1988) also presented evidence that abuse may be associated with early childhood illness. In related work, when recipients of tertiary health care were studied, the important effect of neglect in children with chronic illness has also been identified (e.g., Boxer et al. 1988; Jaudes and Diamond 1986). Although the chronic preexisting illness could occasion neglect, in these studies neglect was seen as exacerbating the chronic illness.

Other child characteristics that have been thought to increase stress and increase risk for abuse or neglect are handicapping conditions. Because handicapping conditions can result in children who are difficult to manage, who evidence significant cognitive impairments, who are communicatively limited, or who are limited in mobility, handicapping conditions can be conceptualized as chronic stressors for child care providers as well as disrupters of the attachment process. Unfortunately, virtually all handicapping conditions or their behavioral manifestations can be occasioned by physical abuse or neglect (e.g., Jaudes and Diamond 1985; Sandgrund et al. 1974; Solomons 1979). As a result, it is often impossible to determine whether the handicapping condition contributes to the occurrence of abuse or whether it is a consequence of abuse. It is therefore not surprising that there is some controversy regarding handicaps as risk factors in abuse.

Some reviews have identified the presence of a handicap as a contributor to abuse (e.g., Friedrich and Boriskin 1976; Gil 1975; Gillespie et al. 1977; Morse et al. 1970); other reviews (e.g., Starr et al. 1984) and studies (e.g., Coon et al. 1980) have questioned the role of handicaps as a factor in the occurrence of abuse. One of the primary criticisms of the position that abuse could be facilitated by handicaps is the lack of solid epidemiological data on handicapping conditions among abused groups as well as problems with sampling biases, retrospective analyses, or an absence of control groups. For example, Ammerman et al. (1989) reported a physical abuse prevalence rate of 19% among a sample of 150 multihandicapped children consecutively admitted to a psychiatric hospital; they concluded that abuse risk was increased by handicaps, especially milder handicaps. However, when contrasted with physical abuse prevalence rates of 24% in other psychiatric facilities (e.g., Zaidi et al. 1989), the data do not suggest a link between handicaps and abuse in child psychiatric populations. Camblin (1982) noted that almost half of the central registries failed to record handicapping conditions. More recent research suggests that many states cannot provide data on handicapping conditions of children in foster care (Hill et al. 1990). Nevertheless, the foster care data that do exist suggest that up to 20% of the children in foster care have some handicapping condition (e.g., Hill et al. 1990). Although such data provide suggestive evidence that handicaps may relate to maltreatment, very few state records indicate whether the handicap played a role in either the placement or the emergence of abuse or neglect.

Other lines of indirect evidence have caused some to argue that it is premature to discard the possible link between handicaps and abuse (Garbarino et al. 1987). For example, research with communicatively impaired and hearing-impaired children has suggested that hearing impairment is a risk factor in physical and sexual abuse (Sullivan et al. 1991). Moreover, related data have suggested that parents of deaf children are more likely to use physical coercion than are parents of hearing children (e.g., Schlesinger and Meadow 1972). In addition, evidence from residential placement facilities suggests that sensorially impaired children may be at greater risk for maltreatment (Brookhouser 1987; Whittaker 1987).

Numerous studies suggest abused and neglected children present with significant developmental delays, although they are as likely to be consequences of abuse as precursors. In one of the few long-term follow-up studies, Elmer (1967) reported that after 13 years, only 2 of 33 abused children evidenced normal development. Similarly, Sandgrund et al. (1974) reported that physically abused and neglected children evidenced significantly lower IQ scores than a comparison group matched on age, sex, and socioeconomic status. Consistent with Sandgrund et al., Tarter et al. (1984) found that physically abused delinquents evidenced lower verbal IQs and particularly lower scores on the comprehension and similarities subtests of the Wechsler Intelligence Scale for Children—Revised than nonabused delinquents referred to the same psychiatric facility. In a study of 42 closed cases served by a family-based services program, 45% of the families had one or more children who presented with a learning disability, mental retardation, emotional disability, or physical handicap (Bribitzer and Verdieck 1988).

In a sample of 260 consecutively referred physically abused or neglected children seen at a single pediatric clinic, 27% had growth problems, and 33% evidenced speech and language or other developmental delays (Taitz and King 1988). Not surprisingly, there was a significant association between the growth problems and the developmental delays. Schor and Holmes (1983) described cases of severe neglect and physical abuse of a preschool child and infant that were characterized by extreme growth delay. Following 4.5 months in foster care, the children had evidenced dramatic compensatory growth rates well beyond what could be expected from normal growth in the period of time elapsed. Cognitive and language delays continued on follow-up, however. Similarly, long-term follow-up studies of 29 NO-FTT children (Singer 1986) indicated persistence of intellectual delays even when weight gain had been maintained. Although rescued children with abuse-dwarfism syndrome evidenced improvements in intelligence that correlated with growth in stature, the longer-term outcome was not uniformly positive (Money et al. 1983a). Based on the same sample, Money et al. (1983b) suggested that the pattern of arrested growth and intellectual development reflected long-term neuroendocrinological consequences of the maltreatment and that the maltreatment may be manifested in health consequences well beyond the acute results of the maltreatment.

A wide range of medical problems characterized 44% of 5,181 children placed in protective custody in Illinois over a 22-month period (Flaherty and Weiss 1990). Of the sample, 30% were placed in foster care because of neglect, 8% because of physical abuse, 3% because of sexual abuse, 3% because of extreme risk of harm, 12% because of being runaways, and 23% because of an imminent move between foster homes. The remaining 23% were voluntary placements occasioned by a wide range of parental circumstances not necessarily associated with maltreatment. Because the runaways in most cases reflect prior abuse (e.g., Janus et al. 1987; McCormack et al. 1986), and because multiple placements in foster care are common among abused children (Pardeck 1985), the sample is primarily composed of abused and neglected children. Most importantly, these children in the custody of the state evidenced a large number of significant medical problems well beyond their usual prevalence. The authors used the data to argue for health screening of children placed in foster care; the data also point to the high probability of significant health difficulties among abused and neglected children.

Another study (Karp et al. 1989) demonstrated adverse health consequences of physical abuse beyond the immediate results of the abusive incident. Based on a total sample of 196 urban day-care recipients, growth indices of 53 abused children were compared with those of nonabused children, with the data adjusted for age, sex, and ethnicity. The body mass index of the abused children was significantly less than that of the comparison group; 16.3% of the abused children evidenced wasting, compared with only 0.7% of the nonabused children. Although there was clearly more wasting among abused children, that difference only approached statistical significance. These data are not inconsistent with those reported by R. C. Herrenkohl and Herrenkohl (1981), in which a link between physical abuse and neglect and adverse health consequences was noted.

Appearance has also been considered a factor in the emergence of abuse. Although some studies (e.g., Dion 1974; Roscoe et al. 1985) have suggested that attractiveness may affect punitive interactions, more recent work (e.g., R. C. Herrenkohl and Herrenkohl 1981; Starr et al. 1984) failed to support the position that physical anomalies contribute significantly to abuse. There are, however, data that implicate unattractive physical appearance in the disruption of attachment, which may have an indirect influence on the emergence of abuse. Barden et al. (1989) demonstrated that craniofacial deformity in infants was associated with consistently less nurturant behavior by mothers when compared with the mothers of children without such deformities. Perhaps most importantly, Barden et al. observed that the mothers of the children with deformities were unaware of their less nurturant responses, and they actually rated their interactions with their children more positively than did the mothers of children without deformities. If attachment influences risk for abuse or neglect and if appearance affects attachment, then appearance could influence risk for abuse or neglect. The lack of parental awareness regarding interactions with the child also has obvious implications for the gathering of information from parents when making parent-child relational diagnoses of abuse or neglect.

As noted, research in child abuse poses many methodological difficulties. When the focus of a review is on child attributes that might occasion abuse or might contribute to the continuation of abuse, the relative absence of longitudinal studies or long-term prospective studies is a major problem. Although prospective studies are represented in the child abuse literature (e.g., Egeland and Brunnquell 1979;

Elmer 1977, 1978; Farber and Egeland 1987), such studies are extremely rare. Because retrospective studies are greatly compromised by potential subject selection biases, conclusions regarding causal relationships are greatly compromised. Of course, interpretive problems with follow-back studies are common in research on psychopathology (e.g., Kohlberg et al. 1972). Not only do the cross-sectional studies of abused or neglected children compromise efforts to understand possible antecedents of maltreatment, but they also limit understanding of possible consequences of maltreatment. Thus, considerations of child risk factors in abuse, of the comorbidity of child psychiatric diagnoses and abuse, and of the consequences of abuse are greatly limited at present. Despite these difficulties, some emerging patterns suggest that a broad range of child behavior problems are associated with physical abuse and neglect.

Behavioral characteristics of abused and neglected children. Like health and developmental status, the behavioral characteristics of abused and neglected children may reflect either antecedents or consequences of abuse. In addition, because behavioral characteristics are often observed in a context with a child caretaker, they often reflect interactive processes. Behavioral characteristics of abused and neglected children are most often evaluated through assessments of cognitive attributes or assessments of social behaviors. Further, it has been reported that abusing parents often describe the victim as being a particularly difficult or deviant child (e.g., Coombes 1980; Green et al. 1974; R. C. Herrenkohl and Herrenkohl 1981).

One major problem in studies of child abuse victims is the dependence on parental reports and questions regarding their veracity. Although maltreated children have been described as difficult and demanding, the source of the report is often a perpetrator; thus, the validity of the report must be questioned. Consistent with the attributional research of Brock and Pallak (1969), reports of child deviance by abusive or neglectful parents may merely reflect a rationalization or justification for the maltreatment rather than an accurate appraisal of the child. For example, Gregg and Elmer (1969) reported that physicians could not discern any differences between abused and accidentally injured children from a sample of 146 infants. Yet reports from the mothers of the children suggested that they perceived the children very differently. J. E. Martin and Kourany (1980) reported on a series of cases of abusive adolescent babysitters who described their child victims as being clingy, fearful, manipulative, and oppositional, suggesting that even nonparental perpetrators perceive the physically abused children negatively.

In a study of mothers of physically abused, physically neglected, sexually abused, and control adolescents, Williamson et al. (1991) reported that the mothers of the physically abused adolescents reported more conduct disorder problems on the Revised Behavior Problem Checklist (Quay and Peterson 1987) than did the mothers of neglected or sexually abused adolescents, who in turn reported more conduct disorder problems than the nonmaltreating mothers. Mothers of neglected and physically abused adolescents also reported more socialized aggression than the mothers of nonmaltreated adolescents. These data are, however, somewhat compromised by the fact that the source of the ratings was the mother of the adolescent. Although some studies have suggested that abusive parents view an abused child more negatively and feel less able to influence that child's behavior than the behavior of nonabused children in the same household (e.g., E. C. Herrenkohl and Herrenkohl 1979), other studies have failed to replicate that finding (e.g., Halperin 1983). Moreover, when abusive mothers were compared with other mothers who were experiencing parenting difficulties, the abusive mothers' perceptions of their children were no more negative than those reported by nonabusive mothers (M. S. Rosenberg and Repucci 1983). Such data suggest that parents who have difficulty controlling their children perceive their children negatively, regardless of the use of extreme physical coercion by the parent. Such data are certainly consistent with placing abusive parenting in the broader context of a parent-child relational problem.

Parent information regarding child behavior problems in abusive families might be confounded with the views of the perpetrator and, therefore, might be more an assessment of parent characteristics than of child characteristics. Occasionally, investigators have used ratings by persons outside the family to assess the behavioral attributes of maltreated children. Salzinger et al. (1984) obtained teacher ratings of maltreated children seen in different clinics of a single hospital. Teachers rated the children from abusive families as displaying more negative behavior than control children and differentiated the behavior of the target children and nontarget children from the same abusive household. Targeted children were seen as more likely to display conduct disorder behaviors and hyperactivity, to manifest more attentional problems, and to be more anxious than their nontargeted siblings. Moreover, the nontarget children were also rated as displaying more positive behaviors than the target children. When these same children were rated by maltreating parents, the target children and the nontarget children were not differentiated. Unfortunately, the Salzinger et al. (1984) study aggregated physically abused, sexually abused, emotionally abused, and neglected children in the abused group. Thus, it is impossible to know whether the results reflect the specific influence of physical abuse and neglect.

Reidy (1977) found that abused and neglected children were reported to evidence more behavior problems in school than control children. Teacher ratings did not differentiate between abused and neglected children. The Reidy data suggest it is possible that the negative ratings of the children in the Salzinger et al. (1984)

study could be attributable to the influence of the physically abused and neglected children in the sample. Consistent with that possibility is the observation by Goldston et al. (1988) that the presenting problem of aggressive behavior in a group of sexually abused girls was probably a function of girls who had been both sexually and physically abused. Similarly, Kolko et al. (1988) reported that sexually abused psychiatric inpatients evidenced more sexual and internalizing behaviors than comparison children and physically abused children in the psychiatric facility. The physically abused children did not differ significantly from other hospitalized psychiatric patients. These data of Reidy, Goldston et al., and Kolko et al. imply that the behavioral consequences of abuse might be specifically related to the type of abuse sustained. That is, sexual abuse seems to increase the probability of sexualized behavior, and physically abusive or neglectful parenting seems to increase aggressive behavior. Such a pattern was also noted by Briere and Runtz (1990) in a study of nonclinical university women who reported childhood histories of physical abuse or sexual abuse.

Observational analyses also suggest that physically abused children or children from physically abusive homes are more aggressive than children from nonabusive but distressed homes. George and Main (1979) reported that abused toddlers were more physically and verbally aggressive with peers and caregivers and more avoidant of other children when compared with matched control toddlers from families experiencing stress. Burgess and Conger (1977) also reported that children from abusive families displayed more aggressive behavior than children from either neglectful or control families. Similar data based on home observations of abusive and nonabusive deviant families were reported by Reid and Taplin (1976).

Reid et al. (1981) contrasted home observational data obtained from three types of families: nondistressed families recruited from the community, families referred for child management problems, and families referred for child management problems with evidence of physical abuse. The children from the families characterized by abuse displayed higher levels of aversive behaviors than children from either the community control families or the nonabusive families referred for child management difficulties. Because the child management referrals reflected high levels of aggression, antisocial behavior, and conduct disorder symptoms, the greater level of aggression displayed by the children from the abusive households is indicative of the absolute level of aversive behavior. Furthermore, Reid (1984) reported significant correlations between the aversive acts displayed by the children and the aversive behaviors of the parents. Based on intensive observations of a small number of families, Koverola et al. (1985) described either a pattern of reciprocated coercion or a pattern of randomly coercive exchanges in families characterized by abuse. The data suggesting a pattern of reciprocity of aversiveness in the abusive families are consistent with Patterson's (1982) coercion theory of social aggression.

Moreover, Reid et al. (1982) argued from their observational data that the probability that a parent will abuse, hit, or threaten a child is, in part, influenced by the behavior problems the child presents. Thus, these highly aversive children in physically abusive households might occasion some of the maltreatment because of their high levels of aggressive and aversive behavior. Interestingly, based on a reanalysis of the national survey by Straus et al. (1980), Larzelere (1986) concluded that there was a strong association between the level of spanking in the household and the level of aggression the children directed at their siblings.

Closely related to the aversive and aggressive behaviors identified in abused children is oppositional or noncompliant behavior. Observations of mother-child interactions between physically abusive mothers and their children suggest that the abused children comply less often than do the children observed interacting with nonabusing mothers (George and Main 1979; Schindler and Arkowitz 1986). This pattern of noncompliance could reflect unique interactions between an abused child and a parent. In a naturalistic study of abused or neglected and nonmaltreated children in a day-care setting, Schaeffer and Lewis (1990) noted that the abused children displayed impaired interactions with mothers but did not differ significantly in their interactions with caretakers or with peers drawn from a sample of nonabused preschoolers. Other data, however, suggest that the pattern described by George and Main and Schindler and Arkowitz may reflect a general lack of appropriate response to social overtures. For example, R. S. Jacobson and Straker (1982) videotaped the interactions of child triads that included abused and control children ranging in age from 5 to 10 years. Although the observational records did not indicate any greater hostility or aggression by the abused children, the abused children were less socially interactive than their nonabused peers. Impaired peer interactions by abused or neglected children have been noted in other studies as well (e.g., R. C. Herrenkohl and Herrenkohl 1981; B. Johnson and Morse 1968; Young 1971).

Based on observational analyses of mother-infant dyads from abusing, neglecting, abusing and neglecting, "marginally maltreating," and nonmaltreating samples, Crittenden and DiLalla (1988) identified a pattern of child behavior in the maltreatment groups that they described as compulsive compliance. This behavior pattern is viewed as adaptive in the maltreatment setting, but it is maladaptive in other contexts. The work of Crittenden and DiLalla thus implicates the mother-child interaction in the ontogeny of the inflexible maladaptive patterns of abused children. The description of the test-taking behavior of 30 abused adolescents offered by Hjorth and Harway (1981) suggested a pattern of unquestioning compliance that would be consistent with this compulsive compliance formulation. Although the compulsive compliance might seem inconsistent with the oppositional behavior noted, there is the suggestion that this compulsive compliance is characterized by rigidity across situations that could be seen as oppositional in some contexts.

There have been several studies investigating social-emotional behavior and social cognition in abused and neglected children. Based on a structured assessment procedure, Barahal et al. (1981) found that abused children are more likely to perceive outcomes as being determined by external events and that the abused children are less likely to assume personal responsibility for life events. Moreover, differences between abused and nonabused children in terms of taking the perspective of others, accuracy in labeling the emotions of others, and concepts of social role suggest that impaired social cognitive development could play a mediating role in the aggressive and withdrawn behaviors displayed by abused children. Using a day-camp setting, J. Kaufman and Cicchetti (1989) evaluated peer interactions and self-esteem in children from the full range of maltreatment categories. Impaired prosocial behavior and poor self-esteem characterized all subtypes of maltreated children. Similarly, the day-camp counselors rated all the maltreated children as more withdrawn than the comparison groups. Most importantly, however, the counselors rated the physically abused children as more aggressive than the other subtypes of abused or comparison children. Such data provide another example of the possible specificity of the influence of physical abuse on the emergence of aggressive behavior.

Klimes-Dougan and Kistner (1990) contrasted physically abused and nonabused preschool children in peer interactions at a day-care center. All of the abused children had experienced nonaccidental injury a mean of 24 months (range = 9–41 months) prior to the study, so the data generally reflect long-term behavioral characteristics rather than characteristics proximal to the abusive event. Abused children were more likely to cause distress in their peers, and they were more likely to respond inappropriately to distress displayed by peers regardless of the causative agent. These data are consistent with the findings of Main and George (1985), in which signs of distress displayed by peers evoked aggressive responses from abused children in a day-care setting.

In related research, when abused and neglected children interact with unfamiliar adults, they are described as evidencing wariness and patterns of avoidance (e.g., Aber and Allen 1987). Such impaired response to adults could be a factor in the reports that abused children are less effectively engaged in the school setting (e.g., Hoffman-Plotkin and Twentyman 1984). Interestingly, J. W. Fantuzzo et al. (1988) demonstrated that peers who were trained to increase the social behaviors of abused, neglected, or endangered children were more successful than adult caretakers.

The impaired responsiveness to social overtures and the disrupted social interaction that characterizes some abused children may be a result of their elevated aggressiveness. The work by Dodge et al. (1986) on the formation of friendships in children suggests that children who are inappropriately aggressive in the early stages of peer interaction tend to be rejected. Coie and Kupersmidt (1983) found that peer status based on classroom ratings of children is a stable phenomenon. Moreover, rejected children are more likely to take offense and to draw hostile inferences from their interactions with peers (Dodge 1980; Dodge and Frame 1982; Dodge and Newman 1981). Considering the aggressiveness and poor peer interactions that many abused children tend to display at the preschool level, it seems likely that they are at considerable risk for persistent problems in peer interaction.

The impaired interpersonal interactions that characterize abused and neglected children could reflect disrupted emotional development as well as the acquisition of an aggressive behavioral repertoire. Schneider-Rosen and Cicchetti (1991), using a mirror self-recognition task, demonstrated that maltreatment (involving physical abuse, neglect, or emotional abuse) coupled with lower socioeconomic status was associated with less positive affective reactions to mirror self-recognition. If the emotional development of children contributes to their social development (Cicchetti 1990), then the less positive affective response to self-recognition could represent another vector in the adverse outcome of the abuse and neglect of children by their parents.

Child and adolescent psychopathology. The primary research strategy for assessing an association between abuse or neglect and child psychopathology has been to determine the prevalence of abuse histories in diagnostic groups or among recipients of services from psychiatric clinics. As noted, when clinics assess abuse histories, there is a tendency for the prevalence of maltreatment to exceed that which would be expected on the basis of national incidence studies. Unfortunately, many studies are compromised for our purposes because they do not distinguish among physical abuse, neglect, sexual abuse, emotional abuse, or "high-risk status." Given the link between abuse and aggressive behavior noted, it is not surprising that there is a general tendency in the literature to identify associations between abuse and externalizing disorders.

Attention-deficit/hyperactivity disorder was first identified as a risk factor of abuse by B. Johnson and Morse (1968). More recently, research has suggested that parents are more physically intense and controlling in their interactions with boys with attention-deficit/hyperactivity disorder (e.g., Whalen et al. 1981), as well as less positive in their interactions with children with attention-deficit/hyperactivity disorder (e.g., Campbell 1975; Cunningham and Barkley 1979). Consistent with these studies, Heffron et al. (1987) reported that, among children with attention-deficit disorder referred to a psychiatric outpatient facility, documented physical abuse was more prevalent in those patients diagnosed attention-deficit disorder with hyperactivity than in those diagnosed with just attention-deficit disorder. Similarly, Accardo et al. (1990) reported higher rates of abuse and neglect in children referred for an evaluation of hyperactivity and inattention who did *not* qualify for a diagnosis of attention-deficit disorder than for those who were diagnosed with attention-deficit disorder, suggesting that hyperactivity per se and not attention-deficit disorder may be associated with abuse.

Monane et al. (1984) studied 166 consecutive admissions of children and adolescents to an inpatient psychiatric service. In this study, 42% of the boys and 41% of the girls were rated as having been physically abused; psychiatric diagnosis, perinatal problems, and neurological signs and symptoms did not differentiate abused from nonabused. However, significantly more of the abused group than the nonabused group had suffered accidents or injuries other than those inflicted by the abuse they incurred. Also, significantly more were head and facial injuries that could have resulted in central nervous system damage. Consistent with evidence of elevated aggressiveness noted, based on a review of chart information, the abused group was also rated as more violent than the nonabused group and manifested homicidal ideation more often.

In a similar comparison of abused, neglected, and nonabused children, Rogeness et al. (1986) reported that 16% of the female patients and 24% of the male patients could be categorized within a broad definition of physical abuse, whereas an additional 27% of the boys and 17% of the girls could be categorized within a broad definition of neglect (with and without physical abuse). Significantly more of the abused and neglected boys were diagnosed with conduct disorder, with the neglected boys evidencing more undersocialized conduct disorder than the other two groups. For girls, significantly more of the abused group were diagnosed with socialized conduct disorder than either the neglected group or the nonabused and nonneglected group. Significantly more of the nonabused nonneglected group were diagnosed with dysthymia than the abused or neglected girls. For boys and girls, there were no significant differences among groups with respect to the diagnoses of borderline personality disorder, schizophrenia, or major depression. Investigations based on symptom checklists indicated, however, that abused and neglected boys evidenced more borderline symptoms, conduct disorder symptoms, and concentration symptoms, and fewer anxiety symptoms than the control group boys. Abused and neglected girls manifested more concentration symptoms than control samples. However, abused girls, alone, evidenced more conduct and hyperactivity symptoms than neglected or control samples, suggesting the possibility of an interaction between gender and maltreatment in determining the outcome of the presenting symptoms.

The possible link between conduct disorder and abuse might be mediated somewhat by social class. Behar and Stewart (1984) reported that, although 57% of a sample of children with conduct disorder from social classes IV and V had been physically abused, only 18% of the children with conduct disorder from classes I–III had been abused. Of course, the base rate of abuse in the latter group exceeds that which would be expected in a random sample of children from classes I–III.

Fire setting is a conduct disorder symptom that also has been associated with physical abuse histories. Gruber et al. (1981) identified 90 fire-setting inpatient children from a sample of 544. For 35% of the fire setters, a history of physical abuse was documented in their records. Abandonment and parental neglect were reported to be present in 35% and 54% of the fire setters, respectively. Unfortunately, it is not clear whether the neglect in that study could be classified as physical neglect. Showers and Pickell (1987) contrasted 186 fire-setting psychiatric patients between 4 and 17 years old with a comparison sample based on the next same-sex and same-age admission to the clinic without a history of fire setting. Physical abuse was more prevalent in the histories of the fire-setting group; the groups could not be distinguished on the basis of physical neglect, but emotional neglect was also more prevalent in the fire-setting group.

Addressing particular diagnoses or symptom patterns, it has been suggested that abused or neglected children manifest borderline and multiple personality symptoms. However, most studies of patients with borderline or multiple personality disorder have demonstrated substantial intercorrelations between physical abuse and sexual abuse, suggesting an association between types of child maltreatment and no clear evidence of a specific identified link between type of maltreatment and these disorders. Studies of adolescent girls diagnosed with borderline personality disorder have reported significantly higher rates of physical abuse, neglect, and sexual abuse in the borderline groups than in comparison groups of adolescent female inpatients with diagnoses of depression, eating disorders, or other personality disorders (Ludolph et al. 1990; Westen et al. 1990). Unfortunately, these investigations have not established the independent contributions of maltreatment to borderline personality disorder nor the interactions attributable to the different types of child maltreatment in the borderline personality disorder. Interestingly, however, Westen et al. found significant associations between physical abuse, but not sexual abuse, of biological mothers or first-degree relatives and the borderline personality diagnosis in the adolescent probands studied.

Concerning other psychiatric symptoms, abused and neglected children have also been reported to suffer from depression (Kashani and Carlson 1987; Kazdin et al. 1985) and to exhibit an elevated risk for suicide (Deykin 1989; Deykin et al. 1985; Kosky 1983). Unfortunately, most of these studies defined abuse or neglect as some type of contact with CPS, suggesting that sexual abuse, emotional abuse, or risk for abuse may be included in the samples. Based on a survey of 988 adolescents, G. A. Bernstein et al. (1989) reported that a history of physical abuse was associated with high scores on the Manifest Anxiety Scale (Taylor 1953). In addition to depression and anxiety, research has noted elevated rates of physical abuse in the histories of self-mutilating patients (e.g., Carroll et al. 1980). A study by Burke et al. (1985) failed to find significant differences among physically abused, sexually abused, physically and sexually abused, and matched control children on reported hallucinations.

Parent characteristics. There is very little information about physically abusive or neglecting fathers. J. A. Martin (1984) reviewed 66 studies of abusive "parents" published in the period 1976–1980. Only 2 studied fathers alone, and only 17 provided any data on fathers. The pattern seems not to have changed in more recent research (e.g., Bradley and Lindsay 1987). This lack of attention to fathers is particularly interesting in light of evidence that reports of abuse are more likely if the father is the perpetrator (Hampton and Newberger 1985). Moreover, fathers were involved as perpetrators in 65% of the cases of fatal abuse reviewed over a 3-year period in Texas (Anderson et al. 1983). A study by Greif and Zuravin (1989) of 17 fathers who were awarded custody in the context of deficient parenting presented a bleak picture. Data indicated that this group of fathers were no better than marginally adequate and that most displayed drug and alcohol abuse, physical abuse of their spouses, and a host of antisocial behaviors. Although the perception of an antisocial father as a factor in child abuse or neglect is widely held, the amount of data in support of that position is actually quite limited (e.g., Green 1978; Merrill 1962; S. M. Smith and Hanson 1975). Despite a pressing need, repeated calls for studies of abusive or neglectful fathers seem not to have been heeded.

Early in the research on the "battered child syndrome," there was a search for extreme psychopathology in the parents. Those efforts were decidedly unsuccessful. Efforts to identify *the* abusive personality type have also met with failure. The attempt by J. A. James and Boake (1988) to use cluster analyses of Minnesota Multiphasic Personality Inventory (Hathaway and McKinley 1970) profiles reflects some of the problems that are encountered: 13 different profile clusters were identified in a sample of 178 physically abusive, emotionally abusive, or neglecting parents. Thus, the results do not identify a single, or even a few, personality types associated with abuse or neglect. Although the search for parent variables has focused on nonpsychopathological attributes, some attention has been given to affective disorders or symptoms of depression in the emergence of abuse or neglect.

A possible link between maltreatment and depression is consistent with studies of the parenting behaviors of depressed mothers (e.g., Weissman and Paykel 1974; Weissman et al. 1972). Studies of postpartum depression (e.g., O'Hara et al. 1983, 1984) suggest that depression could disrupt the attachment process and add to the social stress that has been seen as a factor in the emergence of abuse. Data linking maltreatment and depression have been equivocal, however. Of 11 studies of depression and abuse or neglect, only 6 have shown an association between depression and abuse. The many methodological differences among these studies compromise any possibility of reaching an unequivocal conclusion regarding affective disorders and child maltreatment, but the studies do merit some consideration in the context of relational diagnoses.

With the exception of Culp et al. (1989), Green et al. (1980), and Zuravin (1988a), who did not restrict the sample selection to physical abuse and/or neglect, the studies have focused either on physical abuse or on physical abuse and neglect combined into a single category of maltreatment. Because Green et al. (1980) did not support the link between depression and maltreatment, but both Culp et al. (1989) and Zuravin (1988a) were able to document associations between maternal depression and abuse and neglect, this methodological factor does not account for all aspects of the inconsistencies among studies. Various indices of depression have also been used with mixed results. Of the studies using the Minnesota Multiphasic Personality Inventory (Evans 1980; Gabinet 1979; Paulson et al. 1974; Wright 1976), only Evans (1980) reported an association between maternal depression and abuse. One study using the Beck Depression Inventory (Beck 1978) reported no association between abuse and depression (Webster-Stratton 1985), but two other studies using the Beck Depression Inventory reported that depression was linked to abuse (Lahey et al. 1984; Zuravin 1988a). Using an assessment of current and past psychopathology, Green et al. (1980) did not establish a relation between depression and either abuse or neglect. Using the lifetime version of the Schedule for Affective Disorders and Schizophrenia (Endicott and Spitzer 1978), however, Kaplan et al. (1983) did show a relationship between depression and abuse or neglect. In addition, Famularo et al. (1986b) identified a greater incidence of affective disorders among a sample of 50 parents who experienced a court-ordered removal of a child when they were compared with a matched control group from a pediatric clinic. Famularo et al. (1986a) also established a higher rate of depression and alcoholism (Research Diagnostic Criteria [Spitzer et al. 1978]) among court-ordered referrals for evaluation because of severe maltreatment compared with a matched pediatric control sample.

Most of the studies of maltreatment and depression suffer from relatively small sample sizes, control groups that are less than ideal (e.g., psychiatric outpatients or recipients of hospital services), and inadequately operationalized maltreatment groups. In one of the few studies with large samples, Zuravin (1988a) interviewed 118 abusive mothers, 119 neglecting mothers, and 281 control mothers, all of whom were recipients of Aid for Dependent Children (AFDC). In addition to the administration of the Beck Depression Inventory, participants were interviewed about past depressive symptoms, hospitalizations for depression, and professional treatment for depression. Zuravin (1988a) reported that severity of depressed symptoms on the day of the interview was significantly associated with risk for abuse and neglect. Although the degree of depression significantly influenced the degree of risk for neglect, the depression-abuse association seemed to follow an all-or-nothing step function. This study does not have many of the compromising features of other studies of depressed affect and abuse or neglect. It is important to note, however, that it established a link between depressed symptoms and maltreatment, but does not establish a link between a *diagnosis* of depression and abuse. The study did not provide a cohort of subjects meeting Research Diagnostic Criteria or Schedule for Affective Disorders and Schizophrenia—Lifetime or DSM-III-R (American Psychiatric Association 1987) diagnostic criteria for depression. Moreover, the study does not rule out the possibility that the depressed symptoms are a reflection of being identified as a maltreating parent. Thus, it continues to be impossible to conclude that depression is causally linked to either abuse or neglect, although there is some suggestive evidence of depressed symptoms being associated with mothers identified as abusive or neglectful.

If being identified as a deviant parent were the determinant of the depression, it might be expected that other indices of negative emotion would also covary with the detection of maltreatment. Although lower self-esteem has been associated with identified abusive mothers (e.g., Culp et al. 1989; Perry et al. 1983), neglectful mothers were not lower on self-esteem than control mothers (Culp et al. 1989). Thus, merely being identified as a deviant parent does not account for all of the variance in negative emotional state that has been associated with being an identified maltreating mother.

Lahey et al. (1984) suggested that parents under extreme emotional and somatic distress are more reactive to child misbehavior and react more punitively to child transgressions. Thus, the influence of depression on abuse can be seen in the context of parental reactivity to child behaviors. Interestingly, when mothers diagnosed with somatization disorder or Briquet's syndrome were contrasted with patients with major depression, 33% of the mothers with somatization disorder were abusive or neglectful and 10% of the depressed mothers evidenced abuse or neglect (Zoccolillo and Cloninger 1986).

The youth of a parent has been implicated as a risk factor in child maltreatment, with adolescent motherhood often being identified as a significant predictor of physical abuse and neglect. Unfortunately, much of the support for the association between adolescent parenthood and maltreatment (e.g., Bolton et al. 1980; Lynch and Roberts 1982; S. M. Smith 1976) has been based on indirect data and has often failed to account for possible confounding or mediating variables. Comparing 532 physically abusive mothers reported to the Maryland Department of Social Services with a case-matched comparison group derived from state birth records, Benedict et al. (1985) reported that abusive mothers were somewhat younger. Interestingly, in the Benedict et al. study, it was the number of mothers in the 17- to 19-year-old range that distinguished the groups, not the number of mothers in the range under 16 years old. Other research has failed to identify an association between parental age and maltreatment (e.g., Elmer 1967; Gil 1970).

When adolescent parenthood is associated with abuse or neglect, it may reflect the operation of stress factors such as economic disadvantage, premarital conception, and unplanned pregnancies (e.g., R. C. Herrenkohl and Herrenkohl 1981), or marital stress occasioned by unwanted children (e.g., Furstenberg 1976; Russell 1980). Because of the higher rate of prior stillbirths or abortions in the abusive group they identified, Benedict et al. (1985) speculated about a negative approach to pregnancy as a factor in abuse by young parents. Based on a sample of 518 AFDC mothers, Zuravin (1987) indicated that the number of unplanned conceptions was a risk factor for both physical abuse and neglect. Based on multiple logistical regression analyses, unplanned pregnancies that occurred despite contraceptive efforts were more frequently associated with abuse, whereas pregnancies in the absence of contraception were more frequently associated with neglect. Based on an analysis of the NIS-1 data, S. H. Miller (1984) concluded that the children of teenage mothers were more likely to suffer physical neglect, and that teenage mothers and mothers older than 35 were more likely to inflict serious (life-threatening or fatal) abuse. Jason and Andereck (1983) noted that younger impoverished parents are most frequently associated with fatal abuse.

Some evidence suggests that the association of adolescent parenthood and abuse or neglect is a function of disorganization in the family of origin or a combination of disorganized family structure coupled with the effects of poverty (Earp and Ory 1980; Kinard and Klerman 1980). Bolton and Laner (1986) noted that a majority of the abusive adolescent mothers were not receiving public assistance despite eligibility, providing additional evidence of a pattern of disorganization and inability to access resources as well as the presence of poverty.

Related to disorganized family structure, Zuravin (1988b) reported that the number of children in the household completely mediated the association between maternal age and neglect and significantly mediated the association between maternal age and abuse. Further support for the role of family size in the emergence of abuse or neglect comes from data indicating that families with twins are overrepresented in CPS records (Groothius et al. 1982; Robarge et al. 1982). Although families with twins were overrepresented, the twins themselves were not overrepresented as victims, suggesting that twins may add a source of stress that could occasion a generally increased risk for maltreatment within the household. H. B. Nelson and Martin (1985), however, examined abuse registries within a single university teaching hospital and established that twins themselves were overrepresented among abused and neglected children younger than age 4. Moreover, both twins were abused in 60% of the abused twin sets. These authors also invoked notions of stress associated with the presence of twins as the factor that increased risk of maltreatment.

Although family size seems to be implicated as a factor in the occurrence of abuse and neglect, an assessment of 42 closed cases participating over a 6-year period in a program designed to avoid foster placement noted that large family size was among the variables predictive of successful reunification of the family (Bribitzer and Verdieck 1988). Thus, family size does not seem to have a simple influence on either the emergence or the persistence of abuse.

Many of the influential models of physical abuse invoke the notion that some stressful environmental event evokes the abusive episode (e.g., Belsky 1984; Emery 1989; Erlanger 1974; Garbarino 1976; Gelles 1980; Kempe and Helfer 1972; Parke and Collmer 1975). The potentiating influence of stress in the emergence of abuse or neglect is usually considered in the context of socioeconomic factors or the presence of stressful life-change events, such as those measured with the T. H. Holmes and Rahe (1967) scale. As noted earlier in the section on epidemiology, poverty is clearly related to the emergence of abuse. Whether that is a reflection of a stress-maltreatment link is not entirely clear, however. A study by Krugman et al. (1986) reported a significant correlation ($r = .66$) between the number of cases seen by CPSs and the annual state unemployment rate over a 15-year period. An average of 49% of the referred cases involved families characterized by unemployment.

The contribution of parental isolation to abuse or neglect has also been noted in the abuse literature (e.g., Elmer 1977; Morris and Gould 1963; Spinetta and Rigler 1972), yet the evidence linking abuse or neglect to isolation is mixed. To some extent, this is attributable to varying definitions of isolation. Investigators have used an absence of memberships in social organizations (e.g., Young 1971), lack of participation in social and religious groups (e.g., Straus 1980), alienation from one's extended family (Bennie and Sclare 1969), or limited networks of peer and family associations (e.g., Salzinger et al. 1983). Clearly, many of these indices of isolation regress on socioeconomic factors. Wahler (1980) emphasized social participation and use of available resources rather than physical isolation when identifying insularity as a factor in the emergence of deviant parenting and deviant child behavior. Consistent with that position, when mothers lack social networks (Salzinger et al. 1983) or they fail to use available social networks (Egeland et al. 1980), there is a greater risk for physical abuse. The Bolton and Laner (1986) data also call attention to abusive mothers' failure to use available community resources. Thus, the data suggest that the contribution of isolation to abuse or neglect may reflect a parental attribute involving disorganization and lack of engagement rather than an environmental characteristic.

Marital discord or generally negative interactions among family members have also been seen to covary with abusive parenting (e.g., Burgess and Conger 1977; R. C. Herrenkohl and Herrenkohl 1981; Straus et al. 1980). Based on observational work, Burgess and Conger demonstrated that abusive mothers responded positively to other family members less often than nonabusive mothers and that they responded negatively to other family members much more often than nonabusive mothers, suggesting that a generally negative pattern of interactions characterizes abusive families. Similar data were reported by Lahey et al. (1984) in their study of maternal depression and abuse. Perry et al. (1983) found that abusive mothers reported less family cohesion than control-group mothers. Similarly, Bousha and Twentyman (1984) noted recurrent patterns of coercive parenting by abusive mothers.

Although these family studies all point to a generally acrimonious pattern of family interaction within abusive households, Oldershaw et al. (1989) identified three distinct patterns of parent-child interaction on the basis of cluster analyses of coded parent-child interactions obtained from 73 physically abusive mothers and 43 matched control mother-child dyads. In addition to the intrusive and hostile patterns that are consistent with the coercive patterns noted, a pattern of emotionally distant mothering was identified. Schindler and Arkowitz (1986) reported that physically abusive mothers displayed lower overall levels of interacting with their children when compared with matched control mothers. In addition, the abusive mothers provided less contingent praise. Thus, data from these observational studies suggest that a general pattern of more negative but, perhaps, less active parenting (e.g., Dietrich et al. 1980) characterizes physically abusive parents. Interestingly, in a home observation study of 47 NO-FTT infants who were 6 months old and a sample of matched control mother-infant dyads, Drotar et al. (1990) noted that the mothers of NO-FTT infants were less positive in their behavior. Additionally, the mothers of NO-FTT infants terminated the feeding of the infants in a more arbitrary fashion, suggesting either a lack of sensitivity to infant signals or an inadequate recognition of the needs of the child. Haynes (1983) also noted the deviant mother-child interactions in NO-FTT patient dyads.

The interactive aspects of parents with their maltreated children relate closely to the possible diagnosis of abuse or neglect as a parent-child relational problem. An article by Deitrich-MacLean and Walden (1988) reported that a sample of 52 child protection caseworkers could distinguish abusive from nonabusive mothers with a 76% accuracy rate from videotapes of mothers teaching a child to operate a puzzle box. These data strongly suggested that the interactions of abusive mothers with their children are distinguishable. In this study, the experience level of the caseworkers did not affect their accuracy, but it did affect confidence in the ratings offered. Because the interactional quality of the parent-child relation seems distinguishable as a function of the abusive or neglectful status of the parent, considerable research has been directed toward assessing specific parental attributes that could yield these interactions. With the growing importance of cognitive models of behavior, it is not surprising that several investigators have focused on internal representational models (e.g., Crittenden 1988) or parental perceptions or expectations of their children (e.g., M. S. Rosenberg and Repucci 1983; Twentyman and Plotkin 1982) as attributes that may contribute to the emergence of abusive or neglectful parent-child interactions.

Two research strategies have been used to support the hypothesis that abusive or neglectful parents have distorted perceptions or unrealistic expectations of their children or children in general. The first strategy has been to infer perceptions or expectations from the parents' behavior. When young children are left unattended, required to be responsible for siblings at an inappropriately early age, or asked to provide emotional support for parents (e.g., Dubanoski et al. 1978; Elmer 1977; Morris and Gould 1963; Steele 1976), investigators have suggested that the expectations of the parents are the mediating factors in the abuse or neglect. For example, Gladston (1965) reported that abusive parents describe their children as if they were capable of the organized and intentional behavior of adults. Excessively high expectations for the child are then thought to mediate abuse when the child fails to meet the parent's expectation or to mediate the neglect by seeing no need to provide supervision when the child is placed at risk for physical harm. Unfortunately, these unrealistic expectations have generally been inferred from the abusive or neglectful acts themselves or from comments in retrospective clinical interviews. Thus, the evidence of distorted perceptions by abusive or neglectful parents has not been as strong as has been presumed in the clinical literature. There have been attempts, however, to assess perceptions or expectations directly using standardized tests or stimulus materials that are independent of the incident that identified the subject as abusive or neglecting.

In one of the first attempts to assess directly the expectations of 14 abusive, 15 neglecting, and 12 matched control parents, Twentyman and Plotkin (1982) used a questionnaire to assess expectations regarding the attainment of developmental milestones by their own children and "average" children. By basing the questionnaire on the Vineland Social Maturity Scale (Doll 1965), these parental expectations could be contrasted with existing normative data. In general, the group differences were modest. With respect to absolute scores, the abusive group expected their own child to attain developmental milestones at a later age than the "average" child, and the abusive and neglecting groups estimated that the average child would attain developmental milestones later than normative data would suggest. In addition, the abusing and neglecting parents showed a pattern of both overestimating and underestimating the abilities of their youngsters relative to the control group parents. Thus, when overall differences did not obtain, there was the suggestion that it was due to the canceling effects of both overestimating and underestimating within maltreating groups. The data indicated that abusive and neglecting parents were as likely to set low expectations for their children as they were to set high ones. In a follow-up study, Azar and Rohrbeck (1986) contrasted physically abusive mothers with mothers whose partner engaged in physical abuse of a child. The abusive mothers had significantly higher and more unrealistic expectations than the mothers who had an abusive partner. Such data suggest that more unrealistic expectations are specific to perpetrators rather than just a family characteristic.

When Perry et al. (1983) contrasted 55 parents from 37 abusing families with parents from 37 matched nonabusing families, both fathers and mothers from the abusive families expected slower development from their children. With respect to what would be expected of an "average" child, Williamson et al. (1991) reported that physically abusive mothers of adolescents were likely to overestimate when developmental milestones would be met and physically neglecting and control mothers were likely to underestimate when the milestones would be met. Because different instruments were used by Williamson et al. and Twentyman and Plotkin (1982), the apparent inconsistencies cannot be easily reconciled.

Because mere knowledge of developmental milestones might have been an inadequate test of the unrealistic expectations hypothesis, Azar et al. (1984) completed a study in which neglecting and abusive parents were assessed regarding expectations for developmental milestones and expectations regarding more complex family interaction and behavioral events involving children. Parents were also asked to provide solutions to a behavioral problem. Both the neglecting and abusing mothers evidenced more unrealistic expectations in the complex family interaction context, and they evidenced poorer behavioral problem-solving skills than did a group of matched control mothers. The data suggest that it was not just unrealistic expectations in the context of developmental milestones that distinguished maltreating from nonmaltreating mothers, but that it was unrealistic expectations in the context of dealing with normal, but potentially distressing, child behaviors. In related work, Hansen et al. (1989) compared physically abusive parents and neglectful parents with a community control sample and a sample of parents seeking clinical services because of child behavior problems. The abusive and neglectful parents were more deficient in problem-solving skills than either the community sample or the clinic sample.

Rohrbeck and Twentyman (1986) provided data suggesting that abusive and neglecting parents are less able to inhibit their behavior than matched control group parents. Thus, maltreatment could reflect a combination of a lack of inhibitory control coupled with reacting to unrealistic expectations for the child. Interestingly, McCabe (1984) noted that abused children placed in state care and pictures of abused children from police files had smaller cranial-facial proportions than matched control children from a nursery school setting. Based on these data, McCabe argued that cranial-facial information provides apparent age-level specification to a parent that may contribute to unrealistic expectations relative to a child's actual developmental status. Thus, the perception of the child, unrealistic expectations, and poor inhibitory control could yield an abusive interaction.

In addition to the reactions based on unrealistic expectations, distorted negative perceptions of the abused child by the parents have been considered a contributor to abusive interactions (Gladston 1971; Gregg and Elmer 1969). E. C. Herrenkohl and Herrenkohl (1979) contrasted parental perceptions of abused and nonabused children from the same families. Their data suggested that the abusive mothers had more negative perceptions of the abuse victim and felt less able to influence that child's behavior relative to the sibling's. Although distorted negative perceptions could be a precursor to abuse or neglect, they might also reflect derogation of the victim by perpetrators attempting to justify maltreatment (Brock and Pallak 1969). Although Halperin (1983) did not demonstrate differing parental perceptions of abused and nonabused children from the same family, abused children and their siblings were perceived more negatively by their parents than were nonabused children and their siblings from matched control groups. Such data suggest the possibility of a generally negative perception of children by abusing parents.

M. S. Rosenberg and Repucci (1983) did not find that abusing mothers had more negative perceptions. The control group, however, consisted of mothers who were referred because of "parenting difficulties." Thus, the failure of M. S. Rosenberg and Reppucci to obtain group differences might have been due to the fact that both the abusing parents and those having difficulty with their children perceive their youngsters negatively. Consistent with that hypothesis is the work by Holleran et al. (1982), who demonstrated that deviant, but not necessarily abusive, parents were less likely to track positive child responses accurately.

In an attempt to develop a taxonomy of subtypes of abusive mothers, Oldershaw et al. (1989) studied 73 physically abusive mothers and 43 matched comparison group mothers. Based on a coding of parent-child interaction, the authors concluded that there were three subtypes of abusive mothers: hostile, emotionally distant, and intrusive. Regardless of subtype, however, all physically abusive mothers perceived their children more negatively than did the control group mothers. Similarly, Wood-Shuman and Cone (1986) contrasted ratings of videotaped child behaviors by abusive, "at-risk," and control mothers. In terms of the negative ratings, the group of abusive mothers exceeded the group of at-risk mothers who, in turn, exceeded the control group. Moreover, supplementary analyses of combined groups suggested the insular mothers who did not participate socially and made poor use of available resources were more negative in their ratings than the noninsular mothers.

Larrance and Twentyman (1983) contrasted abusive, neglecting, and control group mothers' perceptions of their own child and another child engaging in deviant and nondeviant acts. In this study, the abusing mothers had the most negative expectations for their children, and the control group mothers had the most positive expectations. Perhaps more importantly, the mothers made different attributions regarding the variables determining the children's acts. When negative acts by the child or negative consequences to the child were depicted, abusive mothers made internal child attributions, whereas when positive acts or consequences were depicted, external and capricious attributions were made. The attributions of the mothers in the control group were virtually the opposite of those of the abusive mothers, and the neglecting mothers were in an intermediate position. In a related analog study of parental perceptions, Bauer and Twentyman (1985) compared reactions to stressful audiotapes of parent-child interactions that included either annoying child cries or irritating alarms. They reported that abusive mothers were more likely to perceive the depicted children as purposely acting to annoy adults.

In general, then, there is a growing body of evidence that abusive and neglectful parents have overly negative perceptions of their children and somewhat unrealistic expectations. It is important to note, however, that they may share these attributes with other deviant parents, or parents seeking services for child behavior problems, who may not be characterized as either abusive or neglectful. Thus, a diagnosis of an abusive or neglectful relational problem could not be made exclusively on assessments of expectations or perceptions offered by parents.

Outcome of Abuse and Neglect

There are three aspects of the outcome of physical abuse and physical neglect that are relevant to the inclusion of abuse and neglect as a relational problem in DSM-IV. The most obvious relates to the behavioral, emotional, and psychiatric consequences experienced by the child. Much of that data has already been considered in the section on the characteristics of abused and neglected children. The second important consideration relates to the likely outcome of the parent-child relation; this, of course, relates almost exclusively to a consideration of the parents' response to treatment and recidivism, because identified maltreating families are not typically left unattended. The third important aspect of outcome relates to the long-term consequences of abuse and neglect in the adjustment and psychopathology displayed by adolescents and adults.

Chronicity of maltreatment. As noted, the therapy outcome literature lacks adequate control or comparison groups to document the efficacy of therapy. Although we do not attempt to identify the better interventions in this chapter, we reviewed therapy studies because response to treatment may be a factor to be considered in diagnosis. Evidence of success tends to be associated with efforts on behalf of high-risk families (e.g., Hardy and Streett 1989; Hornick and Clarke 1986; Wolfe et al. 1988). When severely abusive or neglecting families are studied, the chronicity of the problem is readily apparent.

Using recidivism data from a treatment program and contrasting 50 treated families with 47 other recipients of services from the regional CPS office, Lutzker and Rice (1984) reported that the treated group had a 1-year recidivism rate of 10% and the comparison group had a rate of 21%. After 2 years, the prevalence of recidivism was 35% in their treated group and 41.3% in the comparison group (Lutzker and Rice 1987). Because recidivism can reflect risk for severe injury, even a "successful" intervention presents a sobering picture. Interestingly, other data from that same project suggest that engagement of families in treatment was not influenced by whether participation was court ordered or "voluntary" (Irueste-Montes and Montes 1988).

In the context of abuse or neglect as a relational problem, the role of out-of-home placements in outcome data may be important. For example, Leitenberg et al. (1981) presented data suggesting that foster placement resulted in better school attendance and fewer police contacts than group home or natural parent placements among children who were recipients of state services. Unfortunately, differences among jurisdictions in terms of variables that could contribute to placement make overall conclusions difficult. Moreover, there are significant patterns of variability within single jurisdictional areas that compromise our understanding of the outcome of abuse. For example, Runyan et al. (1982) used the central registry data of North Carolina to contrast foster-placed children with those who remained at home. Although severity of abusive acts, need for hospitalization, or abandonment were modest predictors, 83% of the variance in foster placement could not be understood using evidence in the central registry. This does not mean that foster care is capriciously used (Finkelhor 1983), merely that the central registries do not seem to reflect the important variables in the decision process. In terms of outcome, it is the pattern of multiple placements in out-of-home care or continuous out-of-home care that is important as a marker of the chronicity of the problem. Although some of the multiple placements in foster care can be attributed exclusively to the difficult behavioral characteristics of the child (e.g., Cooper et al. 1987; Kagan and Reid 1986; Pardeck 1983, 1985; Runyan et al. 1982), the continued pattern of abusive and neglectful parenting on the child's return home is an important factor in assessing chronicity. Thus, the fact that 25% of the children placed in foster care remain in foster care after 2 years (Lahti and Dvorak 1981) may be seen as a reflection of the chronicity of both physical abuse and physical neglect.

Based on a sample of 172 abused or neglected children, Cooper et al. (1987) associated multiple and disrupted placements with drug- or alcohol-abusing parents who engaged in additional maltreatment. R. C. Herrenkohl and Herrenkohl (1981) reported that 43% of the children placed in foster care and then returned to the care of their parents had experienced additional episodes of abuse and neglect. Rivara (1985) obtained 71 complete case records of physically abused children younger than 25 months old from among some 1,100 CPS cases of abuse. Of these children, 30% experienced further abuse following the abuse-initiated evaluation. Moreover, evidence indicated that 50% of the referred children had experienced multiple episodes of abuse, and 69% of the families with more than one child had abused or neglected a sibling of the referred child. Consistent with the data described by Rivara, D. H. Browne (1986) examined data obtained from 11 projects throughout the United States that had treated 1,874 families involved in physical abuse, neglect, or sexual abuse. Of these families, 30% had committed subsequent acts of maltreatment. Severity of initial assault, income under $5,500, and presence of life stress predicted recidivism in the D. H. Browne study. The highest recidivism risk was among families referred because of physical neglect. Crittenden (1983) completed a 4-year follow-up of 22 children referred by the court for mandatory day care because of maltreating parents: 13 had actually received the service, and 9 had not. Only 3 of the children from each service condition were in home care on follow-up, whereas 12 of the 22 had been removed from their homes and 4 were in foster care.

Based on a review of 107 physical abuse cases in California, Barth et al. (1985–1986) reported that 11 were in permanent out-of-home placement and only 74 had been reunited with their parents. After expanding their sample of permanently placed children to 21, Barth et al. were able to show that severity of abuse and the presence of school behavior problems were important in determining permanent out-of-home placements. Lawder et al. (1986) reviewed cases of 185 children placed in foster care during 1 year by a single agency in Pennsylvania and found that, after 5 years, 34% had been placed for adoption or continued in foster care. In a related study, Segal and Schwartz (1987) examined the case files of 510 children admitted to an emergency shelter for abused and neglected children over a 6-year period. Only 46% were placed with their families on discharge. Of those entering the facility directly from their natural family, 61% were returned home. In an evaluation of the impact of an experimental residential placement for severely neglected infants, Elmer (1986) reported that, at a short-term follow-up assessment, only 3 of 31 infants were with their biological mothers. Continuous family dysfunction precluded return of the children despite the expressed reunification goals of the courts and CPS agencies.

Cohn and Daro (1987) summarized four extensive federally funded program evaluation projects that represented 89 separate research and demonstration projects completed over a decade. Costing approximately $40 million, these 89 projects provided data from 3,253 abusing and neglecting families. As an overview of efforts to intervene in maltreating families, this aggregation of projects underscores the chronic nature of abusive and neglectful parent-child relationships. The overall impression of the authors was that only modest gains were achieved and that the risk for continued maltreatment was high. Indeed, only 40% of the neglectful families could be categorized as "unlikely to repeat." Thus, the available data strongly suggest that abusive and neglectful parent-child relations are not likely to be merely acute episodes nor are they likely to evidence spontaneous remission.

A study by Wolfe et al. (1988) is somewhat optimistic about the prospects of intervening in a prophylactic fashion, although based on families at risk rather than families with documented episodes of abuse. Such data, however, do not really alter the outcome picture of diagnosis and the course of truly abusive or neglecting families.

Criminality. Because of the association between physical maltreatment and aggressive behavior in children, and because of the temporal stability of aggressive behaviors (Huesmann and Eron 1984; Loeber 1982), the possible contribution of physical maltreatment to more extreme antisocial behavior and criminal activity has been investigated in many different contexts. McCord (1983) completed a 40-year tracing of men who had been identified as children prior to World War II in a Massachusetts youth program and who had records that permitted the coding of the parenting to which the men had been exposed. Childhood histories were classified as loving, rejecting, emotionally neglecting, or abusive. Of the 232 families, 49 could be classified as physically abusive. Of the physically abused youth, 39% had been convicted of criminal acts as adults or juveniles, whereas 35% of the emotionally neglected, 53% of the rejected, and 23% of the loved subjects had been convicted. Although compromised by the use of records from decades before mandatory reporting, the McCord study provides suggestive evidence for the association of maltreatment with criminal activity, but it does not suggest that physical abuse is uniquely associated with criminal activity. Similarly, Rosenbaum (1989) reported that 37% of 159 women committed to the California Youth Authority for criminal acts had mothers who had been charged with abuse or neglect.

In a more recent study based on a matched cohorts design, Widom (1989a, 1989c) identified a group of 908 children who met stringent standards for having been physically abused or neglected between 1967 and 1971 and who were younger than age 12 at the time. A nonmaltreated comparison group of 667 was carefully matched on the basis of age, sex, race, and approximate socioeconomic background. The latter was achieved by selecting school-age matches from the elementary school of the abused or neglected subjects. Matches for subjects under school-age were accomplished using records from the subjects' hospital of birth to identify potential matches. Juvenile court records, juvenile probation department records, and the federal, state, and local criminal records were then searched for all identified subjects. With respect to adult criminal activity, 28.6% of the abused or neglected group and 21.1% of the comparison group had a record of nontraffic offenses, a statistically significant difference. Moreover, although stronger in male subjects, there was a higher probability of violent offenses being committed by subjects from the abused and neglected groups. Additionally, relative to the comparison youth who did begin delinquent activity, the abused or neglected children commenced their delinquent activity at an earlier age (Rivera and Widom 1990).

Perhaps associated with the elevated levels of aggression in abused children is the indication of physical abuse and neglect in the histories of individuals convicted of murder. Based on the psychological evaluation of all individuals convicted for homicide in a single county in California, Wilcox (1986) reported that only 7% had known neglect in their childhood. In contrast, Feldman et al. (1986) reported that 8 of 15 convicted murderers sentenced to death had been victims of potential filicide and 4 of the 15 had been physically abused to an extent just short of attempted murder by their caretakers. All of the incidents of physical abuse were corroborated by records, relatives' accounts, or physical evidence. In comparison, Husain et al. (1983) reported on all female murderers who were referred to the forensic service of a state psychiatric hospital over a 2-year span. Of these murderers, 30% reported physical abuse as children, suggesting a much lower incidence rate and a rate not appreciably different from that reported in other psychiatric populations. Finally, in a study of juveniles condemned to death in four states, Lewis et al. (1988) reported that 12 of the 14 youths (86%) had histories of physical abuse, a rate similar to the rates noted in adults convicted of murder and sentenced to death. It is, however, important to note that sentencing decisions many be influenced by the histories of the subjects.

Differential incidence rates themselves are not evidence of a causal link between abuse or neglect and homicide. The only available prospective study of murderers was performed by Lewis (1985). Of 33 youths previously evaluated as juvenile delinquents, 9 were subsequently charged with murder. The rate of physical abuse in the histories of the murderers was not significantly different from the rate of physical abuse in the nonmurder group. However, it was possible to distinguish the murderers from the nonmurdering group based on the combination of five variables: psychotic symptoms, major neurological impairment, a first-degree relative with a psychiatric hospitalization or psychosis, serious violence as a juvenile, and physical abuse in childhood. Of the 8 murderers for whom information was available, 6 had all five characteristics, whereas only 2 of the 22 nonmurderers fit these criteria. The nonmurderers, however, had been followed for only about 6 months.

Consistent with the suggestion of elevated physical abuse incidence rates noted in murderers sentenced to death, Lewis et al. (1980) investigated the violent behavior of 97 boys evaluated at a state correctional school and noted that physical abuse histories were significantly associated with ratings of more severely violent behavior by these juveniles. However, violence was also associated with signs of minor neurological impairment, paranoid symptoms, and impaired and loose thought processes. Thus, the widely assumed link between physical abuse and homicide has not been clearly established by these studies.

Alcohol and drug use. In addition to aggression and criminality, excessive alcohol and drug use has been considered among the delinquent behaviors that may be associated with physical abuse and neglect. Baer and Wathey (1977) reported that 38% of the patients in a residential drug treatment program had been struck by their fathers enough to be bruised, and 29% had experienced bruising from the discipline of their mothers. In a sample of high school seniors, more polydrug users and abusers compared with nonpolydrug users reported that they had been physically abused by at least one parent in the past 3 years. The three groups did not differ on parental drinking or drug problems, parental anger or depression, or parental divorce (Wright 1985). Polydrug use was also significantly correlated with self-ratings of laziness, boredom, and rejection, suggesting the possible influence of self-image as a mediating factor. Modest but significant correlations between parental physical abuse in childhood and drug problems were obtained in a sample of freshman university students by Wright and Moore (1982). The correlations between physical abuse by a parent and reported problems with drug use and abuse were .19 for females and .09 for males. In a study of 178 pregnant alcohol- or drug-dependent women, it was noted that 19% had been severely beaten by a parent (Regan et al. 1987). Because of the higher prevalence of physical abuse in the histories of untreated alcoholics from a general population sample, Holmes and Robins (1988) argued that the less severe forms of physical abuse during childhood were associated with increased risk for alcoholism.

Dembo et al. (1987, 1988a, 1988b, 1989) completed structural analyses and replicated studies of drug use and physical abuse among juveniles incarcerated for delinquency or status offenses (i.e., noncriminal juvenile violations). A physical abuse factor was significantly correlated with reported illicit drug use in samples of 145 detainees (Dembo et al. 1987) and 399 detainees (Dembo et al. 1989). Based on the structural analyses, it was found that reported physical abuse, as well as sexual abuse, had significant direct associations with drug use as well as significant indirect paths through a pattern of self-derogation.

Potter-Efron and Potter-Efron (1985) reported a 28% prevalence rate of physical abuse in a sample of 250 adolescents seen at a treatment center for chemical dependency. In a similar study, Cavaiola and Schiff (1988) obtained a lower prevalence of physical abuse. Cavaiola and Schiff selected a random sample of records of 500 adolescents admitted to an 8-week residential chemical dependency treatment program: 15.2% had experienced injurious physical abuse and another 4.8% had experienced physical abuse and incest. Somewhat inconsistent with general population prevalence estimates, males were overrepresented in the physical abuse category; however, the overrepresentation of females in the sexually abused category is not inconsistent with national data. These groups were contrasted with sexually abused victims, incest victims, or nonabused chemically dependent adolescents from the center, as well as a sample of nonabused and nondrug-dependent adolescents from the community. Within the group of chemically dependent youth, the abused groups tended to begin the use of drugs at an earlier age. The differences among the various abuse groups were largely not significant, except that sexual exploitation was associated with sexual acting out and less aggressiveness than was physical abuse, a pattern consistent with other studies described earlier. It is important to note that most of the abuse experienced by these adolescent subjects had not been reported to the relevant CPS agency prior to admission to the treatment program.

Schaefer et al. (1988) selected 100 Veterans Administration inpatients who met DSM-III (American Psychiatric Association 1980) criteria for alcoholism and who did not evidence a psychosis or organic brain syndrome. Each patient completed the Michigan Alcoholism Screening Test (Selzer 1971), the Severity of Alcohol Dependence Questionnaire (Stockwell et al. 1983), the Symptom Checklist-90—Revised (Derogatis 1977), and a questionnaire assessing physically abusive histories: 31% of the sample reported repeated physical abuse, 4% denied knowledge of abuse, and 2% refused to respond. When the abused and nonabused alcoholic veterans were compared, several significant differences were identified. The nonabused alcoholic veterans reported higher educational attainment than the abused alcoholic veterans. Although there were no differences in severity of alcohol dependence, number of treated episodes, or length of time since last treatment, the higher scores on the Michigan Alcoholism Screening Test of the abused alcoholic veterans suggest they experienced more adverse consequences and more problem behaviors associated with drinking (e.g., fighting, arrests for drunk driving, loss of friends) than the nonabused alcoholic veterans. Moreover, on the Symptom Checklist-90—Revised, the abused alcoholic veterans had significantly higher scores on all of the symptom and global scales. Interestingly, they also reported higher levels of psychopathology during abstinence than the nonabused alcoholic veterans. Thus, the physically abused alcoholic veteran presented a symptom pattern characterized by greater severity of behavioral impairment, greater hostility, and persistent psychopathology during abstinence.

Other psychiatric disorders. Although the data are limited concerning prospective studies of abused and neglected children, there is information concerning the incidence rates of child abuse and neglect within adult, adolescent, and child psychiatric populations. Within adult psychiatric populations, various studies estimate that 26% of female outpatients (Surrey et al. 1990), 37% of female inpatients (Bryer et al. 1987), and 64% of male outpatients (Swett et al. 1990) reported that they had been physically abused as minors. Differences in incidence rates may be partially attributable to different definitions. Bryer et al. specified abuse as that which occurred prior to age 16, whereas Surrey et al. and Swett et al. required that the abuse occur before age 18. Furthermore, the estimates by Surrey et al. and Swett et al. are based on patients that reported only physical abuse and no sexual abuse. An additional 25% of female outpatients and 8% of male outpatients reported that they were victims of both physical and sexual abuse prior to age 18. Using semistructured interviews to assess histories of maltreatment, A. Jacobson (1989) assessed 31 outpatients and A. Jacobson and Richardson (1987) assessed a sample of 100 inpatients: 38% of the outpatients and 49% of the inpatients provided evidence of physical abuse prior to age 16. Pure, retrospective incidence rates, however, do not contribute much to our understanding of the long-term effects of abuse. When Surrey et al. and Swett et al. investigated the association between abusive histories and specific psychiatric illnesses, both studies found that abusive histories were not significantly associated with particular psychiatric diagnoses.

Based on a random sample of 225 adolescent psychiatric inpatients, Mundy et al. (1989) noted a high prevalence of residential instability (5–20 domicile moves). This instability correlated with documented physical abuse (.82) and with neglect (.47). The group of adolescents with higher domicile instability were more likely to present conduct disorder symptoms than the low instability groups. Among the conduct disorder symptoms often attributed to abuse is running away. For example, 43% of 149 adolescents surveyed at a runaway shelter in Toronto, Canada, indicated that physical abuse was an important factor in their leaving home (McCormack et al. 1988).

Several studies have examined the childhood histories of adult patients to determine whether abusive histories might be associated with borderline personality disorders. Herman et al. (1989) contrasted the childhood histories of 21 patients diagnosed with borderline personality disorder with those of 11 patients with borderline traits and with those of patients diagnosed with schizotypal personality disorder, antisocial personality disorder, or bipolar II disorder: 71% of the patients with borderline personality disorder reported physical abuse, whereas only 36% of the patients with borderline traits and 39% of the patients with other diagnoses reported physical abuse. Thus, although the prevalence of physical abuse was higher in all patient groups than in the general population, the prevalence of physical abuse in patients with borderline personality disorder was close to twice that of the other patient groups. In a similar study by Zanarini et al. (1989), 50 patients meeting DSM-III criteria for borderline personality disorder were compared with 29 outpatients diagnosed with antisocial personality disorder and 26 outpatients diagnosed with dysthymia and another Axis II disorder. Although the borderline group reported maltreatment in general, the greater prevalence of physical abuse or physical neglect reported by the borderline group was not statistically significant. When patients diagnosed with borderline personality disorder were contrasted with schizophrenic patients, Byrne et al. (1990) reported that the prevalence of physical abuse resulting in hospital treatment was 33.3% in the borderline group and 7.1% in the schizophrenic group, a statistically significant difference.

Chu and Dill (1990) reported that female inpatients with histories of childhood physical abuse or sexual abuse scored significantly higher on the Dissociative Experiences Scale (E. M. Bernstein and Putnam 1986) than female patients without a childhood history of abuse, although the two abuse groups did not differ significantly from each other. Analyses of dissociative experiences identified significant main effects for both physical abuse and sexual abuse, as well as a significant interaction effect. Dissociative experiences were most prevalent in subjects who revealed both physical and sexual abuse, suggesting an additive or multiplicative effect of maltreatment on dissociative symptoms. Surveys of clinicians treating individuals with multiple personality disorder report extremely high rates of physical abuse, as well as sexual abuse, with 74% of multiple personality clients reporting physical abuse and 79% reporting sexual abuse (Ross et al. 1989b). Other investigators have also reported higher rates of physical abuse, as well as sexual abuse, in female inpatients diagnosed with multiple personality disorder compared with other female inpatients (Coons and Milstein 1986). Based on information obtained from clinicians' surveys, Ross and Norton (1989) reported that multiple personality disorder patients with histories of physical abuse were significantly more likely to have attempted suicide than those without an abusive childhood history, whereas multiple personality disorder patients with a history of sexual abuse were not found to demonstrate an elevated risk of suicide.

Ross et al. (1989a) contrasted patients diagnosed with multiple personality disorder, panic disorder, schizophrenia, or an eating disorder (20 per group) using the Dissociative Disorders Interview Schedule (Heber et al. 1987). Significantly more of the multiple personality disorder group (75%) reported physically abusive childhood histories relative to the three comparison groups (5%–25%). All of these studies use different abuse criteria, and all are based on a relatively small number of patients. Although they do not provide sufficient data to support a clear link between physical abuse or physical neglect and borderline personality disorders, these studies do suggest a high base rate of abuse in the histories of personality disorder patients.

Transgenerational abuse. No other long-term outcome of physical abuse and neglect has been considered in the literature as often as the possible transgenerational pattern of child abuse. For approximately a decade, the position that abused children become the next generation of abusive parents was supported by an extensive, albeit often nonempirical, literature (e.g., Baldwin and Oliver 1975; Blumberg 1974; M. I. Cohen et al. 1966; Gelles 1973; Gil 1970; Green et al. 1974; Justice and Justice 1976; Kempe and Helfer 1972; Oliver and Taylor 1971; Parens 1987; Silver et al. 1969; S. M. Smith 1976; Spinneta and Rigler 1972; Steele and Pollack 1974; Van Stolk 1972; Zalba 1967). These papers were so influential that the notion that child abuse leads to abusive parenting became axiomatic and was uncritically accepted by researchers and clinicians. This uncritical acceptance of the multigenerational hypothesis of abuse, however, was later challenged because of the methodological inadequacies of the research (e.g., Berger 1980; de Lissovoy 1979; Herzberger 1983; Jayaratne 1977; J. Kaufman and Zigler 1987; Rutter 1983; Widom 1989b). Although the methodological challenges have led some to argue that the transgenerational hypothesis is patently false, other reviews have suggested that the literature, although methodologically compromised, supports a more limited transgenerational hypothesis. For example, Widom (1989b) argued that abuse history probably increases risk for abuse, but that the vast majority of abusive parents were not themselves abused. J. Kaufman and Zigler (1987) estimated a 30% transgenerational persistence of child abuse on the basis of their review and reconsideration of three frequently cited studies (B. Egeland and D. Jacobvitz, unpublished data, 1984; E. C. Herrenkohl et al. 1983; Hunter and Kilstrom 1979).

Although the Hunter and Kihlstrom (1979) study was a prospective study of mothers and newborn infants, the 1-year follow-up period was too short to provide a reliable estimate of a transgenerational pattern. E. C. Herrenkohl et al. (1983), however, conducted follow-up assessments of families cited for abuse or neglect over a 10-year period as well as a sample of matched comparison families for which there was no reason to suspect abuse. E. C. Herrenkohl et al. then contrasted the current disciplinary activities of the families with the parenting characteristics of the family of origin. By having a relatively large sample ($N = 529$) and by controlling for social desirability, economic status, and the number of children in the home, the E. C. Herrenkohl et al. research avoided some of the limitations of other studies in this area. Based on a prevalence of abuse histories among the abusive parents of 56% and among the nonabusive parents of 38%, E. C. Herrenkohl et al. concluded that the risk of a parent's using severely punitive discipline was increased by exposure to abusive parenting as a child. Because 53% of those who had been abused as children did not evidence abusive parenting, it was also noted that the transgenerational transmission of abuse does not reflect a simple relation between childhood experience and adult parenting.

Both Widom (1989b) and J. Kaufman and Zigler (1987) described a paper presented by B. Egeland and D. Jacobvitz (unpublished paper, 1984) that was derived from a prospective longitudinal study of mothers and their children developed by Egeland and colleagues (Egeland and Brunnquell 1979; Egeland and Sroufe 1981). Infants and mothers who participated in the original prospective study had been identified to be at high risk for developmental problems because of adolescent pregnancies, poverty, or limited parenting knowledge. Egeland and Jacobvitz evaluated the parenting and disciplinary histories of 160 mothers using semistructured interviews. Although a 70% prevalence rate of severe punishment among the mothers with a history of abusive parenting was reported, this severe punishment group included mothers who used regular spanking as well as those whose children were in the care of someone outside the home. The rate of truly abusive parenting was reported to be 34%. These mother-child dyads continued to be followed for 6 years, with the long-term follow-up outcome being described by Pianta et al. (1989). A 60% maltreatment rate was reported for the 47 mothers who had been physically abused, distributed as follows: 17% physical abuse, 17% neglect, 12% "psychologically unavailable," and 12% having homes in which their child had been sexually abused.

Evidence of an intergenerational pattern of physical abuse was obtained by Zaidi et al. (1989) from both an analog study and a study of parents and children from a tertiary care child psychiatry clinic. Based on a sample of 169 children with two parents providing data who were consecutively admitted to a child psychiatry clinic, Zaidi et al. assessed the childhood disciplinary experiences of the parents using an objective questionnaire; the abuse status of the child was assessed from the social history and medical records of the child. Although the overall rate of physical abuse in the sample of children was 24.3%, of the children who had one parent reporting an abusive childhood, 32% had been abused. Moreover, of the small number of children who had two parents describing an abusive childhood history, 50% had been abused. Although limited like other studies using self-report measures of abuse histories, the data obtained from families in which one parent had been abused are remarkably close to the J. Kaufman and Zigler (1987) estimated rate of transgenerational transmission of physical abuse.

Other studies are not inconsistent with a more limited multigenerational pattern of abuse or neglect. Indirect evidence of a transgenerational pattern was provided by Oates et al. (1985) in a study of abusive and nonabusive mothers. The abusive mothers were more likely to have lived away from their natural parents during the early period of childhood, suggesting a pattern of out-of-home placements in their histories. Haynes et al. (1984) contrasted mothers of hospitalized NO-FTT children with those of thriving children. Although none of the mothers of thriving children described a history of neglect, 22% of the NO-FTT mothers described neglecting childhoods; 4% of the mothers of thriving children and 16% of the mothers of NO-FTT children described physically abusive childhoods. Based on a reanalysis of National Survey Data, Cappell and Heiner (1990) concluded that mothers with a history of physical coercion in their family of origin were more likely to use aggression toward children than mothers whose families of origin were not characterized by coercion.

Although J. Kaufman and Zigler (1987), Pianta et al. (1989), and Zaidi et al. (1989) suggested that the multigenerational pattern of physical abuse may be far from a one-to-one relationship, a 30% persistence cannot be considered trivial. Although childhood abuse histories may exert only a relatively modest influence on the maltreating behaviors of parents (Dubowitz et al. 1987), even a modest influence may be important.

For the transgenerational hypothesis of abuse, and all the other associations between abusive or neglectful histories and later functioning, it is important to reiterate that causal links have not been established. That is, other familial or biological variables (DiLalla and Gottesman 1991) could contribute to both the abuse and the other characteristics of the abused child. Moreover, the contribution of vulnerability or resilience (Garmezy 1985; Garmezy et al. 1984; Mrazek and Mrazek 1987; Rutter 1987) to the emergence of psychopathology in the face of abusive or neglectful experiences is not well understood. However, data such as those offered by Farber and Egeland (1987) suggest that even the presence of resilient attributes may not fully buffer abused children from the adverse consequences of maltreatment. Thus, neither the absence of evidence of a clear causal link between abuse and adverse long-term outcomes nor the limited understanding of the role of vulnerability to the effects of abuse vitiate the possible utility of the diagnosis of abuse or neglect as a parent-child relational problem.

Discussion and Recommendations

Based on the available empirical evidence, it seems uncontroversial to conclude that physical abuse and physical neglect of children by their parent(s) are important public health problems. Even when stringent criteria are used to define abuse or neglect, the base rate of the problem is clearly sufficient to warrant attention. Additionally, the apparent chronicity of the problem strongly suggests that intervention on behalf of maltreated children is needed. Moreover, because of the strong association between the occurrence of abuse or neglect and either the presence of child psychopathology or later behavioral deviance in adulthood, physical abuse and neglect are appropriate areas of interest for psychiatry. Because efforts to understand abuse by focusing on either the child or the parent have been relatively unsuccessful, the available evidence suggests that conceptualizing physical abuse or neglect as a relational problem may be fruitful. Thus, based on the material reviewed here, there is a substantial database that can be used to argue in favor of physical abuse or neglect as a parent-child relational problem, and the case can be made that it would be appropriate to include such a relational problem as a diagnostic category in DSM-IV. Of course, this position has already been strongly advocated by some investigators in the abuse area (e.g., Cicchetti 1990). Yet, there are several issues and complexities that must be considered in the context of adopting parent-child relational diagnoses of abuse and neglect in DSM-IV.

Perhaps the major issue that must be considered is the implication of relational diagnoses in general. Although there is some basis for relational diagnoses in ICD-10 (World Health Organization 1990), relational diagnoses would be a major departure from the tradition of the preceding editions of the DSM. Because the DSM provides a structure for the diagnosis of mental disorders and because mental disorders are conceptualized as residing in individuals, it can be argued that relational diagnoses are outside the domain of diagnosable disorders in the DSM. To a great extent, that was the position adopted by the DSM-IV Task Force in considering relational diagnoses. Yet, because the available evidence underscores the importance of abuse and neglect to psychiatric problems and because available evidence suggests that abuse and neglect diagnoses can best be considered in a relational context, if the DSM-IV is to represent the domain of psychiatrically important events adequately, abuse and neglect as parent-child relational diagnoses would have to be included. The compromise position of the Task Force, as reflected in the *DSM-IV Options Book* (American Psychiatric Association 1991), is to include relational problems within a broad classification of "other clinically significant problems that may be a focus of diagnosis and treatment." These relational problems were then assigned the ICD-10 codes of Y07.11 (Parent-Child Relational Problem With Physical Abuse of Child) and Z62.5 (Parent-Child Relational Problem With Child Neglect).

Although this compromise approach will certainly play to mixed reviews, whether this compromise approach to the inclusion of physical abuse and physical neglect of children in DSM-IV is adequate should be more a function of operational aspects of diagnosis than the code to which they are assigned. That is, if the assessment of physical abuse and physical neglect is acknowledged to be central to the diagnostic process in the context of child psychopathology and if physical abuse and physical neglect are recognized as important targets of mental health services, then the inclusion of these important problems as Y07.11 and Z62.5 should pose no problems. If, however, DSM-IV does not adequately reflect the centrality of abuse and neglect in diagnosis and service delivery, it would be a significant deficiency. In establishing an adequate approach to physical abuse and neglect as relational diagnoses, there are several issues that must be addressed in the course of adopting diagnostic criteria.

One critical issue that must be considered is the diagnostic criteria that would be adopted and the likelihood of diagnostic errors. In all diagnoses, the criteria adopted should maximize accuracy and minimize errors. In abuse or neglect, the consequences of errors can be extreme. False positives are seen as having particularly deleterious effects on parent-child relationships and the social and emotional development of the child (e.g., Parke 1977; S. R. Smith and Meyer 1984); false negatives may be associated with rather severe health consequences to the child. In this context, it is probably important to reiterate that the adoption of diagnostic standards for abuse and neglect in DSM-IV would not supersede the mandatory reporting requirements of clinicians who suspect the occurrence of abuse. Thus, evidence that elicits a suspicion may not be sufficient to merit a diagnosis, but psychiatrists and other mental health professionals who subscribe to the DSM-IV diagnostic standards would still be required to report suspicions of abuse to the appropriate CPS agency. Although this would be a unique and perhaps problematic aspect of all the child maltreatment diagnoses, such circumstances should not preclude the adoption of the diagnostic categories.

In the context of suspicions versus diagnoses, it is important to note that making a psychiatric diagnosis of abuse or neglect may not be critical in the investigatory practices of CPS agencies. Based on the NIS-2 data, mental health agencies account for only 4% of the abuse reports submitted to CPS agencies and only 3% of the total abuse reports submitted. Because it was estimated in NIS-2 that mental health agencies submit reports on approximately 50% of the abuse cases known to them, it is unlikely that the inclusion of diagnostic standards for abuse and neglect in DSM-IV would have a major impact on the overall reporting of suspected abuse. Rather, the adoption of the diagnosis would be more likely to have an impact on the services provided to maltreated children and their families and the research that is conducted.

The pivotal problem in adopting abuse or neglect as a parent-child relational problem is the setting of appropriate diagnostic standards. Those standards will determine the clinical utility of the diagnosis, its acceptability to clinicians and researchers, the reliability of the diagnoses made, and the prevalence estimates that will emerge over the next decade. Thus, diagnostic criteria that are adopted should be as empirically based as possible. There have been several studies of the reporting standards that various professionals apply to circumstances of alleged maltreatment. Although these studies are related to the criteria used by those who submit reports to CPS agencies, they do provide some evidence relevant to establishing diagnostic criteria. Most importantly, several studies have demonstrated that there are significant differences among professionals in their ratings of the severity of various episodes of abuse or neglect (e.g., Gardner et al. 1984; Giovannoni and Becerra 1979; Snyder and Newberger 1986; Turbett and O'Toole 1983), with similarities in professional role yielding similar ratings of abusive events. However, studies have also shown that the caseload that clinicians carry can determine the abuse criteria they apply (e.g., Wolock 1982).

When process analyses have been done to determine the factors that reporters use to rate an event as abusive, the identified variables include recency, severity, surrounding conditions, intentionality, locus of injury, victim age, precipitating events, and frequency (e.g., Gardner et al. 1984; Giovannoni and Becerra 1979; Snyder and Newberger 1986; C. A. Wilson and Gettinger 1989). Similar factors are considered when child protective workers make decisions regarding likely recidivism risk (Meddin 1985). In a study of decisions by 1,196 mandatory reporters (physicians, psychiatrists, psychologists, social workers, school principals, child care workers) representing 15 states, Zellman (1990) demonstrated that judgments regarding the seriousness of the event, understanding of the reporting laws, and perceived efficacy of a report determined a substantial amount of variance in decisions to make a report. Interestingly, in the Zellman study, physical abuse and neglect were less likely to be considered reportable than were instances of sexual abuse. Although these studies of decision making demonstrate considerable variability among professionals in rating events as abusive, there is very little variability among professionals in the ratings of the more severe or blatant forms of maltreatment. That is, the obtained variability is a reflection of differences of opinion on the more subtle forms of abuse or neglect or those that are associated with more modest physical consequences. Thus, if the standards for the diagnosis of abuse or neglect in DSM-IV were reasonably stringent and the criteria were reasonably explicit, it is likely that high interjudge concordance could be obtained and that the diagnoses would be quite reliable.

Although stringent criteria for the diagnosis of physical abuse or neglect can be placed in a behavioral context, it is the injury standard that is most typically considered in setting standards for defining abuse. To a large extent, setting injury criteria for the diagnosis is a major issue that must be confronted. The argument in favor of using an endangerment criterion was advanced in the NIS-2 and by some contributors to the abuse and neglect literature (e.g., Straus 1980). Not surprisingly, an endangerment standard would yield a much higher prevalence of the disorder than an injury standard. Unfortunately, the prevalence of an abuse diagnosis based on endangerment might be so high that it would vitiate the utility of the diagnosis. Using a criterion based on the definition of abuse offered by Straus (1980), a prevalence rate of self-reported abuse among university students of more than 50% was obtained (Berger et al. 1988). Even requiring the occurrence of some injury may result in a prevalence rate that would exceed a reasonable prevalence for a psychiatric diagnosis. For example, based on a sample of 375 undergraduates from two state universities, Milner et al. (1990) reported that 21.1% of the respondents reported physical sequelae from the disciplinary acts of their parents. Berger et al. (1988) reported that 12.1% of 4,695 university students indicated that they had been injured by the discipline meted out by their parents, with bruising being the most frequent form of injury. A 12% prevalence rate in a largely middle-class population would clearly be too high for a psychiatric diagnosis that must necessarily reflect a statistically infrequent pattern of parent-child interaction. As a result, with respect to setting diagnostic criteria on the basis of the consequences of the parental behavior, the DSM-IV standard should emphasize the occurrence of injury and that injury should not be merely minor bruising in the context of physical discipline.

If the injurious standard were to require that the injury be sufficient to result in medical attention, the standard is likely to be too stringent and too many false negatives would occur. Berger et al. (1988) reported that 1.9% of the undergraduates indicated they had required medical services because of the disciplinary acts of their parents. The NIS-2 distinguished among fatal, serious, and moderate injuries, as well as the standards of probable injury and endangerment. Serious injury included loss of consciousness, stopping breathing, broken bones, diagnosed NO-FTT, third-degree burns, or extensive second-degree burns and was estimated to have an annual incidence rate of 2.5 per 1,000 children from all forms of maltreatment. According to the NIS-2, moderate injuries involving pain and impairment included events such as bruising that would persist for 48 hours. Combining fatal, severe, and moderate injurious outcomes of physical abuse, a national annual incidence rate of 4.9 per 1,000 children was established. Comparable standards applied to physical neglect resulted in an annual incidence estimate of 2.9 per 1,000 children. When endangerment is used as a standard, the annual incidence of physical abuse rises to 5.7; the incidence estimate for physical neglect rises to 9.1. It is virtually impossible to project lifetime prevalence rates from these incidence data, but it seems likely that adopting the standard of moderate injury for the diagnosis of physical abuse and a higher standard for endangerment than that adopted by the NIS-2 would be appropriate for a parent-child psychiatric diagnosis that had a childhood through adolescence lifetime prevalence rate in the range of 4%–7%.

If the diagnostic criteria also specify acts of endangerment, those acts should present a clear and present danger of significant injury to the child, and a noninjurious consequence should be less probable than a significant injurious consequence. Of course, the developmental and health status of the child will be an important determinant of whether a disciplinary or neglectful act poses a significant risk to the child. For example, C. F. Johnson and Coury (1988) noted the importance of considering minor bruising as a reflection of abuse or neglect in hemophiliac children.

The developmental status of the child is critically important in setting standards for physical neglect, especially if endangerment is considered. Within NIS-2, the incorporation of endangerment had the greatest effect on the incidence estimates of physical neglect. In the area of physical neglect, the endangerment standard should not be unlike an endangerment standard for physical abuse. That is, the probability of an adverse physical outcome due to inadequate parenting and care should be much greater than a nonpernicious outcome. For example, preschool children left unattended for a weekend in a remote cottage secured from the outside with a padlock may not experience significant adverse physical consequences. If, however, the episode were to be repeated, an injurious outcome might be more likely than not, and it would be on that basis that a neglect diagnosis would be made.

Although it might seem to be desirable to develop a listing of parental acts and injury types that would meet the diagnostic criteria for physical abuse or neglect as a parent-child relational problem, there seems to be an almost infinite array of injurious parental acts (e.g., Ellerstein 1981; Reece 1990). Thus, a diagnostic listing of physically abusive or neglectful acts and consequences would necessarily be incomplete. General standards with exemplars would be more appropriate than a catalogue. Additionally, some consideration of the chronicity of the parenting or repeated instances of moderate injuries should be included.

Another factor in the diagnosis of abuse and neglect as a relational problem that must be considered is the fact that much of the information necessary to make the diagnosis would not be obtained firsthand by the diagnostician. Although other psychiatric diagnoses can be dependent on reports by other parties, it is unlikely that much of the critical information for abuse and neglect will be obtained directly. Thus, persons making a diagnostic decision will be confronted with the task of obtaining information from other parties and assessing the importance and veridicality of the evidence. This is particularly true of evidence regarding physical injury and whether the injury is consistent with a disciplinary act of a parent (abuse) or attributable to an act of omission by a parent (neglect). False-positive errors in the diagnosis of physical abuse do occur (Wheeler and Hobbs 1988), and false accusations of physical abuse are also made (Goodwin et al. 1980; Schuman 1986). Diagnosis will require vigilance on the part of clinicians, and the standards could appropriately recognize the potential source of unreliability stemming from false accusations.

Diagnostic standards of parent-child relational problems will have to consider the possibility of both false accusations and parental denial in the context of reconciling apparent incongruities between acts and consequences. For example, one of the areas in which there has been some controversy regarding the occurrence of a parental act and injurious consequences is the "shaken baby syndrome." Questions have been raised whether shaking in the absence of external signs of injury could account for significant intracranial injury. However, Alexander et al. (1990a) reported that one-half of a sample of 24 shaken baby syndrome patients evidenced no external signs of direct impact, yet computed tomography scan or magnetic resonance imaging was able to establish the presence of significant intracranial injury. Moreover, external signs were not predictive of fatal injuries in this sample. Other studies have demonstrated that shaken infants can often present with central nervous system dysfunction plus a spectrum of other injuries that may require intensive diagnostic efforts to identify. For example, Carter and McCormick (1983) identified shaking-induced retinal hemorrhages only after pupillary dilation, and Levin et al. (1989) reported cerebral hemorrhages identified only by magnetic resonance imaging and subdural hematomas identified only by computed tomography.

Another diagnostic issue relates to intentionality and determinations of accidental events. We do not believe intention to harm should be a determining factor in making a diagnosis. Yet bona fide accidents should not yield a diagnosis of a parent-child relational problem. It has been suggested that differences between abuse-induced injuries and accidental injuries may be reflected in the organs injured. For example, in a study of 156 children younger than age 13 with blunt abdominal injuries, 65% of those who had been abused suffered injury to hollow viscus organs, whereas only 8% of the accidentally injured children experienced such injuries. Additionally, 61% of the accidentally injured children experienced injury to a single solid organ (Ledbetter et al. 1988). A much less clear picture of abdominal injuries was provided by Sivit et al. (1989) on the basis of computed tomography scans and surgical evidence obtained from 14 abused children with lower thoracic or abdominal injury. Although Merten and Carpenter (1990) noted that virtually any injury locus could be due to abuse and that radiological evidence cannot provide definitive evidence that abuse occurred, they argued that combinations of intracranial injury and abdominal injuries should occasion careful evaluations for possible maltreatment. Similarly, Tenenbein et al. (1990) suggested that radiological signs of a midshaft tibial fracture in a toddler may be indicative of physical abuse. Recurrent tympanic membrane lacerations or bilateral auricular hematomas identified by otolaryngological services (Manning et al. 1990) or ocular injury diagnosed by optometrists or ophthalmologists (S. K. Smith 1988) may also reflect abuse.

Burns resulting in injury sufficient to require seeking medical services can result from physical abuse, neglect, or accidents. Delay between the occurrence of the burn and seeking medical assistance is often a basis for suspicions of maltreatment. However, Hammond et al. (1991) and N. M. Rosenberg and Marino (1989) demonstrated that whether or not treatment is sought in less than or more than 24 hours did not distinguish between abuse or accidental burns. Based on a sample of 431 child burn patients assessed in an emergency department, N. M. Rosenberg and Marino demonstrated that old burns, past history of failure to thrive, or past evidence of abuse and neglect distinguished 69% of the abused from the accidentally burned children. Thus, it should be not the type of injury that determines the abuse diagnosis, but the child's history and the context of the injury. Interestingly, based on the characteristics of children hospitalized for severe burns, C. F. Johnson et al. (1990) concluded that children burned while in walkers experienced the most severe injuries, that the use of walkers should be discouraged, and that the use of walkers by parents could be defined as neglectful if the child were to be burned.

Another form of injurious parenting that would be appropriate to include in a diagnostic category of physical abuse is Munchausen syndrome by proxy (McGuire and Feldman 1989; Roth 1990). Although there is not a large and well-established literature in the area, the injurious consequences of the Munchausen syndrome by proxy are documented in several case studies in the literature. It is an example of parental acts that are neither disciplinary nor neglectful, but that result in injurious consequences to the child. The Munchausen syndrome by proxy is an excellent example of the diagnosticians' likely inability to determine unequivocally the intention of the parent who engages in injurious parenting.

One of the major problems that characterizes the abuse and neglect research is the various definitions of maltreatment that are used. By having a DSM-IV standard of abuse or neglect, research on treatment outcome, comorbidity, and the possible causal link between childhood maltreatment and psychopathology will be enhanced. Thus, one advantage associated with including physical abuse and neglect as a parent-child relational problem relates directly to improving clinical research on a very important public health problem.

Although the literature reviewed suggests that abused and neglected children are likely to present with a broad range of behavioral problems, at the present time they are not necessarily mandated to receive psychiatric services. Because abused children are disproportionately represented in economically disadvantaged groups that are dependent on mandated services through Title XIX, the lack of mandated mental health services associated with the occurrence of abuse results in only a relatively small proportion of the abused and neglected children receiving mental health services. The inclusion of abuse and neglect as a relational problem in DSM-IV should have the consequence of increasing the likelihood that such children would be mandated to receive services.

Summary

Although there are many complexities associated with the inclusion of physical abuse and physical neglect as parent-child relational problems, the advantages are clear. First, it is congruent with the large amount of data strongly suggesting that abuse and neglect are interactional problems involving a specific relationship. Second, such a diagnosis should improve the quality of the research relating the occurrence of abuse and neglect to other child and adult psychopathologies. Most important, it should result in an improvement in services provided to children who are clearly at great risk for a host of health and behavioral difficulties. The standards for the diagnosis should be appropriately stringent to preclude prevalence estimates that would exceed a rate appropriate for a diagnosis based on a model of statistical deviance. Thus, for both physical abuse and physical neglect, the diagnostic standards must be based on a consequence of at least moderate injury or high risk for severe or potentially fatal injury. Violations of most standards of endangerment as well as educational neglect, both of which are often included in neglect statistics, would be more appropriately subsumed in a diagnostic category of "parental inadequate discipline." Although some would argue that the intentions of the parents may be pivotal in labeling acts as abusive, the actual intentions of parents are not readily discerned, and few abusive parents express malevolent intentions. Thus, the diagnostic standards should not emphasize efforts to establish the intentionality of the perpetrator. Integration of information from multiple sources will, however, be critical in distinguishing abuse or neglect from other sources of injury. Recognition of the role of abusive fathers is necessary to avoid exclusive focus on mothers. Similarly, it is important that the diagnostic standards permit distinguishing between the perpetrating and nonperpetrating parent. The acts that meet the criteria for abuse or neglect must be related to the age and developmental status of the victim. Additionally, the diagnosis should reflect a recognition of the apparent links between physical abuse or neglect and poverty. Although this may be controversial in some quarters, it would not be the only psychiatric diagnosis with unequal prevalence across the economic spectrum. If physical abuse and neglect is adopted as a parent-child relational problem, it will be important for DSM-IV to include a clear indication that the diagnostic standards are not to be used by clinicians in deciding to submit a mandatory report for a suspicion of abuse, but that the standards would be appropriate for diagnosis in the context of clinical services or clinical research.

References

Aber JL, Allen JP: The effects of maltreatment on young children's socio-emotional development: an attachment theory perspective. Developmental Psychology 23:406–414, 1987

Accardo PJ, Blondis TA, Whitman BY: Disorders of attention and activity level in a referral population. Pediatrics 85:426–431, 1990

Acord LD: Child abuse and neglect in the Navy. Mil Med 142(11):862–864, 1977

Ainsworth MDS, Blehar MC, Waters E, et al: Patterns of Attachment: a Psychological Study of the Strange Situation. Hillsdale, NJ, Lawrence Erlbaum Associates, 1978

Alexander R, Sato Y, Smith W, et al: Incidence of impact trauma with cranial injuries ascribed to shaking. Am J Dis Child 144(6):724–726, 1990a

Alexander R, Crabbe L, Sato Y, et al: Serial abuse in children who are shaken. Am J Dis Child 144(1):58–60, 1990b

Alperstein G, Rappaport C, Flanigan JM: Health problems of homeless children in New York City. Am J Public Health 78(9):1232–1233, 1988

Alter CF: Decision making factors in cases of child neglect. Child Welfare 64(2):99–111, 1985

American Humane Association: Child Protective Services Entering the 1980's: A Nationwide Survey. Englewood, CO, American Humane Association, 1979

American Humane Association: Annual Report 1981: Highlights of Official Child Neglect and Abuse Reporting. Denver, CO, American Humane Association, 1983

American Humane Association: Highlights of Official Child Neglect and Abuse Reporting 1986. Denver, CO, American Humane Association, 1988

American Psychiatric Association: Diagnostic and Statistical Manual of Mental Disorders, 3rd Edition. Washington, DC, American Psychiatric Association, 1980

American Psychiatric Association: Diagnostic and Statistical Manual of Mental Disorders, 3rd Edition, Revised. Washington, DC, American Psychiatric Association, 1987

American Psychiatric Association: DSM-IV Options Book: Work in Progress. Washington, DC, American Psychiatric Association, 1991

Ammerman RT, Van Hasselt VB, Hersen M, et al: Abuse and neglect in psychiatrically hospitalized multihandicapped children. Child Abuse Negl 13(3):335–343, 1989

Anderson R, Ambrosino R, Valentine D, et al: Child deaths attributed to abuse and neglect: an empirical study. Children and Youth Services Review 5(1):75–89, 1983

Augoustinos M: Developmental effects of child abuse: recent findings. Child Abuse Negl 11:15–27, 1987

Ayoub CC, Milner JS: Failure to thrive: parental indicators, types and outcomes. Child Abuse Negl 9:491–499, 1985

Azar ST, Rohrbeck CA: Child abuse and unrealistic expectations: further validation of the parent opinion questionnaire. J Consult Clin Psychol 54:867–868, 1986

Azar ST, Robinson DR, Hekimian E, et al: Unrealistic expectations and problem-solving ability in maltreating and comparison mothers. J Consult Clin Psychol 52:687–691, 1984

Baer AM, Wathey RB: Covert forms of child abuse: a preliminary study. Child Psychiatry Hum Dev 8(2):115–128, 1977

Baldwin JA, Oliver JE: Epidemiology and family characteristics of severely-abused children. British Journal of Preventive Social Medicine 29:205–221, 1975

Barahal RM, Waterman J, Martin HP: The social cognitive development of abused children. J Consult Clin Psychol 49:508–516, 1981

Barden RC, Ford ME, Jensen AG, et al: Effects of craniofacial deformity in infancy on the quality of mother-infant interactions. Child Dev 60:819–824, 1989

Barth RP, Snowden LR, Broeck ET, et al: Contributors to reunification of permanent out-of-home care for physically abused children. Journal of Social Service Research 9(2–3):31–45, 1985–1986

Bauer WD, Twentyman CT: Abusing, neglectful and comparison mothers' responses to child-related and non-child-related stressors. J Consult Clin Psychol 53(3):335–343, 1985

Beck AT: Depression Inventory. Philadelphia, PA, Philadelphia Center for Cognitive Therapy, 1978

Behar D, Stewart MA: Aggressive conduct disorder: the influence of social class, sex, and age on the clinical picture. J Child Psychol Psychiatry 25(1):119–124, 1984

Bell RC: A reinterpretation of the direction of effect in studies of socialization. Psychol Rev 75:81–95, 1968

Belsky J: The determinants of parenting: a process model. Child Dev 55:83–96, 1984

Benedict MI, White RB, Çornely DA: Maternal perinatal risk factors and child abuse. Child Abuse Negl 9(2):217–224, 1985

Bennie EH, Sclare AB: The battered child syndrome. Am J Psychiatry 125:975–979, 1969

Berger AM: The child abusing family, I: methodological issues and parent-related characteristics of abusing families. Am J Family Therapy 8:53–66, 1980

Berger AM: Characteristics of child abusing families, in Handbook of Family Psychology and Therapy, Vol 2. Edited by L'Abate L. Homewood, IL, Dorsey Press, 1985, pp 900–936

Berger AM, Knutson JF, Mehm JG, et al: The self-report of punitive childhood experiences of young adults and adolescents. Child Abuse Negl 12:251–262, 1988

Berkowitz L: Aversively stimulated aggression: some parallels and differences in research with animals and humans. Am Psychol 38:1135–1144, 1983

Bernstein EM, Putnam FW: Development, reliability, and validity of a dissociation scale. J Nerv Ment Dis 174:727–735, 1986

Bernstein GA, Garfinkel BD, Hoberman HM: Self-reported anxiety in adolescents. Am J Psychiatry 146(3):384–386, 1989

Besharov DJ: Toward better research on child abuse and neglect: making definitional issues an explicit methodological concern. Child Abuse Negl 5(4):383–390, 1981

Blumberg ML: Psychopathology of the abusing parent. Am J Psychother 28:21–29, 1974

Blume SB: Public policy issues relevant to children of alcoholics. Adv Alcohol Substance Abuse 6(4):5–15, 1987

Bolton FG, Laner RH: Children rearing children: a study of reportedly maltreating younger adolescents. J Fam Violence 1(2):181–196, 1986

Bolton FG, Laner RH, Kane S: Child maltreatment risk among adolescent mothers: a study of reported cases. Am J Orthopsychiatry 50:489–504, 1980

Bopp J: Protection of disabled newborns: are there constitutional limitations? Issues in Law and Medicine 1(3):173–200, 1985

Bopp J, Balch TJ: The child abuse amendments of 1984 and their implementing regulations: a summary. Issues in Law and Medicine 1(20):91–130, 1985

Bousha DM, Twentyman CT: Mother-child interactional style in abuse, neglect, and control groups: naturalistic observations in the home. J Abnorm Psychol 93:106–114, 1984

Bower M: Classification of disciplinary events and disciplinary choices as a function of childhood history. Unpublished masters thesis, University of Iowa, Iowa City, IA, 1991

Boxer GH, Carson J, Miller BD: Neglect contributing to tertiary hospitalization in childhood asthma. Child Abuse Negl 12:491–501, 1988

Bradley EJ, Lindsay RC: Methodological and ethical issues in child abuse research. J Fam Violence 2(3):239–255, 1987

Bribitzer MP, Verdieck MJ: Home-based family-centered intervention: evaluation of a foster care prevention program. Child Welfare 67(3):255–266, 1988

Briere J, Runtz M: Differential adult symptomatology associated with three types of child abuse histories. Child Abuse Negl 14(3):357–364, 1990

Brock TC, Pallak MS: The consequences of choosing to be aggressive: an analysis of the dissonance model and review of relevant research, in The Cognitive Control of Motivation. Edited by Zimbardo PG. Glenview, IL, Scott Foresman, 1969, pp 185–200

Bromley MA, Riolo JA: Complying with mandated child protective reporting: a challenge for treatment professionals. Alcoholism Treatment Quarterly 5(3–4):83–96, 1988

Brookhouser PE: Ensuring the safety of deaf children in residential schools. Otolaryngol Head Neck Surg 97:361–368, 1987

Brown SE: Social class, child maltreatment, and delinquent behavior. Criminol Interdisciplinary J 22(2):259–278, 1984

Browne A, Finkelhor D: Impact of child sexual abuse: a review of the research. Psychol Bull 99:66–77, 1986

Browne DH: The role of stress in the commission of subsequent acts of child abuse and neglect. J Fam Violence 1(4):289–297, 1986

Browne D, Saqi S: Mother-infant interaction and attachment in physically abusing families. J Reprod Infant Psychol 6:163–182, 1988

Browne EW, Penny L: The Non-Delinquent Child in Juvenile Court: a Digest of Case Law. Reno, NV, National Council of Juvenile and Family Court Judges, 1974

Bryer JB, Nelson BA, Miller JB, et al: Childhood sexual and physical abuse as factors in adult psychiatric illness. Am J Psychiatry 144(11):1426–1430, 1987

Burgess R, Conger R: Family interaction patterns related to child abuse and neglect: some preliminary findings. Child Abuse Negl 1:269–277, 1977

Buriel R, Loya P, Gonda T, et al: Child abuse and neglect referral patterns of Anglo and Mexican Americans. Hispanic J Behav Sciences 1(3):215–227, 1979

Burke P, DelBeccaro M, McCauley E, et al: Hallucinations in children. Journal of the American Academy of Child Psychiatry 24(1):71–75, 1985

Buss AH: The Psychology of Aggression. New York, John Wiley, 1961

Bussiere A: Prosecution OK'd when prayer healing ineffective, child dies. Youth Law News 9–10, November-December 1988

Byrne CP, Velamoor VR, Cernovsky ZZ, et al: A comparison of borderline and schizophrenic patients for childhood life events and parent-child relationships. Can J Psychol 35(7):590–595, 1990

Caffey J: On the theory and practice of shaking infants. Am J Dis Child 124:161–169, 1972

Camblin LD: A survey of state efforts in gathering information on child abuse and neglect in handicapped populations. Child Abuse Negl 6(4):465–472, 1982

Campbell SB: Mother-child interactions: a comparison of hyperactive, hearing disabled, and normal boys. Am J Orthopsychiatry 45:51–57, 1975

Cappell C, Heiner RB: The intergenerational transmission of family aggression. J Fam Violence 5:135–147, 1990

Carlson V, Barnett D, Cicchetti D, et al: Disorganized/disoriented attachment relationships in maltreated infants. Developmental Psychology 25(4):525–531, 1989

Carroll J, Schaffer C, Spensley J, et al: Family experiences of self-mutilating patients. Am J Psychiatry 137(7):852–853, 1980

Carter JE, McCormick AQ: Whiplash shaking syndrome: retinal hemorrhages and computerized axial tomography of the brain. Child Abuse Negl 7(3):279–286, 1983

Cavaiola AA, Schiff M: Behavioral sequelae of physical and/or sexual abuse in adolescents. Child Abuse Negl 12(2):181–188, 1988

Christophersen RJ: Public perception of child abuse and the need for intervention: are professionals seen as abusers? Child Abuse Negl 7(4):435–442, 1983

Chu JA, Dill DL: Dissociative symptoms in relation to childhood physical and sexual abuse. Am J Psychiatry 147(7):887–892, 1990

Cicchetti D: The organization and coherence of socioemotional, cognitive, and representational development: illustrations through a developmental psychopathology perspective on Down Syndrome and child maltreatment, in Nebraska Symposium of Motivation 1988, Vol 36: Socioemotional Development. Edited by Dienstbier R, Thompson RA. Lincoln, NE, University of Nebraska Press, 1990, pp 259–366

Cohen MI, Raphling DL, Green PE: Psychological aspects of the maltreatment syndrome in childhood. J Pediatr 69:279–284, 1966

Cohen S, Warren RD: The intersection of disability and child abuse in England and the United States. Child Welfare 69:253–262, 1990

Cohn AH, Daro D: Is treatment too late: what ten years of evaluative research tell us. Child Abuse Negl 11(3):433–442, 1987

Coie JD, Kupersmidt JB: A behavioral analysis of emerging social status in boys' groups. Child Dev 54:1400–1416, 1983

Connors ET: Student Discipline and the Law. Bloomington, IN, Phi Delta Kappa Educational Foundation, 1979

Coombes P: Are we protecting children? an approach to measuring impact in protection services. Child Abuse Negl 4:105–113, 1980

Coon KB, Beck FW, Coon RC: Implications for evaluating abused children: an independent study of the frequency of abused children referred to and enrolled in special education classes in a major southeastern United States metropolitan area. Child Abuse Negl 4:153–156, 1980

Coons PM, Milstein V: Psychosexual disturbances in multiple personality: characteristics etiology and treatment. J Clin Psychiatry 47(3):106–110, 1986

Cooper CS, Peterson NL, Meier JH: Variables associated with disrupted placement in a select sample of abused and neglected children. Child Abuse Negl 11(1):75–86, 1987

Creighton SJ: An epidemiological study of abused children and their families in the United Kingdom between 1977 and 1982. Child Abuse Negl 9(4):441–448, 1985

Crittenden PM: The effect of mandatory protective daycare on mutual attachment in maltreating mother-infant dyads. Child Abuse Negl 7(3):297–300, 1983

Crittenden PM: Distorted patterns of relationship in maltreating families: the role of internal representation models. J Reprod Infant Psychol 6:183–199, 1988

Crittenden PM, DiLalla DL: Compulsive compliance: the development of an inhibitory coping strategy in infancy. J Abnorm Child Psychol 16(5):585–599, 1988

Culp RE, Culp AM, Soulis J, et al: Self-esteem and depression in abusive, neglecting, and nonmaltreating mothers. Infant Mental Health J 10(4):243–251, 1989

Cunningham CE, Barkley RA: The interactions of normal and hyperactive children with their mothers in free play and structured tasks. Child Dev 50:217–224, 1979

Daley MR, Piliavin I: "Violence against children" revisited: some necessary clarification of findings from a major national study. J Soc Serv Research 5(1–2):61–81, 1982

Deitrich-MacLean MG, Walden T: Distinguishing teaching interactions of physically abusive from nonabusive parent-child dyads. Child Abuse Negl 12(4):469–479, 1988

de Lissovoy V: Toward the definition of "abuse provoking child." Child Abuse Negl 3:341–350, 1979

Dembo R, Dertke M, la-Voic L, et al: Physical abuse, sexual victimization, and illicit drug use: a structural analysis among high risk adolescents. J Adolescence 10(1):13–34, 1987

Dembo RM, Williams L, Berry E, et al: The relationship between physical and sexual abuse and illicit drug use: a replication among a new sample of youths entering a juvenile detention center. Int J Addict 23(11):1101–1123, 1988a

Dembo R, Dertke M, Borders S, et al: The relationship between physical and sexual abuse and tobacco and alcohol use. Int J Addictions 23(4):351–378, 1988b

Dembo RM, Williams L, la-Voie L, et al: Physical abuse, sexual victimization, and illicit drug use: replication of a structural analysis among a new sample of high-risk youths. Violence and Victims 4(2):121–138, 1989

Derogatis LR: SCL-90-R: Administration and Scoring Procedures, Manual I. Baltimore, MD, Johns Hopkins University School of Medicine, Clinical Psychometrics Research Unit, 1977

Deykin EY: The utility of emergency room data for record linkage in the study of adolescent suicidal behavior. Suicide Life Threat Behav 19(1):90–98, 1989

Deykin EY, Alpert JJ, McNamara JJ: A pilot study of the effect of exposure to child abuse or neglect on adolescent suicidal behavior. Am J Psychiatry 142:1299–1303, 1985

Dietrich KN, Starr RH, Kaplan MG: Maternal stimulation and care of abused infants, in High Risk Infants and Children: Adult and Peer Interaction. Edited by Field TM, Goldberg S, Stern D. New York, Academic Press, 1980, pp 25–41

DiLalla LF, Gottesman I: Biological and genetic contributors to violence: Widom's untold tale. Psychol Bull 109:125–129, 1991

Dion KK: Children's physical attractiveness and sex as determinants of adult punitiveness. Developmental Psychology 10:722–778, 1974

Dodge KA: Social cognition and children's aggressive behavior. Child Dev 51:162–170, 1980

Dodge KA, Frame CL: Social cognitive biases and deficits in aggressive boys. Child Dev 53:620–635, 1982

Dodge KA, Newman JP: Biased decision-making processes in aggressive boys. J Abnorm Psychol 90:375–379, 1981

Dodge KA, Pettit GS, McClaskey CL, et al: Social competence in children. Monogr Soc Res Child Dev 51(2):Serial No. 213, 1986

Doek JE: Policy options on child abuse and neglect. Child Abuse Negl 8(4):385–386, 1984

Doll EA: Vineland Social Maturity Scale. Circle Pines, MN, American Guidance Services, 1965

Dollard J, Doob LW, Miller NE, et al: Frustration and Aggression. New Haven, CT, Yale University Press, 1939

Drotar D, Eckerle D, Satola J, et al: Maternal interactional behavior with nonorganic failure-to-thrive infants: a care comparison study. Child Abuse Negl 14(1):41–51, 1990

Dubanoski RA, McIntosh SR: Child abuse and neglect in military and civilian families. Child Abuse Negl 8(1):55–67, 1984

Dubanoski RA, Evans IM, Higuchi AA: Analysis and treatment of child abuse: a set of behavior propositions. Child Abuse Negl 2:153–172, 1978

Dubowitz H, Hampton RL, Bithoney WG, et al: Inflicted and noninflicted injuries: differences in child and familial characteristics. Am J Orthopsychiatry 57(4):525–535, 1987

Dukes RL, Kean RB: An experimental study of gender and situation in the perception and reportage of child abuse. Child Abuse Negl 13(3):351–360, 1989

Earp JA, Ory MG: The influence of early parenting on child maltreatment. Child Abuse Negl 4:237–245, 1980

Eckenrode J, Powers J, Doris J, et al: Substantiation of child abuse and neglect reports. J Consult Clin Psychol 56(1):9–16, 1988

Egeland B, Brunnquell D: An at-risk approach to the study of child abuse. Journal of the American Academy of Child Psychiatry 18:219–235, 1979

Egeland B, Sroufe LA: Attachment and early maltreatment. Child Dev 52:44–52, 1981

Egeland B, Vaughn B: Failure of "bond formation" as a cause of abuse, neglect, and maltreatment. Am J Orthopsychiatry 51:78–84, 1981

Egeland B, Breitenbucher M, Rosenberg D: Prospective study of the significance of life stress in the etiology of child abuse. J Consult Clin Psychol 48:195–205, 1980

Ellerstein NS: Child Abuse and Neglect: a Medical Reference. New York, John Wiley, 1981

Elliott D: State intervention and childhood multiple personality disorder. J Psychiatry Law 10(4):441–456, 1982

Elmer E: Children in Jeopardy. Pittsburgh, PA, University of Pittsburgh Press, 1967

Elmer E: Fragile Families, Troubled Children: the Aftermath of Infant Trauma. Pittsburgh, PA, University of Pittsburgh Press, 1977

Elmer E: Effects of early neglect and abuse on latency age children. J Pediatr Psychol 3:14–19, 1978

Elmer E: Outcome of residential treatment for abused and high-risk infants. Child Abuse Negl 10(3):351–360, 1986

El-Sheikh M, Cummings M, Goetsch VL: Coping with adults' angry behavior: behavioral, physiological, and verbal responses in preschoolers. Developmental Psychology 25:490–498, 1989

Emery RE: Family violence. Special Issue: Children and their development: Knowledge base, research agenda, and social policy application. Am Psychol 44(2):321–328, 1989

Endicott J, Spitzer RL: A diagnostic interview: the Schedule for Affective Disorders and Schizophrenia. Arch Gen Psychiatry 35:837–844, 1978

Erlanger HS: Social class differences in parents' use of physical punishment, in Violence in the Family. Edited by Steinmetz SK, Straus MA. New York, Harper & Row, 1974, pp 150–158

Evans AL: Personality characteristics and disciplinary attitudes of child abusing mothers. Child Abuse Negl 4:179–187, 1980

Faller KC: Unanticipated problems in the United States child protection system. Child Abuse Negl 9(1):63–69, 1985

Famularo R, Stone K, Barnum R, et al: Alcoholism and severe child maltreatment. Am J Orthopsychiatry 56(3):481–485, 1986a

Famularo R, Barnum R, Stone K: Court-ordered removal in severe child maltreatment: an association to parental major affective disorder. Child Abuse Negl 10(4):487–492, 1986b

Fantuzzo JH: Behavioral treatment of the victims of child abuse and neglect. Behav Modif 14(3):316–339, 1990

Fantuzzo JW, Jurecic L, Stovall A, et al: Effects of adult and peer social initiations on the social behavior of withdrawn maltreated preschool children. J Consult Clin Psychol 56(1):34–39, 1988

Faranoff AA, Kennell JH, Klaus MH: Follow-up of low birth-weight infants: the predictive value of maternal visiting patterns. Pediatrics 49:287–290, 1972

Farber EA, Egeland B: Invulnerability among abused and neglected children, in The Invulnerable Child. Edited by Anthony EJ, Cohler BJ. New York, Guilford, 1987, pp 253–288

Feldman M, Mallouh K, Lewis DO: Filicidal abuse in the histories of 15 condemned murderers. Bull Am Acad Psychiatry Law 14(4):345–352, 1986

Feshbach S: Dynamics and morality of violence and aggression: some psychological considerations. Am Psychol 26:281–292, 1971

Finkelhor D: Removing the child – prosecuting the offender in cases of sexual abuse: evidence from the National Reporting System for Child Abuse and Neglect. Child Abuse Negl 7:195–205, 1983

Finkelhor D, Hotaling GT: Sexual abuse in the National Incidence Study of Child Abuse and Neglect: an appraisal. Child Abuse Negl 8:23–33, 1984

Finkelhor D, Korbin J: Child abuse as an international issue. Child Abuse Negl 12(1):3–23., 1988

Flaherty EG, Weiss H: Medical evaluation of abused and neglected children. Am J Dis Child 144(3):330–334, 1990

Flango CR: State Courts' Jurisdiction and Terminology for Child Abuse and Neglect Cases. Williamsburg, VA, National Center for State Courts, 1988

Flango VE, Casey P, Dibble T, et al: Central Registries for Child Abuse and Neglect: A National Review of Records Management, Due Process Safeguards and Data Utilization. Williamsburg, VA, National Center for State Courts, 1988

Flowers RB: Withholding medical care for religious reasons. J Religion Health 23(4):268–282, 1984

Fontana VJ, Besharov DJ: The Maltreated Child. Springfield, IL, Charles C Thomas, 1979

Fosarelli PD: Latchkey children. J Dev Behav Pediatr 5(4):173–177, 1984

Franks CM: Behavior theory with children and adolescents. Annu Rev Behav Therapy Theory Practice 8:273–304, 1982

Friedrich WN, Boriskin JA: The role of the child in abuse: a review of the literature. Am J Orthopsychiatry 46:580–590, 1976

Frodi AM: Contributions of infant characteristics to child abuse. Am J Ment Defic 85:341–349, 1981

Frodi AM, Lamb ME, Leavitt LA, et al: Fathers' and mothers' responses to the faces and cries of normal and premature infants. Developmental Psychology 14:490–498, 1978

Frodi AM, Lamb ME, Wille D: Mothers' responses to the cries of normal and premature infants as a function of the birth status of their own child. J Res Personality 15:122–133, 1981

Furstenberg FF Jr: Premarital pregnancy and marital instability. J Soc Issues 40:580–590, 1976

Gabinet L: MMPI profiles of high-risk and outpatient mothers. Child Abuse Negl 3:373–379, 1979

Gaines R, Sandgrund A, Green AH, et al: Etiological factors in child maltreatment: a multivariate study of abusing, neglecting, and normal mothers. J Abnorm Psychol 87:531–540, 1978

Garbarino J: A preliminary study of some ecological correlates of child abuse: the impact of socioeconomic stress on mothers. Child Dev 47:178–185, 1976

Garbarino J, Crouter A: Defining the community context for parent-child relations: the correlates of child maltreatment. Child Dev 49(3):604–616, 1978

Garbarino J, Gillian G: Understanding Abusive Families. Lexington, MA, Lexington Books, 1980

Garbarino J, Sherman D: High-risk neighborhoods and high-risk families: the human ecology of child maltreatment. Child Dev 51(1):188–198, 1980

Garbarino J, Stocking SH: Protecting Children From Abuse and Neglect: Developing and Maintaining Effective Support Systems for Families. San Francisco, CA, Jossey-Bass, 1980

Garbarino J, Brookhouser PE, Authier KJ: Special Children, Special Risk: The Maltreatment of Children With Disability. New York, Aldine De Gruyter, 1987

Gardner GM, Schadler M, Kemper S: Classification strategies used by mandated reporters in judging incidents of child abuse. J Clin Child Psychol 13(3):280–287, 1984

Garfield SL: Suggested recommendations for publication in the area of depression (editorial). J Consult Clin Psychol 51:807–808, 1983

Garmezy N: Stress-resistant children: the search for protective factors, in Recent Research in Developmental Psychopathology (Journal of Child Psychology and Psychiatry Book Suppl 4). Edited by Stevenson JE. Oxford, England, Pergamon, 1985, pp 213–233

Garmezy N, Mastern AS, Tellegen A: The study of stress and competence in children: a building block for developmental psychopathology. Child Dev 55:97–111, 1984

Gelles RJ: Child abuse as psychopathology: a sociological critique and reformulation. Am J Orthopsychiatry 43:611–621, 1973

Gelles RJ: A profile of violence towards children in the United States, in Child Abuse: An Agenda for Action. Edited by Gerbner G, Ross CJ, Zigler E. New York, Oxford University Press, 1980, pp 82–105

Gelles RJ: Toward better research on child abuse and neglect: a response to Besharov. Child Abuse Negl 6:487–496, 1982

George C, Main M: Social interactions of young abused children: approach, avoidance, and aggression. Child Dev 50:306–318, 1979

Gil DG: Violence Against Children. Cambridge, MA, Harvard University Press, 1970

Gil DG: Unraveling child abuse. Am J Orthopsychiatry 45:346–356, 1975

Gillespie D, Seaberg J, Berline S: Observed causes of child abuse. Victimol 2:342–349, 1977

Giovannoni J: Overview of issues on child neglect, in Child Neglect Monograph: Proceedings from a Symposium, November 10, 1985. Washington, DC, Clearinghouse on Child Abuse and Neglect Information (Department of Health and Human Services), 1985, pp 1–6

Giovannoni JM, Becerra RM: Defining Child Abuse. New York, Free Press, 1979

Gladston R: Observations on children who have been physically abused and their parents. Am J Psychiatry 122:440–443, 1965

Gladston R: Violence begins at home: The Parents' Center project for the study and prevention of child abuse. Journal of the American Academy of Child Psychiatry 10:336–350, 1971

Goldberg S: Premature birth: consequences for the parent-infant relationship. Am Sci 67:214–220, 1979

Goldston DB, Turnquist DC, Knutson JF: Presenting problems of sexually abused girls receiving psychiatric services. J Abnorm Psychol 98:314–317, 1988

Goodman RS: The battered child–too little too late: the historical development of a legal diagnosis. Legal Aspects of Medical Practice 17(1): 5–6, 1989

Goodwin J, Cauthorne CG, Rada RT: Cinderella syndrome: children who simulate neglect. Am J Psychiatry 137(1):1223–1225, 1980

Green AH: Child-abusing fathers. Journal of the American Academy of Child Psychiatry 18:270–282, 1978

Green AH, Gaines RW, Sandgrund D: Child abuse: pathological syndrome of family interaction. Am J Psychiatry 131:882–886, 1974

Green AH, Liang V, Gaines R, et al: Psychological assessment of child-abusing neglecting and normal mothers. J Nerv Ment Dis 168:356–360, 1980

Gregg GS, Elmer E: Infant injuries: accident or abuse? Pediatrics 44:434–439, 1969

Greif GL, Zuravin SJ: A placement resource for abused and neglected children? Child Welfare 68(5):479–490, 1989

Groothius JR, Altemeier WA, Robarge JP, et al: Increased child abuse in families with twins. Pediatrics 70:769–773, 1982

Gruber AR, Heck ET, Mintzer E: Children who set fires: some background and behavioral characteristics. Am J Orthopsychiatry 51(3):484–488, 1981

Guyer MJ: Child abuse and neglect statutes: legal and clinical implications. Am J Orthopsychiatry 52(1):73–81, 1982

Hallett C: Research in child abuse: some observations on the knowledge base. J Reprod Infant Psychol 6(3):119–124, 1988

Halperin SM: Family perceptions of abused children and their siblings. Child Abuse Negl 7:107–115, 1983

Hammond J, Perez-Stable A, Ward CG: Predictive value of historical and physical characteristics for the diagnosis of child abuse. South Med J 84(2)166–168, 1991

Hampton RL: Race, class, and child maltreatment. J Comp Fam Studies 18(1):113–126, 1987

Hampton RL, Newberger EH: Child abuse incidence and reporting by hospitals: significance of severity, class, and race. Am J Public Health 75:56–60, 1985

Hampton RL, Gelles RJ, Harrop JW: Is violence in black families increasing? A comparison of 1975 and 1985 national survey rates. J Marriage Fam 51:969–980, 1989

Hansen DJ, Pallotta GM, Tishelman AC, et al: Parental problem-solving skills and child behavior problems: a comparison of physically abusive, neglectful, clinic and community families. J Fam Viol 4(4):353–368, 1989

Hardy JB, Streett R: Family support and parenting education in the home: an effective extension of clinic-based preventive health care services for poor children. J Pediatrics 115(6):927–931, 1989

Hart SN, Brassard MR: A major threat to children's mental health: psychological maltreatment. Am Psychol 42(2):160–165, 1987

Hartley EK: American state intervention in the parent-child legal relationship. Child Abuse Negl 5:141–145, 1981

Hathaway SR, McKinley JC: Minnesota Multiphasic Personality Inventory, Revised. Minneapolis, MN, University of Minnesota, 1970

Haynes CF: Non-organic failure to thrive: decision for placement and videotaped evaluations. Child Abuse Negl 7(3):309–319, 1983

Haynes CF, Cutler C, Gray J, et al: Hospitalized cases of nonorganic failure to thrive: the scope of the problem and short-term lay health visitor intervention. Child Abuse Negl 8(2):229–242, 1984

Heber S, Ross CA, Norton GR, et al: The Dissociative Disorder Interview Schedule: a structured interview, in Proceedings of the 4th International Conference on Multiple Personality/Dissociative States. Edited by Braun BB. Chicago, IL, Rush-Presbyterian Medical Center, 1987, p 141

Heffron WM, Martin CA, Welsh RJ, et al: Hyperactivity and child abuse. Can J Psychiatry 32(5):384–386, 1987

Hegar RL, Yungman JJ: Toward a causal typology of child neglect. Children and Youth Services Review 11(3):203–220, 1989

Herman JL, Perry JC, van der Kolk BA: Childhood trauma in borderline personality disorder. Am J Psychiatry 146(4):490–495, 1989

Herrenkohl EC, Herrenkohl RC: A comparison of abused children and their nonabused siblings. Journal of the American Academy of Child Psychiatry 18:260–269, 1979

Herrenkohl EC, Herrenkohl RC, Toedter LJ: Perspectives on the intergenerational transmission of abuse, in The Dark Side of Families: Current Family Violence Research. Edited by Finkelhor D, Gelles RJ, Hotaling GT, et al. Beverly Hills, CA, Sage, 1983, pp 305–316

Herrenkohl RC, Herrenkohl EC: Some antecedents and developmental consequences of child maltreatment. New Directions for Child Development 11:57–76, 1981

Herzberger SD: Social cognition and the transmission of abuse, in The Dark Side of Families: Current Family Violence Research. Edited by Finkelhor D, Gelles RJ, Hotaling GT, et al. Beverly Hills, CA, Sage, 1983, pp 317–329

Hibbard RA, Ingersoll GM, Orr DP: Behavioral risk, emotional risk, and child abuse among adolescents in a nonclinical setting. Pediatrics 86(6):896–901, 1990

Hill BK, Hayden MF, Lakin CK, et al: State-by-state data on children with handicaps in foster care. Child Welfare 69:447–462, 1990

Hillard JR, Slomowitz M, Deddens J: Determinants of emergency psychiatric admission for adolescents and adults. Am J Psychiatry 145(11):1416–1419, 1988

Hjorth CW, Harway M: The body-image of physically abused and normal adolescents. J Clin Psychol 37(4):863–866, 1981

Hoffman-Plotkin D, Twentyman CT: A multimodal assessment of behavioral and cognitive deficits in abused and neglected preschoolers. Child Dev 55:794–802, 1984

Holleran PA, Littman DC, Freund RD, et al: A signal detection approach to social perception: identification of negative and positive behaviors by parents of normal and problem children. J Abnorm Child Psychol 10:547–558, 1982

Holmes SJ, Robins LN: The role of parental disciplinary practices in the development of depression and alcoholism. Psychiatry 51(1):24–36, 1988

Holmes TH, Rahe RH: The Social Readjustment Rating Scale. J Psychosom Res 11:213–218, 1967

Hornick JP, Clarke ME: A cost/effectiveness evaluation of play therapy treatment for child abusing and high risk parents. Child Abuse Negl 10(3):309–318, 1986

Hudgins HC Jr, Vacca RS: Law and Education: Contemporary Issues and Court Decisions, 2nd Edition. Charlottesville, VA, The Mitchie Company, 1985

Huesmann LR, Eron LD: Cognitive processes and the persistence of aggressive behavior. Aggressive Behavior 10:243–251, 1984

Hunter RS, Kilstrom N: Breaking the cycle in abusive families. Am J Psychiatry 136(10):1320–1322, 1979

Husain A, Anasseril DE, Harris PW: A study of young-age and mid-life homicidal women admitted to a psychiatric hospital for pre-trial evaluation. Can J Psychiatry 28(2):109–113, 1983

Irueste-Montes AM, Montes F: Court-ordered vs. voluntary treatment of abusive and neglectful parents. Child Abuse Negl 12(1):33–39, 1988

Jacobson A: Physical and sexual assault histories among psychiatric outpatients. Am J Psychiatry 146(6):755–758, 1989

Jacobson A, Richardson B: Assault experiences of 100 psychiatric inpatients: evidence for the need for routine inquiry. Am J Psychiatry 144:908–913, 1987

Jacobson RS, Straker G: Peer group interaction of physically abused children. Child Abuse Negl 6:321–327, 1982

James JA, Boake C: MMPI profiles of child abusers and neglecters. Int J Fam Psychiatry 9(4):351–371, 1988

James KK, Furukawa TP, James NS, et al: Child abuse and neglect reports in the United States Army Central Registry. Mil Med 149(4):205–206, 1984

Janus MD, McCormack A, Burgess AW, et al: Adolescent Runaways: Causes and Consequences. Lexington, MA, Lexington Books, 1987

Jason J, Andereck ND: Fatal child abuse in Georgia: the epidemiology of severe physical child abuse. Child Abuse Negl 7(1):1–9, 1983

Jaudes PK, Diamond LJ: The handicapped child and child abuse. Child Abuse Negl 9:341–347, 1985

Jaudes PK, Diamond LJ: Neglect of chronically ill children. Am J Dis Child 140:655–658, 1986

Jayaratne S: Child abusers as parents and children: a review. Social Work 22:5–9, 1977

Johnson B, Morse HA: Injured children and their parents. Children 15:147–152, 1968

Johnson CF: Inflicted injury versus accidental injury. Pediatr Clin North Am 37(4):791–814, 1990

Johnson CF, Coury DL: Bruising and hemophilia: accident or child abuse? Child Abuse Negl 12(3):409–415, 1988

Johnson CF, Ericson AK, Caniano D: Walker-related burns in infants and toddlers. Pediatric Emergency Care 6(1):58–61, 1990

Junewicz WJ: A protective posture toward emotional neglect and abuse. Child Welfare 62:243–252, 1983

Justice B, Justice R: The Abusing Family. New York, Human Services Press, 1976

Kagan RM, Reid WJ: Critical factors in the adoption of emotionally disturbed youths. Child Welfare 65(1):63–73, 1986

Kaplan SJ, Pelcovitz D, Salzinger S, et al: Psychopathology of parents of abused and neglected children and adolescents. Journal of the American Academy of Child Psychiatry 22:238–244, 1983

Karp RJ, Scholl TO, Decker E, et al: Growth of abused children: contrasted with the non-abused in an urban poor community. Clin Pediatr 28(7):317–320, 1989

Kashani JH, Carlson GA: Seriously depressed preschoolers. Am J Psychiatry 144(3):348–350, 1987

Kaufman H: Aggression and Altruism. New York, Holt Rinehart & Winston, 1970

Kaufman J, Cicchetti D: Effects of maltreatment on school-age children's socioemotional development: assessments in a day-camp setting. Developmental Psychology 25:516–524, 1989

Kaufman J, Zigler E: Do abused children become abusive parents? Am J Orthopsychiatry 57(2):186–192, 1987

Kazdin AE, Moser J, Colbus D, et al: Depressive symptoms among physically abused and psychiatrically disturbed children. J Abnorm Psychol 94(3):298–307, 1985

Kempe CH, Helfer RE: Helping the Battered Child and His Family. Philadelphia, PA, JB Lippincott, 1972

Kempe CH, Silverman FN, Steele BF, et al: The battered child syndrome. JAMA 181:17–24, 1962

Kessel JA, Robbins SP: The Indian Child Welfare Act: dilemmas and needs. Child Welfare 63(3):225–232, 1984

Kinard EM, Klerman LV: Teenage parenting and child abuse: are they related? Am J Orthopsychiatry 50:481–488, 1980

Klein M, Stern L: Low birth weight and the battered child syndrome. Am J Dis Child 122:15–18, 1971

Klimes-Dougan B, Kistner J: Physically abused preschoolers' responses to peers' distress. Developmental Psychology 26(4):599–602, 1990

Knudsen DD: Duplicate reports of child maltreatment: a research note. Child Abuse Negl 13(1):41–43, 1989

Knutson JF: Aggression as manipulable behavior, in Control of Aggression: Implications From Basic Research. Edited by Knutson JF. Chicago, IL, Aldine-Atherton, 1973, pp 253–295

Knutson JF: Child abuse research as an area of aggression research. Pediatr Psychol 3:20–27, 1978

Knutson JF: Physical abuse and sexual abuse of children, in Handbook of Pediatric Psychology. Edited by Routh DK. New York, Guilford, 1988, pp 32–70

Knutson JF, Mehm JG: Transgenerational patterns of coercion in families and intimate relationships, in Violence in Intimate Relationships. Edited by Russell GW. New York, PMA Publishing, 1988, pp 67–90

Knutson JF, Schartz HA, Zaidi LY: Victim risk factors in the physical abuse of children, in Targets of Violence and Aggression. Edited by Baenninger R. Amsterdam, Elsevier/North Holland, 1991, pp 103–157

Kohlberg L, LaCrosse J, Ricks D: The predictability of adult mental health from childhood behavior, in Manual of Child Psychopathology. Edited by Wolman BB. New York, McGraw-Hill, 1972, pp 1217–1284

Kolko DJ, Moser JT, Weldy SR: Behavioral/emotional indicators of sexual abuse in child psychiatric inpatients: a controlled comparison with physical abuse. Child Abuse Negl 12(4):529–541, 1988

Kosky E: Childhood suicidal behaviour. J Child Psychol Psychiatry 24(3):457–468, 1983

Kotch JB, Thomas LP: Family and social factors associated with substantiation of child abuse and neglect reports. J Fam Viol 1(2):167–179, 1986

Koverola C, Manion I Wolfe D: A microanalysis of factors associated with child-abusive families: identifying individual treatment priorities. Behav Res Ther 23(5): 499–506, 1985

Krugman RD, Lenherr M, Betz L, et al: The relationship between unemployment and physical abuse of children. Sixth International Congress of the International Society for Prevention of Child Abuse and Neglect. Child Abuse Negl 10(3):415–418, 1986

Kufeldt D, Nimmo M: Youth on the street: abuse and neglect in the eighties. Child Abuse Negl 11(4):531–543, 1987

Kupfer DJ, Rush AJ: Recommendations for depression publications. Arch Gen Psychiatry 40:1031, 1983

Lahey BB, Conger RD, Atkeson BM, et al: Parenting behavior and emotional status of physically abusive mothers. J Consult Clin Psychol 52(6):1062–1071, 1984

Lahti J, Dvorak J: Coming home from foster care, in The Challenge of Partnership: Working with Parents of Children in Foster Care. Edited by Maluccio AN, Sinanoglu PA. New York, Child Welfare League of America, 1981, pp 52–66

Lally JR: Three views of child neglect: expanding visions of preventive intervention. Child Abuse Negl 8(2):243–254, 1984

Lamb ME (ed): The Role of the Father in Child Development. New York, John Wiley, 1981

Larrance DT, Twentyman CT: Maternal attributions and child abuse. J Abnorm Psychol 92:449–457, 1983

Larson OW, Doris J, Alvarez WF: Child maltreatment among U.S. east coast migrant farm workers. Child Abuse Negl 11(2):281–291, 1987

Larson OW, Doris J, Alvarez WF: Migrants and maltreatment: comparative evidence from central register data. Child Abuse Negl 14(3):375–385, 1990

Larzelere RE: Moderate spanking: model or deterrent of children's aggression in the family? J Fam Viol 1:27–36, 1986

Lawder EA, Poulin JE, Andrews RG: A study of 185 foster children 5 years after placement. Child Welfare 65(3):241–251, 1986

Leal CA: Treatment of abused and neglected preschool children in a city hospital. Psychiatric Annals 6(5):216–226, 1976

Ledbetter DJ, Hatch EI Jr, Feldman KW, et al: Diagnostic and surgical implications of child abuse. Arch Surg 123(9):1101–1105, 1988

Leitenberg H, Burchard JD, Healy D, et al: Nondelinquent children in state custody: does type of placement matter? Am J Community Psychol 9(3):347–360, 1981

Leonard CH, Clyman RI, Piecuch RE, et al: Effect of medical and social risk factors on outcome of prematurity and very low birth weight. J Pediatr 116(4):620–626, 1990

Leventhal JM: Risk factors for child abuse: methodologic standards in case-control studies. Pediatrics 68:684–690, 1981

Leventhal JM: Research strategies and methodologic standards in studies of risk factors for child abuse. Child Abuse Negl 6:113–123, 1982

Leventhal JM: Can child maltreatment be predicted during the perinatal period: evidence from longitudinal cohort studies. J Reprod Infant Psychol 6:139–161, 1988

Leventhal JM, Graber RB, Brady CA: Identification during the postpartum period of infants who are at high risk of child maltreatment. J Pediatr 114(3):481–487, 1989

Levin AV, Magnusson MR, Rafto SE, et al: Shaken baby syndrome diagnosed by magnetic resonance imaging. Pediatric Emergency Care 5(3):181–186, 1989

Lewis DO: Biopsychosocial characteristics of children who later murder: a prospective study. Am J Psychiatry 142(10):1161–1167, 1985

Lewis DO, Shanock SS, Pincus JH, et al: Violent juvenile delinquents: psychiatric, neurological, psychological, and abuse factors. Annual Progress in Child Psychiatry and Child Development 591–603, 1980

Lewis DO, Pincus JH, Bard B, et al: Neuropsychiatric, psychoeducational, and family characteristics of 14 juveniles condemned to death in the United States. Am J Psychiatry 145(5): 584–589, 1988

Light R: Abuse and neglected children in America: a study of alternative policies. Harvard Educational Review 43:556–598, 1973

Loeber R: The stability of antisocial and delinquent child behavior: a review. Child Dev 53:1431–1446, 1982

Ludolph PS, Westen D, Misle B, et al: The borderline diagnosis in adolescents: symptoms and developmental history. Am J Psychiatry 147(4) 470–476, 1990

Lutzker JR, Rice JM: Project 12-ways: measuring outcome of a large in-home service for treatment and prevention of child abuse and neglect. Child Abuse Negl 8(4):519–524, 1984

Lutzker JR, Rice JM: Using recidivism data to evaluate project 12-ways: an ecobehavioral approach to the treatment and prevention of child abuse and neglect. J Fam Viol 2(4):283–290, 1987

Lynch MA: Ill-health and child abuse. Lancet 2:317–319, 1975

Lynch MA, Roberts J: Consequences of Child Abuse. New York, Academic Press, 1982

Lyons-Ruth K, Connell DB, Zoll D, et al: Infants of social risk: relations among infant maltreatment maternal behavior and infant attachment behavior. Developmental Psychology 23:223–232, 1987

Main M, George C: Response of abused and disadvantaged toddlers to distress in age mates: a study in the day care setting. Developmental Psychology 21:407–412, 1985

Manning SC, Casselbrant M, Lammers D: Otolaryngologic manifestations of child abuse. Int J Pediatr Otorhinolarynogoly 20(1):7–16, 1990

Margolin L: Fatal child neglect. Child Welfare 69:309–319, 1990

Marshall WM, Puls T, Davidson G: New child abuse spectrum in an era of increased awareness. Am J Dis Child 142(6):664–667, 1988

Martin HP: Which children get abused: high risk factors in the child, in The Abused Child: a Multidisciplinary Approach to Developmental Issues and Treatment. Edited by Martin HP. Cambridge, Ballinger Press, 1976, pp 27–41

Martin JA: Neglected fathers: limitations in diagnostic and treatment resources for violent men. Child Abuse Negl 8(4):387–392, 1984

Martin JE, Kourany RFC: Child abuse by adolescent babysitters. Child Abuse Negl 4:15–22, 1980

McCabe V: Abstract perceptual information for age level: a risk factor for maltreatment? Child Dev 55(1):267–276, 1984

McCluney RS: The legal aspects of corporal punishment in American public schools. Doctoral dissertation, University of North Carolina, Greensboro, NC, 1987

McCord J: A forty year perspective on effects of child abuse and neglect. Child Abuse Negl 7:265–270, 1983

McCormack A, Janus MD, Burgess AW: Runaway youths and sexual victimization: gender differences in an adolescent runaway population. Child Abuse Negl 10:387–395, 1986

McCormack A, Burgess AW, Hartman C: Familial abuse and post-traumatic stress disorder. Journal of Traumatic Stress 1(2):231–242, 1988

McGuire TL, Feldman KW: Psychologic morbidity of children subjected to Munchausen syndrome by proxy. Pediatrics 83(2):289–292, 1989

Meddin BJ: The assessment of risk in child abuse and neglect case investigations. Child Abuse Negl 9(1):57–62, 1985

Mele-Sernovitz S: Some problems of vagueness and overbreadth in criminal child abuse statutes, in Advocacy for the Legal Interests of Children. Edited by Bross DC. Denver, CO, National Association of Counsel for Children, 1980, pp 375–380

Merrill EJ: Physical abuse of children: an agency study, in Protecting the Battered Child. Edited by DeFrancis V. Denver, CO, American Humane Association, 1962

Merten DF, Carpenter BL: Radiologic imaging of inflicted injury in the child abuse syndrome. Pediatr Clin North Am 37(4):815–837, 1990

Miller KA, Miller EK: Self-reported incidence of physical violence in college students. J Am Coll Health 32(2):63–65, 1983

Miller SH: The relationship between adolescent childbearing and child maltreatment. Child Welfare 63(6):553–557, 1984

Milner JS, Robertson KR, Rogers DL: Childhood history of abuse and adult child abuse potential. J Fam Viol 5(1):15–34, 1990

Misener TR: Toward a nursing definition of child maltreatment using seriousness vignettes. Advances in Nursing Science 8(4):1–14, 1986

Monane M, Leichter D, Lewis DO: Physical abuse in psychiatrically hospitalized children and adolescents. Journal of the American Academy of Child Psychiatry 23(6):653–658, 1984

Money J, Annecillo C, Kelley JF: Abuse-dwarfism syndrome: after rescue, statural and intellectual catchup growth correlate. J Clin Child Psychol 12:279–283, 1983a

Money J, Annecillo C, Kelley JF: Growth of intelligence: failure and catchup associated respectively with abuse and rescue in the syndrome of abuse dwarfism. Psychoneuroendocrinology 8(3):309–319, 1983b

Morris MG, Gould RW: Role reversal: a concept in dealing with the neglected battered child syndrome, in The Neglected Battered Child Syndrome. Edited by Child Welfare League of America. New York, Child Welfare Leagues of America, 1963, pp 26–46

Morse C, Sahler O, Friedman S: A three-year follow-up of abused and neglected children. Am J Dis Child 120:439–446, 1970

Mrazek PJ, Mrazek DA: Resilience in child maltreatment victims: a conceptual exploration. Child Abuse Negl 11:357–366, 1987

Mundy P, Robertson J, Greenblatt M, et al: Residential instability in adolescent inpatients. Journal of the American Academy of Child Adolesc Psychiatry 28(2):176–181, 1989

Myers JEB, Carter LE: Proof of physical child abuse. Missouri Law Review 53:189–225, 1988

Myers SS: Child abuse and the military community. Mil Med 144(1):23–25, 1979

National Center on Child Abuse and Neglect: Child abuse and neglect: state reporting laws (DHHS Publ No OHDS-80-30265). Washington, DC, U.S. Government Printing Office, 1980

Nelson BJ: Making an Issue of Child Abuse: Political Agenda Setting for Social Problems. Chicago, IL, University of Chicago Press, 1984

Nelson HB, Martin CA: Increased child abuse in twins. Child Abuse Negl 9(4):501–505, 1985

Newman SA: Baby Doe, Congress and the states: challenging the federal treatment standard for impaired infants. Am J Law Med 15(1):1–60, 1989

Nixon J, Pearn J, Wilkey I, et al: Social class and violent child death: an analysis of fatal non-accidental injury, murder, and fatal child neglect. Child Abuse Negl 5:111–116, 1981

Oates RK, Forrest D, Peacock A: Mothers of abused children: a comparison study. Clin Pediatr 24(1):9–13, 1985

Office of Human Development Services: Study findings: study of national incidence and prevalence of child abuse and neglect: 1988 (Department of Health and Human Services). Washington, DC, U.S. Government Printing Office, 1988

O'Hara MW, Rehm LP, Campbell SB: Postpartum depression: a role for social network and life stress variables. J Nerv Ment Dis 171:336–341, 1983

O'Hara MW, Neunaber DJ, Zekoski EM: Prospective study of postpartum depression: prevalence, course, and predictive factors. J Abnorm Psychol 93:158–171, 1984

Oldershaw L, Walters CC, Hall DK: A behavioral approach to the classification of different types of physically abusive mothers. Merrill Palmer Quarterly 35(3):255–279, 1989

Oliver JE, Taylor A: Five generations of ill-treated children in one family pedigree. Br J Psychiatry 119:473–480, 1971

Olsen LJ, Holmes WM: Youth at risk: adolescents and maltreatment. Children and Youth Services Review 8(1):13–35, 1986

O'Toole R, Turbett P, Nalepka C: Theories, professional knowledge, and diagnosis of child abuse, in The Dark Side of Families: Current Family Violence Research. Edited by Finkelhor D, Gelles RJ, Hotaling GT, et al. Beverly Hills, CA, Sage Publications, 1983, pp 349–362

Pardeck JT: An empirical analysis of behavioral and emotional problems of foster children as related to replacement in care. Child Abuse Negl 7:75–78, 1983

Pardeck JT: A profile of the child likely to experience unstable foster care. Adolescence 20(79):689–695, 1985

Parens H: Cruelty begins at home. Child Abuse Negl 11:331–338, 1987

Parke RD: Socialization into child abuse: a social interactional perspective, in Law, Justice, and the Individual in Society: Psychological and Legal Issues. Edited by Tapp JL, Levine FJ. New York, Holt Rinehart & Winston, 1977, pp 1–49

Parke RD, Collmer CW: Child abuse: an interdisciplinary analysis, in Review of Child Development Research, Vol 5. Edited by Hetherington EM. Chicago, IL, University of Chicago Press, 1975, pp 1–102

Patterson GR: Coercive Family Process. Eugene, OR, Castalia Publishing Company, 1982

Paulson MJ, Afifi AA, Thomason ML, et al: The MMPI: a descriptive measure of psychopathology in abusive parents. J Clin Psychol 30:387–390, 1974

Pelton LH: Child abuse and neglect: the myth of classlessness. Am J Orthopsychiatry 48(4):608–617, 1978

Perry MA, Wells EA, Doran LD: Parent characteristics in abusing and nonabusing families. J Clin Child Psychol 12(3):329–336, 1983

Pianta R, Egeland B, Erickson MF: The antecedents of maltreatment: results of the Mother-Child Interaction Research Project, in Child Maltreatment: Theory and Research on the Causes and Consequences of Child Abuse and Neglect. Edited by Cicchetti D, Carlson V. Cambridge, MA, Cambridge University Press, 1989, pp 203–253

Pieterse JJ, Van-Urk H: Maltreatment of children in the Netherlands: an update after ten years. Child Abuse Negl 13(2):263–269, 1989

Pless IB, Sibald AD, Smith MA, et al: A reappraisal of the frequency of child abuse seen in pediatric emergency rooms. Child Abuse Negl 11(2):193–200, 1987

Plomin R: Childhood temperament, in Advances in Clinical Child Psychology, Vol 6. Edited by Lahey B, Kazdin A. New York, Plenum, 1983, pp 45–92

Plotkin RC, Azar S, Twentyman CT, et al: A critical evaluation of the research methodology employed in the investigation of causative factors of child abuse and neglect. Child Abuse Negl 5(4):449–455, 1981

Polansky NA, Hally C, Polansky NF: Profile of neglect: a survey of the state of knowledge of child neglect. Washington, DC, Community Services Administration, Department of Health, Education and Welfare, 1975

Polansky NA, Ammons PW, Weathersby BL: Is there an American standard of child care? Social Work 28(5):341–346, 1983

Potter-Efron RT, Potter-Efron PS: Family violence as a treatment issue with chemically dependent adolescents. Alcoholism Treatment Quarterly 2:1–5, 1985

Powers JL, Eckenrode J: The maltreatment of adolescents. Child Abuse Negl 12(2):189–199, 1988

Powers JL, Eckenrode J, Jaklitsch B: Maltreatment among run away and homeless youth. Child Abuse Negl 14:87–98, 1990

Quay HC, Peterson DR: Manual for the Revised Behavior Problem Checklist. Coral Gables, FL, University of Miami, 1987

Rausch K, Knutson JF: The self-report of personal punitive childhood experiences and those of siblings. Child Abuse Negl 15:29–36, 1991

Reece RM: Unusual manifestations of child abuse. Pediatr Clin North Am 37(4):905–921, 1990

Regan DO, Ehrlich SM, Finnegan LP: Infants of drug addicts: at risk for child abuse, neglect, and placement in foster care. Neurotoxicol Teratol 9(4):315–319, 1987

Reid JB: Social-interactional patterns in families of abused and nonabused children, in Social and Biological Origins of Altruism and Aggression. Edited by Zahn-Waxler C, Cummings M, Radke-Yarrow M. Cambridge, MA, Cambridge University Press, 1984, pp 238–255

Reid JB, Taplin PS: A social interactional approach to the treatment of abusive families. Paper presented at the meeting of the American Psychological Association, Washington, DC, 1976

Reid JB, Taplin PS, Loeber R: A social interactional approach to the treatment of abusive families, in Violent Behavior: Social Learning Approaches to Prediction, Management, and Treatment. Edited by Stewart RB. New York, Brunner/Mazel, 1981, pp 88–101

Reid JB, Patterson GR, Loeber R: The abused child: victim, instigator, or innocent bystander, in Response Structure and Organization. Edited by Berstein D. Lincoln, NE, University of Nebraska Press, 1982, pp 47–68

Reidy TJ: The aggressive characteristics of abused and neglected children. J Clin Psychol 33:1140–1145, 1977

Reitman A: Corporal punishment in the schools: the ultimate violence. Children's Legal Rights Journal 9:6–13, 1988

Ringwalt C, Caye J: The effect of demographic factors on perceptions of child neglect. Children and Youth Services Review 11(2):133–144, 1989

Rivara FP: Physical abuse in children under two: a study of therapeutic outcomes. Child Abuse Negl 9(1):81–87, 1985

Rivera B, Widom CS: Childhood victimization and violent offending. Violence and Victims 5(1):19–35, 1990

Robarge JP, Reynolds ZB, Groothuis JR: Increased child abuse in families with twins. Research in Nursing and Health 5(4):199–203, 1982

Rogeness GA, Amrung SA, Macedo CA, et al: Psychopathology in abused or neglected children. Journal of the American Academy of Child Psychiatry 25(5):659–665, 1986

Rohner RP, Rohner EC: Antecedents and consequences of parental rejection: a theory of emotional abuse. Child Abuse Negl 4:189–198, 1980

Rohrbeck CA, Twentyman CT: Multimodal assessment of impulsiveness in abusing, neglecting, and normal treating mothers and their preschool children. J Consult Clin Psychol 54(2):231–236, 1986

Roscoe B, Callahan JE, Peterson KL: Physical attractiveness as a potential contributor to child abuse. Education 105(4):349–353, 1985

Rosenbaum JL: Family dysfunction and female delinquency. Special Issue: Women and Crime. Crime and Delinquency 35(1):31–44, 1989

Rosenberg MS, Repucci ND: Abusive mothers: perceptions of their own and their children's behavior. J Consult Clin Psychol 51:674–682, 1983

Rosenberg NM, Marino D: Frequency of suspected abuse/neglect in burn patients. Pediatric Emergency Care 5(4):219–221, 1989

Rosenthal JA: Patterns of reported child abuse and neglect. Child Abuse Negl 12(2):263–271, 1988

Ross CA, Norton GR: Suicide and parasuicide in multiple personality disorder. Psychiatry 52(3):365–371, 1989

Ross CA, Heber S, Norton GR, et al: Differences between multiple personality disorder and other diagnostic groups on structured interview. J Nerv Men Dis 177(8):487–491, 1989a

Ross CA, Norton GR, Wozney K: Multiple personality disorder: an analysis of 236 cases. Can J Psychiatry 34(5):413–418, 1989b

Roth D: How "mild" is mild Munchausen syndrome by proxy? Isr J Psychiatry Relat Sci 27(3):160–167, 1990

Runyan DK, Gould CL, Trost DC, et al: Determinants of foster care placement for the maltreated child. Child Abuse Negl 6(3):323–350, 1982

Russell CS: Unscheduled parenthood: transition to "parent" for the teenager. J Soc Iss 36:45–63, 1980

Rutter M: Stress coping and development: some issues and some questions, in Stress, Coping, and Development in Children. Edited by Garmezy N, Rutter M. New York, McGraw-Hill, 1983, 1–41

Rutter M: Psychosocial resilience and protective mechanism. Am J Orthopsychiatry 57:316–331, 1987

Saltzman A: Reporting child abusers and protecting substance abusers. Social Work 31(6):474–476, 1986

Salzinger S, Kaplan S, Artemyeff C: Mothers' personal social networks and child maltreatment. J Abnorm Psychol 92(1):68–76, 1983

Salzinger S, Kaplan S, Pelcovitz D, et al: Parent and teacher assessment of children's behavior in child maltreating families. Journal of the American Academy of Child Psychiatry 23:458–464, 1984

Sandgrund A, Gaines RW, Green AH: Child abuse and mental retardation: a problem of cause and effect. Am J Ment Deficiency 79:327–330, 1974

Sapp AD, Carter DL: Child Abuse in Texas: a Descriptive Study of Texas Residents' Attitudes. Huntsville, TX, Sam Houston State University, 1978

Schaefer MR, Sobieraj K, Hollyfield RL: Prevalence of childhood physical abuse in adult male veteran alcoholics. Child Abuse Negl 12(2):141–149, 1988

Schaeffer S, Lewis M: Social behavior of maltreated children: a naturalistic study of day care. Res Clin Center Child Dev 12:79–117, 1990

Schindler F, Arkowitz H: The assessment of mother-child interactions in physically abusive and nonabusive families. J Fam Viol 1:247–257, 1986

Schlesinger H, Meadow K: Sound and Sign: Child Deafness and Mental Health. Berkeley, CA, University of California Press, 1972

Schmitt BD, Mauro RD: Nonorganic failure to thrive: an outpatient approach. Child Abuse Negl 13(2):235–248, 1989

Schneider-Rosen K, Cicchetti D: The relationship between affect and cognition in maltreated infants: quality of attachment and the development of visual self-recognition. Child Dev 55:648–658, 1984

Schneider-Rosen K, Cicchetti D: Early self-knowledge and emotional development: visual self-recognition and affective reactions to mirror self-images in maltreated and non-maltreated toddlers. Developmental Psychology 27(3):471–478, 1991

Schneider-Rosen K, Braunwald KG, Carlson V, et al: Current perspectives in attachment theory: illustrations from the study of maltreated infants, in Growing Points in Attachment Theory and Research. Edited by Bretherton I, Waters R. Monogr Soc Res Child Dev 209(50):194–210, 1985

Schor DP, Holmes CS: Partial recovery from severe child neglect and abuse. J Dev Behav Pediatr 4(1):70–74, 1983

Schuman DC: False accusations of physical and sexual abuse. 15th Annual Meeting of the American Academy of Psychiatry and the Law. Bull Am Acad Psychiatry Law 14(1):5–21, 1986

Seaberg JR: Predictors of injury severity in physical child abuse. J Soc Serv Res 1(1):63–76, 1987

Sedlak AJ: Technical amendment to the study findings: national incidence and prevalence of child abuse and neglect: 1988. Paper submitted to National Center on Child Abuse and Neglect, Washington, DC. Rockville, MD, Westat, 1990

Segal UA, Schwartz S: Admission discharge patterns of children in emergency treatment shelters: implications for child and youth care practitioners. Child and Youth Care Quarterly 16(4):263–271, 1987

Selzer ML: The Michigan Alcoholism Screening Test: the quest for a new diagnostic instrument. Am J Psychiatry 127:89–94, 1971

Sherrod KB, O'Connor S, Vietze PM, et al: Child health and maltreatment. Child Dev 55:1174–1183, 1984

Showers J, Pickell E: Child firesetters: a study of three populations. Hosp Community Psychiatry 38(5):495–501, 1987

Silver LB, Dublin CC, Lourie RS: Does violence breed violence? contributions from the study of the child abuse syndrome. Am J Psychiatry 126:404–407, 1969

Singer L: Long-term hospitalization of failure-to-thrive infants: developmental outcome at three years. Child Abuse Negl 10(4):479–486, 1986

Sivit CJ, Taylor GA, Eichelberger MR: Visceral injury in battered children: a changing perspective. Radiology 173(3):659–661, 1989

Skolnick A: Religious exemptions to child neglect laws still being passed despite convictions of parents. JAMA 264(10):1226,1229,1233, 1990

Smetana JG, Kelly M, Twentyman CT: Abused, neglected, and nonmaltreated children's conceptions of moral and social-conventional transgressions. Child Dev 55:277–287, 1984

Smith SK: Child abuse and neglect: a diagnostic guide for the optometrist. J Am Optometry Assoc 59(10):760–766, 1988

Smith SM: The Battered Child Syndrome. London, England, Butterworths, 1976

Smith SM: Child abuse: a medico-legal issue. Psychiatr Med 2(3):223–233, 1984

Smith SM, Hanson R: Interpersonal relationships and child-rearing practices in 214 parents of battered children. Br J Psychiatry 127:513–525, 1975

Smith SR, Meyer RG: Child abuse reporting laws and psychotherapy: a time for reconsideration. Int J Law Psychiatry 7(3–4):351–366, 1984

Snyder JC, Newberger EH: Consensus and difference among hospital professionals in evaluating child maltreatment. Violence and Victims 1(2):125–129, 1986

Solomons G: Child abuse and developmental disabilities. Dev Med Child Neurol 21:101–105, 1979

Spearly JL, Lauderdale M: Community characteristics and ethnicity in the prediction of child maltreatment rates. Child Abuse Negl 7(1):91–105, 1983

Spinetta JJ, Rigler D: The child-abusing parent: a psychological review. Psychol Bull 77:296–304, 1972

Spitzer RL, Endicott J, Robins E: Research Diagnostic Criteria: rationale and reliability. Arch Gen Psychiatry 35:773–782, 1978

Starr RH: Pre- and perinatal risk and physical abuse. J Reprod Infant Psychol 6:125–138, 1988

Starr RH, Dietrich KN, Fischhoff J, et al: The contribution of handicapping conditions to child abuse. Topics of Early Childhood Special Education 4:55–69, 1984

Steele BF: Violence within the family, in Child Abuse and Neglect: The Family and the Community. Edited by Helfer RE, Kempe CH. Cambridge, MA, Ballinger, 1976, pp 3–23

Steele BF, Pollack CB: A psychiatric study of parents who abuse infants and small children, in The Battered Child, 2nd Edition. Edited by Helfer RE, Kempe CH. Chicago, IL, University of Chicago Press, 1974, pp 89–133

Stiffman AR: Physical and sexual abuse in run away youths. Child Abuse Negl 13:417–426, 1989

Stockwell T, Murphey D, Hodgson R: The Severity of Alcohol Dependence Questionnaire: its use, reliability and validity. Br J Addict 78:145–155, 1983

Straus MA: Measuring intrafamily conflict and violence: the Conflict Tactics (CT) Scales. Journal of Marriage and the Family 41:75–88, 1979

Straus MA: Stress and physical child abuse. Child Abuse Negl 4:75–88, 1980

Straus MA, Gelles RJ: Societal change and change in family violence from 1975 to 1985 as revealed by two national surveys. Journal of Marriage and the Family 48(3):465–479, 1986

Straus MA, Gelles RJ, Steinmetz SK: Behind Closed Doors: Violence in the American Family. Garden City, NJ, Anchor/Doubleday, 1980

Sullivan PM, Brookhouser PE, Scanlon JM, et al: Patterns of physical and sexual abuse of communicatively handicapped children. Ann Otol Rhinol Laryngol 100(3):188–194, 1991

Surrey J, Swett C, Michaels A, et al: Reported history of physical and sexual abuse and severity of symptomatology in women psychiatric outpatients. Am J Orthopsychiatry 60(3):412–417, 1990

Swett C, Surrey J, Cohen C: Sexual and physical abuse histories and psychiatric symptoms among male psychiatric outpatients. Am J Psychiatry 147(5):632–636, 1990

Taitz LS, King JM: A profile of abuse. Arch Dis Child 63(9):1026–1031, 1988

Tarter RE, Hegedus AM, Winsten NE, et al: Neuropsychological personality and familial characteristics of physically abused delinquents. Journal of the American Academy of Child Psychiatry 23(6):668–674, 1984

Taylor JA: A personality scale of manifest anxiety. Journal of Abnormal and Social Psychology 48:285–290, 1953

Tenenbein M, Reed MH, Black GB: The toddler's fracture revisited. Am J Emergency Med 8(3):208–211, 1990

Tertinger DA, Greene BF, Lutzker JR: Home safety: development and validation of one component of an ecobehavioral treatment program for abused and neglect children. J Appl Behav Anal 17(2):159–174, 1984

Turbett JP, O'Toole R: Teachers' recognition and reporting of child abuse. J Sch Health 53(1):605–609, 1983

Twentyman CT, Plotkin RC: Unrealistic expectations of parents who maltreat their children: an educational deficit that pertains to child development. J Clin Psychol 38(3):497–503, 1982

U.S. Department of Health and Human Services: Executive Summary: Study of National Incidence and Prevalence of Child Abuse and Neglect: 1988. Washington, National Center on Child Abuse and Neglect, 1988

Van Dyke H: Corporal punishment in our schools. Phi Delta Kappa 65:287–292, 1983

Van Stolk M: The battered child in Canada. Toronto, Canada, McClelland & Stewart, 1972

Wahler RG: The insular mother: her problems in parent-child treatment. J Appl Behav Anal 13:207–219, 1980

Wald MS: State intervention on behalf of neglected children: a search for realistic standards. Stanford Law Review 27:985, 1975

Wald MS: State intervention on behalf of "neglected" children: standards for removal of children from their homes, monitoring the status of children in foster care, and termination of parental rights. Stanford Law Review 28:623–707, 1976

Wald MS: State intervention on behalf of endangered children: a proposed legal response. Child Abuse Negl 6:3–45, 1982

Wasserman S, Rosenfeld A: Decision making in child abuse and neglect. Bull Am Acad Psychiatry Law 13(3):259–271, 1985

Watson-Perczel M, Lutzker JR, Greene BF, et al: Assessment and modification of home cleanliness among families adjudicated for child neglect. Behav Modif 12(1):57–81, 1988

Webster-Stratton C: Comparison of abusive and nonabusive families with conduct-disordered children. Am J Orthopsychiatry 55:59–69, 1985

Weissman MM, Paykel ES: The Depressed Woman. Chicago, IL, University of Chicago Press, 1974

Weissman MM, Paykel ES, Klerman GL: The depressed woman as a mother. Social Psychiatry 7:98–108, 1972

Westen D, Ludolph P, Misle B, et al: Physical and sexual abuse in adolescent girls with borderline personality disorder. Am J Orthopsychiatry 60(1):55–66, 1990

Whalen CK, Henker B, Dotemoto S: Teacher response to methylphenidate versus placebo status of hyperactive boys in the classroom. Child Dev 52:1005–1014, 1981

Wheeler DM, Hobbs CJ: Mistakes in diagnosing non-accidental injury: 10 years' experience. BMJ 296:1233–1236, 1988

White RB, Cornely DA: Navajo child abuse and neglect study: a comparison group examination of abuse and neglect of Navajo children. Child Abuse Negl 5(1):9–17, 1981

Whittaker JK: The role of residential institutions, in Special Children, Special Risk: the Maltreatment of Children With Disabilities. Edited by Garbarino J, Brookhouser PE, Authier KJ. New York, Aldine De Gruyter, 1987, pp 83–100

Wichlacz CR, Wechsler JG: American Indian law on child abuse and neglect. Child Abuse Negl 7(3):347–350, 1983

Widom CS: Sampling biases and implications for child abuse research. Am J Orthopsychiatry 58(2):260–270, 1988

Widom CS: Child abuse, neglect, and adult behavior: research design and findings on criminality, violence, and child abuse. Am J Orthopsychiatry 59(3):355–367, 1989a

Widom CS: Does violence beget violence? a critical examination of the literature. Psychol Bull 106(1):3–28, 1989b

Widom CS: The cycle of violence. Science 244:160–166, 1989c

Wilcox DE: Characteristics of seventy-one convicted murderers. Am J Forensic Psychiatry 7:48–52, 1986
Williamson J, Borduin C, Howe B: The ecology of adolescent maltreatment: a multilevel examination of adolescent physical abuse, sexual abuse, and neglect. J Consult Clin Psychol 59 449–457, 1991
Wilson AL: The state of South Dakota's child: 1989. S D J Med 43(1):5–10, 1990
Wilson CA, Gettinger M: Determinants of child-abuse reporting among Wisconsin school psychologists. Professional School Psychology 4(2):91–102, 1989
Wissow LW, Wilson MH: The use of consumer injury registry data to evaluate physical abuse. Child Abuse Negl 12(1)25–31, 1988
Wolfe DA, Edwards B, Manion I, et al: Early intervention for parents at risk of child abuse and neglect: a preliminary investigation. J Consult Clin Psychol 56(1):40–47, 1988
Wolock I: Community characteristics and staff judgments in child abuse and neglect cases. Social Work Research and Abstracts 18(2):9–15, 1982
Wolock I, Horowitz B: Child maltreatment as a social problem: the neglect of neglect. Am J Orthopsychiatry 54(4):530–543, 1984
Wood-Shuman S, Cone JD: Differences in abusive, at risk for abuse, and control mothers' descriptions of normal child behavior. Child Abuse Negl 10(3):397–405, 1986
World Health Organization: ICD-10 Chapter V: Mental and Behavioral Disorders: Diagnostic Criteria for Research. Geneva, Switzerland, World Health Organization, 1990
Wright L: "The sick but slick" syndrome: a personality component of parents of battered children. J Clin Psychol 32:41–45, 1976
Wright LS: High school polydrug users and abusers. Adolescence 20(80):853–861, 1985
Wright LS, Moore R: Correlates of reported drug abuse problems among college undergraduates. Journal of Drug Education 12(1):65–73, 1982
Young L: Wednesday's Children: a Study of Child Neglect and Abuse. New York, McGraw-Hill, 1971
Zaidi LY, Knutson JF, Mehm JB: Transgenerational patterns of abusive parenting: analog and clinical tests. Aggressive Behavior 15:137–152, 1989
Zalba SR: The abused child, II: a typology for classification and treatment. Social Work 12:70–79, 1967
Zanarini MC, Gunderson JG, Marino MF, et al: Childhood experiences of borderline patients. Compr Psychiatry 30(1):18–25, 1989
Zellman GL: Report decision-making patterns among mandated child abuse reports. Child Abuse Negl 14:325–336, 1990
Zigler E: Controlling child abuse in America: an effort doomed to failure? in Critical Perspectives on Child Abuse. Edited by Bourne R, Newberger EH. Lexington, MA, Lexington Books, 1979, pp 171–213
Zoccolillo M, Cloninger CR: Somatization disorder: psychologic symptoms, social disability, and diagnosis. Compr Psychiatry 27(1):65–73, 1986
Zuravin SJ: Unplanned pregnancies, family planning problems, and child maltreatment. Family Relations 36:135–139, 1987
Zuravin SJ: Child abuse, child neglect, and maternal depression: is there a connection? in National Center on Child Abuse and Neglect: Research Symposium on Child Neglect. Washington, DC, U.S. Department of Health and Human Services, 1988a, pp D23–D48
Zuravin SJ: Child maltreatment and teenage first births: a relationship mediated by chronic sociodemographic stress? Am J Orthopsychiatry 58(1):91–103, 1988b

Zuravin SJ: The ecology of child abuse and neglect: review of the literature and presentation of data. Violence and Victims 4(2):101–120, 1989

Zuravin SJ, Watson B, Ehrenschaft M: Anonymous reports of child physical abuse: are they as serious as reports from other sources? Child Abuse Negl 11(4):521–529, 1987

Chapter 40

Incest

Sandra Kaplan, M.D., and
David Pelcovitz, Ph.D.

Statement of the Issues

In this chapter, we assess the evidence for including incest as a parent-child relational diagnosis in DSM-IV. Incest is defined as the sexual abuse of a child under age 18 years by a family member. The National Center on Child Abuse and Neglect (Kempe and Kempe 1984) defines child sexual abuse as contacts or interactions between a child and an adult when the child is being used for the sexual stimulation of that adult or another person. For the purposes of this chapter, the parent-child relational disorder of child sexual abuse as defined is discussed from a family perspective, because the research literature has focused almost exclusively on a family-system approach to incest.

In the last decade, there has been increasing awareness that incest is far more prevalent than had previously been imagined, thereby making it a major public health problem. In only a few decades, we have gone from estimates of prevalence that were as low a one per million in the United States to estimates as high as the 21% involving physical contact reported by Wyatt and Peters (1986). Parallel with this knowledge has come increasing recognition that the emotional sequelae of incest are pervasive and often permanent. Despite this, there are no diagnostic categories in DSM-III-R (American Psychiatric Association 1987) that specifically address incest. Even more than is the case with physical child abuse and neglect, the clinical literature on incest has often portrayed intrafamilial sexual abuse as stemming primarily from major pathology in the family. The purpose of this review is to address the question of whether a category of incest should be included under parent-child relational diagnoses. The following areas are reviewed.

1. Family studies: Controlled studies that directly assess functioning in incestuous families are reviewed with an emphasis on examining the empirical support that exists for assertions in the clinical literature that incest is generally characterized by a specific type of family structure.

2. The child or adolescent victim: Studies of child sexual abuse victims during childhood and adolescence. As the area where most of the empirical research has been done, this section confines itself to comparative studies of the emotional and behavioral difficulties of incest victims. Also included are controlled studies of the emotional, cognitive, behavioral, and social functioning of adult survivors of incest.
3. The nonoffending parent: Studies that evaluate how "collusive" the nonoffending parent is in incestuous families. Empirical studies of the role of the mother (most often the nonabusive parent) in incestuous families are contrasted with the clinical literature that often describes the nonabusive family member as the "cornerstone" of the pathological family process in intrafamilial sexual abuse.
4. The offending parent: Studies that evaluate the psychological, sexual, and interpersonal functioning of the perpetrator of incest. In this section, we focus on whether the victimization of the child in incestuous families reflects a pattern that is reactive to family pathology or exists outside of the family system as well.
5. Methodological criticisms of studies of incestuous families and the implications of these difficulties for including incest as a parent-child relational diagnosis are considered.

Significance of the Issues

Prevalence of Child and Adolescent Sexual Abuse

As mentioned earlier, in the past two decades, it has become increasingly recognized that the incidence of incest is far greater than had been previously recognized. The following is a review of the major American studies of the prevalence of child and adolescent sexual abuse.

Studies of Adults Who Were Sexually Abused as Children

The only national study of the prevalence among adults of previous child and adolescent sexual abuse experiences has been the *Los Angeles Times* Poll study of 2,626 American men and women, ages 18 years or over, recruited by the *Los Angeles Times* Survey Research organization from residential telephone numbers throughout the United States using a random digit dialing procedure (Finkelhor et al. 1990). Respondents who were included encompassed those with both intrafamilial or extrafamilial experiences of sexual abuse. The survey found that 27% of the women and 16% of the men had sexual abuse experiences prior to age 18. The median age of abuse for boys was 9.9 years; for girls the median age was 9.6 years. Boys were more likely to have been abused by strangers than were girls (40% versus 21%); girls were more likely than boys to have been abused by family members (29% versus 11%). Of the female victims, 6% had been abused by a father or stepfather; 83% of the perpetrators of the sexual abuse of boys and 98% of the perpetrators of the sexual abuse of girls were males. Most perpetrators were at least 10 years older than their victims. As part of their child sexual abuse, 62% of male victims and 49% of female victims had experienced actual or attempted intercourse. Force was involved in 15% of the abuse of boys and 19% of the abuse of girls. The sexual abuse lasted longer than a year for 8% of the boys and 11% of the girls; 42% of males and 33% of females had never disclosed their child sexual abuse to anyone.

Risk factors for child sexual abuse in this study were unhappy family life during childhood, the absence of one biological parent in the home during childhood, Pacific regional residence as an adult, English or Scandinavian ancestry for males, females reporting inadequate sexual education, and age of female respondent of 40–49 years.

Wyatt and Peters (1986) studied the prevalence of child and adolescent sexual abuse in a multistage stratified probability sample of 126 African American and 122 white women in Los Angeles County, California. Sexual abuse in this study referred to contact of a sexual nature involving a female under age 18 years by a perpetrator of any age, but at least 5 years older than the female victim. Coercive sexual experiences (those not agreed to by the victim) were considered sexual abuse in those age 13 and older, even if there was not a 5-year age difference between perpetrator and victim. All sexual experiences reported as having occurred at age 12 or younger, even if reported as having involved consent, were considered as sexually abusive. Interviews were conducted in person. One-third of the women reported child sexual abuse with an adult partner; 9% reported child sexual abuse with an adolescent partner; and 26% reported sexual abuse by adult partners during adolescence. Wyatt and Peters reported intrafamilial abuse (incest) involving physical contact in 17% of women respondents up to age 13 and in 21% of women respondents up to age 17 and extrafamilial contact abuse in 23% up to age 13 and in 29% up to age 17. When contact and noncontact intrafamilial and extrafamilial sexual abuse were combined, 47% of women in this study reported sexual abuse up to age 13, and 53% up to age 17. Physical coercion was involved in the fondling of 38% of black victims and in 29% of white victims. Of the women who reported intercourse, coercion was involved for 65% of white women and 42% of black women. In more than one-third of sexual abuse incidents, both white and African American women reported that they had told no one of the abuse. African American women reported that they were sexually abused by extended family members more often than white women, whereas white women were more likely than black women to have told either peers or authority figures. White and African American women reported that 70% of the undisclosed incidents had involved contact abuse.

Russell (1988) conducted a probability study of 930 women residents of San Francisco, California. Sexual abuse was defined in this study as any exploitive sexual contact or attempt at contact between the respondent and a relative (incest) prior to the victim's 18th birthday. Of the respondents, 17% of white women and 16% of African American women reported incest (intrafamilial abuse). In this study, 56% of the incestuous sexual abuse experiences reported by African Americans and 18% of those reported by whites involved intercourse or attempted intercourse. That the perpetrators of their incestuous experiences were fathers or stepfathers was reported by 28% of the African American women and 24% of the white women. The mean age at onset of incest was 10.7 years for white women and 12.6 years for African American women.

The Los Angeles Epidemiological Catchment Area Study (Stein et al. 1988) involved in-person interviews of a randomly generated sample of 3,132 adults who resided in two Los Angeles mental health catchment areas. Child sexual abuse was defined in this study as coercive sexual contact occurring before age 16. Age of perpetrators at the time of sexual abuse was not obtained. Child sexual abuse prior to age 16 was reported by 82 respondents, which represented a prevalence rate of 5.3%. Non-Hispanic whites reported 8.7%, Hispanics 3.0%, men 3.8%, and women 6.8%. This study did not include sexual abuse occurring between ages 16 and 18.

A more recent study using a probability sample of 2,004 adult women living in Charleston County, South Carolina, was done by Saunders et al. (1992). Child sexual abuse (sexual assault) was defined in this study as sexual experiences that were not wanted by the victim, that involved the use of threat or of force, and that occurred prior to age 18. Child sexual abuse was categorized as rape if penetration of the vagina, mouth, or anus by the perpetrator's genitalia or finger or by an object had occurred during the respondent's childhood. Molestation was considered contact without penetration, and noncontact abuse was defined as not involving any physical contact. In this study, 33.5% reported sexual assault experiences; 24.6% reported physical contact; 15.6% had been molested; and 10% had been penetrated. Fathers or stepfathers perpetrated 7.2% of the abuse.

Prevalence of Child Sexual Abuse Studied During Childhood

In contrast to surveys based on interviews of adult survivors of child sexual abuse, there have been far fewer systematic studies of the prevalence of child sexual abuse based on samples of children or adolescents. The most comprehensive study in the United States was the 1988 federally funded National Incidence and Prevalence of Child Abuse and Neglect (U.S. Department of Health and Human Services 1988). Child Protective Services records were sampled in 29 counties across the country.

Results indicated that 2.5 per 1,000 children under age 18 years were reported to have been sexually abused, which represented 155,900 cases.

The incidence of incest described above is alarmingly high. The significance of considering a relational disorder diagnosis for incest is that it would take into account the family dynamics that, from a standpoint of face validity, are a major contributor to the process of a child being victimized by a parent. It is noteworthy that virtually every major book addressing the treatment needs of incest victims includes family treatment as a major component (e.g., Sgroi 1982; Trepper and Barrett 1989). The purpose of this review is to determine if the empirical database supports inclusion of such a diagnosis.

Method

We conducted a computer-assisted search on PsychLit and Medline covering the period 1970–1991 and using all descriptors relevant to relational aspects of intrafamilial sexual abuse. References were also obtained from the National Clearinghouse for Child Abuse and Neglect. We reviewed the comprehensive bibliography of sexual abuse prepared by the Family Violence Bulletin and searched their computer database for relevant citations. The following family violence journals were also systematically reviewed: *Victimology, Journal of Interpersonal Violence, Journal of Family Violence,* and *The International Journal of Child Abuse and Neglect.* We included only articles that were peer reviewed and used comparison groups. Although dissertations were not reviewed, we did include books that were authored by reputable researchers in the field.

Results

Family Studies

Clinical reports of incestuous families describe systems characterized by a high level of enmeshment (James and Nasjleti 1983), rigidity (Alexander and Lupfer 1987), traditional family values and sexual stereotyping (Herman and Hirschman 1981), a tendency for at least one child to assume a parent's role (Blick and Porter 1982), and social isolation (Williams and Finkelhor 1990). The family dynamic most frequently described is that of a poor marital relationship in which the mother is absent or emotionally unavailable and the father is rigid and controlling. The vacuum left by the mother's unavailability is filled by the daughter, who assumes her mother's role both emotionally and sexually (Lustig et al. 1966). The results from most studies in the abuse literature are difficult to generalize because they fail to include controls or use inappropriate control groups and because they fail to differentiate psychopathology after disclosure from psychopathology before disclosure.

A number of controlled studies have been published that empirically address the characteristics of incestuous families (Table 40–1). These studies include two that use direct observations, five that rely on established self-administered questionnaires, and three that rely on interviews or questionnaires designed by their authors. Six of the studies directly investigate incestuous families, and four rely on retrospective data provided by adult survivors of childhood incest. A clear consensus regarding the incestuous family does not emerge from these studies.

In the first study of its kind, Madonna et al. (1991) compared the families of 30 referred incest victims with the families of 30 children attending an outpatient psychiatry clinic. Independent raters found that the incestuous families were significantly more likely to have diffuse boundaries, dysfunctional parental coalitions, rigid belief systems, and emotional unavailability. Although the previous clinical literature had led to a prediction that there would be an unbalanced power structure, this hypothesis was not confirmed. This important study lends some empirical support to clinical observations that incestuous families are characterized by dysfunctional coalitions, rigidity, and a failure of parental empathy. Unfortunately, the failure to use raters who were blind to the status of the subjects makes the objectivity of the results suspect.

The only other observational study of incest victims investigated interactional communication patterns in seven incestuous families, seven families with oppositional children, and seven control families (Levang 1989). Findings did not directly support much of the clinical speculation regarding the structure of incestuous families: role-reversals were not seen more often in mothers of incest victims than in the others; signs of belittling, attacking, or ignoring were not more prevalent in the incestuous families, nor were incestuous fathers seen as more controlling. The author did comment, however, that incest victims communicated less with their mothers. Major flaws in this study include its small number of subjects and the use of a rating system that does not seem to lend itself readily to direct comparisons with the family constructs described in the incest literature.

The remaining studies relied on questionnaires and clinical interviews administered to members of incestuous families or to survivors of childhood sexual abuse. Although there is consensus on some of the family variables associated with incest, findings regarding other family characteristics are contradictory.

Incestuous families are described as less cohesive in one study that compares victims of incest with victims of extrafamilial abuse (Alexander and Lupfer 1987) and another that compares college-age incest survivors with control subjects whose

Table 40–1. Summary of family interaction studies

Alexander and Lupfer 1987
Subjects: Recruited from a survey of 586 female undergraduates: 40 incest survivors, 53 sexually abused by a member of the extended family, 56 victims of extrafamilial sexual abuse.
Measures: FACES II, traditional family ideology scale, self-concept scale.
Results: Incest victims saw family as more traditional in parent-child or mother-father relationships. All victims saw family as less cohesive and adaptable. Uniformly low family self-concept in three victim groups.

Cole and Woolger 1989
Subjects: 21 survivors of incest, 19 of extrafamilial child abuse recruited through media.
Measures: Children's report of parental behavior inventory; parental attitudes research instrument.
Results: Incestuous fathers were less accepting, more negatively controlling, stricter disciplinarians. Incest mothers were less involved, more negatively controlling. Sex abuse survivors as mothers were more indulgent, less accepting.

Harter et al. 1988
Subjects: 29 undergraduate child sexual abuse survivors; 59 nonabused undergraduates.
Measure: FACES II, family perception grid.
Results: Decreased cohesion and adaptability in family of origin. Increased social isolation. Paternal sexual abuse significantly contributed to social maladjustment even when nonabuse family variables were controlled for.

Herman and Hirschman 1981
Subjects: 40 incestuous child sexual abuse survivors in treatment versus 20 women in treatment whose fathers were seductive but not incestuous.
Measure: Semistructured clinical interview.
Results: Incest survivors were more likely to be ill, disabled, or battered. Fathers were described as violent. Daughters were described as filling in impaired mother's vacuum by assuming maternal role (e.g., housework and child care).

Levang 1989
Subjects: 7 incest referred for treatment; 7 oppositional/conduct disorder in treatment; 7 nonclinical.
Measures: Structural analysis of social behavior, analyzing interactional communication patterns.
Results: Incest families talked in more parent-like way to fathers than nonclinicals. More role reversal was not seen in incest families, nor were there greater signs of attacking or ignoring. Incest fathers were not more controlling. Significantly lower communication rates between incest mothers and daughters.

(continued)

Table 40–1. Summary of family interaction studies *(continued)*

Madonna et al. 1991
Subjects: 30 referred for treatment from incest families versus 30 nonabused child psychiatry clinic outpatients.
Measures: Direct observations on Beavers-Timberlawn.
Results: Incestuous families were more likely to have weak, dysfunctional coalitions, emotional unavailability, less autonomy, and diffuse boundaries. Dominance-submission power structure not found.

Milner and Robertson 1990
Subjects: 15 intrafamilial sex abusers, 30 physical child abusers, and 30 child neglecters, all subjects indicated by Department of Social Services and/or referred for treatment.
Measures: Child Abuse Potential Inventory.
Results: Compared with neglect and physical abuse groups, sexual child abusers report more positive views of their children, fewer problems with children, and fewer family problems.

Paveza 1988
Subjects: 34 father-daughter incest families referred for treatment, versus 68 random community controls.
Measures: Self-administered questionnaire.
Results: Risk factors for incest include poor marital satisfaction (7 times greater risk), violence between abuser and spouse (6 times greater risk), distant mother-daughter relationship (11 times greater risk), low income (6 times greater risk than middle income and 40 times greater risk than high income).

Sagatun and Prince 1988
Subjects: 56 male incest offenders referred for therapy; 36 spouses; 43 victims.
Measures: Questionnaire regarding perception of family relations.
Results: Fathers rate father-daughter relationship as good before therapy. Victims rate father-daughter relationship as bad before therapy. Mother-daughter relationship rated as neutral by all the family. Daughter continues to rate family relations as bad after therapy.

White et al. 1988
Subjects: 17 victims of sexual abuse (mixed incestuous and otherwise) referred for treatment; 18 victims of neglect referred for treatment; 23 nonreferred recruited from hospital personnel.
Measures: Minnesota Child Development Inventory revised for sexual abuse.
Results: Sexually abused boys had poorer relationships with their fathers. Sexually abused girls and neglected girls had poorer relationships with their fathers. Relationship with mother described as good by 86% of sexually abused boys and 90% of abused girls.

fathers were seductive but not incestuous (Harter et al. 1988). Both studies used the FACES II scale (Olson et al. 1983). Reports of lower levels of cohesiveness are not consistent with the clinical literature's description of enmeshed incestuous families. However, recent research suggests that a high level of "cohesiveness" in

FACES III, the family measure used in these studies, does not necessarily signify enmeshment, but may be associated with closeness that is more typical of "healthy" families (Perosa and Perosa 1990).

High levels of rigidity were also reported in the two studies using FACES II (Alexander and Lupfer 1987; Harter et al. 1988). Incest survivors described their families as more "traditional" than did victims of extrafamilial sexual abuse (Alexander and Lupfer 1987). Incestuous families have also been found to use discipline in a more rigid manner than families of victims of extrafamilial sexual abuse (Cole and Woolger 1989). Studies that find a high level of social isolation in incestuous families (e.g., Harter et al. 1988) attribute this inflexibility to a lack of exposure to the child-rearing behaviors of neighbors and friends.

Data on the quality of mother-child relationships in incestuous families are contradictory. Although White et al. (1988) found that 86% of sexually abused boys and 90% of sexually abused girls describe a good mother-child relationship, other researchers have characterized the mother-child dyads they studied as "distant" (Levang 1989; Paveza 1988), impaired (Herman and Hirschman 1981), or "neutral" (Cole and Woolger 1989; Sagatun and Prince 1988).

These studies are more consistent on the nature of the incestuous father-daughter relationship. Victims of incest consistently describe poorer relationships with their fathers on questionnaires (Sagatun and Prince 1988) than do victims of child neglect (White et al. 1988) or victims of extrafamilial abuse (Coles and Woolger 1989). In contrast, incestuous fathers rate the father-daughter relationship as "good" (Sagatun and Prince 1988) and their families as free of parenting and family problems. In light of the clinical descriptions of incest perpetrators as being prone to misrepresent their views on emotionally laden issues (Milner and Robertson 1990; Williams and Finkelhor 1990), it is not surprising that they deny the family difficulties described by the victims.

Clinical descriptions of dysfunctional marriages in incestuous families are supported by Paveza (1988), who found that poor marital satisfaction placed families at seven times greater risk for incest. High levels of spouse abuse have also been reported (Herman and Hirschman 1981). H. Parker and Parker (1986), however, found no significant differences in marital quality in incestuous families compared with other clinical families.

In summary, there have been virtually no empirical investigations of family dynamics in incest until relatively recently. Although this recent literature provides some limited support for the presence of rigidity, poor parent-child relationships, and dysfunctional marriages, there is no evidence that the majority of incestuous families have these characteristics. Well-designed studies have also failed to document whether the difficulties attributed to incestuous families are unique to this population or are also characteristic of other pathological families.

Victims

The literature has reported that the victims of childhood incest experience a wide range of behavioral and emotional difficulties. The majority of studies of the mental health problems associated with child or adolescent sexual abuse deal with victims of incest. The findings of these studies are presented in Tables 40–2 through Table 40–8, grouped according to the age of the victim at the time of the study. These tables present definitional issues, study samples, identities of perpetrators (if mentioned), measures, and results.

Studies of incest victims and survivors under 12 years old.   We reviewed 21 comparative studies of the mental health of sexually abused children under 12 years old (Table 40–2 and Table 40–3). The samples were all recruited from their treatment sites. The type of sexual abuse varied in these studies: 11 studies involved only contact child sexual abuse; 9 involved either contact or noncontact child sexual abuse; 3 studies involved only incest; and 17 involved either incest or extrafamilial sexual abuse. In 15 studies, subjects had been legally documented as child sexual abuse victims; 5 studies did not report legal or medical documentation of abuse. None of the studies reported analyses of risk factors for child mental health problems, nor did any report the dates of the onset, cessation, or disclosure of the abuse or of legal events or the onset of mental health problems.

The symptoms and disorders reported in these studies, in descending order of frequency, were depressive symptoms and/or depressive diagnoses (10 studies), aggressive behavior (9 studies), anxiety (9 studies), sexualized behavior problems (8 studies), cognitive and/or social functional impairment (5 studies), low self-esteem (5 studies), somatization (3 studies), posttraumatic stress disorder (PTSD) symptomatology (1 study), and dissociation (1 study).

The severity of the symptomatology reported in these studies was associated with a lack of family and adult support, the frequency and types of sexual abuse, family dysfunction, use of physical restraint or bribery during abuse, denial of abuse by the perpetrator, and the perpetrator being a close relative (Conte and Schuerman 1987). Increased family conflict, increased duration of abuse, and lack of family support were associated with the development of sexualized problems. Severity of sexual abuse and family conflict were associated with the development of externalized behaviors. Family conflict and the time that had elapsed since the abuse (Friedrich et al. 1987), the duration of abuse, the age of the child when abused, and the severity of abuse (Gomez-Schwartz et al. 1985) were also associated with increased symptomatology in the victim.

Studies of adolescent victims and survivors.   We reviewed 12 comparative studies of the mental health of sexually abused adolescents 12–18 years old (Table 40–4,

Table 40–2. Studies of children under age 12 years: behavioral and emotional/somatic symptoms

August and Forman 1989
Type of abuse: Unspecified; for medical evaluation of abuse.
Subjects: 32 females, ages 5–8, mean age 6 years.
Victims: 16 females referred for evaluation and treatment.
Control subjects: 16 females from public school.
Perpetrators: Unspecified.
Measure: Play with anatomically detailed dolls.
Results: Sexually abused < nonabused in free play. With interviewer present, sexually abused > nonabused in avoidance. With interviewer absent, sexually abused > nonabused in private parts reference and aggression.

Conte and Schuerman 1987
Type of abuse: All contact, documented.
Victims: 296 female, 73 male sex abuse victims in treatment. For most, time lapsed < 6 months. Mean age 8.8 years.
Control subjects: 181 nonabused females, 137 nonabused males. Mean age 8.1 years.
Perpetrators: Unrelated acquaintances, parents, other relatives, strangers.
Measures: Symptom impact checklist; clinical assessment; child behavioral profile.
Results: Sexually abused > control subjects in poor self-esteem, depression, fear, withdrawal, concentration problems, aggression, somatic problems, behavioral regression, personality problems. Factors associated with increased impact of abuse: lack of family support, family dysfunction, use of physical restraint or bribery, denial of abuse by perpetrator, relation to perpetrator otherwise close or positive.

Fagot et al. 1989
Type of abuse: Unspecified, legally documented.
Victims: 11 sexually abused females, 4 sexually abused males; median age 3.5 years; source: private agency.
Control subjects: 8 physically abused females, 3 physically abused males; median age 3 years 7 months; source: state agency. 5 nonabused females, 5 nonabused males; median age 3 years, 8 months; source: community.
Perpetrators: Unspecified.
Measures: Observation of free play.
Results: Sexually abused > control subjects in passivity, female-type activity. Sexually abused < control subjects in interaction.

Friedrich and Einbender 1989
Type of abuse: All contact, legally documented.
Victims: 46 females, time elapsed ≤ 4 years, ages 6–14 years, mean age 10.3 years. Source: treatment or state agency.
Control subjects: 46 nonabused females. Source: community.
Perpetrators: Unspecified.
Measures: Wechsler Intelligence Scale for Children—Revised, Wide Range Achievement Test—Revised, Rorschach, Thematic Apperception Test, CBCL, Piers-Harris.
Results: Sexually abused > nonabused in sexual preoccupation, poor cognitive and social functioning, and internalizing and externalizing behavior problems.

(continued)

Table 40–2. Studies of children under age 12 years: behavioral and emotional/somatic symptoms *(continued)*

Friedrich et al. 1987
Type of abuse: Fondling, penetration, some noncontact. Legally documented.
Victims: 58 sexually abused females and 35 sexually abused males in treatment. Mean time lapsed 11.2 months. Mean age 7.2 years.
Control subjects: 41 nonabused female and 23 nonabused male psychiatric outpatients; mean age 7.4 years. 47 nonabused females and 31 nonabused males undergoing no treatment; mean age 7.1 years.
Perpetrators: Father or father figure, other relative, nonrelative.
Measures: Revised child behavioral profile, clinical assessment of family.
Results: Sexually abused > all control subjects in sexual problems. Sexually abused and psychiatric control subjects > nonabused in anxiety, depression, hyperactivity, delinquent aggression, and total behavioral problems. Increased duration of abuse and decreased family support associated with increased external problems. Conflict, less cohesion, and increased time elapsed associated with internal problems.

Friedrich et al. 1988
Type of abuse: Penetration, fondling. Legally/medically documented.
Victims: 31 sexually abused males, ages 3–8, mean age 5.6 years, mean time elapsed 6.34 months. Source: treatment.
Control subjects: 32 nonsexually abused males with conduct or oppositional disorder, ages 4–8, mean age 5.7 years.
Perpetrators: Father or father figure, other male relative, mother, nonrelative.
Measures: CBCL.
Results: Sexually abused > nonabused psychiatric control subjects in sex problems and social competence. Sexually abused < nonabused psychiatric control subjects in external behavior problems and aggression.

Gale et al. 1988
Type of abuse: Fondling, penetration. Legally documented.
Victims: 28 sexually abused females, 9 sexually abused males, all younger than 7 years old. Source: treatment.
Control subjects: 18 physically abused females and 17 physically abused males; 54 nonabused females and 76 nonabused males with behavior problems; all younger than 7 years old. Source: treatment.
Perpetrators: 50% incest.
Measures: Symptom Checklist; chart review.
Results: Sexually abused > all control subjects in sex problems. Sexually abused and physically abused > nonabused in depression, anxiety, and withdrawal.

(continued)

Table 40–2. Studies of children under age 12 years: behavioral and emotional/somatic symptoms *(continued)*

Gomez-Schwartz et al. 1985
Type of abuse: Penetration, fondling, some noncontact. 1–5 years duration. Medically documented.
Victims: 87 sexually abused females and 25 sexually abused males, ages 4–18 years. Time elapsed less than 6 months for most. Source: treatment.
Control subjects: Normative sample of published Louisville Checklist scores.
Perpetrators: 67% incest.
Measures: Louisville Behavior Checklist.
Results: Sexually abused ages 4–6 > normative sample in cognitive disability, social immaturity, and neurotic behavior. Sexually abused ages 7–13 > normative sample on all Louisville scales except somatic complaints and prosocial deficit. Most disturbance in internal/external patterns, aggression, and fear of sex. Sexually abused ages 14–18 significantly > in neuroticism and dependent/inhibited. Sexually abused ages 7–13 > ages 4–6 and 14–18 in overall pathology.

Jampole and Weber 1987
Type of abuse: Unspecified, legally documented.
Victims: 8 sexually abused females, 2 sexually abused males, in state custody.
Control subjects: 8 females and 2 males with unspecified nonsexual abuse (some physically abused, some neglected). In state custody or from community.
Perpetrators: Unspecified.
Measures: Observed play with anatomically detailed dolls.
Results: Sexually abused > control subjects in demonstrated sexual behavior with dolls.

Kolko et al. 1988
Type of abuse: Contact and noncontact.
Victims: 5 females and 2 males who were sexually abused; 10 females and 12 males who were sexually and physically abused. Ages 5–14, mean 9.9 years. All psychiatric inpatients, mostly with conduct or adjustment disorder.
Control subjects: 5 females and 25 males who were physically abused; 8 females and 36 males who were not abused. Ages 5–14, mean 9.9 years. All psychiatric inpatients, mostly with conduct or adjustment disorder.
Perpetrators: Nonrelatives and parents.
Measures: Sexual Abuse Symptom Checklist; chart review.
Results: Sexually abused > physically abused and nonabused in sexual problems, fear, anxiety, depression, and withdrawal.

(continued)

Table 40–2. Studies of children under age 12 years: behavioral and emotional/somatic symptoms *(continued)*

Lipovsky et al. 1989
Type of abuse: Penetration and fondling. Legally documented.
Victims: 81 females and 7 males who were sexually abused. Mean age 11.2 years. Time elapsed < 2 months for most.
Control subjects: 44 female and 57 male nonabused siblings of victims, mean age 9.5 years.
Perpetrators: Fathers or father figures.
Measures: CBCL Parent Form; Beck Children's Depression Inventory; index of self-esteem.
Results: Sexually abused > nonabused siblings in both parent reported behavior problems and self-reported depression. Both sexually abused and nonabused siblings had very low self-esteem.

Mannarino et al. 1989
Type of abuse: All contact, legally documented.
Subjects: Ages 6–12, mean age 9.38 years.
Victims: 94 sexually abused females. Time elapsed ≤ 6 months. Source: treatment.
Control subjects: 89 nonabused female psychiatric outpatients; 75 females who were not abused and not undergoing treatment.
Perpetrators: father or father figure, known nonrelative, or stranger.
Measures: CBCL; Piers-Harris.
Results: Sexually abused > nonabused and psychiatric control subjects in state anxiety and sexual problems. Sexually abused and psychiatric control subjects > nonabused in poor social competence, internalizing, externalizing, and total behavior problem scales.

Miller-Perrin et al. 1990
Type of abuse: Fondling, penetration, some noncontact. Legally documented. Frequency 3 times or more for most.
Subjects: 32 females and 18 males, ages 5–12, mean age 7.96 years.
Victims: 16 sexually abused females and 9 sexually abused males. Source: treatment program.
Control subjects: 16 females, 9 males, no sex abuse.
Perpetrators: Father, another relative or nonrelative.
Measures: Questionnaire on 3 safety vignettes, 1 involved sex (children's perception questionnaire).
Results: Both sexually abused and nonabused were able to define incident in story as sex abuse and describe perpetrator in psychiatric terms. Subjects recommended that perpetrators be rehabilitated, attributed victim compliance to fear, and wanted victim as a friend.

(continued)

Table 40–2. Studies of children under age 12 years: behavioral and emotional/somatic symptoms *(continued)*

Rimsza et al. 1988
Type of abuse: Penetration or fondling, all legally or medically documented, 6 months to 2 years duration.
Subjects: 144 females ages 2–17, mean age 10 years.
Victims: 72 females in treatment. Mean time elapsed 2 years.
Control subjects: 72 nonabused females in medical treatment.
Perpetrators: Fathers or father figures, known relatives, other relatives, strangers.
Measures: Chart review, interview with patient.
Results: Sexually abused > nonabused in muscle tension, gastrointestinal and genitourinary symptoms, emotional problems, running away and other behavioral problems. Those abused 7–24 months showed increased genitourinary symptoms; those abused more than 24 months showed increased gastrointestinal symptoms.

Shapiro et al. 1990
Type of abuse: Penetration, fondling. Legally documented. Mean duration 5 months. Frequency > biweekly for most.
Victims: 53 females in treatment, ages 5–16, mean age 8.9 years, time elapsed < 6 months.
Control subjects: 32 nonabused female medical patients.
Perpetrators: Mostly adult male relatives and known nonrelatives.
Measures: CBCL; Rorschach.
Results: CBCL: sexually abused > control subjects in internalization. Rorschach: sexually abused > control subjects in constrained affect, damaged self, and depression.

Stovall and Craig 1990
Type of abuse: Penetration, fondling. Legally documented.
Victims: 20 sexually abused females, all subjects ages 7–12. Time elapsed 1–6 months for most. Source: social services.
Control subjects: 20 physically abused females. Source: hospital or social services. 20 nonabused females in psychotherapy for behavioral problems.
Perpetrators: Father or father figure.
Measures: Thematic Apperception Test; Piers-Harris.
Results: Sexually and physically abused > nonabused in splitting negative perceptions from consciousness.

Tong et al. 1987
Type of abuse: Unspecified, medically documented.
Victims: 37 sexually abused females, 12 sexually abused males. Mean time elapsed 2.6 years. Source: treatment.
Control subjects: 37 females and 12 males. Source: community.
Perpetrators: Relatives, known nonrelatives, strangers.
Measures: Interview with Piers-Harris; CBCL: parent, teacher, and youth.
Results: Sexually abused females > nonabused females in poor self-esteem, parent- and teacher-reported behavior problems (externalizing and internalizing) and self-reported internalizing problems. Sexually abused males > nonabused males in parent-, teacher-, and self-reported problems (mostly internalizing). Sexually abused males and females showed increased sexual awareness and social withdrawal.

(continued)

Table 40–2. Studies of children under age 12 years: behavioral and emotional/somatic symptoms *(continued)*

White et al. 1988
Type of abuse: Unspecified.
Victims: 10 sexually abused females and 7 sexually abused males. Source: treatment.
Control subjects: 6 neglected females and 12 neglected males. Source: treatment. 16 nonabused females and 7 nonabused males. Source: community. Both victims and control subjects ages 2–6.8 years.
Perpetrators: Unspecified.
Measures: Minnesota Child Development Inventory.
Results: Sexually abused males > nonabused and neglected in sexual problems, poor relationship with fathers, somatic and safety problems, pseudosophistication, friendliness to adult strangers, and low self-esteem. Sexually abused females > neglected females in friendliness to adult strangers.

Note. CBCL = Child Behavior Checklist.

Table 40–5, Table 40–6). Of these studies, 10 consisted of samples recruited from treatment sites, 1 study consisted of a sample recruited from a child welfare agency and comprised adolescents in and out of foster placement, and another study consisted of a sample recruited from a shelter for runaway youth.

Types of sexual abuse varied in the adolescent studies. Of the 12 studies, 7 involved contact child sexual abuse, whereas 4 involved both contact and noncontact child sexual abuse; 4 studies involved only incest; 6 involved incest or extrafamilial sexual abuse, and 2 study reports did not mention the type of sexual abuse. Three cases were legally documented by state social services, whereas in 9 cases no medical or legal documentation of sexual abuse was mentioned. Seven studies included both male and female victims, whereas 5 included only female victims. None of the studies reported analyses of the temporal relationships between onset, disclosure, and cessation of sexual abuse and the onset of symptomatology.

Symptoms and disorders reported by these studies, in descending order of frequency, were sexualized behavior and/or gender identity disturbance (8 studies), aggressive behavior (7 studies), substance abuse (6 studies), suicidal behavior (3 studies), depression (3 studies), low self-esteem (3 studies), and impairment in social functioning (2 studies).

Studies of adults reporting sexual abuse during childhood. We reviewed 31 studies of the mental health problems of adults who reported having been sexually abused as children when they were younger than age 18 years. Table 40–7 and Table

Table 40–3. Child studies based on psychiatric diagnosis

Adams-Tucker 1982
Type of abuse: All contact, medically or legally documented.
Victims: 22 sexually abused females and 6 sexually abused males in treatment, ages 2½–15½, mean age approximately 10 years.
Control subjects: None.
Perpetrators: Father or father figure, other relative, some peers.
Measures: Louisville Behavior Checklist, clinical evaluation.
Results: Most diagnoses: depressive, anxiety, adjustment, and behavioral disorders. Factors associated with more severe diagnosis and behavior problems: sexual abuse by father, penetration, onset of abuse by age 6–7, and lack of support by a significant adult.

Deblinger et al. 1989
Type of abuse: All contact, medically documented.
Subjects: 41 female and 46 male psychiatric inpatients, ages 3–13, mean age 8.8 years.
Victims: 29 sexually abused (20 also physically abused).
Control subjects: 29 physically abused only, 29 nonabused.
Perpetrators: Nonrelatives, relatives, parents.
Measures: Symptom checklist based on DSM-III-R posttraumatic stress disorder criteria.
Results: Sexually abused > physically abused and nonabused in meeting posttraumatic stress disorder criteria. Reexperiencing: sexually abused > physically abused and nonabused. Avoidance/dissociative: sexually abused and physically abused > nonabused. Hyperarousal: sexually abused and nonabused > physically abused.

Livingston 1987
Type of abuse: Unspecified, some legally documented.
Subjects: Psychiatric inpatients, ages 6–12.
Victims: 13 sexually abused.
Control subjects: 15 physically abused, 72 nonabused.
Perpetrators: Parent, other relative, nonrelative.
Measures: Diagnostic Interview for Children and Adolescents, child version.
Results: Sexually abused > physically abused and nonabused in major depressive disorder, anxiety disorders, somatic complaints, and psychosis. Sexually abused > control subjects in conduct disorder. Sexually abused and physically abused > nonabused in oppositional disorder.

40–8 summarize 27 of these studies. Eighteen consisted of samples recruited from mental health or substance abuse treatment sites; 12 consisted of adults recruited from the community; and 1 consisted of women recruited from a gynecological treatment program.

Types of sexual abuse varied. Of the 31 adult comparative studies reviewed, 24 consisted of victims of contact sexual abuse, whereas 7 consisted of victims of both contact and noncontact sexual abuse; 28 studies involved incest alone, whereas 3 studies were of victims of either incest or extrafamilial sexual abuse. No cases

Table 40–4. Adolescent studies: behavioral and emotional symptoms

Aiosa-Karpas et al. 1991
Type of abuse: Penetration and fondling, legally documented.
Victims: 31 females, ages 12–19. Source: residential and outpatient treatment.
Control subjects: 31 nonabused female psychiatric inpatients; 31 nonabused females from community; ages 12–19.
Perpetrators: Father, father figure, other male relative.
Measures: Gender Role Assessment Schedule, Deprivation Enhancement of Fantasy Patterns, Gender Identity Conflict Scale, Personality Assessment Questionnaire self-scale.
Results: Sexually abused > control groups in gender identity conflict (especially distorted body perceptions) and male identity in early childhood play.

Hart et al. 1989
Type of abuse: Nature of sex abuse not specified.
Subjects: 51 psychiatric inpatients, mostly for conduct disorders, ages 14–17, mean age 16 years.
Victims: 10 females and 4 males both physically and sexually abused, mean age at onset 8.7 years, mean duration 3.6 years. 2 females and 1 male sexually abused only, mean onset 11.3 years, mean duration 1.3 years.
Control subjects: 1 female and 10 males physically abused, 3 females and 20 males not abused.
Perpetrators: Fathers, stepfathers, other relatives, 2 extrafamilial, 2 female perpetrators.
Measures: Questionnaire, revised behavior problem checklist.
Results: Victims of concurrent physical and sexual abuse > sexual or physical abuse alone and no abuse in substance use, self-reported emotional symptoms, and interpersonal problems. Sexual abuse alone > other three groups in socialized aggression.

McCormack et al. 1986
Type of abuse: Contact and noncontact.
Victims: 40 females, 34 males, sexually abused, ages 15–20. Source: runaway youth shelter.
Control subjects: 15 females, 55 males, not sexually abused, ages 15–20. Source: runaway youth shelter.
Perpetrators: Unspecified.
Measures: Adolescent checklist.
Results: Sexually abused females > nonabused females in sexual ambivalence, anxiety, suicidal ideation, problems with same-sex violence. Sexually abused males > nonabused males in social withdrawal, problems with friends of both sexes, fear of adult men, anxiety, suicidal ideation, and physical symptoms.

(continued)

Table 40–4. Adolescent studies: behavioral and emotional symptoms *(continued)*

Orr and Downes 1985
Type of abuse: Penetration, fondling, all contact. Legally or medically documented. Duration from a single incident to more than 10 years.
Victims: 20 females, ages 9–15, mean age 12.9 years. Source: treatment.
Control subjects: 20 nonabused, acutely ill females, mean age 14.1 years. Source: treatment.
Perpetrators: Father or father figure, stranger, uncle, acquaintance.
Measures: Offer Self Image Questionnaire.
Results: Sexually abused > acutely ill and "normal" raters to Offer Self Image Questionnaire normative data for problems with external mastery, vocational/educational goals, psychopathology. Sexually abused > Offer Self Image Questionnaire "normal" raters for problems with family relations and sexual attitudes.

Polit et al. 1990
Type of abuse: Fondling and penetration, some legally documented. Onset at approximately 10 years.
Subjects: 90 subjects in foster care, 87 at home; ages 13–18, mean age 15.7 years. Source: child welfare service.
Victims: 76 sexually abused females.
Control subjects: 101 females not sexually abused.
Perpetrators: Unspecified.
Measures: Interview.
Results: Sexually abused > control subjects in frequency of voluntary intercourse, early age at first intercourse, permissive sexual attitudes. Sexual abused living at home > sexually abused in foster care never reported abuse outside family, abuse an ongoing problem.

Stiffman 1989
Type of abuse: Unspecified.
Subjects: 207 females and 84 males, ages 12–18. Source: shelter.
Victims: 141 abused runaways, of whom 128 had been physically abused, 28 sexually abused.
Control subjects: 150 nonabused runaways, 98 female and 52 male.
Perpetrators: Incest.
Measures: Child Behavior Checklist self-report; Beck Depression Inventory.
Results: Abused > nonabused in internalizing and externalizing scores. Abused > emotionally disordered nonabused in depression before controlling for gender.

---

reported sexual abuse that had been legally or medically documented, nor did any provide temporal analyses of onset, cessation, and disclosure of child sexual abuse and onset of symptomatology. Of the 31 studies, 5 included both male and female victims, 2 included only male subjects, and 24 included only female subjects.

Symptoms and disorders reported in studies of adults, in descending order of frequency, were sexual behavioral problems (including sexual dysfunction and

Table 40–5. Adolescent studies: sexual abuse and substance use

Cavaiola and Schiff 1988, 1989
Type of abuse: Contact. Onset usually between 10 and 12 years.
Victims: 77 females and 73 males, ages 13–18, mean age 15 years. 45 were victims of incest, of whom 24 were also physically abused; 29, mostly female, were victims of extrafamilial sexual abuse; 76, mostly male, were only physically abused. Source: chemical dependency treatment program.
Control subjects: 24 nonabused females and 36 nonabused males in chemical dependency treatment, mean age 16 years. 35 nonabused females and 25 nonabused males from the community.
Perpetrators: For incest, father, stepfather, or other relative.
Measures: Chart review, Tennessee Self Concept Scale, data gathering.
Results: All abused groups > control subjects in early onset of drug use, low self-esteem, running away, promiscuity, and other acting-out behavior. Incest victims > other abused groups and control subjects in suicide attempts, poor identity. Sexually abused > physically abused and control subjects in running away and promiscuity.

Edwall et al. 1989
Type of abuse: Unspecified.
Subjects: 444 females in chemical dependence treatment. Mean age 15.6 years.
Victims: 47 incest, 120 extrafamilial sexual abuse, 43 both incest and extrafamilial sexual abuse.
Control subjects: 234 not sexually abused.
Perpetrators: Unspecified.
Measures: Semistructured interview, checklist.
Results: Incest > extrafamilial and control subjects in suicide attempts, shame, early onset of alcohol use, substance use to escape family problems, stimulant and minor tranquilizer use. Incest and extrafamilial > control subjects in agitation, sleep problems, early onset of substance use, stimulant, minor tranquilizer, and hallucinogen use.

Singer and Petchers 1989
Type of abuse: Unspecified. Mean onset at 10.9 years.
Subjects: 64 females, 32 males, mean age 15.6 years.
Victims: 48 sexually abused psychiatric inpatients.
Control subjects: 48 nonsexually abused psychiatric inpatients.
Perpetrators: Fathers, other relatives, nonrelatives; adults and peers.
Measures: Questionnaire, interviews, records.
Results: Sexually abused > control subjects in regular cocaine and stimulant use and frequent substance use.

gender identity disturbance) (13 studies), depressive symptomatology or disorders (9 studies), substance abuse (7 studies), somatic concerns (7 studies), suicidal and/or other self-destructive behavior (6 studies), PTSD symptomatology (6 studies), dissociation (5 studies), social impairment (5 studies), anxious behavior (5 studies), aggressive behavior (5 studies), low self-esteem (2 studies), borderline

Table 40–6. Adolescent studies based on psychiatric diagnosis

Emslie and Rosenfeld 1983
Type of abuse: Penetration, fondling. Age at onset 4–14 years. Duration: single incident to 4 years.
Victims: 9 female, 3 male sexually abused psychiatric inpatients.
Control subjects: 17 female, 36 male nonsexually abused psychiatric inpatients.
Perpetrators: Father, other relative, or nonrelative.
Measures: Questionnaire, chart review, patient observation.
Results: Sexually abused > nonsexually abused in nonpsychiatric diagnoses, sexual acting-out.

Sansonnet-Hayden et al. 1987
Type of abuse: Penetration, fondling. Age at onset 4–14 years. Duration: single incident to more than 6 years.
Victims: 11 female and 6 male sexually abused psychiatric inpatients. Time elapsed mostly less than 1 year.
Control subjects: 19 female and 18 male nonsexually abused psychiatric inpatients.
Perpetrators: Father or father figure, uncle, brother, other relative, nonrelative.
Measures: Diagnostic Interview Schedule, interviews.
Results: Sexually abused females > nonsexually abused females in major depression, schizoid/psychotic symptoms, somatic complaints. Sexually abused males > nonsexually abused males in conduct disorders. Sexually abused > nonsexually abused in sex problems, long hospitalization, treatment with neuroleptics.

Westen et al. 1990
Type of abuse: Penetration, fondling. Age at onset 5–10 years.
Subjects: Psychiatric inpatients, ages 14–18.
Victims: 27 females with borderline personality disorder.
Control subjects: 23 females with nonborderline diagnoses.
Perpetrators: Fathers, nonrelatives, siblings, other relatives.
Measures: Diagnostic Interview for Borderlines, chart review.
Results: Borderline personality disorder > nonborderline personality disorder in sex abuse, concurrent physical abuse and neglect, sex abuse by father. Sexually abused borderline personality disorder > nonsexually abused borderline personality disorder in substance abuse, promiscuity and other impulsivity, paranoia, pathological objective relations, avoidance of being alone. All sexually abused subjects > nonsexually abused in anger, < in verbal IQ.

---

personality disorder (4 studies), and eating disorders (2 studies). Wyatt and Newcomb (1990) reported that severity of symptomatology was associated with severity of abuse (i.e., with or without penetration and force), close relationship between perpetrator and victim (as in incest), and older age of victim at the time of abuse.

Sexualized behavioral problems, dysfunctions, and gender identity disturbance have been reported in comparative studies of incest victims regardless of their

Table 40–7. Adult studies of behavioral, emotional, and somatic symptoms

Briere and Runtz 1987
Type of abuse: Fondling and penetration. Onset before age 15. Undocumented.
Subjects: 152 walk-ins to crisis center, ages 14–54, average age 27.3 years.
Victims: 67 females with a history of sex abuse.
Control subjects: 85 females with no history of sex abuse.
Perpetrators: All perpetrators were at least 5 years older than victims.
Measures: Crisis Symptom Checklist.
Results: Victims > control subjects in use of psychoactive medication, history of substance abuse, suicide attempts, revictimizing relationships in adulthood, dissociative experiences, anxiety and fear, isolation, anger, self-destructiveness, and problems with sleep and sex.

Briere and Runtz 1988
Type of abuse: All contact, 7.3% intercourse. Average age at onset 9 years. 41.4% single incident, average of 7.2 incidents. Duration > 1 year for 12.2%. Undocumented.
Subjects: 224 subjects from the community, ages 17–40, average age 19.8 years.
Victims: 33 abused females.
Control subjects: 191 nonabused females.
Perpetrators: 12.2% parental incest. Most perpetrators male. All at least 5 years older than victims.
Measures: SCL-90-R, Family Experiences Questionnaire.
Results: Victims > control subjects in acute and chronic dissociation, somatization, chronic anxiety, and depression. Parental incest associated with increased rates of somatization, anxiety, and dissociation. Older perpetrators associated with increased anxiety and dissociation.

Briere and Runtz 1989
Type of abuse: All contact, 77% penetration. Mean age at onset 8 years. Mean duration 5.9 years.
Victims: 133 females from treatment, mean age 29.6 years.
Control subjects: 62 females from treatment, mean age 26.3 years.
Perpetrators: 61% incest.
Measures: Trauma Symptom Checklist 33.
Results: Victims > control subjects in trauma symptoms (i.e., dissociative symptoms, sleep problems, self-destructive ideation, and interpersonal problems).

(continued)

Table 40–7. Adult studies of behavioral, emotional, and somatic symptoms *(continued)*

Briere and Zaidi 1989

Type of abuse: All contact, 74% penetration. Mean onset at 8.6 years, mean duration 4.4 years.

Subjects: 50 charts randomly selected from emergency room files at start of study including 35 sexually abused females.

Perpetrators: 74% incest. All perpetrators at least 5 years older than victims.

Measures: Chart review.

Results: Only 3 (6%) of victims in the first 50 cases had spontaneously reported sexual abuse. When the 50 patients in the second group were directly asked about sexual molestation, 70% reported a history of such abuse. A history of sexual abuse was associated with greater rates of suicidality, substance abuse, sexual problems, multiple psychiatric diagnoses, and Axis II traits or disorders, especially borderline personality.

Bryer et al. 1987

Type of abuse: All contact, onset before age 16. Undocumented.

Subjects: Psychiatric inpatients, ages 18–64, mean age 31.8 years.

Victims: 14 sexually abused females, 10 physically abused females, 15 female victims of both types of abuse.

Control subjects: 27 nonabused females.

Perpetrators: Mostly fathers and brothers.

Measures: SCL-90-R, Millon Clinical Multiaxial Inventory.

Results: Severity of symptoms increased in victims of physical or sexual abuse and were greatest in victims of both types of abuse. Physically abused had higher scores than sexually abused on most SCL-90-R subscales. Sexually abused had higher scores than physically abused on most Millon Clinical Multiaxial Inventory subscales. Victims of both physical and sexual abuse scored higher than all other subjects on narcissistic, compulsive, and histrionic scales. Victims of only one type of abuse scored lower than control subjects on narcissistic and compulsive scales. No difference was found between sexually abused women and control subjects in mean scores on histrionic subscale.

Chu and Dill 1990

Type of abuse: All childhood onset, mostly prepuberty. Frequency > 10 incidents. Undocumented.

Subjects: Psychiatric inpatients ages 18–60, mean age 34 years.

Victims: 12 sexually abused, 23 sexually and physically abused, and 27 physically abused females.

Control subjects: 36 nonabused females.

Perpetrators: 27 intrafamilial, 8 extrafamilial, 11 both.

Measures: Dissociative Experiences Scale, SCL-90-R, Life Experiences Questionnaire.

Results: 83% of all subjects had dissociative symptom scores above norms and 24% had scores at or above the median for posttraumatic stress disorder. Victims of both sexual and physical abuse had highest dissociative and SCL-90-R global severity scores. Intrafamilial > extrafamilial sex abuse victims in dissociative symptoms.

(continued)

Table 40–7. Adult studies of behavioral, emotional, and somatic symptoms *(continued)*

Hunter 1991
Type of abuse: All contact. For females, mean age at onset 7.4 years, for males 8.1 years. For females mean duration 67.2 months, for males 31.4 months. Undocumented.
Subjects: From community.
Victims: 28 females, mean age 29.3 years. 24 males, mean age 34.2 years.
Control subjects: 28 females, 24 males.
Perpetrators: For female victims, in descending order of frequency, fathers, other adult relatives, nonrelatives. For male victims, nonrelatives (50% extrafamilial), relatives (other than fathers), fathers. All perpetrators were at least 3 years older than their victims.
Measures: Structured interview, MMPI, Rosenberg self-esteem, Dyadic Adjustment, Derogatis Sexual Functioning, Body-Self Relations Questionnaire.
Results: Sexually abused females > female control subjects on MMPI scales for hypochondriasis, depression, hysteria, psychopathic deviate, paranoia, psychasthenia, schizophrenia, mania, and social introversion. The sexually abused females showed increased sexual functioning symptomatology and fantasy scores, and less dyadic satisfaction, and rated themselves in poor health, less attentive to physical fitness, and as having better physical appearance. Sexually abused males > male control subjects on MMPI scales for hypochondriasis, depression, hysteria, psychopathic deviate, paranoia, psychasthenia, schizophrenia, and masculinity/femininity; sexual symptomatology, more feminine role definition, less dyadic consensus and satisfaction, lower self-esteem, and less positive affect.

Hunter et al. 1990
Type of abuse: Unspecified, undocumented.
Subjects: Ages 19–57, mean age 37.5 years. Source: treatment.
Victims: 33 male incestuous perpetrators with a history of childhood sexual abuse.
Control subjects: 55 male incestuous perpetrators with no history of sexual abuse.
Perpetrators: Mostly male adults.
Measures: MMPI, questionnaire.
Results: Offenders with a history of sexual abuse evidenced more pathology on every MMPI subscale than nonvictimized offenders, with particular elevations on depression and psychopathic deviate, and were significantly more likely to have molested more than one victim.

(continued)

Table 40–7. Adult studies of behavioral, emotional, and somatic symptoms *(continued)*

Jackson et al. 1990
Type of abuse: 59% penetration, 91% fondling. Average onset at 7.82 years. Duration up to 10 years for 32%; single incident for 14%. Undocumented.
Victims: 22 females, ages 18–33, mean age 23.14 years. Source: community.
Control subjects: 18 nonabused females, mean age 21.94 years. Source: community.
Perpetrators: 45% fathers or stepfathers, 36% brothers or stepbrothers, all others male relatives. 23% multiple perpetrators.
Measures: BDI, Social Adjustment Scale, DSFI, Rosenberg self-esteem, Family Environment Scale, semistructured interview.
Results: Sexually abused subjects < control subjects in social adjustment, self-esteem, body-image, and sexual satisfaction; > control subjects in depression. 65% of abused sample met DSM-III criteria for one or more sexual dysfunctions. Sexual abuse families reported as less cohesive and more controlling than control subjects' families.

Murphy et al. 1988
Type of abuse: Mostly fondling of children and adolescents, mostly penetration of victims 18 and older, some victims noncontact. Undocumented.
Subjects: Age range 18 to over 50, most between 30 and 49 years. Source: community.
Victims: 38 females abused before age 12, mean time lapsed 36.8 years. 48 females abused at ages 12–17, mean time lapsed 21.7 years. 81 females abused at age 18 or over, mean time lapsed 14.8 years. 34 females abused before and after age 18, mean time lapsed 12.6 years.
Control subjects: 184 nonabused females.
Perpetrators: Unspecified.
Measures: SCL-90-R, Modified Fear Survey, Impact of Event scale.
Results: Victims had a pattern of increased hostility, interpersonal sensitivity, obsessive-compulsive symptoms, anxiety, and paranoid ideation. Women abused during adolescence had increased symptoms. Women abused during childhood had more anxiety as adults and more symptoms on the SCL global severity measure than nonvictims. Revictimization with abuse occurring both before and after age 18 was associated with the highest level of symptomatology.

Owen 1984
Type of abuse: Penetration and fondling. Mean onset at 8.1 years. Mean duration 5.6 years. Undocumented.
Victims: 17 females receiving outpatient psychotherapy, mean age 36.1 years.
Control subjects: 17 females receiving outpatient psychotherapy, ages matched with victims within 5 years.
Perpetrators: Mostly fathers, all incestuous.
Measures: Rorschach.
Results: Victims more often gave Rorschach responses that indicated a denial of a need for affection, lack or rejection of conventionality, minimized social involvement, lack of self-concern, and a high level of aggression.

(continued)

Table 40–7. Adult studies of behavioral, emotional, and somatic symptoms *(continued)*

S. Parker and Parker 1991
Type of abuse: All contact, onset at less than 16 years. Undocumented.
Victims: 134 females from the community, ages 18–63, mean age 33 years.
Control subjects: 357 females from the community, mean age 25 years.
Perpetrators: 20 parent or stepparent, 114 other relatives or extrafamilial. All over age 18.
Measures: Sexual Adjustment Inventory, Eysenck Subscale, Texas Social Behavior Inventory.
Results: Only the Texas Social Behavior Inventory yielded significant differences between samples. Significant social maladjustment in incestuously abused samples. Perception of treatment by parents ("bad" or "good") had a greater impact on social functioning of abused sample than of control subjects.

Roland et al. 1989
Type of abuse: Contact and noncontact. Onset before adolescence. Undocumented.
Subjects: From community.
Victims: 20 female victims of abuse by their fathers or stepfathers, mean age 31.4 years. 32 female victims of abuse by other family members or nonrelatives, mean age 30.9 years.
Control subjects: 119 nonabused females, mean age 29.6 years.
Perpetrators: Fathers, stepfathers, uncles, brothers, other male relatives, and family friends. All perpetrators at least 5 years older than their victims.
Measures: MMPI.
Results: Victims of father-daughter incest > nonabused and victims of abuse by other than father on the following MMPI scales: validity (F), depression, psychopathic deviate, psychasthenia, and schizophrenia. Victims of abuse by other relatives and nonrelatives had elevated scores on the following MMPI scales: psychopathic deviate, paranoia, schizophrenia, and hypomania. Both abused groups > control subjects on the following MMPI scales: test-taking attitude (K), hypochondriasis, and social introversion.

Sedney and Brooks 1984
Type of abuse: Contact and noncontact. Age at onset mostly under 12. Duration: 58% single occurrence, 14% more than 1 year. Undocumented.
Subjects: Ages 18–58, mean 19 years, from community.
Victims: 51 females.
Control subjects: 51 females.
Perpetrators: Mostly brothers, other family members, nonrelatives. 10 had multiple perpetrators. Most incidents occurring at age 12 or under were incest; after age 12, more were extrafamilial.
Measures: Questionnaire.
Results: Victims > control subjects in reported depression, anxiety, insomnia, self-destructive ideation, and criminal revictimization of any kind. Victims of incest more often reported learning problems and having seen a doctor and having been hospitalized for anxiety and depression.

(continued)

Table 40–7. Adult studies of behavioral, emotional, and somatic symptoms *(continued)*

Swett et al. 1990
Type of abuse: Contact. Onset mostly before age 18. Mean frequency 3.9 episodes. Undocumented.
Subjects: Psychiatric outpatients, mean age 37.1 years.
Victims: 9 sexually abused males, 7 sexually and physically abused males, 44 physically abused males.
Control subjects: 65 nonabused males.
Perpetrators: Intra- and extrafamilial, mostly all male.
Measures: SCL-90-R, interview.
Results: Victims of sexual and both sexual and physical abuse > victims of physical abuse only and control subjects in SCL-90-R global severity scores and subscale scores. Men with a history of sexual abuse evidenced greater frequency of major affective illness, anxiety, dysthymic, and adjustment disorders.

Wyatt 1990
Type of abuse: Body contact when victim was under age 18. Perpetrators were at least 5 years older. If they used coercion, perpetrators of any age were admitted.
Victims: African American female child sexual abuse victims recruited from the community: 66 noncontact, 79 contact.
Control subjects: White female child sexual abuse victims recruited from the community: 65 noncontact, 93 contact.
Perpetrators: Relatives and nonrelatives.
Measures: Wyatt Sex History Questionnaire.
Results: Reasons for nondisclosure of type of abuse: fear of consequences for family, fear of perpetrator, fear of getting in trouble, desire to forget, uncertainty at the time whether the abuse was right or wrong, abuse was associated with prohibited behavior such as hitchhiking. Victims of both races evidenced sexual problems and avoided men resembling the perpetrator.

Wyatt and Newcomb 1990
Type of abuse: Body contact when victim was under age 18. Perpetrators were at least 5 years older. If they used coercion, perpetrators of any age were admitted.
Subjects: 62 white women and 49 African American women with histories of child sexual abuse recruited from the Los Angeles community.
Perpetrators: Relatives and nonrelatives.
Measures: Wyatt Sex History Questionnaire.
Results: Negative effects: depression, appetite change, sleep problems, impairment of social functioning, preoccupation with the incident, changes in sexual attitudes, and avoidance and mistrust of men. Worst outcomes associated with close relationship with perpetrator, severe abuse, older age of victim.

Note. SCL-90-R = Hopkins Symptom Checklist—90. MMPI = Minnesota Multiphasic Personality Inventory.

Table 40–8. Adult studies based on psychiatric diagnosis

Beck and van der Kolk 1987
Type of abuse: Penetration or fondling; all contact or unspecified. Onset at 2–14 years, duration 1–9 years. Some documented.
Subjects: All psychiatric inpatients, most being treated for schizophrenia, median age 36.5 years.
Victims: 12 sexually abused females.
Control subjects: 11 females not sexually abused.
Perpetrators: Fathers, stepfathers, brothers, mother.
Measures: Chart review, clinical observation, Carmen Checklist.
Results: Victims > control subjects in suspected organicity, sexual delusions, affective symptoms, substance abuse, major medical problems, aggressive behavior toward others, and attempts at social contact.

Becker et al. 1982
Type of abuse: Penetration, fondling, unspecified. All contact. Some documented.
Subjects: 83 female victims of incest or extrafamilial rape.
Victims: Ages 18–60, mean age 29.5.
Control subjects: Victims of extrafamilial sexual abuse.
Perpetrators: Incest and extrafamilial.
Measures: Sexual Arousal Inventory.
Results: More than half of subjects reported at least one sexual dysfunction, especially nonorgasmic and arousal disorder, mostly precipitated by abuse. Incest victims > rape victims in nonorgasmic.

Coons et al. 1989
Type of abuse: 7 female rape victims with PTSD, others unspecified.
Subjects: 71 psychiatric inpatients, 69 outpatients. 97 female, 43 male, ages 17–67, mean age 32.5 years. Diagnostic categories (in descending order): PTSD, multiple personality disorder, bulimia, schizophrenia, affective disorder, borderline personality disorder, psychogenic amnesia, atypical dissociative. No control subjects.
Perpetrators: Unspecified.
Measures: Dissociative Experiences Scale, trauma questionnaire, full clinical assessment.
Results: Only the males with PTSD and factitious PTSD had no history of sex abuse. The most common diagnostic categories of sexually abused patients were multiple personality disorder followed by atypical dissociative and PTSD in females. Patients in these categories experienced sex abuse more than physical abuse, verbal abuse, neglect, or no abuse.

(continued)

Table 40–8. Adult studies based on psychiatric diagnosis *(continued)*

Craine et al. 1988

Type of abuse: Penetration, fondling, noncontact. Mean onset at 10.5 years. Mean duration 2.8 years.
Subjects: All psychiatric inpatients, mostly with schizophrenia or affective disorder, ages 13–81, mean age 34.7 years.
Victims: 54 sexually abused females, 27 of whom were also physically abused.
Control subjects: 51 females with no history of sex abuse, but 10 of whom had been physically abused.
Perpetrators: Incest and extrafamilial.
Measures: Medical records, interview.
Results: Victims > control subjects in personality disorders, adjustment disorder, substance abuse, PTSD, sexual problems, gender identity problems, sadomasochistic fantasy, and family history of chronic fatigue, psychiatric illness, or substance abuse.

Hall et al. 1989

Type of abuse: Penetration, fondling (all contact). Onset: less than 12 years to 16 years old.
Subjects: Patients on eating disorders unit, ages 12–58, average 27.7 years.
Victims: 59 sexually abused females, 1 sexually abused male.
Control subjects: 83 females and 15 males with no history of sex abuse.
Perpetrators: In descending order, fathers or stepfathers, other relatives, parents' lovers, brothers, acquaintances, strangers, uncles.
Measures: Clinical interview.
Results: Victims were given a diagnosis of mixed anorexia/bulimia significantly more often than were the control subjects.

Herman et al. 1989

Type of abuse: Unspecified.
Study sample: 17 females and 4 males with borderline personality disorder.
Control subjects: 12 females and 22 males with borderline traits, bipolar II, antisocial or schizotypal personality disorder.
Perpetrators: Unspecified.
Measures: Semistructured interview, Impact of Event Scale, Dissociative Experiences Scale.
Results: A history of sex abuse was found most often in subjects with borderline personality disorder (67%), followed by those with borderline traits; least in those with no borderline diagnosis. Borderline personality disorder associated with high Dissociative Experiences Scale scores.

(continued)

Table 40–8. Adult studies based on psychiatric diagnosis *(continued)*

Miller et al. 1987, 1988
Type of abuse: Fondling, penetration, noncontact.
Victims: 45 female alcoholics, mean age 39.44 years. Source: treatment.
Control subjects: 40 female nonalcoholics, mean age 30.98 years. Source: community.
Perpetrators: Extrafamilial, all at least 5 years older than victim, and stepfathers or fathers.
Measures: Interview.
Results: Alcoholic females > nonalcoholic females in history of sex abuse. Alcoholic, sexually abused females > nonalcoholic, sexually abused females in variety of sexually abusive experiences, intercourse, violent coercion, duration of abuse, and immediate reaction affecting emotions toward self.

Morrison 1989
Type of abuse: Contact and noncontact. Mean onset at 10 years.
Study sample: 60 females with somatization disorder.
Control subjects: 31 females with unipolar or bipolar affective disorder.
Perpetrators: Nonrelatives, brothers, fathers, other relatives.
Measures: Two interviews, one based on Renard Diagnostic Interview.
Results: Subjects with somatization disorder > subjects with affective disorder in history of sex abuse and inorgasmia with intercourse.

Ogata et al. 1990
Type of abuse: All contact, 41% penetration. Onset mostly before age 12.
Study sample: 19 female and 5 male inpatients with borderline personality, ages 18–60, mean 30 years.
Control subjects: 13 female and 5 male depressed inpatients, mean age 42 years.
Perpetrators: Incest and extrafamilial.
Measures: Diagnostic Interview for Borderlines, Research Diagnostic Criteria to assess depression, Family Experiences Interview.
Results: 71% (16 female and 1 male) of borderline patients reported a history of sex abuse, compared with 22% of depressed patients. More borderline than depressed patients reported multiple perpetrators, physical as well as sexual abuse, and incest. Victims of father-daughter incest had the lowest mean age at onset of abuse, victims of only extrafamilial abuse the highest. The Diagnostic Interview for Borderlines items of derealization and chronic dysphoria were most strongly associated with childhood sexual abuse in borderline patients.

(continued)

Table 40–8. Adult studies based on psychiatric diagnosis *(continued)*

Saunders et al. 1992

Type of abuse: In descending order: fondling, penetration, noncontact. Mean onset at 11.4 years.
Subjects: From the community, mean age 39.9 years.
Victims: 127 sexually abused females, mean time lapsed 29.1 years.
Control subjects: 260 nonsexually abused females.
Perpetrators: Noncontact abuse more by acquaintances and relatives other than the father, and by strangers. Penetration more by fathers.
Measures: Diagnostic Interview Schedule, Incident Report Interview, assessment for PTSD DSM-III criteria.
Results: Victims of penetration > control subjects in major depression, agoraphobia, obsessive-compulsive disorder, social phobia, and sexual disorders. Victims of fondling > control subjects in major depression, obsessive-compulsive disorder, and sexual disorders. Victims of penetration and fondling > in PTSD than victims of fondling. Victims of fondling > in PTSD than victims of noncontact abuse.

Note. PTSD = posttraumatic stress disorder.

age at the time of the study. In contrast, as would be expected from findings of developmental psychopathology, suicidal behavior and substance abuse were reported more frequently in adolescents or adults who had been victims of child or adolescent incest (Rutter 1989). Before firm conclusions can be drawn regarding the effects of incest on mental health, more research needs to be done that uses increased numbers of samples recruited from the community rather than treatment, employs uniform definitions of incest, identifies perpetrators, describes the severity of incest, and analyzes the temporal relationships between onset of symptomatology and onset, cessation, and disclosure of abuse. We also need documentation of sexual abuse, legal proceedings, and medical events that follow the disclosure of incest and analyses that take into account risk factors for psychopathology.

Nonabusive Parent in Incestuous Families

There are few controlled studies that systematically investigate the psychological functioning of the nonabusive parent in incestuous families. The literature consists primarily of clinical descriptions of the role that the nonabusive mother (because a father or stepfather is most frequently the abuser) typically plays in the family structure. In most of these articles, the mother is described as "the cornerstone in the pathological family system" (Lustig et al. 1966), responding to marital tensions by consciously or unconsciously distancing herself from her daughter, while encouraging her to have a closer relationship with her father (Sgroi 1982). The literature is replete with unsubstantiated claims that mothers generally know that their daughters are being abused (e.g., Kempe and Kempe 1978). Macholka et al. (1967) also described the mother in the incestuous family as the cornerstone in the pathological system, because they view her as encouraging the father to take the role of abuser as a way of keeping the family intact. More recent empirical studies, however, indicate that mothers are frequently unaware of the abuse. When they do discover what is happening, the majority of mothers take active steps to stop it (Mannarino et al. 1989). It appears that the early literature's emphasis on maternal psychopathology in incestuous families may, in part, have grown out of the tradition of blaming the victim that is seen in clinical descriptions of other victim groups (Snell et al. 1964).

The clinical literature does indicate a high level of psychological and psychosocial difficulties in incestuous families. In a study of 72 cases of incest, Maisch (1972) reported that 88% of the couples had a high degree of marital conflict, and 41% reported a disturbed sexual relationship. The fathers typically described their wives as "frigid" or "cold." Truesdell et al. (1986) found that 73% of the mothers of incest victims in their sample had been physically abused by their husbands. In light of these stressors, it is not surprising that the clinical literature notes that the mother is at significant risk for depression and suicide (Browning and Boatman 1977). In Finkelhor et al.'s (1990) study of 795 college students, a mother's chronic illness or physical absence from home served as significant risk factors for sexual abuse. It has also been found that female incest victims report more anger and resentment at their mothers than at their abusive fathers (Meiselman 1980; Tsai and Wagner 1978).

Controlled studies of the functioning of mothers in incestuous families, however, are far more inconsistent. Of the six studies we found that systematically evaluated the quality of mother-daughter relationships in incestuous families, three found difficulties (Cole and Woolger 1989; Levang 1989; Paveza 1988), one found a neutral relationship (Sagatun and Prince 1988), and two characterized the relationship as positive (Salt et al. 1990; White et al. 1988). The studies that report problematic relationships describe significantly lower communication rates (Levang 1989), significantly more emotional distance, and more negative control between female incest victims and their mothers (Cole and Woolger 1989; Paveza 1988). Paveza concluded that a distant mother-daughter relationship places girls at 11 times greater risk for sexual abuse. In contrast to these studies, Sagatun and Prince, using a questionnaire administered to family members in therapy for incest, reported that mother-daughter relationships were rated as neutral by all family members. Similarly, White et al. found that 86% of sexually abused boys in their sample and 90% of sexually abused girls rated their relationships with their mothers as good. When mothers were interviewed, 97% had moderate to high nurturing attitudes to the victims, and 77% expressed no hostility to the children (Salt et al.

1990). It is important to note that all of these studies involved small samples (ranging from 7 to 156) and relied on groups referred for treatment, which are likely to overestimate the true incidence of mother-child difficulties.

In recent years, researchers have begun to take a more systematic approach to studying mothers' collusion in incest. Table 40–9 presents a summary of studies that evaluate the nonoffending parent in incestuous families. These studies have for the most part concluded that in most incestuous families there is no collusion. Salt et al. (1990) reported that more than 80% of the mothers in their treatment program for sex abuse victims took some action to protect the child. Similarly, Sirles and Franke (1989) reported that 78% of the 193 mothers of intrafamilial sexual abuse victims in their treatment-referred sample believed the child's report. Everson et al. (1989) reported that 44% of the mothers in their sample of incestuous families referred by the Department of Social Services were consistently supportive after disclosure. Maternal support after disclosure was more forthcoming when the report was made by a younger child (Sirles and Franke 1989) and the abuser was the biological father (Salt et al. 1990; Sirles and Franke 1989). In contrast, Faller (1988) found that the mothers were more collusive when the perpetrator of incest was the biological father. However, she found higher levels of maternal support for the victim when the biological father was not living at home (Faller 1988). Studies of the psychopathology of mothers of incest victims have been contradictory. To date, there have been no systematic studies of DSM-III-R diagnoses in this population. Groff and Hubble (1984) found the Minnesota Multiphasic Personality Inventory (MMPI) (Hathaway and McKinley 1943) scores of the wives of incest offenders to be within normal limits. Salt et al. gave the Millon Clinical Multiaxial Inventory (Millon 1983) to mothers in incestuous families and found that 88% had a passive-submissive pattern, one-fourth had major problems with emotional lability, and 81% showed some signs of social withdrawal. Using the Rorschach, Wald et al. (1990) found that 28 mothers of incest victims had significantly greater weakness in reality testing, more interpersonal guardedness, and higher depression scores than a matched control group taken from Exner's norms. It is not clear, however, whether some of these results could be related to the extraordinarily high levels of tension and disorganization that accompany the disclosure of intrafamilial sexual abuse.

In summary, despite the assertion of clinicians that mothers in incestuous families are often silent partners in the abuse, the empirical literature provides no consistent support for such a dynamic. Although there clearly are some incestuous families where the nonabusive mother makes an important contribution to the abusive process, systematic investigations indicate that the majority of mothers are not collusive; nor do studies consistently confirm a negative mother-child relationship in these families.

Table 40–9. The nonoffending parent

Everson et al. 1989
Subjects: Mothers of 88 Department of Social Services-referred intrafamilial sexual abuse victims.
Measures: Child Assessment Schedule, Child Behavior Checklist, semistructured interview designed for the study.
Results: 44% of the mothers were consistently supportive after disclosure. Lack of maternal support significantly associated with foster placement and higher psychopathology scores.

Faller 1988
Subjects: 171 mothers in incestuous families referred for treatment.
Measures: Chart review.
Results: Mothers married to the victim's biological father most "collusive" and most dependent on the perpetrator. Mothers no longer living with the perpetrator had a "warmer" relationship with the victim.

Groff and Hubble 1984
Subjects: 26 couples—incest offenders and their wives. 23 female control subjects referred for treatment.
Measures: Minnesota Multiphasic Personality Inventory.
Results: Spouses of incestuous fathers had Minnesota Multiphasic Personality Inventory within normal limits. They were not more withdrawn, depressed, dependent, or inadequate.

Salt et al. 1990
Subjects: 156 mothers of victims of incest or extrafamilial sexual abuse referred for treatment.
Measures: Questionnaires designed for the study measuring actions and attitudes, Millon Clinical Multiaxial Inventory.
Results: Almost all the mothers (97%) had moderate to high nurturing attitudes toward the victim. Most (80%) took some action to protect the child; only 18% failed to take any protective action. Mothers were least protective when the abuser was a stepfather. 88% of the mothers showed a passive-submissive pattern on the Millon Clinical Multiaxial Inventory.

Sirles and Franke 1989
Subjects: 193 mothers of victims of intrafamilial sexual abuse referred for treatment.
Measures: Questionnaire designed for the study.
Results: Most of the mothers (78.2%) believed the child's report. If the child reported that the mother was not at home at the time of abuse, the mothers found it more believable. Believability decreased for older children (95% for preschoolers versus 63.2% for adolescents). Spouse abuse was reported in 44.3% of the families; physical child abuse in 30.5%.

(continued)

Table 40–9.   The nonoffending parent *(continued)*

Wald et al. 1990
Subjects: 28 mothers of incest victims referred for treatment compared with a matched control group for Exner's Rorschach norms.
Measures: Rorschach.
Results: Compared with the norms, mothers of incest victims had significantly greater weakness in reality testing, higher depression, and more interpersonal guardedness.

Incest Perpetrators

Table 40–10 summarizes studies of the psychosocial functioning of perpetrators of incest. Although an increasing number of investigators in recent years have been systematically studying incest perpetrators, until the last decade most knowledge of this population came from studies of sex offenders who were incarcerated for offenses of extrafamilial sexual molestation. The recent literature raises questions about the most basic assumptions underlying the clinical literature. For example, most family-based incest treatment programs assume that the father himself usually suffered sexual abuse in childhood, but systematic investigations find that only 10%–20% report childhood histories of sexual abuse (Kirkland and Bauer 1982; Langevin et al. 1978). These percentages are not greater than the incidence of sexual abuse reported in the general population. H. Parker and Parker (1986) reported that 59% of their sample of incest perpetrators reported histories of physical abuse when they were children. This suggests the possibility that the "world of abnormal rearing" (Kempe and Kempe 1978) that typifies families of physical abuse victims may be a more potent risk factor for incest than a history of sexual victimization.

Most studies that use the MMPI to assess psychopathology in incest perpetrators fail to reveal a consistent pattern of psychological disturbance. Scott and Stone (1986) did not find mean scores outside the normal range in their study of 62 outpatient offenders, but other investigators have found as many as two clinically elevated scores (Kirkland and Bauer 1982; Langevin et al. 1978). Using unstructured clinical evaluations, Langevin et al. found that 47% of their sample received a diagnosis of personality disorder, whereas 35% did not qualify for any psychiatric diagnosis. Williams and Finkelhor (1990) reviewed six studies (including unpublished dissertations) of the psychological characteristics of incestuous fathers and found elevated scores on the MMPI that indicate a significant level of psychopathy in this population.

These findings might suggest a high level of antisocial personality in incest offenders, but their domineering behavior with family members and lack of concern for the effects of incest on their children does not necessarily generalize to

Table 40–10.　Child sexual abusers

Ballard et al. 1990
Subjects: 373 incest perpetrators in inpatient and outpatient treatment.
Measures: Self-report questionnaires, clinical interviews, demographic variables.
Results: Approximately 40% reported needing help with relationships with adults; 67% needed help understanding the victim's feelings.

Faller 1990
Subjects: 196 referred incestuous fathers and stepfathers.
Measures: Clinical interviews.
Results: 48% of the marriages where the biological father was the perpetrator were characterized by male dominance. More than a third of the stepfathers were younger than their wives.

Marshall et al. 1986
Subjects: 21 incest offenders and 40 nonfamilial offenders referred for treatment; 27 unemployed control subjects from the community.
Measures: Plethysmograph measuring sexual arousal to various stimuli.
Results: Extrafamilial child molesters showed greater arousal to stimuli involving children than did the incest or control groups. Control subjects showed more arousal to adult stimuli than did the incest group.

Milner and Robertson 1990
Subjects: 15 incest offenders, 30 physical child abusers, and 30 child neglecters and matched control subjects.
Measures: Child Abuse Potential Inventory.
Results: All reported elevated levels of personal distress, unhappiness, loneliness, and rigidity. Incest perpetrators reported more positive views of children and self and fewer problems with children than did the physical abuse and neglect groups. The incest group reported fewer family problems than the physical abuse group.

Panton 1979
Subjects: 35 incarcerated incest offenders, 28 incarcerated extrafamilial sex offenders.
Measures: Minnesota Multiphasic Personality Inventory.
Results: Both groups had mean scale elevations indicative of self-alienation, despondency, rigidity, inhibition, feelings of insecurity, and concerns regarding adequate heterosexual functioning.

H. Parker and Parker 1986
Subjects: 56 incestuous fathers, incarcerated or referred for psychotherapy, versus 54 comparable but nonoffending fathers.
Measures: Questionnaire designed for the study.
Results: The incestuous sample was more socially introverted. Abusing fathers were more likely to have a perception that they had been deprived of parental love and affection, spent less time with their daughters, and were less involved in child care and nurturance.

(continued)

Table 40–10. Child sexual abusers *(continued)*

Prentky et al. 1989
Subjects: 82 sex offenders.
Measures: Structured Clinical Interview.
Results: A history of numerous caregivers and sexual deviation in the family is associated with sexual aggression. A history of institutionalization and child abuse and neglect is associated with general aggression.

Quinsey et al. 1979
Subjects: 9 psychiatric inpatients who had molested their daughters or stepdaughters. Matched nonincestuous child molesters.
Measures: Measure of penile response to slides of various sexual stimuli.
Results: The incest group showed more appropriate age preferences than nonincestuous child molester group.

Scott and Stone 1986
Subjects: 33 natural father incest perpetrators, 29 stepfather perpetrators, 44 nonparticipating mothers, 22 daughter victims. All in therapeutic treatment programs. Compared with matched control subjects.
Measures: Minnesota Multiphasic Personality Inventory.
Results: Mean profiles of father and stepfather groups were not pathological. The mean profile of the daughter victims was more elevated and differed significantly from the other three groups on validity, psychasthenia, and schizophrenia scales.

Truesdell et al. 1986
Subjects: 30 mothers (married to incest perpetrators) attending an incest treatment group.
Measures: Conflict Tactics Scale.
Results: 73% reported at least one incident of some form of physical abuse committed against them as well as some form of psychological abuse.

---

situations outside of the family. Saunders et al. (1992) found that incest offenders are in general significantly more dependent or pathologically unassertive than control or normative samples. Williams and Finkelhor (1990) reviewed five studies that found significant symptoms of anxiety and depression in incest offenders. None of these studies used structured interviews, nor did any include a retrospective analysis of whether these affective symptoms were reactive to or antedated the disclosure of sex abuse. Although a paranoid style has been reported in a number of studies of incest perpetrators, it is not clear whether this style is related to a need to keep the incest secret. No studies are reported that find a higher incidence of psychoses than is seen in the general population.

A number of studies of incest offenders conclude that social isolation and deficient social skills, coupled with a failure to bond with family members, are characteristics of incest offenders. The research findings on the prevalence of alcohol and drug abuse by incest offenders is contradictory. Some studies find a high incidence (Langevin et al. 1978); others do not (H. Parker and Parker 1986). It is clear that substance abuse does not play a major role in many cases of incest. In keeping with the conceptualization of Araji and Finkelhor (1986), there are a number of possible contributors to the disinhibition that leads to incest, and alcohol or drug abuse are only two of many such variables.

Conte (1986), in a critique of the family-oriented views of incest, asserted that most family-based theories of the etiology of incest rest on two assumptions regarding the sexual behavior of incest perpetrators: 1) that fathers and stepfathers do not act out sexually outside the home and 2) that incest is the sexual expression of nonsexual needs. The most commonly cited typology used in the literature on sex offenders is Groth et al.'s (1982) division of sexual offenders into the categories of "fixated" or "regressed." Fixated offenders have no history of appropriate adult sexual functioning, and their primary sexual orientation is to children. In contrast, the primary sexual orientation of regressed offenders (presumably the more common type of offender in incestuous families) is toward adults. However, as a result of stress such as family pathology, children may become temporary sources of sexual gratification. This typology, derived from studies of incarcerated offenders, is based on a group of men with sexual difficulties that are not necessarily representative of patterns seen in sexual offenders who have not been caught, discovered, or incarcerated. When viewed systematically, there is virtually no empirical support for the presence of this type of bimodal distribution in incest perpetrators. In fact, the largest group of offenders appears to consist of a mixed group that combines behaviors of both fixated and regressed offenders (Conte 1990).

The early literature on sexual preference in incest perpetrators comprised investigations of small samples with contradictory findings: one found deviant sexual arousal patterns (Abel et al. 1988), and one did not (Quinsey et al. 1979). More recent studies suggest that, although some incestuous fathers may not have pedophilic preferences, a significant minority do show evidence of deviant arousal and behavior toward young girls (Langevin et al. 1978). Low levels of arousal toward adult females have also been reported (Langevin et al. 1978; Marshall et al. 1986), as have significant difficulties in the sexual relationships of parents of incest victims (Saunders et al. 1986). Abel et al. reported that almost half of the incest perpetrators referred to their treatment program had sexually abused children outside of the family as well as within the family. One in five also reported raping adult women at the same time that they were sexually abusing their own children. Although the definitive study on sexuality in the incest offender has yet to be done, it is clear from the current literature that consideration of a relational disorder diagnosis for incestuous families needs to take into account the fact that, in a significant percentage of incestuous families, the deviant sexual behavior on the part of the father is likely to exist outside of the family situation as well. Clinical descriptions of incest as resulting from dysfunctional family dynamics also need to address the possibility that a significant percentage of incest perpetrators manifested deviant sexual patterns in adolescence, well before the formation of the current family.

Methodological Issues

In the last decade, there has been a significant increase in research on the effects of intrafamilial sexual abuse that has resulted in an improved understanding of the sequelae of incest. However, because of a paucity of systematic investigation of the relational aspects of incest, there has not been a corresponding improvement in our understanding of the interactional aspects of this problem. Those studies that are in the literature are often marked by major methodological flaws, including confusion regarding definitions of sexual abuse, failure to use appropriate control groups, and failure to use adequate measures.

The definitions of child sexual abuse used by the studies cited in this review vary greatly, and their results may in part be a function of the different definitions. Studies frequently do not address the differential effects of definitions of child sexual abuse, including type of sexual abuse (i.e., contact versus noncontact, with or without penetration, with or without photographs), duration, frequency, age of victim at onset and age of victim at disclosure, identity of perpetrator, age of perpetrator at onset and at disclosure of sexual abuse, numbers of perpetrators, victim allegations of rituals during abuse (including the use of substances), and sources of information regarding abuse incidents (i.e., legal, medical, educational, or law enforcement sources). Legal and/or medical substantiation of abuse and the nature of coercion during abuse (including threats and/or force) are also issues related to definition.

We discussed the definitions used in the major American prevalence studies of child sexual abuse earlier in this chapter. Studies of mental health problems in treatment-referred samples have used numerous definitions. Briere and Runtz (1988) (see Table 40–7) defined sexual abuse as sexual contact (fondling to intercourse) experienced prior to age 15 and perpetrated by someone at least 5 years older than the victim. Their consecutive sample of adult female outpatients of mental health clinics showed a 44.1% prevalence rate of child sexual abuse. Conte and Schuerman (1987) (see Table 40–2), in their study of 369 children 4–17 years old who had been referred for treatment of sexual abuse to the Sexual Assault Center of the Harborview Medical Center, Seattle, Washington, defined sexual abuse as any self-reported sexual contact (fondling to intercourse) experienced before the age of 18 and initiated by someone at least 5 years older.

Friedrich and colleagues (Friedrich and Einbender 1989; Friedrich et al. 1987, 1988) (see Table 40–2), in studies of 155 children between the ages of 3 and 12 years who were receiving mental health evaluations and/or treatment, defined child sexual abuse as sexual contact between a child and a perpetrator at least 6 years older than the child. The abuse in this study had to have been documented by two sources: the government agency responsible for investigating it and either a physician or a mental health expert. The abuse had to have occurred within 48 months of the study. Perpetrators in this study were fathers (54%), other male relatives (23%), stepfathers (12%), and, in smaller numbers, neighbors, family friends, and mothers.

It should be noted that those studies based on legally substantiated cases of incest require a definition based on laws that differ from state to state, and these legal definitions of incest may also differ from those used in studies of cases that have not entered the courts. Child protective services use definitions outlined by state laws for case documentation and for criminal prosecution. An example of such a definition is that used by New York State Department of Social Services (1991):

> There is reasonable cause to suspect child sexual abuse or maltreatment when the parent or other person legally responsible for the care of the child, does the following (examples are not all inclusive):
>
> Touches a child's genitals, buttocks, breasts or other intimate parts in a sexual manner; or, forces or encourages the child to touch the genitals, buttocks, breasts or other intimate parts of the parent, or other person legally responsible for the child, in a sexual manner.
>
> Engages or attempts to engage the child in sexual intercourse or deviant sexual intercourse (i.e. contact between penis and anus, mouth and penis, or mouth and vulva).
>
> Forces, encourages or willfully and/or knowingly allows a child to engage in sexual activity (for example, prostitution) with other children or adults.
>
> Uses or permits a child to be used in a sexual performance such as a photograph, play, motion picture or dance, giving rise to impairment or imminent danger of impairment to the child, regardless of whether the material itself is obscene.
>
> Fails to exercise a minimum degree of care when a child is sexually abused (as described above) by a person not legally responsible for the child. (p. 3)

Studies of the relational aspects of incest that use control groups frequently draw conclusions that are not justified by the data. When, in addition to "normal" control subjects, they use psychiatric control subjects or families with maritally discordant parents for comparison, different results often ensue (Aiosa-Karpas et al. 1991). A related difficulty, unique to sex abuse, is the tendency of children to rely heavily on dissociation in response to sexual victimization. This leads to a much higher incidence of amnesia for incest than one might see in other types of victimization (Putnam 1985). Given the high incidence of incest in the general population, one cannot be certain that a family in a "normal" control group does not include sexual abuse victims.

Another major flaw in many studies of incestuous families is the use of inappropriate measures or the failure to include adequate numbers of informants. When measures not specific to sex abuse are used, findings are often spuriously negative. Thus, general measures of self-concept or gender are often not adequate for uncovering difficulties in this population (Mannarino et al. 1989). In contrast, when measures specific to sex abuse are used, such as the Trauma Symptom Checklist (Lanktree and Briere 1990), fewer false negatives result.

Numbers and types of informants also often affect findings. For example, because of legal consequences, perpetrators of sexual abuse are often reluctant to disclose the true nature of underlying psychological and family difficulties, in particular paraphilias. It is therefore not surprising to find that incestuous fathers often report very few family difficulties (see Table 40–1). Furthermore, some of the disorders prevalent in this population, such as alcohol and drug abuse, make it more likely that relying exclusively on self-report measures will lead to an underestimation of true underlying psychopathology.

Parents who face investigations into their fitness may be motivated to hide the true extent of child and parental behavioral and emotional difficulties. The validity of child mental health diagnoses varies with sources and numbers of informants. Studies have found that diagnoses of externalizing behaviors such as attention-deficit/hyperactivity disorder or conduct disorder are more accurate if they include parent and teacher informants. Internalizing symptoms such as depression are most accurately assessed when the child is the main informant. Many studies of sexual abuse victims rely exclusively on the child or parent as the sole informant.

The nature of the sex abuse assault is inextricably intertwined with psychological outcome. Many studies fail to address the multitude of variables that may affect the results of the studies, such as the use of force, the identity of the perpetrator, the frequency and duration of assault, the use of threats and/or violence, the numbers of witnesses and/or victims (e.g., siblings), and where in the continuum of sexually assaultive behaviors the abuse falls (ranging from seductive "courting" behavior to fondling to penetration). The age at onset of abuse and age at disclosure are also major variables that are not often systematically investigated, although abuse of a preschooler likely reflects a different type of family pathology than abuse of an adolescent. The complexities of developmental differences may also result in a preschool child being asymptomatic immediately after the sexual abuse, but manifesting very serious psychosocial difficulties as an adolescent or as an adult.

The overwhelming majority of studies cited in this chapter fail to differentiate between psychopathology before and after disclosure. The immense impact of the disclosure of sexual abuse is felt throughout the family system. Symptoms such as depression, PTSD, anxiety, and marital discord may be a result of either the sexual abuse or its disclosure. Important variables that can greatly affect family functioning include the quality of support for the victim after disclosure, the nature of judicial and law enforcement interventions, whether the abuse was confirmed by child protective services, numbers and types of examinations of the victim, and whether the victim or the perpetrator was removed from the home.

The correlational nature of much of the research on incest makes it difficult to differentiate the effects of incest from these variables. Statistical analyses (such as the semipartial correlation approach) are often used incorrectly in abuse effect research, which leads researchers to draw incorrect conclusions from their data (Briere 1988). Until more prospective studies are completed and reported, it will be difficult to have a firm understanding of the relational aspects of incest.

Discussion

Diagnostic Issues in Incest

As awareness of the extent of incest has increased, there has been increasing dissatisfaction with the failure of DSM-III-R to address the specific psychiatric sequelae that result. Although diagnoses such as PTSD and adjustment disorders describe the effects of incest in a limited group of victims, these disorders fail to take into account a large group of victims who do not respond in a manner consistent with these categories. Furthermore, these diagnoses do not address the complexities of a process that is inextricably associated with family interactions.

One of the most commonly cited systems for organizing the symptoms that result from childhood sexual abuse is Summit's (1983) "child sexual abuse accommodation syndrome." The syndrome describes five commonly observed correlates of childhood sexual abuse: 1) secrecy; 2) helplessness; 3) entrapment and accommodation; 4) delayed, unconvincing disclosure; and 5) retraction. Summit based his "syndrome" on observations made during the course of consultation to sexual abuse treatment programs. He reported that these observations have been corroborated by thousands of professionals who recognized the syndrome when described to them during the course of sexual abuse training symposia. Many clinicians have found this child sexual abuse accommodation syndrome to be a valuable description of the dynamic that frequently results in sexual abuse going unreported and undisclosed. It is also helpful as a description of the process that accounts for much of the damage done to children by incest. However, this syndrome is less an empirically derived constellation of symptoms than it is a clinical description of the process observed during the course of a child's sexual victimization. Furthermore, the syndrome does not include many of the behavioral and affective symptoms often described in victims, such as difficulty with sexual behavior, chronic depression, and difficulties with intimacy.

PTSD is perhaps the most frequently used diagnosis for victims of incest (Deblinger et al. 1989; Goodwin 1985). The reexperiencing, arousal, and avoidance symptoms that make up this disorder have been found to be twice as prevalent in victims of sexual assault as in victims of other crimes (Kilpatrick et al. 1987). When researchers rely on referred samples, very high rates of PTSD are generally found in incest victims. Lindberg and Distad (1985) found PTSD in all of the 17 patients in their study who were survivors of incest, and Donaldson and Gardner (1985) reported PTSD in 96% of 26 women who were receiving therapy for the sequelae of sexual abuse. Similarly, in a referred sample of 31 sexually abused children, McLeer et al. (1988) reported a 48.4% incidence of PTSD (ranging from 75% of children abused by their fathers to 25% of those abused by trusted adults). However, when the relative incidence of PTSD in victims of incest is examined more systematically using nonclinical samples, it is clear that a significant proportion of victims do not meet the criteria for this disorder. Greenwald and Leitenberg (1990) found that 4% of 54 women in a nonclinical sample of sexual abuse victims reported moderate PTSD symptomatology currently and that only 17% might have met criteria in the past. In their investigation of 126 adult survivors of child sexual abuse, Kilpatrick et al. (1987) found that the current incidence of PTSD was 10% and the lifetime history was 36%.

Finkelhor (1988) criticized exclusive reliance on this diagnosis for sexual abuse victims. He noted that PTSD is a more appropriate diagnosis for "events" like crimes or combat and may be a less relevant diagnosis for incest, which is more of a "process" and is frequently not accompanied by violence or threats. Furthermore, symptoms frequently reported in the incest literature, such as self-blame, revictimization, and sexual difficulties, are not addressed. Finally, the few studies that document the incidence of PTSD in incest victims are plagued by methodological difficulties including small sample sizes, retrospective designs, use of referred samples, and/or failure to use structured measures.

Several researchers have proposed the use of more specific models to organize the symptoms associated with childhood sexual abuse. Finkelhor and Browne (1985) proposed a framework of four traumatogenic dynamics as essential features that account for the negative sequelae of sexual abuse: "traumatic sexualization," "betrayal," "stigmatization," and "powerlessness." They suggested that these dynamics are responsible for such symptoms as compulsive sexual behavior, clinging, self-mutilation, and dissociation, respectively. This model for understanding the traumatogenic dynamics of child sexual abuse has proven to be a valuable resource in assessment, treatment, and research. However, it is more a theoretical framework than a diagnostic category.

A National Summit Conference on Diagnosing Child Sexual Abuse was convened in 1985 to determine if there was a consensus among experts regarding a "sexually abused child's disorder" (Corwin 1988). The primary feature of this disorder was age-inappropriate sexual behavior or awareness. In addition, a number of other possible symptoms were identified, including dissociation and/or difficulty discussing the abuse. Nearly 100 professionals who attended the conference, including many experts on child sexual abuse, proposed that the disorder be included in DSM-III-R. Although a general consensus regarding the validity of the symptoms of the disorder was reported, there was disagreement about where in DSM-III-R the diagnosis should be placed (i.e., as a subcategory of PTSD or as a childhood disorder). The architects of DSM-III-R decided not to include this diagnosis in the manual or appendix, and the issue of a special diagnosis for victims of child sexual abuse was referred to committee for further study. There is a growing body of literature supporting age-inappropriate sexual behavior as a core symptom associated with child sexual abuse. Inclusion of such a diagnosis, however, has been criticized as an oversimplification of a complex social phenomenon that cannot be understood by focusing only on the victim without reference to family, cultural, and social forces (Salzinger 1990).

Spitzer et al. (1989) proposed a diagnosis—"disorders of extreme stress, not otherwise specified" (DESNOS)—that would be used to diagnose the prolonged and severe symptomatology that follows extreme stress but does not meet the criteria for any other diagnosis. As a result of extreme stress, alterations in six areas have been hypothesized: 1) regulation of affect and impulses, 2) attention or consciousness, 3) self-perception, 4) perception of the perpetrator, 5) relations with others, and 6) systems of meaning. The criteria for this diagnosis were developed from interviews with clinicians working with victims of extreme stress, systematic literature reviews, and several pilot studies investigating whether various victim groups generally show symptoms consistent with the proposed disorder. The validity of this diagnosis is currently being explored as part of the DSM-IV Field Trials on PTSD (results will appear in Volume IV of the *DSM-IV Sourcebook*). This diagnosis would apply not only to victims of sex abuse but also to victims of other types of extreme stress such as child physical abuse victims, Holocaust survivors, and individuals subject to long-term interpersonal victimization.

Pelcovitz and Kaplan (1990) reported data on the applicability of DESNOS to populations of extrafamilial sexual abuse survivors. In a sample of 35 victims of extrafamilial sexual abuse who were assessed through structured interviews, Pelcovitz and Kaplan found that only 11% met criteria for PTSD but that most of these children exhibited DESNOS symptoms, including difficulty modulating anger, persistent preoccupation with the victimization experience, and persistent shame. Reasons that might explain the low incidence of PTSD in this group include the fact that the evaluations were done very soon after disclosure of the abuse and that the victims were from intact, affluent, and very supportive families. In a related study (Pelcovitz and Kaplan 1991) that relied on therapist interviews, a roughly equal number of incest and extrafamilial victims were assessed. Unlike the first study, the children were evaluated after they had been in individual or group therapy for some time. Results supported a much higher PTSD incidence than the first study (57%). The main findings of this study were that there were significantly more DESNOS symptoms exhibited by the incest victims than by victims of extrafamilial sexual abuse ($P < .01$) and that there were significantly more PTSD than DESNOS symptoms in the combined group of extrafamilial and incest victims. Despite this, most of the victims were seen as having a number of DESNOS symptoms not addressed in the PTSD criteria, including guilt, anger, shame, feeling set apart, and feeling permanently damaged.

The PTSD Field Trials for DSM-IV systematically investigated the incidence of DESNOS symptoms in a group of 500 subjects across five national sites. Many of these subjects had histories of sex abuse, and the results of the Field Trials, which will appear in Volume IV of the *DSM-IV Sourcebook*, should shed light on the relative prevalence of DESNOS symptoms in many types of traumatized populations, including incest victims.

Although an inclusive diagnosis of DESNOS would be more parsimonious than separate diagnoses for each type of extreme violence, such a diagnosis fails to take into account the complex interactional quality of incest. Further, data from systematic investigations of DESNOS symptoms in populations of incest victims are relatively sparse.

Recommendations

It is difficult to envision a DSM-IV diagnosis for incest that does not recognize that incest is a trauma involving relational dysfunction. Unfortunately, there are a number of serious difficulties with including such a diagnosis at this time.

1. The literature does not support a clear-cut family dynamic for incest. Although a very rich clinical literature exists, there is not yet strong empirical support for a specific family structure associated with an increased risk of incest. Future research may justify inclusion of specific criteria for an incestuous family or a

parent-child relational disorder, but the fact that systematic efforts at research in this area began only recently precludes inclusion of such criteria in DSM-IV.
2. Although DSM-III-R has a specific caveat concerning the use of diagnostic categories for forensic purposes, this warning is often ignored (Shuman 1989). An unusually high standard of accuracy is needed in the area of child sexual abuse because, of all diagnostic areas, incest is perhaps the one that is most likely to be misused in forensic settings. Following disclosure, intrafamilial child sex abuse is typically considered by both family and criminal courts. There is increasing recognition that there has been a substantial increase in false allegations of incest in recent years, particularly in custody disputes (Kaplan and Kaplan 1981). In addition, there is increasing civil litigation involving adult survivors of child sexual abuse. Literature describing a subtype of incest in which fathers or stepfathers sexually molest children outside their families as well as their own children implies that many cases of incest may reflect the individual psychopathology of the perpetrator and its effects on other family members, but not a more general family dysfunction. The danger exists that in such situations an allegation of actual incest may be falsely discounted because such a family fails to meet the criteria of incest relational disorder.

In light of the current state of the empirical literature, it is our opinion that it is premature to include specific criteria for incest as a relational disorder in DSM-IV. However, we do feel that considering incest in a relational context has a number of major advantages, including helping to train clinicians to assess and treat all family members affected by intrafamilial sexual abuse. Common sense dictates that, at the very least, incest is a major dysfunction in the parent-child relationship. We recommend that any specific diagnosis of incest take into account knowledge from future studies obtained from dysfunctional family and parent-child relationships. Until the research database warrants formulating specific criteria necessary for a diagnosis of an incest relational disorder, we recommend that DSM-IV consider including incest in two places.

1. As a V code "parent-child relational problem with sexual abuse of child." At this time, operationalized criteria are thought to be premature.
2. Far more is known about the psychiatric symptoms associated with incest victimization on an individual level than on a family level. Including incest in a DSM-IV section that addresses victims of stress, but without specifying specific incest-related criteria, would seem to be warranted given the current state of the art of the incest literature.

References

Abel G, Becker J, Cunningham-Rathner J: Multiple paraphiliac diagnoses among sex offenders. Bull Am Acad Psychiatry Law 16:153–168, 1988

Adams-Tucker C: Proximate effects of sexual abuse in childhood: a report of 28 children. Am J Psychiatry 139:1252–1256, 1982

Aiosa-Karpas CJ, Karpas R, Pelcovitz D, et al: Gender identification and sex role attribution in sexually abused adolescent females. J Am Acad Child Adolesc Psychiatry 30:266–271, 1991

Alexander PC, Lupfer SL: Family characteristics and long-term consequences associated with sexual abuse. Arch Sex Behav 16:235–245, 1987

American Psychiatric Association: Diagnostic and Statistical Manual of Mental Disorders, 3rd Edition, Revised. Washington, DC, American Psychiatric Association, 1987

Araji S, Finkelhor D: Abusers: a review of the research, in A Sourcebook on Child Sexual Abuse. Edited by Finkelhor D, Araji S, Baron L, et al. Newbury Park, CA, Sage Publications, 1986, pp 89–118

August RL, Forman BD: A comparison of sexually abused and nonsexually abused children's behavioral responses to anatomically correct dolls. Child Psychiatry Hum Dev 20:39–47, 1989

Ballard DT, Blair GD, Devereaux S, et al: A comparative profile of the incest perpetrator: background characteristics, abuse history, and use of social skills, in The Incest Perpetrator: a Family Member No One Wants to Treat. Edited by Horton AL, Johnson BL, Roundy LM, et al. Newbury Park, CA, Sage, 1990, pp 43–64

Beck JC, van der Kolk B: Reports of childhood incest and current behavior of chronically hospitalized psychotic women. Am J Psychiatry 144:1474–1476, 1987

Becker JV, Skinner LJ, Abel GG, et al: Incidence and types of sexual dysfunctions in rape and incest victims. J Sex Marital Ther 8:65–74, 1982

Blick LC, Porter FS: Group therapy with female adolescent incest victims, in Handbook of Clinical Intervention in Child Sexual Abuse. Edited by Sgroi SM. Lexington, MA, Lexington Books, 1982, pp 147–176

Briere J: Controlling for family variables in abuse effects research. Journal of Interpersonal Violence 3:80–89, 1988

Briere J, Runtz M: Post sexual abuse trauma. Journal of Interpersonal Violence 2:367–379, 1987

Briere J, Runtz M: Symptomatology associated with childhood sexual victimization in a nonclinical adult sample. Child Abuse Negl 12:51–59, 1988

Briere J, Runtz M: The trauma symptom checklist (TSC-33): early data on a new scale. Journal of Interpersonal Violence 4:151–165, 1989

Briere J, Zaidi LY: Sexual abuse histories and sequelae in female psychiatric emergency room patients. Am J Psychiatry 146:1602–1606, 1989

Browning DH, Boatman B: Incest: children at risk. Am J Psychiatry 134:69–72, 1977

Bryer JB, Nelson BA, Miller JB, et al: Childhood sexual and physical abuse as factors in adult psychiatric illness. Am J Psychiatry 144:1426–1430, 1987

Cavaiola AA, Schiff M: Behavioral sequelae of physical and/or sexual abuse in adolescents. Child Abuse Negl 12:181–188, 1988

Cavaiola AA, Schiff M: Self-esteem in abused chemically dependent adolescents. Child Abuse Negl 13:327–334, 1989

Chu JA, Dill DL: Dissociative symptoms in relation to childhood physical and sexual abuse. Am J Psychiatry 147:887–892, 1990

Cole PM, Woolger C: Incest survivors: the relation of their perceptions of their parents and their own parenting attitudes. Child Abuse Negl 13:409–416, 1989

Conte JR: Sexual abuse and the family: a critical analysis, in Treating Incest: A Multimodal Systems Perspective. Edited by Trepper TS, Ballett MJ. New York, Haworth Press, 1986, pp 113–125

Conte JR: The incest offender: an overview and introduction, in The Incest Perpetrator. Edited by Horton AL, Johnson B, Roundy L, et al. Newbury Park, CA, Sage Publications, 1990, pp 19–28

Conte JR, Schuerman JR: Factors associated with an increased impact of child sexual abuse. Child Abuse Negl 11:201–211, 1987

Coons PM, Bowman ES, Pellow TA, et al: Post-traumatic aspects of the treatment of victims of sexual abuse and incest. Psychiatr Clin North Am 12:325–335, 1989

Corwin D: Early diagnosis of child sexual abuse: diminishing the lasting effects, in Lasting Effects of Child Sexual Abuse. Edited by Wyatt G, Powell G. Newbury Park, CA, Sage Publications, 1988, pp 251–269

Craine LS, Henson CE, Colliver JA, et al: Prevalence of a history of sexual abuse among female psychiatric patients in a state hospital system. Hosp Community Psychiatry 39:300–304, 1988

Deblinger E, McLeer SV, Atkins MS, et al: Post-traumatic stress in sexually abused, physically abused, and nonabused children. Child Abuse Negl 13:403–408, 1989

Donaldson MA, Gardner R: Diagnosis and treatment of traumatic stress among women after childhood incest, in Trauma and its Wake. Edited by Figley CR. New York, Brunner/Mazel, 1985, pp 356–377

Edwall GE, Hoffmann NG, Harrison PA: Psychological correlates of sexual abuse in adolescent girls in chemical dependency treatment. Adolescence 24:279–288, 1989

Emslie GJ, Rosenfeld A: Incest reported by children and adolescents hospitalized for severe psychiatric problems. Am J Psychiatry 140:708–711, 1983

Everson MD, Hunter WM, Runyon DK, et al: Maternal support following disclosure of incest. Am J Orthopsychiatry 59:197–207, 1989

Fagot BI, Hagan R, Youngblade LM, et al: A comparison of the play behaviors of sexually abused, physically abused, and nonabused preschool children. Topics in Early Childhood Special Education 9:88–100, 1989

Faller KC: The myth of the "collusive" mother. Journal of Interpersonal Violence 3:190–196, 1988

Faller KC: Sexual abuse by paternal caretakers: a comparison of abusers who are biological fathers in intact families, stepfathers, and noncustodial fathers, in The Incest Perpetrator: a Family Member No One Wants to Treat. Edited by Horton AL, Johnson BL, Roundy LM, et al. Newbury Park, CA, Sage, 1990, pp 65–73

Finkelhor D: The trauma of child sexual abuse: two models, in Lasting Effects of Child Sexual Abuse. Edited by Wyatt G, Powell G. Newbury Park, CA, Sage Publications, 1988, pp 61–82

Finkelhor D, Browne A: The traumatic impact of child sexual abuse: a conceptualization. Am J Orthopsychiatry 55:530–541, 1985

Finkelhor D, Hotaling G, Lewis IA, et al: Sexual abuse in a national survey of adult men and women: prevalence, characteristics, and risk factors. Child Abuse Negl 14:19–28, 1990

Friedrich WN, Einbender AJ: Psychological functioning and behavior of sexually abused girls. J Consult Clin Psychol 57:155–157, 1989

Friedrich WN, Beilke RL, Urguiza AJ: Children from sexually abusive families. Journal of Interpersonal Violence 2:391–402, 1987

Friedrich WN, Beilke RL, Urguiza AJ: Behavior problems in young sexually abused boys. Journal of Interpersonal Violence 3:21–28, 1988

Gale J, Thompson RJ, Moran T, et al: Sexual abuse in young children: its clinical presentation and characteristic patterns. Child Abuse Negl 12:163–170, 1988

Goodwin J: Post-traumatic symptoms in incest victims, in Post-Traumatic Stress Disorder in Children. Edited by Eth S, Pynoos RS. Los Angeles, CA, American Psychiatric Press, 1985, pp 157–168

Gomez-Schwartz B, Horowitz JM, Sauzier M: Severity of emotional distress among sexually abused preschool, school-age, and adolescent children. Hosp Community Psychiatry 36:503–508, 1985

Greenwald E, Leitenberg H: Posttraumatic stress disorder in a nonclinical and nonstudent sample of adult women sexually abused as children. Journal of Interpersonal Violence 5:217–228, 1990

Groff MG, Hubble LM: A comparison of the father-daughter and stepfather-daughter incest. Criminal Justice and Behavior 11:461–475, 1984

Groth AN, Hobson WF, Gary TS: The child molester: clinical observations. Social Work and Human Sexuality 1:129–144, 1982

Hall R, Tice L, Beresford T, et al: Sexual abuse in patients with anorexia and bulimia. Psychometrics 30:73–79, 1989

Hart LE, Mader L, Griffith K, et al: Effects of sexual and physical abuse: a comparison of adolescent inpatients. Child Psychiatry Hum Dev 20:49–57, 1989

Harter S, Alexander PC, Neimeyer RA: Long-term effects of incestuous child abuse in college women: social adjustment, social cognition, and family characteristics. J Consult Clin Psychol 56:5–8, 1988

Hathaway SR, McKinley JC: Minnesota Multiphasic Personality Inventory. Minneapolis, MN, University of Minnesota, 1943

Herman J, Hirschman L: Families at risk for father-daughter incest. Am J Psychiatry 138:967–970, 1981

Herman JL, Perry JC, van der Kolk BA: Childhood trauma in borderline personality disorder. Am J Psychiatry 146:490–495, 1989

Hunter JA: A comparison of the psychosocial maladjustment of adult males and females sexually molested as children. Journal of Interpersonal Violence 6:205–217, 1991

Hunter JA, Childers SE, Gerald R, et al: An examination of variables differentiating clinical subtypes of incestuous child molesters. International Journal of Offender Therapy and Comparative Criminology 34:95–104, 1990

Jackson JL, Calhoun KS, Amick AE, et al: Young adult women who report childhood intrafamilial sexual abuse: subsequent adjustment. Arch Sex Behav 19:211–221, 1990

James B, Nasjleti M: Treating Sexually Abused Children. Palo Alto, CA, Consulting Psychologists Press, 1983

Jampole L, Weber MK: An assessment of the behavior of sexually abused and nonsexually abused children with anatomically correct dolls. Child Abuse Negl 11:187–192, 1987

Kaplan SL, Kaplan SJ: The child's accusation of sexual abuse during a divorce and custody struggle. Hillside Journal of Clinical Psychiatry 3:81–95, 1981

Kempe R, Kempe CH: Child Abuse. Cambridge, MA, Harvard University Press, 1978

Kempe R, Kempe CH (eds): The Common Secret. New York, WH Freeman, 1984

Kilpatrick DG, Saunders BE, Vernon LJ, et al: Criminal victimization: lifetime prevalence, reporting to police, and psychological impact. Crime and Delinquency 33:479–489, 1987

Kirkland K, Bauer C: MMPI traits of incestuous fathers. Journal of Criminal Psychology 38:645–649, 1982

Kolko DJ, Moser JT, Weldy SR: Behavioral/emotional indicators of sexual abuse in child psychiatric inpatients: a controlled comparison with physical abuse. Child Abuse Negl 12:529–541, 1988

Langevin R, Paitich D, Freeman R, et al: Personality characteristics and sexual anomalies in males. Canadian Journal of Behavioural Science 10:222–238, 1978

Lanktree C, Briere J: Early data on the Trauma Symptom Checklist for Children. Paper presented at the annual meeting of the American Psychological Association, Boston, MA, August 1990

Levang CA: Interactional communication patterns in father/daughter incest families. Journal of Psychology and Human Sexuality 1:53–68, 1989

Lindberg FH, Distad LJ: Post-traumatic stress disorders in women who experienced childhood incest. Child Abuse Negl 9:329–334, 1985

Lipovsky JA, Saunders BE, Murphy SM: Depression, anxiety, and behavior problems among victims of father-child sexual assault and nonabused siblings. Journal of Interpersonal Violence 4:452–468, 1989

Livingston R: Sexually and physically abused children. J Am Acad Child Adolesc Psychiatry 26:413–415, 1987

Lustig N, Dresser JW, Spellman SW, et al: Incest: a family group survival pattern. Arch Gen Psychiatry 14:31–40, 1966

Macholka P, Pittman FS, Flomenhaft K: Incest as a family affair. Fam Process 6:98–116, 1967

Madonna PG, Van Scoyk S, Jones D: Family interactions within incest and nonincest families. Am J Psychiatry 148:46–49, 1991

Maisch H: Incest. New York, Stein & Day, 1972

Mannarino AP, Cohen JA, Gregor M: Emotional and behavioral difficulties in sexually abused girls. Journal of Interpersonal Violence 4:437–451, 1989

Marshall WL, Barbaree HE, Christophe D: Sexual offenders against female children: sexual preferences for age of victims and type of behavior. Canadian Journal of Behavioral Science 18:424–439, 1986

McCormack A, Janus MD, Burgess AW: Runaway youths and sexual victimization: gender differences in an adolescent runaway population. Child Abuse Negl 10:387–395, 1986

McLeer SV, Deblinger E, Atkins MS, et al: Post-traumatic stress disorder in sexually abused children. J Am Acad Child Adolesc Psychiatry 27:650–654, 1988

Meiselman KC: Personality characteristics of incest history psychotherapy patients: a research note. Arch Sex Behav 9:195–197, 1980

Miller BA, Gondoli DM, Downs WR, et al: The role of childhood sexual abuse in the development of alcoholism in women. Violence and Victims 2:157–172, 1987

Miller BA, Gondoli DM, Downs WR: Thematic analyses of female sexual abuse victims: alcoholic women vs comparison group. Violence and Victims 3:248–252, 1988

Miller-Perrin CL, Wurtele SK, Kondrick PA: Sexually abused and nonabused children's conceptions of personal body safety. Child Abuse Negl 14:99–112, 1990

Millon T: Millon Clinical Multiaxial Inventory. Minneapolis, MN, National Computer Systems, 1983

Milner JS, Robertson KR: Comparison of physical abusers, intrafamilial sexual child abusers, and child neglecters. Journal of Interpersonal Violence 5:37–48, 1990
Morrison J: Childhood histories of women with somatization disorder. Am J Psychiatry 146:239–241, 1989
Murphy SM, Kilpatrick DG, Amick-McMullan A, et al: Current psychological functioning of child sexual assault survivors. Journal of Interpersonal Violence 3:55–79, 1988
New York State Department of Social Services: Suspected Child Abuse and Maltreatment: Identification and Management in Hospitals and Clinics. Albany, NY, 1991
Ogata SN, Silk KR, Goodrich S, et al: Childhood sexual and physical abuse in adult patients with borderline personality disorder. Am J Psychiatry 147:1008–1013, 1990
Olson DH, Russel CS, Sprenkle DH: Circumplex model of marital and family systems, VI: theoretical update. Fam Process 22:69–83, 1983
Orr DP, Downes MC: Self-concept of adolescent sexual abuse victims. Journal Youth and Adolescence 14:401–410, 1985
Owen TH: Personality traits of female psychotherapy patients with a history of incest. J Pers Assess 48:606–608, 1984
Panton JH: MMPI profile configurations associated with incestuous and non-incestuous child molesting. Psychol Rep 45:335–338, 1979
Parker H, Parker S: Father-daughter sexual abuse: an emerging perspective. Am J Orthopsychiatry 56:531–549, 1986
Parker S, Parker H: Female victims of child sexual abuse: adult adjustment. Journal of Family Violence 6:183–197, 1991
Paveza GJ: Risk factors in father-daughter child sexual abuse: a case-control study. Journal of Interpersonal Violence 3:290–306, 1988
Pelcovitz D, Kaplan S: Extrafamilial sexual abuse of children: a pilot study of a proposed new diagnosis. Paper presented at the annual meeting of the American Academy of Child Psychiatry, Chicago, IL, October 1990
Pelcovitz D, Kaplan S: DSM-IV PTSD Field Trials update: PTSD in physically abused adolescents, adolescent cancer survivors, and their mothers. Paper presented at the annual convention of the International Society for Traumatic Stress Studies, Washington, DC, October 1991
Perosa L, Perosa S: The uses of a bipolar item format for FACES III: a reconsideration. Journal of Marital and Family Therapy 16:187–199, 1990
Polit DF, White CM, Morton TD: Child sexual abuse and premarital intercourse among high-risk adolescents. Journal Adolescent Health Care 11:231–234, 1990
Prentky RA, Knight RA, Sims-Knight JE, et al: Developmental antecedents of sexual aggression. Development and Psychopathology 1:153–169, 1989
Putnam F: Dissociation as a response to extreme trauma, in Childhood Antecedents of Multiple Personality. Edited by Kluft RP. Washington, DC, American Psychiatric Press, 1985, pp 65–98
Quinsey VL, Chaplin TC, Carrigan WF: Sexual preferences among incestuous and nonincestuous child molesters. Behavior Therapy 10:562–565, 1979
Rimsza ME, Berg RA, Locke A: Sexual abuse: somatic and emotional reactions. Child Abuse Negl 12:201–208, 1988
Roland B, Zelhart P, Dubes R: MMPI correlates of college women who reported experiencing child/adult sexual contact with father, stepfather, or with other persons. Psychol Rep 64:1159–1162, 1989

Russell DEH: The incidence and prevalence of intrafamilial and extrafamilial sexual abuse of female children, in Handbook on Sexual Abuse of Children: Assessment and Treatment Issues. Edited by Walker L. New York, Springer, 1988, pp 19–36

Rutter M: Isle of Wight revisited: twenty-five years of child psychiatric epidemiology. J Am Acad Child Adolesc Psychiatry 28:633–653, 1989

Sagatun IJ, Prince L: Incest family dynamics: family members' perceptions before and after therapy (Special Issue: Treatment of sex offenders in social work and mental health settings). Journal of Social Work and Human Sexuality 7:69–87, 1988

Salt P, Myer M, Coleman L, et al: The myth of the mother as "accomplice" to child sexual abuse, in Child Sexual Abuse: the Initial Effects. Edited by Gomes-Schwartz BG, Horowitz J, Caldorelli A. Newbury Park, CA, Sage Publications, 1990, pp 109–131

Salzinger S: Review of Lasting Effects of Child Sexual Abuse, edited by Wyatt G, Powell G. Child and Family Behavior Therapy 12:87–90, 1990

Sansonnet-Hayden H, Haley G, Marriage K: Sexual abuse and psychopathology in hospitalized adolescents. J Am Acad Child Adolesc Psychiatry 26:753–757, 1987

Saunders B, McClure S, Murphy S: Final report: profile of incest perpetrators indicating treatability, I. Charleston, SC, Crime Victims Research and Treatment Center, 1986

Saunders BE, Villeponteaux LA, Lipovsky JA, et al: Child sexual assault as a risk factor for mental disorders among women: a community survey. Journal of Interpersonal Violence 7:189–204, 1992

Scott RL, Stone DA: MMPI profile constellations in incest families. J Consult Clin Psychol 54:364–368, 1986

Sedney MA, Brooks B: Factors associated with a history of childhood sexual experience in a nonclinical female population. Journal of the American Academy of Child Psychiatry 23:215–218, 1984

Sgroi SM: Family treatment of child sexual abuse. Journal of Social Work and Human Sexuality 1:109–128, 1982

Shapiro JP, Leifer M, Martone MW, et al: Multimethod assessment of depression in sexually abused girls. J Pers Assess 55:234–248, 1990

Shuman DW: The diagnostic and statistical manual of mental disorders in the courts. Bull Am Acad Psychiatry Law 17:25–32, 1989

Singer MI, Petchers MK: The relationship between sexual abuse and substance abuse among psychiatrically hospitalized adolescents. Child Abuse Negl 13:319–325, 1989

Sirles EA, Franke PJ: Factors influencing mothers' reactions to intrafamily sexual abuse. Child Abuse Negl 13:131–139, 1989

Snell JE, Rosenwald RJ, Robey A: The wife-beater's wife. Arch Gen Psychiatry 11:107–112, 1964

Spitzer R, Kaplan S, Pelcovitz D: Victimization Sequelae Disorder: a proposed addition to DSM-IV. Paper presented at the annual meeting of the American Psychiatric Association, San Francisco, CA, May 1989

Stein JA, Golding JM, Siegel J, et al: Long-term psychological sequelae of child sexual abuse, in Lasting Effects of Child Sexual Abuse. Edited by Wyatt GE, Powell GJ. Newbury Park, CA, Sage Publications, 1988, pp 135–154

Stiffman AR: Physical and sexual abuse in runaway youths. Child Abuse Negl 13:417–426, 1989

Stovall G, Craig RJ: Mental representations of physically and sexually abused latency aged females. Child Abuse Negl 14:233–242, 1990

Summit RC: The child sexual abuse accommodation syndrome. Child Abuse Negl 7:177–193, 1983

Swett C, Surrey J, Cohen C: Sexual and physical abuse histories and psychiatric symptoms among male psychiatric outpatients. Am J Psychiatry 147:632–636, 1990

Tong L, Oates K, McDowell M: Personality development following sexual abuse. Child Abuse Negl 11:371–383, 1987

Trepper TS, Barrett MJ: Systemic Treatment of Incest. New York, Brunner/Mazel, 1989

Truesdell DL, McNeil JS, Deschner J: The incident of wife abuse in incestuous families. Social Work 31:138–142, 1986

Tsai M, Wagner NN: Therapy groups for women sexually molested as children. Arch Sex Behav 7:417–427, 1978

U.S. Department of Health and Human Services: Study Findings: Study of National Incidence and Prevalence of Child Abuse and Neglect. Washington, DC, U.S. Department of Health and Human Services, 1988

Wald BK, Archer RP, Winstead BA: Rorschach characteristics of mothers of incest victims. J Pers Assess 55:417–425, 1990

Westen D, Ludolph P, Misle B, et al: Physical and sexual abuse in adolescent girls with borderline personality disorder. Am J Orthopsychiatry 60:55–66, 1990

White S, Halpin BM, Strom GA, et al: Behavioral comparisons of young sexually abused, neglected and nonreferred children. Journal of Clinical Child Psychiatry 17:53–61, 1988

Williams LM, Finkelhor D: The characteristics of incestuous fathers, in Handbook of Sexual Assault. Edited by Marshall WL, Laws DR, Barbaree HE. New York, Plenum, 1990, pp 231–255

Wyatt GE: The aftermath of child sexual abuse of African American and White American women: the victim's experience. Journal of Family Violence 5:61–81, 1990

Wyatt GE, Newcomb MD: Internal and external mediators of women's sexual abuse in childhood. J Consult Clin Psychol 58:758–767, 1990

Wyatt G, Peters S: Issues in the definition of child sexual abuse in prevalence research. Child Abuse Negl 10:231–240, 1986

Section VI

Cultural Issues for DSM-IV

Introduction to Section VI

Cultural Issues for DSM-IV

Juan E. Mezzich, M.D., Ph.D., Arthur Kleinman, M.D.,
Horacio Fabrega Jr., M.D., Delores L. Parron, Ph.D.,
Byron J. Good, Ph.D., Keh-Ming Lin, M.D., M.P.H., and
Spero M. Manson, Ph.D.

In line with Ortega y Gassett's dictum, "I am I and my circumstance," mental disorders do not happen in organismic isolation. Likewise, the proposals for enhancing the cultural validity of DSM-IV have not emerged in a vacuum. Their general circumstance is a biopsychosocial framework that is presently fighting a tough battle with organicist reductionism to remain the weltanschauung of contemporary psychiatry. Curiously, this is happening while some of the most eminent thinkers in general medicine (e.g., Feinstein 1989) are increasingly concerned with adaptive functioning and quality of life, and the scope of the ICD-10 (World Health Organization 1992) has been broadened to incorporate contextual factors to deal more effectively with the complexity of the health field. The need for a biopsychosocial-cultural base is thus, as pointed out by Rogler (1993), an issue of scientific accuracy.

The view that psychiatric diagnosis must be culturally informed (Fabrega 1974) reflects the position that the proper focus of clinical work is the person of the patient. As articulated by Strauss (1992), rather than treating self-contained disorders, psychiatrists and other mental health professionals treat and care for people who happen to experience disorders and other health-related problems.

Furthermore, the importance of culture for all diagnostic work has been made increasingly clear by a new generation of cross-cultural psychiatric research (e.g., Kleinman 1988). Culture has a profound influence on the experience and expression of symptoms, creating idioms of distress and prototypical behavioral patterns that are unique to societies, cultures, and subcultures. As treatments become more specifically linked to diagnosis, giving explicit attention to cultural issues in DSM-IV and in the diagnostic process thus takes on special urgency. These issues are more compelling because the DSM has high international visibility, and multiculturalism is being increasingly recognized as a central feature in the United States. The strong presence of diverse communities of African (or black) Americans, Asian Americans, American Indians (or Native Americans), and Latinos (or Hispanic Americans) is, in fact, growing both in magnitude and in cultural differentiation, and evidence suggests that misdiagnosis occurs more frequently among members of minority populations (Good 1993). The flow of migrants and refugees who are enriching and challenging the fabric of society must also be considered. Even more broadly, there is increasing awareness of multiculturality as a phenomenon that is relevant, one way or another, to all of us.

In 1990, as the process of developing a new edition of the American Psychiatric Association's diagnostic manual took form, the leadership of this serial enterprise decided, for the first time, to explore the possibility of seriously taking culture into consideration. Experts working at the interface of psychiatry and anthropology were contacted. Perceiving an unusual opportunity to advance the field, they responded positively to the overture.

A benchmark Conference on Culture and Psychiatric Diagnosis, held in Pittsburgh, Pennsylvania, in April 1991, offered a forum for a meeting of minds. Under the sponsorship of the National Institute of Mental Health and the American Psychiatric Association, 15 nosologists (members of the DSM-IV Task Force) chaired by Allen Frances, M.D., met with 45 experts in cultural psychiatry (both anthropological scholars and representatives of prominent ethnic minorities) coordinated by Juan Mezzich, M.D., Ph.D. (also a member of the DSM-IV Task Force), Arthur Kleinman, M.D., Horacio Fabrega, M.D., and Delores Parron, Ph.D. Major conclusions of the conference included the identification of specific points for culturally enhancing DSM-IV (i.e., the introduction to the diagnostic manual, cultural considerations pertinent to the various diagnostic categories and the multiaxial schema, and a glossary of culture-bound syndromes), the need to appraise the ethnic representativeness of the DSM-IV field trial samples, and plans to prepare pertinent research documentation and educational materials (e.g., Mezzich et al. 1996), all of this to be potentiated by the formation of a strong study group.

In connection with the last point, the Office for Special Populations of the National Institute of Mental Health accorded crucial sponsorship and funding to make possible the formation of a Culture and Diagnosis Group. This has included 50 cultural experts, both clinicians and scholars, coordinated by a steering committee. (J. E. Mezzich, A. Kleinman, H. Fabrega, D. Parron, B. Good, K.-M. Lin, and S. Manson. G. Johnson-Powell also participated during the initial phase of the project.) For each identified task, this committee designated a writing work group and a primary reader, with advisers and consultants added as needed. Literature reviews were undertaken, and extensive communications, both written and oral (including conference calls), were maintained among the scholars working on the project.

An initial booklet of proposals (Mezzich et al. 1992) was produced and distributed to the DSM-IV Task Force members in the spring of 1992. Further scholarly work involved the expansion of the cultural proposals and the preparation of papers supporting such proposals, which were assembled and submitted to the DSM-IV Task Force in January 1993 (Mezzich et al. 1993a). A workshop on Culture and Psychiatric Diagnosis was then held at Redondo Beach, California, in February 1993 to appraise the early drafts of DSM-IV vis-à-vis the proposals generated up to that point and to discuss how to proceed. Additional literature reviews, written consultations, and conference calls involving the primary writing groups and the steering committee led to the development of revised cultural proposals, which were submitted to the DSM-IV Task Force as the revisions were completed between June and September 1993 (Mezzich et al. 1993b).

The cultural proposals accepted by the DSM-IV Task Force for incorporation into the manual are listed below. The specific wording of these contributions, as is the case with all components of DSM-IV, has been revised extensively throughout 1993.

Cultural Statement for the Introduction to the Manual

This statement alerts the clinician to the challenge of using DSM-IV thoughtfully in a multicultural society. It outlines the concepts of culture and ethnicity, refers to the substantial anthropological research findings underlying the specific recommendations offered, and encourages the clinician to be aware of his or her ethnocentric biases as well as to keep in mind the personal perspectives of the patient being seen.

Cultural Considerations for Various Diagnostic Categories

Paragraphs are included in the text describing specific psychiatric disorders that summarize information on cultural variations in distress idioms, symptom patterns, dysfunctions, correlates, and course of the disorder. The aim of these inclusions is to stimulate a culturally sensitive use of the corresponding diagnostic criteria. As justified by available research findings, statements have been prepared for the following major classes of mental disorders:

1. Child-onset disorders
2. Cognitive impairment disorders
3. Substance related disorders
4. Schizophrenia and other psychotic disorders
5. Mood disorders
6. Anxiety disorders
7. Somatoform disorders
8. Dissociative disorders
9. Sexual disorders
10. Eating disorders
11. Sleep disorders
12. Impulse control disorders
13. Adjustment disorders
14. Personality disorders
15. Other clinically significant conditions

Additionally, some comments were offered for factitious disorders, but given the scarcity of cultural research in this area, no specific cultural considerations were developed.

The inclusion of a category for religious and spiritual problems was proposed for DSM-IV because of its potential utility in diagnosis and treatment. For this reason, the Task Force on DSM-IV solicited a literature review on the topic. Although the proposal was not made in time to be included in the *DSM-IV Options Book* (American Psychiatric Association 1991), the literature review done on this proposed category is included here.

Cultural Annotations for the Multiaxial Schema

Although the multiaxial system embodies most patently the biopsychosocial underpinnings of DSM-IV, proper use of its purportedly standardized typologies and scales requires attention to how cultural factors can influence the standing of the individual being assessed. This applies to all mental disorders on Axis I and especially on Axis II; to general medical disorders (Axis III), which can be differentially distributed across ethnic groups and often display complex interactions with psychopathology; to psychosocial stressors (Axis IV), which are particularly frequent in minority and multi-disadvantaged populations; and to functioning levels (Axis V), the accurate rating of which can be enhanced by considering the individual's reference group.

Cultural Formulation Guideline

This contribution, to be included in the appendix of DSM-IV, evolved relatively recently but has attracted considerable interest. It supplements the nomothetic or standardized diagnostic ratings with an idiographic statement, emphasizing the perspectives of the patient's personal experience and the corresponding cultural reference group. Its components include the cultural identity of the patient, cultural explanations of the individual's illness, cultural factors related to psychosocial environment and functioning, cultural elements of the relationship between the individual and the clinician, and overall cultural assessment for diagnosis and care. Field trials with various ethnic groups have yielded illustrative case formulations.

Glossary of Culture-Bound Syndromes and Idioms of Distress

This collection, to be placed in the DSM-IV appendix, defines some of the folk or popular psychiatric syndromes and idioms (not always pathological) for describing distress that may present in clinical practice in the multicultural United States society. It illustrates the importance of an anthropological framework for understanding any disorder. Culture-bound syndromes are often organized with regard to perceived cause as well as symptom clusters, representing both distinctive forms of illness experience and local approaches to explaining and classifying them. The glossary focuses on items that are widely acknowledged both in non-Western societies and in North America—for example, among African Americans (e.g., *rootwork, falling out*), American Indians (e.g., *ghost sickness, pibloktoq*), Asian Americans (e.g., *shenjing shuairuo, taijing kyofusho*), and Latinos (e.g., *susto, ataque de nervios*). Also recognized are Western culture-bound syndromes, found almost exclusively or in distinctive form in Western countries or Westernized segments of other societies (e.g., anorexia nervosa, multiple personality disorder).

In this section of the *DSM-IV Sourcebook,* a set of short chapters supporting the proposals outlined here is presented. They summarize the pertinent literature and articulate key arguments. As such, they are integral to enhancing the cultural sensitivity and suitability of DSM-IV within a biopsychosocial framework, consistent with an attitude of respect for and interest in the totality, uniqueness, and depth of each patient.

References

American Psychiatric Association: DSM-IV Options Book: Work in Progress. Washington, DC, American Psychiatric Association, 1991

Fabrega H: Disease and Social Behavior: an Interdisciplinary Perspective. Cambridge, MA, MIT Press, 1974

Feinstein AR: ICD, POR, and DRG: unsolved scientific problems in the nosology of clinical medicine. Arch Intern Med 148:2269–2274, 1989

Good BJ: Culture, diagnosis and comorbidity. Cult Med Psychiatry 16:427–446, 1993

Kleinman A: Rethinking Psychiatry: From Cultural Category to Personal Experience. New York, Free Press, 1988

Mezzich JE, Kleinman A, Fabrega H, et al: Cultural Proposals for DSM-IV. Technical report submitted to the DSM-IV Task Force by the Steering Committee of the Group on Culture and Diagnosis. Pittsburgh, PA, National Institute of Mental Health, April 1992

Mezzich JE, Kleinman A, Fabrega H, et al: Cultural Proposals and Supporting Papers for DSM-IV. Technical report submitted to the DSM-IV Task Force by the Steering Committee of the Group on Culture and Diagnosis. Pittsburgh, PA, National Institute of Mental Health, January 1993a

Mezzich JE, Kleinman A, Fabrega H, et al: Revised Cultural Proposals for DSM-IV. Technical report submitted to the DSM-IV Task Force by the Steering Committee of the Group on Culture and Diagnosis. Pittsburgh, PA, National Institute of Mental Health, September 1993b

Mezzich JE, Kleinman A, Fabrega H, et al: Culture and Psychiatric Diagnosis. Washington, DC, American Psychiatric Press, 1996

Rogler LH: Culture in psychiatric diagnosis: an issue of scientific accuracy. Psychiatry 56:324–327, 1993

Strauss JS: The person—key to understanding mental illness: towards a new dynamic psychiatry, III. Br J Psychiatry 161 (suppl 18):19–26, 1992

World Health Organization: ICD-10 Chapter V: Mental and Behavioral Disorders: Diagnostic Criteria for Research. Geneva, Switzerland, World Health Organization, 1992

Chapter 41

Culture in DSM-IV

Arthur Kleinman, M.D., Delores L. Parron, Ph.D.,
Horacio Fabrega Jr., M.D., Byron J. Good, Ph.D., and
Juan E. Mezzich, M.D., Ph.D.

The term *culture,* in its more recent forms, has been employed in psychiatry as a demographic description of populations. The relationship between ethnicity and particular disease profiles, risk factors, or even disorders that are culture-bound to particular groups continues as a useful avenue for epidemiological research (Hahn et al. 1992).

In the 1950s, 1960s, and 1970s, culture was understood more as shared value orientations and beliefs about the body, the self, illness, and treatment (Geertz 1973). That view of culture is apparent in the large number of studies of the illness beliefs and therapeutic practices of different groups or subgroups. Although this approach to culture often fosters "cultural sensitivity," it also suffers from the tendency to stereotype entire groups superficially and to convey the erroneous sense that cultural orientations are conventions, mistaken beliefs that can be taken off and put back on again at will (Helman 1990).

In recent years, a much more sophisticated idea of culture has gained ground in anthropology (Clifford and Marcus 1986; Herzfeld 1987). This is the notion that culture is constituted by, and in turn constitutes, local worlds of everyday experience. That is, culture is the product of daily patterns of activities—common sense, communication with others, and the routine rhythms and rituals of community life that are usually taken for granted. These reciprocally reflect the *patterning* downward of social relations by shared symbolic apparatuses—language, aesthetic sensibility, and core value orientations conveyed by master metaphors. In these local worlds, experience is an interpersonal flow of communication, interaction, and negotiation, which centers on agreement and conflict about what is most at stake and how that which is at stake is to be sought and gained. Gender, age cohort, social role and status, and personal desire all inflect this small moral universe in different ways. The upshot is culture in the making, in the processes that generate action and that justify it. Thus, the locus of culture is not the mind of the isolated person, but the interconnected body/self of groups—families, work settings, networks, and whole communities (Ware and Kleinman 1992).

In this new perspective, culture is more than what is meant when we talk of rates, symptoms, or treatment of psychiatric conditions in exotic places or among special groups: schizophrenia in China, depression among Puerto Ricans, or the mental health system (or lack thereof) in Tanzania. In addition to these culturally salient phenomena, culture is also an influential aspect of North American psychiatry and society (Good 1994; Kleinman 1988).

Cultural processes pattern the diagnostic practices of a psychiatrist in Boston, a psychologist in San Francisco, a psychiatric social worker in Toledo, or a mental health aide in Beijing, as much as they do the forms and patterns of disorder and the coping processes families engage in to deal with afflicted members. DSM, the official diagnostic system of the American Psychiatric Association, and its application by professionals in particular institutional and societal contexts, then, are cultural phenomena: the former, a document that is clothed with cultural commitments; the latter, forms of interaction that are culturally patterned and socially negotiated (Kleinman 1988).

For example, the chief symptom of major depression is said to be the emotion of sadness or depression. Yet in most societies, most people suffering clinical depression do not complain mainly of sadness. Instead they talk about fatigue, headaches, backaches, stomach upset, insomnia, loss of appetite, and so on. For most depressed people, this physical experience is most real. As a result, they visit primary care doctors rather than mental health professionals, and usually their depression is neither diagnosed nor effectively treated (Kleinman 1986; Kleinman and Good 1985).

To define emotions as central to the experience of depression is to make a commitment every bit as "cultural" as the beliefs of Chinese businesspersons, Hindu peasants, or ethnic minorities in the United States (Jenkins et al. 1991). It is characteristic of Western culture to separate the emotional and physical components of depression and give primacy to the former. This cultural bias in favor of a mind-body dichotomy is strengthened by another feature of our society and our medicine—the fact that most research on depression involves patients in psychiatric treatment, who are a special, often self-selected, minority of all depressed persons (Guarnaccia et al. 1990).

Because illness categories reflect cultural principles, we must be careful not to let our own cultural bias exert a hidden, damaging effect on our scientific research and therapies. For example, many Plains Indians hear the voice of a recently deceased relative calling them from the afterworld. The experience is normative and without psychopathological sequelae for members of these communities, and therefore by definition cannot be abnormal. On the other hand, for an adult white North American, it might well be a hallucination with serious mental health consequences (Kleinman 1988).

Of all the adult mental disorders described in DSM-III-R (American Psychiatric Association 1987), besides the organic brain disorders and substance abuse, convincing evidence exists to support the case of only four that are distributed worldwide: schizophrenia, manic-depressive (bipolar) disorder, major depression, and a group of anxiety disorders (including panic anxiety, obsessive-compulsive disorder, and certain phobias). The rest of our mental illness categories are peculiar to North America and Western Europe (Littlewood and Lipsedge 1987).

Schizophrenia is nearly ubiquitous. Although the content of hallucinations, delusions, and thought disorder varies, those symptoms as well as negativity, withdrawal, and impaired reality testing can be demonstrated nearly everywhere—proof, it is claimed, of schizophrenia's strong biological roots. Nevertheless, there are also important cultural differences that may be clues to the causes of schizophrenia. Contrary to conventional assumptions, epidemiological and ethnographic studies show that it is not equally common everywhere (Kleinman 1988). The prevalence ranges from 1 in 1,000 in non-Western societies to more than 1% in the West. Some preliterate hunter-gatherer groups, nomads, and settled horticulturist societies have little or no schizophrenia. Economically and technologically advanced, urbanized, and bureaucratized societies have much higher rates of schizophrenia than peasant societies. Indeed, the disorder seems to be relatively uncommon in any society without a system of wage labor (Warner 1985). The reason remains unclear.

Furthermore, the symptoms and course of schizophrenia vary geographically. One of every fourth or fifth schizophrenic patient in Madras, India, is catatonic, but there are hardly any catatonic patients in Western Europe or North America. More than half of hospitalized Japanese patients with this diagnosis are hebephrenic. Schizophrenia is more likely to have a rapid onset in Nigeria or China than in the United States (Sartorius and Jablensky 1976, 1986).

The practice of the psychiatrist is also culturally patterned. A psychiatric diagnosis, after all, is an interpretation of an interpretation. Contrary to the positivism of most academic psychiatry, there can be no immediate grasping of reality outside of historically derived categories. What the patient reports is itself an interpretation of suffering based on his or her own cultural categories, words, images, and feelings for expressing (and thereby constituting) symptoms. The psychiatrist's view is, then, an interpretation, with its own cultural categories, of that interpretation.

The psychiatrist is influenced as well by what is at stake in a particular institutional setting. The diagnosis in a disability evaluation, in a contested courtroom drama, in a military hospital, or in a politically oppressive system—such as the former Soviet Union's mental hospitals—is inseparable from powerful institutional constraints, which become a normative order that can change absolutely how a diagnosis is applied (Freidson 1986).

Further, the conviction that psychiatric disorders are preprogrammed diatheses out of which unfolds a natural course of the disease process can influence diagnosis. Yet the course of psychiatric disorders has been shown repeatedly and definitively to be inseparable from ongoing social events and coping resources (Moos 1991), from family relationships (Jenkins and Karno 1992; Vaughn and Leff 1976), and from involvement with medical and welfare systems (Katon et al. 1982; Osterweis et al. 1984, 1987). That is, the course of mental illness is social, not natural (Ware and Kleinman 1992). The fact that the outcome of schizophrenia varies inversely with social development of the country in which schizophrenia is experienced—a fact that has been replicated on several occasions—is another piece of evidence in support of this argument (Hopper 1991).

Culturally sensitive application of the DSM diagnostic system means that questions in clinical interviews and in other assessment techniques must be translated into terms that are socially meaningful; it also means, however, that consideration must be given to indigenous conceptualizations, values, and practices. Cultural sensitivity must be given particular attention when clinical work or research is conducted cross-culturally and internationally (Rogler 1989).

For members of ethnic minority groups, such as Puerto Ricans, for whom considerable baseline knowledge is available, common cultural idioms of distress (e.g., *nervios* or *ataques*) that are known to affect mental status assessment should be a focus of special inquiry. Clinicians should be aware that these are common channels of communication and behavior that may express either normal or pathological states (Guarnaccia et al. 1989). There is no one-to-one correlation between a specific DSM diagnostic category and a cultural idiom of distress. The same method could be used to handle other common culture-bound syndromes, such as *susto* ("soul loss") among Hispanics.

Consideration of the cultural blind spot syndrome, which results when patient and practitioner share the same ethnicity or culture, but the practitioner fails to take culture into account (Lin 1984), needs to be articulated as well. In addition, a serious interest in the patient's culture means a more sophisticated and sensitive engagement with religious values than psychiatrists generally demonstrate. Culturally sensitive diagnostic interviewing and culturally valid translation and application of DSM-based diagnostic tests and research instruments must also be explicated (Johnson et al., in press).

For example, clinicians could ask patients to describe their ethnic or cultural identity as well as their perceived degree of acculturation, language fluency, religious affiliation, and any special dietary or other practices that could be used to assess the degree of practicing "behavioral ethnicity" (Harwood 1981). Patients' or families' "explanatory models" would be elicited to assess culturally influential beliefs on illness experience by asking them: What do you call your illness? What do you believe to be its cause? Why did it begin when it did? What do you expect to be the course or outcome? What do you fear most about this condition? What treatment do you expect? What do you fear most about the treatment? Are you following the prescribed treatment? If not, can you explain why? (The last two questions are useful because noncompliance is an especially frequent and predictable problem in cross-cultural care.)

It should be understood that cultural groups are heterogeneous owing to gender, age, subethnic grouping, social class, religion, and lifestyle. Thus, the danger of stereotyping patients must be avoided. Practitioners need to understand how culture, including their professional culture, influences their own perspectives and actions. Cultural beliefs and orientations are, for most people, like natural law, the way things are, and therefore are neither easily negotiated nor abandoned. If the practitioner's focus is on suffering—the felt experience of pain and distress, the bearing or enduring or going through of trials to the body-self and the network—then taking culture into account, including religious values, does not mean changing beliefs regarded as unscientific, but rather affirming, witnessing, and engaging the illness in the embodied and contextualized terms in which it is experienced.

References

American Psychiatric Association: Diagnostic and Statistical Manual of Mental Disorders, 3rd Edition, Revised. Washington, DC, American Psychiatric Association, 1987
Clifford J, Marcus GE: Writing Culture. Berkeley, CA, University of California Press, 1986
Freidson E: Professional Powers. Chicago, IL, University of Chicago Press, 1986
Geertz C: The Interpretation of Culture. New York, Basic Books, 1973
Good B: Medicine, Rationality and Experience: an Anthropological Perspective. Cambridge, Cambridge University Press, 1994
Guarnaccia P, Rubio-Stipec M, Canino G, et al: Ataques de nervios in the Puerto Rican Diagnostic Interview Schedule: the impact of cultural categories on psychiatric epidemiology. Cult Med Psychiatry 13:275–295, 1989
Guarnaccia P, Good B, Kleinman A, et al: A critical review of epidemiological studies of Puerto Rican mental health. Am J Psychiatry 147:11, 1990
Hahn R, Mulinare J, Teutsch S, et al: Inconsistencies in coding of race and ethnicity between birth and death in US infants. JAMA 267:259–263, 1992
Harwood A (ed): Ethnicity and Medical Care. Cambridge, MA, Harvard University Press, 1981

Helman CG: Culture, Health and Illness. London, England, Wright, 1990
Herzfeld M: Anthropology through the looking-glass: critical ethnography in the margins of Europe. Cambridge, Cambridge University Press, 1987
Hopper K: Some old questions for the new cross-cultural psychiatry. Medical Anthropology Quarterly 5:299–330, 1991
Jenkins J, Karno M: Expressed emotion among Mexican-descent families: cultural adaptation of the method and principal findings. Am J Psychiatry 149:9–21, 1992
Jenkins JA, Kleinman A, Good B: Cross-cultural studies of depression, in Psychosocial Aspects of Depression. Edited by Becker J, Kleinman A. Hillsdale, NJ, Lawrence Erlbaum Associates, 1991, pp 67–99
Johnson T, Hardt E, Kleinman A: Cultural factors in the medical interview, in The Medical Interview. Edited by Lipkin M, Putnam S, Lazare A, et al. New York, The Task Force on the Medical Interview, Society of General Internal Medicine (in press)
Katon W, Kleinman A, Rosen G, et al: Depression and somatization, I and II. Am J Med 72:127–135, 241–247, 1982
Kleinman A: Social Origins of Distress and Disease: Depression, Neurasthenia and Pain in Modern China. New Haven, CT, Yale University Press, 1986
Kleinman A: Rethinking Psychiatry. New York, Free Press, 1988
Kleinman A, Good B (eds): Culture and Depression. Berkeley, CA, University of California Press, 1985
Lin EHB: Intraethnic characteristics and patient-physician interaction: cultural blind spot syndrome. J Fam Pract 16:91–98, 1984
Littlewood R, Lipsedge M: The butterfly and the serpent: culture, psycho-pathology and biomedicine. Cult Med Psychiatry 11:289–336, 1987
Moos R: Life stressors, social resources, and the treatment of depression, in Psychological Aspects of Depression. Edited by Becker J, Kleinman A. Hillsdale, NJ, Lawrence Erlbaum Associates, 1991, pp 187–214
Osterweis M, Solomon F, Green M (eds): Bereavement. Washington, DC, National Academy Press, 1984
Osterweis M, Kleinman A, Mechanic D (eds): Pain and Disability. Washington, DC, National Academy Press, 1987
Rogler L: The meaning of culturally sensitive research in mental health. Am J Psychiatry 146:296–303, 1989
Sartorius N, Jablensky A: Transcultural studies of schizophrenia. WHO Chronicle 30:481–485, 1976
Sartorius N, Jablensky A: Early manifestation and first contact incidence of schizophrenia. Psychol Med 16:909–928, 1986
Vaughn C, Leff J: The measurement of expressed emotion in the families of psychiatric patients. British Journal of Social and Clinical Psychology 15:157–165, 1976
Ware N, Kleinman A: Depression in neurasthenia and chronic fatigue syndrome. Psychosom Med 22:202–208, 1992
Warner R: Recovery from Schizophrenia: Psychiatry and Political Economy. New York, Routledge & Kegan Paul, 1985

Chapter 42

Cultural Considerations in the Classification of Mental Disorders in Children and Adolescents

Glorisa Canino, Ph.D., Ian Canino, M.D., and
William Arroyo, M.D.

Introduction

The same symptoms in children may have very different implications for different ages at different developmental levels, as well as for different cultures. Moreover, the comprehensive assessment of children requires multiple sources of data—the school, the parent, and the child—each of which can contribute a different picture of the child's functioning. Contextual variations are important in childhood assessment within a given culture, but they are even more critical when evaluating children from different cultures. Furthermore, the process of acculturation within certain cultural groups has been shown to be an important mediator of self-reported symptoms (Montgomery and Orosco 1985). Yet the task of classifying disorders among children from different cultures is greatly hampered by a lack of consensus on the most valid definitions of childhood psychopathology in general. Specific examples of the challenges facing the clinician under these circumstances are illustrated in this chapter in terms of conditions and factors on the five axes of DSM-IV.

Axes I, II, and III Disorders

Mental Retardation, Learning Disorders, and Pervasive Developmental Disorders

The criteria for these disorders are heavily based on communication, socialization, and intelligence. Patterns and styles of communication (including language) and socialization are strongly determined by cultural influences. The likelihood of making an erroneous diagnosis, either positive or negative, is substantial unless the patterns of the patient's cultural group are understood. In addition, several of these disorders require the use of so-called standardized testing instruments. However, caution must be exercised in the use of instruments that are not standardized to the individual's cultural group. In the case of individuals or their parents whose language is different from that of the testing instrument and from whom data must be collected during the diagnostic process, special caution in the use of such instruments is imperative.

Substance-Related Disorders

Extremely elevated rates of alcohol use disorders are found in both adult (Manson et al. 1992) and adolescent (Oetting and Beauvais 1987) American Indian populations. These high rates have been attributed to prejudice, unemployment, and poverty, as well as to the disruption of the cultural practices of American Indians and their resultant alienation. Alcoholism in American Indian women, although lower than in men, is also very common, affecting about 40% of women in some communities (Fleming and Manson 1990; Manson et al. 1992). Such high rates of alcoholism among American Indian adults often result in family disruption and child abuse and neglect. These and other chronic stressors, common in families of alcoholic persons, place young children at risk of developing psychiatric disorders or symptomatology, particularly suicidal behavior, anxiety, posttraumatic stress disorder, and aggressive or delinquent behavior (Egeland et al. 1988; Gelles and Conte 1990; Siegel and Brown 1988).

American Indian adolescents engage in the same type of pathological patterns of alcohol use as their parents. High suicide rates among American Indian youth have been linked to underlying depression resulting from the chronic burdens they are exposed to as well as from their excessive drinking (Dick et al. 1992; King et al. 1992; Manson et al. 1989). Feelings of helplessness and hopelessness resulting from these chronic stressors make death an acceptable solution for many of these youth (J. W. Thompson and Walker 1990).

Although alcohol-induced disorders are not as common among African American or Hispanic American youth, these groups are overrepresented in clinic samples of individuals addicted to other drugs (e.g., amphetamines, opiates) (De la Rosa et al. 1990; N. Velez and Ungermack 1989). The rate per 100,000 persons of Hispanic clients (adults and adolescents) in drug treatment facilities has been found to be higher than that of white non-Hispanics (National Institute of Drug Abuse 1986). This high rate of seeking help is probably related to the use of heroin, cocaine, and phencyclidine as primary drugs of abuse. Because these drugs cause medical emergencies, these patients are more readily referred to drug treatment facilities.

Disruptive Behavior Disorders

The risk of conduct-oppositional disorders is strongly associated with paternal and maternal substance abuse and antisocial personality (Frick et al. 1992), parental discord, and erratic and severe discipline patterns (Quinton et al. 1990; Robins 1991). Many of these risk factors are present in the families of inner-city minority children, making them vulnerable to the development of these disorders. However, caution should be exercised before determining the presence of a disruptive disorder in minority children. Many of these children exhibit aggressive behavior that is syntonic with environmental demands that emphasize such behavior as a survival skill. Truancy and other types of misbehavior also may be a part of these subcultures' norms. In addition, clinicians should inquire about malnutrition, lead poisoning, and fetal alcohol effects—common risk factors that may be associated with attention-deficit/hyperactivity disorder.

Elective Mutism

Speech disorders in children and adolescents are especially sensitive to stressors and the concomitant anxiety. Maternal overprotection and immigration from a country with a different language from that of the host country are particular risk factors. Maternal overprotection is commonly observed among immigrant mothers who feel fearful of the new and sometimes violent environments in which they live, who lack the language skills to communicate, and who have lost the support systems they had in their country of origin. Clinicians should be aware of the stressors to which parents are subject and assist them in developing problem-solving strategies, including better utilization of community support systems. Helping parents overcome their burdens often alleviates the child's symptomatology.

Reactive Attachment Disorders and Stereotypy Habit Disorder

These disorders are often seen in inner-city and rural areas where the child has been exposed to severe isolation, understimulation, and deprivation. Immigrants who are fearful of exposing their children to inner-city dangers frequently isolate them from contact with the outside world. Deprivation and understimulation typically are experienced by minority children who live in poverty or in rural areas.

Separation Anxiety

Separation anxiety as well as posttraumatic stress disorder are often observed in refugee immigrant children who have been forcefully and suddenly separated from loved ones and who have suffered severe, traumatic experiences, such as the killing of parents and other relatives. Separation anxiety also frequently occurs among immigrants from cultures in which "enmeshed family systems" are part of the cultural norm (Canino and Canino 1982). These family systems rely on extended kin and emphasize mutual dependence and family loyalty. Immigration disrupts these family systems, often leading to symptoms of separation anxiety in the child.

Posttraumatic Stress Disorder

Asian children who escaped from concentration camps and who witnessed or experienced torture and homicide are particularly prone to symptoms of posttraumatic stress disorder and depression (Kinzie et al. 1986). Newly arrived Asian children have to learn a new language to communicate and new ways of behavior and learning. They often cannot count on parents, who may still be grieving and depressed, for the requisite emotional support. To intervene appropriately, clinicians must understand the multiple stressors to which these children are subject and the available support systems. Children who migrated without their nuclear families—most of whom were killed—are at particular risk for posttraumatic stress disorder and depression (Kinzie et al. 1986).

Often children from different ethnic groups live in poor public housing projects or neighborhoods where exposure to homicide and muggings is common. Moreover, multiple stressors impinge on their families, placing them at increased risk for domestic violence and for child abuse. These violent and traumatic events are known risks not only for posttraumatic stress disorder, but also for depression, conduct disorder, and oppositional defiant disorder (Egeland et al. 1988; Rutter 1981; Siegel and Brown 1988).

Culture-Bound Syndromes and Healing

Research on local categories of illness or culture-bound syndromes have tended to overlook children and adolescents. As a result, local syndromes, discussed in more detail in other chapters of this section in the *DSM-IV Sourcebook,* such as "brain fag" (Prince 1985), "ataques de nervios" (Guarnaccia et al. 1989), "nervios" in different settings of Latin America (Low 1985), and "susto" (Simons and Hughes 1985), have not been described in the literature for children and adolescents. Nevertheless, clinicians should be aware that these syndromes or similar manifestations can be found in children, particularly adolescents.

Clinicians should also be alert to the fact that cultural attitudes and beliefs often determine the type of help sought by parents and their children. Indigenous healing practices may be quite active in certain ethnic minority groups. Moreover, some forms of culturally specific treatment can result in physical marks that can lead to a misdiagnosis of child abuse. Perhaps the most widely known example is the practice of "cupping" among Cambodians and Hmong. Cupping is a healing practice consisting of placing a small heated cup on the skin and allowing it to cool, which causes a circular ecchymotic area to appear (Buchwald et al. 1992; Reinhart and Ruhs 1984). Another healing practice common among the Vietnamese, Chinese, and Cambodians, and which is also commonly misdiagnosed, is called "Cao Cíío" or "coin rubbing." This practice consists of rubbing the skin with a coin to alleviate common symptoms and can result in symmetric linear purpura and petechiae (Golden and Duster 1977; Yeatman and Dang 1980). The rubbing is usually done on the back, neck, head, shoulders, and chest. A third healing practice, used almost exclusively by the Mien, is "moxibustion" (Buchwald et al. 1992; Reinhard and Ruhs 1984). This folk remedy consists of the application of heat to the skin in a specific pattern, usually round, by means of a burning object such as incense. Buchwald et al. stated that these healing practices may result in scarring, lesions, false accusations of physical abuse, and unnecessary medical evaluations. Clinicians should therefore inquire about these practices, solicit further information from cultural sources, and be careful in the interpretation given to the facts, before assuming the presence of parental child abuse.

Chronic Illness

Minority children have higher rates of tuberculosis, rheumatic fever, upper respiratory infections, lead poisoning, and other illnesses as a consequence of impoverished conditions such as deteriorated and poorly heated housing and highly contaminated urban environments (Mitchell and Heagarty 1991). Frequent hospitalizations and school absenteeism are thus common in this population, and both factors may affect normal development. High blood levels of lead poisoning may be related to a series of behavior problems such as aggression and hyperactivity (G. O. B. Thompson et al. 1989) and impaired visual-motor and visual-spatial integration (Dietrich et al. 1991; Winneke et al. 1990). Practitioners thus should be aware of the fact that behavioral or learning difficulties in some of these children living under disadvantageous conditions may be related to lead poisoning. In addition, in some cultures (e.g., Mexico), many low-income children are exposed to high levels of lead as part of folk healing. These children may be treated with lead tetroxide ("azarcon"), lead carbonate ("alabayalde"), and lead monoxide ("greta") to cause constipation for "empacho," which is the folk word describing gastrointestinal symptoms and diarrhea (Mushak and Crocetti 1989).

Clinicians should keep in mind that alcoholism is more prevalent among the lower socioeconomic classes (Helzer et al. 1991) and consider the possibility of maternal alcoholism and that the child being evaluated may suffer from fetal alcohol syndrome. Screening for fetal alcohol syndrome is particularly important among some Native American tribes, such as the White Plain Indians, where the prevalence is very high (1 per 102 child births [May et al. 1983]). The risk of fetal alcohol syndrome for African American children is seven times greater than for white children, even after adjusting for maternal alcohol intake, occurrence of chronic alcohol problems, and number of children born (Sokol et al. 1986). Common sequelae of fetal alcohol syndrome relevant to psychiatric risk are learning, attention, and memory problems; hyperactivity and impulsiveness; and speech and auditory problems (Streissguth and La Due 1985; Streissguth et al. 1989).

More recently, it has been noted that many minority children are at increased risk for human immunodeficiency virus seropositivity. In the United States, of those children infected during the prenatal period, 80% are from ethnic minority groups and are also the poorest (Centers for Disease Control 1989). Many of these children experience a decline in language as well as other cognitive and motor deficits, which affect their school performance and emotional stability.

Acculturation Difficulty

This new category is one of several listed in the section titled "Other Conditions That May be a Focus of Clinical Attention." A category that acknowledges a potentially problematic transitional period for individuals who relocate from one country or culture to another is long overdue. Numerous studies (Vega et al. 1993) suggest that immigrants and refugees experience significant stress from the process of adaptation to the new environment of another country or culture. Adolescents may be at higher risk than children of experiencing acculturative stress because of their more advanced developmental level. The degree of severity is probably a function of the degree of dissimilarity between the community of origin and the new local community.

Axis IV

Cultural dislocation and/or underprivileged status subject immigrant and inner-city minority children to multiple stressors. Examples include acculturation stress, prejudice, disruption of support systems, inadequate schooling, poor housing, living in high crime areas, frequent family dysfunction, and poor health care delivery. Such psychosocial conditions and stressful life events are frequently associated with increased risk for psychopathology and poor prognosis in children (Compas et al. 1987, 1988; Goodyear et al. 1988; Rutter 1981).

A checklist of potential psychosocial and environmental problems has both advantages and disadvantages compared with the DSM-III-R (American Psychiatric Association 1987) rating scale for overall level of psychosocial stress. In children coming from a "multiproblem" environment (e.g., inner-city and rural areas), it may be difficult to verify the items endorsed without a detailed inquiry. However, it is critical to determine systematically the existence of problems in areas such as primary support groups, parent-child relationships, education, occupation, and housing to plan adequately for comprehensive service delivery. For this, a checklist would be of considerable clinical utility.

Axis V

The results of several psychiatric epidemiological surveys in different regions of the world (Anderson et al. 1987; Bird et al. 1988; Costello et al. 1988; Offord et al. 1987; C. M. Velez et al. 1989) suggest higher rates of psychiatric disorders for children and adolescents than reported in previous studies (Gould et al. 1980). However, it is difficult to ascertain whether these higher rates are due to a true increase in psychiatric disorders in children over time or to the overinclusiveness of the current psychiatric nosology (Bird et al. 1990). The overinclusiveness of the DSM-III (American Psychiatric Association 1980) classificatory system for children and adolescents is an issue that is currently being debated. Evidence from epidemiological studies carried out among special ethnic populations (e.g., Puerto Ricans and American Indians) suggests the need to consider impairment in functioning as an additional dimension for appropriate classification (Bird et al. 1988, 1990; Canino 1990; Dauphinais et al. 1991).

Data from the Puerto Rico epidemiology study clearly illustrate the need to use the Global Assessment of Functioning in the classification of children from different cultural backgrounds (Bird et al. 1987, 1988). In that study, 49.5% of the population of children and adolescents in the island met criteria for a DSM-III disorder. When the severity criteria of the Children's Global Assessment Scale (Shaffer et al. 1983) were applied, the prevalence rates fell to 18.2%, a much better approximation of clinical reality. If all children meeting DSM-III criteria were viewed as cases, one would be compelled to conclude—improbably—that nearly half the children of Puerto Rico are psychiatrically disturbed (Bird et al. 1990). Further analyses of these data revealed that many children who met diagnostic criteria were not severely impaired and were not considered to be in need of mental health service by the same psychiatrists responsible for the assessments. Apart from the need to account for the potentially overinclusive nature of the diagnostic criteria, the high prevalence of psychiatric morbidity also may be a function of the higher baseline levels of stress intrinsic to these communities.

Conclusion

Because of the complex array of issues that affect culturally diverse, ethnic minority children in the United States, the diagnostic process is fraught with numerous challenges. Child-rearing practices, tolerance of symptomatic behaviors, idioms of distress, and attitudes toward and beliefs about mental illness as well as help-seeking behavior vary along social and cultural lines. Symptom selection, degree of exacerbation and remission of disorder, and prognosis may differ as a consequence.

It is important to distinguish social class from cultural sources of variation in the etiology and expression of symptoms. Furthermore, the clinician must carefully evaluate whether the resulting symptoms are acute or chronic, reactive or inherent in the child, or a reflection of the cultural style of adult informants, typically parents who themselves are highly stressed. In such instances, clinicians should defer a diagnosis until these uncertainties are clarified and adequate historical information has been obtained.

References

American Psychiatric Association: Diagnostic and Statistical Manual of Mental Disorders, 3rd Edition. Washington, DC, American Psychiatric Association, 1980

American Psychiatric Association: Diagnostic and Statistical Manual of Mental Disorders, 3rd Edition, Revised. Washington, DC, American Psychiatric Association, 1987

Anderson JC, Williams S, McGee R, et al: DSM-III disorders in preadolescent children. Arch Gen Psychiatry 44:69–80, 1987

Bird H, Canino G, Rubio-Stipec M, et al: Further measures of the psychometric properties of the Children's Global Assessment Scale. Arch Gen Psychiatry 44:821–824, 1987

Bird HR, Canino G, Rubio-Stipec M, et al: Estimates of the prevalence of childhood maladjustment in a community survey in Puerto Rico. Arch Gen Psychiatry 45:1120–1126, 1988

Bird HR, Yager TJ, Staghezza B, et al: Impairment in the epidemiological measurement of childhood psychopathology in the community. J Am Acad Child Adolesc Psychiatry 29:796–803, 1990

Buchwald D, Panwala S, Hooton TM: Use of traditional health practices by southeast Asian refugees in a primary care clinic. Western Journal of Medicine 156:507–511, 1992

Canino G: Progress report of the Methodological Child and Adolescent Study. Submitted to the Division of Clinical Research, National Institute of Mental Health, 1990

Canino G, Canino I: Culturally syntonic family therapy for migrant Puerto Ricans. Journal of Hospital and Community Psychiatry 39:200–203, 1982

Centers for Disease Control: Update: Acquired immunodeficiency syndrome: United States 1981–1988. MMWR 38:229–237, 1989

Compas BE, Davis GE, Forsythe CJ, et al: Assessment of major and daily stressful events during adolescence: the Adolescent Perceived Events Scale. J Consult Clin Psychol 55:534–541, 1987

Compas BE, Malcarne VL, Focadaro K: Coping with stressful events in older children and young adolescents. J Consult Clin Psychol 56:405–411, 1988

Costello EJ, Costello AJ, Edelbrock C, et al: Psychiatric disorders in pediatric primary care: prevalence and risk factors. Arch Gen Psychiatry 45:1107–1116, 1988

Dauphinais P, Beals J, Jones M, et al: National Center for American Indian and Alaska Native Mental Health Research: flower of two soils reinterview study (supplemental grant from the National Institute for Mental Health and the Indian Health Services to the National Center for American Indians and Alaska Native Mental Health Research core funding from NIMH) (2 R01 MH42473-06). Bethesda, MD, National Institute of Mental Health, 1991

De la Rosa MR, Kholsa JH, Bouse BA: Hispanics and illicit drug use: a review of recent findings. Int J Addict 25:665–691, 1990

Dick RW, Manson SM, Beals J: Alcohol use among American Indian adolescents: patterns and correlates of students' drinking in a boarding school. J Stud Alcohol 54:172–177, 1992

Dietrich KN, Succop PA, Berger OG, et al: Lead exposure and the cognitive development of urban preschool children: the Cincinnati Lead Study Cohort at age 4 years. Neurotoxicol Teratol 13:203–211, 1991

Egeland B, Jacobvitz D, Sroufe LA: Breaking the cycle of abuse. Child Dev 59:1080–1088, 1988

Fleming CM, Manson SM: Indian women and alcohol, in Women, Alcohol, and Other Drugs. Edited by Engs RC. Dubuque, IA, Kendall/Hunt, 1990, pp 143–148

Frick PJ, Lahey BB, Loeber R, et al: Familial risk factors to oppositional defiant disorder and conduct disorder: parental psychopathology and maternal parenting. J Consult Clin Psychol 60:49–55, 1992

Gelles RJ, Conte JR: Domestic violence and sexual abuse of children: a review of research in the eighties. Journal of Marriage and the Family 52:1045–1058, 1990

Golden SM, Duster MC: Hazards of misdiagnosis due to Vietnamese folk medicine. Clin Pediatr (Philadelphia) 16:949–950, 1977

Goodyear IM, Wright C, Altham PM: Maternal adversity and recent stressful life events in anxious and depressed children. J Child Psychol Psychiatry 29:651–667, 1988

Gould MS, Wunsch-Hitzag R, Dohrenwend BP: Formulation of hypotheses about the prevalence, treatment, and prognostic significance of psychiatric disorders in children in the U.S., in Mental Illness in the U.S.: Epidemiological Estimates. Edited by Dohrenwend BP, Gould MS, Link B. New York, Praeger, 1980, pp 9–42

Guarnaccia P, Rubio-Stipec M, Canino G: Ataques de nervios in the Puerto Rican Diagnostic Interview Schedule: the impact of cultural categories on psychiatric epidemiology. Cult Med Psychiatry 13:275–295, 1989

Helzer JE, Burnam A, McEvoy T: Alcohol abuse and dependence in America, in Psychiatric Disorders in America. Edited by Robins R, Regier D. New York, Free Press, 1991, pp 81–115

King J, Beals J, Manson SM, et al: A structural equation model of factors related to substance abuse among American Indian adolescents. Drugs and Society 6:253–268, 1992

Kinzie JD, Sack WW, Angell RH, et al: The psychiatric effects of massive trauma on Cambodian children, I: the children. Journal of the American Academy of Child Psychiatry 25:370–376, 1986

Low SM: Culturally interpreted symptoms or culture-bound syndromes: a cross cultural review of nerves. Soc Sci Med 21:187–196, 1985

Manson SM, Beals J, Dick R, et al: Risk factors for suicide among Indian adolescents at a boarding school. Public Health Reports 104:609–614, 1989

Manson SM, Shore JH, Baron AE, et al: Alcohol abuse and dependence among American Indians, in Alcoholism—North America, Europe and Asia: a Coordinated Analysis of Population Data From Ten Regions. Edited by Helzer J, Canino G. London, England, Oxford University Press, 1992, pp 113–130

May PA, Hymbaugh KJ, Aase JM, et al: Epidemiology of fetal alcohol syndrome in American Indians of the Southwest. Soc Biol 30:374–387, 1983

Mitchell JL, Heagarty M: Special consideration for minorities in pediatric AIDS, in The Challenge of HIV Infection in Infants, Children, and Adolescents. Edited by Pizzo PA, Wilfert CM. Baltimore, MD, Williams & Wilkins, 1991, pp 704–713

Montgomery GT, Orosco S: Mexican American's performance on the MMPI as a function of level of acculturation. J Clin Psychol 41:203–212, 1985

Mushak P, Crocetti AF: Review: determination of numbers of lead exposed American children as a function of lead source: integrated summary of a report to the U.S. Congress on childhood lead poisoning. Environ Res 50:210–229, 1989

National Institute of Drug Abuse: Demographic characteristics and patterns of drug use of clients admitted to drug abuse treatment facilities in selected states: annual data, 1983 (DHHS Publ No AD271-84-7308). Rockville, MD, U.S. Government Printing Office, 1986

Oetting ER, Beauvais F: Epidemiology and correlates of alcohol use among Indian adolescents living on reservations, in Alcohol Use and Abuse among U.S. Ethnic Minorities (National Institute on Alcohol Abuse and Alcoholism Monogr Series No 18) (DHHS Publ No ADM-89-1435). Edited by Spiegler DL, Tate DA, Aitken SS, et al. Washington, DC, U.S. Government Printing Office, 1987

Offord DR, Boyle MH, Szatmari P, et al: Ontario Child Health Study, II: six month prevalence of disorder and rates of services utilization. Arch Gen Psychiatry 44:832–836, 1987

Prince R: The concept of culture-bound syndromes: anorexia nervosa and brain fag. Soc Sci Med 21:197–203, 1985

Quinton D, Rutter M, Gulliver L: Continuities in psychiatric disorders from childhood to adulthood in the children of psychiatric patients, in Straight and Devious Pathways from Childhood to Adulthood. Edited by Robins LN, Rutter M. Cambridge, MA, Cambridge University Press, 1990, pp 259–278

Reinhart MA, Ruhs H: Moxibustion: Another traumatic folk remedy. Clin Pediatr 24:58–59, 1984

Robins LN: Conduct disorder. J Child Psychol Psychiatry 32:193–212, 1991

Rutter M: Stress, coping and development: some questions and some answers. J Child Psychol Psychiatry 22:323–353, 1981

Shaffer D, Gould MS, Brasic J, et al: A Children's Global Assessment Scale (C-GAS). Arch Gen Psychiatry 40:1228–1231, 1983

Siegel JM, Brown JD: A prospective study of stressful circumstances, illness symptoms, and depressed mood among adolescents. Developmental Psychopathology 24:715–721, 1988

Simons RC, Hughes CC: The Culture-Bound Syndromes: Folk Illnesses of Psychiatric and Anthropological Interest. Dordrecht, Netherlands, Reidel, 1985

Sokol RJ, Ager J, Martier S, et al: Significant determinants of susceptibility of alcohol teratogenicity. Ann N Y Acad Sci 447:87–102, 1986

Streissguth AP, La Due RA: Psychological and behavioral effects in children prenatally exposed to alcohol. Alcohol Health and Research World 10:6–12, 1985

Streissguth AP, Sampson PD, Barr HM: Neurobehavioral dose response effects on prenatal alcohol exposure in humans from infancy to adulthood. Ann N Y Acad Sci 562:145–158, 1989

Thompson GOB, Raab GM, Hepburn WS, et al: Blood lead levels and children's behavior: results from the Edinburgh lead study. J Child Psychol Psychiatry 30: 515–528, 1989

Thompson JW, Walker RD: Adolescent suicide among American Indian and Alaskan natives. Psychiatric Annals 20:128–133, 1990

Vega WA, Gil A, Warheit G, et al: Acculturation and delinquent behavior among Cuban American adolescents: toward an empirical model. Am J Community Psychol 21:113–125, 1993

Velez CM, Johnson J, Cohen P: A longitudinal analysis of selected risk factors for childhood psychopathology. J Am Acad Child Adolesc Psychiatry 28:861–864, 1989

Velez N, Ungermack J: Drug use among Puerto Rican youth: an exploration of generational status differences. Soc Sci Med 29:779–789, 1989

Winneke G, Brockhaus A, Ewers V, et al: Results from the European multi-center study on lead neurotoxicity in children: implications for risk assessment. Neurotoxicol Teratol 12:553–559, 1990

Yeatman GW, Dang VV: Cao Gío (coin rubbing): Vietnamese attitudes toward health care. JAMA 244:2748–2749, 1980

Chapter 43

Cultural Considerations on Cognitive Impairment Disorders

Keh-Ming Lin, M.D., M.P.H., and
Horacio Fabrega Jr., M.D.

Introduction

The study of the influence of culture on behavior disturbances has a long history in psychiatry. Attention has principally focused on etiological questions and on how psychiatric illness is handled socially, although there is a tradition that deals with the manifestations of so-called functional psychiatric illnesses. In all of these instances, the methods and rationale of the social sciences have been employed and underlying neurobiological factors neglected. A basic question that is rarely addressed relates to how cultural influences may possibly affect the organization and functioning of the nervous system and, by extension, behavior and its disturbances. The topic of concern, then, is how cultural conventions about space, time, self, and ecological setting come to be represented in cerebral mechanisms and how disturbance of these mechanisms will affect the manifestations and appraisal of "organic" conditions.

Possibly because of the assumption that the pathogenesis of "organic" conditions is biologically based, and hence "universal," relatively less attention has been given by researchers and clinicians to the cultural influences on these disorders. There is thus currently a paucity of information in the professional literature regarding these issues. However, both theoretical considerations and empirical findings derived from existing literature indicate that there are several major ways through which culture and ethnicity could play an important role in the assessment of these conditions.

Epidemiological Considerations

Unlike the majority of psychiatric syndromes, the diagnosis and "subtyping" of cognitive impairment disorders are based on etiology, and the etiologically based subtypes have important therapeutic and prognostic implications. For example, misjudgment regarding the "reversibility" of dementia (e.g., brain abscess versus "senile dementia") could lead to serious consequences including death and a loss of opportunity for potential cure. Knowledge of the prevalence of different types of organic conditions in different groups of patients will help clinicians to avoid misdiagnosing such patients.

Cultural variations as well as historical changes in the prevalence of different types of organic brain syndromes and "organic psychoses" have been well documented. The prevalences of different types of infection, nutritional deficiencies, head injuries, endocrinological abnormalities, cerebrovascular diseases, seizure disorders, brain tumors, and substance abuse vary substantially across cultural groups (Cruickshank and Beevers 1989; Goodman 1979; Polednak 1989). For example, organic brain disorders caused by abscesses, head injuries, and malnutrition may still be relatively more prevalent in preindustrial, less urbanized societies, among refugees (K. M. Lin 1986; Westermeyer 1988, 1989) and in certain ethnic minority groups in the United States (Spector 1979; R. A. Williams 1975). AIDS-related organic mental disorders are expected to be more prevalent among groups with higher risk for AIDS, such as Haitians, Africans, and homosexuals (Kaslow and Francis 1989), and are still less prevalent in most Asian countries, including China, Japan, and Taiwan.

Dramatic differences have been found in the rate of alcoholism among different countries and ethnic groups (Agarwal and Goedde 1990). The same is true of the type and prevalence of drug abuse (Adlaf et al. 1989; Kleinman and Lukoff 1978), which is influenced by a complicated mixture of sociocultural and economic as well as geopolitical forces.

Although apparently rare, culturally related practices have been reported to cause certain types of organic conditions. "Kuru," a condition caused by slow viral infection as a result of ritualistic cannibalism in Papua New Guinea in the context of mourning (Gajdusek 1977), represents a most dramatic example. Other culturally related practices, such as prolonged fasting or dieting, could also conceivably cause organic conditions whose etiology may be difficult to identify without an adequate understanding of the patient's cultural background.

Hypertension and strokes are significantly more prevalent among blacks and certain Asian groups (Cruickshank and Beevers 1989; Spector 1979), leading one to speculate that vascular (multi-infarct) dementia might also be more prevalent among these groups. Several studies have reported data suggesting that this indeed is the case (de la Monte et al. 1989; H. N. Lin et al. 1984).

The possibility of ethnic differences in the prevalence and incidence of dementia of the Alzheimer's type raises interesting theoretical and practical questions. Reports from Taiwan (H. N. Lin et al. 1984), China (Li et al. 1989; Zhang et al. 1990), Singapore, and New York (Serby et al. 1987) have suggested that Alzheimer's disease may be less prevalent among Chinese and Chinese Americans. A study by de la Monte et al. (1989) further suggested that Alzheimer's disease may also be less prevalent among blacks as compared with Caucasians. However, other studies have not been able to demonstrate similar findings (Schoenberg et al. 1985).

Cultural Influences on the Manifestations and Detection of Cognitive Impairment

Although often neglected by health professionals, the cross-cultural research literature clearly demonstrates that cultural factors strongly influence the way in which symptoms of various medical conditions are experienced and expressed (Kleinman 1988). For example, numerous studies have demonstrated that the way a symptom as simple as pain is experienced, interpreted, and reported can vary greatly across cultural groups because of differences in the culturally specific meanings attached to the symptom (Bates 1987; Lipton and Marbach 1984; Streltzer and Wade 1981; Zatzick and Dimsdale 1990; Zborowski 1952). Similar cultural differences could be expected to affect clinical manifestations of the medical conditions responsible for cognitive impairment disorders, as well as the symptoms of the cognitive impairment itself (K. M. Lin, 1996). For example, milder degrees of disorientation and confusion in people of "older age" may not be regarded as pathological in cultures where "role changes" are expected at certain ages, and "older people" are not expected to make major decisions or take care of themselves (Cowgill 1986; Hsu 1981; Ikels 1991).

Acute delirium occurring in the context of a "reactive psychosis" has been reported to be more prevalent in Africa (K. M. Lin and Kleinman 1988; Wittkower and Prince 1974) and other less developed countries. These patients are often diagnosed as suffering from "bouffée délirante" by French-trained psychiatrists in Africa. It is reasonable to expect that this would also be the case with recent immigrants coming from these places to the United States and other industrialized countries. Similarly, catatonia, both with and without organic causes, occurs more commonly in these groups (Mann et al. 1986), posing a particular problem in differential diagnosis for clinicians evaluating such patients.

Biases in the Cross-Cultural Assessment of Cognitive Impairment

Psychiatric evaluations in general are fraught with difficulties and potential mistakes in the face of cultural and language barriers (Westermeyer 1985, 1987). The evaluation of cognitive impairment is no exception. Depending on the situation, difficulties in communication may either conceal signs of cognitive impairment or, on the contrary, give the false impression of such impairment when it does not exist. Similarly, such barriers will make the differential diagnosis between dementia and certain "functional" psychiatric conditions (e.g., late-onset schizophrenia with prominent negative symptoms and major depression with prominent psychomotor retardation) even more difficult.

Numerous studies have documented that severe underestimation routinely occurs when Western-based instruments are used to evaluate the mental capacities of subjects with non-Western backgrounds (C. L. Williams 1987). This is true not only with most intelligence tests but also with relatively more "straightforward" tests such as the Mini-Mental State Exam (Folstein et al. 1975). Community surveys have documented that the Mini-Mental State Exam misclassifies as cognitively impaired a significantly larger portion of Hispanics (Escobar et al. 1986), Taiwanese (Yeh et al. 1990), Chinese (Katzman et al. 1988; Salmon et al. 1989), and Southeast Asians (J. Westermeyer, J. Neider: Mini-Mental State Exam among refugees: a pilot study of its utility as a cross-cultural screening instrument, University of Minnesota, unpublished manuscript, 1987) than Western whites. Differences in level of education explain only part of the discrepancy. Cultural differences in the conceptualization of space and time and in the fund of knowledge, and familiarity with the test method (e.g., the use of paper and pen), can all affect the results of the mental status examinations. For example, Pacific Islanders conceptualize direction in relation to whether it is toward the ocean or the center of the island (Levy 1973). Traditional Pueblo Indians use a system with five instead of four directions, as did the Chinese in classic times. Non-Westerners may not remember their birth dates because they have not been reminded throughout their lives with celebrations (e.g., traditional Chinese celebrate the birthdays only of the elders) or because they may use different calendar systems. Tropical peoples may have two seasons (dry and rainy) instead of four. Geographic and political divisions that appear natural to urban Westerners may be completely foreign to others (e.g., most new immigrants are not able to answer the question regarding the name of the county). Knowledge that is assumed to be essential in one cultural setting may be completely irrelevant in others (e.g., questions frequently asked for the assessment of mental status such as the names of the presidents or the capitals of the states). Fabrega (1979) illustrated how cultural conventions regarding time, self, other, and the behavioral environment can be expected to be reflected more generally in how people behave in the context of quintessential organic conditions.

Summary and Conclusion

The manifestation of classic functional disorders in different cultures is a frequent topic of investigation in psychiatry; a related topic involves the specificity of so-called culture-bound syndromes. In studies of this type, the researcher contends that cultural factors might be operative in the ways a person who is ill behaves and in the way he or she is dealt with in the group. This perspective in psychiatry, and its counterparts in anthropology, culture, and personality theory, examine behavior from a psychological and social point of view. In other words, emphasis is placed on such things as thought content and progression, perceptions, emotional expression, social relations, and conventions about deviance, and these kinds of phenomena are typically approached using the perspectives of the social sciences. Culture, ordinarily defined as a people's system of social symbols and their meanings, is a variable traditionally linked to the methods of these sciences.

The influences of culture may also be approached from a neurobiological point of view. From this standpoint, behavior is seen as the output of an organ consisting of neurological routines that are a product of evolution, but that require an experiential base that is culturally conditioned. In other words, it is assumed that a people's view of the world and their guidelines for operating in it play a key role in the development and maturation of an individual and influence the way the whole nervous system comes to be organized and how it functions (Fabrega 1979). As an example, cultural factors would be held to influence the way sensory stimuli are built into perceptions; the way these come to influence basic motor schemata as well as general programs of action; the way conventions about time, space, and motor expression become neurologically encoded and enter into the formation of key concepts such as object, person, self, other, and ecological setting; the way internal visceral or emotional responses come to be structured and linked to culturally specific mental experiences of the world and of social and physical activity; and the role that language plays in contextualizing this whole system of meaning.

A neurobiological emphasis on culture might, of course, pave the way for new, cross-cultural ways of studying functional psychiatric illnesses such as schizophrenia and depression-mania. However, we have argued here for the fruitfulness of studying cultural influences in brain-behavior relations.

Despite the potential significance of the interplay between culture and brain-behavior relations, relatively little attention has been given to this area of research.

Because of this neglect, this review has been selective and theoretical in nature. We hope that this review will stimulate future studies that will provide more specific information conducive to formulating culturally specific guidelines for the evaluation of cognitive impairment in patients from different cultural backgrounds.

References

Adlaf EM, Smart RG, Tan SH: Ethnicity and drug use: a critical look. Int J Addict 24:1–18, 1989

Agarwal DP, Goedde HW: Alcohol Metabolism, Alcohol Intolerance and Alcoholism. Berlin, Germany, Springer-Verlag, 1990

Bates MS: Ethnicity and pain: a biocultural model. Soc Sci Med 24:47–50, 1987

Cowgill DO: Aging Around the World. New York, Wadsworth Publishing, 1986

Cruickshank JK, Beevers DG: Ethnic Factors in Health and Disease. London, England, Wright, 1989

de la Monte SM, Hutchins GM, Moore GW: Racial differences in the etiology of dementia and frequency of Alzheimer lesions in the brain. J Natl Med Assoc 81:644–652, 1989

Escobar JI, Burnam A, Karno M, et al: Use of the Mini-Mental Status Examination in a community population of mixed ethnicity, cultural and linguistic artifacts. J Nerv Ment Dis 174:607–614, 1986

Fabrega H Jr: Neurobiology, culture, and behavior disturbances, an integrative review. J Nerv Ment Dis 167:467–474, 1979

Folstein MF, Folstein SE, McHugh PR: Mini-Mental State: a practical method for grading the cognitive state of patients for the clinician. J Psychiatr Res 12:189–198, 1975

Gajdusek DC: Unconventional viruses and the origin and disappearance of Kuru. Science 197:943–960, 1977

Goodman R: Genetic Disorders Among the Jewish People. Baltimore, MD, Johns Hopkins University Press, 1979

Hsu FLK: Americans and Chinese: Passage to Differences, 3rd Edition. Honolulu, HI, University Press of Hawaii, 1981

Ikels C: Aging and disability in China: cultural issues in measurement and interpretation. Soc Sci Med 32:649–665, 1991

Kaslow RA, Francis DP: The Epidemiology of AIDS. New York, Oxford University Press, 1989

Katzman R, Zhang M, Qu OY, et al: A Chinese version of the Mini-Mental Status Examination: impact of illiteracy in a Shanghai dementia survey. J Clin Epidemiol 41:971–978, 1988

Kleinman A: Rethinking Psychiatry. New York, Free Press, 1988

Kleinman PH, Lukoff IF: Ethnic differences in factors related to drug use. J Health Soc Behav 19:190–199, 1978

Levy RI: Tahitians' Mind and Experience in the Society Islands. Chicago, IL, University of Chicago Press, 1973

Li G, Shen YC, Chen CH, et al: An epidemiological survey of age-related dementia in an urban area of Beijing. Acta Psychiatr Scand 79:557–563, 1989

Lin HN, Tsai MT, Rin H: Psychiatric disorders among rural elderly: the Hun-Tsun study. Bulletin of Chinese Society of Neurology and Psychiatry, Special Issue 1:65–79, 1984

Lin KM: Psychopathology and social disruption in refugees, in Refugee Mental Health in Resettlement Countries. Edited by Williams CL, Westermeyer J. Washington, DC, Hemisphere Publishing, 1986, pp 61–73

Lin KM: Cultural influences on the diagnosis of psychotic and organic disorders, in Culture and Psychiatric Diagnosis. Edited by Mezzich J, Kleinman A, Fabrega H Jr, et al. Washington, DC, American Psychiatric Press, 1996

Lin KM, Kleinman AM: Psychopathology and clinical course of schizophrenia: a cross-cultural perspective. Schizophr Bull 14:555–567, 1988

Lipton JA, Marbach JJ: Ethnicity and the pain experience. Soc Sci Med 19:1279–1298, 1984

Mann SC, Caroff SN, Bleier HR, et al: Lethal catatonia. Am J Psychiatry 143:1374–1381, 1986

Polednak AP: Racial and Ethnic Differences in Disease. New York, Oxford University Press, 1989

Salmon DP, Riekkinen PJ, Katzman R, et al: Cross-cultural studies of dementia. Arch Neurol 46:769–772, 1989

Schoenberg BS, Anderson DW, Haerer AF: Severe dementia: prevalence and clinical features in a biracial US population. Arch Neurol 41:740–743, 1985

Serby M, Chou JCY, Franssen E: Dementia in an American-Chinese nursing home population. Am J Psychiatry 144:811–812, 1987

Spector RE: Cultural Diversity in Health and Illness. New York, Appleton-Century-Crofts, 1979

Streltzer J, Wade TC: The influence of cultural group on the undertreatment of postoperative pain. Psychosom Med 43:397–401, 1981

Westermeyer J: Psychiatric diagnosis across cultural boundaries. Am J Psychiatry 142:798–885, 1985

Westermeyer J: Clinical considerations in cross-cultural diagnosis. Hosp Community Psychiatry 38:160–165, 1987

Westermeyer J: Some cross-cultural aspects of delusions, in Delusional Beliefs. Edited by Oltmanns TF, Maher BA. New York, John Wiley, 1988, pp 212–222

Westermeyer J: Mental Health for Refugees and Other Migrants: Social and Preventive Approach. Springfield, IL, Charles C Thomas, 1989

Williams CL: Issues surrounding psychological testing of minority patients. Hosp Community Psychiatry 38:184–189, 1987

Williams RA: Textbook of Black-Related Diseases. New York, McGraw-Hill, 1975

Wittkower E, Prince R: A review of transcultural psychiatry, in American Handbook of Psychiatry, Vol 2: Child and Adolescent Psychiatry, Sociocultural and Community Psychiatry. Edited by Caplan G (Editor-in-Chief Avieti S). New York, Basic Books, 1974, pp 535–550

Yeh Ek, Hwu HG, Chang LY, et al: Lifetime prevalence of cognitive impairment by Chinese-modified NIMH Diagnostic Interview Schedule among the elderly in Taiwan communities. J Neurolinguist 5:83–104, 1990

Zatzick DF, Dimsdale JE: Cultural variation in response to painful stimuli. Psychosom Med 52:544–557, 1990

Zborowski M: Cultural components in response to pain. J Soc 8:16–30, 1952

Zhang M, Katzman R, Salmon D, et al: The prevalence of dementia and Alzheimer's disease in Shanghai, China: impact of age, gender and education. Ann Neurol 27:428–437, 1990

Chapter 44

Culture and Substance-Related Disorders

Joseph Westermeyer, M.D., Ph.D., and
Glorisa Canino, Ph.D.

Introduction

The prevalence of substance-related disorders involving alcohol or other drugs varies considerably across cultures, suggesting that cultural norms influence the etiology and manifestation of these disorders (Babor 1986; Helzer and Canino 1992; Westermeyer 1983). Specific factors affecting the degree of risk for substance-related disorders include patterns of use, attitudes toward substance consumption, accessibility of the drug, physiological reactions to the drug, and family norms and patterns. Other associated features of the disorders, such as comorbidity patterns, certain sociodemographic factors, dependence syndromes, and age at onset, as well as laboratory and physical exam results, are less associated with cultural variability. In this chapter, we address the cultural variations in substance-related disorders to help clinicians make more appropriate DSM-IV diagnoses when assessing patients from diverse cultural backgrounds.

Alcohol Disorders

Prevalence Rates

Drinking behavior cannot be fully understood without considering the social and cultural environment in which the individual lives (Babor 1992). Societies differ in how they view alcohol consumption, in its accessibility, and even in physiological tolerance of alcohol. It should therefore not be surprising that prevalence rates of alcoholism as well as the risk for the disorder vary dramatically from one culture to another, even when the same criteria and methods of ascertainment are employed. Comparisons of lifetime prevalence of alcoholism in 10 different regions of the world (as measured by the Diagnostic Interview Schedule [Robins et al. 1984]) showed that the rates fluctuated from a 23% prevalence in an American Indian population and 22% among the Korean population to 3.5% in Taipei and a low of .45% among the population of Shanghai (Helzer and Canino 1992). High rates of alcoholism in some American Indian populations have been attributed to unemployment, prejudice, poverty, lack of optimism about the future, alienation, and peer socialization processes (Manson et al. 1992). Among Koreans, high rates of alcoholism have been associated with the cultural expectation that men drink heavily on some social occasions (Lee 1992). The prevalence of abuse was significantly higher than that of dependence in this population when DSM-III (American Psychiatric Association 1980) criteria were used. This pattern was attributed to the fact that Korean culture is less tolerant than others of solitary drinking. Low rates of alcoholism in many other Asian countries (excluding Korea) have been attributed to the Confucian moral ethic and to biological conditions such as the flushing response.

Pathological Use

Differences in rates of alcoholism among cultures are more dramatic when only pathological use or impairment in functioning is considered in the definition. This is due largely to the fact that definitions of pathological use may vary according to the drinking practices of a given culture. Evidence from the International Study of Alcohol Experiences shows that overall consumption levels in seven European countries were not strongly related to social consequences (Osterberg 1986). For example, the data from this study showed that in both Poland and Finland, the level of overall consumption was very low, yet social conflicts related to drinking were common, and both countries had high rates of arrests for drunkenness. In the Netherlands, the alcohol consumption patterns were similar to those of Poland and Finland, yet there were few signs of conflicts related to alcohol. Thus, it is not surprising that cultural attitudes toward drinking and intoxication to a great extent determine the risk for alcoholism. In societies with a permissive attitude toward heavy drinking in males, as in Puerto Rico, a large percentage of heavy drinkers do not meet criteria, primarily because they are not deemed impaired in their social or occupational functioning (Canino et al. 1992). In patriarchal societies, families are less likely to complain about excessive drinking among men; physicians are also less likely to warn male drinkers about alcohol abuse. In societies with less permissive attitudes toward drinking, such as some United States communities, most heavy drinkers meet criteria for the disorder, because their drinking pattern is usually associated with multiple social or occupational consequences (Helzer et al. 1991).

In a cross-cultural prospective comparison of men from different ethnic groups, Valliant (1986) also found that cultural attitudes are strongly related to the risk of alcoholism. In this study, Valliant found that Irish men were seven times more likely to develop alcohol dependence than men from Italy. Unlike in Italy, Irish drinking practices prohibit alcohol consumption by children but tolerate and encourage heavy drinking and drunkenness in men, particularly in pubs away from the family and from food intake. Italians, on the other hand, educate their children to drink moderately, encourage drinking with family members and around the dinner table, and are strongly opposed to drunkenness.

The difficulties in defining pathological use among people from different cultural backgrounds is compounded by the absence of DSM criteria for quantity-frequency or dosage. Clearly, many drinking patterns (e.g., bottle sharing by peer groups, binge drinking) frustrate the quantification of the amount consumed and the frequency of consumption. However, constant dosages in the range of 3–4 ounces of ethanol per day are associated with pathological organ changes (i.e., brain, liver, pancreas) in vulnerable individuals. Hence, the century-old concept of "Anstie's limit" (Baldwin 1977) may be a useful starting point for purposes of clinical assessment. Particular subgroups or individuals may not be able to consume culturally sanctioned substances and doses safely. Scientifically derived limits, analogous to Anstie's limit for alcohol, should supersede more liberal cultural parameters. "Pathogenic Substance Use" as a V code could be applied to use that is very likely to produce pathology if continued.

Dependence and Other Associated Features

Although pathological use and the social or occupational consequences of drinking, as well as the prevalence of alcohol dependence, are subject to great cultural variability, there are a number of other factors that seem to remain constant across cultures. Dependence symptoms are relatively invariant regardless of cultural influences (Babor 1992; Babor et al. 1987). This relative invariance is also true of the mean age at onset of alcoholism, the duration of the disorder, the relative frequency of symptoms, and the patterns of co-occurrence of alcoholism with other psychiatric disorders (Helzer and Canino 1992). For example, alcoholism is strongly associated with abuse of other drugs, mania and antisocial personality, and, to a moderate degree, depression and anxiety (Anthony and Helzer 1991; Helzer and Canino 1992; Helzer and Pryzbeck 1988; Regier et al. 1990). Helzer and Canino observed a strong correlation between the relative risk rates for antisocial personality disorder and the prevalence rate of alcoholism in diverse populations. In cultures where alcoholism was prevalent, such as Korea and the United States, antisocial personality disorder was five to six times more common among those with alcoholism. Where the rate of alcoholism was low, such as Taipei, antisocial personality was 240 times more common among those with alcoholism, even though there was also a low prevalence rate of antisocial personality in this population. Based on this evidence, the authors concluded that "in cultures where social sanctions against alcoholism are strong, the occurrence of other diagnoses plays a greater role in the development of alcoholism" (Helzer and Canino 1992, p. 304).

The predominance of the disorder in men as compared with women is constant across cultures, but the gender ratio may vary from 2:1 to 40:1 (see Caetano 1986; Canino et al. 1989, 1992; Heok 1987; Lee 1992; Robins et al. 1984; Westermeyer 1981; Yeh and Hwu 1992). Lower exposure to alcohol among women due to strong cultural sanctions and stigmas may account for these sex-ratio differences (Westermeyer 1981). Helzer et al. (1991) equalized the exposure to alcohol between men and women by estimating the prevalence of the disorder only among those of both sexes who were heavy drinkers. The results showed lower and more consistent sex ratios of alcoholism in seven different cultures.

Pathophysiological changes from alcohol are qualitatively similar across cultures, although quantitative differences may exist (Orford 1973). For example, some ethnic groups with a binge-pattern of drinking have more violent deaths (Levy and Kunitz 1974; Westermeyer and Brantner 1972) or alcoholic psychoses (Gottheil et al. 1973). On the other hand, groups with more controlled drinking manifest greater hepatic and gastrointestinal pathology. Types of personal and social impairment (i.e., family discord, interpersonal problems, occupational disability, legal offenses, and financial insecurity) also tend to be qualitatively similar within each group (Westermeyer 1983). However, the quantitative distribution of these problems can vary by ethnicity in association with cultural values and socioeconomic class (Westermeyer and Brantner 1972). Physical and laboratory findings, such as anemia and plasma protein, can also differ considerably, probably because of nutrition and socioeconomic factors (Westermeyer and Brantner 1972).

Drug Disorders

Prevalence

As with alcohol, societies differ regarding their attitudes toward drug use and the accessibility of drugs. In third-world countries where a great part of the population lives at a subsistence level, lack of income may preclude access to drugs. In Latin American countries, such as Mexico and Brazil, the prevalence of drug disorders in the general population is below 2% (Almeida-Filho et al. 1991; Ortiz and Medina-Mora 1988). The prevalence of drug disorders in Asian countries can vary from less than 2% (e.g., Taiwan, Korea, and Shanghai) to around 10% in poppy-producing communities (Lee 1992; Westermeyer 1983; Yeh and Hwu 1992). Attitudes toward drug use can be inversely related to attitudes toward alcohol use. In Puerto Rico, for example, where attitudes toward alcohol use and intoxication are permissive, high rates of heavy drinking and alcoholism are evident (Canino et al. 1989, 1992). Conversely, attitudes toward drug use are punitive and stigmatizing (Szalay et al. 1993), and the prevalence of both drug use (8.2%) as well as drug addiction (1.2%) in the population is significantly lower than that reported for communities in the United States (30.5% and 6.2%, respectively) (Anthony and Helzer 1991; Canino et al. 1993).

Other Associated Features

As with alcohol disorders, some aspects of drug use remain fairly constant across cultural boundaries. For example, the mean time between the onset of heroin addiction and seeking treatment has been observed to be about 3 years in groups from both Asia and North America (Berger and Westermeyer 1979). Cocaine abuse also appears to run a rapid course prior to treatment seeking, whereas the mean course of opium abuse prior to treatment may extend as long as a decade (Westermeyer 1983). Drug-related disorders are more common among males, urban populations, the less educated, and the young (Anthony and Helzer 1991; Canino et al. 1993; Westermeyer 1980). In the United States and Puerto Rico, investigators have reported similar comorbidity rates between drug disorders and antisocial personality, posttraumatic stress disorders, and the use of other substances such as alcohol (Anthony and Helzer 1991; Berk et al. 1989; Canino et al. 1993; Myers et al. 1984; Regier et al. 1990). In most cultures, individuals abuse more than one type of drug. What seems to vary across cultures is the combination of drugs abused. For example, in Peru, the most frequently used drugs are phencyclidine and cocaine or coca paste (Almeida-Filho 1978).

Clinical Recommendations

Based on these findings, a number of recommendations emerge for the clinician working with patients from different cultural backgrounds.

First, an episodic pattern of substance use should be defined as pathological if it indicates physiological tolerance (e.g., repeated consumption of 10 ounces of alcohol in a 24-hour period) or carries significant risk (e.g., cannabis use and piloting an aircraft), even if supported by the social group. In either instance, careful inquiry is necessary to determine the quantity consumed and the context of its consumption.

Second, potentially pathological use of a specific substance (e.g., inhalants, street drugs of unknown composition, illegal use of prescription drugs, driving when intoxicated, parenteral injection of drugs) should be included as 300.9 "Unspecified Mental Disorder (nonpsychotic)" or 799.9 "Diagnosis or Condition Deferred on Axis I," even if it has not yet been associated with a particular problem but has persisted over time (e.g., 2 weeks or a month). This recommendation derives from the high likelihood of subsequent pathology if use continues. Here, clinicians should be alert for substances with which they are unfamiliar (e.g., peyote or betel nut), which may be differentially preferred by other cultures (Ahluwalia and Ponnampalam 1968; Westermeyer 1982). Moreover, careful questioning is required to establish onset and duration of substance use, perhaps even employing a calendar based on social events to facilitate the patient's report.

Third, in some cultures characterized by heavy substance use among subgroups, the "ideal" norm (i.e., that which people are supposed to do) may permit clearly pathological use or may require abstinence. In view of this, clinicians are recommended to ignore ethnic or cultural norms regarding abstinence or pathological use in applying diagnostic criteria (e.g., moderate use in a culture requiring abstinence *may not* warrant a diagnosis, but pathological use within the norms of the culture may warrant a diagnosis if it meets diagnostic criteria).

Lastly, unlike most other disorders, substance-related disorders provide numerous biological indications of abuse and/or dependence. These include clinical signs and symptoms of 1) intoxication, 2) withdrawal, 3) other organic mental disorders (e.g., dementia, amnesia), 4) organic damage (i.e., abnormal liver function, increased red blood cell count), and 5) consumption of substances (i.e., in blood, urine, or breath). These attributes improve the potential for diagnostic reliability and validity across ethnic groups, cultures, and nations. However, the clinician's own biases or ignorance of the patient's sociocultural ecology may operate against this potential (Chappell 1973).

References

Ahluwalia HS, Ponnampalam JT: The socioeconomic aspects of betel-nut chewing. Journal of Tropical Medicine and Hygiene 71:48–50, 1968

Almeida-Filho N: Contribución al estudio de la historia natural de la dependencia a la pasta básica de cocaína. Revista de Neuropsiquiatríca 41:44–45, 1978

Almeida-Filho N, Santana VS, Pinto IM, et al: Is there an epidemic of drug misuse in Brazil? a review of the epidemiologic evidence (1977–1988). Int J Addict 26:355–369, 1991

American Psychiatric Association: Diagnostic and Statistical Manual of Mental Disorders, 3rd Edition. Washington, DC, American Psychiatric Association, 1980

Anthony JC, Helzer JE: Syndromes of drug abuse and dependence in America, in Psychiatric Disorders in America. Edited by Robins L, Regier N. New York, Free Press, 1991, pp 116–154

Babor T: Alcohol and culture: comparative perspectives from Europe and America. Ann N Y Acad Sci 472:1–9, 1986

Babor T: Cross-cultural research on alcohol: a quoi bon? in Alcoholism in North America, Europe and Asia. Edited by Helzer J, Canino G. Oxford, England, Oxford University Press, 1992, pp 60–72

Babor T, Laurerman R, Cooney H: In search of the alcohol dependence syndrome: a cross-national study of its structure and validity, in Cultural Studies on Drinking and Drinking Problems (Report on a Conference). Edited by Paakkaneno P, Sulkunen P. Helsinki, Finland, Social Research Institute of Alcohol Studies, 1987, pp 1–9

Baldwin AD: Anstie's alcohol limit. Am J Public Health 67:679–681, 1977

Berger LJ, Westermeyer J: World traveler addicts in Asia, II: comparison with "stay at home" addicts. American Journal of Drug Abuse 2:495–503, 1979

Berk E, Black J, Locastro J, et al: Traumatogenicity: effects of self-reported noncombat trauma and noncombat veterans treated for substance abuse. J Clin Psychol 45:704–708, 1989

Caetano R: Patterns and problems of drinking among U.S. Hispanics, in Report of the Secretary's Task Force on Black and Minority Health, Vol 7: Chemical Dependency and Diabetes. Washington, DC, U.S. Department of Health and Human Services, 1986, pp 143–186

Canino G, Bird R, Rubio-Stipec M, et al: The prevalence of alcohol abuse and dependence in Puerto Rico, in Alcohol Use Among U.S. Ethnic Minorities (NIAAA Research Monograph No 18) (DHHS Publ No ADM-88-1435). Edited by Spiegler DL, Tate DA, Aitken SS, et al. Washington, DC, U.S. Government Printing Office, 1989, pp 179–190

Canino G, Burham A, Caetano R: The prevalence of alcohol abuse/dependence in two Hispanic communities, in Alcoholism—North America, Europe and Asia: A Coordinated Analysis of Population Data From Ten Regions. Edited by Helzer J, Canino G. London, England, Oxford University Press, 1992, pp 131–155

Canino G, Anthony JC, Freeman D, et al: Drug abuse and illicit drug use in Puerto Rico. Am J Public Health 83:194–200, 1993

Chappell JN: Attitudinal barriers to physician involvement with drug abusers. JAMA 224:1011–1013, 1973

Gottheil E, Alterman AL, Skolada TE, et al: Alcoholics' pattern of controlled drinking. Am J Psychiatry 130:418–422, 1973

Helzer JE, Canino G: Comparative analyses of alcoholism in ten cultural regions, in Alcoholism—North America, Europe and Asia: A Coordinated Analysis of Population Data From Ten Regions. Edited by Helzer JE, Canino G. London, England, Oxford University Press, 1992, pp 131–155

Helzer JE, Pryzbeck TR: The co-occurrence of alcoholism with other psychiatric disorders in the general population, and its impact on treatment. J Stud Alcohol 49:219–224, 1988

Helzer JE, Burnam A, McEvoy T: Alcohol abuse and dependence in America, in Psychiatric Disorders in America. Edited by Robins L, Regier D. New York, Free Press, 1991, pp 81–115

Heok KE: A cross-cultural study of alcohol dependence in Singapore. Br J Addict 82:771–773, 1987

Lee CK: Alcoholism in Korea, in Alcoholism—North America, Europe and Asia: A Coordinated Analysis of Population Data From Ten Regions. Edited by Helzer JE, Canino G. London, England, Oxford University Press, 1992, pp 247–262

Levy JE, Kunitz SJ: Indian Drinking. New York, Wiley Interscience, 1974

Manson SM, Shore JH, Baron AE, et al: Alcohol abuse and dependence among American Indians, in Alcoholism—North America, Europe and Asia: A Coordinated Analysis of Population Data From Ten Regions. Edited by Helzer JE, Canino G. London, England, Oxford University Press, 1992, pp 113–130

Myers JK, Weissman M, Tischler G, et al: Six-month prevalence of psychiatric disorders in three communities. Arch Gen Psychiatry 41:959–967, 1984

Orford J: A comparison of alcoholics whose drinking is totally uncontrolled, and those whose drinking is mainly controlled. Behav Res Ther 11:565–576, 1973

Ortiz A, Medina-Mora ME: Research on drugs in Mexico: epidemiology of drug abuse and issues among Native American populations, in Community Epidemiology Work Group Proceedings (Contract No. 271-87-8321). Washington, DC, U.S. Government Printing Office, December, 1988

Osterberg E: Alcohol-related problems in cross-national perspectives: results of the ISACE study. Ann N Y Acad Sci 472:10–20, 1986

Regier DA, Farmer ME, Rae D, et al: Comorbidity of mental disorders with alcohol and other drug abuse. JAMA 264:2511–2518, 1990

Robins LN, Helzer JE, Weissman MM, et al: Lifetime prevalence of specific psychiatric disorders in three sites. Arch Gen Psychiatry 41:949–958, 1984

Szalay LB, Canino G, Vilov SK: Vulnerabilities and culture change: drug use among Puerto Rican adolescents in the United States. Int J Addict 28:327–354, 1993

Valliant G: Cultural factors in the etiology of alcoholism: a prospective study. Ann N Y Acad Sci 472:142–148, 1986

Westermeyer J: Sex ratio among opium addicts in Asia: influences of drug availability and sampling method. Drug Alcohol Depend 6:131–136, 1980

Westermeyer J: Opium availability and prevalence of addiction in Asia. Br J Addict 76:85–90, 1981

Westermeyer J: Betel nut chewing (letter). JAMA 148:1831–1832, 1982

Westermeyer J: Treatment of opiate addiction in Asia: current practice and recent advances, in Research Advances in Alcohol and Drug Problems. Edited by Smart R, Glaser F. New York, Plenum, 1983, pp 433–455

Westermeyer J, Brantner J: Violent death and alcohol use among the Chippewa of Minnesota. Minn Med 55:749–752, 1972

Yeh EK, Hwu HG: Alcoholism in Taiwan Chinese communities, in Alcoholism—North America, Europe and Asia: A Coordinated Analysis of Population Data From Ten Regions. Edited by Helzer JE, Canino G. London, England, Oxford University Press, 1992, pp 214–246

Chapter 45

Cultural Considerations in the Diagnosis of Schizophrenia and Related Disorders and Psychotic Disorders Not Otherwise Classified

Marvin Karno, M.D., and
Janis H. Jenkins, Ph.D.

Issues

The primary symptoms of schizophrenia and related disorders have been reported from extremely diverse cultures that represent myriad forms of social organization, different levels of economic and industrial development, and divergent religious and other belief systems.

The most reliable cross-cultural data on the symptomatology of schizophrenia and related disorders come from the World Health Organization's (1973, 1979) nine-country International Pilot Study of Schizophrenia. This study was conducted in Colombia, Czechoslovakia, Denmark, India, Nigeria, China, the USSR, the United Kingdom, and the United States. Data from this study are important because of the investigators' use of a systematic diagnostic instrument, the Present State Examination (PSE) (Wing et al. 1974), and a large sample size. The computer-generated CATEGO subtype S+ (a core or "nuclear" syndrome), which was derived from the PSE data, revealed significant similarity of schizophrenic symptom profiles across centers (Kulhara et al. 1987; World Health Organization 1979). On the other hand, when the data from the PSE were analyzed using a broader symptom range, the results showed substantial variation. Insofar as the PSE is both a conservative and reliable cross-cultural instrument, this heterogeneity of symptom profiles is important to an adequate understanding of the phenomenology and manifestation of schizophrenia across settings (Bellak 1975, Shamis 1976). Analysis from the Determinants of Outcome study (Sartorius et al. 1986) has similarly yielded evidence that supports both the cross-cultural similarity (Jablensky et al. 1992) and heterogeneity of symptom profiles (Ndetei and Vadher 1984a).

There is strong evidence for the interpretation drawn from the two major multisite studies of schizophrenia sponsored by the World Health Organization (1973, 1979) that the incidence of a core schizophrenic syndrome is similar worldwide, despite objections that the case has not yet been made (Cohen 1992; Stevens and Wyatt 1987).

The symptomatic presentation of schizophrenia has been found to vary in other clinical studies from different cultural contexts. A high prevalence of visual hallucinations has been reported for schizophrenic patients in Mexico (Krassoievitch et al. 1982) and in Kenya (Ndetei and Singh 1983). Among 593 patients admitted to one London hospital, hallucinations of all types were found to be more prevalent among patients from African, West Indian, and Asian cultural groups than among patients from English and other cultural groups (Ndetei and Vadher 1984b).

Delusions must be carefully evaluated with reference to cultural and religious belief systems (Ndetei and Vadher 1984c). For example, belief in witchcraft or sorcery is common cross-culturally (Murdock et al. 1980; Rubel and Hass 1990). Patients may also participate in culturally specific belief systems that are part of their religious traditions. For example, among some Latino groups in the United States (e.g., Cubans, Puerto Ricans, Dominicans, Salvadorans), the religions of Spiritism and Santeria incorporate active involvement with the dead, spirits, or multiple deities (Gonzales-Wippler 1989; Harwood 1987). Caution should be exercised when probing these domains because patients may be reluctant to divulge their views (Rubel and Hass 1990).

An essential feature of a culturally appropriate diagnosis is that all prodromal, active psychotic, and residual symptoms must be evaluated with reference to the patient's particular cultural context. This context includes beliefs, affects, behavior, and sense of self.

Culture and Affect

Affect must be carefully assessed to avoid misdiagnosis of psychotic disorders. Difficulties in assessment stem from the fact that there are substantial cross-cultural differences in the experience and expression of affect (Briggs 1970; Levy 1973; Myers 1979; Schieffelin 1983). These differences present difficulties for the establishment of normative baselines for flat affect. Some cultures, for example, inhibit the social expression of positive or negative affect of any sort (Briggs 1970; Geertz 1984). What makes affect an essentially cultural phenomenon is the fact that emotions—no less than other attitudes, beliefs, and behaviors—are substantially mediated by culture (Jenkins and Karno 1992; Jenkins et al. 1991; Kleinman and Good 1985; Lutz 1988; Shweder and LeVine 1984). Cultures differentially socialize their members to foster or inhibit affective displays. As Anderson and Holder (1989) summarized, "The symptoms of schizophrenia also tend to vary by gender. Women have a greater affective component while men show more disturbances in the areas of cognition, behavior, and motivation" (p. 392). In addition, cultural styles may vary by gender within cultures, and implicit rules for interaction between men and women may differ. Women in many cultures may be more reluctant to display positive affect in the presence of male interviewers, whereas men may inhibit the display of positive affect in the presence of nonintimate others (Bayes 1981; Broverman et al. 1981; Stephenson and Walker 1981). For these reasons, the presence of "flat affect" must be carefully considered with respect to the patient's gender and cultural background. In diagnostic assessments of schizophrenia, significant variations in flat affect (as assessed through the PSE) have been found (Kulhara et al. 1987; World Health Organization 1979).

Ethnic and Sociocultural Bias in Diagnosis

Bias and stereotyping in the diagnosis of schizophrenia among patients from devalued and ethnic minority groups have been reported in a study of British psychiatrists' responses to case vignettes of African Caribbean and Anglo-white subjects (Lewis et al. 1990), and a study of American psychiatric diagnoses of African American and Puerto Rican bipolar patients (Jones and Gray 1986). Actual differences in the presentation of schizophrenic symptoms as well as delusional disorder and other psychoses have been reported for black versus white patients in the United States (Chu et al. 1985; Mukherjee et al. 1983). These studies did not rule out potential bias nor, more importantly, did they consider the fact that in certain sociocultural contexts mental disorder may have to reach a more advanced degree of overt and threatening expression before the patient is brought to clinical attention. This had been the conclusion of an earlier study in Texas that demonstrated a more florid degree of psychotic symptoms among Mexican American than non-Hispanic white schizophrenic patients on initial psychiatric evaluation (Fabrega et al. 1968).

In addition to the cautions mentioned, a reverse phenomenon also needs to be stressed in cross-cultural situations of diagnostic assessment. Psychotic symptoms that are psychopathological may be mistakenly interpreted as culturally normative because of limited cultural familiarity (Chandrasena 1983).

Gender and cultural variations in the expression of affect that are sufficient to confound an appropriate psychiatric diagnosis have been reported from Brazil (Nations et al. 1988) and New Guinea (Herdt 1986), as well as among Asian cultures (Clancy 1986; Marcella et al. 1985).

Culture and Sense of Self

Cross-cultural studies note that disturbances in the sense of self often thought to be characteristic of schizophrenia must also be evaluated with respect to a patient's cultural background. For example, not all cultural groups socialize their members to regard themselves as ideally unique, independent, or autonomous. Some cultures are more likely to foster a socially based, interdependent sense of self that is intimately bound up with others (Fabrega 1989a, 1989b; Geertz 1984; Jenkins et al. 1991; Kleinman 1988; Shweder and Bourne 1985).

Culture and Course of Schizophrenia

The evidence that schizophrenia is characterized by a shorter course and more complete resolution in developing compared with developed societies derives from a series of studies carried out in the 1960s and 1970s (Murphy and Raman 1971; Rin and Lin 1962; Waxler 1977). This finding has been substantially buttressed by the two World Health Organization (1973, 1979) collaborative multisite studies mentioned earlier. This finding from the World Health Organization International Pilot Study of Schizophrenia was further confirmed by the ongoing Determinants of Outcome study (Sartorius et al. 1986), which greatly strengthens the evidence.

Numerous studies have demonstrated that the course of schizophrenia is associated with the "expressed emotion" factors (Karno et al. 1987; Leff et al. 1987; Vaughn and Leff 1976; Vaughn et al. 1984). The expressed emotion factors (criticism, hostility, and emotional overinvolvement) have been found to vary cross-culturally. Moreover, a comparative approach reveals that the construct of expressed emotion is essentially cultural in nature (Jenkins and Karno 1992).

Cultural Factors and Psychotic Disorders Not Otherwise Classified

Socially sanctioned and culturally valued hallucinatory experiences are apparently common among the American Plains Indians (Hultkrantz 1979; LaBarre 1972) and among some Caribbean and Latin American cultures (Gonzales-Wippler 1989;

Harwood 1987). Psychotic symptoms experienced in settings where cultural expectations may render such symptoms nonpathological have been reported in a recent psychiatric community epidemiological study in Puerto Rico (Guarnaccia et al. 1992) and anthropologically informed clinical studies from India (Andrade et al. 1988, 1989) and Australia (Cheng 1985). The experience of psychotic but apparently nonpathological delusions in response to sorcery has been reported in Puerto Rican (Griffith 1982) and Polish (Freedman 1988) subjects.

References

Anderson C, Holder D: Women and serious mental disorders, in Women and Mental Health. Edited by Howell E, Bayes M. New York, Basic Books, 1989, pp 381–405

Andrade C, Srinath S, Andrade AC: True hallucinations as a culturally sanctioned experience. Br J Psychiatry 152:838–839, 1988

Andrade C, Srinath S, Andrade AC: True hallucinations in non-psychotic states. Can J Psychiatry 34:704–706, 1989

Bayes M: The prevalence of gender-role bias in mental health services, in Women and Mental Health. Edited by Howell E, Bayes M. New York, Basic Books, 1981, pp 83–85

Bellak L: Intercultural studies in search of a disease. Schizophr Bull 12:6–9, 1975

Briggs J: Never in Anger: Portrait of an Eskimo Family. Cambridge, MA, Harvard University Press, 1970

Broverman I, Broverman D, Clarkson F, et al: Sex-role stereotypes and clinical judgments of mental health, in Women and Mental Health. Edited by Howell E, Bayes M. New York, Basic Books, 1981, pp 86–97

Chandrasena R: Culture and clinical psychiatry. Revue de Psychiatrie de l'Université d'Ottawa 8:16–19, 1983

Cheng SK: Cultural explanation of a "psychosis" in a Chinese woman living in Australia. Aust N Z J Psychiatry 19:190–194, 1985

Chu CC, Sallach HS, Zakeria SA, et al: Differences in psychopathology between black and white schizophrenics. Int J Soc Psychiatry 31:252–257, 1985

Clancy P: The acquisition of communicative style in Japanese, in Language Socialization Across Cultures. Edited by Schieffelin B, Ochs E. Cambridge, MA, Cambridge University Press, 1986, pp 213–250

Cohen A: Prognosis for schizophrenia in the third world: a reevaluation of cross-cultural research. Cult Med Psychiatry 16:53–75, 1992

Fabrega H: On the significance of an anthropological approach to schizophrenia. Psychiatry 52:45–65, 1989a

Fabrega H: The self and schizophrenia. Schizophr Bull 15:277–290, 1989b

Fabrega H, Swartz JD, Wallace CA: Ethnic differences in psychopathology, II: specific differences with emphasis on the Mexican American group. Psychiatr Res 6:221–235, 1968

Freedman J: Cross cultural intervention: the case of the hexed hair. Clin Soc Rev 6:159–166, 1988

Geertz C: From the native's point of view: on the nature of anthropological understanding, in Culture Theory: Essays on Mind, Self, and Emotion. Edited by Shweder RA, LeVine RA. Cambridge, MA, Cambridge University Press, 1984, pp 123–136

Gonzales-Wippler M: Santeria: The Religion. New York, Crown Publishers, 1989

Griffith E: The impact of culture and religion on psychiatric care. J Natl Med Assoc 74:1175–1179, 1982

Guarnaccia PJ, Luz MG-R, Gonzalez G, et al: Cross-cultural aspects of psychotic symptoms in Puerto Rico. Res Commun Ment Health Annual 7:99–110, 1992

Harwood A: Rx: Spiritist As Needed: A Study of a Puerto Rican Community Mental Health Resource. Ithaca, NY, Cornell University Press, 1987

Herdt G: Madness and sexuality in the New Guinea highlands. Soc Res 53:349–367, 1986

Hultkrantz A: The Religions of the American Indians. Berkeley, CA, University of California Press, 1979

Jablensky A, Sartorius N, Ernberg G, et al: Schizophrenia: Manifestations, Incidence and Course in Different Cultures: A World Health Organization Ten-Country Study. Psychol Med Monograph Supplement 20, 1992, pp 1–97

Jenkins JH, Karno M: The meaning of expressed emotion: theoretical issues raised by cross-cultural research. Am J Psychiatry 149:9–21, 1992

Jenkins JH, Kleinman A, Good B: Cross-cultural studies of depression, in Psychosocial Aspects of Depression. Edited by Becker J, Kleinman A. Hillsdale, NJ, Lawrence Erlbaum Associates, 1991, pp 67–99

Jones BE, Gray BA: Problems in diagnosing schizophrenia and affective disorders in blacks. Hosp Community Psychiatry 37:61–65, 1986

Karno M, Jenkins JH, de la Selva A, et al: Expressed emotion and schizophrenic outcome among Mexican-American families. J Nerv Ment Dis 175:143–151, 1987

Kleinman A: Rethinking Psychiatry: From Cultural Category to Personal Experience. New York, Free Press, 1988

Kleinman A, Good BJ (eds): Culture and Depression: Studies in the Anthropology and Cross-Cultural Psychiatry of Affect and Disorder. Berkeley, CA, University of California Press, 1985

Krassoievitch M, Perez-Rincon H, Suarez P: Correlation entre les hallucinations visuelles et auditives dans une population de schizophrènes Mexicains. Confrontations Psychiatriques 15:149–162, 1982

Kulhara P, Mattoo S, Awasthi A, et al: Psychiatric manifestations of CATEGO Class S+ schizophrenia. Indian J Psych 29:307–313, 1987

LaBarre W: The Ghost Dance: The Origins of Religion. New York, Delta Publishers, 1972

Leff J, Wig N, Ghosh A, et al: Expressed emotion and schizophrenia in north India, III: influence of relatives' expressed emotion on the course of schizophrenia in Chandigarh. Br J Psychiatry 151:166–173, 1987

Levy R: Tahitians: Mind and Experience in the Society Islands. Chicago, IL, University of Chicago Press, 1973

Lewis G. Croft-Jeffreys C, Anthony D: Are British psychiatrists racist? Br J Psychiatry 157:410–415, 1990

Lutz CA: Unnatural Emotions: Everyday Sentiments on a Micronesian Atoll and Their Challenge to Western Theory. Chicago, IL, University of Chicago Press, 1988

Marcella A, DeVos G, Hsu F: Culture and Self: Asian and Western Perspectives. New York, Tavistock, 1985

Myers FR: Emotions and the self: a theory of personhood and political order among Pintupi Aborigines. Ethos 7:343–370, 1979

Mukherjee S, Shukla S, Woodle J, et al: Misdiagnosis of schizophrenia in bipolar patients: a multiethnic comparison. Am J Psychiatry 140:1571–1574, 1983

Murdock G, Wilson SF, Frederick V: World distribution of theories of illness. Transcult Psych Res Rev 17:37–74, 1980

Murphy HBM, Raman AC: The chronicity of schizophrenia in indigenous tropical peoples: results of a 12-year follow-up on Mauritius. Br J Psychiatry 118:489–497, 1971

Nations MK, Rebuhn LA, Scheper-Hughes N: Angels with wet wings won't fly: maternal sentiment in Brazil and the image of neglect. Cult Med Psychiatry 12:141–200, 1988

Ndetei DM, Singh A: Hallucinations in Kenyan schizophrenic patients. Acta Psychiatr Scand 67:144–147, 1983

Ndetei DM, Vadher A: A comparative cross-cultural study of the frequencies of hallucination in schizophrenia. Acta Psychiatry Scand 70:545–549, 1984a

Ndetei DM, Vader A: A cross-cultural study of the frequencies of Schneider's first rank symptoms of schizophrenia. Acta Psychiatry Scand 70:540–544, 1984b

Ndetei DM, Vadher A: Frequency and clinical significance of delusions across cultures. Acta Psychiatry Scand 70:73–76, 1984c

Rin H, Lin T: Mental illness among Formosan aborigines as compared with Chinese in Taiwan. J Ment Sci 108:134–146, 1962

Rubel AJ, Hass C: Ethnomedicine, in Medical Anthropology: Contemporary Theory and Method. Edited by Johnson T, Sargent C. New York, Praeger, 1990, pp 115–131

Sartorius N, Jablensky A, Korten A, et al: Early manifestations and first contact incidence of schizophrenia in different cultures: a preliminary report on the initial evaluation phase of the WHO collaborative study on determinants of outcome of severe mental disorders. Psychol Med 16:909–928, 1986

Schieffelin E: Anger and shame in the tropical forest: on affect as a cultural system in Papua, New Guinea. Ethos 11:181–191, 1983

Shamis S: Linguistic relativity and the diagnosis of schizophrenia. Schizophr Bull 4:503–504, 1976

Shweder RA, Bourne EJ: Does the concept of the person vary cross-culturally? in Culture Theory: Essays on Mind, Self, and Emotion. Edited by Shweder RA, LeVine RA. Cambridge, MA, Cambridge University Press, 1985, pp 158–199

Shweder RA, LeVine RA (eds): Culture Theory: Essays on Mind, Self, and Emotion. Cambridge, MA, Cambridge University Press, 1984

Stephenson A, Walker G: The psychiatrist-woman patient relationship, in Women and Mental Health. Edited by Howell E, Bayes M. New York, Basic Books, 1981, pp 113–130

Stevens JR, Wyatt RJ: Similar incidence worldwide of schizophrenia: case not proven. Br J Psychiatry 151:131–132, 1987

Vaughn C, Leff J: The influence of family and social factors on the course of psychiatric illness: a comparison of schizophrenic and depressed neurotic patients. Br J Psychiatry 129:125–137, 1976

Vaughn C, Snyder K, Jones S, et al: Family factors in schizophrenic relapse: replication in California of British research on expressed emotion. Arch Gen Psychiatry 41:1169–1177, 1984

Waxler N: Is outcome for schizophrenia better in nonindustrialized societies? the case of Sri Lanka. J Nerv Ment Dis 167:144–158, 1977

Wing JK, Cooper JE, Sartorius N: The Description and Classification of Psychiatric Symptoms: An Instructional Manual for the PSE and CATEGO System. London, England, Cambridge University Press, 1974

World Health Organization: The International Pilot Study of Schizophrenia. Geneva, Switzerland, World Health Organization, 1973

World Health Organization: Schizophrenia: An International Follow-Up Study. New York, John Wiley, 1979

Chapter 46

Cultural Considerations in the Diagnosis of Mood Disorders

Spero M. Manson, Ph.D.

Introduction

In this chapter, I examine the mood disorders within a cross-cultural context. I focus on the operational characteristics of the major diagnostic criteria that 1) encompass specific symptoms and assign greater importance to some than others; 2) reflect different dimensions or clusters of cognitive, affective, behavioral, and somatic experiences; 3) assume critical thresholds by requiring certain minimums in both the number and duration of symptomatology; and 4) define relationships between disorders, particularly in terms of relative priority for subsequent diagnosis. The discussion draws selectively from the available literature to illustrate the manner and extent to which these criteria may be extended to other cultural populations.

Separation of Mind and Body

The most salient feature of the mood disorders is a distinction between psyche and soma that reflects a long Western intellectual history of mind-body dualism. This distinction is particularly evident in the formulation of major and minor depressive episodes as well as dysthymia, which revolve around particular affects (e.g., dysphoria, represented by depressed mood or loss of interest or pleasure) and associated somatic symptoms, notably appetite and weight change, sleep disturbances, psychomotor agitation or retardation, fatigue, difficulty concentrating, recurrent thoughts of death, motor tension, and autonomic hyperactivity. The somatic symptoms, like many physical experiences, are relatively easy to ascertain across cultures, although eliciting them poses a special set of problems to which

I return later. The greatest difficulty lies in determining the presence of dysphoria as defined by Western experience, largely because of the attendant assumptions about emotion and its phenomenology.

Attitudes toward the nature of emotions have the potential to polarize discussions about the cross-cultural applicability of DSM. To the extent that emotions appear to be shared or common experiences of people from diverse cultural groups, many assume that this similarity is a function of universal, innate human propensities (Ekman 1982; Izard 1977; Wierzbicka 1986). Others argue that they are essentially cultural artifacts (C. Geertz 1973; Rosaldo 1984).

It seems plausible that culture at least organizes the stimulus, manifestation, and interpretation of emotions like dysphoria (Myers 1979). This conclusion follows from the rapidly growing body of evidence on cultural variations in the phenomenology of these experiences (C. Geertz 1980; B. J. Good and Good 1982; B. J. Good and Kleinman 1985; Kinzie et al. 1982; Kleinman and Good 1985; Lutz 1985, 1988; Manson et al. 1985; Marsella et al. 1985; Myers 1979; Rosaldo 1983, 1984; Shweder and LeVine 1984). As Jenkins et al. (1990) pointed out, key elements to understanding this variation involve definitions of selfhood, indigenous categories of emotion, emphases on particular aspects of emotional life, patterning of relationships among emotions, precipitating social situations, and ethnophysiological accounts of bodily experiences of emotions.

Definitions of Self and Loci of Emotion

Definitions of the self vary along a continuum between "egocentric" and "sociocentric" (Shweder and Bourne 1984). Egocentric conceptions, best exemplified in Western, industrialized populations, characterize the person as unique, separate, and autonomous. Sociocentric conceptions, found in many non-Western cultural traditions, depict the person in relational terms as part of an interdependent collective defined by kinship and myth (C. Geertz 1984). In the United States, such differences are thought to distinguish Hispanics (Murillo 1976), American Indians and Alaskan natives (Trimble et al. 1984), and Asian Americans (Kleinman and Lin 1981; Tseng and Hsu 1969) from white, middle-class Americans. It should not be surprising, then, that the locus and experience of emotions vary along similar lines (Lutz 1985, 1988; Toussignant 1984). In other words, they are not necessarily just intrapsychic phenomena. Hence, diagnostic criteria that depend on eliciting individualistically oriented self-statements of dysphoria (e.g., "*I* feel blue," "These things no longer mean anything to *me*") or worry (e.g., "*I* am bothered by things that usually do not bother *me*," "*I* fear things that *I* do not normally fear") that are unrelated to context may be constrained, intrinsically, from discovering other ways of feeling and expressing the same affect.

Variation in the Language of Affect

Numerous studies underscore the rich and varied lexicons of emotion in non-Western cultures (Chang 1985; H. Geertz 1959; B. J. Good 1977; B. J. Good and Good 1982; B. J. Good et al. 1985; Guarnaccia et al. 1990; Kinzie et al. 1982; Lutz 1985, 1988; Marsella and White 1982; White and Kirkpatrick 1985). Establishing the semantic equivalence of the terms by which people from different cultures refer to the same affect is typically approached through a translation/backtranslation process. One bilingual speaker of languages A and B answers the question: "What is the word or phrase for '_____' in language B?" Presented with that answer, another bilingual speaker of the same two languages is asked: "What is the word or phrase for '_____' in language A?" The results are seldom unequivocal, reflecting the indeterminacy of meaning that typifies human language (B. J. Good and Good 1986; Robins 1989). For example, guilt, shame, and sinfulness are often closely linked in Western experience and, indeed, make up a single question on the Diagnostic Interview Schedule (Robins et al. 1981) intended to assess feelings of worthlessness. These terms can be translated into Hopi but are conceptualized quite differently and evoke attributions that are both distinct from one another and distinct from those implied by their English counterparts within a Judeo-Christian framework (Manson et al. 1985). In another example, Chinese offers a wealth of terms that convey sadness and despair. One, *you-yu* (Zhihai 1957), closely approximates the affective aspect of depression (Chang 1985). It describes a prevailing sadness, despair, and listlessness combined with a tendency toward crying, much like the statement "I feel downhearted and blue." However, as Chang pointed out, this mood is treated and reported quite differently by the Chinese than by their Western counterparts.

Then, too, an equivalent for the word *depressed* is absent from the languages of some cultures (Marsella 1980), including certain American Indians and Alaskan natives (Manson et al. 1985; Terminsen and Ryan 1970) and Southeast Asian refugee groups (Kinzie et al. 1982). However, its absence does not, in and of itself, preclude the existence of related affect or even analogous categories of illness. Manson et al. (1985) demonstrated that the DSM-III (American Psychiatric Association 1980) formulation of major depressive disorder does not correspond directly to any of the categories of illness indigenous to the Hopi. Instead, DSM-III symptoms of major depressive disorder are distributed differentially across the Hopi categories, which are characterized by distinct etiologies and treatments. This particular example depicts the problem of category validity described by B. J. Good and Good (1986).

Selective Elaboration of Emotional Experience

Such variation in the phenomenology as well as the language of emotion suggests that cultures selectively emphasize and elaborate these experiential domains. Drawing from the ethnographic literature on anger, Jenkins et al. (1990) illustrated the dramatic degree to which different cultures may contrast with one another in this regard. Whereas Eskimos (Briggs 1970) and Tahitians (Levy 1973) seldom display anger, the Kaluli of New Guinea (Schieffelin 1983, 1985) and the Yanamamo of Brazil (Chagnon 1977) employ elaborate and complex means of expressing anger. Likewise, Iranian culture encourages displays of extreme sadness and sorrow (B. J. Good and Good 1982; B. J. Good et al. 1985), whereas Navajo culture discourages displays of these emotions (Miller and Schoenfeld 1971; Witherspoon 1977).

Differences within groups are also evident along these lines, most notably in terms of social class and gender, and especially for dysphoria. This appears to be true among mainstream Americans (Hirschfeld and Cross 1982; Weissman and Klerman 1977) as well as among ethnic minorities (Ackerson et al. 1990; Baron et al. 1990; Canino et al. 1987; Manson et al. 1990; Mendes de Leon 1988; Vega et al. 1984, 1986; Zavalla 1984). Similar dynamics have been observed around the world, for example in Ghana (Field 1960), Kenya (Abbott and Klein 1979; Mitchell and Abbott 1987; Ndetei and Vadher 1982), Uganda (Orley and Wing 1979), and India (Ullrich 1987, 1988).

Culture not only may place differential emphasis on particular emotions, but can also assign unique attributions to the intensity of their experience as well as their expression. Vietnamese refugees, for instance, distinguish states of sadness by the frequency of their feelings, as well as by the degree and duration (Kinzie et al. 1982). Culture also shapes the general tone of emotional life to which a person should aspire, ranging from the tumultuous involvement of the Yanamamo (Chagnon 1977) to the serenity of the Javanese (C. Geertz 1973).

Thus, distinguishing among mood, symptom, and disorder, which are presumed to vary along a continuum, is not as simple as it might seem (Kleinman and Good 1985). Although there is no empirical evidence to this effect, current diagnostic operations assume that such experiences are unidimensional, linear, and additive in nature, not unlike a ruler. The cross-cultural literature suggests that the "markers" on the ruler may vary from one group to another, akin to the difference between metric and nonmetric systems of measurement. Not only may the scale of measurement differ in terms of minimal units (e.g., millimeter versus $1/32$ of an inch), but also the significant categories of aggregation may also not correspond (e.g., centimeter and meter versus inch, foot, and yard). Assessing the degree to which subjective conditions like dysphoria and mania are present in cross-cultural settings, then, is not straightforward, as elegantly demonstrated by McNabb (1990), in his article on determining the accuracy and meaning of self-reported "satisfaction" among the Eskimo, and by Iwata et al. (1989), in their report on the Japanese use of the Center for Epidemiologic Studies Depression Scale (CES-D) (Radloff 1977) scaler values.

Even if ways are developed to translate from one "ruler" to another, by no means an easy task even in the simplest form of the problem, this accomplishment does not take into account the normative uncertainty of psychiatric ratings (Chance 1963; B. J. Good and Good 1986; Guarnaccia et al. 1990; Jenkins 1988a, 1988b; Manson et al. 1985; Murphy and Hughes 1965; Robins 1989). Specifically, the literature indicates that the threshold at which "normal" is demarcated from "abnormal" may vary by gender and cultural group. For example, the persistently higher prevalence of depressive *symptoms* reported among females compared with males and among Puerto Ricans compared with white, middle-class Americans (Guarnaccia et al. 1990) may represent culturally patterned variations in the experiential levels of these phenomena and not necessarily higher rates of *disorder*. Consequently, such normative differences imply different "cutoff points" for distinguishing common, unremarkable episodes of mood from those that are unusual and noteworthy. Returning to the "ruler" analogy, if such cutoff points were solely a function of intensity or severity, then female and Yanamamo thresholds between normal and abnormal dysphoria, for example, might fall much further along (or "out" or "up," depending on its orientation) the ruler than male and Javanese thresholds. Current DSM debate over the number of symptoms required to meet criterion C (persistent avoidance or psychic numbing) for posttraumatic stress disorder reflects an analogous struggle to establish a viable cutoff point.

DSM, however, employs more than just intensity or severity in rendering such judgments. Duration often figures into the diagnostic calculus (e.g., 2 weeks of persistent dysphoria to meet criteria for major depressive episode or 1 month of symptoms for posttraumatic stress disorder). Nevertheless, the same logic applies. For example, among the Hopi, sadness is so common and widespread that periods of 1 month or more may be required to reach a level of significance for the individual and fellow community members equivalent to that presupposed by DSM (Manson et al. 1985). Even then, it appears as if duration is only a "proxy" measure of functional impairment: the sadness or worry experienced by a Hopi person becomes a concern when she or he begins to fail to meet deeply ingrained social expectations.

The developers of DSM-IV are dealing with a similar issue in their attempt to clarify earlier distinctions between major depressive syndrome and major depressive episode and between major depression and dysthymia. This may explain, at least in part, why other criteria (i.e., Feighner criteria [Feighner et al. 1972] and Research Diagnostic Criteria [Spitzer et al. 1978]) have only slowly been discarded. The very same definitional quandary emerges and multiplies in complexity as one moves across different cultures.

Dimensions of Depression and Mania

Further insight into the gender as well as cultural patterning of affect—in this case, symptoms of depression and mania—can be obtained from studies involving the CES-D. The CES-D is a composite measure that includes items from previously established scales and was developed by researchers at the National Institute for Mental Health for use in epidemiological studies of depressive symptomatology (Radloff 1977). The 20-item scale assesses the occurrence and persistence of the following symptoms in the past week: depressed mood, feelings of guilt and worthlessness, psychomotor retardation, loss of appetite, and sleep disturbance. The scale has been shown to be psychometrically sound in terms of its reliability across diverse populations: adults (Radloff 1977; Zich et al. 1990), adolescents (Radloff 1991; Roberts et al. 1990), and different racial and ethnic groups (Radloff 1977; Roberts 1980; Ying 1988). Radloff (1977) described factor analyses by gender and ethnicity (white versus black) that yielded a consistent dimensional structure comprising four factors that she labeled *depressed affect, somatic complaints, positive affect,* and *interpersonal difficulties.* Other researchers have subsequently reported important differences in the factor structures across gender and ethnic groups.

Four studies have examined the CES-D factor structure across gender. Clark et al. (1981) performed principal components factor analysis with varimax rotation on data provided by a sample of mixed ethnicity. The authors reported a factor structure generally consistent with Radloff's (1977) when the full sample was included. However, when factor analyses were performed by gender, the factor structure for females was quite different. Using the Kaiser criterion, Clark et al. found only three factors; the items making up Radloff's depressed affect dimension were distributed across the factors of somatic complaints, positive affect, and interpersonal difficulties. Guarnaccia et al. (1989) and Garcia and Marks (1989) examined factor structures across gender within Hispanic Health and Nutrition Examination Survey samples, and both reported gender differences. Roberts et al. (1990) used confirmatory factor-analytic methods to examine differences in an adolescent sample. Although the Radloff model fit the data adequately for the overall sample, analyses across gender indicated that an assumption of factorial invariance was not warranted.

The possibility of different factor structures across ethnic groups has been considered among Chinese Americans and Hispanics. Both Kuo (1984) and Ying (1988) conducted principal components analyses of CES-D data from samples of Chinese Americans. Using the Kaiser criterion, they reported finding three factors in which Radloff's depressed affect and somatic complaints factors were combined. The majority of the work in this area has examined the performance of the CES-D among Mexican American subsamples. Although Roberts (1980) reported finding no differences between Mexican American and Anglo samples, others using exploratory methods found that the somatic complaints and depressed affect factors formed a single factor (Garcia and Marks 1989; Guarnaccia et al. 1989). In another study, Golding and Aneshensel (1989), using Los Angeles Epidemiologic Catchment Area data, first performed a maximum likelihood exploratory factor analysis with the complete sample and found that the four-factor solution closely corresponded to Radloff's and encompassed all 20 items. They then conducted a confirmatory factor analysis across non-Hispanic whites, United States-born Mexican Americans, and Mexican-born Mexican Americans. Their results failed to support an assumption of factorial invariance.

Three studies have examined the performance of the CES-D among American Indian samples. Manson et al. (1990) performed factor analyses on data collected from Indian adolescents attending a boarding school. They obtained a three-factor solution with a strong "general" factor that included items from Radloff's depressed affect, somatic complaints, and interpersonal factors. The remaining two factors encompassed additional items from the somatic complaints factor, as well as a distinct positive affect factor. In a study of older American Indians with chronic physical illnesses, Baron et al. (1990) reported obtaining a four-factor solution, again with a strong general factor that included both depressed affect and somatic complaints. The remaining three factors were not well defined. Beals et al. (1991) examined the viability of the model tested by Golding and Aneshensel (1989) in which all 20 CES-D items were proposed to load on one of four factors. This model is essentially equivalent to that of Radloff if the criteria are loosened to include each item as an indicator of the factor on which it had the highest loading. Three alternative models were tested for the full sample: the original four-factor model, a three-factor model in which the somatic complaints and depressed affect factors were collapsed, and a single-factor model. The three-factor model was based on the studies of ethnic minority samples described earlier, and which the literature on American Indians supports, specifically, that depressed affect and somatic complaints are not as differentiated in these populations as in others. The justification for the single-factor model stemmed from the frequent use of the overall CES-D score rather than the subscales. The fit of these models was also tested across gender to determine whether the factor structure can be assumed to be equivalent. The correlations between the four factors proved to be moderate in size (.44–.64) with one exception: the correlation between the depressed affect and somatic complaints factors was .90. Although the four-factor and three-factor models provided comparable fits to the data, it was apparent that the depressed affect and somatic complaints factors correlated so highly that for the purpose of application they should be considered indistinguishable. The three-factor model, therefore, was deemed the most appropriate for these data.

A number of studies have shown that the factor structures for similar self-report measures of symptoms of depression and anxiety (e.g., Brief Symptom Index [Derogatis and Spencer 1982], Zung Self-Rating Depression Scale [Zung 1965], Beck Depression Inventory [Beck 1978]) also vary significantly by cultural populations (Chang 1985; B. J. Good et al. 1985; Marsella et al. 1973; Tashakkori et al. 1989), although the evidence for the convergence of depressed affect and somatic complaints in these studies is not as strong as that which has emerged in the context of the CES-D.

The high correlation between depressed affect and somatic complaints is relevant to the ongoing debate about the somatization of depressed mood (Lipowski 1990), especially with regard to the role of sociocultural factors, and returns us to the discussion on epistemological differences in the relationship of mind and body. One view holds that non-Western populations are predisposed to report depressive affect in somatic rather than psychological terms. Explanations include communicational style and socialization (Katon et al. 1982). A popular extension of this view is that non-Western populations do not differentiate somatic from affective complaints. However, as noted earlier, many non-Western populations clearly possess elaborate vocabularies to describe emotional states. The levels at which the respondents in the studies cited earlier endorsed the items subsumed under depressed affect confirm their salience for these populations. Yet, the degree of association between the depressed affect and somatic complaints factors suggests significant overlap that may be either conceptual or artifactual in nature. This issue deserves close attention, especially to determine how the diagnostic criteria for a disorder like major depression, which emphasizes affective problems over concomitant somatic complaints, can be applied in the absence of similar distinctions or priorities (Eysenck et al. 1983).

Differences in Narrative Context

The expression of emotion also varies by the cultural contexts in which such experiences are discussed. Individuals selectively report the elements they believe to be situationally relevant (Beiser 1985; Cheung 1982; Kinzie and Manson 1983;

Tseng and Hsu 1969; Wu 1982). Disclosures of physical and psychological states differ in form as well as content between patient and physician, husband and wife, parent and child, and men and women (M.-J. Good and Good 1988; Jenkins 1988a; Kleinman 1986). This dynamic is a specific corollary of the more general observation that cultural systems provide guidelines for matching behavior to social events and circumstances (Cole et al. 1971; Labov 1970; LeVine 1970). Consequent differences in rules for the display of emotion in non-Western cultures may frustrate the elicitation of relevant criteria and assignment of diagnosis.

Ethnophysiology of Somatic Experience

Lastly, diagnoses of mood disorders also hinge on the presence of somatic complaints: rapid, unintended weight loss or gain; significant changes in appetite; marked disturbances of sleep patterns; fatigue; exaggerated startle responses; motor tension; or autonomic hyperactivity. Although more easily observed and ascertained than affective states, such physical experiences are likewise mediated by social and cultural conventions. The medical literature recognized early that the manner in which pain is described, and even potential sites for its occurrence in the body, may vary from one population to another (Kleinman 1986). In cross-cultural settings, it is not unreasonable to inquire about the somatic complaints detailed by DSM. Indeed, the endorsement of these symptoms by the patient should encourage more aggressive investigation of the possible presence of the disorder of interest to the clinician. At this point, the diagnostic endeavor must broaden to include the discovery and elimination of alternative causes of the complaints in question (e.g., infectious disease, malnutrition, parasites, and other organic conditions that may be common to the local ecology).

The absence of these symptoms, however, is not equally as informative. Somatic distress can be expressed in diverse ways not anticipated by DSM. Consider, for example, Ebigbo's (1982) observation of such complaints as "heat in the head," "crawling sensation of worms and ants," "heaviness sensation in the head," and "biting sensation all over the body" (p. 9) among Nigerian patients, or Jenkins' (1988a) description of *nervios* among Mexican Americans, which includes "brain ache," or the sensation that the brain is "exploding" or "uncontrollable." These and other indigenous means of describing bodily experiences may represent the physiological equivalent of the somatic symptom specified by DSM, which would not have been elicited on direct inquiry. They also may represent different bodily experiences that either co-occur with or even denote the criterion affect (e.g., dysphoria or excessive worry) and thus are as clinically meaningful as those designated in DSM.

This growing body of evidence in regard to cross-cultural variation in the identification, elicitation, and meaning of the diagnostic criteria for the mood disorders poses a major challenge for present-day psychiatry. Maser et al. (1991) surveyed 146 mental health professionals, primarily psychiatrists and psychologists, from 42 countries excluding the United States, on international uses of and attitudes toward DSM-III and DSM-III-R (American Psychiatric Association 1987). Their study revealed that the mood disorders, often in conjunction with anxiety and other disorders, were perceived to be problematic and in need of revision by nearly a quarter of the respondents. Although it was not possible to determine the genesis of these perceptions, Maser et al. concluded by emphasizing the cross-cultural deficiencies of DSM and the need to reflect a broader range of experience in the nosology and diagnostic formulation.

References

Abbott S, Klein R: Depression and anxiety among rural Kikuyu in Kenya. Ethos 7:161–188, 1979

Ackerson LM, Dick RW, Manson SM, et al: Depression among American Indian adolescents: psychometric characteristics of the Inventory to Diagnose Depression. J Am Acad Child Adolesc Psychiatry 29:601–607, 1990

American Psychiatric Association: Diagnostic and Statistical Manual of Mental Disorders, 3rd Edition. Washington, DC, American Psychiatric Association, 1980

American Psychiatric Association: Diagnostic and Statistical Manual of Mental Disorders, 3rd Edition, Revised. Washington, DC, American Psychiatric Association, 1987

Baron AE, Manson SM, Ackerson LM, et al: Depressive symptomatology in older American Indians with chronic disease: some psychometric considerations, in Screening for Depression in Primary Care. Edited by Attkinsson C, Zich J. New York, Routledge Chapman & Hall, 1990, pp 217–231

Beals J, Manson SM, Keane KM, et al: The factorial structure of the Center for Epidemiologic Studies Depression Scale among American Indian college students. J Consult Clin Psychol 3:623–627, 1991

Beck AT: Depression Inventory. Philadelphia, PA, Philadelphia Center for Cognitive Therapy, 1978

Beiser M: A study of depression among traditional Africans, urban North Americans, and Southeast Asian refugees, in Culture and Depression: Studies in the Anthropology and Cross-Cultural Psychiatry of Affect and Disorder. Edited by Kleinman A, Good B. Berkeley, CA, University of California Press, 1985, pp 272–298

Briggs J: Never in Anger: Portrait of an Eskimo Family. Cambridge, MA, Harvard University Press, 1970

Canino GJ, Bird H, Shrout P, et al: The prevalence of specific psychiatric disorders in Puerto Rico. Arch Gen Psychiatry 38:381–389, 1987

Chagnon N: Yanomamo: the Fierce People. New York, Holt, Rinehart, & Winston, 1977

Chance N: Conceptual and methodological problems in cross-cultural health research. Am J Public Health 52:410–417, 1963

Chang WC: A cross-cultural study of depressive symptomatology. Cult Med Psychiatry 9:295–317, 1985

Cheung FM: Psychological symptoms among Chinese in urban Hong Kong. Soc Sci Med 16:1339–1344, 1982

Clark VA, Aneshensel CS, Frerichs RR, et al: Analysis of effects of sex and age in response to items on the CES-D scale. Psychiatry Res 5:171–181, 1981

Cole M, Gay J, Glick JA, et al: The Culture Context of Learning and Thinking. New York, Basic Books, 1971

Derogatis LP, Spencer MS: The Brief Symptom Inventory (BSI): Administration, Scoring, and Procedures Manual. Baltimore, MD, Clinical Psychometric Research, 1982

Ebigbo P: Development of a culture specific (Nigeria) screening scale of somatic complaints. Cult Med Psychiatry 6:29–44, 1982

Ekman P: Emotion in the Human Face. Cambridge, MA, Cambridge University Press, 1982

Eysenck HJ, Wakefield JA, Friedman AF: Diagnosis and clinical assessment: the DSM-III, Third Edition. Annu Rev Psychol 34:167–194, 1983

Feighner JP, Robins E, Guze SB, et al: Diagnostic criteria for use in psychiatric research. Arch Gen Psychiatry 16:57–63, 1972

Field MJ: Search for Security: An Ethnopsychiatric Study of Rural Ghana. Evanston, IL, Northwestern University Press, 1960

Garcia M, Marks G: Depressive symptomatology among Mexican-American adults: an examination of the CES-D scale. Psychiatry Res 27:137–148, 1989

Geertz C: The Interpretations of Cultures. New York, Basic Books, 1973

Geertz C: Negara: the Theater State in Nineteenth-Century Bali. Princeton, NJ, Princeton University Press, 1980

Geertz C: For the native's point of view: on the nature of anthropological understanding, in Culture Theory: Essays on Mind, Self, and Emotion. Edited by Shweder R, LeVine R. Cambridge, MA, Cambridge University Press, 1984, pp 123–136

Geertz H: The vocabulary of emotion: a study of Javanese socialization processes. Psychiatry 22:225–237, 1959

Golding JM, Aneshensel CS: Factor structure of the Center for Epidemiologic Studies Depression Scale Among Mexican Americans and Non-Hispanic Whites. Psychological Assessment 1:163–168, 1989

Good BJ: The heart of what's the matter. Cult Med Psychiatry 1:25–38, 1977

Good BJ, Good M-J: Toward a meaning-centered analysis of popular illness: categories "fright illness" and "heart distress" in Iran, in Cultural Conceptions of Mental Health and Therapy. Edited by Marsella A, White G. Boston, MA, D Reidel, 1982, pp 141–166

Good BJ, Good M-J: The cultural context of diagnosis and therapy: a view from medical anthropology, in Research and Practice in Minority Communities. Edited by Miranda M, Kitano H. Washington, DC, U.S. Government Planning Office, National Institute of Mental Health, 1986, pp 1–27

Good BJ, Kleinman A: Epilogue: culture and depression, in Culture and Depression: Studies in the Anthropology and Cross-Cultural Psychiatry of Affect and Disorder. Edited by Kleinman A, Good B. Berkeley, CA, University of California Press, 1985, pp 491–505

Good BJ, Good M-J, Moradi R: The interpretation of Iranian depressive illness and dysphoric affect, in Culture and Depression: Studies in the Anthropology and Cross-Cultural Psychiatry of Affect and Disorder. Edited by Kleinman A, Good B. Berkeley, CA, University of California Press, 1985, pp 369–428

Good M-J, Good BJ: Ritual, the state, and the transformation of emotional discourse in Iranian society. Cult Med Psychiatry 12:43–63, 1988

Guarnaccia PJ, Angel R, Worobey JL: The factor structure of the CES-D in the Hispanic Health and Nutrition Examination Survey: the influences of ethnicity, gender and language. Soc Sci Med 29:85–94, 1989

Guarnaccia PJ, Good BJ, Kleinman A: A critical review of epidemiological studies of Puerto Rican mental health. Am J Psychiatry 147:1449–1456, 1990

Hirschfeld RM, Cross C: Epidemiology of affective disorders: psychosocial risk factors. Arch Gen Psychiatry 39:35–46, 1982

Iwata N, Okuyama Y, Kawakami Y, et al: Prevalence of depressive symptoms in a Japanese occupational setting: a preliminary study. Am J Public Health 70:1486–1489, 1989

Izard C: Human Emotions. New York, Plenum, 1977

Jenkins JH: Conceptions of schizophrenia as a problem of nerves: a cross-cultural comparison of Mexican-Americans and Anglo-Americans. Soc Sci Med 26:1233–1244, 1988a

Jenkins JH: Ethnopsychiatric interpretations of schizophrenic illness: the problem of nervios within Mexican-decent families. Cult Med Psychiatry 12:302–318, 1988b

Jenkins JH, Kleinman A, Good BJ: Cross-cultural studies of depression, in Advances in Mood Disorders. Edited by Becker J, Kleinman A. New York, Lawrence Erlbaum Associates, 1990, pp 67–99

Katon W, Kleinman A, Rosen G: Depression and somatization, a review: part I. Am J Med 72:127–135, 1982

Kinzie JD, Manson SM: Five years of experience in the Indochinese Psychiatric Clinic: what have we learned? Journal of Operational Psychiatry 14:105–111, 1983

Kinzie JD, Manson SM, Do TV, et al: Development and validation of a Vietnamese-language depression rating scale. Am J Psychiatry 139:1276–1281, 1982

Kleinman A: Social Origins of Distress and Disease: Depression, Neurasthenia, and Pain in Modern China. New Haven, CT, Yale University Press, 1986

Kleinman A, Good BJ (eds): Epilogue, in Culture and Depression: Studies in the Anthropology and Cross-Cultural Psychiatry of Affect and Disorder. Berkeley, CA, University of California Press, 1985, pp 491–505

Kleinman A, Lin TY: Normal and Abnormal Behavior in Chinese Culture. Boston, MA, D Reidel Publishing Co, 1981

Kuo W: Prevalence of depression among Asian Americans. J Nerv Ment Dis 172:449–457, 1984

Labov W: The logic of non-standard English, in Language and Poverty. Edited by Williams F. Chicago, IL, Markam Publishing, 1970, pp 153–189

LeVine RA: Cross-cultural study in child psychology, in Carmichael's Manual of Child Psychology, Vol 2. Edited by P. Mussen. New York, John Wiley, 1970, pp 559–614

Levy R: Tahitians: Mind and Experience in the Society Islands. Chicago, IL, University of Chicago Press, 1973

Lipowski ZJ: Somatization and depression. Psychosomatics 31:13–71, 1990

Lutz C: Depression and the translation of emotional worlds, in Culture and Depression Studies in the Anthropology and Cross-Cultural Psychiatry of Affect and Disorder. Edited by Kleinman A, Good B. Berkeley, CA, University of California Press, 1985, pp 63–100

Lutz C: Unnatural Emotions: Everyday Sentiments on a Micronesian Atoll and Their Challenge to Western Theory. Chicago, IL, University of Chicago Press, 1988

Manson SM, Shore JH, Bloom JD: The depressive experience in American Indian communities: a challenge for psychiatric theory and diagnosis, in Culture and Depression. Edited by Kleinman A, Good B. Berkeley, CA, University of California Press, 1985, pp 331–368

Manson SM, Ackerson LM, Dick RW, et al: Depressive symptoms among American Indian adolescents: psychometric characteristics of the Center for Epidemiologic Studies Depression Scale (CES-D). Psychological Assessment 2:231–237, 1990

Marsella AJ: Depressive experience and disorder across cultures, in Handbook of Cross-cultural Psychology, Vol 5: Psychopathology. Edited by Triandis H, Draguns J. Boston, MA, Allyn & Bacon, 1980, pp 132–156

Marsella AJ, White GM (eds): Cultural Conceptions of Mental Health and Therapy. Boston, MA, D Reidel Publishing, 1982

Marsella AJ, Kinzie JD, Gordon P: Ethnocultural variations in the expression of depression. Journal of Cross Cultural Psychology 4:453–458, 1973

Marsella AJ, DeVos G, Hsu F: Culture and Self: Asian and Western Perspectives. New York, Tavistock Publications, 1985

Maser JD, Kaelber C, Weise RE: International use and attitudes toward DSM-III (-III-R): growing consensus in psychiatric classification. J Abnorm Psychol 100:271–279, 1991

McNabb SL: Self-reports in cross-cultural contexts. Human Organization 49:291–299, 1990

Mendes de Leon C-F: Depressive symptoms among Mexican Americans: a three-generation study. Am J Epidemiol 127:150–160, 1988

Miller SI, Schoenfeld LS: Suicide attempt patterns among the Navajo Indians. Int J Soc Psychiatry 17:189–193, 1971

Mitchell S, Abbott S: Gender and symptoms of depression and anxiety among Kikuyu secondary school students in Kenya. Soc Sci Med 24:303–316, 1987

Murillo N: The Mexican-American family, in Chicanos: Social and Psychological Perspectives. Edited by Vega W. St. Louis, MO, CV Mosby, 1976, pp 97–108

Murphy JM, Hughes CC: The use of psychophysiological symptoms as indicators of disorder among Eskimos, in Approaches to Cross-Cultural Psychiatry. Edited by Murphy JM, Leighton AH. Ithaca, NY, Cornell University Press, 1965, pp 108–160

Myers F: Emotions and the self: a theory of personhood and political order among Pintupi Aborigines. Ethos 7:343–370, 1979

Ndetei D, Vadher A: A study of some psychological factors in depressed and non-depressed subjects in a Kenyan setting. Br J Med Psychol 55:235–239, 1982

Orley J, Wing JK: Psychiatric disorders in two African villages. Arch Gen Psychiatry 36:513–557, 1979

Radloff LS: The CES-D scale: a self-report depression scale for research in the general population. Applied Psychological Measurement 1:385–401, 1977

Radloff LS: The use of the Center for Epidemiologic Studies Depression Scale in adolescents and young adults. Journal of Youth and Adolescence 20:149–166, 1991

Roberts RE: Reliability of the CES-D scale in different ethnic contexts. Psychiatry Res 2:125–134, 1980

Roberts RE, Andrews JA, Lewinsohn PM, et al: Assessment of depression in adolescents using the Center for Epidemiologic Studies Depression Scale. Psychological Assessment 2:122–128, 1990

Robins LN: Cross-cultural differences in psychiatric disorder. Am J Public Health 79:1479–1480, 1989

Robins LN, Helzer JE, Croughan J, et al: The National Institute of Mental Health Diagnostic Interview Schedule: its history, characteristics, and validity. Arch Gen Psychiatry 38:381–389, 1981

Rosaldo M: The shame of headhunters and the autonomy of self. Ethos 11:135–151, 1983

Rosaldo M: Toward an anthropology of self and feeling, in Culture Theory: Essays on Mind, Self, and Emotion. Edited by Shweder RA, LeVine RA. Cambridge, MA, Cambridge University Press, 1984, pp 137–157

Schieffelin EL: Anger and shame in the tropical forest: on affect as a cultural system in Papua, New Guinea. Ethos 11:181–191, 1983

Schieffelin EL: The cultural analysis of depressive affect: an example from New Guinea, in Culture and Depression. Edited by Kleinman A, Good B. Berkeley, CA, University of California Press, 1985, pp 101–133

Shweder R, Bourne E: Does the concept of the person vary cross-culturally?, in Culture Theory: Essays on Mind, Self, and Emotion. Edited by Shweder R, LeVine R. Cambridge, MA, Cambridge University Press, 1984, pp 158–199

Shweder R, LeVine R (eds): Culture Theory: Essays on Mind, Self, and Emotion. Cambridge, MA, Cambridge University Press, 1984

Spitzer RL, Endicott J, Robins E: Research Diagnostic Criteria: rationale and reliability. Arch Gen Psychiatry 35:773–782, 1978

Tashakkori A, Barefoot J, Mehryar AH: What does the Beck Depression Inventory measure in college students? evidence from a non-Western culture. J Clin Psychology 45:595–602, 1989

Terminsen J, Ryan J: Health and disease in a British Columbian community. Canadian Psychiatric Association Journal 15:121–127, 1970

Toussignant M: Pena in the Ecuadorian Sierra: a psychoanthropological analysis of sadness. Cult Med Psychiatry 8:381–398, 1984

Trimble JE, Manson SM, Dinges NG, et al: American Indian concepts of mental health: reflections and directions, in Mental Health Services: The Cross-cultural Content. Edited by Pedersen PB, Sartorius N, Marsella AJ. Beverly Hills, CA, Sage Publications, 1984, pp 199–220

Tseng WS, Hsu J: Chinese culture, personality formation, and mental illness. Int J Soc Psychiatry 6:5–14, 1969

Ullrich HE: A study of change and depression among Havik Brahmin women in a south Indian village. Cult Med Psychiatry 11:261–287, 1987

Ullrich HE: Widows in South India society: depression as an appropriate response to cultural factors. Sex Roles 19:169–188, 1988

Vega W, Warheit G, Buhl-Auth J, et al: The prevalence of depressive symptoms among Mexican Americans and Anglos. Am J Epidemiol 120:592–607, 1984

Vega W, Kolody B, Valle R, et al: Depressive symptoms and their correlates among immigrant Mexican women in the United States. Soc Sci Med 22:645–652, 1986

Weissman M, Klerman G: Sex differences and the epidemiology of depression. Arch Gen Psychiatry 34:98–111, 1977

White GM, Kirkpatrick J: Person, Self, and Experience: Exploring Pacific Ethnopsychologies. Berkeley, CA, University of California Press, 1985
Wierzbicka A: Human emotions: universal or culture-specific? American Anthropologist 88:584–594, 1986
Witherspoon G: Language and Art in the Navajo Universe. Ann Arbor, MI, University of Michigan Press, 1977
Wu DHY: Psychotherapy and emotion in traditional Chinese medicine, in Culture Conceptions of Mental Health and Therapy. Edited by Marsella AJ, White GM. Boston, MA, D Reidel Publishing, 1982, pp 202–220
Ying Y: Depressive symptomatology among Chinese-Americans as measured by the CES-D. J Clin Psychol 44:739–746, 1988
Zavalla I: Depression among women of Mexican descent, University of Massachusetts, Department of Psychology, unpublished Ph.D. dissertation, 1984
Zhihai: Zhihai (Ocean of words and terms). Taipei, Shangwu (Commercial) Printing House, 1957
Zich J, Attkisson C, Greenfield T: Screening for depression in primary care clinics: the CES-D and the BDI. Int J Psychiatry Med 20:259–277, 1990
Zung WWK: A self-rating depression scale. Arch Gen Psychiatry 12:63–70, 1965

Chapter 47

Culture and the Anxiety Disorders

Peter J. Guarnaccia, Ph.D., and
Laurence J. Kirmayer, M.D.

Statement and Significance of the Issues

In this review, we examine cultural issues in applying the diagnostic criteria for the anxiety disorders to individuals from different cultural groups, both within the United States and across the globe. A key issue in the cross-cultural application of anxiety diagnostic criteria is whether excessive worry and apprehension are necessarily the predominant symptoms and whether these emotional symptoms should be given priority over the range of somatic symptoms and rich bodily idioms of anxiety that, as shown in the cross-cultural literature, are often of concern to people experiencing these disorders. In examining the specific diagnostic categories within the anxiety disorders section of DSM-III-R (American Psychiatric Association 1987), a number of concerns were identified with specific diagnoses. Some concerns arose out of the need for clinicians to have considerable cultural knowledge to make the differential diagnostic decisions required by the DSM-III-R criteria; others arose out of the need for the expansion of diagnostic categories or the creation of new categories to encompass culture-specific syndromes identified by cross-cultural researchers.

The importance of examining the interface between culture and anxiety was thoroughly reviewed by Good and Kleinman (1985). This chapter takes that review as a starting point and builds on their findings. Good and Kleinman's review poses a number of questions and issues that remain unresolved. The purpose of the current review is to update progress on these issues and to specify areas for further research. There has been less attention to the anxiety disorders than to either schizophrenia or depression in cross-cultural research. There has not been a major World Health Organization study for anxiety disorders as there has been for schizophrenia (World Health Organization 1973, 1979) and depression (World

Health Organization 1983). Even in the Epidemiologic Catchment Area (ECA) studies (Regier et al. 1984), there has been limited focus on the anxiety disorders despite their high prevalence in the population (Brown et al. 1990; Karno et al. 1989).

There are five major questions examined in this review:

1. Does the prevalence of anxiety disorders differ among ethnic and cultural groups?
2. Do the risk factors for developing anxiety differ among ethnic and cultural groups?
3. What are the differences in symptom pattern of the different expressions of anxiety across cultures?
4. What culture-specific syndromes and idioms of distress might fit, at least in part, within the anxiety disorders section of DSM-IV, and what questions do these categories raise about the proposed diagnostic criteria?
5. Is the diagnosis of posttraumatic stress disorder appropriate for categorizing the experience of refugees from Southeast Asia and Central America, and do the criteria for posttraumatic stress disorder need to be modified for these groups?

Method

We selected studies for this chapter that 1) updated findings in the review by Good and Kleinman (1985), 2) focused on psychiatric diagnosis (i.e., for their assessment of anxiety disorders) rather than psychological assessment (i.e., anxiety as a continuous dimension of personality), and 3) provided insights into the major anxiety categories listed in DSM-IV.

Results

Prevalence of Anxiety Disorders in Multicultural Settings

Two epidemiological reports of anxiety disorders using the ECA data indicate that there are important similarities and differences in the prevalence of selected anxiety disorders among different ethnic and cultural groups. In an analysis by Karno et al. (1989) of the prevalence of the full range of anxiety disorders in the Los Angeles ECA site, similar prevalences of panic disorder, social phobia, and obsessive-compulsive disorder were found among non-Hispanic whites and Mexican Americans born in both the United States and Mexico. Differences were found for the diagnoses of simple phobia, agoraphobia, and generalized anxiety disorder. A major finding of this study was that Mexicans born in Mexico had lower rates of anxiety (and other disorders) than Mexican Americans born in the United States. The authors suggested selective migration as a key factor in the differences in rates. From the perspective of cross-cultural psychiatry, much research is needed to explore in detail the nature of the migration experience and the effects of long-term residence in the urban United States to understand the source of these differences and to identify preventive interventions for the children of these migrants.

Brown et al. (1990) reviewed data on phobias from the Baltimore, Maryland, and St. Louis, Missouri, ECA sites, both with large numbers of African American respondents. The authors found that African Americans had higher rates of phobias than whites, even when sociodemographic factors were controlled. They suggested that greater numbers of stressful life events and that higher stress from marginal minority group status may account for the higher rates of phobias among African Americans.

Both of the ECA studies highlight important ethnic differences in rates of anxiety disorders and offer hypotheses relating to different sociocultural experiences as explanations, because analyses demonstrated that social class factors alone were not sufficient to explain the differences. Yet measures of these social experiences of marginality and stress are lacking and are greatly needed to further mental health research generally and cross-cultural research in particular. Neither study addressed the validity of using the anxiety questions, particularly the phobia questions, as measures of psychiatric disorder rather than as measures of social stress. Considerable research is needed to establish whether elevated symptoms of anxiety, particularly phobia, are signs of a disordered individual or a disordered social environment.

A clinical study by Friedman and Paradis (1991), which compared 15 African American patients with panic and agoraphobia to 15 white patients with panic and agoraphobia, specified some of the life events that may be related to higher rates of anxiety disorders among African Americans. Although both groups had similar symptom profiles, the authors found that the African Americans with panic and agoraphobia had experienced more separations from parents and more traumatic events in childhood than the white patients; they also experienced worse treatment outcome. Despite the small samples, the study provides a direction for examining in more detail the different risk factors for the development of anxiety disorders across ethnic and cultural groups.

Cross-Cultural Differences in Patterns of Anxiety Symptoms

Although ethnic comparisons within the United States have not identified major symptom differences for the anxiety disorders, cross-cultural studies have indicated that there are significant differences in the ways anxiety is described and, potentially, experienced. Key implications of this work are that the range of symptoms included in DSM-IV needs to be expanded to make the manual applicable across cultures and that diagnostic criteria need to be modified in some cases. Of particular concern is the primary emphasis on the emotional experiences of excessive worry or apprehension as the key to diagnosis and the lack of emphasis on somatic forms or presentations of anxiety.

Many of these cross-cultural studies have come from Africa and include clinical studies of both culture-specific syndromes (Makanjuola 1987) and anxiety (Awaritefe 1988) and the development of the Enugu Somatization Scale by Ebigbo (1986). Several of the studies indicated that a core symptom of anxiety, at least as experienced in Nigeria, was a sensation of an insect crawling through the head and sometimes other parts of the body (Awaritefe 1988; Ebigbo 1986; Makanjuola 1987). More broadly, these studies demonstrated that when symptoms were freely listed by those suffering anxiety and were systematically studied (see Ebigbo 1986), new criterial symptoms emerged for the anxiety disorders. These studies call into question findings in the United States that symptom patterns are not significantly different among ethnic groups. Studies in the United States all used structured instruments that allowed for response to only a limited set of symptom items that were originally derived from European American populations.

Culture-Specific Syndromes and Their Relationship to Anxiety Disorders

A brief discussion of some culture-specific syndromes that have been proposed for inclusion in the anxiety disorders highlights the following issues: 1) the need for an expanded set of symptoms for the anxiety disorders; 2) the issue of the boundary between anxiety, affective, somatoform, and dissociative disorders; and 3) the need to expand the broader anxiety category to include cultural expressions that do not fit easily into existing anxiety diagnoses. Three syndromes, about which we have considerable information allowing comparison with DSM-III-R diagnoses, highlight these issues: *ataques de nervios* (Guarnaccia et al. 1989, 1993), *koro* (Bernstein and Gaw 1990), and *taijin kyofusho* (Kirmayer 1991).

Guarnaccia et al. (1993) reported on an epidemiological study of the mental health of Puerto Rican adults in Puerto Rico. The study included a question on ataque de nervios, a syndrome most widely studied among Puerto Ricans but common to the Hispanic Caribbean and reported in other areas of Latin America. The most common symptom reported for experiences of ataques de nervios was "screaming uncontrollably," a symptom that does not appear in DSM-III-R. "Attacks of crying" was the next most prominent symptom, which appears in the somatization section of the Diagnostic Interview Schedule (Robins et al. 1981) and is most often associated with affective disorders. Although the symptom profile of an ataque de nervios is closest to the DSM-III-R description of a panic attack, a major difference is that ataques are almost always provoked by an upsetting event, whereas panic attacks occur in situations that are not inherently upsetting or frightening. In looking at the association between experiencing an ataque de nervios and meeting criteria for psychiatric disorders, Guarnaccia et al. found significant associations not only with anxiety but also with affective disorders.

The defining feature of koro is "acute anxiety associated with the fear of genital retraction and is usually accompanied by the thought that complete disappearance of the organ into the abdomen will result in death" (Bernstein and Gaw 1990, p. 1670). It has been reported in several Asian cultural groups and has been described in both Eastern and Western medical texts for centuries. In proposing a DSM-IV classification for the syndrome, Bernstein and Gaw noted the dilemmas involved in fitting koro into current diagnostic categories. Although acute anxiety is a core feature of the syndrome, arguing for its inclusion as an anxiety disorder, the defining feature is concern over a physical symptom (genital retraction) with no physiological basis, arguing for inclusion as a somatoform disorder.

Kirmayer (1991) analyzed how taijin kyofusho fits into DSM criteria as part of a broader cultural critique of psychiatric diagnosis. Taijin kyofusho is a syndrome particular to Japan that involves anxiety or fears that certain features of personal style or of one's physical self will give offense to others. Taijin kyofusho reverses the usual definitions of social phobia (anxiety of being scrutinized or embarrassed by others in social situations) found in DSM-III-R. Kirmayer noted that fear of blushing, fear of eye-to-eye contact, and fear of emitting body odor, all symptoms of taijin kyofusho, are absent from DSM-III-R. Kirmayer argued that the different subtypes of taijin kyofusho described in Japanese psychiatry would, in DSM-III-R, range from adjustment disorders in childhood to psychotic disorders.

Posttraumatic Stress Disorder in Refugees

Posttraumatic stress disorder has received considerable recent attention from cross-cultural researchers in the United States and elsewhere because of its high prevalence among refugees fleeing from violence and state terror in Southeast Asia and Central America (Eisenbruch 1991; Jenkins 1991; Mollica et al. 1987, 1990). Although posttraumatic stress disorder is considered an anxiety disorder, clinicians and researchers working with these refugees have found a high co-occurrence with posttraumatic stress disorder of major depressive disorder (Jenkins 1991; Kinzie et al. 1990; Mollica et al. 1987) and of dissociative experiences (Carlson and Rosser-Hogan 1991). Eisenbruch (1991) proposed a new category, "cultural bereavement," as a diagnosis that more fully captures the nature of the syndrome of traumatic losses experienced by Southeast Asian refugees. The recent introduction of the posttraumatic stress disorder diagnosis and its even more recent application to groups who are culturally different and whose trauma experience is unique suggest a need for considerable research before conclusions can be reached about the applicability of posttraumatic stress disorder to these populations or the place of posttraumatic stress disorder within the diagnostic system.

Discussion

The issues discussed here highlight major concerns about the cross-cultural applicability of the anxiety disorders section of DSM-III-R and raise challenges for DSM-IV. The current lists of criterial symptoms in DSM-III-R are a limited palette of the cross-cultural experience of anxiety. Some culture-specific syndromes may fit within the anxiety disorders with some modification of criteria or additions of subcategories. Many of the culture-specific syndromes challenge the current nosology, which rigidly separates the anxiety disorders from affective and somatoform disorders. Although the mixed anxiety-depression category proposed for DSM-IV is a start, we need a more interactive and integrated view of these disorders.

Recommendations

In light of the comments in this chapter, the following recommendations are made for examining cross-cultural issues in the anxiety disorders section of DSM-IV:

1. More systematic research is needed to identify the range of symptoms prominently associated with anxiety disorders in different cultural groups and different cultural contexts.
2. For those culture-specific syndromes about which we have considerable detailed information from clinical and/or epidemiological research, multidisciplinary research efforts between psychiatric and cross-cultural researchers are needed to assess the relationship of these syndromes with current diagnostic categories and the need for new categories or subcategories of disorder.
3. For culture-specific syndromes about which our level of knowledge is currently insufficient to assess their relationship to DSM-IV categories, research efforts to describe and assess more fully the epidemiology of the disorders and their impact on those who suffer from them are needed.
4. Recognition of the interplay among the anxiety, affective, somatoform, and dissociative disorders is needed to open the possibility for research that would examine the appropriateness of these categories and the place of cultural forms of expressing distress and culture-specific syndromes within them.

References

American Psychiatric Association: Diagnostic and Statistical Manual of Mental Disorders, 3rd Edition, Revised. Washington, DC, American Psychiatric Association, 1987

Awaritefe A: Clinical anxiety in Nigeria. Acta Psychiatr Scand 77:729–735, 1988

Bernstein RL, Gaw AC: Koro: proposed classification for DSM-IV. Am J Psychiatry 147:1670–1674, 1990

Brown DR, Eaton WW, Sussman L: Racial differences in prevalence of phobic disorders. J Nerv Ment Dis 178:434–441, 1990

Carlson EB, Rosser-Hogan R: Trauma experiences, post-traumatic stress, dissociation, and depression in Cambodian refugees. Am J Psychiatry 148:1548–1551, 1991

Ebigbo PO: A cross sectional study of somatic complaints of Nigerian females using the Enugu Somatization Scale. Cult Med Psychiatry 10:167–186, 1986

Eisenbruch M: From post-traumatic stress disorder to cultural bereavement: diagnosis of Southeast Asian refugees. Soc Sci Med 33:673–680, 1991

Friedman S, Paradis C: African-American patients with panic disorder and agoraphobia. Journal of Anxiety Disorders 5:35–41, 1991

Good BJ, Kleinman AM: Culture and anxiety: cross-cultural evidence for the patterning of anxiety disorders, in Anxiety and the Anxiety Disorders. Edited by Tuma AH, Maser J. Hillsdale, NJ, Lawrence Erlbaum Associates, 1985, pp 297–324

Guarnaccia PJ, Rubio-Stipec M, Canino G: Ataques de nervios in the Puerto Rican Diagnostic Interview Schedule. Cult Med Psychiatry 13:275–295, 1989

Guarnaccia PJ, Canino G, Rubio-Stipec M, et al: The prevalence of ataques de nervios in the Puerto Rico Disaster Study. J Nerv Ment Dis 181:157–165, 1993

Jenkins JH: The state construction of affect: political ethos and mental health among Salvadoran refugees. Cult Med Psychiatry 15:139–165, 1991

Karno M, Golding JM, Burnham MA, et al: Anxiety disorders among Mexican Americans and Non-Hispanic Whites in Los Angeles. J Nerv Ment Dis 177:202–209, 1989

Kinzie JD, Boehnlein JK, Leung PK, et al: The prevalence of post-traumatic stress disorder and its clinical significance among Southeast Asian refugees. Am J Psychiatry 147:913–917, 1990

Kirmayer LJ: The place of culture in psychiatric nosology: Taijin Kyofusho and DSM-III-R. J Nerv Ment Dis 179:19–28, 1991

Makanjuola ROA: "Ode Ori": a culture-bound disorder with prominent somatic features in Yoruba Nigerian patients. Acta Psychiatr Scand 75:231–236, 1987

Mollica RF, Wyshak G, Lavelle J: The psychosocial impact of war trauma and torture on Southeast Asian refugees. Am J Psychiatry 144:1567–1572, 1987

Mollica RF, Wyshak G, Lavelle J, et al: Assessing symptom change in Southeast Asian refugee survivors of mass violence and torture. Am J Psychiatry 147:83–88, 1990

Regier DA, Myers JK, Kramer M, et al: The NIMH Epidemiologic Catchment Area program. Arch Gen Psychiatry 41:934–941, 1984

Robins LN, Helzer JE, Croughan J, et al: National Institute of Mental Health Diagnostic Interview Schedule: its history, characteristics, and validity. Arch Gen Psychiatry 38:381–389, 1981

World Health Organization: The International Pilot Study of Schizophrenia. Geneva, Switzerland, World Health Organization, 1973

World Health Organization: Schizophrenia: An International Follow-up Study. Chichester, England, John Wiley, 1979

World Health Organization: Depressive Disorders in Different Cultures. Geneva, Switzerland, World Health Organization, 1983

Chapter 48

Cultural Considerations for Somatoform Disorders

Laurence J. Kirmayer, M.D., and
Mitchell Weiss, M.D., Ph.D.

Introduction

In a survey of international use of DSM-III (American Psychiatric Association 1980) and DSM-III-R (American Psychiatric Association 1987), somatoform disorders were reported to be among the more problematic diagnoses (Maser et al. 1991). Worldwide, somatic symptoms are the most common clinical presentation of major affective and anxiety disorders as well as of milder forms of emotional and social distress (Kirmayer 1984). This raises three issues for current and proposed nosology:

1. The category of somatoform disorders distinguishes somatic syndromes from other disorders with which they may be closely associated. Although the distinctness of mood, anxiety, and somatoform disorders, even when they coexist as "comorbid" conditions, is an accepted premise of American and international psychiatry, the mixture of symptoms that characterizes many patients with somatoform disorders indicates the importance of considering alternative categories that include both somatic and mood symptoms as integral features (Angel and Thoits 1987; Kleinman 1988).
2. High levels of medically unexplained symptoms are found in some ethnic groups (Escobar 1987). However, somatic symptoms are common features of many cultural "idioms of distress." The application of North American criteria for somatoform disorders may pathologize individuals who are using such culturally sanctioned patterns of distress to express or negotiate personal and social predicaments.
3. The DSM symptom lists do not include many of the most common somatic symptoms reported in other parts of the world (Ebigbo 1986; Mumford et al.

1991). The presence of culturally distinctive somatic symptoms that are not noted in current diagnostic criteria may lead to underrecognition or misdiagnosis of a wide range of culture-specific syndromes documented by ethnographic research (Good 1977; Guarnaccia et al. 1989; Kleinman 1986; Lock and Dunk 1987; Simons and Hughes 1985).

Somatization and the Somatoform Disorders

Most epidemiological studies find that somatic symptoms, anxiety, and depression are highly intercorrelated, contradicting the clinical assumption that somatic distress is expressed in place of other forms of distress and raising questions about the distinctness of depressive, anxiety, and somatoform syndromes (Beiser and Fleming 1986; Simon and Von Korff 1991). Ethnographic and clinical work also provides much evidence for mixed somatic-affective syndromes. The most prominent example is neurasthenia, which presents a mix of depressive and somatoform symptoms, predominantly fatigue and weakness (Costa e Silva and Girolamo 1990). Neurasthenia remains an extremely common diagnosis in neuropsychiatric settings in China, where Kleinman (1986) found that 87 of a series of 100 patients with neurasthenia met DSM-III criteria for major depression and 69 met criteria for an anxiety disorder. Despite the overlap with depression and anxiety, many clinicians argue that neurasthenia is a distinct syndrome (T.-Y. Lin 1989; Young 1989; Zhang 1989). Related syndromes with prominent symptoms of fatigue and weakness include brain-fag in Nigeria (Prince and Tcheng-Laroche 1987) and "ordinary" *shinkeishitsu* in Japan (Suzuki 1989); these syndromes are also often associated with anxiety (Morakinyo 1985; Russell 1989). Prince (1991) noted that a therapeutic response to antidepressant medication is insufficient to establish that a disorder is equivalent to depression and argued on phenomenological grounds that neurasthenia is more properly viewed as a distinct somatoform disorder.

Other culturally defined somatoform disorders include both psychological and somatic symptoms. Culturally based concerns about semen loss—notably the South Asian *dhat* syndrome and its East Asian analogs—typically present with physical symptoms including weakness and fatigue associated with depression, obsessional anxiety, or phobia (Bhatia and Malik 1991). *Nervios* in Latino communities links depressive, anxiety, somatoform, and dissociative symptoms (Angel and Guarnaccia 1989; Guarnaccia et al. 1990). *Nevra* among Greek immigrants links grief, depression, anxiety, and somatic symptoms (Lock and Dunk 1987). *Hwabyung*, a culturally defined disorder in Korea, includes a mix of somatic and psychological symptoms associated with anger that patients attribute to physical, emotional, and interpersonal causes (K.-M. Lin 1983; Pang 1990). These syndromes are heterogeneous with respect to DSM-III-R and may meet criteria for a variety of Axis I disorders (e.g., Saxena et al. 1988).

Level of Somatic Symptomatology

A legacy of cross-cultural research, now controversial, has suggested that somatized presentations of depression and anxiety are more common among Asians than Westerners (Kirmayer 1984). This impression is largely based on ethnographic and clinical studies that compare community and medical clinic settings in non-Western cultures with psychiatric settings in the West. Krause et al. (1990) reported a relative predominance of somatoform symptoms among Punjabi immigrants and of depressive symptoms among white British in England using the General Health Questionnaire (Goldberg and Williams 1988). Other research with cross-cultural samples in similar settings, however, suggests that the prominence of somatization in Asians relative to Westerners has been exaggerated (Bhatt et al. 1989; Cheng 1989; Mumford 1989; Yamamoto et al. 1985). Recent data make it clear that medically unexplained symptoms and somatoform disorders are also extremely frequent presentations in primary care and other medical settings in Britain and North America (Goldberg and Bridges 1988; Katon et al. 1991; Kirmayer and Robbins 1991). Observed ethnic differences may reflect socially determined patterns of seeking help and symptom presentation rather than differences in underlying psychopathology.

Comparatively high levels of medically unexplained symptoms were found among blacks in the United States and Puerto Ricans in the Epidemiologic Catchment Area study (Swartz et al. 1991). These differences may reflect specific cultural idioms of distress, including *ataques de nervios* among Hispanics (Guarnaccia et al. 1989, 1990) and "falling out" or *indisposition* among blacks (Lefley 1979; Weidman 1979).

Culture may also influence the sex ratio of the somatoform disorders. For example, although somatization disorder is reported to be up to 10 times as frequent in women as in men in North America, in the Puerto Rico Epidemiologic Catchment Area study, the prevalence of somatization disorder (and somatization syndrome) was approximately the same for men and women (Swartz et al. 1991).

Conversion symptoms appear to be more common in rural, less educated, and non-Western populations (Swartz et al. 1991; Tomasson et al. 1991). They may be more common in family or social structures that allow few opportunities for protest (Nichter 1981). Nandi et al. (1992) attributed the observed decrease in prevalence of conversion disorders in a rural Indian population over a 10- to 15-year period to the improved social and economic status of women.

Culture-Specific Symptoms

Culturally transmitted schemata of illness shape individuals' search for and report of symptoms (Angel and Thoits 1987). Consequently, somatic symptoms also vary in their content, and there are many culture-specific medically unexplained somatic symptoms, such as burning hands and feet in Pakistani or Indian patients (Mumford 1989; Mumford et al. 1991), a hot or peppery sensation in the head or a sensation of something crawling in the head in African patients (Ebigbo 1986), and tightness in the chest in Iranian or Turkish patients (Good 1977; Mirdal 1985). These symptoms may occur sporadically or in association with culture-specific somatoform syndromes. For example, the complaint that the penis is retracting into the body is a core symptom of *koro* (Bernstein and Gaw 1990). Loss, or altered state, of consciousness with falling and paralysis occurs in the syndromes of "falling-out" or indisposition among American and Caribbean blacks (Philippe and Romain 1979; Weidman 1979). Many culture-specific somatic syndromes, however, are clusters of symptoms grouped together by a common causal explanation in ethnophysiological terms rather than by a consistent natural history (Prince and Tcheng-Laroche 1987). Examples include dhat in India (Bhattia and Malik 1991), *ode ori* in Nigeria (Makanjuola 1987), and "high blood" or "low blood" among African Americans (Weidman 1979).

Although certain nonspecific symptoms, including weakness, fatigability, dizziness, and pain, are widespread (e.g., Srinivasan and Suresh 1991), the symptom lists in DSM-III-R for somatization disorder, generalized anxiety disorder, panic disorder, and so on are inadequate for cross-cultural comparisons. Expanded inventories of somatic distress are more sensitive to cultural differences (Ebigbo 1986; Mumford et al. 1991), but as yet few cross-cultural comparisons have been done using these measures.

Discussion

Although there are many useful ethnographic studies of somatic idioms of distress, there is still a paucity of comparative cross-cultural data on the symptomatology, course, and outcome of somatoform disorders. Needs for further research identified by this review include the following:

1. The development of culturally sensitive somatic symptom inventories with expanded pools of items to compare the prevalence of somatic symptoms. Latent variable statistical methods can be used to explore the underlying patterns of symptoms and their association with depression, anxiety, and cultural models of illness.

2. Study of the natural history and treatment response of somatoform disorders, including culture-specific syndromes that are currently classified as "somatoform disorder not otherwise specified."
3. Determination of whether high levels of somatic symptoms found in some cultures indicate comparable levels of psychopathology or whether diagnostic thresholds must be altered to avoid inappropriately labeling low levels of distress as psychiatric disorder or similarly misconstruing patterns of help seeking.
4. Study of the extent to which the somatic expression of distress alters the natural history of other coexisting or underlying disorders.

Although there are no definitive studies, the literature does allow the following tentative conclusions:

1. In cultural settings where the distinction between depression, anxiety, and somatoform disorders is difficult to make, simply reporting comorbidity between somatoform and other disorders may be misleading in that it implies that patients are suffering from multiple problems rather than a single disorder that is culturally coherent. If future studies demonstrate that certain patterns of comorbidity have wide prevalence and a distinctive natural history, it may be appropriate to recognize their validity by including them as discrete diagnostic entities. For example, neurasthenia may be a useful diagnosis, and its inclusion may encourage much-needed research on the natural history and outcome of syndromes that cut across the depressive, anxiety, and somatoform categories.
2. In cultures in which high levels of somatic symptoms are commonly reported, patients may be overdiagnosed with somatoform disorders. The same symptom threshold that identifies a relatively homogeneous pathological group in one culture may lead clinicians to misinterpret common idioms of distress as indicative of somatoform pathology in another. Considering disability and outcome in different cultural settings will help to distinguish subclinical distress from clinically significant symptoms.
3. On the other hand, somatoform disorders may be missed if a wide range of symptoms are not canvassed. Locally adapted symptom lists may improve the recognition of somatoform disorders as well as make it possible to examine the status of a variety of culture-specific somatic syndromes with distinctive natural histories (Ebigbo 1986; Mumford et al. 1991). For example, symptoms related to male reproductive function may be more prevalent in cultures where there is widespread concern about semen loss (e.g., dhat syndrome in India).
4. Complaints associated with specific popular illness categories (e.g., ataques de nervios) may account in large measure for cultural differences in the preva-

lence of somatoform disorders. In some cases, recognition of such categories may facilitate reanalysis of data derived from standard instruments (such as the Diagnostic Interview Schedule [Robins et al. 1981]), allowing more culturally sensitive analysis of prevalence, care seeking, and course of illness (Guarnaccia et al. 1989).

Many cultural variations reflect idioms of distress rather than disorders likely to have a distinctive pathophysiology and psychopathology. Rather than adding new diagnostic categories, an axis for cultural diagnosis—or emphasis on a cultural formulation as part of a complete evaluation—would be helpful.

The review also identified issues relevant to the diagnosis of specific somatoform disorders.

Somatization Disorder

The requirement that somatoform symptoms be medically unexplained (or in excess of what is medically expected) is problematic in settings where parasitic and infectious diseases, poor nutrition, and recurrent low-grade medical illnesses are endemic. This may result in overdiagnosis if organic causes are not identified or underdiagnosis if organic explanations are uncritically accepted for systemic illness.

Conversion Disorder

Dissociative or conversion symptoms are common aspects of religious and healing rituals (Griffith et al. 1980). Diagnosis thus requires familiarity with culture-specific aspects of social context. Although proposed criterion D in the *DSM-IV Options Book* (American Psychiatric Association 1991)—"the symptom is not a culturally sanctioned response pattern" (p. I:4)—alerts the clinician to the need to assess the pathological significance of such symptoms in social context, it may introduce ambiguity about symptoms that are culturally sanctioned, yet still have pathological consequences. Disability, role impairment, and distress must be considered with cultural sanctioning to determine the pathological significance of symptoms.

Hypochondriasis

The diversity of alternative health care providers and the relative value and emphasis placed on seeking medical help vary widely across cultural groups. This variation may complicate efforts to determine how appropriate health concerns are with respect to local norms. Proposed criterion B in the *DSM-IV Options Book*—"the preoccupations persist despite appropriate medical reassurance" (American Psychiatric Association 1991, p. I:7)—must therefore be considered in the larger context of help providers. Culturally consistent ideas about disease cannot be summarily replaced by authoritative medical opinions.

Body Dysmorphic Disorder

Certain culturally defined disorders may emphasize concerns about body image similar to those found in body dysmorphic disorder (e.g., *taijin kyofusho* [Russell 1989]). Cultural concerns about the importance of proper physical self-presentation may amplify anxiety or lend delusional rigidity to imagined physical deformity (Kirmayer 1991; Osman 1991).

Somatoform Disorder Not Otherwise Specified

Certain culture-specific syndromes involve anxiety about abnormal bodily function or predominantly somatic distress attributed to bodily dysfunction (e.g., koro, dhat). Although better conceptualized as anxiety disorders (cf., Tseng et al. 1992), these syndromes should be mentioned as illustrative examples in the not otherwise specified category.

References

American Psychiatric Association: Diagnostic and Statistical Manual of Mental Disorders, 3rd Edition. Washington, DC, American Psychiatric Association, 1980

American Psychiatric Association: Diagnostic and Statistical Manual of Mental Disorders, 3rd Edition, Revised. Washington, DC, American Psychiatric Association, 1987

American Psychiatric Association: DSM-IV Options Book: Work in Progress. Washington, DC, American Psychiatric Association, 1991

Angel R, Guarnaccia PJ: Mind, body, and culture: somatization among Hispanics. Soc Sci Med 28:1229–1238, 1989

Angel R, Thoits P: The impact of culture on the cognitive structure of illness. Cult Med Psychiatry 11:465–494, 1987

Beiser M, Fleming JAE: Measuring psychiatric disorder among Southeast Asian refugees. Psychol Med 16:627–639, 1986

Bernstein RL, Gaw AC: Koro: proposed classification for DSM-IV. Am J Psychiatry 147:1670–1674, 1990

Bhatia MS, Malik SC: Dhat syndrome: a useful diagnostic entity in Indian culture. Br J Psychiatry 159:691–695, 1991

Bhatt A, Tomenson B, Benjamin S: Transcultural patterns of somatization in primary care. J Psychosom Res 33:671–680, 1989

Cheng TA: Symptomatology of minor psychiatric morbidity: a crosscultural comparison. Psychol Med 19:697–708, 1989

Costa e Silva JA, Girolamo G: Neurasthenia: history of a concept, in Psychological Disorders in General Medical Settings. Edited by Sartorius N, Goldberg D, de Girolamo G, et al. Toronto, Canada, Hogrefe & Huber, 1990, pp 69–81

Ebigbo PO: A cross-sectional study of somatic complaints of Nigerian females using the Enugu somatization scale. Cult Med Psychiatry 10:167–186, 1986

Escobar JI: Cross-cultural aspects of the somatization trait. Hosp Community Psychiatry 38:174–180, 1987

Goldberg DP, Bridges K: Somatic presentations of psychiatric illness in primary care setting. J Psychosom Res 32:137–144, 1988

Goldberg DP, Williams P: A User's Guide to the General Health Questionnaire. Berkshire, England, Basingstoke Press, 1988

Good BJ: The heart of what's the matter: the semantics of illness in Iran. Cult Med Psychiatry 1:25–58, 1977

Griffith EEH, English T, Mayfield V: Possession, prayer, and testimony: therapeutic aspects of the Wednesday night meeting in a black church. Psychiatry 43:120–128, 1980

Guarnaccia PJ, Rubio-Stipec M, Canino G: Ataques de nervios in the Puerto Rican Diagnostic Interview Schedule: the impact of cultural categories on psychiatric epidemiology. Cult Med Psychiatry 13:275–295, 1989

Guarnaccia PJ, Good BJ, Kleinman A: A critical review of epidemiological studies of Puerto Rican mental health. Am J Psychiatry 147:1449–1456, 1990

Katon WJ, Lin E, Von Korff MV, et al: Somatization: a spectrum of severity. Am J Psychiatry 148:34–40, 1991

Kirmayer LJ: Culture, affect and somatization. Transcultural Psychiatric Research Review 21:159–188 and 237–262, 1984

Kirmayer LJ: The place of culture in psychiatric nosology: taijin kyofusho and DSM-III-R. J Nerv Ment Dis 179:19–28, 1991

Kirmayer LJ, Robbins JM: Three forms of somatization in primary care: prevalence, co-occurrence and sociodemographic characteristics. J Nerv Ment Dis 179:647–655, 1991

Kleinman A: Social Origins of Distress and Disease. New Haven, CT, Yale University Press, 1986

Kleinman A: Rethinking Psychiatry. New York, Free Press, 1988

Krause IB, Rosser RM, Khianai ML, et al: Psychiatric morbidity among Punjabi medical patients in England measured by General Health Questionnaire. Psychol Med 20:711–719, 1990

Lefley HP: Prevalence of potential falling-out cases among the black, Latin and non-Latin white populations of the city of Miami. Soc Sci Med 13B:113–114, 1979

Lin K-M: Hwa-Byung: a Korean culture-bound syndrome? Am J Psychiatry 140:105–107, 1983

Lin T-Y: Neurasthenia revisited: its place in modern psychiatry. Cult Med Psychiatry 13:105–130, 1989

Lock M, Dunk P: My nerves are broken: the communication of suffering in a Greek-Canadian community, in Health and Canadian Society: Sociological Perspectives. Edited by Cobrun D, D'Arcy T. Markham, Ontario, Canada, Fitzhenry & Whiteside, 1987, pp 295–313

Makanjuola ROA: "Ode Ori": a culture-bound disorder with prominent somatic features in Yoruba Nigerian patients. Acta Psychiatr Scand 75:231–236, 1987

Maser JD, Kaelber C, Weise RE: International use and attitudes toward DSM-III and DSM-III-R: growing consensus in psychiatric classification. J Abnorm Psychol 100:271–279, 1991

Mirdal GM: The condition of "tightness": the somatic complaints of Turkish migrant women. Acta Psychiatr Scand 71:287–296, 1985

Morakinyo O: Phobic states presenting as somatic complaints syndromes in Nigeria: sociocultural factors associated with diagnosis and psychotherapy. Acta Psychiatr Scand 71:356–365, 1985

Mumford DB: Somatic sensations and psychological distress among students in Britain and Pakistan. Soc Psychiatry Psychiatr Epidemiol 24:321–326, 1989

Mumford DB, Bavington JT, Bhatnagar KS, et al: The Bradford Somatic Inventory: a multiethnic inventory of somatic symptoms reported by anxious and depressed patients in Britain and the Indo-Pakistan subcontinent. Br J Psychiatry 158:379–386, 1991

Nandi DN, Banerjee G, Nandi S, et al: Is hysteria on the wane? a community survey in West Bengal, India. Br J Psychiatry 160:87–91, 1992

Nichter M: Idioms of distress: alternatives in the expression of psychosocial distress: a case study from India. Cult Med Psychiatry 5:379–408, 1981

Osman AA: Monosymptomatic hypochondriacal psychosis in developing countries. Br J Psychiatry 159:428–431, 1991

Pang KYC: Hwabyung: the construction of a Korean popular illness among Korean elderly immigrant women in the United States. Cult Med Psychiatry 14:495–512, 1990

Philippe J, Romain JB: Indisposition in Haiti. Soc Sci Med 13B:129–133, 1979

Prince RH: Somatic complaint syndromes, depression and DSM-III-R, in Psychiatry: A World Perspective. Edited by Stefanis CN, Rabavilas AD, Soldatos CR, et al. Amsterdam, Netherlands, Elsevier, 1991, pp 462–466

Prince R, Tcheng-Laroche F: Culture-bound syndromes and international disease classification. Cult Med Psychiatry 11:3–20, 1987

Robins LN, Helzer JE, Croughan J, et al: National Institute of Mental Health Diagnostic Interview Schedule: its history, characteristics, and validity. Arch Gen Psychiatry 38:381–389, 1981

Russell JG: Anxiety disorders in Japan: a review of the Japanese literature on shinkeishitsu and taijinkyofusho. Cult Med Psychiatry 13:391–403, 1989

Saxena S, Nepal MK, Mohan D: DSM-III Axis I diagnoses of Indian psychiatric patients with somatic symptoms. Am J Psychiatry 145:1023–1024, 1988

Simon GE, Von Korff M: Somatization and psychiatric disorder in the NIMH Epidemiologic Catchment Area study. Am J Psychiatry 148:1494–1500, 1991

Simons RC, Hughes CC (eds): The Culture Bound-Syndromes: Folk Illnesses of Psychiatric and Anthropological Interest. Dordrecht, Netherlands, D Reidel, 1985

Srinivasan K, Suresh TR: The nonspecific symptom screening method: detection of nonpsychotic morbidity based on nonspecific symptoms. Gen Hosp Psychiatry 13:106–114, 1991

Suzuki T: The concept of neurasthenia and its treatment in Japan. Cult Med Psychiatry 13:187–202, 1989

Swartz M, Landerman R, George LK, et al.: Somatization disorder, in Psychiatric Disorders in America: The Epidemiologic Catchment Area Study. Edited by Robins LN, Regier DA. New York, Free Press, 1991, pp 220–257

Tomasson K, Dent D, Coryell W: Somatization and conversion disorders: comorbidity and demographics at presentation. Acta Psychiatr Scand 84:288–293, 1991

Tseng W-S, Kan-Ming M, Li-Shuen L, et al: Koro epidemics in Guangdong China: a questionnaire survey. J Nerv Ment Dis 180:117–123, 1992

Weidman HH: Falling-out: a diagnostic and treatment problem viewed from a transcultural perspective. Soc Sci Med 13B:95–112, 1979

Yamamoto J, Yeh EK, Loya F, et al: Are American psychiatric outpatients more depressed than Chinese outpatients? Am J Psychiatry 142:1247–1351, 1985

Young D: Neurasthenia and related problems. Cult Med Psychiatry 13:131–139, 1989

Zhang M-Y: The diagnosis and phenomenology of neurasthenia: a Shanghai study. Cult Med Psychiatry 13:147–162, 1989

Chapter 49

Impact of Culture on Dissociation: Enhancing the Cultural Suitability of DSM-IV

Carlos A. González, M.D., Roberto Lewis-Fernández, M.D.,
Ezra E. H. Griffith, M.D., Roland Littlewood, M.B.,
D. Phil., M.R.C. Psych., and Richard J. Castillo, Ph.D.

Introduction

DSM-III-R (American Psychiatric Association 1987) does not account for various dissociative disorders commonly found in the "non-Western" world (Karp 1985; Kleinman 1977, 1987; Saxena and Prasad 1989; Yap 1967). This chapter is meant to provide a framework with which to describe these poorly addressed syndromes and present an organized view of their clinical features to inform the development of DSM-IV.

We do not think it helpful to add to the existing system dissociative states that are seen as part of a normal individual's usual cultural experience. There is no evidence, in the first place, that trance or dissociative states that are part of a culturally sanctioned ceremony or ritual should be regarded as pathological. Examples of such culturally accepted dissociative states include those occurring in African American prayer meetings (Griffith et al. 1980), Puerto Rican spiritist sessions (Comas-Díaz 1981; Garrison 1977; Koss 1975), Native American rituals (Jilek 1982), and in many other societies as healing rituals, as culturally accepted facets of social intercourse (Constantinides 1985; Crapanzano 1977; Lambek 1981), or as states sought by those employing meditative techniques (Castillo 1990). Secondly, syndromes ought to be considered pathological only if they cause significant distress and dysfunction and thereby lead to help-seeking behavior.

It is also not helpful to equate mere belief in the supernatural with actual dissociation, seen as a "disruption in the normal integration of experience" and characterized by "derealization, depersonalization, amnesia, identity confusion, and identity alteration" (Kirmayer 1991, p. 21). Individuals from a number of cultures may attribute the incidence of mental illness or physical complaints to supernatural causes, such as spirits, even in the absence of any discernible signs of dissociation (Bourguignon 1968; Saunders 1977). Bourguignon (1976) made the important distinction between "possession belief" and "possession trance," stating that only the latter involves dissociation as described earlier.

Brief Literature Review

Review of the psychiatric and anthropological literature reveals several groups of syndromes from around the world that have dissociation as a key feature.

Possession Trance Syndromes

There are numerous reports of possession trance syndromes, characterized by the belief that the victim's body is taken over by a spirit and manifested by identity confusion, an apparent loss of self-control, a temporary change in the personality of the victim, and partial or total amnesia for the episode (Akhtar 1988; Chandrashekar 1989; Gussler 1973; Kleinman 1980; Stoller 1989; Suryani 1984; Suwanlert 1976). In India, this disorder appears to be more prevalent among women (Chandrashekar 1989) and among those who have experienced chronic or acute interpersonal conflict or a recent loss. It is often reversible, with the longest episodes lasting days to weeks. In many cases, an episode of possession trance makes the sufferer more likely to be possessed again in the future.

The various accounts of possession trance reveal substantial differences from multiple personality disorder as described in DSM-III-R. The association with childhood abuse has hardly been mentioned with regard to pathological possession trance, but it has also not been systematically studied. Instead, several accounts (Constantinides 1985; Lewis 1989; Littlewood and Lipsedge 1987) have linked the occurrence of possession trance to the degree of stratification and inequality between the sexes in a given society. Although both multiple personality disorder and possession trance involve the coexistence within a person of different personalities, the presumed origin of alternate personalities in multiple personality disorder is internal, whereas the possessed person views the phenomenon as the effect of an external, supernatural entity. In addition, cases of pathological possession trance are often episodic and remitting, in contrast to the chronic nature of multiple personality disorder.

The relationship between pathological possession trance and multiple personality disorder is presently uncertain, with several authors (Adityanjee et al. 1989;

Varma et al. 1981) suggesting that these two syndromes, although clinically dissimilar, may share common mechanisms whereas "the pathoplastic influence of the prevailing culture may be important in causing [the] differences" (Adityanjee et al. 1989, p. 1610) in presentation.

"Fleeing" or "Running" Syndromes

Another subcategory of dissociative syndromes includes *pibloktoq* among the native peoples of the Arctic (Gussow 1960), *chakore* in the Ngawbere of Panama (Bletzer 1985), *grisi siknis* among the Miskito of Nicaragua (Dennis 1985), and Navajo "frenzy" witchcraft (Neutra et al. 1977). Because these disorders are characterized by wandering or fleeing aimlessly, the term *running taxon* has been given to some of them (Simons 1985). In *grisi siknis, pibloktoq,* and *chakore,* there is a documented prodromal period that may last several days and that is characterized by feelings of lethargy, depression, and anxiety. In all four syndromes, there is a sudden onset of a high level of activity; a trance-like state; running or fleeing behavior; and ensuing exhaustion, sleep, and amnesia for the episode. Prevalence and demographic data are scarce. Although these disorders present in both sexes, they appear to have higher prevalence among women.

Amok in Malayo-Indonesia (Arboleda-Flores 1979; Carr 1978; Schmidt et al. 1977; Tan and Carr 1977) is similar to the syndromes described earlier, but three features warrant separate discussion: 1) it is characterized by extreme violence and threat of injury or death to self and/or others, 2) it has been observed almost exclusively among men, and 3) it has been associated with psychotic disorders (Tan and Carr 1977). As in the "fleeing" syndromes, there is a prodromal period of brooding, followed by trance-like "running" that is accompanied by the apparently indiscriminate and brutal assault of nearby persons or animals. If the "runner" survives the episode, there is subsequent exhaustion, sleep, and amnesia for the episode.

Using the current DSM, it is difficult to classify these "running" syndromes, although their principal symptoms are dissociative in character. Although dissociative fugue does not fully capture the essence of the syndrome, it appears to be the only alternative outside of dissociative disorder not otherwise specified—hardly a fitting description. Amok presents additional nosological difficulties, given the central role of violence in the disorder and the suggested relationship with chronic psychosis. Spiegel and Cardeña (1991) view the syndrome as a variant of intermittent explosive disorder, and this may at present be the most adequate diagnosis, with the reservation that this would put it in a class of disorders whose "unifying" theme is that of being "not elsewhere classified." Evidence of psychotic features in an individual would, of course, lead to consideration of a psychotic or mood disorder.

Trance Syndromes

Weidman (1979) described a syndrome among Southern blacks and Bahamians referred to as "falling-out" or "blacking-out," respectively. This syndrome typically occurs in response to a high degree of emotional excitement, such as may be seen in the setting of a religious ceremony, during an argument, in situations producing fear, or in "profound sexual conflict" (Weidman 1979, p. 99). It is characterized by the affected individual falling down in an altered state of consciousness and not being able to move, despite being able to hear and understand surrounding events. Philippe and Romain (1979) described a strikingly similar syndrome in Haitians, known locally as *indisposition*. Available data reveal prevalences of 10% and 23% for falling-out and blacking-out, respectively (Weidman 1979); a Haiti opportunity sample (Philippe and Romain 1979) yielded a prevalence rate for *indisposition* of 43%. Although these high prevalence rates do not distinguish between normative and pathological cases, the numbers do suggest a significant rate of dissociative pathology.

The syndrome *ataque de nervios,* which is described in many Hispanic groups (Guarnaccia et al. 1989a, 1989b), also refers to a socially sanctioned display of grief or great conflict characterized by "difficulty moving limbs, loss of consciousness or mind going blank, memory loss, [symptoms of hyperventilation] . . . the person begins to shout, swear and strike out at others, [then] falls to the ground and either experiences convulsive body movements or lies 'as if dead'" (Guarnaccia et al. 1989a, p. 280). Approximately 12% of a probability sample in Puerto Rico reported suffering from ataques de nervios and either suffering some functional impairment or seeking professional help as a consequence of the syndrome (Canino et al. 1990). Of subjects with ataques, 63% also met diagnostic criteria for one or more anxiety or depressive disorders. People reporting ataques de nervios were more likely to be female, older than age 45, with less than a high school education, formerly married, and out of the labor force. Those subjects exposed to a natural disaster exhibited a higher rate of ataques relative to the unexposed population (Guarnaccia et al. 1993).

DSM-III-R relegates these heterogeneous phenomena to the realm of dissociative disorder not otherwise specified. Clearly, the principal symptoms and signs are those of dissociation. The associated elements of falling and temporary loss of voluntary motion, as well as the amnesia and loss of consciousness described in some cases, would not be taken into account by a diagnosis of depersonalization disorder. Prevalence data indicate that these are not uncommon phenomena, that they are often pathological conditions associated with other psychiatric diagnoses, and that recurrence of such a phenomenon in an individual is seen as illness behavior by the victim's cultural peers.

Conclusions

Although most dissociative syndromes found globally should not be viewed as pathological, a small but significant proportion of these do seem to be distressing to the individual and are viewed as illness behaviors within the individual's culture. The current classification scheme applies poorly to these dissociative syndromes and results in ill-fitting diagnoses.

The data examined support consideration of trance/possession trance disorder as a diagnostic entity separate from multiple personality disorder.

In addition, the literature describes various "running" syndromes that, on further investigation, may serve to enrich future diagnostic manuals. It may make sense to include phenomenological descriptions of these syndromes in the section of DSM-IV relevant to dissociative fugue. Some episodes of amok not fulfilling criteria for a psychotic or mood disorder may be diagnosable as intermittent explosive disorder or as dissociative fugue. It would therefore be useful to include a clinical description of *amok* as part of the "Cultural Considerations" section under intermittent explosive disorder and dissociative fugue.

Finally, the available literature indicates that trance phenomena are heterogeneous entities, and pathological cases of these might be diagnosed under two categories: 1) acute stress disorder/brief reactive dissociative disorder, when the precipitating stressor is of the magnitude described in this DSM category; and 2) trance and possession trance disorder, when a stressor of sufficient magnitude is not identified.

References

Adityanjee MD, Raju GSP, Khandelwal SK: Current status of multiple personality disorder in India. Am J Psychiatry 146:1607–1610, 1989

Akhtar S: Four culture-bound psychiatric syndromes in India. Int J Soc Psychiatry 34:70–74, 1988

American Psychiatric Association: Diagnostic and Statistical Manual of Mental Disorders, Third Edition, Revised. Washington, DC, American Psychiatric Association, 1987

Arboleda-Flores J: Amok. Bull Am Acad Psychiatry Law 7:286–295, 1979

Bletzer KV: Fleeing hysteria (chakore) among Ngawbere of northwestern Panama: a preliminary analysis and comparison with similar illness phenomena in other settings. Med Anthropol 9:297–318, 1985

Bourguignon E: World distribution and patterns of possession states, in Trance and Possession States. Edited by Prince R. Montreal, Canada, RM Bucke Memorial Society, 1968, pp 3–34

Bourguignon E: Possession. San Francisco, CA, Chandler & Sharp, 1976

Canino G, Bravo M, Rubio-Stipec M, et al: The impact of disaster on mental health: prospective and retrospective analyses. Int J Mental Health 19:51–69, 1990

Carr JE: Ethno-behaviorism and the culture-bound syndromes: the case of amok. Cult Med Psychiatry 2:269–293, 1978

Castillo RJ: Depersonalization and meditation. Psychiatry 53:158–168, 1990

Chandrashekar CR: Possession syndrome in India, in Altered States of Consciousness and Mental Health. Edited by Ward CA. Newbury Park, CA, Sage, 1989, pp 79–95

Comas-Díaz L: Puerto Rican espiritismo and psychotherapy. Am J Orthopsychiatry 51(4):636–645, 1981

Constantinides P: Women heal women: spirit possession and sexual segregation in a Muslim society. Soc Sci Med 21(6):685–692, 1985

Crapanzano V: Mohammed and Dawia: possession in Morocco, in Case Studies in Spirit Possession. Edited by Crapanzano V, Garrison V. New York, John Wiley, 1977, pp 141–176

Dennis PA: Grisi Siknis in Miskito culture, in The Culture-Bound Syndromes: Folk Illnesses of Psychiatric and Anthropological Interest. Edited by Simons RC, Hughes CC. Dordrecht, Netherlands, D Reidel, 1985, pp 289–306

Garrison V: The "Puerto Rican Syndrome" in psychiatry and espiritismo, in Case Studies in Spirit Possession. Edited by Crapanzano V, Garrison V. New York, John Wiley, 1977, pp 383–449

Griffith EEH, English T, Mayfield V: Possession, prayer, and testimony: therapeutic aspects of the Wednesday night meeting in a black church. Psychiatry 43:120–128, 1980

Guarnaccia PJ, Rubio-Stipec M, Canino G: Ataques de nervios in the Puerto Rican Diagnostic Interview Schedule: the impact of cultural categories on psychiatric epidemiology. Cult Med Psychiatry 13:275–295, 1989a

Guarnaccia PJ, de la Cancela V, Carrillo E: The multiple meanings of ataques de nervios in the Latino community. Med Anthropol 11:47–62, 1989b

Guarnaccia PJ, Canino G, Rubio-Stipec M, et al: The prevalence of ataques de nervios in the Puerto Rican Disaster Study: the role of culture in psychiatric epidemiology. J Nerv Ment Dis 181:157–165, 1993

Gussler J: Social change, ecology and spirit possession among the South African Nguni, in Religion, Altered States of Consciousness, and Social Change. Edited by Bourguignon E. Columbus, OH, Ohio State University Press, 1973, pp 88–126

Gussow Z: Pibloktoq (hysteria) among the polar Eskimo. The Psychoanalytic Study of Society 1:218–236, 1960

Jilek WG: Altered states of consciousness in North American Indian ceremonials. Ethos 10:326–343, 1982

Karp I: Deconstructing culture-bound syndromes. Soc Sci Med 21:221–228, 1985

Kirmayer LJ: Pacing the void: concepts and measures of dissociation. Paper presented at the MacArthur Foundation Mind-Body Network Workshop on Dissociation, Stanford, CA, October 1991

Kleinman AM: Depression, somatization, and the "New Cross-Cultural Psychiatry." Soc Sci Med 11:3–10, 1977

Kleinman AM: Patients and Healers in the Context of Culture. Berkeley, CA, University of California Press, 1980

Kleinman AM: Rethinking Psychiatry: From Cultural Category to Personal Experience. New York, Free Press, 1987

Koss JD: Therapeutic aspects of Puerto Rican cult practices. Psychiatry 38:160–171, 1975

Lambek M: Human Spirits: A Cultural Account of Trance in Mayotte. New York, Cambridge University Press, 1981
Lewis IM: Ecstatic Religion: A Study of Shamanism and Spirit Possession. London, England, Routledge, 1989
Littlewood R, Lipsedge M: The butterfly and the serpent: culture, psychopathology and biomedicine. Cult Med Psychiatry 11:289–335, 1987
Neutra R, Levy JE, Parker D: Cultural expectations versus reality in Navajo seizure patterns and sick roles. Cult Med Psychiatry 1:255–275, 1977
Philippe J, Romain JB: Indisposition in Haiti. Soc Sci Med 13B:129–133, 1979
Saunders LW: Variants in Zar experience in an Egyptian village, in Case Studies in Spirit Possession. Edited by Crapanzano V, Garrison V. New York, John Wiley, 1977, pp 177–191
Saxena S, Prasad KVSR: DSM-III subclassification of dissociative disorders applied to psychiatric outpatients in India. Am J Psychiatry 146:261–262, 1989
Schmidt K, Hill L, Guthrie G: Running amok. Int J Soc Psychiatry 23:264–274, 1977
Simons RC: Sorting the culture-bound syndromes, in The Culture-Bound Syndromes: Folk Illnesses of Psychiatric and Anthropological Interest. Edited by Simons RC, Hughes CC. Dordrecht, Netherlands, D Reidel, 1985, pp 25–38
Spiegel D, Cardeña E: Cultural diversity of dissociative and somatoform disorders. Paper presented at the NIMH Conference on Culture and Diagnosis, Pittsburgh, PA, 1991
Stoller P: Fusion of the Worlds. Chicago, IL, University of Chicago Press, 1989
Suryani LK: Culture and mental disorder: the case of bebainan in Bali. Cult Med Psychiatry 8:95–113, 1984
Suwanlert S: Neurotic and psychotic states attributed to Thai "Phii Pob" spirit possession. Aust N Z J Psychiatry 10:119–23, 1976
Tan EK, Carr JE: Psychiatric sequelae of amok. Cult Med Psychiatry 1:59–67, 1977
Varma VK, Bouri M, Wig NN: Multiple personality in India: comparison with hysterical possession state. Am J Psychotherapy 35:113–120, 1981
Weidman HH: Falling-out: a diagnostic and treatment problem viewed from a transcultural perspective. Soc Sci Med 13B:95–112, 1979
Yap PM: Classification of the culture-bound reactive syndromes. Aust N Z J Psychiatry 1:172–179, 1967

Chapter 50

Cultural Issues and Sexual Disorders

Dona Davis, Ph.D., and
Gilbert Herdt, Ph.D.

Statement and Significance of the Issues

The sexual disorders of the DSM are divided into three categories: paraphilias, sexual dysfunctions, and other sexual disorders. The significance of this condensed review is limited by several factors, including an appalling lack of contemporary data and a preponderance of poorly designed studies, as well as the fact that the major American ethnic minorities do not seek medical treatment for this class of complaint (Johnson 1977; Kendell 1991; Wyatt 1982). Given these limitations, the literature indicates that 1) cultural features can and do affect the experience and diagnosis of all three categories; 2) the categories are culture-bound and difficult to apply cross-culturally; and 3) the "culture-bound sexual disorders" such as *d'hat* and *koro* are best subsumed under other DSM-IV categories.

Results and Discussion

The Paraphilias

Although the cross-cultural literature on the nature and incidence of the paraphilias is thought-provoking, the paraphilias so described bear limited resemblance to the paraphilias of DSM. For example, exposing the genitals as a form of sexual invitation has been called exhibitionism (Rooth 1973), and biting in lovemaking has been labeled sadomasochism (Ford and Beach 1951). The DSM specifications that a paraphilia must be a matter of preference or a habitual, recurrent, compelling, and intense sexual urge or fantasy have not been incorporated into cross-cultural analyses. An exception is Gregersen (1992), who eschewed issues of cultural relativism and advocated characterizing paraphilias in terms of specificity of sexual interest, regardless of social acceptability.

Cross-cultural studies that have focused on DSM-III-R (American Psychiatric Association 1987) diagnostic categories conclude that the DSM paraphilias should be viewed as unique to Western society and inseparable from the United States legal system (Ames and Houston 1990). Rooth (1973) and Weatherford (1986) related the Western paraphilias to a lack of partners and the primacy of masturbation as a sexual outlet in North America. Gebhard (1971) suggested that paraphilias are unique to complex societies where individuals can evade social sanctions through anonymity. In their discussion of "love maps," Money and Lamacz (1989) viewed paraphilias as interpsychically determined, but encoded in ethnic customs and conventions.

In any discussion of the paraphilias, it is important to remember that what is considered deviant in one culture or at one time may be regarded as nonproblematic in another culture or time (Rubin 1984). For example, Herdt and Stoller (1989) provided a sophisticated cultural analysis of a New Guinea cultural group to demonstrate how man/boy sexual relations have no relevance to the concept of pedophilia as listed in DSM.

Sexual Dysfunctions

The DSM sexual dysfunction categories are characterized by a biological essentialism (Irvine 1990; Tiefer 1987) that maintains that sexual response is unaffected by ethnicity and culture (Christopher 1982). This position is supported by a few suggestive clinical studies that found similar rates of female orgasmic dysfunction (Fisher 1980; Frank et al. 1978) and male impotency (Finkle and Finkle 1978) in small, regional samplings of white and African American populations. Yet there are also clinical reports suggesting that ethnicity may affect the nature of sexual dysfunctions. Data from clinical case studies by Johnson (1977), Mokuau (1986), and Wyatt (1982) suggest that a tendency for some African American men and women to internalize racist stereotypes of male hypersexuality and female hyposexuality can result in sexual dysfunctions. It has also been suggested that among Latin Americans the madonna/whole complex, machismo, and the eroticization of forbidden acts (Espin 1984; Parker 1991) may affect the nature of sexual dysfunctions.

There is more literature on sexual dysfunction among Asians than for any other cultural group. The tendency to somatize depression or emotional complaints provides the focus for analysis of sexual problems and impotence among two clinical samples of Chinese men (Leih-Mak and Ng 1981; Mollica et al. 1987). Several authors have mentioned how important Asian men consider semen retention to be for robust health (Dewaraja and Sasaki 1991; Leih-Mak and Ng 1981).

Ballard (cited in d'Ardenne 1986) stated that concerns about potency loom large in Asian men because potency is related to a comprehensive cosmology and because Asian men expect to exert a greater degree of personal dominance over their wives.

Bhugra and Cordle (1988) and d'Ardenne (1986) both reported that ejaculatory problems were a primary presenting complaint for Asians originating on the Indian subcontinent and that women tended to complain of vaginal discharge rather that painful intercourse. As with the Chinese sample of Leih-Mak and Ng (1981), problems with conception among Indians reflect the enormous social pressure on young couples to conceive and are cited as the major factor bringing young people to clinics specializing in the treatment of sexual problems (Bhugra and Cordle 1988).

From the literature cited, we see that cultural considerations such as the equation of sexual disorders with anxiety about fertility and the tendency to somatize mood disorders (both noted among Asians) can affect the diagnosis of sexual dysfunction. Moreover, it is important to note that different cultural groups may have different social constructions for sexuality (Vance 1991) and, therefore, different standards of sexual performance (Irvine 1990; Leiblum and Rosen 1988; Tiefer 1987), with further distinctions for males and females as well as for different age and marital status groups. Marmor's (1971) often-cited characterization of healthy sex as tender, affectionate, seeking to give and receive pleasure, discriminating as to partner, and triggered by erotic needs would have limited applicability across many ethnic and cultural groups (Davis and Whitten 1987; Leavitt 1991).

In addition, recent research suggests not only that sexual desire and preference is influenced by sociocultural factors, but also that a life-course developmental perspective is necessary to understand more complex interactions between the individual and the social context. Gagnon (1988) systematically reviewed individuals' life-course adjustments in sexual scripts, goals, social roles, and networks in the United States. Social and developmental "time" and age affect particular inputs of individual experience and sexual expression in childhood, adolescence, adulthood, and later years. Historical and age-cohort differences affect not only stages of life-course adjustment and sexual identity development, but also the influence of historical changes on cohorts and subcultures (Herdt and Boxer 1992).

Other Sexual Disorders

The category "Other Sexual Disorders" includes a number of different behaviors such as sexual addiction, dissatisfaction with physical self or sexual competence, and problematic sexual orientation. This category has received a great deal of criticism. The ethnographic literature clearly shows that standards for sexual competence differ markedly across the cultural spectrum (Davis and Whitten 1987). For example, Asian Americans living in the United States may be prone to feelings of physical inadequacy and low sexual self-image because they live within a dominant culture that values tall muscular men and large blonde women (Mokuau 1986).

Many societies are characterized by a far more flexible approach to issues of sexual orientation than supposed by DSM (Bolin 1988; Ernst et al. 1991; Herdt 1990; Jacobs and Roberts 1989; Petersen 1992; Williams 1986). The range of same-sex and opposite-sex attraction and sexual behavior obviously varies greatly across groups (Greenberg 1988; Herdt 1990). The general category "homosexual" must now be seen as a bundle of different behaviors that vary by social pressure, opportunity structure, and the reward and prestige system, as well as individual desire (Green 1987; Herdt 1981). For example, Herdt (1990) proposed a schema of four types of same-sex practice based on 1) age structures, 2) gender structures, 3) class or role structures, and 4) modern egalitarian structures of social influence on individual desire.

Culture-Bound Sex Syndromes

A number of so-called culture-bound sex syndromes can be found in the ethnographic and medical literature (Simons 1985), which demonstrate that not all sexual cosmologies are similar to those of Western medicine. These syndromes include koro (India, Southeast Asian, Malaysia, China) and d'hat (India). Koro refers to a sudden and intense anxiety that the penis will recede into the body. D'hat refers to marked obsession with or anxiety over excessive loss of semen. Bernstein and Gaw (1990) proposed that koro be designated as a culture-specific genital retraction syndrome in DSM-IV and classified under the somatoform disorders. Others object to the culture-specific status, claiming that genital retraction syndrome is more universally experienced (Edwards 1985; Simons 1985). The same arguments are cited for d'hat (Bhatia and Malik 1991; Bottero 1991). Although there is a lack of agreement on what symptoms define these syndromes, there is substantial agreement that koro or d'hat should not be overdiagnosed as schizophrenia or a delusional disorder (Bernstein and Gaw 1990; Chadda and Shome 1991). Mood disorder (depression or anxiety) (Bhatia and Malik 1991; Bottero 1991) or somatoform disorder (Bernstein and Gaw 1990) have been offered as more appropriate diagnoses.

Conclusion

There is a much larger literature on the culture/ethnicity and treatment of sexual disorders than there is on their diagnosis. Criticisms of the DSM sexual disorders echo criticism of sexology in general, which is disparaged for its lack of "rigor" as well as for the very constructs that guide it (Tiefer 1991; Vance 1991). It is said that the vast majority of ethnic minorities who seek treatment for sexual dysfunctions turn to folk practitioners and folk cures (d'Ardenne 1986; Wyatt 1982). This not only reflects the politics of research and the alienation of these people from modern medicine but must also be viewed as reflecting the cultural essence of their problems.

The several changes that have been proposed for DSM-IV have little importance in terms of enhancing culturally sensitivity. However, the notion that self-conceived "marked distress" must be a condition for a sexual desire disorder implies cultural sensitivity, as does the consideration of the context of a person's life. We would note that culture plays an important part in shaping that context, and the cultural contexts of the clinician and client may be quite distinct.

References

American Psychiatric Association: Diagnostic and Statistical Manual of Mental Disorders, 3rd Edition, Revised. Washington, DC, American Psychiatric Association, 1987

Ames AM, Houston DA: Legal, social, and biological definitions of pedophilia. Arch Sex Behav 19:333–345, 1990

Bernstein R, Gaw A: Koro: proposed classification for DSM-IV. Am J Psychiatry 147:1670–1674, 1990

Bhatia MS, Malik SC: D'hat syndrome: a useful diagnostic entity in Indian culture. Br J Psychiatry 159:691–695, 1991

Bhugra D, Cordle C: A case control study of sexual dysfunction in Asian and non-Asian couples 1981–1985. Sexual and Marital Therapy 3:71–76, 1988

Bolin A: In Search of Eve: Transsexual Rites of Passage. South Hadley, MA, Bergin & Garvey, 1988

Bottero A: Consumption by semen loss in India and elsewhere. Cult Med Psychiatry 15:303–320, 1991

Chadda RK, Shome RL: Koro: classification and case reports (letter). Am J Psychiatry 148:1766–1767, 1991

Christopher E: Psychosexual medicine in a mixed racial community. British Journal of Family Planning 7:115–119, 1982

d'Ardenne P: Sexual dysfunction in a transcultural setting: assessment, treatment and research. Sexual and Marital Therapy 1:23–34, 1986

Davis DL, Whitten RG: The cross-cultural study of human sexuality. Annual Review of Anthropology 16:69–98, 1987

Dewaraja R, Sasaki J: Semen-loss syndrome: a comparison between Sri Lanka and Japan. Am J Psychotherapy 55:14–20, 1991

Edwards JW: Indigenous Koro, a genital retraction syndrome of insular Southeast Asia: a critical review, in The Culture-Bound Syndromes. Edited by Simons RC, Hughes CC. Dordrecht, Netherlands, D Reidel, 1985, pp 169–191

Ernst F, Francis R, Lench C, et al: Black men and women's response to homosexuality. Arch Sex Behav 20:579–586, 1991

Espin OM: Cultural and historical influences on sexuality in Hispanic/Latin women: implications for psychotherapy, in Pleasure and Danger: Exploring Female Sexuality. Edited by Vance C. Boston, Routledge & Kegan Paul, 1984, pp 149–164

Finkle A, Finkle C: Sexual impotency: counseling of 388 private patients from 1954 to 1982. Urology 23:25–30, 1978

Fisher S: Personality correlates of sexual behavior in black women. Arch Sex Behav 9:27–35, 1980

Ford CS, Beach FA: Patterns of Sexual Behavior. New York, Harper & Brother, 1951

Frank E, Anderson C, Rubenstein D: Frequency of sexual dysfunction in "normal couples." N Engl J Med 299:111–115, 1978

Gagnon J: Sexuality across the life-course in the United States, in AIDS. Edited by Turner C, Miller H, Moses L. Washington, DC, National Academy Press, 1988, pp 33–46

Gebhard PH: Human sexual behavior: a summary statement, in Human Sexual Behavior. Edited by Marshall DS, Suggs RC. New York, Basic Books, 1971, pp 206–217

Green R: The Sissy Boy Syndrome. New Haven, CT, Yale University Press, 1987

Greenberg D: The Construction of Homosexuality. Chicago, IL, University of Chicago Press, 1988

Gregersen E: The World of Sexuality. New York, Irvington Publishers, 1992

Herdt GH: Guardians of the Flutes. New York, McGraw-Hill, 1981

Herdt GH: Developmental continuity as dimension of sexual orientation across cultures, in Homosexuality and Heterosexuality. Edited by McWhirter D, Reinisch J, Sanders P. New York, Oxford University Press, 1990, pp 108–238

Herdt GH, Boxer A: Introduction, in Gay Culture in America. Edited by Herdt G. Boston, MA, Beacon, 1992, pp 1–28

Herdt GH, Stoller RJ: Commentary to "The socialization of homosexuality and heterosexuality in a non-Western society." Arch Sex Behav 18:31–34, 1989

Irvine JM: Disorders of Desire: Sex and Gender in Modern American Sexology. Philadelphia, PA, Temple University Press, 1990

Jacobs S, Roberts C: Sex, sexuality and gender variance, in Gender and Anthropology: Critical Reviews for Research and Teaching. Edited by Morgan S. Washington, DC, American Anthropological Association, 1989, pp 438–462

Johnson LB: Blacks, in The Sexually Oppressed. Edited by Gochros HL, Gochros J. New York, Association Press, 1977, pp 173–191

Kendell R: Relationship between DSM-IV and ICD-10. J Abnorm Psychol 100:297–301, 1991

Leavitt S: Sexual ideology and experience in a Papua New Guinea society. Soc Sci Med 33:897–907, 1991

Leiblum SR, Rosen RC: Introduction: changing perspectives on sexual desire, in Sexual Desire Disorders. Edited by Leiblum SR, Rosen RC. New York, Guilford, 1988, pp 1–17

Leih-Mak F, Ng ML: Ejaculatory incompetence in Chinese men. Am J Psychiatry 138:685–686, 1981

Marmor J: "Normal" and "deviant" sexual behavior. JAMA 217:165–170, 1971

Mokuau N: Ethnic minorities, in Helping the Sexually Oppressed. Edited by Gochros HL, Gochros JS, Fischer J. Englewood Cliffs, NJ, Prentice-Hall, 1986, pp 141–161

Mollica RF, Wyshak G, deMarneffe D, et al: Indochinese versions of the Hopkins Symptom Checklist-25: a screening instrument for the psychiatric care of refugees. Am J Psychiatry 144:497–500, 1987

Money J, Lamacz M: Vandalized Love Maps. Buffalo, NY, Prometheus, 1989
Parker R: Bodies, Pleasures and Passions: Sexual Culture in Contemporary Brazil. Boston, MA, Beacon Press, 1991
Petersen J: Black men and same sex desires and behaviors, in Gay Culture in America. Edited by Herdt G. Boston, MA, Beacon, 1992, pp 147–164
Rooth G: Exhibitionism outside Europe and America. Arch Sex Behav 2:351–363, 1973
Rubin G: Thinking sex: notes for a radical theory of the politics of sexuality, in Pleasure and Danger: Exploring Female Sexuality. Edited by Vance C. Boston, MA, Routledge & Kegan Paul, 1984, pp 267–319
Simons RC: Introduction: the Genital Retraction Taxon, in The Culture-Bound Syndromes. Edited by Simons RC, Hughes CC. Dordrecht, Netherlands, D Reidel, 1985, pp 151–153
Tiefer L: Social constructionism and the study of human sexuality, in Sex and Gender. Edited by Shaver P, Hendrick C. Newbury Park, CA, Sage Publications, 1987, pp 70–94
Tiefer L: New perspectives in sexology: from rigor (mortis) to richness. Journal of Sex Research 28:593–602, 1991
Vance C: Anthropology rediscovers sexuality: a theoretical comment. Soc Sci Med 33:875–884, 1991
Weatherford JM: Porn Row. New York, Arbor House, 1986
Williams W: The Spirit and the Flesh: Sexual Diversity in American Indian Culture. Boston, MA, Beacon Press, 1986
Wyatt GE: Identifying stereotypes of Afro-American sexuality and their Impact on sexual behavior, in The Afro-American Family. Edited by Bass BA, Wyatt GE, Powell G. New York, Grune & Stratton, 1982, pp 334–339

Chapter 51

Eating Disorders: A Cross-Cultural Review

Cheryl Ritenbaugh, Ph.D., M.P.H., Catherine Shisslak, Ph.D.,
Nicolette Teufel, Ph.D., Tina K. Leonard-Green, M.S., R.D., and
Raymond Prince, Ph.D.

Statement of the Issues

Anorexia nervosa and bulimia nervosa have been considered to be the prototypical "culture-bound syndromes" of Western society. Both have been examined intensively from the perspectives of psychology, medical anthropology, and feminist theory, with considerable attention to the interaction of cultural norms and individual pathology. The pathologic fear of fatness is pathognomonic among Western anorexic persons, and it is incorporated into the DSM-III-R (American Psychiatric Association 1987) definition of anorexia nervosa. Bulimia has been associated with the years from late teens to early adulthood and with normal body weight. Eating disorders may currently be underdiagnosed in minority or non-Western populations if these features vary in their expression or are altogether absent.

Significance of the Issues

Review of the literature indicates that patients with eating disorders have now been diagnosed in many Western and non-Western countries and among several important United States minority groups, including American blacks, Puerto Ricans, Mexican Americans, Asian Americans, and some American Indian groups. In the United States, some individuals present with features that do not conform to the standard diagnostic criteria for anorexia nervosa or bulimia nervosa (Shisslak et al. 1989), and these individuals' disorders are often missed by the health care system.

Bulimic features may be common among older and heavier minority women, and recognition of this trend may increase identification and appropriate treatment. The information presented below suggests that practitioners need to be aware of eating disorders across a broader ethnic spectrum of individuals.

Method

We have reviewed a representative sample of the literature on anorexia nervosa and bulimia nervosa in non-Caucasians in both the United States and other countries. We paid particular attention to reports that include data on specific individuals, whether identified through questionnaire-based surveys in communities or chart review of diagnosed cases in hospitals or clinics. Medline and *Index Medicus* were searched for the years 1985–1991, and references in these articles were tracked until no new articles were found. The search yielded 28 potentially relevant reports. We summarize the 14 with data: 8 that focused primarily on United States minority groups and the remainder covering eating disorders among populations in Canada, England, Europe, Africa, and Asia (Table 51–1).

Results

Blacks

In college student surveys, American black women were found to be significantly less likely than Caucasian women to indicate fear and discouragement regarding their weight and control of food intake (Gray et al. 1987). In three series with a total of 40 cases, a greater number of American black males were identified than would have been expected from the sex ratio usually observed in whites, and bulimic features were common in both sexes (Anderson and Hay 1985; Hsu 1987; Silber 1986). In one United States series (Anderson and Hay 1985), American black patients with eating disorders were shown to be essentially similar to other American black nonpsychotic psychiatric patients in the same institution, except that the eating disorder patients were from a significantly higher social class.

Hispanics

Case series include individuals from a number of Latin American countries, as well as Mexican Americans born in the United States. Diagnoses of eating disorders were unusually delayed for recent immigrants from upper-income families who were experiencing the pressures of rapid acculturation, perhaps because health care

Table 51–1. Summary of studies on anorexia and bulimia among United States minorities and for other countries, 1980–1991

Study	Country	Number by ethnic group	Number anorexic	Number bulimic	Number other	Survey	Case study	Measures
Anderson and Hay 1985	United States	7 black females 1 black male 110 Caucasian females 10 Caucasian males	4 1 }98{	3 }22{			X	
Gray et al. 1987	United States	341 black females 166 black males 220 Caucasian females 119 Caucasian males		10 (3%) 3 (2%) 29 (13%) 5 (4%)		X		Questionnaire (designed to DSM-III)
Hiebert et al. 1988	United States	19 Caucasian females 1 Caucasian male 9 Hispanic females 1 Hispanic male	19 1 9 1				X	Chart review (outcome comparison)

(continued)

Table 51–1. Summary of studies on anorexia and bulimia among United States minorities and for other countries, 1980–1991 (*continued*)

Study	Country	Number by ethnic group	Number anorexic	Number bulimic	Number other	Survey	Case study	Measures
Hsu 1987	United States	6 black females	2	3	1 anorexia nervosa with bulimia		X	
		1 black male			1 anorexia nervosa with bulimia			
Kope and Slack 1987	Canada	3 Vietnamese refugee females	1	1	1 anorexia nervosa with bulimia		X	
Lee 1991	China (Hong Kong)	16 Chinese females (lower social class)	16 (few had bulimic symptoms)				X	
Lee et al. 1989	China (Hong Kong)	3 Chinese females	1		1 bulimic anorexia nervosa; 1 atypical anorexia nervosa		X	
Lee et al. 1991	China (Hong Kong)	35 Chinese females	32	3			X	

Study	Country	Sample					Method
Mumford and Whitehouse 1988	United States	204 Asian females 355 Caucasian females	1 0	7 (3.4%) 2 (0.6%)		X	Eating Attitudes Test, Body Shape Questionnaire and Interview
Nasser 1986	Egypt	50 Arab females at universities in London 60 at universities in Cairo (reported in previous 1986 study by author)		6 0		X	
Rosen et al. 1988	United States	85 American Indian females			> 50% were dieting and using potentially hazardous methods; 24% used one or more purging methods	X	Questionnaire (not designed to DSM-III diagnoses)
Silber 1986	United States	5 Hispanic females 2 black females	5 2			X	DSM-III criteria
Snow and Harris 1989	United States	56 American Indian (51 female) 37 Hispanics (31 female)		5 female (10%) 4 female (13%)		X	Questionnaire (DSM-III based)

(*continued*)

Table 51–1. Summary of studies on anorexia and bulimia among United States minorities and for other countries, 1980–1991 *(continued)*

Study	Country	Number by ethnic group	Number anorexic	Number bulimic	Number other	Survey	Case study	Measures
Suematsu et al. 1985	Japan	1,011 Japanese (970 females) (41 males)	1,011 970 41			X		DSM-III

personnel had a low index of suspicion for the condition (Silber 1986). In a treatment outcome study, Hiebert et al. (1988) observed no differences attributable to ethnic group. In a DSM-III-R-based questionnaire survey of 31 Hispanic females in a rural New Mexico high school (Snow and Harris 1989), increased weight was related to indications of disordered eating and the use of potentially harmful weight-control techniques. The authors considered concerns about weight, body shape, and dieting to be similar to responses seen in Caucasian American populations, although the risk of anorexia appeared to be low.

American Indians

Surveys of American Indian high school and college students show anorexia to be rare, but bulimic symptoms to be common and associated with greater-than-average weight (Rosen et al. 1988; Snow and Harris 1989). Among older Chippewa women, Rosen et al. found widespread use of purging and other deleterious weight-loss strategies associated with eating disorders: 74% had dieted; 55% had used pathogenic weight-loss techniques (e.g., fasting, purging); 12% reported vomiting; and 6% reported use of laxatives and diuretics. Women reporting dieting were significantly heavier than those who did not, and among the dieters, those who used pathogenic dieting techniques were heavier than those who did not. Women reporting more severe dieting tended to be older than the sample average. Anorexia did not seem to be a problem.

Immigrant Studies

Immigrants appear to be adopting the normative values and fear of fatness associated with the country to which they immigrate (Kope and Slack 1987; Mumford and Whitehouse 1988; Nasser 1988a, 1988b). In three female Vietnamese refugees in Canada with anorexia nervosa, the onset of the illness appeared to be related to the loss of family contacts, traumatic escapes, and coping with the problems of living under the control of older siblings. The classic features of the condition, including disturbed body image and fear of fatness, were all present. Nasser's (1986) survey of 50 Egyptian females at London universities and 60 Egyptian females at Cairo universities showed no evidence of eating disorders in the Cairo sample, but 12% of the sample in England met DSM-III-R criteria by questionnaire. Mumford and Whitehouse (1988) surveyed Asian and Caucasian girls in a school in England. Asian girls scored significantly higher than Caucasian girls on the Eating Attitudes Test: 3.6% of the Asian and 0.6% of the Caucasian girls met the criteria for bulimia nervosa on interview; one Asian girl but no Caucasian girls met the criteria for anorexia nervosa. The authors attributed the high rate of bulimia nervosa among the Asian girls in part to acculturation.

Non-Western Countries

Anorexic individuals from the lower socioeconomic classes in Hong Kong have been described (Lee 1991; Lee et al. 1989, 1991). In these cases, all DSM-III-R criteria were met except for the fear of fatness. In traditional Chinese culture, some degree of fatness is highly valued, and cultural prescriptions of beauty focus on the face rather than the body. Acne was reported as a precipitant of anorexia nervosa in this group (Lee et al. 1991). These patients explained their refusal to eat as secondary to feelings of fullness or epigastric pain. Family dynamics conformed to patterns seen in anorexic families in the United States. In Japan, Suematsu et al. (1985) reported on more than 2,000 cases of anorexia based on a survey of physicians at more than 1,000 institutions. Diagnostic criteria included distorted body image and denial of illness, but not fear of fatness per se.

Discussion

Much has been written in the popular and lay press about the extreme cultural value that Western society places on thinness and the concurrent negative valuation of fatness (e.g., Callaway 1990; Nichter and Nichter 1991; Ritenbaugh 1982; Seid 1989). High rates of anorexia nervosa in Western societies and increasing rates of anorexia nervosa found among their immigrant groups and rapidly acculturating ethnic minorities attest to this cultural obsession with thinness. Individuals from groups that traditionally had a low prevalence of eating disorders (such as United States minorities, immigrants, and populations of developing countries) may be particularly vulnerable to the development of such disorders when faced with the stresses of rapid Westernization, acculturation, and social assimilation. The studies reviewed here point to the need for clinicians to have a heightened suspicion of anorexia nervosa when dealing with underweight patients from virtually any population having contact with or adapting to Western society.

The review also pointed toward the association of Western cultural values with bulimia nervosa. Bulimic behaviors and bulimia nervosa are found among persons of all body sizes. Three of the papers reviewed here suggest that clinicians should be alert to these types of behaviors among older and heavier Hispanic, American Indian, and American black women; all of these populations have a high prevalence of obesity. With growing attention to the negative consequences of obesity in these populations, an increasing incidence of pathogenic attempts at weight loss would not be surprising. Further research into the etiology and prevalence of bulimia in these minority populations would be desirable.

The cross-cultural studies presented here suggest that "atypical anorexia" may be more widespread than previously recognized and may be the category of choice when dealing with some cultural groups. Shisslak et al. (1989) described a series of 15 individuals with atypical anorexia in the United States, of whom only three had distorted body image. Publication of more case series of atypical anorexia from varied cultural contexts could provide important insights into the roles of cultural norms in the chosen idioms of distress (Nichter 1981). An alternative, and more international, approach comes from Lee (1991), who argued that diagnostic criteria for anorexia nervosa that allow a level of cultural variability may be particularly useful in encouraging cross-cultural and multiethnic studies. He proposed replacing "intense fear of gaining weight" with the use of rigid complaints such as fear of fatness, abdominal fullness, or distaste for food to account for the severe restriction of food intake or other weight-losing behaviors. This recommendation does not deny the higher rates of eating disorders in cultures where fear of fatness is the norm, but rather suggests the use of diagnostic criteria that lend themselves more readily to international and cross-cultural situations. Careful international and cross-cultural studies addressing the characteristics of anorexic and bulimic individuals are needed to move these issues toward resolution.

Recommendations

A major step in the diagnosis of bulimia nervosa and anorexia nervosa is a heightened awareness among practitioners of the possibility of both conditions among minority and non-Western populations. Diagnosis of bulimia nervosa is currently relatively culture-free in that it focuses on behavior rather than attribution. Future research in populations of non-European extraction may show that "fear of fatness" is a frequent feature of anorexia nervosa but not a required diagnostic criterion. The important message to health professionals is that individuals of all backgrounds are potentially at risk for eating disorders and may require intervention.

References

American Psychiatric Association: Diagnostic and Statistical Manual of Mental Disorders, 3rd Edition, Revised. Washington, DC, American Psychiatric Association, 1987

Anderson AE, Hay A: Racial and socioeconomic influences in anorexia nervosa and bulimia. International Journal of Eating Disorders 4:479–487, 1985

Callaway CW: The Callaway Diet: Successful Permanent Weight Control for Starvers, Stuffers, and Skippers. New York, Bantam Books, 1990

Gray JJ, Ford K, Kelly LM: The prevalence of bulimia in a black college population. International Journal of Eating Disorders 6:733–740, 1987

Hiebert KA, Felice ME, Wingard DL, et al: Comparison of outcome in Hispanic and Caucasian patients with anorexia nervosa. International Journal of Eating Disorders 7:693–696, 1988

Hsu LKG: Are the eating disorders becoming more common in blacks? International Journal of Eating Disorders 6:113–124, 1987

Kope TM, Slack WH: Anorexia nervosa in Southeast Asian refugees: a report on three cases. J Am Acad Child Adolesc Psychiatry 26:795–797, 1987

Lee S: Anorexia nervosa in Hong Kong: a Chinese perspective. Psychol Med 21:703–711, 1991

Lee S, Chiu HFK, Chen C: Anorexia nervosa in Hong Kong: why not more in Chinese? Br J Psychiatry 154:683–688, 1989

Lee S, Leung CM, Wing YK, et al: Acne as a risk factor for anorexia nervosa in Chinese. Aust N Z J Psychiatry 25:134–137, 1991

Mumford D, Whitehouse A: Increased prevalence of bulimia nervosa among Asian schoolgirls. BMJ 297:718, 1988

Nasser M: Comparative study of the prevalence of abnormal eating attitudes among Arab female students of both London and Cairo Universities. Psychol Med 16:621–625, 1986

Nasser M: Culture and weight consciousness. J Psychosom Res 32(6):573–577, 1988a

Nasser M: Eating disorders: the cultural dimension. Soc Psychiatry Psychiatr Epidemiol 23:184–187, 1988b

Nichter M: Idioms of distress: alternatives in the expression of psychosocial distress: a case study from South India. Cult Med Psychiatry 5:379–408, 1981

Nichter M, Nichter M: Hype and weight. Medical Anthropology 13:249–284, 1991

Ritenbaugh C: Obesity as a culture-bound syndrome. Cult Med Psychiatry 6:347–361, 1982

Rosen LW, Shafer CL, Dummer GM, et al: Prevalence of pathogenic weight-control behaviors among Native American women and girls. International Journal of Eating Disorders 7:807–811, 1988

Seid R: Never Too Thin: Why Women Are at War With Their Bodies. New York, Prentice Hall, 1989

Shisslak CM, Crago M, Yates A: Typical patterns in atypical anorexia nervosa. Psychosomatics 30:307–311, 1989

Silber TJ: Anorexia nervosa in blacks and Hispanics. International Journal of Eating Disorders 5:121–128, 1986

Snow JR, Harris MB: Brief report: disordered eating in Southwestern Pueblo Indians and Hispanics. Journal of Adolescence 12:329–336, 1989

Suematsu H, Ishikawa H, Kuboki T, et al: Statistical studies on anorexia nervosa in Japan: detailed clinical data on 1,011 patients. Psychother Psychosom 43:96–103, 1985

Chapter 52

Culture and the Diagnosis of Adjustment Disorders

Janis H. Jenkins, Ph.D., and
J. David Kinzie, M.D.

Cultural Issues

Although adjustment disorders are not severe enough to qualify for other DSM-IV diagnoses, such as mood or anxiety disorders, their presenting symptoms may include subclinical manifestations of mood disorders and anxiety disorders (Fabrega et al. 1987). Therefore, it is useful to review the principles of mood and anxiety disorders for cultural consideration of adjustment disorders (Jenkins et al. 1991; Kleinman and Good 1985). In adjustment disorders, culture plays an important role both in the *appraisal* of the psychosocial stressor in a particular cultural context (Dressler 1991; Monat and Lazarus 1977) and by providing members of a cultural group with behavioral and emotional *repertoires of response* to distressing events and circumstances).

Assessment of the particular psychosocial stressor(s) preceding the symptomatic response must be made in light of the patient's particular sociocultural background (Dressler 1991; Kleinman 1980). A cultural judgment must be made as to the nature and meaning of the potential inventory of stressors. Although some stressors (e.g., divorce, serious accident or injury, rape or sexual assault, natural disaster) may invariably invoke symptoms of adjustment disorder in most individuals, other precipitating events (e.g., witchcraft or religious transgression) may be culturally specific (Fabrega and Mezzich 1987). Individuals of lower socioeconomic status frequently experience a disproportionately greater number of distressing life events (e.g., accident, assault, poverty, inadequate housing) (Brown and Harris 1978).

The judgment of what constitutes clinically significant symptoms or a *maladaptive response* to the particular psychosocial stressor must also be considered in relation to what exceeds the cultural norms of response to that particular stressor

(Fabrega and Mezzich 1987; Kleinman 1988). This judgment may be difficult because few systematic data on culturally normative responses to stressors are currently available. Nevertheless, failure to consider a patient's sociocultural context adequately may result in misdiagnosis.

Migration and Adjustment Disorder

Migrants are typically considered to be either immigrants or refugees. Adjustment disorders with mixed emotional features are apparently common among both immigrants and refugees. Immigrants of lower socioeconomic status may encounter multiple psychosocial stressors, including cultural differences, language barriers, employment and housing difficulties, family breakdown, and prejudice and discrimination (Jenkins 1991; Westermeyer 1989). Refugees often face these same stressors, and their distress is frequently compounded by their experience of extreme poverty, terror, or political violence in war-torn countries. Symptomatic distress associated with such conditions can endure for many years, exacerbated by concurrent sociopolitical and familial conditions in the countries from which they have fled (Beiser 1991; Kinzie et al. 1984, 1990).

Although the designation of "immigrant" implies some degree of choice in leaving one's native country, the designation of "refugee" signals that one's migration is forced, and repatriation often impossible. Although the flight of refugees is not a new social phenomenon, the extent of the problem has recently increased. In a report from the U.S. Committee for Refugees (1990), it is estimated that today there are more than 15 million refugees worldwide. In the last 5 years alone, the worldwide refugee population has increased by 50%. Many of these refugees leave their homelands under the press of conditions that threaten their personal, familial, and cultural survival (Jenkins 1991; Kinzie and Manson 1983; Kinzie et al. 1984).

The symptomatic distress commonly observed among refugees is arguably a normal human response to abnormal (i.e., pathological) human conditions. Sustained exposure to sociopolitical turmoil in the context of war-related violence or terror is likely to produce symptomatic distress in nearly anyone. Such distress should not therefore be taken as evidence of individual failure to cope with or adapt to adverse life conditions. Nevertheless, epidemiological work has suggested the prevalence of psychiatric symptoms among refugees. Using the Cornell Medical Index with Vietnamese, Lin et al. (1979) found widespread symptoms of depression, anxiety, and somatic preoccupation. These symptoms continued to increase over 3 years after resettlement (Masuda et al. 1980). Westermeyer (1989), using self-rating scales to study the Hmong longitudinally, found evidence of acculturation and reduced symptoms of depression, phobias, and somatization over time, but anxiety, hostility, and paranoia changed little. Beiser (1988) reported on a study of depressive symptoms among Vietnamese and Laotian refugees in Vancouver. In general, the longer the refugee had been in Canada, the fewer the depressive symptoms. However, those who were unmarried and without relatives had the highest level of depression 10–12 months after arrival. Beiser (1987) suggested that refugees alter their perception of time as an adaptive strategy to adjustment. During the acute stress, refugees focus on the present to the relative exclusion of past and future. Later, when conscious awareness of past and future reemerges, there is a risk of depression.

A study in California using a psychological well-being scale showed marked differences in depressive symptoms among the various ethnic refugee groups (Rambaut 1985). The Cambodians showed the highest rates of depression and the least adjustment of all groups from Indochina. Gong-Guy (1987) performed a thorough community study to determine the mental health needs of Southeast Asians in America. She found a moderate-to-severe need for psychiatric services among 31% of Vietnamese, 54% of the Hmong, 50% of the Laotians, and 48% of Cambodians. Extremely high rates of posttraumatic stress disorder and depression were also found in one community sample of Cambodian adolescents (Kinzie et al. 1986). Many of the disorders were still present in a follow-up study 3 years later (Kinzie et al. 1989).

The results of epidemiological studies on refugees have documented the presence of many disorders and the concomitant need for services. Some of the disorders meet Axis I criteria for major disorders, but others would classify as adjustment disorders.

Popular Folk Categories and Adjustment Disorder

Some adjustment disorders in migrants may be expressed through specific cultural idioms of distress, such as *nervios* among Latin American patients or explanations like yin-yang imbalance in East Asian cultures. Such examples reflect diverse indigenous explanatory models (Kleinman 1980), but these are not restricted to adjustment disorders. These terms may be popularly employed for what are professionally diagnosed as adjustment disorders, but may also describe what would be diagnosed as schizophrenia or major depression, for example. There apparently is no direct one-to-one correspondence between popular cultural categories and professional psychiatric cultural categories, owing to the often complex and multiple forms of "cultural work" entailed in the former (Good 1977; Kleinman 1988).

The purpose of professional psychiatric categories is to systematically describe syndromes of particular symptomatology for classification and treatment. The purpose of popular folk categories, particularly at the family level of analysis, is to reflect the moral standing, social relations, role functioning, and emotional and physical well-being of the ill person and the person's family (Jenkins 1988, p. 323; but see also Fabrega 1970). The meanings of folk categories of illness represent a complex set of interrelations, as Good (1977) wrote in his classic article on "heart distress" in Iran:

> The meaning of a disease category cannot be understood simply as a set of defining symptoms. It is rather a "syndrome" of typical experiences, a set of words, experiences, and feelings which typically "run together" for the members of a society. Such a syndrome is not merely a reflection of symptoms linked in natural reality, but a set of experiences associated through networks of meaning and social interactions in a society. (p. 27)

Thus, the cultural work of folk categories is different from the cultural work of psychiatric diagnostic classification (Fabrega 1970; Gaines 1992; Good 1977). For example, Latin American families and patients alike employ the term *nervios* for everything from everyday stress to major depression and schizophrenia (Jenkins 1988). The purposely vague and fluid boundaries of this folk category are maintained for a different kind of cultural work, including management of stigma, family bonds, and culturally preferred styles of affective communication (Jenkins and Karno 1992).

References

Beiser M: Changing time perspective in mental health among Asian refugees. Cult Med Psychiatry 11:437–464, 1987
Beiser M: Influence of time, ethnicity and attachment of depression in Southeast Asian refugees. Am J Psychiatry 145:46–51, 1988
Beiser M: Adjustment disorder in DSM-IV: cultural considerations. Paper presented at the NIMH Conference on Culture and Diagnosis, Pittsburgh, PA, 1991
Brown G, Harris T: The Social Origins of Depression. New York, Free Press, 1978
Dressler W: Stress and Adaptation in the Context of Culture. Albany, NY, State University of New York Press, 1991
Fabrega H: On the specificity of folk illnesses. Southwest J Anthrop 26:305–314, 1970
Fabrega H, Mezzich J: Adjustment disorder and psychiatric practice: cultural and historical aspects. Psychiatry 50:31–49, 1987
Fabrega H, Mezzich J, Mezzich A: Adjustment disorder as a marginal or transitional illness category in DSM-III. Arch Gen Psychiatry 44:567–572, 1987
Gaines A (ed): Ethnopsychiatry: The Cultural Construction of Professional and Folk Psychiatries. Albany, NY, State University of New York Press, 1992

Gong-Guy E: The California Southeast Asian Mental Needs Assessment (Contract Number 85-7628-28-2). Sacramento, CA, California State Department of Mental Health, 1987

Good B: The heart of what's the matter: the semantics of illness of Iran. Cult Med Psychiatry 1:25–58, 1977

Jenkins JH: Ethnopsychiatric interpretations of schizophrenic illness. the problem of *nervios* within Mexican-American families. Cult Med Psychiatry 12:303–331, 1988

Jenkins JH: The state construction affect: political ethos and mental health among Salvadoran refugees. Cult Med Psychiatry 15:139–157, 1991

Jenkins JH, Karno M: The meaning of expressed emotion: theoretical issues raised by cross-cultural research. Am J Psychiatry 149:9–21, 1992

Jenkins J, Kleinman A, Good B: Cross-cultural studies of depression, in Psychological Aspects of Depression. Edited by Becker J, Kleinman A. Hillsdale, NJ, Lawrence Erlbaum Associates, 1991, pp 67–99

Kinzie JD, Manson S: Five years experience with Indochinese refugee psychiatric patients. J Operational Psych 14:1005–1111, 1983

Kinzie JD, Fredrickson RH, Ben R, et al: Posttraumatic stress disorders among survivors of Cambodian concentration camps. Am J Psychiatry 141:645–650, 1984

Kinzie JD, Sack WH, Angell RH, et al: The psychiatric effects of massive trauma on Cambodian children, I: the children. J Am Acad Child Adolesc Psychiatry 25:370–376, 1986

Kinzie JD, Sack WH, Angell RH, et al: A three-year follow-up of Cambodian young people traumatized as children II. J Am Acad Child Adolesc Psychiatry 28:501–505, 1989

Kinzie JD, Boehnlein JK, Leung PK, et al: The prevalence of posttraumatic stress disorder and its clinical significance among Southeast Asian refugees. Am J Psychiatry 147:913–917, 1990

Kleinman A: Patients and Healers in the Context of Culture: An Exploration on the Borderland between Anthropology, Medicine, and Psychiatry. Berkeley, CA, University of California Press, 1980

Kleinman A: Rethinking Psychiatry: From Cultural Category to Personal Experience. New York, Free Press, 1988

Kleinman A, Good BJ (eds): Culture and Depression: Studies in the Anthropology and Cross-Cultural Psychiatry of Affect and Disorder. Berkeley, CA, University of California Press, 1985

Lin KM, Tazuma L, Masuda M, et al: Adaptational problems of Vietnamese refugees: health and mental health status. Arch Gen Psychiatry 36:955–961, 1979

Masuda M, Lin KM, Tazuma L, et al: Adaptational problems of Vietnamese refugees, II: life changes and perception of life events. Arch Gen Psychiatry 37:447–450, 1980

Monat A, Lazarus R (eds): Stress and Coping: An Anthology. New York, Columbia University Press, 1977

Rambaut RG: Mental health and the refugee experience: a comparative study of Southeast Asian refugees, in Southeast Asian Mental Health: Treatment, Prevention, Service Training, and Research. Edited by Owan TC. Rockville, MD, National Institutes of Mental Health, 1985, pp 433–486

U.S. Committee for Refugees: World Refugee Survey: 1989 in Review. Washington, DC, U.S. Committee for Refugees, 1990

Westermeyer J: Psychiatric Care of Migrants. Washington, DC, American Psychiatric Press, 1989

Chapter 53

Cultural Factors and Personality Disorders

Renato D. Alarcon, M.D., M.P.H., and
Edward F. Foulks, M.D., Ph.D.

Introduction

Psychiatric diagnosis attempts to define particular behavioral states, relationships, or processes in a way that will reliably allow their recognition and identification as particular clinical entities and will therefore lead to more standard approaches in therapeutic management. The unique human experience of mental disorder has to do in many ways with the socioculture in which such behavior evolves. Culture will influence diagnostic categorizations, treatment, prognosis, prevention, and research (Westermeyer 1985). The area of personality disorders is no exception.

In an attempt to stress the etiopathogenic relevance of sociocultural factors in the occurrence of personality disorders and the value of the current diagnostic criteria for the personality disorders from a cultural vantage point, we conducted three literature searches, using specific item codes such as *personality, personality disorders and culture,* and *personality disorders and cultural factors.* The PsychInfo database yielded 40 references for the years 1980–1991; the PsychLit database yielded 70 references for 1974–1991; and the Medline database yielded 276 references for the years 1966–1991. We also conducted our own search on pertinent sections of *Index Medicus* and collected 46 additional papers.

Cultural Etiopathogenesis of Personality Disorders

Personality disorders have lower levels of diagnostic validity and reliability than any other mental disorders (Millon 1981). In part, this is due to the ubiquitous role of social and cultural factors in the determination of the clinical profiles of these disorders. Cultural factors are involved in determining personality through child-rearing practices, family-based customs and traditions, and the defensive postures provided by societal norms (Dunham 1976). Those who study child development have well documented the reinforcing character of cultural factors in the formation of personality (Apprey 1985; Battan 1983; Clements 1982; Hamilton 1971; Morrison 1973).

As an etiopathogenic agent, culture is consensually understood to be one of several factors involved in determining personality disorders. Indirect evidence comes, for example, from the near absence of antisocial behavior among the Hutterites, an ethnic enclave living for more than a century in the United States and Canada (Favazza 1985). This finding illustrates that psychiatric diagnostic categories may be universal in presentation but different in distribution and that cultural factors may be a preventive element in the occurrence of personality disorders. The content of the symptomatology (pathoplasty) also varies as a function of culture and other factors such as social class.

Personality as a cultural product plays a role in the way Puerto Ricans, in contrast to blacks, Jews, and the Irish, tend to express psychological distress, although it should be emphasized here that variations of personality within ethnic groups are perhaps as great as those found between different ethnic groups (Harwood 1981). In addition, many cultural factors, such as prevailing social attitudes toward psychopathology, competition, and the impersonalization brought about by living in disenfranchised social settings, affect the occurrence and the manifestations of psychiatric conditions (Dohrenwend and Dohrenwend 1974; U. H. Peters 1989). It is therefore necessary to apply the principle of cultural contextualization during the diagnostic process. Contextualizing means to "put in perspective" all criteria, evaluative techniques, or clinical approaches to the assessment of a given personality disorder category. The context has to be derived from some understanding of the culture from which the individual comes to the clinician. Contextualization would prevent stereotyping and misidentification of behaviors that may express native cultural styles or the individual's attempts to acculturate to the host culture (DeLeon et al. 1976). Labeling such behaviors as clinical entities may, in fact, interfere with a healthy process of contextualization and enhance the negative meaning of behaviors that the psychiatric profession identifies as pathological. In addition, it should be noted that in many societies, in contrast to our own, the self is not perceived as manifesting an individual personality separate from family and society.

Dana (1984) asserted that personality disorders have become a typical psychopathological reaction to changing social conditions and advocated an assessment that includes awareness of the effects of modernization and acculturation. Clear distinctions between etic and emic observations (coming from outside and inside the individual's group of reference, respectively) can reduce assessor bias and enhance fairness in descriptions of culturally different persons. Prejudices induced by lack of awareness of cultural factors and buttressed by fear of "unknown" minority persons may result in an unrealistic appraisal of their aspirations and motivations. It is therefore important to apply "moderator variables in the personality assessment of minority persons in order to assess degree of acculturation, and hence, the suitability of available norms" (Dana 1984, p. 52). This point is also argued by Neligh (1988) in relation to the American Indian population. On the basis of an epidemiological comparison of psychiatric inpatients in Saskatchewan, Fritz (1976) found Indians to be 20% and Metis 76% more frequently diagnosed with personality and behavior disorders than were non-Native patients. Indian females were hospitalized much more frequently than non-Indian females, whereas Indian males were hospitalized for these disorders less frequently than non-Native males.

In a study of Eskimo villagers in Alaska and Yoruba villagers in Nigeria, Leighton and colleagues (Leighton 1981; Leighton et al. 1963) found that cultural factors influenced the frequency of affective and personality disorders, but that it was "hard to disentangle them from the much more powerful effects of age and sex, and of situational factors such as poverty" (Leighton 1981, p. 526). Leighton considered culture and personality as sets of more or less independent variables that interact with each other in particular ways in the life of each particular patient. Personality disorders occur when the coping guidelines of culture that have been passed down from previous generations are no longer relevant to the new context of living.

Studies Relating to Specific Personality Disorders

Antisocial Personality Disorder

The lifetime prevalence of antisocial personality disorder (the only personality disorder investigated in the Epidemiologic Catchment Area [ECA] [Regier et al. 1984] study) was found to be 2.1% in New Haven, Connecticut; 2.6% in Baltimore, Maryland; 3.3% in St. Louis, Missouri (Robins et al. 1984); 3.0% in Los Angeles, California, whites, and 3.6% in Los Angeles Mexican Americans (Karno et al. 1987). The ECA-related Puerto Rico Island Study found that there was no major difference between rates in Puerto Rico and the five sites of the ECA study in the mainland United States (Guarnaccia et al. 1990). If the possibility of cultural bias is disregarded, these findings suggest that culturally unique factors may not play an important role in the formation of antisocial personality disorder among such ethnically diverse groups as Mexican Americans, Puerto Ricans, and non-Hispanic

Americans, and that social class may be the more important determinant.

Rates of neuroses and personality disorders are higher in the urban than in the rural setting, likely due to the particular effects of stress in enclaves of urban poverty or to the migration of a pathological subset of rural people to cities (Dohrenwend and Dohrenwend 1974). Another formulation relates the source of the stress in disadvantaged groups to environmentally induced disjunctions between goals and the means to achieve them (Dohrenwend and Dohrenwend 1974) and to related discrepancies between aspirations (a culturally relevant variable of personality) and achievements (U. H. Peters 1989).

Reid (1985) discussed the role of the family in antisocial personality disorder, emphasizing a "chronicle of purported injustices" (p. 832). He returned to the old comparison between antisocial and asocial and made the suggestive point that underprivileged persons with antisocial characteristics may be "highly adaptive in the context of no alternative opportunities or resources" (p. 835), a point also stressed by Levine and Shaiova (1974). It should be noted that as many as half of inner-city ethnic youths may meet the criteria for antisocial personality disorder, indicating that a personality diagnosis may be unfeasible or inappropriate for settings in which learning to be oppositional and suspicious is a protective strategy for life on the streets. It is the value system and behavioral styles of such broken communities that lead to behaviors easily diagnosed as antisocial personality disorder, but a community diagnosis rather than a personality diagnosis is needed.

Histrionic Personality Disorder

Lucchi and Gaston (1990) presented histrionic and antisocial personalities as two phenomenological expressions of a single character disorder, differing only on the basis of culturally established sex roles. On the other hand, Van Moffaert and Vereecken (1989) did not find an excess of histrionic personalities among adolescent and adult Mediterranean immigrants to Belgium (despite a predominance of somatization symptom patterns) and prevailing stereotypes of Mediterranean women as having traits of emotionality, dramatic interpersonal style, demonstrativeness, and subjection to authority figures.

Standage et al. (1984) applied a 54-item questionnaire to assess role-taking in people with histrionic personality disorder. Role-taking, as defined by Gough (1948), is the ability to perceive and evaluate one's own behavior as it is perceived and evaluated by others in the same culture. Experimental subjects were 20 women seen in a general hospital psychiatric unit with the diagnosis of histrionic personality disorder, compared with 20 control female inpatients, hospitalized for treatment of depressions of all kinds. The socialization scores (aptly considered a cultural dimension) of the women with histrionic personalities were significantly lower, indicating impaired role-taking. Although these authors conceded that the specificity of their findings for the histrionic personality is not well established, they made some persuasive comments about the clear distinction between histrionic personality disorder and other personality disorders.

Borderline Personality Disorder

Borderline personality disorder has been found in some instances to be the result of rapid cultural changes faced by individuals who lack adaptive skills (Hisama 1980; Murphy 1982) or to be a clinical cradle for cross-cultural variants such as the "negative possession trance" (L. G. Peters 1988). Similarly, identity problems, emptiness, abandonment, absence of autonomy, and low anxiety threshold have been found in child and adult immigrants (Laxenaire et al. 1982; Skhiri et al. 1982). Behaviors resembling borderline features have also been observed in different non-Western cultures, although seemingly at much lower prevalence (Jilek-Aall 1988).

Other Personality Disorders

Prevalence studies of other personality disorders in general populations have not been performed. Zimmerman and Coryell (1989) reported that the overall point (5-year) prevalence rate for any personality disorder was low (antisocial personality disorder = 3.3%, passive-aggressive personality disorder = 3.3%, histrionic personality disorder = 3%, schizotypal personality disorder = 2.9%, avoidant personality disorder = 1.3%, paranoid-schizoid personality disorders = 1.8%). Hyler et al. (1990) suggested that these personality disorders may have accounted for a considerable portion of the population in the ECA study who sought mental health services but had no disorder according to the Diagnostic Interview Schedule (Robins et al. 1981).

Paris (1991) reported on a cross-cultural survey of the incidence of personality disorders that was conducted by the World Health Organization. The survey used the Personality Disorder Examination (Loranger et al. 1983), which was designed according to the criteria for personality disorders in ICD-10 (World Health Organization 1990). Clinical populations in 15 sites in North America, Asia, Africa, and Europe were evaluated, and findings suggest that most of the personality disorders recognizable in the West could be identified in the other sites as well. The study populations were all urban, however, and the general community prevalence rates of personality disorders in rural, underdeveloped countries have yet to be determined. Of note is Smith's (1990) finding of lower narcissism scores among Asian American women when compared with Caucasian and Hispanic American women. Shepherd and Sartorius (1974) recognized the inadequacy of the subdivisions of personality disorders in the ICD, whether because of imprecise criteria, lack of mention of severity and relationship to other illnesses, or an ill-defined notion of normality. Finally, it should be noted that certain personality styles may be peculiar to, or receive greater emphasis in, unique cultural settings. Such traits may deserve discussion as a separate category of personality disorder when they are recognized to be extreme or dystonic within their cultural context. Machismo in Latin American males and "religious scrupulosity" in traditional people are two examples of the types of traits that may require special diagnostic consideration.

Discussion

The incorporation of cultural factors in DSM-IV should make clear the need to culturally contextualize the assessment of personality characteristics. Impairment may be the result of maladjustment to a majority or new dominant cultural perspective or may be related to dysfunction with respect to the reference group itself (Littlewood 1984). The clinician should take into account aspects of everyday behavior in the person's ethnic, minority, and immigrant groups and realize that he or she may be following deeply ingrained cultural rules and customs to prevent the "pathologization" of such culturally sanctioned behaviors. At the same time, the combination of emic and etic approaches in actual clinical contact is imperative to avoid mislabeling or, what is worse, strengthening behaviors that, if unduly prolonged, may evolve into true psychopathologies.

From our review of the literature, it is evident that there is not enough heuristic evidence to justify the proposal of socioculturally derived criteria to identify specific personality disorders. In fact, it would be inappropriate to do so, because it would open a Pandora's box of labeling, counterlabeling, and other damaging prospects for cultural psychiatry and its tenets. Rather, we suggest adopting a general exclusion criterion in the actual listing of diagnostic criteria pertaining to each personality disorder in DSM-III-R (American Psychiatric Association 1987) and DSM-IV. Such an exclusion criterion would serve as a continuous reminder to clinicians and other mental health workers who exercise diagnostic judgment to consider the impact of cultural factors on the behavior that they examine and evaluate.

Recommendations for DSM-IV

We offer three general recommendations based on the preceding discussion:

1. Inclusion of a discussion of Cultural Considerations as part of the introductory text to the Personality Disorders section of DSM-IV.
2. Inclusion of specific paragraphs on the same subject for each personality disorder.

3. Addition of a general exclusion criterion for each of the personality disorder categories, noting exclusionary cultural factors.

References

American Psychiatric Association: Diagnostic and Statistical Manual of Mental Disorders, 3rd Edition, Revised. Washington, DC, American Psychiatric Association, 1987

Apprey M: C.R. Badcock and the problem of adaptation. Journal of Psychoanalytic Anthropology 8:189–196, 1985

Battan JF: The "new narcissism" in 20th century America: the shadow and substance of social change. Journal of Social History 17:199–220, 1983

Clements CV: Misusing psychiatric models: the culture of narcissism. Psychoanal Rev 69:283–295, 1982

Dana RH: Personality assessment practice and teaching for the next decade. J Pers Assess 48:46–57, 1984

DeLeon O, Sevilla E, Salas G: Cross cultural aspects of somatic complaints: social and personality factors. Revista de Neuro-Psiquiatria 39:10–23, 1976

Dohrenwend BP, Dohrenwend BS: Social and cultural influences on psychopathology. Annu Rev Psychol 25:417–452, 1974

Dunham HW: Society, culture and mental disorder. Arch Gen Psychiatry 33:147–156, 1976

Favazza AR: Anthropology and psychiatry, in Comprehensive Textbook of Psychiatry, Vol 4. Edited by Kaplan HI, Sadock JD. Baltimore, MD, Williams & Wilkins, 1985, pp 247–265

Fritz WB: Psychiatric disorders among natives and non-natives in Saskatchewan. Canadian Psychiatric Association Journal 21:393–400, 1976

Gough HG: A sociological theory of psychopathy. American Journal of Sociology 53:359–366, 1948

Guarnaccia P, Good B, Kleinman A: A critical review of epidemiological studies of Puerto Rican mental health. Am J Psychiatry 147:1449–1455, 1990

Hamilton JW: Some cultural determinants of intrapsychic structure and psychopathology. Psychoanal Rev 58:279–294, 1971

Harwood A (ed): Ethnicity and Medical Care. Cambridge, MA, Harvard University Press, 1981

Hisama T: Minority group children and behavior disorders: the case of Asian-American children. Behavioral Disorders 5:186–196, 1980

Hyler S, Skodol A, Kellman D, et al: Validity of the personality diagnostic questionnaire revised: comparison with two structured interviews. Am J Psychiatry 147:1043–1047, 1990

Jilek-Aall L: Suicidal behavior among youth: a cross-cultural comparison. Transcultural Psychiatric Research Review 25:87–105, 1988

Karno M, Hough R, Burnham M, et al: Lifetime prevalence of specific psychiatric disorders among Mexican Americans and Non-Hispanic whites in Los Angeles. Arch Gen Psychiatry 44:695–701, 1987

Laxenaire M, Ganne-Vevònec M, Streiff O: Les problèmes d'identité chez les enfants des migrants. Ann Med Psychol 140:602–605, 1982

Leighton AH: Culture and psychiatry. Can J Psychiatry 26:522–529, 1981

Leighton DC, Harding JS, Macklin DB, et al: The Character of Danger: Psychiatric Symptoms in Selected Communities. New York, Basic Books, 1963

Levine EM, Shaiova CH: Biology, personalities and culture: a theoretical comment on the etiology of character disorders in industrial society. Israel Annals of Psychiatry and Related Disciplines 12:10–28, 1974

Littlewood R: The irritation of madness: the influence of psychopathology upon culture. Soc Sci Med 19:705–715, 1984

Loranger AW, Oldham JM, Russokoff LM, et al: Personality Disorder Examination: A Structured Interview for Making DSM-III Axis II Diagnoses. White Plains, NY, New York Hospital—Cornell Medical Center, Westchester Division, 1983

Lucchi N, Gaston A: Cultural relativity of hysteria as a nosographic entity: hysteria and antisocial behavior. Minerva Psichiatrica 31:151–154, 1990

Millon T: Disorders of Personality. New York, John Wiley, 1981

Morrison SD: Intermediate variables in the association between migration and mental illness. Int J Soc Psychiatry 19:60–65, 1973

Murphy HBM: Comparative Psychiatry: The International and Intercultural Distribution of Mental Illness. New York, Springer-Verlag, 1982

Neligh G: Major mental disorders and behavior among American Indians and Alaska natives. American Indian and Alaska Native Mental Health Research 1:116–150, 1988

Paris J: Personality disorders, parasuicide and culture. Transcultural Psychiatric Research Review 28:25–39, 1991

Peters LG: Borderline personality disorder and the possession syndrome: an ethno psychoanalytic perspective. Transcultural Psychiatric Research Review 25:5–46, 1988

Peters UH: Psychological sequelae of persecution: the survivor syndrome. Fortschr Neurol Psychiatr 57:169–191, 1989

Regier DA, Myers JK, Kramer M, et al: The NIMH Epidemiologic Catchment Area program. Arch Gen Psychiatry 41:934–941, 1984

Reid WH: The antisocial personality: a review. Hosp Community Psychiatry 36:831–837, 1985

Robins LN, Helzer JE, Croughan J, et al: National Institute of Mental Health Diagnostic Interview Schedule: its history, characteristics, and validity. Arch Gen Psychiatry 38:381–389, 1981

Robins L, Helzer J, Weissman M, et al: Lifetime prevalence of specific psychiatric disorders in three sites. Arch Gen Psychiatry 41:949–958, 1984

Shepherd M, Sartorius N: Personality disorder and the international classification of diseases. Psychol Med 4:141–146, 1974

Skhiri D, Annabi S, Bi S, et al: Enfants d'immigrés: facteurs de liens ou de rupture? Ann Med Psychol 140:197–202, 1982

Smith BM: The measurement of narcissism in Asian, Caucasian, and Hispanic American women. Psychol Rep 67:779–785, 1990

Standage M, Bilsbury C, Jain S, et al: An investigation of role taking in histrionic personalities. Can J Psychiatry 29:407–411, 1984

Van Moffaert M, Vereecken A: Somatization of psychiatric illness in Mediterranean migrants in Belgium. Cult Med Psychiatry 13:297–313, 1989

Westermeyer J: Psychiatric diagnosis across cultural boundaries. Am J Psychiatry 142:798–805, 1985

World Health Organization: ICD-10 Chapter V: Mental and Behavioral Disorders. Diagnostic Criteria for Research. Geneva, Switzerland, World Health Organization, 1990

Zimmerman M, Coryell W: DSM-III personality disorder diagnosis in a non-patient sample. Arch Gen Psychiatry 46:682–689, 1989

Chapter 54

On Culturally Enhancing the DSM-IV Multiaxial Formulation

Juan E. Mezzich, M.D., Ph.D., and
Byron J. Good, Ph.D.

Introduction

The need for a culturally sensitive and cross-culturally valid DSM-IV, including its multiaxial schema, is primarily based on the multicultural reality of the United States. The substantial and growing presence of African Americans, Asian Americans, Native Americans, and Latinos is impressive and presents special problems for diagnosis. So too the flow of migrant refugees to the United States and the growth of special populations such as the homeless create particular difficulties for making valid and reliable diagnoses using uniform criteria. The international visibility expected of DSM-IV, predicated on the worldwide impact of the DSM-III (American Psychiatric Association 1980), noted by Mezzich (1987), provides an added impetus for making cultural considerations explicit within the structure of the manual.

The emerging comprehensive concepts of health status, which encompass physical health, mental condition, functioning levels, and quality of life, are also important here. As Patrick et al. (1985) pointed out, each of these aspects is influenced by cultural factors. Consequently, assessment in multicultural settings requires particular clinician sensitivity, and both reliability and validity of assessments depend on a systematic recognition of difficulties in using diagnostic categories and rating scales across cultures.

Cultural considerations offered for the multiaxial system of DSM-IV are discussed here axis by axis and then with regard to a complementary cultural formulation.

Axes I and II: Mental Disorders

The impact of cultural factors on the various aspects of psychopathology and its professional appraisal and diagnostic categorization has been a focal point of sustained anthropological and cross-cultural psychiatric research, as summarized by Fabrega (1987), Hopper (1991), Kleinman (1988), and Mezzich et al. (1996). Specific recommendations for according a measure of cultural sensitivity to the judgments and ratings corresponding to Axes I and II are for the most part contained in proposals to be inserted in the pertinent sections of the main body of DSM-IV. We also recommend that specific attention be drawn to relevant cultural issues in the section of the manual that discusses the multiaxial structure.

Axis III: General Medical Disorders

The differential distribution of certain medical diseases across ethnic groups, reflected in epidemiological findings and literature on illness behavior (for a summary, see Harwood 1981), is one consideration for sensitive diagnoses on this axis. Such variations may reflect genetic factors (as in the case of sickle-cell anemias and African ethnicity), social and environmental factors (as in the distribution of a wide variety of infectious diseases), and risk behaviors.

Of special importance to psychiatric diagnosis is the fact that general medical diseases interact with psychiatric illness in complex ways. For example, Kleinman (1988) pointed out that several of the primary criteria for major depressive disorder (weakness, tiredness, and appetite disturbance) are common symptoms of many parasitic and infectious diseases, making diagnosis of depression more difficult in populations in which such conditions are endemic. Weiss (1985) has shown that culture strongly influences both normal and pathological responses to such highly stigmatizing illnesses as leprosy, presenting significant difficulties for assessment. Similar considerations may be applicable to AIDS.

Cultural factors also powerfully influence the emergence, meaning, and ramifications of those health problems that are ill defined and difficult to diagnose, such as those often seen in primary care. Culturally distinctive somatic idioms for expressing distress and illness add to the difficulty of making valid and reliable diagnoses across cultures.

Axis IV: Psychosocial Stressors and Supports

The importance of this area has been widely recognized since the proposals of Rutter et al. (1975), despite the modest success reported with the specific procedures developed for assessment of this axis. The importance of this domain appears to be significant not only for psychiatric conditions but also for general health, as documented by House et al. (1988). Options are being formulated for shifting the focus of Axis IV from overall severity of psychosocial stressors to a list of specific stressors and/or a procedure focused on the appraisal of support factors. Because the scaling of stressors and supports assumes an implicit cultural norm, and because any list of stressors and supports will be culturally specific, it will be a challenge to make Axis IV assessments valid across social and cultural subgroups in our society or cross-culturally.

Nonetheless, the need to consider general environmental factors, specific precipitating events, and levels of support as well as the cultural factors influencing them is widely recognized. For example, Tseng (1985) emphasized the need to understand the anthropology of the family to effectively assess pertinent stressors and coping patterns. Pierloot and Ngoma (1988) documented that psychosocial stressors tend to originate in large group interactions in the case of African patients as compared with more restricted family interactions in patients with a European background. Vargas-Willis and Cervantes (1987) discussed the loss of family relations and cultural change faced by Latino immigrants to the United States.

The meaning of the stressors for the affected individuals may have a decisive etiopathogenic role. Furthermore, cultural factors may influence both the structure of social supports and the evaluation of the effectiveness of such support (Guarnaccia 1996).

To furnish information on feasibility and fit, diagnostic proposals on psychosocial factors should be empirically validated through field trials in the major American ethnic groups and minority populations.

Axis V: Functioning

The structure and content of Axis V are subject to a number of competing perspectives. One of them refers to focusing this aspect on adaptive functioning only, without considering symptomatology. This is based on the argument that symptomatology is most relevant to the clinical syndromic axes and the inclusion of symptoms in the functioning axis heavily shifts the clinician's attention to them to the detriment of the role of social performance. Furthermore, the severity of symptoms may be best handled by severity guidelines furnished for psychopathological (Axes I and II) diagnoses.

Another proposal involves separate assessment of key functioning areas such as occupational and interpersonal performance. It has been widely demonstrated that cultural factors can have crucial effects on the design and application of measurement instruments in this area, as indicated by Alarcon (1983), particularly for personality disorders. To illustrate further, Kunce and Vales (1984) discussed the need for sensitivity in the assessment of the functioning of Mexican Americans, taking into consideration differences in behavioral expectations, values, and styles. Good and Good (1986) and Good and Kleinman (1985) summarized the difficulties in adapting psychometric instruments for cross-cultural use.

As in the case of Axis IV, it seems clear that the cultural relevance of measurement instruments or of clinician ratings must be empirically examined and that sensitivity to cultural diversity is required in their administration. In addition to assessing functioning in terms of the norms of the broader society, it should be useful to base it on the evaluation of significant others close to the patient (Guarnaccia 1996).

Complementary Cultural Formulation

The need for dedicated attention to the cultural dimensions of diagnoses has been argued by Hughes (1985) and others. Empirical proposals for culture-relevant axes are exemplified by the octaxial schema conceptualized and implemented in the Puerto Rican mental health care system by H. Ramirez (personal communication, April 2, 1989). Critical perspectives and elements for organizing a cultural axis have been articulated by Good and Good (1986).

Key informants for a cultural formulation would be the patient and his or her primary social group (Good and Good 1986). This represents an emic perspective or "the native point of view" (Geertz 1983).

A major instrumental issue involves language abilities and preferences (Irvine 1985; Marcos and Alpert 1976). A new critical perspective in this regard is multilingualism, prompted by recent observations of Latin American immigrants (Guarnaccia 1996). These considerations are connected to the importance of acculturation and biculturalism. Work in this area has tended to portray an individual's affiliation on a continuum from totally involved in the culture of origin to totally assimilated into the host culture (Cuellar and Roberts 1984). Alternative perspectives have focused on the parallel appraisal of involvement in both the culture of origin and the host culture (Santisteban and Szapocznik 1982). There is a growing literature on the contribution of acculturation stress to the emergence of psychopathology and on the adaptive value of biculturalism (Guarnaccia 1996).

The constitutive elements of a prospective cultural formulation, as initially proposed by Good and Good (1986), would include the meaning of and explanatory models for the diagnoses made, the recognition of culture-specific syndromes and illness idioms, perceived levels of adaptive functioning, care-seeking patterns, and expectations of illness outcome and quality of life.

The proposed cultural formulation could be presented within the framework of a comprehensive psychiatric evaluation, in line with the tradition of familial-genetic and psychodynamic formulations. Further research may lead to the standardization, at least in part, of this formulation, the establishment of more solid connections with other elements of psychiatric assessment, and its effective use for treatment and prognosis.

At the 1991 Conference on Culture and Diagnosis in Pittsburgh, Pennsylvania, sponsored by the National Institute of Mental Health, there was clearly wide interest in some form of cultural statement to complement the standard diagnostic ratings in DSM-IV. The conceptual and consultation work carried out in the following years led to the development of a Cultural Formulation Guideline, growing out of wide empirical research and clinical experience (Mezzich et al. 1993). The guideline consists of the following five components.

Cultural Identity of the Individual

The clinician should specify the individual's cultural reference groups. Attend particularly to language abilities, use, and preferences (including multilingualism). For immigrants and ethnic minorities, note separately the degree of involvement with both the culture of origin and the host or majority culture.

Cultural Explanations of the Individual's Illness

Identify the following:

1. The predominant idioms of distress through which symptoms are communicated (e.g., "nerves," possessing spirits, somatic complaints, inexplicable misfortune).
2. The meaning and perceived severity of the individual's symptoms in relation to norms of the cultural reference group.
3. Any local illness category used by the individual's family and community to identify the condition.
4. The perceived causes or explanatory models that the individual and the reference group employ to explain the illness.
5. Current preferences for and past experience with professional and popular sources of care.

Cultural Factors Related to Psychosocial Environment and Functioning

Note culturally relevant interpretations of social stressors, available social supports, and levels of functioning and disability. Special attention should be given to stresses in the local social environment and to the role of religion and kin networks in providing emotional, instrumental, and informational support.

Cultural Elements of the Relationship Between the Individual and the Clinician

Indicate differences in culture and social status between the individual and the clinician and problems that these differences may cause in diagnosis and treatment (e.g., difficulty in communicating in the individual's first language, in eliciting symptoms or understanding their cultural significance, in negotiating an appropriate relationship or level of intimacy, in determining whether a behavior is normative or pathological).

Overall Cultural Assessment for Diagnosis and Care

The formulation should conclude with a discussion of how these cultural considerations specifically influence comprehensive diagnosis and care.

Field trials were conducted on clinical cases corresponding to prominent ethnically identified minorities in the United States, supporting the feasibility and usefulness of the cultural formulation. We would urge researchers and clinicians, especially those in minority clinics and minority mental health research centers, to develop this cultural formulation further and systematically investigate its utility for clinical description and care.

A properly framed and annotated multiaxial schema, supplemented by an idiographic cultural formulation, would represent a qualitatively enhanced comprehensive diagnostic formulation, one that is not only culturally valid but aimed at appraising the totality of the patient's clinical condition, including the uniqueness of his or her personal experience.

References

Alarcon RD: Latin American perspectives on DSM-III. Am J Psychiatry 140:102–105, 1983
American Psychiatric Association: Diagnostic and Statistical Manual of Mental Disorders, 3rd Edition. Washington, DC, American Psychiatric Association, 1980
Cuellar I, Roberts RE: Psychological disorders among Chicanos, in Chicano Psychology. Edited by Martinez JL, Mendoza RH. Orlando, FL, Academic Press, 1984
Fabrega H: Psychiatric diagnosis: a cultural perspective. J Nerv Ment Dis 175:383–394, 1987
Geertz C: Local Knowledge. New York, Basic Books, 1983
Good BJ, Good M-JD: The cultural context of diagnosis and therapy: a view from medical anthropology, in Mental Health Research and Practice in Minority Communities (DHHS Publ No ADM-86-1466). Edited by Miranda MR, Kitano HHL. Washington, DC, U.S. Government Printing Office, 1986

Good BJ, Kleinman A: Culture and anxiety: cross-cultural evidence for the patterning of anxiety disorders, in Anxiety and the Anxiety Disorders. Edited by Tuma AH, Maser J. Hillsdale, NJ, Lawrence Erlbaum Associates, 1985, pp 297–323

Guarnaccia P: Cultural comments on multiaxial issues, in Culture and Psychiatric Diagnosis. Edited by Mezzich JE, Kleinman A, Fabrega H, et al. Washington, DC, American Psychiatric Press, 1996

Harwood A: Ethnicity and Medical Care. Cambridge, MA, Harvard University Press, 1981

Hopper K: Some old questions for the new cross-cultural psychiatry. Medical Anthropology Quarterly 5:299–330, 1991

House JS, Landis KR, Umberson D: Social relationships and health. Science 241:540–545, 1988

Hughes CC: "Culture-bound or construct-bound?" in The Culture Bound Syndromes. Edited by Simons RC, Hughes CC. Dordrecht, Netherlands, D Reidel, 1985, pp 3–24

Irvine J: Status and style in language. Annual Review of Anthropology 14:557–581, 1985

Kleinman A: Rethinking Psychiatry: From Cultural Category to Personal Experience. New York, Free Press, 1988

Kunce JT, Vales LF: The Mexican American: implications for cross-cultural rehabilitation counseling. Rehabilitation Counseling Bulletin 28:97–108, 1984

Marcos LR, Alpert M: Strategies and risks in psychotherapy with bilingual patients. Am J Psychiatry 133:1275–1281, 1976

Mezzich JE: International use and impact of DSM-III, in An Annotated Bibliography of DSM-III. Edited by Skodol AE, Spitzer RL. Washington, DC, American Psychiatric Press, 1987, pp 37–46

Mezzich JE, Good BJ, Lewis-Fernandez R, et al: Cultural formulation guidelines, in Revised Cultural Proposals for DSM-IV: Technical Report submitted to the DSM-IV Task Force by the Steering Committee, Group on Culture and Diagnosis. Edited by Mezzich JE, Kleinman A, Fabrega H, et al. Pittsburgh, PA, National Institute of Mental Health, 1993, pp 163–168

Mezzich JE, Kleinman A, Fabrega H, et al: Culture and Psychiatric Diagnosis. Washington, DC, American Psychiatric Press, 1996

Patrick DL, Sittampalam Y, Somerville SM, et al: A cross-cultural comparison of health status values. Am J Public Health 75:1402–1407, 1985

Pierloot TA, Ngoma M: Hysterical manifestations in Africa and Europe: a comparative study. Br J Psychiatry 152:112–115, 1988

Rutter M, Shaffer D, Shepherd M: A Multiaxial Classification of Child Psychiatric Disorders. Geneva, Switzerland, World Health Organization, 1975

Santisteban D, Szapocznik J: Substance use disorders among Hispanics, in Mental Health and Hispanic Americans. Edited by Becerra RM, Karno M, Escobar JI. New York, Grune & Stratton, 1982

Tseng W-S: Cultural aspects of family assessment. International Journal of Family Psychiatry 6:19–31, 1985

Vargas-Willis G, Cervantes RC: Consideration of psychosocial stress in the treatment of the Latina immigrant. Special Issue: Mexican immigrant women. Hispanic Journal of Behavioral Sciences 9:315–329, 1987

Weiss M: The interrelationship of tropical disease and mental disorder. Cult Med Psychiatry 9:121–200, 1985

Chapter 55

The "Culture-Bound Syndromes" and DSM-IV

Charles C. Hughes, Ph.D., Ronald C. Simons, M.D., and
Ronald M. Wintrob, M.D.

Evaluating the *culture-bound syndromes* with respect to inclusion in DSM-IV poses problems qualitatively different from those confronting the other working papers, for the challenge is not a matter of simply adding a cultural dimension to an already established DSM diagnostic category. Rather, it is that of laying the groundwork for a conceptual bridge between one *set* of diagnostic categories and concepts (Western nosology) and a heterogeneous array of indicators of disorder found in "folk" societies around the world.

Although the term *culture-bound syndrome* has been seen in the psychiatrically oriented anthropological literature for a number of years, in psychiatry it has come into currency only since cultural dimensions of mental disorders began to be seriously considered. The phenomena referred to as culture-bound syndromes have also been called "ethnic psychoses," "ethnic neuroses," "atypical psychoses," and "culture-reactive syndromes," among other terms (Hughes 1985a). Such collective labels evolved in the clinical as well as ethnographic literature to represent episodes of unusual behavior strikingly different from that known in Western, Europeanized society—different even from such deviant behaviors as conventional and familiar forms of mental illness. From a Euro-American point of view, such behavior patterns were frequently interpreted as not simply different but abnormal, yet they did not seem to accord with Western conceptions of "conventional" ways in which disorder is exhibited. There was something askew, something troubling, when a simplistic translation into Western categories was considered (Simons and Hughes 1985, 1993).

Amok, a classic culture-bound syndrome, can be taken as prototypical of this class of disorders and the conceptual complexities involved in trying to make sense of it. Out of his experience in then Dutch-controlled Indonesia three-quarters of a century ago, the Dutch psychiatrist and neurologist van Loon (1926–1927) expressed the difficulty he experienced attempting to understand what were to him bizarre behavior patterns known locally as *amok* and *lattah*. In inadvertent anticipation of this chapter's assignment (i.e., to argue the case for inclusion of the culture-bound syndromes in DSM-IV in such a fashion as not to violate their nature and at the same time to assess their possible value in enlightening a DSM approach to psychiatric understanding), he cautioned against falling prey to "the fundamental mistake, commonly made, to try and explain all the psychic abnormalities of primitive races according to Western diagnostics, to classify them according to Western schemes, only considering the similarity with the familiar syndromes and classifications of Western pathology" (van Loon 1926–1927, p. 434). But it was not only colonialists' exposure to diverse peoples with different customs and beliefs that brought the culture-bound syndromes to wider attention; the ethnocentrism expressed in writings of travelers, explorers, government officials, missionaries, and others also contributed to giving such syndromes a place in the anthropological and psychiatric literature.

Even though most authors who use the term *culture-bound syndrome* have no problem agreeing on a general sense of what is being talked about—the cultural labeling and folk etiological explanation of nonnormative experience—agreement on a specific and consistent meaning poses numerous semantic and clinical perplexities, for the term is much like a projective test. It has been applied somewhat indiscriminately to a wide range of often disparate biological and psychological phenomena, with some of the purported syndromes referring to fairly straightforward behavioral expressions of particularly salient cultural beliefs and values (e.g., *taijin kyofusho, dhat*), whereas others are labels applied to heterogeneous symptom clusters that include a variety of elements that in Western nosology have no "natural" fit (e.g., *aire*); still others appear to function as explanatory rationalizations for misfortune (e.g., *susto*). Such definitional ambiguities can lead to a scattering of intellectual effort, miscommunication about the nature of the empirical phenomena being discussed, and stultification of effective analysis of the relationships between cultural context and behavioral abnormality. (One could compare the situation to the six blind men touching the elephant in different places and then defining the animal's structure and habits on the basis of such selective data.)

Other ambiguities arise when readers from different perceptual and cultural backgrounds are tempted to project into the phrase their own particular understanding of the term *culture* as well as the word *bound*. The original usage connoted a finite and delimited list of psychiatric disorders, each of which could theoretically be singled out as unique to a particular sociocultural setting. The implication was that such disorders constituted a *distinctive and theretofore unknown class* of psychiatric phenomena found outside the range of those included in such formal diagnostic compilations as DSM.

But closer review of the ethnographic data showed that there were resemblances in the clinical picture among a number of the culture-bound syndromes found in different cultural settings, even those not closely related geographically. Commentators began to note, for example, that X syndrome—which had been thought unique to a particular society—is called Y in an entirely different cultural setting (Hughes 1985b). Hence the question of purported uniqueness has been raised for more penetrating analysis, and the task now is to base distributional statements on symptomatic evidence, not abstract categorical speculation, and to search for etiology in the particular cultural/psychodynamic context in which a given disorder is displayed. For example, *amok*, referred to earlier, is an indigenous term from southeast Asia that has become accepted even in the English language to refer to an episode of spontaneous, indiscriminate violence and/or aggression no matter where it is found, even in the industrialized world.

A second semantic issue relates to the descriptor "-bound." This aspect of the overall phrase points to the kinds of possible etiological relationships hypothesized to exist between a particular cultural setting and forms of pathology (e.g., psychodynamics and social stress points, role definitions, salient values). In that analytic sense, a given syndrome may be construed as "bound" or linked to a particular cultural context but not necessarily unique to it. Based on his long experience in Malaya, Sir Hugh Clifford, a British official, made critical observations on the relationship between a particular bizarre behavior—in this case *amok*—and salient cultural values in the social context. Such comments provide the core conceptual meaning of this different class of disorders called "culture-bound syndromes." Commenting on a particular case of an *amok*-runner, Clifford noted that

> By far the greater number of Malay *amok* results from a condition of mind which is described in the vernacular by the term *sakit hati*—sickness of the liver—that organ, and not the heart, being regarded as the center of sensibility. The states of feeling which are described by this phrase are numerous, complex, and differ widely in degree, but they all imply some measure of anger, excitement, and mental irritation. . . . [Speaking of a particular case of an *amok*-runner . . .] his father had died a natural death. . . . He had no quarrel with the people of Pahang, but his "liver was sick," and to run *amok* was, in his [i.e., the runner's] opinion, the natural remedy. This is merely one instance of many which might be cited, and serves to illustrate my contention that *amok* is caused, in most cases, by a condition of mind, which may result from either serious or comparatively trivial causes, but which, while it lasts, makes a native weary of life. At such times, he is doubtless to some extent a madman—just as all suicides are more or less insane—but the state of feeling which drives a European to take his own life makes a Malay run *amok*. All

> Malays have the greatest horror of suicide, and I know of no properly authenticated case in which a male Malay has committed such an act, but I have known several who ran *amok* when a white man, under similar circumstances, would not improbably have taken his own life. (Clifford 1895/1927, p. 80)

In his culturally insightful comment, Clifford provided the germ of a psychodynamic hypothesis pertaining to this particular culture-bound syndrome that has been much discussed in the literature and may be taken as paradigmatic of the theoretical relationship between a disorder and its cultural context. He suggested a behavioral process that serves as a linkage or articulation between culture and personality. In this case, the cultural value is the "abhorrence of suicide"; how better, then, to effect one's own death than by indiscriminately killing others in the community so that they, out of a sense of self-protection, will kill the *amok*-runner. Thus the salient cultural value—abhorrence of suicide—is accommodated at the same time that the psychodynamic need to efface shame and hurt is also satisfied.

Finally there is the issue of *syndrome*. Insofar as relative stability in observable behavioral pattern, persistence over time, and explicit labeling are key defining features of the generic concept of syndrome, some of the culture-bound syndromes may qualify at least as quasi-syndromes in the medical sense. Certainly they are "folk syndromes." However, there is rarely even an approximation of a match in overall pattern between a given culture-bound syndrome and one from DSM; in fact, there is considerable variance. Further, even as in DSM, a given symptom may appear in different culture-bound syndromes.

Indeed, the data on which the designation culture-bound syndromes is based—variegated cognitive, affective, behavioral, and somatic symptoms—appear not to be unique or exclusive to that putative class. Rather, they are shared with the symptomatic primary data of DSM. It is the packaging into designated conceptual entities that is different. An example is provided by Amering and Katschnig (1990). They compared the symptoms operationalizing a DSM diagnosis of panic attack with the two culture-bound syndromes of *koro* and *kayak-angst*, a comparison that may suggest a useful model for further systematic research into ways to link such folk diagnoses with DSM categories and in so doing find something of a common conceptual ground.

Edwards et al. (1982), in a review of culture-bound syndromes among the Zulu, provided another example of the need to go beyond simplistic Western-based diagnostic assignment for this class of disorders and reach into the cultural matrix of symptoms. The Zulu distinguish 15 different "folk" syndromes (collectively called *ukufa kwabantu*), which the authors grouped into 6 categories of folk etiology (sorcery; environmental, ecological, or atmospheric health hazards; spirit possession; ancestral wrath or displeasure for various reasons; asocial behavior or flouting of cultural norms; pollution). The syndromes themselves are constituted differentially from these etiological influences. The Zulus believe that these syndromes "are unique or peculiar to their people in the sense that their aetiology, diagnosis and treatment are all inextricably bound up with the traditional Zulu and African world views of sickness and health" (p. 82). Regarding diagnosis and treatment by Western professionals, they are

> Commonly diagnosed on the basis of their symptomatology as: various neurotic or psychosomatic conditions, conversion disorders, fictitious disorders, acute psychotic or confusional states, hysterical psychoses. It is obviously essential for treatment with modern Western medicine to correctly diagnose the relative aetiological contributions of biological, psychological and social factors in the patient's illness. However whether, for example primary aetiology is psychogenic e.g., umeqo,[1] presenting in the form of conversion disorder, or organic e.g. prostatic enlargement culturally attributed to sorcery, the specific cultural factors should be taken into account in treatment as the patient has to return to his cultural environment after discharge. (Edwards et al. 1982, p. 85)

The article by Edwards et al. can be cited as an outstanding example of the manner in which an indigenous diagnostic and treatment protocol, which in itself is firmly rooted in cultural belief systems, can articulate with Western psychiatric "culture."

An analogous set of "folk" diagnostic syndromes, their lay etiology, and appropriate treatment in another African group—the Yoruba of Nigeria—is found in Leighton et al. (1963).

Trance or dissociative symptoms are often found listed in any inventory of the culture-bound syndromes. In a study of contemporary Canadian society far removed from the "exotic" locale of many of the so-called culture-bound syndromes, Ross et al. (1990), using a 28-item self-report structured questionnaire with a random sample of 1,539 households, concluded that

> Dissociative disorders, including multiple personality disorder, may be relatively common, with a prevalence that may be in the range of 5%–10% of the general population. If this prediction is borne out, it will be clear that a major form of psychopathology in North America has been almost entirely missed by most mental health professionals. Since dissociative experiences are common in the general population, we suspect that dissociative symptoms may occur in a wide

---

[1] Edwards et al. (1982) described umeqo as "a condition culturally attributed to having stepped over dangerous tracks. ... Alternatively umeqo is often attributed to sorcery" (p. 84).

range of psychiatric disorders, just as anxiety and depression can be components of many different diagnostic entities. (Ross et al. 1990, p. 1552)

Addressing the same point from India, Wig noted that although

In Third World countries one does see definite cases of somatization disorder, conversion disorder, and psychogenic pain disorder that meet DSM-III criteria, there is a still larger number of cases that present a mixture of many of these symptoms and do not fit neatly into any one of the categories. (Wig 1983, p. 85)

Further, with respect to dissociative disorders:

A major difficulty experienced by psychiatrists in Third World countries ... is the problem of classifying so-called "hysterical fits," one of the most common presentations of patients in these countries ... Many of the patients with this disorder show classic features of dissociation, and logically should be included in the dissociative disorders category. But there are other cases in which the predominant underlying phenomenon seems to be acute anxiety, and one wonders whether it is correct to put such cases in the category of dissociation. Moreover, there are many patients who have "hysterical fits" along with other symptoms of somatization disorder.... [There] is a need for more and better clinical studies in Third World countries to clarify these issues. (Wig 1983, p. 86)

Supporting the need for more detailed clinical studies of symptoms in their cultural context, Chakraborty noted that, with

The exception of trance and possession states (listed under "Dissociative Disorders" in ICD-10), local culture-bound syndromes have not found a place in any classification. They are not felt to be worthy of psychiatric attention except as curiosities. Yet "these episodic and dramatic reactions specific to a particular community ... locally identified ... consistent over time and embedded for each generation in a continuing cultural tradition," remain central to an understanding of how cultures recognise and resolve individual and communal tensions. (Chakraborty 1991, p. 1206)

Why are these considerations important? What difference might awareness of culture-bound syndromes make in clinicians' behavior, assessment, and therapeutic plans? Isn't all that they need to know already incorporated in recent editions of the DSM?

No. The phenomena of the culture-bound syndromes do not constitute discrete, bounded entities that can be directly translated into conventional Western categories. Rather, when examined at a primary level, they interpenetrate established diagnostic entities with symptoms that flood across numerous parts of the DSM nosologic structure.

At base, the clinical encounter involves an interaction between two phenomenological worlds comprising culturally structured language symbolism and implicit assumptions about and interpretations of normal and abnormal thought content, verbal expression, and manifest behavioral patterns—all of which have critical implications for interpretation and intervention. Moreover, in an increasingly diverse United States society, the clinical encounter is often one between two persons from cultural traditions with differing definitions of reality. Such different "life-worlds" can be based on ethnic groups or socioeconomic or educational status, or they can be situationally structured (the latter illustrated, for example, when a clinician becomes the patient and experiences the episode from a patient's perspective).

Underlying the clinical encounter, of course, is the question of whether "different" necessarily equates with "disordered" or pathological. That question becomes especially critical with the culture-bound syndromes (which, in more neutral phrasing, are coming to be called "folk diagnoses"), because the challenge for the clinician is to tap into the private phenomenological world of the patient. The difficulty of doing this is compounded when the very parameters of what is defined as a disorder, as well as its precipitants, course, and meaning, are different from conventional professional understanding. This is specifically the case when one is dealing with the culture-bound syndromes, which provide naturally occurring experiments in highly diverse culturally patterned ways of defining reality and normality/abnormality. In a patient-centered approach, the culture-bound syndromes constitute reality in the minds of the patients (with all that implies for the possibility of therapeutic intervention and treatment compliance). The operative question is therefore: "Where does 'normality' lie?" If in the eye of the beholder, which beholder? Is the fixed point of reference to be those categories currently conceptualized in DSM? Or can there be some defensible means within that structure to accommodate world views that do not fit existing niches?

What should be done if the behavior of a particular patient is *not* considered pathological by those of his or her cultural group, and yet might be so judged by an inflexible application of the DSM diagnostic categories—as can happen when the typical clinician treats patients from cultural backgrounds markedly different from his or her own? The obvious can be suggested: namely, that the most effective clinical outcome will result from a microdetailed analysis of the patient's culturally structured definitions of "normality" before rushing to match such behavior with existing DSM categories, and that such an analysis should be informed by data and interpretations from the patient's own family or cultural acquaintances.

Such understanding and clinical effectiveness would be greatly enhanced by some type of structural reminder built into DSM-IV's assessment protocol to allow the culture-bound syndromes as a category of interest to lose their parochial reputation and demonstrate the major contributions they make to understanding the general nature of cultural influences in psychiatric disorders. Optimally, that structural reminder would take the form of a cultural axis, but short of that, some other device for assessing the extent and pervasiveness of cultural factors in the etiology and course of a disorder seems essential. This would enable the clinician to turn the question of the culture-bound syndromes into a working concept that refers not exclusively to faraway cultural groups distant from oneself, but also to the culturally familiar, such as (for many clinicians) current United States society.

Therefore, in attempting to incorporate the culture-bound syndromes into DSM-IV, we suggest a direction of thinking and some type of analytic mechanism that will bring such syndromes into conceptual alignment with centralist professional understanding, perhaps divest them of their exotic nature, and prompt further analysis of their clinical import. One can first look, for example, at mainstream United States society and the crude categories and labels used by the person in the street to communicate lay ideas of deviance to the clinician—in effect, "folk" psychiatric diagnoses. Such categorizing is conceptually equivalent to, but not as institutionalized or fixed as, the *amok, latah, koro,* or other conventional culture-bound syndromes discussed earlier. It is, nonetheless, a comparable "standardized language of distress" (Helman 1990), a folk cultural process in the mainstream population in terms of which abnormal or at least nonnormal behavioral episodes or fixed traits are perceived and labeled in everyday life. Witness such terms as *crazy, moody, blue, down in the dumps, nervous, depressed, wacko, flaky, spacy, grumpy, edgy, off the rocker, out of it, nuts, strange, queer, touchy, wild, weird* and the rest, which convey a general sense of a problem to peers as well as professionals.

But beyond such a street-level vocabulary for recognizing and naming disorders in contemporary United States society, there are other folk-perceived patterns that, in their structure and derivation, are beginning to be thought of as structurally comparable to traditional culture-bound syndromes—that is, their symptomatology expresses a patterned relationship to particular and salient cultural values in a given society. Through usage, such patterns are beginning to move further along the continuum toward professional diagnostic acceptability. Examples frequently suggested in the literature are "type A behavior" ("up-tight," "hard-driving," a morbid actualization of the cultural value of "conquering" time, of impatience with delay) and anorexia nervosa (a fetishistic preoccupation with appearance, with slimness in body form).

The challenge for the clinician, therefore, is to discover or construct an effective semantic bridge between the language and conceptual world of the patient and that of the professional, especially but not limited to the domain of what have been called the culture-bound syndromes. Such bridging is important not only for enhancing patient care and fostering compliance, but also for exposing the cultural biases and limitations of the DSM system itself, which is deeply rooted in Western cultural evolution. In this regard, consideration of the culture-bound syndromes enriches the range of conceptualization and theoretical development of psychiatry as a clinical discipline.

References

Amering M, Katschnig H: Panic attacks and panic disorder in cross-cultural perspective. Psychiatric Annals 20:511–516, 1990

Chakraborty A: Culture, colonialism, and psychiatry. Lancet 337:1204–1207, 1991

Clifford H: In Court and Kampong, Being Tales and Sketches of Native Life in the Malay Peninsula (1895). London, England, Richards Press Ltd, 1927

Edwards SD, Cheetham RWS, Majozi E, et al: Zulu culture-bound psychiatric syndromes. South African Journal of Hospital Medicine, April 1982, pp 82–86

Helman CG: Culture, Health and Illness: An Introduction for Health Professionals. London, England, Wright, 1990

Hughes CC: "Culture-bound or construct-bound"? the syndromes and DSM-III, in The Culture-Bound Syndromes: Folk Illnesses of Psychiatric and Anthropological Interest. Edited by Simons RC, Hughes CC. Dordrecht, Netherlands, D Reidel, 1985a, pp 3–24

Hughes CC: Glossary of "culture-bound" or folk psychiatric syndromes, in The Culture-Bound Syndromes: Folk Illnesses of Psychiatric and Anthropological Interest. Edited by Simons RC, Hughes CC. Dordrecht, Netherlands, D Reidel, 1985b, pp 469–505

Leighton AH, Adeoye Lambo T, Hughes CC, et al: Psychiatric Disorder Among the Yoruba: A Report From the Cornell-Aro Mental Health Research Project in the Western Region, Nigeria. Ithaca, NY, Cornell University Press, 1963

Ross CA, Joshi S, Currie R: Dissociative experiences in the general population. Am J Psychiatry 147:1547–1552, 1990

Simons RC, Hughes CC (eds): The Culture-Bound Syndromes: Folk Illnesses of Psychiatric and Anthropological Interest. Dordrecht, Netherlands, D Reidel, 1985

Simons RC, Hughes CC: The culture-bound syndromes, in Culture, Ethnicity, and Mental Illness. Edited by Gaw AC. Washington, DC, American Psychiatric Press, 1993, pp 75–99

van Loon FHG: Amok and lattah. Journal of Abnormal and Social Psychology 21:434–444, 1926–27

Wig NN: DSM-III: a perspective from the third world, in International Perspectives on DSM-III. Edited by Spitzer RL, Williams JB, Skodol AE. Washington, DC, American Psychiatric Press, 1983, pp 79–89

Further Readings

Apple D: How laymen define illness. Journal of Health and Human Behavior 1:219–225, 1960

Bourhis RY, Roth S, MacQueen G: Communication in the hospital setting: a survey of medical and everyday language use amongst patients, nurses and doctors. Soc Sci Med 28:339–346, 1989

Cantor N, Smith EE, French RD, et al: Psychiatric diagnosis as prototype categorization. J Abnorm Psychol 89:181–193, 1980

Hughes CC: The "Culture-bound syndromes" and DSM-IV: to be or not to be?, in Culture and Psychiatric Diagnosis. Edited by Mezzich JE, Kleinman A, Fabrega H, et al. Washington, DC, American Psychiatric Press, 1996

Katz MM, Cole JO, Lowery HA: Studies of the diagnostic process: the influence of symptom perception, past experience, and ethnic background on diagnostic decisions. Am J Psychiatry 125:109–119, 1969

Kendell RE, Pichot P, von Cranach M: Diagnostic criteria of English, French, and German psychiatrists. Psychol Med 4:187–195, 1974

Ness RC, Wintrob RM: Folk healing: a description and synthesis. Am J Psychiatry 138:1477–1481, 1981

Scott N, Weiner MF: "Patientspeak": an exercise in communication. Journal of Medical Education 59:890–893, 1984

Schwartz MA, Wiggins OP: Diagnosis and ideal types: a contribution to psychiatric classification. Compr Psychiatry 28:277–291, 1987

van Wulfften Palthe PM: Psychiatry and neurology in the tropics, in Clinical Textbook of Tropical Medicine, 1st Edition. Edited by de Langen CD, Lichenstein A, Hamilton AH. Batavia, Netherlands, G Kolff & Co, 1936, pp 525–538

Chapter 56

Religious or Spiritual Problems

Francis G. Lu, M.D., David Lukoff, Ph.D., and
Robert Turner, M.D.

Statement of the Issues

The purpose of this review is to consider the literature and research that would be relevant to the question of whether religious or spiritual problems should be included in some form in DSM-IV, either as a mental disorder diagnosis, as a V Code (a condition that may be the focus of clinical attention), or in the appendix for proposed conditions needing further study.

Significance of the Issues

The religious and spiritual dimensions of culture are considered by some to be among the most important factors that structure human experience, beliefs, values, and behavior, as well as illness patterns (Browning et al. 1990; James 1961; Krippner and Welch 1992). Yet psychiatry, in its diagnostic classification systems as well as its theory, research, and practice, has tended either to ignore or pathologize the religious and spiritual dimensions of life.

The V Code section of DSM-III-R (American Psychiatric Association 1987)

This chapter was revised and adapted from an article published in the *Journal of Nervous and Mental Disease* 180:673–682, 1992 (Lukoff et al. 1992).

The authors wish to acknowledge the assistance of Bruce Flath, M.L.S., head librarian at the California Institute of Integral Studies, and Lisa Dunkel, M.L.S., University of California, San Francisco, in conducting computer bibliographic searches.

excluded many important reasons for presentation to mental health practitioners. The distressing problems related to religious and spiritual experience not attributable to a mental disorder may be among the most significant of these omissions. The proposal to include a new category for religious or spiritual problems in DSM-IV is based on a number of factors, including clinical usefulness, reliability, acceptability to clinicians and researchers from a variety of theoretical orientations, and empirical support for its validity (Spitzer and Williams 1985). However, Kass et al. (1989) pointed out that, in practice, "it is often necessary to recommend for general use a diagnosis for which only face validity can be demonstrated" (p. 1025). Although empirical research on religious and spiritual problems is limited, the existing studies supplemented by the extensive clinical literature could be sufficient to establish the face validity of this proposed diagnostic category. Four types of religious problems and two types of spiritual problems are well documented and are discussed in this chapter.

Although there is no consensus about the boundaries between religiosity and spirituality, a frequently drawn distinction in the literature (which we adopted) uses the term *religiosity* to refer to "adherence to the beliefs and practices of an organized church or religious institution" (Shafranske and Maloney 1990, p. 72). The term *spirituality* is used to describe the transcendental relationship between the person and a Higher Being, a quality that goes beyond a specific religious affiliation (Peterson and Nelson 1987). The clinical literature documents that distressing experiences related to religious and spiritual beliefs and values occur in the life course of some patients in both acute and long-term treatment (Lovinger 1984). Surveys show that patients bring these religious and spiritual issues into treatment, yet psychiatrists are poorly trained to address them (Sansone et al. 1990). This lack of training, combined with the "religiosity gap" between the religious beliefs and practices of mental health professionals and their patients, may complicate the accurate differential diagnosis of presenting complaints with religious and spiritual content. Some of these complaints may not be associated with psychopathology. The absence in DSM-III-R of a category for religious and spiritual problems exemplifies the need for a more culturally sensitive psychiatric classification system (Brody 1990; Fabrega 1987, 1992; Kleinman 1988; Mezzich et al. 1992). Misdiagnosis based on lack of sensitivity to the patient's cultural, religious, or spiritual background has been reported in the clinical literature (Barnhouse 1986; Lukoff 1985). The traditional meaning and significance of diagnosis rests on distinguishing between illness and nonillness (Fabrega et al. 1987). A nonillness diagnostic category for religious and spiritual problems would serve to anchor the nonpathological end of the diagnostic spectrum. This would alert clinicians to the possibility that people may have problems in these areas without necessarily having a mental disorder.

Method

The literature review was directed toward obtaining research and clinical articles concerning the incidence, assessment, treatment, and differential diagnosis of religious and spiritual problems and concerning training and cultural sensitivity issues related to such problems. We followed the method of Larson et al. (1992) for conducting a literature review, which ensures that the review accurately reflects the most up-to-date and accurate research on the issue being studied. We conducted several computerized literature searches.

Our first search was confined to the empirical research published from 1978 to 1988 on mystical experience, which can be distressing and hence viewed as a spiritual problem. Because mystical experiences are designated by a number of different terms in different studies, the first computer search included *mystic$* (the $ ending tells the computer to select any word containing mystic, e.g., mystical, mysticism), *religious, peak experiences, transcendent, transpersonal, spiritual, visions,* and *ecstasy.* To select the research articles, the key words used were *research, variable, experiment$, rating$, test$, scale$, statistic$, methodolo$, data,* and *empirical.* An article had to contain key words relevant to both empirical methodology and mystical experiences to be selected. The PsychInfo, Medline, Religion Index, *Sociological Abstracts,* and ERIC databases were searched. We then conducted a more extensive search of the research literature on *religio$* and *spirit$* in the PsychInfo, Medline, and Religion Index databases because they had yielded the most relevant articles. We conducted some additional searches on Medline to obtain clinical articles that were not research based. Finally, the American Psychiatric Association Library conducted a search for us on "religion and psychiatric treatment." Following the systematic review method of Larson et al. (1992), we then studied the reference lists of these articles to identify additional potentially relevant articles until we reached a saturation point where no new articles were being identified. Finally, we contacted many experts in the field, informing them of our intention to make a proposal for a new diagnostic category for religious and spiritual problems and soliciting additional references for pertinent literature. Those contacted included the following: the American Psychiatric Association Committee on Religion and Psychiatry (R. Thurrell, M.D., Chair), the DSM-IV Advisory Group on Cultural Issues (J. Mezzich, M.D., Chair), and 15 experts in the field (including B. Greyson, M.D., S. Krippner, Ph.D., K. Ring, Ph.D., R. Walsh, M.D., G. Gabbard, M.D., E. Shafranske, Ph.D., S. Waldofel, M.D., D. Larson, M.D., and J. Mack, M.D.). Overall, approximately 300 journal articles, chapters, and books were located through this systematic literature review, although only about 50 of these were empirical and clinical studies of specific religious or spiritual problems.

Results

The small number of research articles on religious and spiritual problems uncovered during the searches corroborates the finding of Larson et al. (1986) that psychiatry has largely ignored religion as a variable. Their study of articles published in four psychiatric journals during a recent 5-year period showed that only 2.5% (59 of 2,348) included religious variables, and these primarily involved the psychopathological uses of religion by patients.

From the literature searches, several factors emerged that help explain the limited exploration of religious and spiritual problems. Because the same factors also impinge on clinical treatment of these problems, we review them below starting with historical factors. This is followed by a discussion of the "religiosity gap" between psychiatrists and the general population, as well as findings on the training (or lack thereof) provided psychiatrists in diagnosing and treating these problems.

Historical Data and Theory

Historically, many of the leading theorists have pathologized religious and spiritual experience (e.g., Freud, Skinner, Ellis; see Lukoff et al. 1992). Yet their negative views of religion and spirituality should perhaps be challenged, because recent studies have found no association between religiosity and psychopathology in the nonpatient population. In fact, a meta-analysis of religiosity and mental health found them to be positively related (Bergin 1983). Church-affiliated individuals showed greater happiness and satisfaction with marriage, work, and life in general. Studies of the self-reported relationship between quality of relationships with divine others (e.g., Christ, God, Mary) and several measures of well-being also found a significant positive association (Pollner 1989). Although there does seem to be a relationship between religiosity and psychopathology in the seriously mentally ill (Feldman and Rust 1989), religiosity may, in fact, be associated with positive characteristics of mental health for much of the population.

This historical trend to pathologize religious and spiritual experience is also evident in the literature on mystical experience. Freud (1930/1959) reduced the "oceanic feeling" of mystics to "infantile helplessness" and the seeking of "the regression to limitless narcissism" (p. 72). The 1976 report by the Group for the Advancement of Psychiatry entitled "Mysticism: Spiritual Quest or Mental Disorder" took a similar stance, describing the mystical experience as an escape and a projection on the world of a primitive infantile state. However, studies have found that people reporting mystical experiences scored lower on psychopathology scales and higher on measures of psychological well-being than control subjects (Caird 1987; Hood 1976, 1977; Spanos and Moretti 1988). Allman et al. (1992) found that most clinical psychologists do not currently view mystical experiences as pathological. In addition, other theorists have challenged the trend to pathologize religion, viewing mystical experiences as a sign of health and a powerful agent for transformation (Hood 1974, 1976; James 1961; Jung 1973; Maslow 1962, 1971; Stace 1960; Underhill 1955).

Religious Problem

Robinson (1986) reported that "some patients have troublesome conflicts about religion that could probably be resolved through the process of therapy" (p. 22). In one survey, psychologists estimated that at least one in six of their patients presented issues that involve religion or spirituality, and 72% indicated they had addressed religious or spiritual issues in treatment (Shafranske and Malony 1990). Although comparable data on the prevalence of religious issues in psychiatry practice are not available, Anderson and Young (1988) observed that "all clinicians inevitably face the challenge of treating patients with religious troubles and preoccupations" (p. 532). In the research literature on religious problems, which is limited to case studies, the most common problems described were loss or questioning of a firmly held faith, change in denominational membership, conversion to a new faith, and intensification of adherence to religious practices and orthodoxy.

Both religious and psychiatric issues are associated with the loss of a firmly held faith. Shafranske (1991) described a man of professional accomplishment whose life was founded on the conservative bedrock of Roman Catholic Christianity. He came to doubt the tenets of his religion and, in so doing, declared he had lost the vitality to live.

Another type of religious problem involves patients who intensify their adherence to religious practices and orthodoxy. If the patient is newly religious, the psychotherapist needs to help determine what potential conflicts exist between his former and current lifestyle, beliefs, and attitudes. Spero (1987) described the case of a 16-year-old adolescent from a Reform Jewish family who underwent a sudden religious transformation to orthodoxy. The dramatic changes in her life, including long hours studying Jewish texts, avoidance of friends, and sullenness at meals, led to her referral to a psychoanalyst. A mental status examination determined that neither schizophrenia nor any other Axis I or II disorders were present. The analysis then dealt with the impact of religious transformation on her identity and object relations. The process of religious change challenges important areas of stability, and "to some degree the sense of historical dislocation represents a crisis for all nouveau-religionists" (Spero 1987, p. 69). Converting to a new faith and changing denominational membership raise similar treatment issues focused on reestablishing stable identity and object relations (Salzman 1985).

The American Psychiatric Association Committee on Religion and Psychiatry (1990) prepared a series of guidelines urging that psychiatrists respect patients' religious beliefs and values and "not impose their own religious, antireligious, or ideologic systems of belief on their patients" (p. 542). These guidelines would be applicable to clinical situations exemplified by the distressing religious problems described.

Spiritual Problem

Numerous clinical phenomena have been conceptualized as spiritual problems, particularly in the field of transpersonal psychology. These include mystical experience (Lukoff 1985), near-death experience (Greyson and Harris 1987), spiritual emergency (Grof and Grof 1989), shamanistic initiatory crisis (Lukoff et al. 1992), and kundalini awakening (Greenwell 1990). However, only the first two types—mystical experience and near-death experience—had a substantial body of research and clinical literature (Greyson and Harris 1987; Lukoff and Lu 1988). A survey by Allman et al. (1992) demonstrated that the number of patients who bring mystical experiences into treatment is not insignificant. Psychologists in full-time practice estimated that 4.5% of their clients over the past 12 months brought a mystical experience into therapy. This challenges the Group for the Advancement of Psychiatry (1976) report, which stated that "mystical experiences are rarely observed in psychotherapeutic practice" (p. 799). One example is the case study from this report that illustrates how a mystical experience can become the focus of treatment. The patient was a woman in her early 30s who sought out therapy to deal with unresolved parental struggles and guilt over a younger brother's psychosis. Approximately 2 years into her therapy, she underwent a typical mystical experience, including a state of ecstasy, a sense of union with the universe, a heightened awareness transcending space and time, and a greater sense of meaning and purpose to her life. This experience increasingly became the focus of her continued treatment, as she worked to integrate the insights and attitudinal changes that followed. As the study reported:

> Her mood was ecstatic (if you prefer a theological term) or euphoric (if you prefer psychiatric vocabulary); it persisted for about ten days. She felt that everything in her life had led up to this momentous experience and that all her knowledge had become reorganized during its course. For her, the most important gain from it was a conviction that she was a worthwhile person with worthwhile ideas, not the intrinsically evil person, "rotten to the core," that her mother had convinced her she was. (Group for the Advancement of Psychiatry 1976, p. 804)

Because of the rapid alteration in her mood and her unusual ideation, the authors considered diagnoses of mania, schizophrenia, and hysteria, but rejected these because many aspects of her functioning were either unchanged or improved, and overall her experience seemed to be "more integrating than disintegrating" (p. 806). They concluded that "while a psychiatric diagnosis cannot be dismissed, her experience was certainly akin to those described by great religious mystics who have found a new life through them" (p. 806). Her subsequent treatment focused on expanding the insights she had gained and on helping her to assimilate the mystical experience.

The near-death experience research is noteworthy for its methodological rigor in the study of an intense and sometimes distressing spiritual experience that is often associated with phenomenologically complex clinical phenomena. Standardized scales have been employed, as well as new ones developed to facilitate assessment of associated features. Outcome and treatment have also been addressed in studies that document the nonpathological nature of near-death experience (Flynn 1982; Greyson 1981, 1983; Ring 1984). Both medical research (Ring 1990; Sabom 1982) and a nationwide poll (Gallup 1982) indicate that about one-third of all individuals who have had a close encounter with death have experienced a near-death experience. People who have had a near-death experience consistently report 1) an increased appreciation for life, self-acceptance, concern for others, and sense of purpose; 2) a decreased concern for personal status and material possessions; and 3) an overall shift toward universalistic spiritual values regardless of previous religious affiliations or lack thereof (Ring 1984). Unfortunately, there are reports of individuals who have shared their experiences with professionals and received negative reactions. One woman stated, "I tried to tell my minister, but he told me I had been hallucinating, so I shut up" (Moody 1975, p. 86). A hospitalized patient recounted that, "I tried to tell my nurses what had happened when I woke up, but they told me not to talk about it, that I was just imagining things" (p. 87). Yet sequelae involving anger, depression, and interpersonal difficulties occur so frequently that they should be considered normal and expectable reactions to the stressor (Greyson and Harris 1987).

In the searches on Medline, more articles on clinical dimensions of religious and spiritual experiences were located in the nursing journals than in the psychiatry journals. The nursing profession's awareness of the spiritual dimension in caring for patients was particularly apparent in the accepted nursing diagnostic classification system, which includes categories for spiritual concerns, spiritual distress, and spiritual despair (Carpenito 1983). For example, the diagnostic category of spiritual distress covers two treatment situations: 1) when religious or spiritual beliefs conflict with a prescribed health regimen, and 2) when there is distress associated with a patient's mental or physical inability to practice religious or spiritual rituals (Carpenito 1983). In addition to numerous articles addressing guidelines for spiritual assessment (Peterson and Nelson 1987; Soeken and Carson 1987; Stoll 1979), there has even been research examining the extent to which nurses assess their patients' spiritual needs (Boutell and Bozett 1990).

Religiosity Gap

Surveys conducted in the United States consistently show a "religiosity gap." Both the general public and psychiatric patients report that they are more highly religious and attend church more frequently than mental health professionals. In a 1975 survey conducted by the American Psychiatric Association Task Force on Religion and Psychiatry, about half of the psychiatrists surveyed described themselves as agnostics or atheists. This contrasts with between 1% and 5% of the general population who consider themselves atheists or agnostics (Gallup 1985). Studies have also found that psychiatrists are relatively uninvolved in organized religion. More than half of psychiatrists reported that they attended church "rarely" or "never" (American Psychiatric Association Task Force on Religion and Psychiatry 1975). In contrast, Gallup (1985) found that one-third of the population consider religion to be the most important dimension of their life, and another third consider it very important. A study of psychiatrically hospitalized patients (Kroll and Sheehan 1989) found that religious beliefs and practices also assumed an important and often central place in the lives of many patients. Some 95% professed a belief in God, and 75% reported the belief that the Bible refers to daily events. Almost two-thirds were church members, and more than half attended church weekly. Based on their findings from the survey, the authors concluded: "Belief in God, and in the teachings of the Bible, the sense of an afterlife, and involvement with a church community are relevant dimensions of our patients' lives that certainly deserve more consideration than the psychiatric profession has customarily provided" (Kroll and Sheehan 1989, p. 72).

The spiritual beliefs and practices of psychiatrists have not been researched to the same extent. But the limited data available do not suggest the existence of a "spirituality gap." A survey of psychiatrists, psychologists, social workers, and marriage and family counselors found that 68% endorsed the item indicating that they: "Seek a spiritual understanding of the universe and one's place in it." The authors concluded: "There may be a reservoir of spiritual interests among therapists that is often unexpressed due to the secular framework of professional education and practice" (Bergin and Jensen 1990, p. 3). They named this phenomenon "spiritual humanism" and indicated that it could provide the basis for bridging the cultural gap between clinicians and the more religious public.

Training

Despite the importance of religion and spirituality in most patients' lives, it may be the case that psychiatrists are not given adequate training to prepare them to deal with issues that arise in these realms. In a survey of members of the American Association of Directors of Psychiatric Residency Training on the role of religion in psychiatric education, didactic instruction on all aspects of religion was infrequent (Sansone et al. 1990). The study concluded that the significance of religion for psychiatry warrants greater consideration, including recognition of the full spectrum of religious experience from unhealthy to healthy. Certain issues in differential diagnosis require knowledge of the patient's religious subgroup (Lovinger 1984) and/or the nature of acceptable expressions of subculturally validated forms of religious expression. For example, discussing one of the cases in the *DSM-III-R Casebook*, Spitzer et al. (1989) noted that "the central question in the differential diagnosis in this case is whether or not the visions, voices, unusual beliefs, and bizarre behavior are symptoms of a true psychotic disorder . . . [or] Can this woman's unusual perceptual experiences and strange notions be entirely accounted for by her religious beliefs?" (pp. 245–246).

Many religious and spiritual experiences are not distressing to the individual. When brought into treatment, these situations simply call for the psychiatrist to treat the individual's beliefs and values with respect and perhaps make a referral to a religious professional or spiritual teacher. Yet, Post (1992) noted that few psychiatrists are trained to understand religion, much less treat it sympathetically. Peck (1993) attributed this oversight to "three hundred years of historical tradition pronouncing that religion is totally out of their domain, and having been trained in this tradition, psychiatrists are ill-equipped indeed to deal with either religious pathology or religious health" (p. 237). Barnhouse (1986) pointed out that "sex and religion are, in some form, universal components of human experience. . . . Psychiatrists who know very little about religion would do well to study it" (p. 103). Potentially, this lack of training may result in an intolerance of religion and subtle forms of bias-related incidents deplored by the American Psychiatric Association Council on National Affairs (1993). In summary, some psychiatrists may be operating outside the boundaries of their professional training, which raises clinical and ethical concerns.

Discussion and Recommendations

There are five options for addressing these issues in the DSM-IV. The first option is not to acknowledge religious and spiritual problems that are not attributable to a mental disorder. In support of this option is the view that this diagnostic category could be an example of "psychiatric imperialism" because it implies greater expertise in diagnosing and treating religious and spiritual problems than most psychiatrists possess. However, the risk of harm related to "psychiatric imperialism" seems minimal compared with the benefit to patients of a more culturally sensitive diagnostic system. Continuing to neglect religious and spiritual issues would perpetuate the predicaments that are related to psychiatry's traditional neglect of these issues: "occasional, devastating misdiagnosis; not infrequent mistreatment; an increasingly poor reputation; inadequate research and theory; and a limitation of psychiatrists' own personal development" (Peck 1993, p. 243). Similarly, much of the recent clinical literature has either understated the incidence and significance of spiritual experiences or ignored studies that indicate their positive impact on mental health (Lukoff et al. 1992).

In addition, the need to expand the context of contemporary Western psychiatry has been noted: "It is incumbent upon us as psychiatrists to be thoroughly familiar with the range and breadth of human experience, whether pathological or healthy. We must respect and differentiate unusual but integrating experiences from those which are . . . disorganizing" (Gabbard et al. 1982, p. 368). Accordingly, it may be important to have a diagnostic category available for unusual religious and spiritual experiences that cause distress, because inappropriately diagnosing them as mental disorders can negatively influence their outcome (Greyson and Harris 1987). The clinician's response can determine whether the experience is integrated and used as a stimulus for personal growth, or whether it is repressed as a bizarre event that may be a sign of mental instability: "Attempts to classify the experience as a pathological entity are neither accurate nor helpful" (Greyson and Harris 1987, pp. 44–45). A category for religious or spiritual problem could provide psychiatry with a more complete diagnostic system for persons who present with complaints that have religious or spiritual content, thereby reducing the potential for misdiagnosis.

A second option would be to subsume religious and spiritual problems under existing diagnostic categories for mental disorders. For example, the Group for the Advancement of Psychiatry (1976) report described the mystical experience as a projection on the world of a primitive infantile state, implying it would warrant treatment as a mental disorder. Adjustment disorder is one diagnostic category in particular that merits consideration in this regard because it is a "transitional illness" between nonillness and more severe mental disorders (Fabrega et al. 1987). This option would not contribute to the proliferation of new diagnostic categories, which the Task Force on DSM-IV has committed itself to avoiding. However, adjustment disorders require a clearly defined stressor, and many religious and spiritual problems have no external stressor. In addition, adjustment disorder is appropriate only when symptoms are in excess of what would be a normal and expectable reaction to a stressor. In the case of the near-death experience, a spiritual problem for which there is an obvious stressor, the sequelae of anger, depression, and interpersonal difficulties occur so frequently that they should be considered normal and expectable reactions (Greyson and Harris 1987). The literature review did not uncover any clinical or research literature supporting this option. In addition, the adjustment disorder label would not guide the clinician toward the relevant diagnostic or treatment literature involving religious and spiritual problems.

A third option would be to subsume religious and spiritual problems under existing V Code categories for conditions that are not mental disorders. This option would not contribute to the proliferation of new diagnostic categories. Phase-of-life problem and identity problem are two candidates that should be considered, because religious and/or spiritual concerns often are part of the phenomenology of these conditions. However, both phase-of-life problem and identity problem are conceptualized as developmental in nature, whereas religious and spiritual problems occur at all developmental stages. Furthermore, subsuming religious and spiritual problems under these developmentally based categories would constitute a form of psychological reductionism. Finally, the use of these existing categories would not guide the clinician toward the relevant diagnostic or treatment literature involving religious and spiritual problems.

A fourth option would be to include a new diagnostic category in the appendix for proposed new diagnostic categories needing further study. The advantage of this option would be to facilitate systematic clinical research in this area by listing it as a proposed new category. However, there may already exist sufficient clinical literature to document the face validity of several specific types of religious and spiritual problems. The opinions of the experts we consulted also strongly supported the creation of a new diagnostic category of religious or spiritual problem.

A fifth option would be to add a separate new diagnostic category in DSM-IV. In 1991, we submitted a proposal for a V Code category entitled "psychoreligious or psychospiritual problem" to the Task Force on DSM-IV. (It was too late to include it in *DSM-IV Options Book* [American Psychiatric Association 1991].) One rationale for including a nonmental-disorder category for distressing religious and spiritual problems in DSM-IV was based on an analogy with the DSM-III-R category of uncomplicated bereavement. Just as individuals who meet the diagnostic criteria for major depression are not given that diagnosis if their symptoms are seen as "a normal reaction to the death of a loved one" (American Psychiatric Association 1987, p. 361), individuals in the midst of an intense, distressing religious or spiritual experience may display certain symptoms that could be misconstrued as due to a mental disorder if viewed out of their cultural context (Lukoff 1985; Lukoff and Everest 1985).

The following is our proposal for a DSM-IV V Code entitled "psychoreligious or psychospiritual problem":

> *Psychoreligious problems* are experiences that a person finds troubling or distressing and that involve the beliefs and practices of an organized church or religious

institution. Examples include loss or questioning of a firmly held faith, change in denominational membership, conversion to a new faith, and intensification of adherence to religious practices and orthodoxy.

Psychospiritual problems are experiences that a person finds troubling or distressing and that involve that person's relationship with a transcendent being or force. These problems are not necessarily related to the beliefs and practices of an organized church or religious institution. Examples include near-death experience and mystical experience. This V Code category can be used when the focus of treatment or diagnosis is a psychoreligious or psychospiritual problem that is not attributable to a mental disorder.

An alternative suggestion is to shorten the title to "religious or spiritual problem" because there are no V Codes that utilize similar terminology. For example, there is no psychoacademic problem, but rather academic problem. In addition, the clinical and research literature does not use psychoreligious and psychospiritual, which might hinder attempts to conduct literature reviews on this diagnosis. However, the proposal had drawn a distinction between "pure" religious/spiritual problems and psychoreligious/psychospiritual problems. The "pure" religious and spiritual problems could be addressed by religious professionals or spiritual teachers without any clinical training (e.g., conflicts over faith and doctrine). Many religious problems, for example, are dealt with in a church setting by a religious counselor who typically does not have training in psychotherapy (Young and Griffith 1989). In contrast, psychoreligious and psychospiritual problems may involve distress that requires assessment and treatment by a mental health professional (e.g., sequelae following a near-death experience). The name change to "religious or spiritual problem" might result in the loss of conceptual clarity that could aid the differential diagnosis and referral process.

We recommend the adoption of this new category because it would result in the following benefits: 1) increasing the accuracy of diagnostic assessments when religious and spiritual issues are involved; 2) reducing the occurrence of iatrogenic harm from misdiagnosis of religious and spiritual problems; 3) improving treatment of such problems by stimulating clinical research; and 4) improving treatment of such problems by encouraging psychiatric centers to address the religious and spiritual dimensions of human experience in their training.

Religious and spiritual problems need to be subjected to more research to better understand their prevalence, clinical presentation, differential diagnosis, outcome, treatment, relationship to the life cycle, ethnic factors, and predisposing intrapsychic factors. Although there is a wealth of clinical literature on these problems, the clinical research on religious and spiritual problems is minimal, with the previously noted exception of the many well-designed studies of near-death experience. Defining discrete religious and spiritual problems for study clearly presents difficulties, but the near-death experience research can serve as a model demonstrating that the obstacles are not insurmountable. Finally, many religious and spiritual experiences are not distressing to the individual and simply call for the psychiatrist to treat the individual's beliefs and values with respect.

When the proposal for psychoreligious or psychospiritual problem was written in 1991, the focus was on the need for a nonmental-disorder category for these conditions. However, the Task Force on DSM-IV is planning a number of important changes in their conceptualization of the section called V Codes. In DSM-III-R, these diagnoses were called "Conditions Not Attributable to a Mental Disorder." In DSM-IV, the section for these problems is entitled "Other Conditions That May Be A Focus of Clinical Attention," and the definition specifically notes the possibility that an individual can have a mental disorder that is related to the problem, as long as the problem is sufficiently severe to warrant independent clinical attention. Thus, for example, religious or spiritual problem could be assigned along with bipolar disorder for manic episodes that include spiritual preoccupations, or with obsessive-compulsive disorder that includes religious scrupulosity, if the treatment addresses these significant dimensions of the patient's experience. This greatly expands the potential usage of this category, because the symptoms and treatment of many mental disorders include religious and spiritual aspects (Robinson 1986).

References

Allman LS, De La Roche O, Elkins DN, et al: Psychotherapists' attitudes towards clients reporting mystical experiences. Psychotherapy 29:564–569, 1992

American Psychiatric Association: Diagnostic and Statistical Manual of Mental Disorders, 3rd Edition, Revised. Washington, DC, American Psychiatric Association, 1987

American Psychiatric Association: DSM-IV Options Book. Washington, DC, American Psychiatric Association, 1991

American Psychiatric Association Committee on Religion and Psychiatry: Guidelines regarding possible conflict between psychiatrists' religious commitments and psychiatric practice. Am J Psychiatry 147:542, 1990

American Psychiatric Association Council on National Affairs: Position statement on bias-related incidents. Am J Psychiatry 150:686, 1993

American Psychiatric Association Task Force on Religion and Psychiatry: Psychiatrists' Viewpoint on Religion and Their Services to Religious Institutions and the Ministry. Washington, DC, American Psychiatric Association, 1975

Anderson RG, Young JL: The religious component of acute hospital treatment. Hosp Community Psychiatry 39:528–555, 1988

Barnhouse RT: How to evaluate patients' religious ideation, in Psychiatry and Religion: Overlapping Concerns. Edited by Robinson L. Washington, DC, American Psychiatric Press, 1986, pp 89–106

Bergin A: Religiosity and mental health: a critical reevaluation and meta-analysis. Professional Psychology 24:270–284, 1983

Bergin A, Jensen J: Religiosity of psychotherapists: a national survey. Psychotherapy 27:3–7, 1990

Boutell KA, Bozett FW: Nurses' assessment of patients' spirituality: continuing education implications. Journal of Continuing Education in Nursing 21:172–176, 1990

Brody EB: The new biological determinism in sociocultural context. Aust N Z J Psychiatry 24:464–469, 1990

Browning D, Gobe T, Evison I: Religious and Ethical Factors in Psychiatric Practice. Chicago, IL, Nelson-Hall, 1990

Caird D: Religion and personality: are mystics introverted, neurotic, or psychotic? Br J Soc Psychol 26:345–346, 1987

Carpenito L: Nursing Diagnosis: Application to Clinical Practice. Philadelphia, PA, JB Lippincott, 1983

Fabrega H: Psychiatric diagnosis: a cultural perspective. J Nerv Ment Dis 175:383–394, 1987

Fabrega H: Diagnosis interminable: toward a culturally sensitive DSM-IV. J Nerv Ment Dis 177:415–425, 1992

Fabrega H, Mezzich J, Mezzich A: Adjustment disorder as a marginal or transitional illness category in DSM-III. Arch Gen Psychiatry 44:567–572, 1987

Feldman J, Rust J: Religiosity, schizotypal thinking, and schizophrenia. Psychol Rep 65:587–593, 1989

Flynn CP: Meanings and implications of NDEr transformations: some preliminary findings and implications. Anabiosis 2:3–14, 1982

Freud S: Civilization and Its Discontents (1930), in The Standard Edition of the Complete Psychological Works of Sigmund Freud, Vol 21. Translated and edited by Strachey J. London, Hogarth Press, 1959

Gabbard GO, Twemlow SW, Jones FC: Differential diagnosis of altered mind/body perception. Psychiatry 45:361–369, 1982

Gallup G: Adventures in Immortality: A Look Beyond the Threshold of Death. New York, McGraw-Hill, 1982

Gallup G: Fifty years of Gallup surveys on religion. The Gallup Report (Report No 236). New York, Gallup, 1985

Greenwell B: Energies of Transformation: A Guide to the Kundalini Process. Cupertino, CA, Shakti River Press, 1990

Greyson B: Near-death experiences and attempted suicide. Suicide Life Threat Behav 11:10–16, 1981

Greyson B: Near-death experience and personal values. Am J Psychiatry 140:618–620, 1983

Greyson B, Harris B: Clinical approaches to the near-death experience. J Near-Death Studies 6:41–52, 1987

Grof S, Grof C (eds): Spiritual Emergency: When Personal Transformation Becomes a Crisis. Los Angeles, CA, Jeremy Tarcher, 1989

Group for the Advancement of Psychiatry: Mysticism: Spiritual Quest or Mental Disorder. New York, Group for Advancement of Psychiatry, 1976

Hood RW: Psychological strength and the report of intense religious experience. J Sci Study Religion 13:65–71, 1974

Hood RW: Conceptual criticisms of regressive explanations of mysticism. Rev Religious Res 17:179–188, 1976

Hood RW: Differential triggering of mystical experience as a function of self-actualization. Rev Religious Res 18:264–270, 1977
James W: The Varieties of Religious Experience. New York, MacMillan, 1961
Jung CG: Psychology and Religion. Princeton, NJ, Princeton University Press, 1973
Kass F, Spitzer R, Williams J, et al: Self-defeating personality and DSM-III-R: development of the diagnostic criteria. Am J Psychiatry 146:1022–1026, 1989
Kleinman A: Rethinking Psychiatry. New York, Free Press, 1988
Krippner S, Welch P: Spiritual Dimensions of Healing. New York, Irvington Publishers, 1992
Kroll J, Sheehan W: Religious beliefs and practices among 52 psychiatric inpatients in Minnesota. Am J Psychiatry 146:67–72, 1989
Larson DB, Pattison M, Blazer DG, et al: Systematic analysis of research on religious variables in four major psychiatric journals, 1978–1982. Am J Psychiatry 143:329–334, 1986
Larson DB, Pastro LE, Lyons J, et al: The systematic review: an innovative approach to reviewing research. Washington, DC, Department of Health & Human Services, April 1992
Lovinger R: Working with Religious Issues in Therapy. New York, Jason Aronson, 1984
Lukoff D: The diagnosis of mystical experiences with psychotic features. Journal of Transpersonal Psychology 17(2):155–181, 1985
Lukoff D, Everest HC: The myths in mental illness. Journal of Transpersonal Psychology 17:123–153, 1985
Lukoff D, Lu F: Transpersonal psychology research review topic: mystical experience. Journal of Transpersonal Psychology 20:161–184, 1988
Lukoff D, Lu F, Turner R: Toward a more culturally sensitive DSM-IV: psychoreligious and psychospiritual problems. J Nerv Ment Dis 180:673–682, 1992
Maslow A: Toward a Psychology of Being. Princeton, NJ, Van Nostrand, 1962
Maslow A: The Farther Reaches of Human Nature. New York, Viking, 1971
Mezzich J, Fabrega H, Kleinman A: Editorial: cultural validity and DSM-IV. J Nerv Ment Dis 180:4, 1992
Moody RA: Life after Life. New York, Bantam, 1975
Peck S: Further Along the Road Less Traveled. New York, Simon & Schuster, 1993
Peterson EA, Nelson K: How to meet your clients' spiritual needs. J Psychosoc Nurs 25:34–39, 1987
Pollner M: Divine relations, social relations, and well-being. J Health Soc Behav 30:92–104, 1989
Post SG: DSM-III-R and religion. Soc Sci Med 35:81–90, 1992
Ring K: Heading Toward Omega: In Search of the Meaning of the Near-Death Experience. New York, William Morrow, 1984
Ring K: Life at Death: A Scientific Investigation of the Near-Death Experience. New York, Coward, McGann & Geoghegan, 1990
Robinson L: Psychoanalysis and religion: a comparison, in Psychiatry and Religion: Overlapping Concerns. Edited by Robinson L. Washington, DC, American Psychiatric Press, 1986, pp 208–230
Sabom MB: Recollections of Death: A Medical Investigation. New York, Harper & Row, 1982
Salzman L: Religious conversion and paranoid states as issues in the psychotherapy process, in Psychotherapy of the Religious Patient. Edited by Spero MH. Springfield, IL, Charles C Thomas, 1985, pp 208–230
Sansone RA, Khatain K, Rodenhauser P: The role of religion in psychiatric education: a national survey. Academic Psychiatry 14:34–38, 1990

Shafranske E: Beyond countertransference: on being struck by faith, doubt, and emptiness. Paper presented at the annual conference of the American Psychological Association, New Orleans, 1991

Shafranske E, Maloney HN: Clinical psychologists' religious and spiritual orientations and their practice of psychotherapy. Psychotherapy 27:72–78, 1990

Soeken KL, Carson VJ: Responding to the spiritual needs of the chronically ill. Nurs Clin North Am 22:603–611, 1987

Spanos NP, Moretti P: Correlates of mystical and diabolical experiences in a sample of female university students. J Sci Study Religion 27:105–116, 1988

Spero MN: Identity and individuality in the nouveau-religious patient: theoretical and clinical aspects. Psychiatry 50:55–71, 1987

Spitzer R, Williams J: Classification in psychiatry, in Comprehensive Textbook of Psychiatry, 4th Edition, Vol 1. Edited by Kaplan HI, Sadock BJ. Baltimore, MD, Williams & Wilkins, 1985, pp 591–612

Spitzer R, Gibbon M, Skodol A, et al: DSM-III-R Casebook. Washington, DC, American Psychiatric Press, 1989

Stace WT: Mysticism and Philosophy. Philadelphia, PA, JB Lippincott, 1960

Stoll RI: Guidelines for spiritual assessment. American Journal of Nursing 79:1574–1577, 1979

Underhill E: Mysticism: A Study in the Nature and Development of Man's Spiritual Consciousness. New York, Meridian, 1955

Young JL, Griffith EE: The development and practice of pastoral counseling. Hosp Community Psychiatry 40:271–276, 1989

Index

Page numbers printed in **boldface** *type refer to tables or figures.*

Abuse. *See* Child abuse and neglect; Partner relational problems with physical abuse
"Abuse or oppression artifact disorder," 679
Academic performance
  of children with attention-deficit/hyperactivity disorder and attention-deficit disorder without hyperactivity, 177–178
  related to parent inadequate discipline, 593–596
Accidents
  differentiation from child abuse, 779–780
  parent inadequate discipline and, 597
Acculturation difficulty, 878. *See also* Cultural issues
Acquired immunodeficiency syndrome (AIDS), 878
Acute Physiology and Chronic Health Evaluation (APACHE II), 494, **495**
Adaptation to illness, 428
Adaptive functioning. *See* Axis V
Adjustment
  impact of social support on, 427
  to sibling's death, 703–704
Adjustment disorder
  of childhood and adolescence, 105, 291–299
    comorbidity of, 296
    definition of, 291
    with depressed mood, 292, **294**, 295, 296
    discriminant validity of, 298
    distinction from posttraumatic stress disorder, 291

  evidence for seriousness of, 297
  nature of symptomatology in, 292, **294**, 295
  prevalence of, 292, **293**
  problems with diagnosis of, 292
  recommended changes in criteria for, 298–299
  reliability of criteria for, 295, 298
  review of studies on, 292
  stability and outcome of, 295–296
  stressor criterion for, 291–292, 296–297
  subtypes of, 291–292
  suicidality and, 295
  temporal characteristics of, 296, 298
culture and, 969–972
  assessment of stressors, 969
  judgment of maladaptive response to stressors, 969–970
  migrants, 970–971
  popular folk categories, 971–972
with depressed mood, 490
Affective expression. *See also* Expressed emotion
  cultural variations in, 902–903
    language differences, 911–912
    narrative context, 916–917
  parent/child, **644**, 647–649
  spouse/spouse, **635**, 637–639
Age at onset of illness, 463, **471–472**, 474
Aggressive behavior
  child abuse and neglect, 526–527, 713–781
  in conduct disorder, 202
  cultural considerations regarding, 875
  in intermittent explosive disorder, 676

1017

Aggressive behavior *(continued)*
  partner relational problems with physical abuse, 525, 673–689
  related to parent inadequate discipline, 573, 587–589
  in sadistic personality disorder, 676–677
  sibling, 525–526, 694–697. *See also* Sibling relational problems
Aid for Families With Dependent Children (AFDC), 754
Aire, 992
Alcohol use. *See also* Substance-related disorders
  among abused or neglected children, 767–769
  culture and disorders of, 893–896
    antisocial personality disorder and, 895–896
    in children and adolescents, 874–875
    dependence and other associated features of, 895–896
    gender distribution of, 896
    pathological use of, 894–895
    pathophysiological changes due to, 896
    prevalence rates for, 893–894
  among lower socioeconomic classes, 877–878
  parental
    children's conduct disorder and, 149
    fetal alcohol syndrome and, 878
    sibling rivalry and, 693
    related to inadequate discipline during childhood, 579–580
  in restrictor and bulimic subtypes of anorexia nervosa, 340, **346**
  spouse abuse and, 684–685
Alzheimer's disease, cultural factors and, 887
Amenorrhea, in anorexia nervosa, 348, **349**
Amok, 945, 947, 991–994
Angina, 428–429

Anorexia nervosa, 97, 101, 335–336. *See also* Eating disorders
  "atypical," 966–967
  bulimia nervosa with and without history of, 365, 367, 372
  bulimic and nonbulimic subtypes of, 335–336, 339–352
    demographic data on, 340, **343–345**
    developmental history, sexual history, and menarche for, 348, **349**
    impulsivity measures in, 340, **346**
    parental psychopathology, parental obesity, and premorbid obesity associated with, 348, **350**
    personality traits and, 340, **347**, 348
    recommended changes in criteria for, 352
    review of studies on, 339–340, **341–342**
  criterion C for, 336
  as culture-bound syndrome of Western society, 865, 959, 966–967
  historical subtypes of, 339
Antisocial personality disorder
  alcoholism and, 895–896
  conduct disorder and oppositional defiant disorder among children of parents with, 149–150, **198**, 198–199
  culture and, 977–978
  defense mechanisms associated with, 512
  parent inadequate discipline and, 580, 599–600
Anxiety
  among abused children, 753
  in purging versus nonpurging bulimic patients, 362–363
  in restrictor versus bulimic anorectic patients, **347**, 348
Anxiety disorders
  of childhood and adolescence, 96, 102–103, 221–235

attention-deficit/hyperactivity
disorder and, **148**, 152–153,
176, 229
avoidant disorder, 226–227
distinction from normal anxiety,
232
distinctness from each other, 234
elective mutism and, 249
overanxious disorder, 227–229
rates in community based on
diagnostic interviews, **234**
recommended changes in criteria
for, 234–235
reliability of criteria for, 229–232,
230–231
review of studies on, 222
separation anxiety disorder,
222–226, **224**
trichotillomania as, 304, 311
culture and, 925–930
culture-specific syndromes, 928–929
posttraumatic stress disorder in
refugees, 929–930
prevalence rates, 926–927
recommendations regarding, 930
review of studies on, 926
symptomatology, 927–928
symptomatology, somatization,
934–935
defense mechanisms associated with,
512
Aphasia, 11, 80, 83–89
Appearance of child, abuse and neglect
related to, 744
Asperger's syndrome, 7–8, 50
clinical course of, 8
clinical features of, 45
differential diagnosis of, 8
autism, 7–8
etiological markers for, 48–49
outcome of, 49
prevalence of, 47
speech in, 47
Ataque de nervios, 865, 870, 876, 928–929,
946
Attachment problem, child abuse and
neglect related to, 740

Attention-deficit disorder, 165–173
cluster analytic studies of, 172–173
factor analyses of symptoms of, 165,
170–172, **171**
Attention-deficit disorder without
hyperactivity, 97–98, 112, 114,
163–185
comparison with ADHD, 173–184
academic underachievement,
177–178
cognitive/neuropsychological
functioning, 179–182
effects of stimulant medication,
182–183
emotional and behavioral
correlates, 173–176
patterns of inattention and
cognitive style, 178–179
peer relationships, 176–177
in DSM-III and DSM-III-R,
163–164
recommendations for DSM-IV
regarding, 184–185
review of studies on, 165, **166–169**
validity of, 183–184
Attention-deficit/hyperactivity disorder
(ADHD), 96–99, 111–140
among abused children, 750–751
in adults, 98
applicability of symptoms throughout
life span, 113
clinical threshold and functional
impairment for diagnosis of,
114–115
comorbidity of, 145–156
anxiety disorders, **148**, 152–153,
176, 229
borderline personality disorder,
155
conduct disorder, 99, 145, 147–150,
148, 175–176
effect on outcome, 146
family-genetic data on, 156
hypotheses about patterns of, 146
learning disabilities, 153–154
mental retardation, 154–155
mood disorders, **148**, 151–152

Attention-deficit/hyperactivity disorder (ADHD)
   comorbidity of *(continued)*
      oppositional defiant disorder, 99, 117, **148**, 150–151
      review of studies on, 146
      significance of, 145–146
      Tourette's syndrome, 155
   controversy about validity of, 146–147
   in DSM-III-R, 97–98, 112
   exclusion criteria for, 115–116
   overdiagnosis of, 98–99
   primary versus secondary status of symptoms of, 115–116
   risk factors for, 875
   situational presentation of symptoms of, 99, 115, 116, 122, 138–140
      parent versus teacher reports, 122
      pervasive versus situational hyperactivity, 122, **123–137**, 138–140
   symptom grouping for diagnosis of, 112–113, 116, 139
      factor analyses of symptoms, 117–122, **118–121**
      symptom cutoffs by age, 122, 139
   tests of new symptoms proposed for diagnosis of, 113–114
Autistic disorder, 4–5, 15–23
   atypical, 8–9
   differential diagnosis of
      Asperger's syndrome, 7–8
      childhood disintegrative disorder, 39
      early-onset schizophrenia, 62, 64
      pervasive developmental disorder not otherwise classified, 49–50
      Rett's syndrome, 6, 28–29
   DSM-III-R criteria for, 4, 15
      age at onset, 4, 15
      diagnostic validity of, 20–22, **21**
      evaluation of psychometric properties of, 15–20, **17**
      recommendations related to, 22–23
   in DSM-IV, 4–5
   pica and, 101, 212, 213

Avoidant disorder, 102, 226–227
   comparison with adult anxiety disorders, 227
   definition of, 226
   differential diagnosis of, 226–227
      depression, 227
      other anxiety disorders, 226
   duration of, 226
   rates in community based on diagnostic interviews, **233**
   recommended changes in criteria for, 235
   reliability of criteria for, 229–232, **230–231**
Avoidant personality disorder, 102, 227
Axis I disorders, 394
   Axis V ratings of persons with, 441, 490
   culture and, 984
   proposals for qualifying course of, 399, 459–482
   proposals for qualifying severity of, 399, 487–500
   relationship of Axis III disorders with, 394–395, 401, 404
Axis II disorders, 394
   culture and, 984
Axis III, 394–395, 401–407. *See also* Medical illness, comorbid with mental disorder
   culture and, 984
   indications for use of, 404–405
   proposals regarding, 405
   relationship with Axis I disorders, 394–395, 401, 404–407
      causative, 406
      coexisting, 406
      exacerbating, 406
      treatment relevant, 406
   underuse of, 394, 404
Axis IV, 395–397, 409–420
   clinical use of, 411–412
   culture and, 878–879, 984–985
   options for changes in, 416–417
   proposals regarding, 396–397
   reasons for inclusion in multiaxial system, 409–410

Index

recommendations for, 417, 420
refocusing on social support, 423–434.
    See also Social support
  benefits of, 424, 431
  personal resources scale of,
      431–434, **432–433**
  rationale for, 424–425
  recommendations for, 431–434
  review of studies on, 425
reliability of, 395, 412–413
  sources of error, 412–413
review of studies on, 410
underutilization of, 395, 396, 410, 423, 424
  reasons for, 424
validity of, 396, 413–416
  evaluation of Axis IV severity ratings, 414–415
  identifying psychosocial stressors using Axis IV, 415–416
  relationship to treatment planning and predictive validity, 416
  stressor theory and Axis IV severity ratings, 413–414
Axis V, 397, 439–454
  background of, 439
  culture and, 879, 985–986
  in DSM-III-R, 442–443
  predictive validity of ratings on, 442, 490
  proposed modifications of, 450–451, **452–453**
  recommendations for, 451, 454, 493
  relationship of treatment status to ratings on, 442
  reliability of ratings on, 440–441
  review of social functioning measures that might be used as models for, 444–450, **445, 447–449**
  review of studies on adaptive functioning, 440
  strengths and weaknesses of, 443–444
  validity of ratings on, 441–442

Baby Doe regulations, 716, 719
Baker v. Owen, 719

Battered child syndrome, 257, 716, 753.
    See also Child abuse and neglect
Battered woman syndrome, 680–681.
    See also Partner relational problems with physical abuse
  essential features of, 680
  legal status of, 680–681
Beck Depression Inventory, 754
Behavior of children
  with attention-deficit/hyperactivity disorder and attention-deficit disorder without hyperactivity, 173–176
  child abuse and neglect related to, 745–750
Behavior Problem Checklist, 173
Behavior Problem Checklist, Revised, 746
Bereavement, 427, 429
  "cultural," 929
Binge eating
  in anorexia nervosa, 335, 351
  in bulimia nervosa, 336, 355
  definition of, 336–337
  frequency of, 337, 355, 357
  "objective" versus "subjective," 356
  other psychopathology and, 357, 358
  in persons who do not meet DSM-III-R criteria for bulimia nervosa, 338, 379–389. *See also* Pathological overeating
  threshold for, 356
Binge eating disorder, 389
Bipolar disorder, 490
  comorbid with childhood attention-deficit/hyperactivity disorder and mood disorders, 152
  defense mechanisms associated with, 512
  impact of social support on outcome of, 428
Birth order, 693
Blacking-out, 946
Body dysmorphic disorder, culture and, 939

Borderline personality disorder
  attention-deficit/hyperactivity
    disorder and, 155
  culture and, 979
  defense mechanisms associated with, 512
  among persons who were abused during childhood, 752, 769–770
  relationship with identity disorder, 107–108
Brain fag, 876, 934
Brief Psychiatric Rating Scale, 551
Briquet's syndrome, 755
Bulimia nervosa, 97, 101, 336–337. *See also* Eating disorders; Pathological overeating
  as culture-bound syndrome of Western society, 959, 966
  diagnostic criteria for, 336–337, 355–358
    binge-eating threshold, 355, 356
    frequency of binge eating, 337, 355, 357
    importance of attitudes regarding shape and weight to diagnosis of, 337, 375–377
      advantages to retaining criterion, 377
      normal women with no history of eating disorder, 376
      prevalence of weight and shape concerns, 376
      recommendations regarding criterion, 377
      restrained eaters, 376–377
  prevalence of, 379
  review of studies on, 355–356
  subtyping of, 337, 361–373
    bulimia with and without history of anorexia nervosa, 365, 367, 372
    bulimia with and without history of obesity, 367–369, **368**, 372
    obese versus normal-weight bulimia, 369–372, **371**
    options for, 361
    purging versus nonpurging bulimia, 362–365, **364–366**, 372
    anxiety, 362–363
    body weight, 362, 363
    recommendations regarding, 372–373
    review of studies on, 361–362
Burn injuries, 780

Camberwell Family Interview (CFI), 532–534, 550–555, 662
  alternatives to, 555–557
  time to administer, 555
Catatonic schizophrenia, 57, **60, 61**
Center for Epidemiologic Studies—Depression Scale (CES-D), 581, 914–916
Chakore, 945
Child Abuse Amendments of 1984, 716, 719
Child abuse and neglect, 526–527, 713–781. *See also* Incest
  characteristics of children and their families, 738–762
    child and adolescent psychopathology, 750–753
      anxiety, 753
      attention-deficit/hyperactivity disorder, 750–751
      borderline and multiple personality disorders, 752
      conduct disorder, 751–752
      depression, 752
      fire setting, 752
    child characteristics as contributing factors, 739–745
      appearance, 744
      attachment style, 740
      developmental delays, 742–743
      handicapping conditions, 741–742
      medical problems, 741, 743–744
      prematurity and low birth weight, 739–741
    children's behavioral characteristics, 745–750

parent characteristics, 753–762
  adolescent parents, 755–756
  distorted negative perceptions of
    child, 761–762
  impact of family size and twins,
    755–756
  isolation, 757
  lack of inhibitory control,
    760–761
  marital discord or acrimonious
    family interactions, 758
  maternal depression, 753–755
  parent-child relational problems,
    758–759
  somatic complaints, 755
  unrealistic expectations of child,
    759–760
cultural influences and, 714–715
definitions of, 713, 720–725
  neglect, 723–725
  physical abuse, 720–723
differentiation from accidents, 779–780
epidemiology of, 730–738
  ethnicity and, 735–736
  homelessness and, 737
  National Incidence Studies, 731–736
  self-report data, 737–738
  socioeconomic status and, 734–735,
    757
  substantiation rates, 737
false accusations of, 778–779
in ICD-10, 774–775
intentionality of, 721–722, 779
issues regarding diagnostic standards
  for, 775–780
lack of mandated mental health
  services for, 780–781
methodological problems in research
  on, 725–729
  dependency on referral source to
    define abuse or neglect,
    726–727
  lack of long-term follow-up
    research, 729
  lack of research involving group
    designs, 728–729
  limited original data, 727–728

limited research utility of state
    registries, 729
  poorly defined samples, 726
  sampling bias, 727
  treatment studies, 728
outcomes of, 762–773
  alcohol and drug use, 767–769
  chronicity of maltreatment and,
    762–765
  criminality and homicide, 765–767
  other psychiatric disorders, 769–771
  role of out-of-home placement on,
    763–764
  transgenerational abuse, 771–773
parent inadequate discipline and, 574
public policy and, 716–720
  Baby Doe regulations, 716, 719
  corporal punishment in schools,
    719–720
  inconsistencies between laws and
    clinical service statutes, 717
  legislation, 716–717
  mandatory reporting statutes, 717,
    775
  religious exemptions to child neglect
    laws, 717–718, 724–725
  standards for diagnosis, 718
  statutory definitions of abuse and
    neglect, 718
reactive attachment disorder and,
    255–261
recommendations regarding, 781
review of studies on, 714–715
significance of, 773–774
Child Abuse Prevention, Adoption, and
  Family Services Act of 1988, 716
Child Abuse Prevention and Treatment
  Act of 1974, 716
Child Behavior Checklist, 267
Child Behavior Checklist—Teacher
  Report Form, 179
Child protective service (CPS) agencies,
  717, 721, 775
Child sexual abuse
  definition of, 805
  incest, 527–529, 805–850
  sibling, 525–526, 697–701

Child sexual abuse *(continued)*
    prevalence of, 806–809
        based on samples of children and adolescents, 808–809
    risk factors for, 807
Child sexual abuse accommodation syndrome, 846–847
Childhood and adolescent disorders
    adjustment disorder, 105, 291–299
    anxiety disorders, 96, 102–103, 221–235
    attention-deficit disorder without hyperactivity, 163–185
    attention-deficit/hyperactivity disorder, 96–99, 111–140
        comorbidity of, 145–156
    correlation of expressed emotion with, 550
    cultural considerations in classification of, 873–880
        acculturation difficulty, 878
        Axis IV, 878–879
        Axis V, 879
        chronic illness, 877–878
        culture-bound syndromes and healing, 876–877
        disruptive behavior disorders, 875
        elective mutism, 875
        mental retardation, learning disorders, and pervasive developmental disorders, 874
        posttraumatic stress disorder, 876
        reactive attachment disorders and stereotypy habit disorder, 875
        separation anxiety, 876
        substance-related disorders, 874–875
    early-onset schizophrenia, 9–10, 55–64
    elective mutism, 103, 241–251
    elimination disorders, 108
    feeding and eating disorders, 97, 101–102, 211–219
    gender identity disorder, 96–97, 106–107, 317–324
    identity disorder, 107–108
    mood disorders, 96, 104
        depression, 265–274
    oppositional defiant disorder and conduct disorder, 99–101, 189–207
    organization of DSM-IV section on, 95–97
        advantages and disadvantages of, 96
    parent inadequate discipline and, 523–524, 584–587
    pervasive developmental disorders, 3–9
        Asperger's syndrome, 7–8
        atypical autism, 8–9
        autistic disorder, 4–5, 15–23
        childhood disintegrative disorder, 6–7, 35–40
        not otherwise specified, 7, 43–52
        Rett's syndrome, 5–6, 25–32
    reactive attachment disorder, 104, 255–261
    sibling rivalry, 107, 327–331
    social skills deficits within learning disorders, 10–11, 67–74
    speech and language disorders, 11–12, 79–89
    suicidality, 105, 279–286
    tic disorders, 108
    trichotillomania, 105–106, 303–313
Childhood disintegrative disorder, 6–7, 35–40
    age at onset of, 36, **37**
    clinical course of, 7, 38
    clinical features of, 37, **37**
    differential diagnosis of
        autism, 39
        Rett's syndrome, 6
    in DSM-IV, 39–40
    epidemiology of, 38
    gender distribution of, **37**
    historical descriptions of, 6, 35
    in ICD-10, 36, 39, 40
    neurological findings in, 38
    prevalence of, 38
    prognosis for, 38
    review of studies on, 36–37
    terminology for, 35
Children's Global Assessment Scale, 292
Children's Reports of Parental Behavior Inventory, 581

Cluttering, 11, 12, 79–80, 82, 85–88
Coalition on Family Diagnosis, 398
Coercive behavior
 within family, **645,** 652–654
  criteria for, 654
  measurement of, 652
  validity of, 652–654
 of perpetrators of spouse abuse, 676
Cognitive competence. *See also* Mental retardation
 of children with attention-deficit/hyperactivity disorder and attention-deficit disorder without hyperactivity, 179–182
 cultural considerations in cognitive impairment disorders, 885–890
  biases in cross-cultural assessment, 888–889
  epidemiology, 886–887
  symptoms and detection, 887
 related to parent inadequate discipline, 593–596
"Coin rubbing," 877
Communication deviance, 642–647, **644**
 criteria for, 646–647
 definition and measurement of, 642–646
Communication problems. *See also* Marital and family communication difficulties
 parent/child, 642–657
  after sibling's death, 703–704
 spouse/spouse, 632–642
Community Adaptation Schedule (CAS), **445,** 446, **448**
Community Adjustment Profile System (CAPS), **445,** 446, **449**
Community Living Assessment Scale (CLAS), **445,** 446, **448**
Compliance of children, 589–591
 compulsive, 748
Conduct disorder, 100–101, 189–207
 among abused children, 751–752
 age-appropriate criteria for, 205
 attention-deficit/hyperactivity disorder and, 99, 145, 147–150, **148,** 175–176
 cultural considerations in diagnosis of, 875
 definition of, 189
 depression and, 269
 in DSM-III-R, 189
 family studies of, 149–150
 gender differences in, 204–205
 in girls, 101
 parent inadequate discipline and, 523
 relationship with oppositional defiant disorder, 100, 189–200, 205–207
  age at onset of symptoms, 192–194, **194,** 205
  comparison of correlates, 197–200, 205–206
  developmental, 195–197, 205
  differences in severity, 200–201, 206
  hierarchical, 195, 205
  impairment, **198,** 199–200, 206
  socioeconomic status and family psychopathology, 197–199, **198**
  statistical covariation among symptoms, 191–192, 205
 subtypes of, 101, 201–204, 206–207
  aggressive versus nonaggressive, 202
  based on comorbid conditions, 203
  childhood- versus adolescent-onset, 202–203, 206
  group versus solitary, 201
  possible redundancy of, 203–204
  utility of diagnostic criteria and possible new criteria for, 204
Conflict resolution in marriage, **636,** 640–641
Conflict Tactics Scale, 640, 686–687, 732–733
Conners Parent Questionnaire, 182
Conners Teacher Rating Scale, 181
Constipation, 108
Conversion disorder, culture and, 935, 938
Coping mechanisms. *See* Defense mechanisms
Coronary heart disease, 428–429
Cost containment, 487

Course of illness, 399, 459–482, 533
  culture and, 869–870
  diagnostic importance of, 460
  in DSM-III-R, 481–482
  individual variables of, 463, 471–473, 482
    age at onset, 463, **471–472**, 474
    duration, 471, 474, 475, **475–477**
    episodicity, 471, 473, 474, **477–479**, 479
    mode of onset, 463, 471, **473–474**, 474, 479
    progression, 473–475, 479, **479–480**
  methods to include variables in DSM-IV, 475, 479, 481
    additional diagnostic character across diagnostic categories, 475, 479, 481
    consideration of course by disorder, 481
    recommendations regarding, 481–482
  review of studies on, 460–461
    DSM-III-R, 463
    empirical papers, 463, **464–470**
    overview papers, **462**, 462–463
    time-frame variables in published multiaxial systems, 459–460, **460**
Criminality
  related to child abuse and neglect, 765–767
  related to parent inadequate discipline, 523, 579–582
Cross-dressing, 320. *See also* Gender identity disorder
Cultural issues, 861–871
  in adjustment disorders, 969–972
  in anxiety disorders, 925–930
  avoiding cultural bias in diagnosis, 868–869
  in child abuse and neglect, 714–715
  in cognitive impairment disorders, 885–890
  conceptualizations of culture, 867–868
  cultural annotations for multiaxial schema, 864
  cultural blind spot syndrome, 870
  cultural statement for introduction to DSM-IV, 863
  culturally enhancing DSM-IV multiaxial formulation, 865, 983–988
  culturally sensitive diagnostic interviewing, 870–871
  culture-bound syndromes, 865, 876–877, 991–999
  in diagnosis of mood disorders, 868, 909–918
  in diagnosis of schizophrenia and related disorders and psychotic disorders not otherwise classified, 901–905
  diagnostic significance of, 861–862
  in dissociation, 943–947
  in eating disorders, 959–967
  expressed emotion and, 553, 904
  idioms of distress, 865, 870
  in personality disorders, 975–981
  related to classification of mental disorders in children and adolescents, 873–880
  related to various diagnostic categories, 863–864
  religious or spiritual problems, 1001–1013
  in sexual disorders, 951–955
  in somatoform disorders, 933–939
  in substance-related disorders, 893–898
Culture-bound syndromes, 865, 876–877, 991–999
  culture-specific somatic symptoms, 936
  dissociative symptoms and, 943–947, 995–996
  evaluation for inclusion in DSM-IV, 991
  recommendations regarding, 998–999
  relationship to anxiety disorders, 928–929
  resemblances in different cultural settings, 993
  semantic ambiguities in meaning of, 992–994
  sexual, 954
  terminology for, 991

"Cupping," 877
Current and Past Psychopathology Scale (CAPPS), **445**, 446, **447**
Cyclothymic disorder, 490

Daydreaming, 179, 184
Death
  children's understanding of, 701
  near-death experiences, 1006, 1007
  sibling, 526, 701–704. *See also* Sibling relational problems
  social support and, 429–430
Defense Mechanism Inventory, 505
Defense Mechanism Rating Scales (DMRS), 506, 509
Defense mechanisms, 398, 503–515
  assessment methods for, 505–506
    clinical interview, 505
    Rorschach test, 506
    self-report questionnaires, 505–506
  associated with personality disorders, 512
  clinical utility of measurements of, 510–511
  consensus on, 507, 514
  definition of, 507
  degree of complexity of axis on, 508–509
  factors affecting proposed axis for, 503–504, 513–515
  field testing of proposed axis for, 513–514
  general applicability of axis on, 507
  hierarchy of, 510–511, 514
  lack of coverage in DSM-III multiaxial system, 504–505
  recommendations regarding, 515
  relationship of proposed axis with other axes, 511–513
  reliability of scales measuring, 509–510
  review of studies on, 505
  support for axial rating of, 507–508
Defense Style Questionnaire (DSQ), 505–506, 510, 512
Delinquency
  conduct disorder, 100–101, 189–207
  parent inadequate discipline and, 575, 584–586
Delirium
  Axis V ratings of persons with, 441, 443
  cultural factors and, 887
Delusions, 9, 57, **60**, 63
  cultural factors and, 902
Dementia, 490
  cultural factors and, 886–887
  infantalis, 6, 35. *See also* Childhood disintegrative disorder
Denver Community Mental Health Questionnaire (DCMHQ), **445**, 445–446, **447**
Depression
  among abused children, 752
  Axis IV severity ratings in, 415
  Axis V ratings of persons with, 441
  of childhood and adolescence, 104, 265–274
    attention-deficit/hyperactivity disorder and, **148**, 151–152
    clinical description of, 266–269, 272
      age-dependent changes in depressive symptomatology, 267–269
      depressed mood and irritability, 266
      duration of depressed mood, 266–267
      syndromic aggregation of depressive symptoms, 267
    conduct disorder and, 269
    delimitation from other disorders, 269, 272
    differences from adult depression in criteria for, 265–266, 269
    family studies of, 271–273
    follow-up studies of, 270–271, 273
    laboratory studies of, 269–270, 272–273
    parent inadequate discipline and, 586–587
    psychosocial dwarfism and, 215
    recommendations regarding criteria for, 273–274
    separation anxiety disorder and, 225

Depression
　of childhood and adolescence
　　(continued)
　　　sleep abnormalities and, 268, 270
　　　social withdrawal associated with, 227
　　　suicidality and, 267, 281
　　　treatment studies of, 271
　　culture and, 909–918. *See also* Mood disorders
　　　somatic symptoms, 868, 917, 934–935
　　versus dysthymia, 490
　　impact of social support on outcome of, 428
　　marital conflict and, 640
　　maternal
　　　child abuse or neglect and, 753–755
　　　parent inadequate discipline and, 597–599
　　　related to inadequate discipline during childhood, 580–582
　　in restrictor and bulimic subtypes of anorexia nervosa, 347, 348
　　Western notion of mind-body dichotomy, 868, 909–910
Developmental delays, 742–743
Developmental Trends Study, 193, 196, 198–200
Dexamethasone suppression test, 270
Dhat, 934, 936, 954, 992
Diagnosis-related groups (DRGs), 487, 494
Diagnostic Interview for Children and Adolescents—Revised, 9
Diagnostic Interview Schedule, 928, 938, 979
Diagnostic Interview Schedule for Children, 170, 172
Discipline problems. *See* Parent inadequate discipline
Disorder of written expression, 10
Disruptive behavior disorders of children and adolescents
　attention-deficit disorder without hyperactivity, 163–185
　attention-deficit/hyperactivity disorder, 96–99, 111–140
　comorbidity of, 145–156
　culture and, 875
　oppositional defiant disorder and conduct disorder, 99–101, 189–207
Dissociation
　culture and, 943–947, 995–996
　"fleeing" or "running" syndromes, 945
　possession trance syndromes, 944–945
　trance syndromes, 946
　among persons who were abused during childhood, 752, 770–771
Dissociative Disorders Interview Schedule, 770
Dissociative Experiences Scale, 770
Dopamine beta-hydroxylase, 270
DRGs (diagnosis-related groups), 487, 494
DSM-IV multiaxial system, 393–399. *See also* specific axes
　Axes I and II, 394
　　proposals for qualifying course of, 399, 459–482
　　proposals for qualifying severity of, 399, 487–500
　Axis III, 394–395, 401–407
　Axis IV, 395–397, 409–420, 423–434
　Axis V, 397, 439–454
　cultural considerations for, 863–865, 867–871, 983–988
　　Axes I and II, 984
　　Axis III, 984
　　Axis IV, 878–879, 984–985
　　Axis V, 879, 985–986
　　complementary cultural formulation, 865, 986–988
　　cultural elements of relationship between individual and clinician, 988
　　cultural explanations of illness, 987
　　cultural factors related to psychosocial environment and functioning, 987–988

cultural identity of individual, 987
    overall cultural assessment for
        diagnosis and care, 988
methods to increase use of, 424
proposals for additional axes, 397–398
    defense or coping axis, 398, 503–515
    relational functioning, 398
reasons for proposed elimination or
    revision of, 393
underutilization of, 393, 424
Duration of illness, 471, 474, 475, **475–477**
Dwarfism
    nonorganic, 211, 212, 215–216
    psychosocial, 211, 212, 215–216
        clinical features of, 215
        comorbidity with, 216
        in ICD-10, 215, 216
        nonorganic failure to thrive and,
            214–216
        reactive attachment disorder and,
            215
        recommended changes in criteria
            for, 218–219
Dyadic Adjustment Scale, 634, 637, 640
Dysthymia, 490

Eating Attitudes Test, 362, 363
Eating disorders, 97, 335–338. *See also*
    Feeding and eating disorders of
    infancy or early childhood
    anorexia nervosa, 335–336, 339–352
    bulimia nervosa, 336–337
        diagnostic criteria for, 355–358
        importance of attitudes regarding
            shape and weight to
            diagnosis of, 375–377
        subtyping of, 361–373
    culture and, 959–967
        American Indians, 965
        blacks, 960
        clinical recommendations
            regarding, 967
        Hispanics, 960, 965
        immigrants, 965
        non-Western countries, 966
        review of studies on, 960, **961–964**
        significance of, 959–960

defense mechanisms associated with, 512
pathological overeating, 337–338,
    379–389
sibling relational problems and, 693
Eating Disorders Examination, 356, 376,
    377
Eating Disorders Inventory, 348, 362–363
Eating Disorders Questionnaire, 365
Education of the Handicapped Act, 10, 68
Ejaculatory problems, 953
Elderly persons, cultural expectations
    about cognitive deficits among, 887
Elective mutism, 11, 12, 80, 85, 87, 89,
    103, 241–251
    associated features of, 248–249
    characteristics of studies on, 242,
        245–247
    comorbidity with enuresis and
        encopresis, 249
    cultural considerations in diagnosis of,
        875
    designing study of, 249–250
    essential features of, 244, 248
    prevalence of, 248
    problems with grouping with speech
        and language disorders, 241
    recommendations regarding, 250–251
    relationship with anxiety disorders, 249
    review of studies on, 241–242, **243–244**
Elimination disorders, 108
Emotional experience, cultural variations
    in definitions and elaboration of,
    910, 912–914
Emotional overinvolvement, 532, **644,**
    649–651
Emotional support. *See* Social support
Emotionally intense interpersonal
    relationship, 522, 558. *See also*
    Expressed emotion
"Empacho," 877
Encopresis, 249
Enuresis, 249
Environmental resources scale, **432–433,**
    433–434
Epidemiologic Catchment Area (ECA)
    study, 579, 808, 926–927, 935, 977,
    979

Episodicity of illness, 471, 473, 474, **477–479**, 479
Ethnicity, 867. *See also* Cultural issues
  "behavioral," 871
  child abuse and neglect related to, 735–736
  expressed emotion and, 553, 904
  parent inadequate discipline and, 602
  sexual dysfunction and, 952
Expressed emotion (EE), 521–522, 531–563. *See also* Affective expression
  characteristics and determinants of, 532, 551–555
    culture, ethnicity, and family constellation, 553, 904
    stability, 554–555
    transactional processes, 551–553
  correlation with childhood disorders, 550
  family communication dysfunction and, 662
  generalizability of, 532, 550–551
  implications of including relevant category in DSM-IV, 557–559
  measurement and clinical criteria for, 532, 555–557
    alternative measures, 555–557
    recommendations for, 561–563
    reliability, 555
  positive and negative attitudes reflected in, 532
  as predictor of schizophrenic relapse, 522, 532, 534–549, 557–558
    influence of variation in relapse criteria across studies, 548–549
    measures of predictive power, 540–541, **542–543**
    naturalistic and special population studies, 535–539, **536–537**
    relationship with patient characteristics, 541, 544, **545–547**
    reliability across studies, 544, 548
    statistical analysis methods, 539–540
    trends in relapse rates, 540–541

recommendations regarding inclusion in DSM-IV, 559–561
review of studies on, 533–534
significance of, 532–533
studies of, 647–648

FACES II scale, 812–813
Failure to thrive, nonorganic (NO-FTT), 102, 211–214
  child neglect and, 725, 758, 773
  complications of, 214
  definition of, 214
  in ICD-10, 214
  psychosocial factors in, 214
  reactive attachment disorder and, 213–214
  recommended changes in criteria for, 217–218
Falling-out, 865, 936, 946
Family
  expressed emotion and constellation of, 553
  incest in, 527–529, 805–850
    sibling, 525–526, 697–701
  violence in. *See* Child abuse and neglect; Partner relational problems with physical abuse
Family Adjustment Measure, 637
Family Assessment Measure, 634, 641
Family Environment Scale, 637, 640, 641
Family Interaction Coding System, 652
Family studies
  of conduct disorder, 149–150
  of depression of childhood and adolescence, 271–273
  of family interactions, 648–649
  of incest, 528, **805–806, 809–813**, 811–812
  of oppositional defiant disorder, 150–151
  of suicidality in children and adolescents, 284
Family/relational problems, 521–530
  child abuse and neglect, 526–527, 713–781
  incest, 527–529, 805–850

Index 1031

marital and family communication
  difficulties, 524, 631–663
options for inclusion in DSM-IV,
  529–530
parent inadequate discipline, 523–524,
  569–616
partner problems with physical abuse,
  525, 673–689
related to mental disorder or general
  medical condition, 521–522,
  531–563. *See also* Expressed
  emotion
among siblings, 525–526, 693–708
Federal Alcohol and Drug Abuse
  Confidentiality Act, 717
Feeding and eating disorders of infancy or
  early childhood, 101–102, 211–219
  in ICD-10, 211
  limitations of studies on, 211
  nonorganic failure to thrive, 213–214,
    217–218
  pica, 212–213, 216–217
  psychosocial dwarfism, 215–216,
    218–219
  rumination disorder, 213, 217
Feighner criteria, 463
Female orgasmic dysfunction, 952
Fetal alcohol syndrome, 878
Fire setting, 752
Five-Minute Speech Sample (FMSS),
  550–552, 554–557
"Fleeing" syndromes, 945
"Folk syndromes," 994-995. *See also*
  Culture-bound syndromes
Foster care, 763–764
Fractures, 779

Gender identity disorder, 96–97, 106–107,
  317–324
  adult issues regarding, 320–321
    exclusion of fetishistic
      cross-dressers, 320
    intersexuality and gender
      dysphoria, 321
    subtypes of disorder, 320–321
  child issues regarding, 319–320

desire to be of opposite sex as
  distinct criterion, 319–320
diagnostic criteria for boys and
  girls, 106–107, 319
in children versus adults, 106
placement in nomenclature, 319
recommended changes in criteria for,
  321–322, **323**
review of studies on, 317–318
severity and natural history of, 318
types of, 318
Gender issues
  battered woman syndrome, 680–681
  in child abuse and neglect, 733
  in conduct disorder and oppositional
    defiant disorder, 204–205
  discipline strategies for boys versus
    girls, 613
  in gender identity disorder, 106–107
  gender-role traditionality and parent
    inadequate discipline, 602
  sibling aggression, 695
  sibling incest, 699–700
  in spouse abuse, 675–677
  in trichotillomania, 306, 309
General Health Questionnaire, 348
Generalized anxiety disorder, 229, 232
Genital ambiguity, 321
Genital retraction syndrome, 929, 936, 954
Ghost sickness, 865
Global Assessment of Functioning Scale
  (GAFS), 397, 423, 439–440, 493.
  See also Axis V
  for children of different cultural
    backgrounds, 879
  defense mechanisms and, 512–513
  limitations of, 450
  proposed modifications of, 450–451,
    452–453
  review of instruments that might be
    used as alternatives to, 444–450,
    445, 447–449
Global Assessment of Relational
  Functioning Scale, 398
Global Assessment Scale, 439–440, 444,
  450, 513, 646
Goodness-of-fit concept, 597

Grief reaction to sibling's death, 701–704
Grisi siknis, 945
Guilt reaction to sibling's death, 702

Hallucinations, 9–10, 57, **60**, 63
　cultural factors and, 868–869, 902
Handicapping conditions, child abuse and neglect related to, 741–742
Healing practices, indigenous, 877
Health. *See also* Medical illness
　relationship between social support and, 428–429
Health Sickness Rating Scale, 511
Heart disease, 428–429
Heller's syndrome. *See* Childhood disintegrative disorder
"High blood," 936
High expressed emotion. *See* Expressed emotion
Histrionic personality disorder, culture and, 978–979
Home Observation for Measurement of the Environment Inventory, 598
Homelessness, child abuse and neglect related to, 737
Homicide
　by persons who were abused during childhood, 766–767
　sibling, 694
Homosexuality, 954
Hopkins Symptom Check List, 340
Human immunodeficiency virus infection, 878
Hwa-byung, 934
5-Hydroxytryptamine (5-HIAA), 284
Hypertension, 886
Hypochondriasis, culture and, 938

Identity disorder, 107–108
Idioms of distress, 865, 870
Impotency, 952
Impulsivity
　in bulimic and restrictor subtypes of anorexia nervosa, 340, **346**, 351
　trichotillomania, 311

Incest, 527–529, 805–850
　behavioral and emotional problems in victims of, 528
　definitions of, 527, 805, 843–844
　diagnostic issues in, 846–849
　　child sexual abuse accommodation syndrome, 846–847
　　disorders of extreme stress, not otherwise specified, 848–849
　　posttraumatic stress disorder, 847–849
　　traumatogenic dynamics, 847–848
　difficulties with inclusion in DSM-IV, 849–850
　family studies of, 528, 805–806, 809–813, **811–812**
　maternal psychopathology and, 528
　methodological problems in studies of, 529, 843–846
　prevalence of, 806–809
　　based on interviews of adult survivors, 806–808
　　based on samples of children and adolescents, 808–809
　psychopathology in perpetrators of, 528–529
　recommendations regarding, 529, 849–850
　review of studies on, 809
　sibling, 525–526, 697–701
　　age and type of onset of, 700
　　course of, 701
　　definition of abusive activity, 697–698
　　factors affecting destructiveness of, 698
　　familial patterns of, 701
　　as nonabusive activity, 697
　　power differential in, 698
　　prevalence and risk of, 699
　　sex ratio and impact of, 699–700
　　versus sexual play, 697
　　short- and long-term consequences of, 698–699
　studies of nonabusive parent in incestuous families, 835–837, **838–839**

studies of perpetrators of, 839–843, 840–841
  fixated versus regressed offenders, 842
  sexual preferences, 842
victims of, 814–835
  studies of adolescent victims and survivors, 814, 820, **822–825**
  studies of adults reporting sexual abuse during childhood, 820–825, **826–835**, 835
  studies of victims and survivors under 12 years old, 814, **815–821**
Inconsistent discipline, 572–573. *See also* Parent inadequate discipline
Indian Child Welfare Act, 717
Indisposition syndrome, 946
Individuals With Disabilities Education Act, 68
Inflexible and rigid discipline, 576–578. *See also* Parent inadequate discipline
Ingraham v. Wright, 719, 720
Intelligence testing, cultural biases in, 888
Interagency Committee on Learning Disabilities, 67–68, 74
Intermittent explosive disorder, 676
  compared with spouse abuse, 676
  DSM-III-R definition of, 676
International Classification of Diseases, 10 Edition (ICD-10)
  avoidant disorder, 227
  child abuse and neglect, 774–775
  childhood disintegrative disorder, 36, 39, 40
  feeding and eating disorders of infancy or early childhood, 211
  nonorganic failure to thrive, 214
  overanxious disorder, 229
  pica, 101, 211–213
  psychosocial dwarfism, 215, 216
  reactive attachment disorder, 104, 255, 259–261
  Rett's syndrome, 6, 25
  rumination disorder of infancy, 211
  separation anxiety disorder, 226, 234
  sibling rivalry, 327–328, 330
  Z codes, 417, **418–419**

International Classification of Health Problems in Primary Care, 417, **418–419**
International Rett Syndrome Association (IRSA), 26
Intersexuality, 321
Interview Schedule for Social Interaction (ISSI), **445**, 446, **448**
Irritable and explosive discipline, 574. *See also* Parent inadequate discipline
Israeli Ischemic Heart Disease Study, 428

Kategoriensystem für Partner-Schafliche Interactions (KPI), 634, 640, 647
Katz Adjustment Scale (KAS), **445**, 446, **447**
KDS-15 Marital Questionnaire (KDS-15), **445**, 445–446, **447**
Kiddie Schedule for Affective Disorders and Schizophrenia, 9
Klein-Levin syndrome, 212, 217
Koro, 929, 936, 954
Kuru, 886

Landau-Kleffner syndrome, 84–85, 89
Language disorders. *See* Speech and language
Lattah, 992
Laxative abuse, 362–365, **364–366**, 372. *See also* Bulimia nervosa
Lead poisoning, 877
Learning disorders, 10–11
  attention-deficit/hyperactivity disorder and, 153–154
  cultural considerations in diagnosis of, 874
  definition of, 10, 68
  Interagency Committee on Learning Disabilities, 67–68, 74
  language disorders and, 80, 85, 87, 89
  serious emotional disturbance and, 10, 68
  social skills deficits and, 10–11, 67–74
Longitudinal Interval Follow-up Evaluation (LIFE), 446, **449**

Low birth weight, child abuse and neglect related to, 739–741
"Low blood," 936
Low supervision and involvement, 575–576. *See also* Parent inadequate discipline
Luria-Nebraska Neuropsychological Battery Children's Revision, 182

Machismo, 980
Mania, culture and, 914–916
Manifest Anxiety Scale, 753
Marital and family communication difficulties, 524, 631–663
　comparison of spouse/spouse and parent/child difficulties, 657–659, **658**
　considerations for inclusion in DSM-IV, 631
　criteria for, 661–662
　in DSM-III and DSM-III-R, 631
　expressed emotion and, 661
　options for inclusion in DSM-IV, 524, 659–661
　　considered as a disorder, 659–663
　　　arguments against, 660–661
　　　arguments for, 659–660
　　considered as V code, 661
　　creation of axis for general family disruption, 661
　parent/child difficulties, 642–657
　　affective communication, 647–648
　　coercive family processes, 652–654
　　communication deviance, 642–647
　　deficits in family problem solving, 654–657
　　emotional overinvolvement, 649–651
　　family interaction studies, 648–649
　　studies of, **644–645**
　relationship with Axis I and II disorders, 524
　relationship with individual disorders, 632
　review of studies on, 632
　spouse/spouse difficulties, 632–642
　　communication of information, 633–637, **635**
　　conflict and conflict resolution, **636**, 640–641
　　deficient problem solving, **635–636**, 639
　　expression of affect, **635**, 637–639
　　structure, **636**, 641–642
　　studies of, **635–636**
　threshold for consideration as disorder, 661
　validity of, 631
Marital Attitude Survey, 637
Marital discord
　child abuse and neglect related to, 758
　incest and, 813, 836
　parent inadequate discipline and, 601
　partner relational problems with physical abuse related to, 685
Marital Satisfaction Inventory, 637, 639, 640
Marital violence. *See* Partner relational problems with physical abuse
Masochism, 679
Matching Familiar Figures Test, 181
Maternal deprivation, 256
Mathematics disorder, 10
Medical illness
　child abuse and neglect related to, 741, 743–744
　comorbid with mental disorder, 401–407. *See also* Axis III
　on Axis III, 394–395, 402
　causal effect of, 403, 405, 406
　incidence of, 401, 403–404
　review of studies on, 402
　screening for, 401
　significance of, 401–402
　cultural considerations in diagnosis of chronic illness in children and adolescents, 877–878
　defense mechanisms and, 512
　indices of severity of, 494, **495**
　relational problem related to, 521–522, 531–563

relationship between social support and, 428–429
sibling, 526, 704–707. *See also* Sibling relational problems
Melatonin, 270
Mental retardation. *See also* Cognitive competence
  attention-deficit/hyperactivity disorder and, 154–155
  childhood disintegrative disorder and, 37
  cultural considerations in diagnosis of, 874
  effects on siblings of child with, 705, 706
  pervasive developmental disorder not otherwise specified and, 44–45
  pica and, 101
  rating severity of, 490
  Rett's disorder and, 31
  rumination disorder and, 213, 217
Methylphenidate, 182–183
Michigan Alcoholism Screening Test, 768
Millon Clinical Multiaxial Inventory, 685, 837
Mind-body dichotomy, 868, 909–910
Mini-Mental State Exam, 888
Minnesota Multiphasic Personality Inventory (MMPI), 348, 599, 753, 754, 837, 839
Minorities. *See* Cultural issues
Mixed receptive/expressive language disorder, 12
Mode of onset of illness, 463, 471, **473–474,** 474, 479
Mood disorders
  of childhood and adolescence, 96, 104
    attention-deficit/hyperactivity disorder and, **148,** 151–152
    depression, 265–274
  culture and, 868, 909–918
    definitions of self and loci of emotion, 910–911
    differences in narrative context, 916–917
    dimensions of depression and mania, 914–916

ethnophysiology of somatic experience, 917–918
  selective elaboration of emotional experience, 912–914
  variation in language of affect, 911–912
  Western notion of mind-body dichotomy, 868, 909–910
Mood lability, in anorexia nervosa, **347**
Mood-dependent discipline, 578–579. *See also* Parent inadequate discipline
"Moxibustion," 877
Multiaxial system. *See* DSM-IV multiaxial system
Multiple personality disorder. *See also* Dissociation
  compared with possession trance syndromes, 944–945
  among persons who were abused during childhood, 752, 770–771
  as Western culture-bound syndrome, 865
Munchausen syndrome by proxy, 780
Mutism, elective, 11, 12, 80, 85, 87, 89, 103, 241–251
  associated features of, 248–249
  characteristics of studies on, 242, **245–247**
  comorbidity with enuresis and encopresis, 249
  cultural considerations in diagnosis of, 875
  designing study of, 249–250
  essential features of, 244, 248
  prevalence of, 248
  problems with grouping with speech and language disorders, 241
  recommendations regarding, 250–251
  relationship with anxiety disorders, 249
  review of studies on, 241–242, **243–244**
Myocardial infarction, 428
Mystical experiences, 1004–1007

National Center on Child Abuse and Neglect, 715, 731, 805
National Incidence and Prevalence of Child Abuse and Neglect, 808

National Incidence Study (NIS)
    NIS-1, 731
    NIS-2, 724, 731–736, 777
National Survey of Physical Violence in American Families, 583
Near-death experiences, 1006, 1007
Neglect. *See* Child abuse and neglect
Nephrotic syndrome, 705–706
Nervios, 928–929, 934, 971
Neurasthenia, 934
Neuropsychological testing, of children with attention-deficit/hyperactivity disorder and attention-deficit disorder without hyperactivity, 179–182
Nevra, 934
Night eating syndrome, 384, **388**
Noncompliance of children, 589–591
Nonorganic failure to thrive (NO-FTT), 102, 211–214, 214
    child neglect and, 725, 758, 773
    complications of, 214
    definition of, 214
    in ICD-10, 214
    psychosocial factors in, 214
    reactive attachment disorder and, 213–214
    recommended changes in criteria for, 217–218
Nonpsychiatric medical conditions, 394–395, 401–407. *See also* Medical illness, comorbid with mental disorder
Norbeck Social Support Questionnaire, 431

Obesity
    binge eating and, 380, **381–383**
    bulimia nervosa with and without history of, 367–369, **368**, 372
    in children, 212
    night eating syndrome and, 384, **388**
    obese versus normal-weight bulimia nervosa, 369–372, **371**
    related to bulimic and restrictor subtypes of anorexia nervosa, 348, **350**

Obsessive-compulsive disorder
    relationship with trichotillomania, 305–306, 311–312
    divergent biological characteristics, 306
    divergent character and personality traits, 306
    gender ratio, 306
    symptom specificity, 305–306
    in restrictor and bulimic subtypes of anorexia nervosa, **347**
Ode ori, 936
Oppositional defiant disorder, 99–101, 189–207
    attention-deficit/hyperactivity disorder and, 99, 117, **148,** 150–151
    cultural considerations in diagnosis of, 875
    definition of, 189
    differentiation from normal oppositional behavior, 100–101
    in DSM-III-R, 189
    family studies of, 150–151
    gender differences in, 204–205
    parent inadequate discipline and, 523
    relationship with conduct disorder, 100, 189–200, 205–207
        age at onset of symptoms, 192–194, **194,** 205
        comparison of correlates, 197–200, 205–206
        developmental, 195–197, 205
        differences in severity, 200–201, 206
        hierarchical, 195, 205
        impairment, **198,** 199–200, 206
        socioeconomic status and family psychopathology, 197–199, **198**
        statistical covariation among symptoms, 191–192, 205
        utility of diagnostic criteria and possible new criteria for, 204
Oregon Youth Study, 592, 594
Overanxious disorder, 102–103, 227–229
    attention-deficit/hyperactivity disorder and, 176

characteristic anxious concerns in, 227
comorbidity with generalized anxiety
    disorder, 229, 232
comparison with adult anxiety
    disorders, 229
compatibility with ICD-10, 229
differential diagnosis of, 228–229
    separation anxiety disorder, 225
duration of, 228
lack of syndromal specificity of, 228
rates in community based on
    diagnostic interviews, **233**
recommended changes in criteria for,
    235
reliability of criteria for, 229–232,
    230–231
Overeaters Anonymous, 379
Overeating. *See* Binge eating; Bulimia
    nervosa; Pathological overeating

Paranoid personality disorder, 512
Paranoid schizophrenia, 57, **61**
Paraphilias, culture and, 951–952
Parent inadequate discipline, 523–524,
    569–616
    adult disorders associated with,
        597–600
        antisocial behavior, 599–600
        maternal depression and
            schizophrenia, 597–599
    assessment of, 615
    for boys versus girls, 613
    familial patterns associated with, 612
    inclusion as diagnostic category,
        613–616
        previous work on, 613–614
        pros and cons of, 614–615
        recommendations regarding,
            615–616
    methodological considerations and,
        523–524, 610–612
        bias associated with parent reports,
            611–612
        interparent agreement, 610–611
        multiagent, multimode versus
            single-agent-mode reports,
            612

reliability, 610
stability, 610
other child correlates of, 587–597
    academic achievement, cognitive
        competence, and school
        adjustment, 593–596
    accidents, 597
    aggressive and antisocial behavior,
        587–589
    compliance and noncompliance,
        589–591
    difficult temperament, 596–597
    poor peer relationships, 591–593
parent-child interactional patterns
    associated with, 602–604
    conditional probability studies, 604
    parent versus child determination
        of discipline, 603–604
past conceptualizations of, 570
predictive validity of, 523, 579–587
relationship to childhood disorders,
    523, 584–587
    delinquency, 575, 584–586
    depression, 586–587
review of studies on, 571–572
    aggregation of findings, 572
    inclusion/exclusion criteria, 571
    sources, 571–572
significance of problems associated
    with, 569–571
social and contextual factors
    associated with, 600–602
    gender-role traditionality, 602
    marital conflict, 601
    race, 602
    socioeconomic status, 601–602
    stress, 600–601
social validity of various types of
    discipline, 605–609
studies of long-term effects of, 579–584
    criminality, 582
    impact of problem discipline in
        family of origin on current
        parenting, 583–584
    problem discipline and adult
        psychiatric or criminal
        status, 579–582

Parent inadequate discipline *(continued)*
    types of, 523, 571–579
        inconsistent discipline, 572–573
            child conduct problems and, 573
            interparent inconsistency, 573, 601
            intraparent inconsistency, 572–573
        inflexible and rigid discipline, 576–578
            influence on moral development, 577
            types of, 576
            versus variations of discipline strategies, 577–578
        irritable and explosive discipline, 574
            family factors associated with, 574
            parental characteristics associated with, 574
            pathognomic effects on children, 574
            types of, 574
        low supervision and involvement, 575–576
            delinquency and, 575
            parental characteristics associated with, 575
            with younger children, 576
        mood-dependent discipline, 578–579
            definition of, 578
            impact of developmental stage of child on, 578
            versus proactive strategies, 578–579
Parental Bonding Instrument, 650
Parental psychopathology
    child abuse and, 753–755
    conduct disorder, oppositional defiant disorder and, 149–150, **198**, 198–199
    inadequate discipline and, 597–600
        antisocial parents, 599–600
        maternal depression and schizophrenia, 597–599
        in incestuous families, 837, 839–841
        restrictor and bulimic subtypes of anorexia nervosa and, 348, **350**
        sibling aggression and, 696
Parent/child communication difficulties, 642–657
    affective communication, 647–649
        criteria for, 649
        definition and measurement of, 647
        family interaction studies of, 648
        self-report studies of, 648–649
        validity of, 647–648
    coercive family processes, 652–654
        criteria for, 654
        measurement of, 652
        validity of, 652–654
    communication deviance, 642–647
        criteria for, 646–647
        definition and measurement of, 642–646
    comparison with spouse/spouse difficulties, 657–659, **658**
    criteria for, 663
    deficits in family problem solving, 654–657
        criteria for, 657
        definition of, 654–655
        measurement of, 655
        validity of, 655–657
    emotional overinvolvement, 649–651
        criteria for, 651
        definition and measurement of, 649–650
        validity of, 650–651
    features associated with, 663
    studies of, **644–645**
Parent-child relational problem with high expressed emotion, 561. *See also* Expressed emotion
Partner relational problems with physical abuse, 525, 673–689
    adequacy of assessments for, 686–687
    alcohol use and, 684–685
    complications of, 684
    course of, 683
    definition of, 686
    differential diagnosis of, 684–686

Index   1039

familial patterns of, 684
head injury among perpetrators of,
    685–686
injuries due to, 682
issues regarding, 673
marital discord and, 685
onset of, 683
perpetrator diagnoses associated with,
    675–677
    intermittent explosive disorder, 676
    sadistic personality disorder, 676–677
personality disorders among
    perpetrators of, 685
prevalence of, 674, 681, **682**
recommendations regarding inclusion
    in DSM-IV, 687–689
    arguments against, 688–689
    arguments for, 687
responsibility for, 683
review of studies on, 675
self-reports of, 681
sex ratio and impact of, 682–683
significance of, 674–675
subcategories of, 675
victim diagnoses associated with,
    677–681
    battered woman syndrome, 680–681
    posttraumatic stress disorder,
        679–680
    self-defeating personality disorder,
        677–679
Pathological overeating, 337–338,
    379–389. *See also* Bulimia nervosa
in children, 212
night eating syndrome, 384, **388**
among obese persons, 380, **381**–383
prevalence of, 384
recommendations regarding, 384, 389
review of studies on, 380, **381**–383,
    385–388
without weight control, 384, **385**–387
Pedophilia, 952
Peer relationships of children
    with attention-deficit/hyperactivity
        disorder and attention-deficit
        disorder without hyperactivity,
        176–177

behavioral characteristics and, 749–750
with conduct disorder and
    oppositional defiant disorder,
    198, 199–200
impact of parent inadequate discipline
    on, 591–593
Pemoline, 182
Performance anxiety, 102, 227
Person in Environment System, 417,
    418–419
Personal Adjustment and Role Skills Scale
    (PARS), **445,** 446, **447**
Personal Resources Inventory (PRI), **445,**
    446, **448**
Personal resources scale, 431–434, **432–433**
Personality, 490
    in bulimic and restrictor subtypes of
        anorexia nervosa, 340, **347,** 348
    cultural influences on formation of,
        975–976
    parental traits associated with child
        abuse, 753, 754
Personality Disorder Examination, 979
Personality disorders, 490. *See also*
    specific personality disorders
    on Axis II, 394
    culture and, 975–981
        antisocial personality disorder,
            977–978
        borderline personality disorder, 979
        etiopathogenesis, 975–977
        histrionic personality disorder,
            978–979
        other personality disorders, 979–980
        recommendations regarding,
            980–981
        review of studies on, 975
    defense mechanisms associated with,
        512
    among perpetrators of spouse abuse,
        685
    point prevalence of, 979
Pervasive developmental disorder not
    otherwise specified (PDDNOS), 7,
    43–52
    clinical features of, 44–47
    in DSM-IV, 4, 51–52

Pervasive developmental disorder not otherwise specified (PDDNOS) *(continued)*
  etiological markers for, 48–49
  outcome of, 49
  prevalence of, 47–48
  review of studies on, 44
  subtypes of, 50
Pervasive developmental disorders, 3–9
  Asperger's syndrome, 7–8
  atypical autism, 8–9
  autistic disorder, 4–5, 15–23
  childhood disintegrative disorder, 6–7, 35–40
  cultural considerations in diagnosis of, 874
  definition of, 30–31
  in DSM-III and DSM-III-R, 3
  in DSM-IV, 3–4, 394
  not otherwise specified, 7, 43–52
  Rett's syndrome, 5–6, 25–32
Phonological disorder, 12, 79, 82
Physical abuse. *See also* Aggressive behavior
  child abuse and neglect, 526–527, 713–781
  partner relational problems with, 525, 673–689
  sibling, 694–697
Pibloktoq, 865, 945
Pica, 101, 211–213
  autism and, 101, 212, 213
  complications of, 213
  definition of, 212
  exclusionary criteria for, 212, 217
  in ICD-10, 101, 211–213
  recommended changes in criteria for, 216–217
Pilot Study of Schizophrenia, 901
Polydipsia, 215
Polyphagia, 215
Positron-emission tomography, 306
Possession belief, 944
Possession trance syndromes, 944–945
  compared with multiple personality disorder, 944–945
  reversibility of, 944

Posttraumatic stress disorder (PTSD)
  compared with adjustment disorder, 291
  compared with spouse abuse, 679–680
  cultural considerations for diagnosis in children and adolescents, 876
  diagnostic criteria for, 679
  due to incest, 847–849
  in refugees, 929–930
Power distribution in marriage, 641–642
Prematurity, child abuse and neglect related to, 739–741
Present State Examination (PSE), 463, 549, 551, 901
Primary Communication Inventory, 634
Problem-solving deficits
  within family, 645, 654–657
  between spouses, **635–636**, 639
Progression of illness, 473–475, 479, **479–480**
Psychiatric Epidemiology Research Interview (PERI), 441, 446, **449**
Psychiatric Evaluation Form (PEF), **445**, 446, **447**
Psychiatric Severity of Illness Index, 494
Psychiatric Status Schedule (PSS), **445**, 446, **447**
Psychosocial dwarfism, 211, 212, 215–216
  clinical features of, 215
  comorbidity with, 216
  in ICD-10, 215, 216
  nonorganic failure to thrive and, 214–216
  reactive attachment disorder and, 215
  recommended changes in criteria for, 218–219
Psychosocial problem checklist, 396–397
Psychotic disorders. *See also* Schizophrenia
  cultural considerations in diagnosis of, 901–905
Public Law 93-247, 716
Public Law 94-142, 68
Public Law 95-266, 716
Public Law 95-608, 717
Public Law 98-457, 716, 719
Public Law 99-401, 717

Index 1041

Public Law 100-294, 716
Purging, 362–365, **364–366**, 372. *See also* Bulimia nervosa

Race. *See also* Cultural issues; Ethnicity
  eating disorders and, 959–965
  parent inadequate discipline and, 602
Reactive attachment disorder, 104, 255–261
  cultural considerations in diagnosis of, 875
  definition of, 258
  difference from other relational problems, 257–258
  essential features of, 258–259
  exclusion criteria for, 258, 260
  in ICD-10, 104, 255, 259–261
  nature versus nurture debate and, 256
  nonorganic failure to thrive and, 213–214
  pathological care and, 104, 255–261
  psychosocial dwarfism and, 215
  recommended changes in criteria for, 261
  reliability of criteria for, 259–260
  review of studies on, 255–256
Reading disorder, 10
Rehabilitation Evaluation of Baker and Hall (REHAB), **445**, 446, **448**
Relational functioning, 398
Relational problem related to mental disorder or general medical condition, 521–522, 531–563
  high expressed emotion and, 521–522, 531–532
Relational problems, 521–530
  child abuse and neglect, 526–527, 713–781
  incest, 527–529, 805–850
  marital and family communication difficulties, 524, 631–663
  parent inadequate discipline, 523–524, 569–616
  partner problems with physical abuse, 525, 673–689
  proposals regarding, 529–530
  related to mental disorder or general medical condition, 521–522, 531–563. *See also* Expressed emotion
  among siblings, 525–526, 693–708
Religion
  evaluating delusions with reference to cultural beliefs about, 902
  exemptions to child neglect laws based on, 717–718, 724–725
  positive mental health effects of, 1004
  "religious scrupulosity," 980
Religious or spiritual problems, 1001–1013
  clinician training about, 1008–1009
  definitions of religiosity and spirituality, 1002
  DSM-IV options for, 1009–1011
  historical data and theory about, 1004–1005
  recommendations regarding, 1011–1013
  religiosity gap between clinicians and patients, 1002, 1008
  religious problem, 1005–1006
    impact of religious transformation, 1005
    loss of faith, 1005
  research needs related to, 1012–1013
  review of studies on, 1003
  significance of, 1001–1002
  spiritual problem, 1006–1007
    mystical experiences, 1006–1007
    near-death experiences, 1006, 1007
    nursing diagnoses for, 1007
Repression-Sensitization Scale, 506
Research Diagnostic Criteria, 463, 754, 755
Rett's syndrome, 5–6, 25–32
  clinical course of, 6, 26–27
  diagnostic criteria for, 26–28
  differential diagnosis of, 6
    autism, 6, 28–29
  in DSM-IV, 32
  exclusion criteria for, 27–28
  external validity of, 28–29
  forme fruste, 32

Rett's syndrome *(continued)*
    gender distribution of, 6, 27
    hand stereotypies in, 6, 27, 29, 30
    in ICD-10, 6, 25
    incidence of, 28
    internal validity of, 26–28
    mental retardation of, 31
    plasma glycosphingolipids in, 29
    prevalence of, 6, 28
    relationship with pervasive
        developmental disorders, 29–30
    social withdrawal of, 6, 31–32
    stages of, 30, 31
    variant forms of, 32
Revised Behavior Problem Checklist, 746
Role Activity Performance Scale, 446
Rootwork, 865
Rorschach Test, 506, 643
Rumination disorder of infancy, 101, 102, 211, 213
    age distribution of, 213
    complications of, 213
    definition of, 213
    gender distribution of, 213
    in ICD-10, 211
    mental retardation and, 213, 217
    recommended changes in criteria for, 217
    voluntariness of, 213
"Running" syndromes, 945

Sadistic personality disorder, 676–677
    clinical utility of, 676
    compared with spouse abuse, 677
    diagnostic criteria for, 677
    potential for misuse of diagnosis, 676–677
Santeria, 902
Schedule for Affective Disorders and Schizophrenia, 463
Schedule for Affective Disorders and Schizophrenia—Lifetime, 754, 755
Schizoaffective disorder, 63, 533
Schizoid personality disorder, 512
Schizophrenia
    Axis V ratings of persons with, 441, 442
    course of, 533
    cultural considerations in, 869, 901–905
        affect, 902–903
        course of illness, 904
        ethnic and sociocultural bias in diagnosis, 903–904
        sense of self, 904
        symptomatology, 901–902
    defense mechanisms associated with, 512
    early-onset, 9–10, 55–64
        age at onset of, **58–59**, 62
        clinical features of, 57, **60–61**
        comparison with adult schizophrenia, 9–10, 57, 63
        diagnosis in nonverbal children, 62, 64
        differential diagnosis of, 62
            Asperger's syndrome, 8
            autism, 62, 64
        gender distribution of, 10, **58**
        modification of criteria for, 57, 62
        review of studies on, 55–56, **58–61**
        structured diagnostic interviews for, 9
        subcategorization of, 57, **61**
    effects on siblings of young adults with, 705
    family communication deviance and, 643, 646
    geographic variations in prevalence, symptoms, and course of, 869
    high expressed emotion as predictor of relapse, 522, 532, 534–549, 557–558
        influence of variation in relapse criteria across studies, 548–549
        measures of predictive power, 540–541, **542–543**
        naturalistic and special population studies, 535–539, **536–537**
        relationship with patient characteristics, 541, 544, **545–547**
        reliability across studies, 544, 548

statistical analysis methods, 539–540
trends in relapse rates, 540–541
maternal, parent inadequate discipline and, 597–599
parental overinvolvement and, 650–651
worldwide distribution of, 869
Schizophreniform disorder, 533
Schizotypal personality disorder, 63, 394
School
 corporal punishment in, 719–720
 parent inadequate discipline and adjustment to, 593–596
 performance of children with attention-deficit/hyperactivity disorder and attention-deficit disorder without hyperactivity, 177–178
School phobia, 223–225, **224**. *See also* Separation anxiety disorder
Secondary disorders, 405, 406
Seizures
 childhood disintegrative disorder and, 38
 Rett's syndrome and, 27
Selective mutism, 103, 241. *See also* Elective mutism
Self, cultural variations in definition of, 910
Self-Assessment Guide (SAG), **445**, 446, **448**
Self-defeating personality disorder, 677–679
 compared with spouse abuse, 678–679
 diagnostic criteria for, 678
 DSM-III-R definition of, 677
Separation anxiety disorder, 103, 222–226, **224**
 age and gender distribution of, 223
 clinical features of, 222–223, **224**
 comparison with adult anxiety disorders, 225–226
 cultural considerations in diagnosis of, 876
 depression comorbid with, 225
 differential diagnosis of, 225
  overanxious disorder, 225

in DSM-III and DSM-III-R, 223
duration of, 223, 225, 235
exclusionary criteria for, 226
in ICD-10, 226, 234
rates in community based on diagnostic interviews, **233**
recommended changes in criteria for, 234–235
reliability of criteria for, 229–232, **230–231**
Serious emotional disturbance, 10, 68
Serotonin (5-HT), 284
Severity of Alcohol Dependence Questionnaire, 768
Severity of illness, 399, 487–500
 clinical importance of, 487
 conceptualizations of, 488–489
 indices in general medicine and surgery, 494, **495**
 measures of, 488–489
  comorbid severity, 489, 490
  functional impairment, 489
  overall severity, 489
  syndromic severity, 488–489
 proposals for ratings of, 494–499
  comparison of, 499
  criterion-based severity, 497
  generic versus specific measurement of syndromic severity, 499
  hybrid criterion/symptom severity, 498–499
  symptom-based severity, 498
  syndromic severity, 494–496
 in psychiatric multiaxial systems, 489–494, **491–492**
 reasons for interest in, 487
 recommendations for noting, 500
 review of studies on, 488
Severity of Illness Index (SII), 494, **495**
Sex reassignment surgery, 318–319
Sexual abuse
 child sexual abuse accommodation syndrome, 846–847
 definition of child sexual abuse, 805, 808
 incest, 527–529, 805–850
  sibling, 525–526, 697–701

Sexual abuse *(continued)*
  prevalence of, 806–809
    based on interviews of adult
      survivors, 806–808
    based on samples of children and
      adolescents, 808–809
Sexual disorders
  culture and, 951–955
    culture-bound sex syndromes, 954
    other sexual disorders, 953–954
    paraphilias, 951–952
    sexual dysfunctions, 952–953
  DSM classification of, 951
Sexual orientation, 954
Sexual play, 697
Shenjing shuairuo, 865
Shinkeishitsu, 934
Short stature. See Psychosocial dwarfism
Sibling relational problems, 525–526,
    693–708
  aggression, 525–526, 694–697
    age and type of onset of, 695–696
    course of, 696
    familial patterns of, 696–697
    homicide, 694
    influence of parental punishment
      on, 697
    prevalence and risk of, 695
    sex ratio and impact of, 695
    symptoms of, 694
  categories of, 525, 694
  cause of, 525
  of children with conduct disorder and
    oppositional defiant disorder,
    198, 200
  death, 526, 701–704
    age and type of onset of reactions
      to, 702–703
    course of adjustment to, 703
    effects on family structure, 702
    familial patterns of grief and
      adjustment after, 703–704
    guilt reactions after, 702
    psychological reactions to, 701–702
    sex ratio and impact of, 702
  illness, 526, 704–707
    age and type of onset of, 707
    course of, 707
    effects of sibling with mental
      retardation, 705, 706
    effects of sibling with nephrotic
      syndrome, 705–706
    effects of sibling with serious
      emotional disturbance, 705
    familial patterns of, 707
    prevalence and risk of problems
      due to, 706
    psychological reactions to, 704–705
    sex ratio and impact of, 706–707
  incest, 525–526, 697–701
    age and type of onset of, 700
    course of, 701
    definition of abusive activity,
      697–698
    factors affecting destructiveness of,
      698
    familial patterns of, 701
    as nonabusive activity, 697
    power differential in, 698
    prevalence and risk of, 699
    sex ratio and impact of, 699–700
    versus sexual play, 697
    short- and long-term consequences
      of, 698–699
  recommendations regarding, 708
  review of studies on, 694
  significance of, 693
Sibling rivalry, 107, 327–331
  coercive behavior toward target child,
    330
  definition of, 327
  distinction from normal sibling
    interactions, 329
  family functioning and, 329, 330
  in ICD-10, 327–328, 330
  impact of parental intervention on,
    329–330
  recommendations related to, 330–331
  review of studies on, 328
  validity of diagnosis of, 329
Sleep disturbance
  depression of childhood and
    adolescence and, 268, 270
  psychosocial dwarfism and, 215

Social Adjustment Scale (SAS), 442, **445**, 446, **449**
Social Behavior and Adjustment Scale (SBAS), **445**, 446, **448**
Social Functioning Schedule (SFS), **445**, 446, **449**
Social phobia, 102, 227, 234
Social skills deficits
 among abused children, 749–750
 within learning disorders, 10–11, 67–74
  extent of, 71–72
  hypotheses relating to nature of, 69–71
  relationship of, 10–11, 68
  review of studies on, 69
  serious emotional disturbance and, 10, 68
  treatment of, 72–73
 related to parent inadequate discipline, 591–593
Social Stress and Functioning Inventory for Psychotic Disorders (SSFIPD), **445**, 446, **449**
Social support, 423–434
 conceptualizations of, 425–426
 definition of, 425
 hypotheses regarding contribution to well-being, 425–426
 instruments for assessment of, 430–431
 mortality and, 429–430
 perceived versus enacted, 425
 physical health and, 428–429
 proposal to refocus Axis IV on, 423–434. *See also* Axis IV
 psychiatric morbidity and, 426–428
 quantitative and qualitative properties of, 425
 rating scale for measurement of, 431–434, **432–433**
Social withdrawal
 Asperger's syndrome and, 45
 avoidant disorder and, 226–227
 depression and, 227
 elective mutism and, 249
 Rett's syndrome and, 6, 31–32

Socioeconomic status
 alcohol use and, 877–878
 child abuse and neglect and, 734–735, 757
 children's chronic illness and, 877–878
 conduct disorder, oppositional defiant disorder and, 197–199, **198**
 parent inadequate discipline and, 601–602
Somatoform disorders
 child abuse related to parental somatization, 755
 culture and, 933–939
  body dysmorphic disorder, 938
  clinical recommendations, 937–938
  conversion disorder, 935, 938
  correlation of somatic symptoms, depression, and anxiety, 934
  culture-specific symptoms, 936
  hypochondriasis, 938
  level of somatic symptomatology, 935
  problems with DSM nosology, 933–934
  research needs, 936–937
  somatization disorder, 938
  somatoform disorder not otherwise specified, 938
 somatization in restrictor and bulimic subtypes of anorexia nervosa, **347**, 348
Speech and language
 in Asperger's syndrome, 47
 in autistic disorder, 5
 disorders of, 11–12, 79–89
  age at identification of, 80, 83, 86
  comorbidity with learning disorders, 80, 85, 87, 89
  in DSM-III-R, 11
  elective mutism and, 241, 248
  inclusionary criteria for, 80, 84, 86–88
  review of studies on, 81
  terminology for, 79, 80, 82, 86, 88
 in early-onset schizophrenia, 57, 62, 63
 in Rett's syndrome, 27
Spiritism, 902, 943

Spiritual problems, 1006–1007. *See also*
	Religious or spiritual problems
	mystical experiences, 1006–1007
	near-death experiences, 1006, 1007
	nursing diagnoses for, 1007
Spouse abuse. *See* Partner relational
	problems with physical abuse
Spouse/spouse communication
	difficulties, 632–642
	communication of information,
		633–637, **635**
		criteria for, 637
		definition and measurement of,
			633–634
		validity of, 634–637
	comparison with parent/child
		difficulties, 657–659, **658**
	conflict and conflict resolution, **636**,
		640–641
		criteria for, 641
		definition and measurement of, 640
		validity of, 640–641
	criteria for, 662
	deficient problem solving, **635–636**, 639
		criteria for, 639
		definition and measurement of, 639
		validity of, 639
	expression of affect, **635**, 637–639
		criteria for, 639
		definition and measurement of,
			637
		low self-disclosure, 638
		validity of, 638
	features associated with, 662
	structure, **636**, 641–642
		definition and measurement of,
			641–642
		validity of, 642
	studies of, **635–636**
Standardized Interview to Assess Social
	Maladjustment (SIASM), **445**, 446,
	449
Stereotypies
	in childhood disintegrative disorder,
		7
	in Rett's syndrome, 6, 27, 29, 30
	stereotypy habit disorder, 875

Stimulants, 182–183
Stonybrook High-Risk Project, 598
"Strain ratio," 442
Stress
	adjustment disorder and, 291–292,
		296–297
	disorders of extreme stress, not
		otherwise specified, 848–849
	Holmes and Rahe severity scores for,
		414
	parent inadequate discipline and,
		600–601
	rating on Axis IV, 395–397, 409–420.
		See also Axis IV
	social support as buffer against,
		427
Stroke, 886
Structured and Scaled Interview to Assess
	Maladjustment (SSIAM), **445**, 446,
	449
Stuttering, 12, 79, 81
Substance-related disorders. *See also*
	Alcohol use
	among abused or neglected children,
		767–769
	in anorexia nervosa, 340, **346**
	biological indications of, 898
	conduct disorder and oppositional
		defiant disorder among
		children of parents with, 149,
		198, 198–199
	culture and, 893–898
		alcohol disorders, 893–896
		clinical recommendations,
			897–898
		diagnosis in children and
			adolescents, 874–875
		drug disorders, 896–897
	among incest offenders, 842
	reporting of child abuse by persons
		receiving services for, 717
Suicidality
	in children and adolescents, 105, 267,
		279–286
		adjustment disorder and, 295
		definition of, 279
		depression and, 267, 281

limitations of DSM-III-R approach to, 279–283
    failure to identify important focus of clinical attention, 282
    lack of adequate coverage in diagnostic studies of suicidal persons, 281–282
    obstacles to recordkeeping and research, 282
as potential diagnostic criteria, 280, 283–285
    biological correlates, 284
    exposure to suicidal persons, 284
    family factors, 284
    genetic factors, 284
    predictive validity, 285
    psychological concomitants, 283
    specifications for validity, 280, 283
proposed supplementary code for, 285–286
related to comorbid attention-deficit/hyperactivity disorder and mood disorders, 152
review of studies on, 280
in restrictor and bulimic subtypes of anorexia nervosa, **346**
Susto, 865, 870, 876, 992
Symptom Checklist-90 (SCL-90), 512, 768

Taijing kyofusho, 865, 929, 992
Tecumseh, Michigan, Community Health Study, 430
Temperament of child
    goodness-of-fit conceptualization of, 597
    parent inadequate discipline and, 596–597
Test anxiety, 228
Thematic Apperception Test, 643
Therapeutic Intervention Scoring System (TISS), 494, **495**
Thought disorder, 57, **60,** 62
Tic disorders, 108
Tourette's syndrome, 155

Trance syndromes, 946, 995–996
    possession trance syndromes, 944–945
Transsexualism, 106, 318
Trichotillomania, 105–106, 303–313
    definition of, 303
    early childhood onset versus adolescent/adult onset of, 303, 308–310, **309,** 312
        associated pathology, 310
        gender ratio, 309
        severity, duration, and prognosis, 309
    maintenance as psychiatric diagnosis, 312–313
    placement in DSM-IV, 303, 310–313
        anxiety disorders, 304, 311
        disorders usually first evident in infancy, childhood, or adolescence, 310
        impulse control disorders not elsewhere classified, 311
    relationship with obsessive-compulsive disorder, 305–306, 311–312
        divergent biological characteristics, 306
        divergent character and personality traits, 306
        gender ratio, 306
        symptom specificity, 305–306
    review of studies on, 305
    as symptom of other primary conditions rather than independent diagnosis, 303, 307–308, **307–308,** 312
Tricyclic antidepressants, 271

Ukufa kwabantu, 994–995
Umego, 995
Urinary incontinence, 108

Vineland Social Maturity Scale, 759
Violence. *See* Aggressive behavior; Child abuse and neglect; Partner relational problems with physical abuse
Voice disorder, 11, 12, 79–83, 86, 88

Vomiting, self-induced, 362–365, **364, 366,** 372. *See also* Bulimia nervosa

Ways of Coping Scale, 506
Wechsler Intelligence Scale for Children—Revised, 182
Wernicke's aphasia, 11, 80, 83–84, 86, 88
Widowhood, 427, 429

Wife abuse. *See* Partner relational problems with physical abuse

Yale Children's Inventory, 114
Yin-yang imbalance, 971

"Zone of proximal development" concept, 579